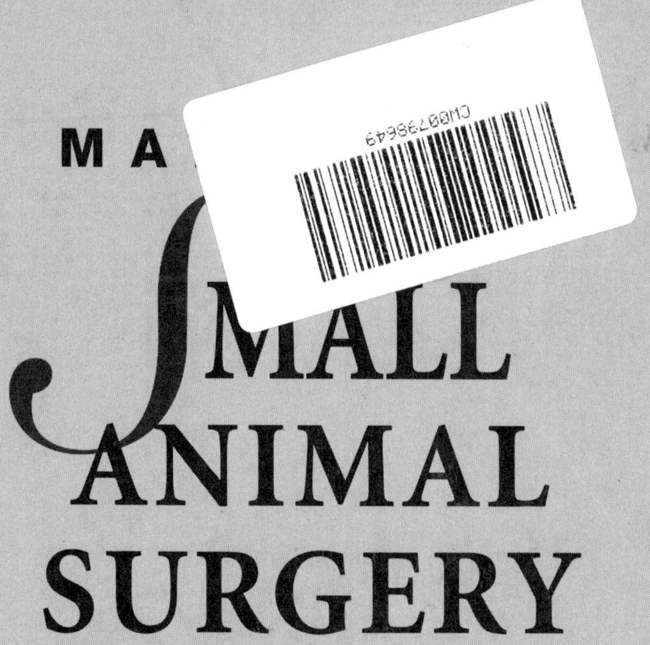
MA
SMALL
ANIMAL
SURGERY

MANUAL OF SMALL ANIMAL SURGERY

Theresa Welch Fossum,
DVM, MS, PhD, Diplomate ACVS
Professor and Chief of Surgery
Department of Small Animal Medicine and Surgery
College of Veterinary Medicine
Texas A&M University
College Station, Texas

With:
Cheryl S. Hedlund
Donald A. Hulse
Ann L. Johnson
Howard B. Seim III
Michael D. Willard
Gwendolyn L. Carroll

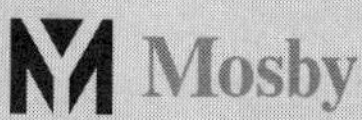

St. Louis Baltimore Boston Carlsbad Chicago Minneapolis New York Philadelphia Portland
London Milan Sydney Tokyo Toronto

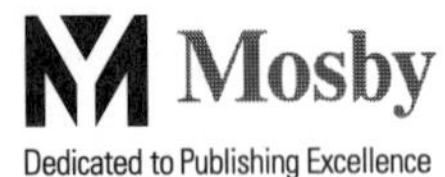

Dedicated to Publishing Excellence

Editor in Chief: John A. Schrefer
Executive Editor: Linda L. Duncan
Project Manager: John Rogers
Production Editor: Beth Hayes
Designer: Kathi Gosche

NOTICE

Pharmacology is an ever-changing field. Standard safety precautions must be followed, but as new research and clinical experience broaden our knowledge, changes in treatment and drug therapy may become necessary or appropriate. Readers are advised to check the most current product information provided by the manufacturer of each drug to be administered to verify the recommended dose, the method and duration of administration, and contraindications. It is the responsibility of the treating physician, relying on experience and knowledge of the patient, to determine dosages and the best treatment for each individual patient. Neither the publisher nor the editor assume any liability for any injury and/or damage to persons or property arising from this publication.

Mosby, Inc.
A Harcourt Health Sciences Company
11830 Westline Industrial Drive
St. Louis, Missouri 63146

Printed in United States of America
Composition by Graphic World, Inc.
Printing/binding by Quebecor

Library of Congress Cataloging in Publication Data

Fossum, Theresa Welch.
Manual of small animal surgery / Theresa Welch Fossum.
p. cm.
Includes bibliographical references.
ISBN 0-323-00562-4
1. Veterinary surgery Handbooks, manuals, etc. I. Title.
SF911.F67 1999
636.089'7—dc21 99-26587
CIP

99 00 01 02 03 / 9 8 7 6 5 4 3 2 1

EDITOR IN CHIEF

Theresa Welch Fossum, DVM, MS, PhD, Diplomate ACVS
Associate Professor and Chief of Surgery
Department of Small Animal Medicine and Surgery
College of Veterinary Medicine
Texas A&M University
College Station, Texas

SECTION EDITORS

Cheryl S. Hedlund, DVM, MS, Diplomate ACVS
Professor of Surgery and Chief, Companion Animal Surgery and Anesthesia
School of Veterinary Medicine
Louisiana State University
Baton Rouge, Louisiana

Donald A. Hulse, DVM, Diplomate ACVS
Professor
Department of Small Animal Medicine and Surgery
College of Veterinary Medicine
Texas A&M University
College Station, Texas

Ann L. Johnson, DVM, MS, Diplomate ACVS
Professor
Department of Veterinary Medicine
University of Illinois
1008 Hazelwood Drive
Urbana, Illinois

Howard B. Seim III, DVM, Diplomate ACVS
Professor and Chief of Small Animal Surgery
Department of Clinical Sciences
Colorado State University
Fort Collins, Colorado

Medical Consultant
Michael D. Willard, DVM, MS, Diplomate ACVIM
Professor
Department of Small Animal Medicine and Surgery
College of Veterinary Medicine
Texas A&M University
College Station, Texas

Anesthesia Consultant
Gwendolyn L. Carroll, DVM, MS, Diplomate ACVA
Assistant Professor, Anesthesiology
Department of Small Animal Medicine and Surgery
College of Veterinary Medicine
Texas A&M University
College Station, Texas

Contributor
Christopher E. Orton, DVM, MS PhD, Diplomate ACVS
Professor
Department of Clinical Sciences
Colorado State University
Fort Collins, Colorado

PREFACE

Manual of Small Animal Surgery is designed as a handy, current reference for use by veterinarians, veterinary students, veterinary technicians, and other clinic staff. The goal of this manual is to provide readers with fast, helpful information on medical conditions for which surgical intervention in the dog and cat may be indicated. The manual contains 37 chapters organized in four parts: General Surgical Principles, Soft Tissue Surgery, Orthopedics, and Neurosurgery. Chapters in the last three sections are organized logically and consistently. General principles are presented first, including preoperative concerns, anesthesia, surgical anatomy, general techniques, wound healing, postoperative care, and age considerations. Specific diseases follow, with discussions of pathophysiology, diagnosis, medical management, and surgical technique. Information is presented in easy outline form and surgical techniques are highlighted throughout for easy access. Valuable appendixes guide readers to common anesthetic and antibiotic drug protocols for a variety of conditions.

In no way is this manual an exhaustive work; it addresses the most common surgeries taught in schools of veterinary medicine and performed in general practices. It is best used in conjunction with *Small Animal Surgery* (referred to in the text as *SAS*), in which the reader will find more detailed discussions of relevant anatomy and physiology, pathophysiology, diagnostic testing, procedures, and underlying rationales for treatment options, and, perhaps most important, hundreds of supporting surgical illustrations and extensive reference lists. Helpful page cross-references to the parent text have been provided throughout the manual to direct readers to more detailed information.

Theresa Welch Fossum

CONTENTS

IV. Neurosurgery

PART

I

General Surgical Principles

1

Principles of Surgical Asepsis (*SAS*, pp. 1-6)

I. Rules of Aseptic Technique

A. Bacteria contaminating surgical wounds may gain entrance from several sources.
1. **Exogenous** (i.e., air, surgical instruments, surgical team, patient).
2. **Endogenous** (i.e., organisms originating from within the patient's body).

B. Contaminating bacteria most commonly originate from the patient's endogenous flora, operating room personnel, and environment.

C. *Aseptic technique* is defined as methods and practices that prevent cross-contamination in surgery and involve proper preparation in the following areas.
1. Facilities and environment (Chapters 3 and 4).
2. Surgical site (Chapter 6).
3. Surgical team (Chapter 7).
4. Surgical equipment (Chapters 2 and 8).

II. Preparation of Surgical Packs

A. Clean instruments manually or with ultrasonic cleaning equipment and appropriate disinfectants as soon after surgery as possible (see Chapter 8). Launder linens. Before packing, separate instruments and place them in order of their intended use.

B. Packing **instruments** (for steam, gas, and plasma sterilization).
1. Organize instruments on a lint-free (huck) towel placed on the bottom of a perforated metal instrument tray.
2. Autoclave instruments with box locks with the box lock open.
3. Separate instruments with a 3- to 5-mm space between them for proper steam/gas circulation.
4. Disassemble complex instruments when possible and lubricate power equipment before sterilization.
5. Flush items with a lumen with a small amount of water immediately before steam sterilization because water vaporizes and forces air out of the lumen.
6. Do not leave moisture in tubing placed in a gas sterilizer because it may decrease the action of the gas below the lethal point.

7. Place containers (e.g., saline bowl) with the open end facing up or horizontal; containers with lids should have the lid slightly ajar.
8. Stack multiple basins with a towel between each.
9. Include a standard count of radiopaque surgical sponges in each pack.
10. Center a sterilization indicator in the center of each pack before wrapping.
11. Steam sterilize solutions separately from instruments using the slow exhaust phase (see Chapter 2).

C. Packing **linens.**
1. The maximum size and weight of linen packs that can be effectively steam sterilized is 12 × 12 × 20 inches and 6 kg, respectively.
2. Pack closely woven table drapes separately.
3. Alternate layers of linen in their orientation to permit steam penetration.

D. Wrapping materials for packs.
1. Selected wraps should be penetrable by steam/gas, impermeable to microbes, durable, and flexible.
2. Packing materials available, advantages and disadvantages of each, and appropriate sterilization techniques are listed in *SAS,* Table 1-2.
3. *Presterilization* wraps for steam comprise two thicknesses of two-layer muslin or nonwoven (i.e., paper) barrier materials. *Poststerilization* wraps (i.e., after sterilization and proper cooldown period) consist of a waterproof, heat-sealable plastic dust cover; this wrap is not necessary if the item is to be used within 24 hours of sterilization.
4. For **steam** sterilization, small items may be wrapped, sterilized, and stored in heat-sealable paper/plastic peel pouches.
5. For **gas** sterilization, use heat-sealable plastic peel pouches or tubing or muslin wrap.
6. For **plasma** sterilization, wrap items in a heat-sealable Tyvek/Mylar pouch or polypropylene wrap.

E. Wrapping instrument packs.

Wrap the instrument pack in a clean huck towel and place a large unfolded wrap diagonally in front of you. Place the instrument tray in the center of the wrap so that an imaginary line drawn from one corner of the wrap to the opposite corner is perpendicular to the two sides of the instrument tray. Fold the corner of the wrap that is closest to you over the instrument tray and to its far edge. Fold the right corner over the pack. Then, fold the left corner similarly. Turn the pack around and fold the final corner of the wrap over the tray, tucking it tightly under the previous two folds. Fold the tip of the final fold so that it is exposed for easy unwrapping. Wrap the pack in a second layer of cloth or paper in a similar manner. Secure the last corner of the outer wrap with masking tape; fold one end of the tape on itself so it can be easily grasped and removed. Place a small piece of heat-sensitive indicator tape over the masking tape. Label the tape with the current date, date of expiration, contents, and whether it is to be gas or steam sterilized.

F. Folding and wrapping gowns.

Place the gown on a clean flat surface with the front of the gown facing up. Fold the sleeves neatly toward the center of the gown with the cuffs of the sleeves facing the bottom hem. Fold the sides to the center so that the side seams are aligned with the sleeve seams. Then, fold the gown in half longitudinally (sleeves will be inside the gown). Ties should be placed so that they can be touched without contaminating the gown. Starting with the bottom hem of the gown, fanfold it toward the neck. Fold a hand towel in half

horizontally and fanfold it into about four folds. Place it on top of the folded gown, leaving one corner turned back to allow it to be easily grasped. Wrap the gown and towel in two layers of paper or cloth wrap as described above.

G. Folding and wrapping drapes.

Fold drapes so that the fenestration can be properly positioned over the surgical site without contaminating the drape. Lay the drape out flat with the ends of the fenestration parallel and the sides of the fenestration perpendicular to you. Grasp the ends of the drape closest to you and fanfold one half of the drape toward the center. Make sure the edge of the drape is dorsal to allow it to be easily grasped during unfolding. Then, turn the drape around and fanfold the other half toward the center, similarly. Next, fanfold one end of the drape to the center; repeat with the other end. Note that when the drape is properly folded, the fenestration is on the ventral outermost aspect of the drape. Fold the drape in half and wrap it in two layers of paper or cloth wrap as described above.

III. Handling and Storage of Sterilized Instruments/Equipment

A. Allow packs to cool and dry individually on racks when removed from the autoclave.

B. Store sterile packs when they are completely dry in waterproof dust covers in closed cabinets (as opposed to uncovered on open shelves).

C. Discourage excessive handling of sterile supplies, especially if items are pointed or have sharp edges. Handle sterile items gently; protect them from bending, crushing, or compression forces that could break a seal or puncture the package.

D. Store sterile packs away from ventilation ducts, sprinklers, and heat-producing light.

E. Sterile shelf life.

1. **Time-related expiration**–Published expiration dates for sterilized items wrapped in various types of wrappers (*SAS,* Table 1-3) have become controversial. The reason for disputing time-related expiration is that events, not time, contaminate products.
2. **Event-related expiration**–If items are packaged, sterilized, and handled properly, they remain sterile unless the package is opened, wet, torn, has a broken seal, or is damaged in some other way.
    a. On sterile packs, place the date on which the item was sterilized and a control lot number to trace an unsterile item.
    b. Place heat-sealed waterproof dust covers on items not routinely used. Remove plastic dust covers or wipe them clean before reaching the surgical area.
3. Do not use a sterile pack that has been damaged (i.e., wraps that have moisture present; packs that have been placed in a dusty environment or stored near an air current source; items that have been dropped, bent, crushed, compressed, torn, or punctured; or packs that have a broken seal).

IV. Unwrapping/Opening Sterile Items

A. Wrap sterile items in a manner that allows operating room personnel to unwrap the item without contaminating it (see above).

1. Unwrapping large sterile linen/paper/polypropylene packs that cannot be held during distribution.
   a. If the pack is too large, cumbersome, or heavy to be held during distribution, place the pack on the center of the Mayo stand or back table and open each folded layer by pulling it toward you. Handle only the edge and underside of the wrap. Follow the same procedure for each fold. When the pack is opened, have a sterile team member place it on the sterile table.
   b. To open double-wrapped sterile packs two techniques may be used (i.e., open the outer layer only or both layers).
      i. *Remove only the outer layer.* This eliminates the risk of microbial shedding from the circulating nurse's hands and arms onto the sterile package.
      ii. *Remove both wraps.* When the outer surface of the inner wrapper is opened, it may become contaminated via dust particles and debris from the outer wrapper. If this wrapper is opened by the circulating nurse, the possibility of contamination is decreased.
2. Unwrapping sterile linen/paper packages that can be held during distribution.

If you are right-handed, hold the pack in your left hand. Using the right hand, unfold one corner of the outside wrap at a time, being careful to secure each corner in the palm of the left hand to keep them from recoiling and contaminating the contents. Hold the final corner with your right hand. When the pack is fully exposed and all corners of the wrap secured, gently drop the pack onto the sterile field being careful to not allow your hand and arm to reach across or over the sterile field. Alternately, have a sterile team member grasp the item and place it on the instrument table.

3. Unwrapping sterile items in paper/plastic or plastic peel-back pouches.

Identify the edges of the peel-back wrapper and carefully separate them. Peel the edges of the wrapper back slowly and symmetrically to ensure the sterile item does not contact the torn edge of the wrapper (the torn edge of a peel-back wrapper is nonsterile). If the item is small, place it on the sterile area as described above, being careful not to lean across the sterile table. If the item is long or cumbersome have a sterile team member grasp it and gently pull it from the peel-back wrapper, taking care not to brush the item against the peeled edge of the wrapper. Open scalpel blades and suture similarly.

V. Pouring Solutions into Basins

Have a sterile team member hold the basin away from the surgical table to prevent the nonsterile assistant's hand and arm from extending over the sterile area. Pour the solution carefully and without splashing into the bowl so that it does not drip down the container onto the sterile person's hand. Do not allow the solution container to touch the sterile basin.

2

Sterilization and Disinfection (*SAS*, pp. 7-10)

I. Definitions

A. **Sterilization** is destruction of all microorganisms (bacteria, viruses, spores) on objects that come in contact with sterile tissue or enter the vascular system.

B. **Disinfection** is destruction of most pathogenic microorganisms on inanimate (i.e., nonliving) objects.

C. **Antisepsis** is destruction of most pathogenic microorganisms on animate (i.e., living) objects.

D. **Antiseptics** are used to kill microorganisms during patient skin preparation and surgical scrubbing (see Chapters 6 and 7); however, the skin is not sterilized.

II. Disinfection

A. Liquid disinfectants are most commonly used.

B. Common disinfectants, their usefulness, and necessary precautions are listed in Table 2-1.

III. Steam Sterilization

A. Mechanism of action–destroys microbes via coagulation and cellular protein denaturation.

B. Loading of an autoclave or gas sterilizer container.
   1. Position instrument packs vertically (i.e., on edge) and longitudinally in an autoclave.
   2. Place heavy packs at the periphery where steam enters the chamber.
   3. Allow a small amount of air space between each pack to facilitate steam flow (1 to 2 inches between each pack and surrounding walls).
   4. Load linen packs so the fabric layers are oriented vertically (i.e., on edge). Do not stack them.

Table 2-1
Common disinfectants used in veterinary practice

Agent	Practical use	Disinfectant properties	Antiseptic properties	Mechanisms of action	Precautions
Alcohol: isopropyl alcohol (50%-70%); ethyl alcohol (70%)	Spot cleaning; injection site preparation	Good	Very good	Protein denaturation, metabolic interruption, and cell lysis	Corrosive to stainless steel; volatile
Chlorine compounds: hypochlorite	Cleaning floors and countertops	Good	Fair	Release of free chlorine and oxygen	Inactivated by organic debris; corrosive to metal
Iodine compounds: iodophors (7.5%) scrub solution	Cleaning dark colored floors and countertops	Good	Good	Iodination and oxidation of essential molecules	Stains fabric and tissue
Glutaraldehyde: 2% alkaline solution	Disinfection of lenses and delicate instruments	Good; sterilizes	None	Protein and nucleic acid alkylation	Tissue reaction; odor (rinse instruments well before using)

C. Types of steam sterilizers/sterilization.
   1. Gravity ("downward") displacement sterilizer.
      a. Most commonly used steam sterilizer in veterinary practice (*SAS*, Fig. 2-1).
      b. Minimum temperature/time standard is 10 to 25 minutes at 270° to 275° F (132° to 135° C) or 15 to 30 minutes at 250° F (121° C).
      c. See Table 2-2 for recommended sterilization times for commonly sterilized items.
   2. Prevacuum sterilizer.
      a. Provides greater steam penetration in a shorter time than the gravity displacement sterilizer.
      b. The minimum temperature/time standard is 3 to 4 minutes at 270° to 275° F (132° to 135° C).
   3. Flash sterilization.
      a. Performed using a gravity sterilizer when an unwrapped, nonsterile item needs to be sterilized quickly.
      b. Place the item unwrapped in a perforated metal tray and sterilize

Table 2-2
Exposure periods for sterilization in gravity displacement sterilizers

Item	Minimum time required 250°-254° F (121°-123° C)
Scrub brushes (in dispensers, cans, individually wrapped)	30
Dressings (wrapped in muslin or paper)	30
Glassware (empty, inverted)	15
Instruments (wrapped in double-thickness muslin)	30
Instruments combined with suture, tubing, porous materials (wrapped in muslin or paper)	30
Metal instruments only (unwrapped)	15
Linen—maximum size 12 × 12 × 20 inches (6 kg wrapped)	30
Needles (individually packaged in glass vials or paper, lumens moist)	30
Needles (unwrapped, lumens moist)	15
Rubber catheters, drains, tubing (wrapped in muslin or paper; lumens moist)	30
Rubber catheters, drains, tubing (unwrapped; lumens moist)	20
Utensils (wrapped in muslin or paper, on edge)	20
Utensils (unwrapped, on edge)	15
Syringes (unassembled, individually packaged in muslin or paper)	30
Syringes (unassembled, unwrapped)	15
Suture—silk, cotton, nylon (wrapped in paper or muslin)	30
Solutions: 75-250 ml	20 (slow exhaust)
500-1000 ml	30 (slow exhaust)
1500-2000 ml	40 (slow exhaust)

it according to the manufacturer's time and temperature recommendations.

c. Use only in emergency situations when no other alternative is available.

d. Minimum temperature/time standard for a gravity flash sterilizer is 4 minutes at 270° to 275° F (132° to 135° C).

IV. Chemical (Gas) Sterilization

A. Ethylene Oxide

1. Mechanism of action–kills microorganisms and their spores by alkylation.
2. Safe for endoscopes, cameras, plastics and power cables that cannot be steam sterilized. Not safe for acrylics, some pharmaceutical items, and solutions.
3. Length of time required for sterilization depends on concentration of ethylene oxide, humidity, temperature, and density and type of materials to be sterilized. Strictly follow manufacturers' recommendations for ethylene oxide exposure time.
4. All materials sterilized with ethylene oxide must be aerated in a well-ventilated area for a minimum of 7 days, or 12 to 18 hours in an aerator. Otherwise cutaneous burns (i.e., vesicant), nausea, vomiting, headaches, weakness, upper and lower respiratory irritation, destruction of red blood cells (i.e., when improperly aerated items come in contact with the circulatory system), and birth defects may occur.
5. Clean and dry items first; moisture and organic material bonds with ethylene oxide and leaves a toxic residue.
6. Disassemble and clean all surfaces of the item; items that cannot be disassembled cannot be sterilized.
7. Pack items and load them loosely to allow gas circulation.

V. Plasma Sterilization

A. Mechanism of action–uses reactive ions, electrons, and neutral atomic particles to sterilize items.

B. *Vapor phase hydrogen peroxide sterilization* is a form of plasma sterilization that uses hydrogen peroxide to process instruments quickly and efficiently.

C. Instruments can be sterilized in 75 minutes and are immediately available because aeration is not required.

D. Items for sterilization must be wrapped in polypropylene, nonwoven fabric (*SAS,* Table 1-2).

E. *Can* be used for stainless steel, aluminum, brass, silicone, Teflon, latex, ethyl vinyl acetate, polycarbonate, polyethylene, polypropylene, polyvinyl chloride, and polymethylmethacrylate.

F. *Cannot* be used for linen, gauze sponges, wood products (including paper), some plastics, liquids, items that cannot be disassembled, items with copper or silver solder or using disphenole A epoxy, tubes and catheters greater than 12 inches, and tubes and catheters less than 3 mm in diameter.

VI. Ionizing Radiation

A. Restricted to commercial use because of expense.

B. Items commonly sterilized with ionizing radiation include suture material, sponges, disposable items (i.e., gowns, drapes, table covers), powders, and petroleum goods.

C. Do not resterilize prepackaged, irradiated items that have been opened but not used by other means because this could damage the item and be a health hazard.

VII. Cold Chemical Sterilization

A. Two percent glutaraldehyde.
1. Noncorrosive and provides a safe means for sterilizing delicate lensed instruments (i.e., endoscopes, cystoscopes, bronchoscopes).
2. Clean and dry items before immersion. Organic matter (e.g., blood, saliva) may prevent penetration of crevices or joints, and residual water causes chemical dilution.
3. Disassemble complex instruments.
4. Adhere to immersion times suggested by the manufacturer (e.g., 2% glutaraldehyde: 10 hours at 20° to 25° C for sterilization; 10 minutes at 20° to 25° C for disinfection).
5. Rinse items thoroughly with sterile water and dry with sterile towels to avoid damaging the patient's tissues.

VIII. Sterilization Indicators

A. Undergo either a chemical or biologic change in response to some combination of time and temperature.

B. Chemical indicators.
1. Do not indicate sterility–only that certain conditions for sterility have been met.
2. Are available for steam, gas, and plasma sterilization and are placed in the center of each pack and on the outside of the item to be sterilized (see *SAS,* pp. 9-10).

C. Biologic indicators.
1. Surest way to test the effectiveness of the sterilization process. Use at least weekly.
2. Use a strain of highly resistant, nonpathogenic, spore-forming bacteria contained in a glass vial or a strip of paper placed within the pack.
3. After the sterilization cycle is complete, the vial or strip is recovered and cultured; growth of the organism documents inadequate sterilization.

3

Surgical Facilities, Equipment, and Personnel (*SAS*, pp. 11-14)

I. Structure and Design of the Surgical Area

A. Divide the surgical area to clearly delineate "clean," "mixed," and "contaminated" areas.

1. Clean areas–operating rooms, scrub sink areas, sterile supply rooms.
2. Mixed areas–hallways between operating rooms and nurses' stations, instrument and supply processing areas, storage areas, utility rooms.
3. Contaminated areas–anesthesia preparation rooms, dressing rooms, lounges, offices.

B. Don proper surgical attire before entering a clean area from a contaminated area (see Chapter 7). When leaving a clean area and entering a contaminated area, cover clothing before leaving and discard these items when returning to the clean area.

C. Keep doors between clean and contaminated areas closed at all times.

D. Clip and vacuum patients in a contaminated area before transporting to a clean area (e.g., operating room).

II. Description and Function of Rooms in the Surgical Area

A. Dressing Room

1. Used by surgical personnel to change into proper surgical attire.
2. Should have closed cabinets for storing scrub suits, shoe covers, masks, and caps and a separate area for hanging street clothes.

B. Anesthesia and Surgical Preparation Room

1. Locate it adjacent to the surgical area, but out of major hospital traffic patterns.
2. Stock with equipment and medications that may be necessary in the event of an emergency (i.e., defibrillator, laryngoscopes, endotracheal tubes, suction, oxygen, crash cart).
3. Use preparation counters and surfaces that are impervious and easily cleaned and disinfected. Have gas-scavenger systems present at each anesthesia preparation table.

4. Maintain room temperature between 62° and 68° F and humidity at 50% or less to reduce microbial growth.
5. Use an adhesive microfilm dust pad at the doorway between the anesthesia preparation room and surgical area to collect dust, hair, and other particulates on gurney rollers, shoes, and anesthetic equipment.

C. Anesthesia Supply Room

1. Locate it adjacent to the anesthesia and surgical preparation room.
2. Store equipment necessary to keep anesthesia machines working properly, extra endotracheal tubes, anesthetic monitoring equipment, oxygen "E" tanks, hoses, catheters, and airway connectors here.

D. Nurses' Work Station

1. Locate it centrally within the surgical area (i.e., clean area).
2. Keep an autoclave (for flash sterilization), incubator/blanket warmer (e.g., irrigation fluids and towels to wrap patients postoperatively), refrigerator (e.g., medications, solutions), and formalin containers here.

E. Sterile Instrument Room

1. Houses all sterilized and packaged instruments and supplies. Surgery personnel assemble items needed for a particular case from supplies located in this room.

F. Equipment Room

1. Store large pieces of equipment (e.g., anesthetic machines, lasers, monitoring equipment, operating microscopes) here.

G. Housekeeping Supply Room

1. Store supplies used to decontaminate and clean surgical suites here.
2. Restrict use of these items to within the operating room to prevent cross-contamination from other hospital areas.

H. Scrub Sink Area

1. Have antiseptic soap in an appropriate dispenser (e.g., foot activated), scrub brushes, and fingernail cleaners located within easy reach at each scrubbing station.
2. Locate the scrub sink area away from wrapped sterile supplies because of possible contamination by water droplets and spray from the sinks.
3. Never use scrub sinks to clean equipment or instruments or dispose of body fluids.

I. Gowning and Gloving Area

1. Gowning and gloving can commence outside or inside the operating room.

J. Operating Room

1. Room size should be large enough to allow personnel to move around sterile equipment without contamination and to accommodate large pieces of equipment.
2. Use smooth, nonporous, fireproof materials for floors, ceilings, and other surfaces.
3. Design ventilation systems to provide positive air pressures within the operating room and lower air pressures within adjoining corridors. Ideal ventilation systems deliver a minimum of 15 to 20 air exchanges per hour.
4. Install scavenging systems that pull anesthetic gases out of operating room.

5. Keep operating room environments at a constant humidity (ideal humidity is 50% or less) and temperature (62° to 68° F).
6. Install main overhead fluorescent lights supplemented by the use of one, or preferably two, halogen spotlights. Mount surgical spotlights in the ceiling directly over the operating table.
7. Use stainless steel operating tables that are fully adjustable for height (hydraulic mechanism) and degree of tilt and that have tabletops that are either flat, one-piece surfaces or have V-trough capabilities.
8. Instrument tables should be made of stainless steel and should be adjustable in height.
9. Provide kick buckets to discard soiled sponges during surgery and suction (portable or piped in) in each operating room. Each operating room should also have a radiographic view box and wall clock.
10. Use supply cabinets with tight-fitting doors (to minimize dust accumulation) to store suture material, dressings, sponges, scalpel blades, and frequently used instruments.

K. Postoperative Recovery Area

1. Should be adjacent to the surgical area yet separate from areas used to house other hospitalized patients.
2. Have warming cabinets with a supply of warm fluids and blankets available.

L. Minor Procedures Surgery Room

Designate a separate room adjacent to the anesthesia preparation area for minor, contaminated surgical procedures (e.g., lacerations, biopsies, wound management, dental procedures, endoscopy). Equip this room with an operating table, spotlight, gas and suction lines for anesthesia equipment, suture, antiseptic preparation materials, and minor surgical instrument packs.

III. Personnel

A. Define Responsibilities and Functions of Every Member of the Surgical Team in Writing

1. The surgeon guides the flow and scope of what happens in the operating room during surgery.
2. Surgical assistants should have a working knowledge of the procedure being performed, provide retraction and hemostasis, and manipulate instruments and tissues into proper position to complete the surgical task.

4

Care and Maintenance of the Surgical Environment (*SAS*, pp. 15-17)

I. Daily Cleaning Routines

A. Operating Room

1. **Mornings**–damp dust with a lint-free cloth and hospital-grade disinfectant all horizontal surfaces, lights, operating room equipment, and furniture (Table 4-1).
2. **After each surgical procedure**–clean/disinfect areas contaminated by organic debris (e.g., floors, doors, counters, equipment, operating table).
3. **Evenings**–clean/disinfect operating tables, counters, lights, equipment, floors, windows, cabinets, and doors. Collect linen and waste bags. Disinfect kick buckets and replace plastic bags. Clean/disinfect surgical lights, monitoring equipment, and anesthesia equipment following manufacturers' specific guidelines. Clean/disinfect wheels and coasters of all movable equipment and gurney. Restock the operating room with commonly used instruments, suture, gauze sponges, needles, and syringes, and wet vacuum (preferred) or damp mop the floor.

B. Scrub Sinks

1. Clean frequently throughout the day (i.e., mop floors, remove used scrub brushes and fingernail cleaners, clean soap dispensers, wash sinks and walls) and disinfect it at the end of the day.

C. Anesthesia and Surgical Preparation Rooms

1. Keep sinks, vacuum, canisters, trash buckets, gurneys, and anesthesia preparation tables clean of organic debris and disinfect as needed throughout the day (*SAS*, Table 4-3).
2. Clean/disinfect plumbing fixtures, floors, cabinets, anesthesia equipment, utility rooms, furniture, and other equipment daily.
3. At the end of the day, disinfect the sink and pour a cup of disinfectant solution down the drain. Disinfect the inner surface of garbage containers.
4. Remove the bag and filter from portable vacuums and replace as needed; wipe and disinfect the outside surfaces of the vacuum (including hose and nozzle).
5. Clean clippers according to manufacturer's instructions.
6. Wet vacuum or damp mop the floor and restock supplies.

Table 4-1
Daily care and maintenance of the operating room

At the Beginning of Each Day

- Wipe flat surfaces of furnishings and lights with a cloth dampened with a disinfectant solution.

After Each Surgical Procedure

- Collect used instruments and place them in a cool water and detergent or enzymatic solution.
- Collect waste materials and soiled linens and place in proper containers.
- Wipe instrument and surgical tables, stands, kick buckets, and heating pads with a disinfectant.
- If necessary, clean the floor (move the surgical table and clean under it if body fluids have collected there).

After the Last Surgical Procedure of the Day

- Clean and disinfect kick buckets.
- Check ceilings, walls, cabinet doors, counter surfaces, and all furniture and clean as necessary.
- Clean/care for individual items (i.e., monitoring devices, anesthesia equipment, surgical lights) according to the manufacturer's instructions.
- Wipe counter surfaces and cabinet doors with a disinfectant solution.
- Wipe instrument and surgical tables, stands, heating pads, and light fixtures with a disinfectant solution. Disassemble the surgical table if necessary to thoroughly clean it.
- Check supplies and restock as necessary.
- Roll wheeled equipment (e.g., surgical table, monitoring devices) through a small amount of disinfectant solution placed on the floor.
- Wet vacuum or damp mop the floor.

D. Recovery Room

1. Clean cages, sinks, trash buckets, and gurneys of organic debris and disinfect as needed throughout the day.
2. Clean/disinfect plumbing fixtures, floors, cabinets, anesthesia equipment, utility rooms, furniture, and other equipment daily, as described above.
3. Disinfect cages between patients.

II. Weekly and Monthly Cleaning Routines

A. Empty surgical suites of moveable equipment and thoroughly clean once a week.

B. Clean/disinfect shelves of supply cabinets, walls, windows, windowsills, ceilings, light fixtures, surgical tables, utility and supply carts and castors, utility rooms, equipment storage areas, and infrequently used equipment.

C. Wet vacuum operating room floors and vacuum ventilation duct grills at least once a week. Once a month mop the walls, floors, and ceilings and lubricate moveable parts of equipment and gurneys.

5

Preoperative Assessment of the Surgical Patient (*SAS*, pp. 18-21)

I. History Taking

A. The history should include the presenting complaint, signalment, diet, exercise, environment, past medical problems, and present treatment. It is particularly important to detect acute or chronic corticosteroid or antimicrobial therapy, as well as evidence of infection elsewhere in the patient's body.

B. Frame questions to avoid vague responses and obtain specific information (e.g., "When was your dog last vaccinated?" vs. "Is your dog current on his vaccinations?"). Note any vomiting, diarrhea, altered appetite, exposure to toxins/foreign bodies, coughing, exercise intolerance, or other abnormalities. Animals with a history of seizures must be identified to avoid drugs that precipitate seizures (e.g., acepromazine). Ascertain the severity, duration, and progression of the specific disease or presenting complaint.

II. Physical Examination

A. Note the animal's general condition (body condition, attitude/mental status). See Chapter 33 for details on performing a neurologic exam and Chapter 28 for details on orthopedic examination.

B. Preanesthetic physical status (Table 5-1).

III. Laboratory Data

A. Recommended Minimum Laboratory Data

1. Young, healthy animals undergoing elective procedures and healthy animals with localized disease (e.g., patellar luxation)–hematocrit, total protein (TP), and urine specific gravity.
2. Animals 5 to 7 years of age, surgical times greater than 1 to 2 hours, animals with physical status of I or II (see Table 5-1)–CBC, serum biochemistry panel, and urinalysis.

Table 5-1
Physical status in surgical patients

Physical status	Animal condition	Examples
I	Healthy with no discernible disease	Elective procedure being performed (e.g., ovariohysterectomy, declaw, castration)
II	Healthy with localized disease or mild systemic disease	Patellar luxation, skin tumor, cleft palate without aspiration pneumonia
III	Severe systemic disease	Pneumonia, fever, dehydration, heart murmur, anemia
IV	Severe systemic disease that is life threatening	Heart failure, renal failure, hepatic failure, severe hypovolemia, severe hemorrhage
V	Moribund; patient is not expected to live longer than 24 hours with or without surgery	Endotoxic shock, multiorgan failure, severe trauma

3. Animals with systemic signs (e.g., dyspnea, heart murmur, anemia, ruptured bladder, gastric dilatation-volvulus, shock, hemorrhage)–CBC, serum biochemistry profile, and urinalysis.
4. Additional laboratory data are dictated by the animal's presenting signs and underlying disease.

IV. Determination of Surgical Risk

A. **Excellent** prognosis–minimal potential for complications and a high probability that the patient will return to normal after surgery.

B. **Good** prognosis–high probability for a good outcome, but some potential for complications.

C. **Fair** prognosis–serious complications are possible but uncommon, recovery may be prolonged, or the animal may not return to its presurgical function.

D. **Guarded** prognosis–the underlying disease or surgical procedure is associated with many or severe complications, recovery is expected to be prolonged, likelihood of death during or after the procedure is high, or the animal is unlikely to return to its presurgical function.

V. Client Communication

A. Inform owners before surgery of the diagnosis, surgical or nonsurgical options, potential complications, postoperative care, and cost.

B. Keep owners apprised of the animal's status and procedures that may affect the initial cost estimate.

C. If the disease is hereditary, recommend neutering.

VI. Patient Stabilization

A. Replace fluid deficits and correct acid-base and electrolyte abnormalities before anesthetic induction, if possible.

1. Normal blood volume of dogs and cats is approximately 90 and 70 ml/kg, respectively.
   a. Transfusions (i.e., whole blood, packed red cells) may be necessary in anemic patients. Animals with preoperative packed cell volumes (PCVs) of less than or equal to 20% usually benefit from blood transfusions.
   b. The amount of donor blood needed can be estimated by the formula given in Appendix A.
2. Generally, give patients in shock 60 to 90 ml/kg of polyionic isotonic fluid intravenously in the first hour; however, consider that patients with pulmonary, cardiovascular, or renal disease may be less tolerant of rapid fluid administration. If hemodilution is not a concern, give balanced electrolyte solutions (i.e., lactated Ringer's solution, Normosol-R). Hypertonic saline solutions are beneficial in reducing total fluid requirements, limiting edema, and increasing cardiac output (see Appendix B).
3. See Appendix C for the formula for calculating bicarbonate.

B. Intravenous fluids are indicated in all animals undergoing general anesthesia and surgery, including elective procedures in healthy animals.

C. See Chapter 10 for recommendations for antibiotic prophylaxis and therapy.

D. See Chapter 11 for preoperative parenteral or enteral hyperalimentation recommendations.

6

Preparation of the Operative Site (*SAS*, pp. 22-25)

I. Dietary Restrictions

A. Restrict food intake 6 to 12 hours before anesthesia to avoid intraoperative or postoperative emesis and aspiration pneumonia. Do not curtail access to water unless the animal is vomiting.

B. To avoid hypoglycemia, do not withhold food for long periods (i.e., >4 to 6 hours) in young animals.

II. Preparation Before Moving the Animal to the Surgery Room

A. If possible, bathe the animal the day before the surgical procedure to remove loose hair, debris, and external parasites. Allow the animal to defecate and urinate shortly before anesthesia. If the animal does not urinate voluntarily, manually express the bladder after anesthetic induction.

B. Verify the patient's identity, the surgical procedure being performed, and the surgical site before anesthetizing the animal.

C. After anesthetic induction, clip hair liberally around the proposed incision site so that the incision can be extended within a sterile field. Clip at least 20 cm on each side of the incision. Consider using depilatory creams in irregular areas where adequate hair removal is difficult. Razors are occasionally used for hair removal (e.g., around the eye), but cause microlacerations in skin that may increase irritation and promote infection. Remove loose hair with a vacuum.

D. For limb procedures, if exposure of the paw is unnecessary, exclude the paw from the surgical area by placing a latex glove over the distal extremity and securing it to the limb with tape. Cover the glove with tape or Vetrap. Drape the foot out of the sterile field (see below). A "hanging-leg" preparation may be done to enhance manipulation of limbs. This requires that the limb be circumferentially clipped; the limb is hung from an IV pole during prepping to allow all sides to be scrubbed.

E. Before transporting the animal to the surgical suite, perform a general cleansing scrub and place ophthalmic antibiotic ointments or lubricants on the cornea and conjunctiva. In male dogs undergoing abdominal procedures, flush the prepuce with an antiseptic solution.

III. Positioning

A. Move the animal to the operating room and position it so that the operative site is accessible to the surgeon. Secure the animal with ropes, sandbags, troughs, tape, or vacuum-activated positioning devices and connect monitoring devices.

B. Position the ground plate under the animal if electrocautery is being used.

C. If a hanging-leg preparation is being done, suspend the limb with tape from an IV pole.

IV. Sterile Skin Preparation

A. Sterilize gauze sponges in a pack along with bowls into which the germicides can be poured. Handle sponges with sterile sponge forceps or a gloved hand using aseptic technique. Use the dominant hand to perform the sterile preparation and the less dominant hand to retrieve sponges from the preparation bowl.

B. Begin scrubbing at the incision site. Use a circular scrubbing motion, moving from the center to the periphery. Do not return sponges from the periphery to the center; discard sponges after reaching the periphery.

C. Blot excess solution on the table or in body "pockets" with a sterile towel or sponges.

V. Draping

A. Draping is performed by a gowned and gloved surgical team member. If an abdominal incision extends to the pubis in male dogs, clamp the prepuce to one side with a sterile towel clamp.

B. Begin with placement of field drapes (quarter drapes) to isolate the unprepared portion of the animal. Place these towels one at a time at the periphery of the prepared area. Do not flip, fan, or shake drapes because rapid movement of drapes creates air currents on which dust, lint, and droplet nuclei can migrate. Once the towels are placed, do not readjust them toward the incision site because this carries bacteria onto the prepared skin. Secure towels at the corners with Bachhaus towel clamps. Once placed through the skin, the tips of the towel clamps are considered nonsterile.

C. When the animal and incision site are protected by field drapes, perform final draping. Place a large drape over the animal and the entire surgical table to provide a continuous sterile field.

D. To drape a limb, place field drapes and secure as described above to isolate the surgical site or the proximal aspect of the limb if the leg is hung. Have a nonsterile surgical team member hold the nonprepared area of the limb and cut the tape holding the elevated limb. Present the limb to the sterile surgical member so that it may be taken with a hand in a sterile stockinette or towel. If a stockinette is used, carefully unroll it down the limb and secure it with towel clamps. If a sterile towel is used, carefully wrap the limb with the towel before securing it to skin with a towel clamp. Cover water-impermeable (disposable) towels (plus the towel clamp) with sterile Kling. If a cloth towel is used, cover it (and the towel clamp) with sterile Vetrap. Place the limb through a fenestration of a lap or fanfold drape and secure the drape. Wrap the end of the stockinette with sterile Vetrap.

E. To reduce skin exposure and subsequent contamination during the surgery, additional skin draping, or "toweling-in," can be performed after the skin incision is made. Alternatively, apply plastic adhesive drapes to the skin and surrounding drapes for the same purpose.

7

Preparation of the Surgical Team (*SAS*, pp. 26-32)

I. Surgical Attire

A. All persons entering the operating room suite, regardless of whether a surgery is in progress or not, should wear scrub clothes rather than street clothes. If a scrub suit is worn outside the surgery room, wear a lab coat or single-use gown to cover it.

B. Hair is a significant carrier of bacteria, thus complete coverage is necessary. Even when surgery is not in progress, wear caps and masks in the surgical suite. Ensure that caps completely cover all head and face hair, and that masks cover the mouth and nostrils. Wear hoods to completely cover sideburns and beards. Do not wear skullcaps that fail to cover the side hair above the ears and hair at the nape of the neck.

C. Don shoe covers when first entering the surgical area and wear them when leaving it to keep shoes clean. Don new shoe covers upon returning to the surgical area.

D. Wear masks whenever entering a sterile area. Fit masks over the mouth and nose and secure the dorsal aspect of the mask by shaping the reinforcing top edge tightly around the nose.

E. Surgical gowns may be reusable and made of woven materials (usually cotton), or they may be disposable. The number of microorganisms isolated from the surgical environment is lower when disposable (single-use), nonwoven materials are used for gowns.

II. Surgical Scrub

A. All sterile surgical team members perform a hand and arm scrub before entering the surgical suite. Do not rely on gloves alone (without a surgical scrub) to prevent microbial contamination; up to 50% of surgical gloves contain holes at the completion of surgery. This number may increase with long or difficult surgeries.

B. Antimicrobial soaps or detergents used for scrubbing should be rapid-acting, broad-spectrum, and nonirritating substances and should inhibit rapid-rebound microbial growth. The most commonly used surgical scrub solutions are chlorhexidine gluconate, povidone-iodine, and hexachlorophene (Table 7-1).

Table 7-1
Common antimicrobial soaps available for surgical scrubs

Antimicrobial soap	Mechanism of action	Properties
Chlorhexidine gluconate	Disruption of cell wall and precipitation of cell proteins	• Broad spectrum (more effective against gram-positive than gram-negative bacteria or fungi) • Good virucide • Residual activity because it binds to keratin • Not inactivated by organic material • May be less irritating to skin than iodophors
Hexachlorophene	Disruption of cell wall and precipitation of cell proteins	• Bacteriostatic for gram-positive cocci • Minimal activity against gram-negative bacteria, fungi, or viruses • Not inactivated by organic material • Cumulative (nullified by alcohol) • May be neurotoxic
Iodophors	Cell wall penetration, oxidation, replaces microbial contents with free iodine	• Broad spectrum (gram-negative and gram-positive bacteria, fungi, and viruses) • Some activity against spores • Inactivated by organic material • Requires minimum of 2 minutes of skin contact
Parachloromethaxylenol (PCMX)	Disruption of cell wall and enzyme inactivation	• Broad spectrum (more effective against gram-positive than gram-negative bacteria, fungi, or viruses) • Slow onset of action
Triclosan	Disruption of cell wall	• Broad spectrum (ineffective against many *Pseudomonas* spp.) • Minimally affected by organic material

C. Two accepted methods of performing a surgical scrub are the anatomic timed scrub (i.e., 5-minute scrub) and counted brush stroke methods (strokes per surface area of skin). Each method is described in Table 7-2. An initial 5- to 7-minute scrub for the first case of the day, followed by a 2- to 3-minute scrub between additional surgical operations, is generally adequate.

D. Before scrubbing, remove all jewelry (including watches) from the hands and forearms. Do not wear fingernail polish or artificial nails. Once the scrub has been started do not handle nonsterile items. After scrubbing procedures, keep the hands higher than the elbows.

E. Dry the hands and arms with a sterile towel. Pick up the sterile towel from the table taking care not to drip water on the gown beneath it and step back from the sterile table. Hold the towel lengthwise and dry one hand and arm working from hand to elbow with one end of the towel; use a blotting motion. Bend over at the waist when drying the arms so the end of the towel will not brush against your scrub suit. Once the hand and arm are dry bring the dry hand to the opposite end of the towel. Dry the other hand and arm in a similar manner. Drop the towel into the proper receptacle or on the floor if a receptacle is not provided. Do not lower your hands below waist level.

III. Gowning

Grasp the gown firmly and gently lift it away from the table. Step back from the sterile table to allow room for gowning. Hold the gown at the shoulders and allow it to gently unfold. Do not shake the gown because this increases the risk of contamination. Once the gown is opened identify the armholes and guide each arm through the sleeves. Keep your hands within the cuffs of the gown. Have an assistant pull the gown up over your shoulders and secure it by closing the neck fasteners and tieing the inside waist tie. If a sterile-back gown is used, do not secure the front tie until you have donned sterile gloves.

IV. Gloving

A. Use gloves in which the inner surfaces are lubricated with an adherent coating of hydrogel.

B. Closed gloving.
   1. Ensure that the hand never comes in contact with the outside of the gown or glove.

Working through the gown sleeve, pick up one glove from the wrapper. Lay the glove palm down over the cuff of the gown with the thumb and fingers of the glove facing toward your elbow. Grasp the cuff of the glove with your index finger and thumb. With the index finger and thumb of the other hand (within the cuff), take hold of the opposite side of the edge of the glove. Lift the cuff on the glove up and over the gown cuff and hand. Turn loose and come to the palm side of the glove and take hold of the gown and glove, pulling them toward the elbow while pushing the hand through the cuff and into the glove. Proceed with the opposite hand using the same technique.

Table 7-2
Surgical scrub procedure

- Locate scrub brushes, antibacterial soap, nail cleaners.
- Remove watches and rings.
- Wet hands and forearms thoroughly.
- Apply 2-3 pumps of antimicrobial soap to hands and wash hands and forearms.
- Clean nails and subungual areas with a nail cleaner under running water.
- Rinse arms and forearms.
- Apply 2-3 pumps of antimicrobial soap to hand and forearm.
- Apply 2-3 pumps of antimicrobial soap to the sterile scrub brush.

Anatomic timed method	Counted brush stroke method
Note starting time; scrub each side of each finger, between fingers, and back and front of the hand for 2 minutes. Proceed to scrub the arms, keeping the hand higher than the arm. Scrub each side of the arm to 3 inches above the elbow for 1 minute. Total scrub time is 2 to 3 minutes per hand and arm.	Apply 30 strokes (one stroke consists of up and down or back and forth motion) to the very tips of your fingers and thumb. Divide each finger and thumb into four parts and apply 20 strokes to each of the four surfaces, including the finger webs. Scrub from the tip of the finger to the wrist when scrubbing the thumb, index, and small fingers. Divide your forearms into four planes and apply 20 strokes to each surface.

- Rinse the scrub brush well under running water and transfer the brush to your scrubbed hand. Do not rinse the scrubbed hand and arm at this time.
- Repeat the process on your other hand and arm.
- When both hands and arms have been scrubbed, drop the scrub brush in the sink.
- Starting with the fingertips of one hand, rinse under water by moving your fingertips up and out of the water stream and allowing the rest of your arm to be rinsed off on the way out of the stream.
- Always allow the water to run from your fingertips to your elbows.
- Never allow your fingertips to come below the level of your elbows.
- Never shake your hands to get rid of excess water; allow the water to drip from your elbows.
- Rinse off your other hand similarly.
- Hold your hands upright and in front of you so that they can be seen, and proceed to the gowning and gloving area.

C. Open gloving.

1. Use when only the hands need to be covered (e.g., urinary catheterization, bone marrow biopsy, sterile patient preparation) or during surgery when one glove becomes contaminated and must be changed. *Do not* use routinely for gowning and gloving.
2. Open gloving when one hand is sterile.

Open the glove wrapper and pick up the correct glove at the folded edge with your sterile hand. Gently put your hand into the glove until your fingers are in the fingers of the glove. Place your thumb inside or near the thumb of the glove and hook the cuff of the glove over your thumb. Let go of the glove. Place the finger of your sterile hand under the cuff at the palm of the glove and bend the wrist of the hand being gloved 90 degrees. Gently walk your fingers around the cuff until they are at the front of the cuff and at the same time pull the cuff up and over.

3. Open gloving when neither hand is sterile.

Pick up one glove by its inner cuff with the opposite hand. Slide the glove onto the opposite hand; leave the cuff down. Using the partially gloved hand, slide your fingers into the other side of the opposite glove cuff. Slide your hand into the glove and unfold the cuff: do not touch your bare arm as the cuff is unfolded. With the gloved hand, slide your fingers under the outside edge of the opposite cuff and unfold it.

D. Assisted gloving.

1. Primarily used when one glove becomes contaminated during surgery, but may be used to don gloves initially.

Have an assistant pick up one glove and place his or her fingers and thumb under the cuff of the glove. With the thumb of the glove facing you, slip your hand into the glove. Then, have the assistant bring the cuff of the glove up and over the cuff of your gown and gently let it go. Have the assistant pick up the other glove. Assist by holding the cuff of the glove open with the fingers of your sterile hand, while putting your ungloved hand into the open glove. Have the assistant keep his or her thumbs under the cuff while you thrust your hand into it.

E. Removing gloves aseptically.

Have a nonsterile assistant grasp the glove near the cuff (being careful not to touch the gown) and pull it gently from the fingertips.

V. Maintaining Sterility of Surgical Personnel

A. Once gowned, always face the sterile field. Do not lean over or touch an unsterile area. Keep arms and hands above the waist and below the shoulders. Do not fold the arms; clasp them in front of the body, above the waist. Sit only when the entire surgical procedure will be performed seated.

B. Consider the front of the gown sterile from the chest to the level of the sterile field; the back of the gown is not considered sterile (even if a sterile-back or wraparound gown is used). The sleeves are sterile from 2 inches above the elbow to the stockinette cuff. Because the stockinette cuff collects moisture (making it an ineffective microbial barrier), it is considered unsterile and should be covered by sterile gloves at all times. The neckline, shoulders, and area under the arms should also be considered unsterile because they may be contaminated by perspiration or by collar and shoulder surfaces rubbing together during head and neck movements.

8

Surgical Instrumentation (*SAS*, pp. 33-41)

I. Instrument Categories

A. Scalpels

1. Reusable scalpel handles (No. 3 and 4) with detachable blades are most commonly used in veterinary medicine. Blades are available in various sizes and shapes; a No. 10 blade is most commonly used in small animal surgery.
2. Use scalpels in a "slide cutting" fashion where the direction of pressure applied to the knife blade is at a right angle to the direction of scalpel pressure. When incising skin, keep the scalpel blade perpendicular to the skin surface.
3. Scalpels can be held using a pencil grip, fingertip grip, or palmed grip (*SAS*, pp. 33).

B. Scissors

1. Scissors are generally classified according to the type of point (e.g., blunt-blunt, sharp-sharp, sharp-blunt), blade shape (e.g., straight, curved), or cutting edge (plain, serrated). Metzenbaum or Mayo scissors are most commonly used in surgery; the former scissors are more delicate and should be reserved for fine, thin tissues. Mayo scissors are used for cutting heavy tissues (e.g., fascia).
2. Hold scissors with the tips of the thumb and ring finger through the finger rings and with the index finger resting on the shanks near the fulcrum. Do not allow the ring finger or thumb to "fall through" the handle.
3. Use the end of the blade to cut tissue or suture. This stabilizes the tissue more securely and results in a more precise cut.

C. Needle Holders

1. Needle holders are used to grasp and manipulate curved needles. Mayo-Hegar needle holders are commonly used in veterinary medicine when medium to coarse needles are being manipulated. Olsen-Hegar needle holders are used similarly but have scissor blades allowing suture to be tied and cut with the same instrument.
2. Place needles perpendicular to the needle holder because this allows the greatest maneuverability. Generally grasp needles near their center because this allows the needle to be advanced through tissue with greater force and less risk of needle breakage.

3. Needle holders may be held using the following grips.
   a. Palmed grip.
      i. No fingers are placed in the rings; upper ring rests against the ball of the thumb.
      ii. Best when tough tissue is being sutured that requires a strong needle-driving force; however, suturing is less precise than with other grips.
   b. Thenar grip.
      i. Upper ring rests on the ball of the thumb, ring finger is inserted through the lower ring.
      ii. Allows the needle to be released and regrasped for extraction without changing grips. Although it enhances mobility, releasing the needle holder causes the handles of the needle holder to "pop" apart, allowing some movement of the needle.
   c. Thumb-ring finger grip.
      i. Thumb is placed through the upper ring and ring finger through the lower ring.
      ii. Allows precision when releasing a needle–preferred when tissue is delicate or when precise suturing is required.
   d. Pencil grip.
      i. Index finger and thumb rest on the shafts of the needle holders; used with Castroviejo needle holders.

D. Tissue Forceps

1. Brown-Adson, the most commonly used tissue forceps (tweezerlike, nonlocking instruments used to grasp tissue), have small serrations on the tips that cause minimal trauma but facilitate holding tissue securely.
2. Use in the nondominant hand. Hold so that one blade functions as an extension of the thumb and the other blade functions as an extension of the opposing fingers (pencil position). When not in use, palm them and hold with the ring and little fingers, leaving the index and middle fingers free.
3. Use to stabilize tissue or expose tissue layers during suturing. When grasping needles during suturing, grasp the needle perpendicular to the shaft.

E. Hemostatic Forceps

1. Crushing instruments used to clamp blood vessels.
   a. Mosquito–small (3-inch) hemostats with transverse jaw serrations.
   b. Kelly–transverse (i.e., horizontal) serrations extend only over the distal portion of the jaws.
   c. Crile–have transverse serrations that extend the entire jaw length.
   d. Rochester-Carmalt–large crushing forceps that have longitudinal grooves with cross grooves at the tip ends to prevent tissue slippage.
   e. Satinsky–allow occlusion of only a portion of a vessel.
2. Place curved hemostats on tissue with the curve facing up. Grasp as little tissue as possible to minimize trauma, and use the smallest hemostatic forceps that will accomplish the job.
3. Place fingertips on the finger rings or insert fingers into the rings only as far as the first joint.

F. Retractors

1. Handheld and self-retaining retractors are used to retract tissue and improve exposure. The ends of handheld retractors may be hooked, curved, spatula shaped, or toothed.
   a. Malleable–handheld retractors that may be bent to conform to the structure or area of the body being retracted.
   b. Senn (rake) retractors–double-ended retractors; one end has three fingerlike, curved prongs, the other end is a flat, curved blade.

c. Gelpi, Weitlaner, Balfour, Finochietto–self-retaining retractors that maintain tension on tissues and are held open with a box lock or other device (e.g., set screw).

II. Instrument Care and Maintenance

A. Rinse instruments in cool water immediately after the surgical procedure to prevent blood, tissue, saline, or other foreign matter from drying on them. Use distilled or deionized water. If tap water is used, dry instruments thoroughly to avoid staining. Dissasemble instruments with multiple components before cleaning and clean and sterilize delicate instruments separately.

B. Ultrasonic cleaners.
   1. Before putting soiled instruments in an ultrasonic cleaner, wash them in cleaning solution to remove all visible debris. Do not mix dissimilar metals (e.g., chrome and stainless steel) in the same cycle. Place instruments in the ultrasonic cleaner with the ratchets and box locks open. Do not pile instruments on top of each other. Remove instruments from the cleaner and rinse and dry at the completion of the cycle.
   2. If an ultrasonic cleaner is not available, clean instruments as thoroughly as possible, paying particular attention to box locks, serrations, and hinges. Rasps and serrated areas may require a wire brush. Use a cleaning solution with a neutral pH to avoid staining.

C. Lubricating and autoclaving.
   1. Before autoclaving, lubricate power equipment and instruments with box locks and hinges with instrument milk or surgical lubricants. Do not use industrial oils.
   2. Wrap instruments in cloth or place them on a cloth inside a fenestrated pan to absorb moisture. Sterilize instruments with the box locks or hinges open.
   3. Avoid overloading the chamber and do not stack instruments. Add a monitor (e.g., OK sterilization indicators, Sterrad chemical indicator strip) to the pack before double wrapping and sealing it with tape (e.g., Auto Clave Tape).
   4. To prevent condensation, avoid rapid cooling of instruments. See Chapter 2 for additional information regarding autoclaving and other methods of sterilization.

III. Draping and Organizing the Instrument Table

A. Instrument tables should be height adjustable to allow them to be positioned within reach of surgical personnel. Do not open the instrument table until the animal has been positioned on the surgical table and draped.

B. Use large, water-impermeable table drapes that cover the entire instrument table. Once the drape has been opened, do not allow nonsterile personnel to reach over it. Instrument layout is generally determined by surgeon's preference, but grouping similar instruments (e.g., scissors, retractors) facilitates their use.

C. Whenever a body cavity is opened, count sponges at the beginning of the procedure (before making the incision) and again before closure to ensure that none have been inadvertently left in the body cavity. Do not place contaminated instruments or soiled sponges back on the instrument table.

9

Biomaterials, Suturing, and Hemostasis (*SAS*, pp. 42-56)

I. Sutures and Suture Selection

A. Suture Characteristics

1. Suture size.
   a. Use the smallest-diameter suture that will adequately hold the mending wounded tissue.
   b. The most commonly used standard for suture size is the United States Pharmacopeia (USP), which denotes dimensions from fine to coarse, according to a numerical scale; 10-0 is the smallest and 7 is the largest. The USP uses different standards for surgical gut and for other materials (Table 9-1). The smaller the suture size, the less its tensile strength.
   c. Stainless steel wire is usually sized according to the metric or USP scale or by the Brown and Sharpe (B and S) wire gauge.
2. Flexibility.
   a. The flexibility of suture is determined by its torsional stiffness and diameter, which influence its handling and use. Flexible sutures are indicated when ligating vessels or performing continuous suture patterns.
   b. Nylon and surgical gut are relatively stiff compared with silk suture; braided polyester sutures have intermediate stiffness.
3. Surface characteristics and coating.
   a. The surface characteristics of a suture influence the ease with which it is pulled through tissues ("drag") and the amount of trauma doing so causes. Smooth surfaces are particularly important in delicate tissues such as the eye. However, sutures with smooth surfaces require increased tension to ensure good apposition of tissues, and they have reduced knot security.
   b. Braided materials have more friction or drag than do monofilament sutures. Braided materials are often coated with Teflon, silicone, wax, paraffin-wax, and calcium stearate to decrease capillarity and yield a smooth surface.
4. Capillarity.
   a. Capillarity is the process by which fluid and bacteria are carried into the interstices of multifilament fibers.
   b. All braided materials (e.g., silk) are capillary; monofilament sutures are less capillary. Capillary suture materials should not be used in contaminated or infected sites.
5. Knot tensile strength.
   a. Measured by the force (in pounds) that the suture strand can withstand before it breaks when knotted.

Table 9-1
Suture sizes

Actual size (mm)	Metric gauge	Synthetic suture materials (USP)	Surgical gut (USP)	Brown and Sharpe wire gauge
0.02	0.2	10-0		
0.03	0.3	9-0		
0.04	0.4	8-0		
0.05	0.5	7-0	8-0	41
0.07	0.7	6-0	7-0	38-40
0.1	1	5-0	6-0	35
0.15	1.5	4-0	5-0	32-34
0.2	2	3-0	4-0	30
0.3	3	2-0	3-0	28
0.35	3.5	0	2-0	26
0.4	4	1	0	25
0.5	5	2	1	24
0.6	6	3,4	2	22
0.7	7	5	3	20
0.8	8	6	4	19
0.9	9	7		18

6. Knot security.
   a. **Relative knot security** is the holding capacity of a suture expressed as a percent of its tensile strength.
   b. **Knot-holding capacity** of a suture material is the strength required to untie or break a defined knot by loading the part of the suture that forms the loop, whereas the suture material's tensile strength is the strength required to break an untied fiber with a force applied in the direction of its length.

B. Suture Materials

1. Monofilament sutures.
   a. Made of a single strand of material.
   b. Have less tissue drag than multifilament suture material and do not have interstices that may harbor bacteria.
2. Multifilament sutures.
   a. Consist of several strands of suture that are twisted or braided together.
   b. Are generally more pliable and flexible than monofilament sutures. They may be coated to decrease tissue drag and enhance handling characteristics.
3. Absorbable suture materials.
   a. Lose most of their tensile strength within 60 days and eventually disappear from the tissue implantation site because they are phagocytized or hydrolyzed (Table 9-2). Examples include surgical gut, polyglycolic acid, polyglactin 910, polydioxanone, and polyglyconate.
   b. Catgut (surgical gut).
      i. Made from the submucosa of sheep intestine or the serosa of bovine intestine and is approximately 90% collagen.
      ii. Broken down by phagocytosis and elicits a marked inflammatory reaction, compared with other sutures.

Table 9-2
Characteristics of suture materials commonly used in veterinary medicine

Generic name	Trade name	Manufacturer	Suture characteristics	Reduction in tensile strength*	Complete absorption (days)	Relative knot security†	Tissue reaction‡
Chromic surgical gut (catgut)	—	—	Absorbable Multifilament	33% at 7 days 67% at 28 days	60	– wet + dry	+++
Polyglactin 910	Vicryl	Ethicon	Absorbable Multifilament	35% at 14 days 60% at 21 days	60	++	+
Polyglycolic acid	Dexon "S" (uncoated) Dexon II (coated)	Davis & Geck	Absorbable Multifilament	35% at 14 days 65% at 21 days	60-90	++	+
Polydioxanone	PDS II	Ethicon	Absorbable Monofilament	14% at 14 days 31% at 42 days	180	++	+
Polyglyconate	Maxon	Davis & Geck	Absorbable Monofilament	30% at 14 days 45% at 21 days	180	++	+
Silk	Perma-Hand	Ethicon Davis & Geck	Nonabsorbable Multifilament	30% at 14 days 50% at 1 year	>2 years	–	+++
Polyester	Mersiline (uncoated) Ethibond (coated) Dacron (uncoated) Ti•cron (coated)	Ethicon Ethicon Davis & Geck Davis & Geck	Nonabsorbable Multifilament		–	++	
Polyamide (Nylon)	Ethilon (monofilament) Nurolon (multifilament) Dermalon (monofilament) Surgilon (multifilament)	Ethicon Ethicon Davis & Geck Davis & Geck	Nonabsorbable Monofilament Multifilament	30% at 2 years (mo) 75% at 180 days (mu)		+	–
Polypropylene	Prolene Surgilene Fluorofil	Ethicon Davis & Geck Mallinckrodt Veterinary	Nonabsorbable Monofilament			+++	–

Polybutester	Novafil	Davis & Geck	Nonabsorbable Monofilament	++	–
Polymerized caprolactum	Supramid Braunamid Vetcassette II	S. Jackson B. Braun Melsungen Ag Mallinckrodt Veterinary	Nonabsorbable Multifilament	++	++ (if coating breaks)
Stainless steel wire	Flexon (multifilament)	Davis & Geck Ethicon	Nonabsorbable Monofilament Multifilament	+++	–

*Values given are approximate. Actual loss of tensile strength may vary depending on suture and tissue.
†(–) = poor (<60%); (+) = fair (60% to 70%); (++) = good (70% to 85%); (+++) = excellent (>85%).
‡(–) = minimal to none; (+) = mild, (++) = moderate; (+++) = severe.

   iii. "Tanning" (cross-linking of collagen fibers), by exposure with chrome or aldehyde, slows absorption.
   iv. Rapidly removed from infected sites or areas where it is exposed to digestive enzymes and is quickly degraded in catabolic patients.
 c. Synthetic absorbable materials (e.g., polyglycolic acid, polyglactin 910, polydioxanone, polyglyconate)
   i. Are generally broken down by hydrolysis. See Table 9-2 for information regarding tensile strength and degradation of the synthetic absorbable suture materials.
   ii. Elicit minimal tissue reaction and time for loss of strength, and absorption is fairly constant in different tissues.
   iii. Infection or exposure to digestive enzymes does not significantly influence the rates of absorption.
4. Nonabsorbable suture materials.
 a. Silk.
   i. A braided multifilament suture, marketed as uncoated or coated.
   ii. Excellent handling characteristics but does not maintain significant tensile strength after 6 months.
   iii. Avoid in contaminated sites.
 b. Synthetic nonabsorbable materials (e.g., polyester, coated caprolactam, polypropylene, polyamide, polyolefins, polybutester).
   i. Typically strong and induce minimal tissue reaction.
   ii. Do not bury nonabsorbable suture materials that consist of an inner core and an outer sheath (e.g., Supramid) because they may predispose to infection and fistulation.
 c. Metallic sutures.
   i. Stainless steel is available as a monofilament or multifilament twisted wire.
   ii. Reaction to stainless steel is generally minimal; however, the knot ends evoke an inflammatory reaction.
   iii. Has a tendency to cut tissue and may fragment and migrate.

C. Surgical Needles

1. Most are made from stainless steel wire because it is strong, corrosion free, and does not harbor bacteria.
2. Eyed needles.
 a. Must be threaded and creates a larger hole than when swaged suture material is used.
 b. May be closed (i.e., round, oblong, or square) or French eyed.
 c. Thread eyed needles from the inside curvature.
3. Needle body.
 a. Straight (Keith) needles are generally used in accessible places where the needle can be manipulated directly with the fingers (e.g., placement of purse-string sutures in the anus).
 b. Curved needles are manipulated with needle holders.
   i. One-fourth (¼) circle needles are primarily used in ophthalmic procedures.
   ii. Three-eighths (⅜) and one-half (½) circle needles are the most commonly used surgical needles in veterinary medicine.
4. Needle point.
 a. Cutting needles.
   i. Generally have two or three opposing cutting edges.
   ii. Designed to be used in tissues that are difficult to penetrate (e.g., skin).
   iii. *Conventional cutting needles*–the third cutting edge is on the inside (i.e., concave) curvature of the needle.
   iv. *Reverse cutting needles*–have a third cutting edge located on the

outer (i.e., convex) curvature of the needle, which reduces the risk of tissue cut-out.

v. *Side-cutting needles* (i.e., spatula needles)–are flat on the top and bottom. Generally used in ophthalmic procedures.

b. Taper needles (i.e., round needles).
   i. Have a sharp tip that pierces and spreads tissues without cutting them.
   ii. Generally used in easily penetrated tissues (e.g., intestine).
   iii. *Taper-cut needles*–are a combination of a reverse cutting edge tip and a taper-point body.
   iv. Blunt-point needles have a rounded, blunt point that can dissect through friable tissue without cutting. They are occasionally used for suturing soft, parenchymal organs (e.g., liver or kidney).

D. Suture Selection

1. Important points to consider.
   a. How long will the suture be required to help strengthen the wound or tissue?
   b. What is the risk of infection?
   c. What is the effect of the suture material on wound healing?
   d. What dimension and strength of suture is required?
2. Abdominal closure.
   a. *Skin*–use monofilament sutures in skin to prevent wicking or capillary transport of bacteria to deeper tissues. Nonabsorbable sutures are generally used. If absorbable sutures are used in skin they should be removed because absorption requires contact with body fluids.
   b. *Subcutaneous sutures*–use to obliterate dead space and decrease tension on skin edges; absorbable suture material (e.g., PDS or Maxon) is preferred.
3. Parenchymal organs and vessels.
   a. Suture parenchymal organs (e.g., liver, spleen, and kidney) with absorbable, monofilament sutures.
   b. Avoid multifilament sutures in areas of contamination.
4. Hollow viscus organs.
   a. Use absorbable sutures in hollow viscus organs (e.g., trachea, gastrointestinal tract, or bladder) to prevent tissue retention of foreign material once the wound is healed.
   b. Avoid nonabsorbable suture in the urinary bladder or gallbladder because they may be calculogenic.
5. Infected or contaminated wounds.
   a. Avoid sutures if possible in highly contaminated or infected wounds.
   b. Do not use multifilament nonabsorbable sutures (e.g., silk or polyester) in infected tissues because they potentiate infection and may fistulate.
   c. Avoid surgical gut because its absorption in infected tissue is unpredictable.

II. Other Biomaterials

A. Tissue Adhesives

1. Cyanoacrylates (e.g., *n*-butyl and isobutyl-2-cyanoacrylate) are commonly used for tissue adhesion during some procedures (e.g., declaws, tail docking, and ear cropping).
2. Persistence of the glue in the dermis may result in granuloma formation or dehiscence, and placement in an infected site may be associated with fistulation.

B. Staples and Ligating Clips

1. Clips (e.g., Hemoclips or Ligaclips) may be used for vessel ligation when the vessels are less than 11 mm in diameter. The vessel should be one third to two thirds of the size of the clip.
2. Staples (e.g., Michel clips, Proximate plus skin staples) are used to appose wound edges or attach drapes to skin.

C. Surgical Mesh

1. Surgical mesh may be used to repair hernias (e.g., perineal hernias) or reinforce traumatized or devitalized tissues (abdominal hernias).
2. Available in nonabsorbable (e.g., Mersilene [polyester] fiber mesh and Prolene [polypropylene] mesh) or absorbable (e.g., Vicryl [polyglactin 910] and Dexon [polyglycolic acid]) forms.
3. When nonabsorbable mesh is placed in contaminated wounds it may extrude or fistulate so remove it when the tissue has healed and the mesh is no longer required for support.

III. Common Suture Techniques

A. Suture Patterns

1. Appositional, inverting, everting sutures.
   a. *Appositional sutures* (e.g., simple interrupted sutures)–bring the tissue in close approximation.
   b. *Everting sutures* (e.g., continuous mattress suture)–turn the tissue edges outward, away from the patient and toward the surgeon.
   c. *Inverting sutures* (e.g., Lembert, Connell, Cushing)–turn tissue away from the surgeon, or toward the lumen of a hollow viscus organ.
2. Subcutaneous and subcuticular sutures.
   a. Subcutaneous sutures are placed to eliminate dead space and provide some apposition of skin so that less tension is placed on skin sutures.
   b. Subcuticular sutures may be used in place of skin sutures to reduce scarring or eliminate the need for suture removal (e.g., fractious animals or castrations).
3. Interrupted suture patterns.
   a. Simple interrupted.
      i. Place by inserting the needle through tissue on one side of an incision or wound, pass it to the opposite side, and tie.
      ii. Place sutures approximately 2 to 3 mm away from the skin edge.
      iii. Right-handed surgeons place sutures from right to left in a horizontal fashion; left-handed surgeons do the opposite.
   b. Horizontal mattress.
      i. Place by inserting the needle on the far side of the incision, pass it across the incision, and exit it on the near side, as described for a simple interrupted suture. Advance the needle 6 to 8 mm along the incision and reintroduce it through the skin on the near side. Then cross the incision, exit from the skin on the far side, and tie the knot.
      ii. Generally separate horizontal mattress sutures by 4 to 5 mm.
      iii. Use in areas of tension.
   c. Vertical mattress.
      i. Introduce the needle approximately 8 to 10 mm from the incision edge on one side, pass across the incision line, and exit at an equal distance on the opposite side of the incision. Reverse the needle and insert it through skin on the same side, approximately 4 mm from the skin edge, and tie the knot.
      ii. *Halsted suture*–when two vertical mattress sutures are placed in a parallel fashion before tieing.

d. Gambee.
   i. Introduce the needle as for a simple interrupted suture from the serosa through muscularis and mucosa to the lumen. Then return it from the lumen through the mucosa to muscularis, before it crosses the incision. After crossing the incision introduce it in the muscularis and continue through the mucosa to the lumen. Reintroduce the needle through the mucosa and muscularis, to exit from the serosal surface, and tie the suture.
   ii. Use in intestinal surgery to reduce mucosal eversion.

4. Continuous suture patterns.
   a. Simple continuous.
      i. A series of simple interrupted sutures, with a knot on either end; the suture is continuous between the knots. To begin a simple continuous suture line, place and knot a simple interrupted suture but cut only the end that is not attached to the needle. Direct the needle through skin, perpendicular to the incision. To end a continuous suture, tie the needle end of the suture to the last loop of suture that is exterior to the tissues.
      ii. Provide maximal tissue apposition and are relatively airtight and fluidtight, when compared with a series of simple interrupted sutures.
   b. Ford interlocking.
      i. Modifications of a simple continuous pattern, in which each passage through the tissue is partially locked. To terminate, introduce the needle in the opposite direction from that used previously (near to far) and hold the end on that side. Tie the loop of suture formed on the opposite side to the single end.
   c. Lembert.
      i. Penetrate the serosa and muscularis with the needle approximately 8 to 10 mm from the incision edge and exit near the wound margin on the same side. After passing over the incision, penetrate with the needle approximately 3 to 4 mm from the wound margin and exit 8 to 10 mm away from the incision. Repeat the pattern along the length of the incision.
      ii. An inverting pattern that is often used to close hollow viscera.
   d. Connell and Cushing.
      i. Connell and Cushing patterns are similar, except that a Connell pattern enters the lumen, whereas a Cushing pattern extends only to the submucosal area.
      ii. Begin the suture line with a simple interrupted or vertical mattress suture. Advance the needle parallel to the incision and introduce into the serosa, passing through the muscular and mucosal surfaces. From the deep surface (lumen with a Connell), advance the needle parallel along the incision and return through the tissues to the serosal surface. Once outside the viscera, pass the needle and suture across the incision and introduce it at a point that corresponds to the exit point on the contralateral side. Repeat the suture. Be sure the suture crosses the incision perpendicularly.
      iii. Frequently used to close hollow organs because they cause tissue inversion and provide a watertight seal.

5. Tendon sutures.
   a. Three-loop pulley suture.
      i. Made with three loops oriented approximately 120 degrees to each other. Place the initial loop perpendicular to the long axis of the tendon ends, in a near-far fashion. Place the second loop in a plane 120 degrees from the first, at a point midway between the near and far positions. Place the final loop in a far-near pattern, 120 degrees from the first two sutures.

b. Bunnell's suture.
   i. Pass the needle from one side of the proximal end of the severed tendon and cross diagonally across the tendon to the opposite side, where it exits. Reintroduce the suture approximately 1 mm distal to the exit site and cross diagonally to the other side of the tendon, and exit from the severed end. Introduce the suture into the distal portion of the severed tendon from the cut end, and place two cruciate sutures. Exit the suture at the severed end of the distal portion of the tendon and reintroduce it into the proximal tendon. Repeat the pattern in this portion of the tendon, with the suture exiting near the original entrance site. Appose the tendon ends and tighten the suture.

c. Far-near-near-far.
   i. Pass the needle through the tendon, perpendicular to, and 5 mm from, the severed tendon end. Enter the distal section of the severed tendon in the same vertical plane, 2 mm from the tendon edge. Loop back to the proximal section of tendon and enter 2 mm from the severed edge. Again loop the suture back to the distal section of tendon, to enter 5 mm from the severed tendon edge. Pull the suture ends taut and tie using a surgeon's knot.

IV. Hemostatic Materials

A. Bone Wax

1. A sterile mixture of semisynthetic beeswax and a softening agent (e.g., isopropyl palmitate).
2. May be pressed into cavities in bone (e.g., mandibular foramen) or applied to the bone surface to inhibit bleeding.
3. Is poorly resorbed and should be used sparingly because it may act as a physical barrier to healing and promote infection.

B. Surgicel

1. Is made of oxidized regenerated cellulose.
2. When saturated with blood it becomes a gelatinous mass that provides a substrate for clot formation. It is not activated by tissue fluids other than blood; therefore use only at sites of hemorrhage.

C. Gelfoam

1. Is an absorbable gelatin sponge that may be used in a similar fashion to Surgicel. When applied to an area of hemorrhage, it swells and exerts pressure on the wound.

10

Surgical Infections and Antibiotic Selection (*SAS*, pp. 57-63)

I. Mechanisms of Antibiotic Action

A. Definitions

1. **Bacteriostatic** antibiotics–inhibit bacterial growth.
2. **Bactericidal** antibiotics–kill bacteria.
3. **Minimal inhibitory concentration** (MIC)–the lowest concentration of antibiotic that inhibits visible bacterial growth. It represents the concentration necessary for bacterial inhibition in the patient's plasma or tissues.
4. **Minimal bacteriocidal concentration** (MBC)–the lowest concentration that kills 99.9% of bacteria in plasma or tissues.

B. Destroy Bacterial Cell Walls

1. Penicillins.
   a. Effective against gram-positive aerobes and gram-positive and gram-negative anaerobes.
   b. Some are inactivated by bacterial penicillinases (a type of β-lactamase), and some bacteria are impermeable to them (e.g., methicillin-resistant staphylococci).
   c. Penicillinase inhibitors (e.g., clavulanic acid) may be combined with penicillins (e.g., amoxicillin or ticarcillin plus clavulanic acid) to enhance their activity.
2. Cephalosporins.
   a. Are more effective than penicillins against gram-negative rods (e.g., *Enterobacteriaceae*), but may be inactivated by cephalosporinases (a type of β-lactamase). Most are poorly effective against anaerobes (cefoxitin is an exception).
   b. First-generation cephalosporins are effective against most gram-positive and some gram-negative organisms.
   c. Second-generation cephalosporins have greater activity against gram-negative bacteria and anaerobes, but have no additional efficacy against gram-positive organisms.
   d. Third-generation cephalosporins are highly effective against more than 90% of gram-negative bacteria, but are often less active against gram-positive organisms than first-generation cephalosporins. Some third-generation cephalosporins have specific gram-negative spectra.
3. Imipenem and aztreonam.
   a. Are as effective against gram-negative organisms as aminoglycosides, but are not nephrotoxic.

b. Imipenem has the broadest antibacterial spectrum of any systemic antimicrobial and is effective against virtually all clinically relevant bacterial species, including gram-negative and gram-positive anaerobes and aerobes.
c. Aztreonam is unaffected by bacterial β-lactamase. It is highly effective against many gram-negative aerobes, but has little activity against anaerobes. It has no activity against gram-positive bacteria and must be used in combination to achieve broad-spectrum activity.

C. Inhibit Protein Synthesis

1. Chloramphenicol
   a. Has broad-spectrum activity against streptococci, staphylococci, *Brucella, Pasteurella,* and anaerobes; activity against *Pseudomonas* is poor.
   b. Is highly lipophilic and readily enters cells, the central nervous system, and the eye.
   c. May be poorly absorbed in fasted cats.
   d. May cause idiosyncratic, fatal anemia in humans, but dogs and cats usually only experience mild, transient anemia (if even that).
2. Tetracyclines.
   a. Effective against many gram-positive and gram-negative bacteria, *Chlamydia, Rickettsia,* spirochetes, *Mycoplasma,* bacterial L-forms, and some protozoa.
   b. Usually ineffective against staphylococci, enterococci, *Pseudomonas,* and *Enterobacteriaceae.*
   c. Calcium-containing products chelate tetracyclines and interfere with oral absorption. Binding of calcium can be a problem in young or pregnant animals, and tooth discoloration and inhibited bone growth can occur.
3. Erythromycin.
   a. Very effective against gram-positive bacteria, but has relatively little effect against gram-negative organisms. It is effective against *Streptococcus* spp., *Staphylococcus* spp., *Bacillus anthracis, P. multocida, Helicobacter* spp., and clostridia.
4. Azithromycin.
   a. Achieves extremely high tissue concentrations and needs to be given only once daily.
5. Clindamycin.
   a. Is active against gram-positive pathogens, including *Staphylococcus, Streptococcus, Clostridium,* several *Actinomyces,* and some *Nocardia,* and is extremely effective against many anaerobic bacteria.
   b. Often used when treating infections that are resistant to penicillins and erythromycin, or in patients that cannot tolerate these drugs.
6. Aminoglycosides (e.g., amikacin, gentamicin, and tobramycin).
   a. Effective against gram-negative and gram-positive bacteria, including *Enterobacteriaceae* and pseudomonads, and have a synergistic effect with b-lactam antibiotics.
   b. Their activity is reduced in necrotic tissue because of free nucleic acid material.
   c. Anaerobes are resistant to them because they lack the receptor necessary for transport into the bacterial cell.
   d. Are polar and thus lipid insoluble, resulting in limited distribution in extracellular fluid and cerebrospinal fluid. Distribution into pleural fluid, bone, joints, and peritoneal cavity is good.
   e. Are nephrotoxic.
      i. Giving higher doses at longer intervals (e.g., once daily), maintains effectiveness but decreases renal toxicity.

ii. Dehydration, electrolyte loss, and preexisting renal disease increase their nephrotoxicity.

D. Inhibit DNA Synthesis

1. Fluoroquinolones (e.g., enrofloxacin, norfloxacin, ciprofloxacin, ofloxacin).
   a. Inactivate DNA gyrase, preventing uncoiling of the DNA molecule during DNA replication and transcription to mRNA.
   b. Rapidly bactericidal and are effective for soft tissue infections, pneumonia, osteomyelitis, and urinary tract infections caused by gram-negative organisms and staphylococci. They are also effective against *R. rickettsiae* and possibly L-forms, but are variably effective against streptococci and ineffective against most anaerobes.
   c. Potential side effects include vomiting, central nervous system effects in animals of all ages, and cartilage lesions in developing animals.
2. Trimethoprim-sulfonamide combinations.
   a. Are effective for the treatment of osteomyelitis, prostatitis, pneumonia, tracheobronchitis, pyoderma, and urinary tract infections.
   b. When used in combination they are bactericidal and function by inhibiting sequential steps in folate synthesis.
   c. Trimethoprim-sulfonamide combinations have a broad spectrum of activity, including most streptococci, many staphylococci, and *Nocardia.* They have relatively little activity against anaerobes, and none against *Pseudomonas.*
   d. Potential side effects include keratoconjunctivitis sicca, thrombocytopenia, anemia, vomiting, hypersensitivity (i.e., vasculitis or arthritis), and hepatic disease. Some breeds (e.g., Doberman pinschers and rottweilers) and some families of dogs seem more likely to have side effects.

II. Causes of Antibiotic Failure and Mechanisms of Antibiotic Resistance

A. Antibiotic Failure

1. Factors that contribute to antibiotic failure include the following.
   a. Inappropriate dose (i.e., excessive or suboptimal), frequency, or route of administration.
   b. Inadequate length of treatment.
   c. Inappropriate antibiotic selection (i.e., not based on culture and sensitivity).
   d. Inability of the antibiotic to reach the cause of infection (i.e., foreign body or implant).
   e. Inability of the antibiotic to reach the target tissue in sufficient dosages (e.g., cross blood-brain barrier).
   f. Antibiotic resistance by bacteria (see below).
   g. Depressed host immunity (i.e., concurrent severe or debilitating illness).
   h. Pharmacokinetics of the drug.
   i. Drug reactions.
   j. Antibiotic antagonism.
   k. Incorrect diagnoses (i.e., viral diseases or foreign bodies).

B. Antibiotic Resistance

1. May be the result of one or more of the following.
   a. Enzymatic destruction of the antibiotic.
   b. Alteration of bacterial permeability to the antibiotic.

c. Alteration of the structural target for the antibiotic.
d. Development of alternative metabolic pathways that bypass the reaction antagonized by the particular antibiotic.

III. Surgical Infection

A. Classification of Surgical Wounds

1. Clean wounds.
   a. Nontraumatic wounds without inflammation or infection, in which breaks in aseptic technique do not occur (or are not identified) and luminal organs are not entered.
   b. Published infection rates range from 0% to 3.5%.
   c. Antibiotic prophylaxis is not indicated unless a prolonged procedure is anticipated or when inexperienced personnel are performing the surgery.
2. Clean-contaminated wounds.
   a. When nonsterile luminal organs are entered without significant spillage of contents such as the following.
      i. Gastrointestinal or respiratory tracts, oropharynx, or vagina is entered.
      ii. Urinary or biliary tracts are entered in the absence of infected urine or bile.
      iii. Minor break in aseptic technique occurs (e.g., perforation of a surgical glove).
   b. Published infection rate is 4.5%.
   c. Antimicrobial prophylaxis is indicated; base antibiotic selection on anticipated flora.
3. Contaminated wounds.
   a. Involve a major break in surgical technique, gross spillage of gastrointestinal contents, fresh traumatic wounds, or entrance of the urinary or biliary tract when gross infection is present.
   b. Published infection rates vary from 5.8% to 14.6%.
   c. Antibiotic prophylaxis is indicated; base drug selection initially on anticipated bacterial flora and modify based on culture and sensitivity results.
   d. The fate of contaminated wounds can be markedly altered by early management. Delicate debridement, copious lavage, and antibiotic therapy can convert these wounds to "clean" ones, whereas inadequate therapy often results in a dirty, infected wound.
4. Dirty wounds.
   a. Wounds in which gross infection is present (e.g., traumatic wounds with retained devitalized tissue, foreign bodies, or fecal contamination) at the time of surgical intervention.
   b. Management requires antibiotic therapy (base initial selection on anticipated flora, later modify by bacterial culture and sensitivity), copious lavage, debridement, drainage, and potentially wet-to-dry bandages (to further debride the wound during the early postoperative period).

IV. Prevention of Surgical Infection

A. Factors That Determine Whether Infection Occurs in a Surgical Wound Include the Following

1. Host factors (e.g., age, physical condition, nutritional status, diagnostic procedures, concurrent metabolic disorders, and nature of the wound).

Table 10-1
Considerations for selection and administration of prophylactic antibiotics

Considerations/action
Antibiotic Selection
Determine system involved and most likely organism
Cefazolin attains appropriate concentrations to prevent bacterial growth of the most common contaminants.
Timing of Antibiotic Administration
Beginning of surgery (at anesthetic induction)
Cefazolin Dose
20 mg/kg
Routes of Antibiotic Administration
Intravenously at induction; may repeat in 2-3 hours depending on length of surgery
Duration of Antibiotic Administration
Discontinue immediately after surgical wound closure

2. Operating room practice.
   a. Principles of aseptic technique; sterilization and disinfection; preparation of the surgical environment; gowning and gloving; and preparation of the surgical patient, operative site, and surgical team.
   b. See Chapters 1 through 7.
3. Characteristics of bacterial contaminants.
   a. Infections that occur during hospitalization are referred to as nosocomial infections.
   b. Prevention of nosocomial infections requires control of endogenous flora (i.e., patient preparation [see Chapter 6]), decreased bacterial transmission (i.e., hand washing, gloves, disinfection, and sterilization [see Chapters 2, 7, and 8]), control of the hospital environment (i.e., maintaining proper cleaning, disinfection, and hospital sterilization protocols [see Chapter 4]), and rational antibiotic use (i.e., based on patient need and culture and sensitivity results).

V. Therapeutic and Prophylactic Antibiotic Use

A. Prophylactic Antibiotics

1. Must be present at the surgical site during the time of potential contamination to prevent growth of contaminating pathogens (Table 10-1).
2. Antibiotics are not a substitute for proper aseptic technique, meticulous and atraumatic tissue handling, careful hemostasis, judicious use of sutures, preservation of blood supply, elimination of dead space, and anatomic apposition of tissues.
3. Rational selection of antibiotics for antimicrobial prophylaxis requires that the most likely contaminating microorganism(s) is identified and that the microorganism is susceptible to the drug used.
   a. Pathogens usually responsible for postoperative wound infection in small animal surgical patients are *Staphylococcus* spp. (especially *S. aureus*), *E. coli, Pasteurella* spp. (especially in cats), and *Bacteroides fragilis* (anaerobic).

B. Therapeutic Antibiotics

1. Indicated in surgical patients with overwhelming systemic infection (i.e., septicemia or bacteremia), infection present at the surgical site or in a

Table 10-2
Considerations for selection and administration of therapeutic antibiotics

Considerations/action
Antibiotic Selection
• Determine system involved and most likely pathogen, to establish primary therapy
• Obtain representative samples for Gram's stain, cytology, and culture and susceptibility testing (e.g., fluid, tissue, implants, necrotic debris)
• Ensure antibiotic reaches target tissue
• If several antibiotics are effective, select the one that is least expensive, least toxic, and most convenient to administer
Timing of Antibiotic Administration
As soon as samples have been obtained, begin empirical antibiotic therapy
Dose
Follow recommended doses carefully
Routes of Antibiotic Administration
Treat for a minimum of 3 days; assess animal's condition; if improving, continue therapy; if no improvement, reevaluate
Duration of Antibiotic Administration
Duration depends on effect of antibiotic, toxicity, and disorder being treated; give for at least 2 to 3 days after resolution of all signs

body cavity (i.e., wound infection, pyothorax, or abdominal abscess), or any contaminated or dirty surgical procedure.

2. Generally, antibiotic therapy is instituted before surgery and continued for at least 2 to 3 days after resolution of all clinical signs; maximum duration of therapy depends on drug toxicity and the disease being treated (Table 10-2).

11

Postoperative Care of the Surgical Patient (*SAS*, pp. 64-85)

I. Initial Postoperative Management

A. Hydration

1. Maintain geriatric patients, ill or debilitated patients (e.g., renal dysfunction, hepatic disease, vomiting, diarrhea), and patients undergoing long surgeries on intravenous fluids until they are able to eat and drink.
2. Pay close attention to fluid rate and urinary losses to prevent volume depletion, severe electrolyte imbalances, and acid-base disorders.

B. Temperature

1. Monitor temperature, pulse, and respiration at least every hour (more frequently in critical patients) until the temperature is normal and the animal is alert.
2. Actively rewarm hypothermic animals with heated cages, hot water bottles or gloves, or warmed blankets. However, be careful not to burn these patients.

C. Positioning

1. Alternate recumbent animals between left and right lateral recumbency or place in sternal recumbency until they are able to sit or stand without assistance.

D. Ventilation, Cardiac Status, and CNS

1. Evaluate blood gases, blood pressure, and oxygen saturation as necessary.
2. Consider oxygen supplementation via an oxygen cage, nasal insufflation, or mask for hypoxemic (P_aO_2 less than 60 mm Hg) animals.
3. Evaluate patients with delayed recovery from anesthetic episodes for increased intracranial pressure, particularly if there was preexisting CNS disease or trauma.
4. Consider mechanical ventilation in some animals (i.e., severe hypoxemia [P_aO_2 less than 50 to 60 mm Hg], severe hypercarbia [P_aCO_2 greater than 50 to 60 mm Hg], increased intracranial pressure).
   a. Adjust respiratory rate and tidal volume to maintain P_aCO_2 between 30 and 40 mm Hg and P_aO_2 levels greater than 60 mm Hg.
   b. P_aO_2 is generally five times that of the F_IO_2 (fractional concentration of inspired oxygen); values less than this may suggest gas exchange

impairment (e.g., if a patient is breathing in 40% O_2, the expected P_aO_2 level is 200 mm Hg).

E. Hemorrhage

1. Monitor the hematocrit postoperatively.
2. Observe for pale mucous membranes, slow capillary refill time, weak pulses, and a high heart rate, which are nonspecific signs of hemorrhage.
3. For severe bleeding, if hemodilution is not a concern, use balanced electrolyte solutions (e.g., Normosol). Give up to two to three times the volume of blood lost rapidly (not to exceed 60 to 90 ml/kg). Monitor central venous pressures to assess volume replacement.
4. If blood products are needed consider the following.
   a. Fresh, whole blood–use to replace red cell mass, plasma proteins, platelets, and clotting factors.
   b. Packed red cells–consider if the animal is not hypoproteinemic.
5. If protein is needed (PCV is satisfactory) consider plasma or other colloidal solutions (e.g., hetastarch, dextrans) to increase plasma oncotic pressure.

Nutritional Management of the Surgical Patient

II. Definitions

A. **Hyperalimentation**–the administration of adequate nutrients to malnourished patients or those at risk.

B. **Enteral hyperalimentation**–provides nutrients to a functional gastrointestinal tract.

C. **Parenteral hyperalimentation**–provides nutrients intravenously.

D. **Monomeric diets**–are usually composed of crystalline amino acids as the protein source, glucose and oligosaccharides as the carbohydrate source, and safflower oil as the essential fatty acid source.

E. **Polymeric diets**–contain large molecular weight proteins, carbohydrates, and fats.

F. **Blenderized diets**–diets made from prescription pet food or homemade diets blended with water or another liquid.

III. Oral Feeding

A. Is preferred if adequate nutrients can be consumed to meet protein and calorie requirements.

B. Drugs that may stimulate anorexic animals to eat include the following.
   1. Cyproheptadine (Periactin).
      a. Cats–2 mg/cat PO.
   2. Diazepam (Valium).
      a. Cats–2.5 mg/cat PO or 0.2 mg/kg IV.
      b. Dogs–0.2 mg/kg IV.

3. Oxazepam (Serax).
   a. Cats–2.5 mg/cat PO.

IV. Total Parenteral Nutrition

Insert a 16-gauge, 18-cm, single-lumen, silicone elastomer catheter in the right or left external jugular vein of a tranquilized or anesthetized patient. Position the catheter tip in the cranial vena cava and create a subcutaneous tunnel such that the catheter hub emerges on the dorsum of the neck. Anchor the catheter to the vein, subcutaneous tissue along the tunnel, and skin at the exit point with 4-0 to 5-0 nonabsorbable monofilament suture. Attach an extension set to the catheter hub and bandage the catheter in place with sterile gauze, cast padding, and self-adherent wrap. Flush the catheter with heparinized saline (0.9% sterile saline with 1 IU/ml heparin) after each use.

A. Administer 50% of the calculated nutrient requirements the first day and 100% the second day. Give the predetermined nutrient formulation using an infusion pump.

B. Monitor serum electrolytes, glucose, total protein, serum lipids, PCV, and blood urea nitrogen (BUN) daily. Measure body weight and temperature twice daily.

C. Remove the neck bandage every 2 days, clean the catheter entrance site, change the extension and administration sets, and apply a new bandage.

D. Complications associated with TPN include catheter kinking and displacement, phlebitis, thrombosis, sepsis, hyperglycemia, hyperlipidemia, azotemia, and electrolyte imbalances.

V. Enteral Hyperalimentation

A. Nasoesophageal Intubation

1. Indication.
   a. Use in patients with protein-calorie malnutrition that will not undergo oral, pharyngeal, esophageal, gastric, or biliary tract surgery. The patient can drink and swallow around the tube.
2. Tube placement.

Instill proparacaine hydrochloride (0.5 to 1 ml; 0.5%) into the nasal cavity and elevate the head to encourage the local anesthetic to coat the nasal mucosa. Repeat application of local anesthetic. Select an appropriate-size feeding tube (Table 11-1). Estimate length of tube to be placed in the esophagus by placing the tube from the nasal planum, along the side of the patient, to the seventh or eighth intercostal space. Place a tape marker on the tube once the appropriate

Table 11-1
Tube diameter based on route of administration of enteral diets

5 French Diameter Tubes	8 French or Larger Diameter Tubes
• Nasoesophageal	• Pharyngostomy
• Enterostomy (jejunostomy)	• Esophagostomy
	• Gastrostomy

measurement has been taken. Do not pass the feeding tube through the lower esophageal sphincter because this may cause sphincteric incompetence, esophageal reflux of hydrochloric acid, and esophagitis. Lubricate the tip of the tube with 5% lidocaine viscous before passage, and hold the patient's head in a normal functional position (i.e., avoid hyperflexion or hyperextension). Place the tube in the ventrolateral aspect of the external nares and pass it in a caudoventral and medial direction into the nasal cavity. After the prominent alar fold is identified, direct the tube from a ventrolateral location in the external nares to a caudoventral and medial direction as it enters the nasal cavity. Push the external nares dorsally to facilitate opening the ventral meatus. Elevate the proximal end of the tube and advance it into the oropharynx and esophagus. Confirm esophageal placement by injecting 3 to 5 ml of sterile saline through the tube and seeing if a cough is elicited, or by injecting 6 to 12 ml of air and auscultating for borborygmus at the xiphoid. Suture the tube to the nose and head to prevent removal by the patient. Do not allow the tube to contact the whiskers of cats. Secure the tube with a Chinese finger-trap suture. Place an Elizabethan collar immediately postoperatively until it is determined whether the patient will tolerate the tube. Place a column of water in the tube before capping it to prevent air intake, reflux of esophageal contents, and/or tube occlusion by diet.

B. Esophagostomy Tube

1. Indications and contraindications.
   a. Esophagostomy tubes are indicated in anorexic patients with disorders of the oral cavity or pharynx and in anorexic patients with a functional gastrointestinal tract distal to the esophagus.
   b. They are contraindicated in patients with primary or secondary esophageal dysfunction (e.g., esophageal stricture, after esophageal foreign body removal or esophageal surgery, esophagitis, mega-esophagus).
2. Tube placement.

Anesthetize and place the animal in right lateral recumbency. Prepare the midcervical area from the angle of the mandible to the thoracic inlet for aseptic surgery. Place a speculum to hold the mouth open, and premeasure a 20 to 24 French polyvinyl chloride feeding tube from its insertion point to the level of the seventh and eighth intercostal space and mark it (ensuring midesophageal to caudal-esophageal placement). Enlarge the two lateral openings of the feeding tube to encourage smoother flow of blended diet. An Eld feeding tube placement device or large right-angle clamp may be used. Place the oblique tip of the instrument into the oral cavity to the level of the midcervical region (i.e., equal distance between the angle of the mandible and thoracic inlet). Palpate the tip as it bulges through the cervical skin. Make a small skin incision over the tip of the instrument. If using an Eld feeding tube device, activate the spring-loaded instrument blade until it is visible through the skin incision. With the tip of a scalpel blade, carefully enlarge the incision in the subcutaneous tissues, cervical musculature, and esophageal wall to allow penetration of the instrument tip or shaft. Clamp the feeding tube in the clamp or place a 2-0 nonabsorbable suture through the side holes of the feeding tube and the hole in the Eld instrument blade. Tighten the suture until the tip of the instrument blade and feeding tube tip are in close apposition. Retract the instrument blade into the instrument shaft so the feeding tube tip enters the instrument shaft (i.e., deactivating the instrument blade), and place lubricant on the tube and instrument shaft. Retract the Eld device or the clamp and pull the feeding tube into the oral cavity to its predetermined measurement. Remove the suture to free the feeding tube from the Eld instrument blade and place a stylet through one of the side holes of the feeding tube and against its tip. Lubricate the tube and advance it into the esophagus until the entire oral portion of the feeding

tube disappears and the tube passes down the esophagus without twisting or bending. Retract the stylet from the oral cavity, with care to ensure its release from the tube. Secure the tube to the cervical skin with a Chinese finger-trap suture of No. 1 nonabsorbable suture. Leave the exit point of the tube exposed or loosely bandage the neck. Place a column of water in the tube and cap the exposed end with a 3-cc syringe.

C. Pharyngostomy Tubes

1. Indications and contraindications.
   a. Indicated to provide nutritional supplementation to an anorexic patient or to patients that are unable or reluctant to ingest food orally.
   b. Do not use in patients with esophageal disorders (i.e., esophagitis, esophageal stricture, recent esophageal surgery or esophageal foreign body removal, esophageal neoplasia).
2. Tube placement.

Anesthetize the patient and position in lateral recumbency with the incision site uppermost. Aseptically prepare a 4-cm-square area just caudal to the angle of the mandible. Hold open the mouth with a mouth speculum. Premeasure a 24 French, polyvinyl chloride feeding tube from the insertion point to the level of the seventh or eighth intercostal space and mark it, ensuring midesophageal placement. Position an index finger into the pharynx, near the base of the tongue, and palpate the epiglottis, arytenoid cartilages, and hyoid apparatus. Flex the orally located index finger toward the lateral aspect of the neck to identify the junction of the intrapharyngeal ostium and laryngopharynx (this is the proper location for pharyngostomy tube exit). Apply enough pressure to the lateral pharyngeal wall to create an externally visible bulge. Substitute large, curved forceps (e.g., curved Rochester-Carmalt forceps) for the index finger to maintain the bulge. Make a 1- to 2-cm skin incision over the bulge, and use the curved forceps to bluntly dissect subcutaneous tissue, pharyngeal muscle, and pharyngeal mucosa until the index finger or forceps becomes visible. Grasp the tip of the pharyngostomy tube and pull it through the incision, into the oral cavity, and out of the mouth. Reinsert the tip of the tube into the mouth and pass it into the midesophagus (i.e., premarked location on the feeding tube). Secure the tube at its exit point with a Chinese finger-trap suture and to the patient's neck to encourage the tube to remain dorsally. Place a column of water in the tube and cap it with a 3-cc syringe.

D. Gastrostomy Tubes

1. Indications and contraindications.
   a. Gastrostomy tubes are indicated in anorexic patients with a functional gastrointestinal tract distal to the stomach or in patients undergoing operations of the oral cavity, larynx, pharynx, or esophagus.
   b. Contraindicated in patients with primary gastric disease (e.g., gastritis, gastric ulceration, gastric neoplasia).
2. Percutaneous placement of a gastrostomy tube with gastropexy.

Place the animal under general anesthesia and prepare the skin of the left side and flank for aseptic surgery. Drape the area and have an unsterile assistant pass a large-bore, stiff, plastic tube into the stomach. Have the sterile surgeon palpate the left flank area until the end of the stomach tube can be palpated and grasped. Hold the tube stable and make a skin incision over the end of the stomach tube. Bluntly dissect the subcutaneous tissues and abdominal muscles to expose the wall of the stomach over the tube; use care not to enter the lumen of the stomach. Place a purse-string suture in the stomach wall around the tube. Use a No. 11 scalpel blade to puncture the

stomach wall by punching the blade into the lumen of the tube. Place a 20 French to 24 French Foley catheter into the lumen of the stomach and into the tube. Place traction on the purse-string suture as the stomach tube is slowly withdrawn. Once the Foley catheter is out of the lumen of the stomach tube, inflate the bulb and apply gentle traction on the catheter to bring it against the stomach wall. Snug the purse-string suture around the Foley catheter. Place three to four simple interrupted sutures of 2-0 absorbable suture (i.e., PDS, Maxon) from the stomach wall to the body wall to firmly pexy the stomach in place. Close subcutaneous tissues and skin around the existing Foley catheter and secure the tube to skin with a Chinese finger-trap suture of No. 1 nonabsorbable suture.

3. Percutaneous gastrostomy tube placement without gastropexy.

Prepare and position the patient as described above. Prepare a 20 French Pezzer urinary catheter as follows. Cut off and discard the dilated proximal end of the tube. Cut off 1.5 cm of the remaining tube and set aside for use as an external flange. Cut the remaining proximal end of the tube at a sharp angle. Cut a strand of No. 1 Braunamid to the length of the prepared feeding tube. Pass a stiff, large-bore stomach tube or feeding tube placement device into the stomach until it can be palpated bulging against the left body wall 1 to 2 cm caudal to the last rib and 2 to 3 cm distal to the transverse spinous processes of lumbar vertebrae two or three. If a stomach tube is being used, pass an 18-gauge hypodermic needle through skin and into the lumen of the stomach tube. Place a strand of No. 1 suture through the needle, into the stomach tube, and out through the mouth. Remove the stomach tube. If a feeding tube placement device is being used (see esophagostomy tube placement above), activate the device and thread the No. 1 suture through the hole in the instrument blade. Retract the blade into the instrument shaft and withdraw the instrument out through the mouth. Thread the end of the suture exiting the oral cavity through the narrow end of an 18-gauge sovereign catheter and tie it to the proximal end of the prepared Pezzer urinary catheter (i.e., feeding tube). Pull the Pezzer catheter tightly into the flange of the catheter and lubricate it. Pull the No. 1 suture exiting the left flank until the catheter tip exits the skin. Enlarge the skin incision to 3 to 4 mm, allowing easy delivery of the catheter. Pull the catheter until the mushroom tip is snugly against the body wall, ensuring a seal between the stomach wall and body wall. Secure the catheter to the skin with a Chinese finger-trap suture using No. 1 nonabsorbable suture (e.g., Novafil).

4. Percutaneous endoscopic gastrostomy tube placement.

Perform as described for percutaneous placement without gastropexy with the exception that the No. 1 suture is placed from the left flank out through the oral cavity with the aid of an endoscope. Pass the endoscope into the stomach and insufflate the stomach with air. Make a 1-mm skin incision in the left flank 1 to 2 cm caudal to the last rib and 2 to 3 cm distal to the transverse spinous processes of lumbar vertebrae two or three. Thrust an 18-gauge needle through the skin incision and into the stomach lumen. Pass the strand of No. 1 suture through the needle and into the stomach, retrieve it endoscopically, and bring it out through the mouth. Once the strand of suture is entering the left flank and exiting the oral cavity, placement of the feeding tube is as described for percutaneous surgical placement without gastropexy.

5. Gastrostomy tube placement via laparotomy.

Place the distal end of a 20 French Foley or Pezzer catheter (i.e., bulb or mushroom tip) into the abdominal cavity through a stab incision in the left body

wall. Exteriorize the ventral surface of the stomach and place a purse-string suture in the ventrolateral body wall. Make a stab incision in the center of the purse-string suture with a No. 11 scalpel blade and place the distal end of the feeding catheter in the lumen of the stomach. Tighten the purse-string suture around the catheter and inflate the bulb of the catheter (i.e., Foley) with saline. Place gentle traction on the catheter to bring the body of the stomach in close apposition to the left body wall. Pexy the stomach wall to the abdominal wall with four 2-0 synthetic absorbable sutures. Secure the feeding tube to the skin with a Chinese finger-trap suture of No. 1 nonabsorbable suture (e.g., Novafil). Perform routine abdominal closure.

E. Enterostomy Tube

1. Indications and contraindications.
   a. Enterostomy tubes are indicated in patients with gastric, intestinal, or pancreatic disease and in patients having biliary tract surgery in which the intestinal tract distal to the disease or surgical site is functional.
   b. If there are no contraindications to larger tubes placed higher in the gastrointestinal tract (i.e., severe vomiting) they are preferred over enterostomy tubes because blenderized diets can be used with them versus liquid diets required for enterostomy tubes.
2. Tube placement.

Perform a celiotomy. Bring the distal tip of a 5 French, 36-inch, infant feeding tube into the abdominal cavity through a 2- to 3-mm stab incision on the right or left body wall using a No. 11 scalpel blade or 10-gauge hypodermic needle. Select a segment of small intestine that can be easily mobilized to the feeding tube entrance location on the body wall. Make a 1- to 1.5-cm linear incision in the seromuscular layers of the antimesenteric border of the selected intestinal segment. Use a No. 11 scalpel blade to enter the lumen of the jejunum at the most aboral end of the incision. Insert the distal end of the feeding tube through the incision and pass 10 to 12 inches of the tube in an aboral direction into the lumen. Position the exiting portion of the tube in the 1- to 1.5-cm seromuscular incision and suture it in this "tunnel" by inverting the seromuscular layer over the tube with three or four Cushing sutures of 4-0 absorbable suture material (i.e., Maxon, PDS). Pexy the jejunal tube exit site to the exit site at the body wall with four to five simple interrupted sutures of 4-0 absorbable suture, and secure the feeding tube to skin using a Chinese finger-trap suture of 2-0 nonabsorbable material (e.g., Novafil). Alternatively, from a laparotomy approach, pass a 10-gauge needle through the abdominal wall from peritoneum to skin. Introduce the feeding tube into the abdominal cavity through the needle and remove the needle, leaving the feeding tube with its hub outside the abdominal cavity. Introduce the needle at an acute angle into the jejunal lumen and exit at an oblique angle, creating a seromuscular tunnel. Advance the catheter into the beveled end of the needle and remove the needle, leaving the catheter in the jejunal lumen. Thread the catheter into the jejunal lumen and suture the jejunum to the body wall and secure it to skin with a Chinese finger-trap friction suture.

VI. Calculation of Rate and Volume of Feeding

A. Feeding into the Stomach

1. The quantity of diet fed is determined by the patient's stomach capacity. Normal canine and feline gastric capacity is approximately 80 ml of fluid/kg of body weight. However, anorexic patients can

Table 11-2
Guidelines for feeding via an enterostomy tube

- Calculate total caloric requirement.
- Give ¼ of the calculated volume during the first 24 hours; a minimum of four to five feedings/day is recommended.*
- Give ½ of the calculated volume during the second 24 hours in four to five feedings.*
- Give ¾ of the calculated volume during the third 24 hours in four to five feedings.*
- Give the entire calculated volume during the fourth 24 hours in four to five feedings.*

*Continuous feeding via infusion pump is preferred.

accommodate only 30 to 40 ml of fluid/kg of body weight when feeding begins.

2. Use a minimum of three feedings daily; however, if vomiting and abdominal distention occur, reduce the volume and increase the number of feedings per day.

B. Feeding into the Small Intestine

1. A guideline for feeding via enterostomy tube is outlined in Table 11-2. These are guidelines only; some patients require a longer adjustment time (5 to 7 days), while others allow total volume feeding in 2 to 3 days.
2. Signs of overfeeding include vomiting, diarrhea, abdominal distention, and cramping. Diluting diet concentration and decreasing the rate and volume of administration generally resolve these complications.

12

Treatment of Perioperative Pain (*SAS*, pp. 86-90)

Pain Assessment

I. Physiologic Parameters

A. Identify changes in heart rate, peripheral circulation, and breathing patterns that may indicate pain, distress, or discomfort.

B. Do not use physiologic parameters exclusively for assessing pain because other variables (e.g., drug administration, hypovolemia) may alter them.

II. Behavioral Parameters

A. The most recognized behavioral manifestation of pain is vocalization (e.g., crying, howling, barking, growling, purring, moaning). However, not all patients in pain vocalize; many animals suffer quietly.

B. Changes in posture or facial expression; guarding or protecting a limb; self-mutilation; dilated pupils; salivation; muscle rigidity or weakness; and changes in sleeping, eating, or elimination patterns also suggest pain.

C. Activity level may change; patients may be either restless or reluctant to move.

D. There may also be attitude alterations (e.g., a previously gentle dog may become aggressive; a previously social animal may become timid). Cats are particularly difficult to assess, but one of the most consistent (albeit not specific) indicators of pain in cats is cessation of grooming.

Pain Management and Postoperative Patient Evaluation

I. General Considerations

A. Comfortable patients are no more likely to injure a surgical site than patients in pain. Use tranquilization, not pain, to restrict movement.

B. Environmental manipulations may facilitate patient comfort. Familiarize the patient with the environment preoperatively and induce and recover the patient in a dry, warm, quiet environment.

C. Do not use tranquilizers such as acepromazine or diazepam alone in patients with pain. Good postoperative pain management begins preoperatively. To be most effective, inhibit nociception with analgesics before the initiation of the painful stimulus.

II. Opioids (Appendix D)

A. Morphine

1. The prototype opioid agonist–indicated for moderate to severe pain.
2. Onset of action is 15 to 30 minutes; duration of action is about 4 hours.
3. Cardiovascular effects include vagally induced bradycardia, direct depression of the sinoatrial node, and slowed atrioventricular (AV) conduction. It does not sensitize the myocardium to catecholamines.
4. Ventilation is directly depressed (dose dependent) by inhibiting central respiratory centers. It also alters the rhythm of breathing. Hypoventilation may cause increased intracranial pressure as a result of elevated P_aCO_2.
5. Nausea and vomiting result from chemoreceptor trigger zone stimulation.
6. May cause hypothermia and miosis in dogs and mydriasis and hyperthermia in cats. Histamine may be released when administered intravenously; slow intravenous administration minimizes this risk.
7. It is frequently used for epidural administration (see later in this section and Appendix E).

B. Oxymorphone

1. Is similar to morphine, but does not cause histamine release.
2. Appropriate for moderate to severe pain and is particularly useful in managing critically ill patients that require intraoperative analgesic supplementation to decrease the amount of inhalant required.
3. It causes sedation, panting, and sometimes hypothermia.

C. Fentanyl

1. Fentanyl, a synthetic opioid, has a more rapid onset of action than morphine.
2. In veterinary medicine fentanyl is used for intraoperative management of critically ill patients in balanced anesthetic techniques but is not used extensively for pain management unless administered transdermally.
3. May cause bradycardia, ventilatory depression, and skeletal muscle rigidity.

D. Buprenorphine

1. Is a partial opioid agonist.
2. Its onset is about 30 minutes and its duration is 4 to 6 hours.
3. Its affinity for mu receptors causes prolonged duration of action and difficulty associated with antagonism.
4. It is used for mild to moderate pain in veterinary patients.
5. Causes little sedation or dysphoria in dogs and cats. Its prolonged duration of action makes it useful if redosing is problematic.

E. Butorphanol

1. A mixed agonist-antagonist.
2. It has a low affinity for mu receptors (not a complete antagonist), a

moderate affinity for kappa receptors (produces analgesia), and minimal affinity for sigma receptors (decreased incidence of dysphoria).

3. Has minimal effects on the biliary and gastrointestinal tracts and is particularly effective for visceral pain such as bile peritonitis and pancreatitis.
4. Produces analgesia with minimal ventilatory depression.

F. Opioid Antagonists

1. Ventilatory depression and sedation caused by opioids may be reversed with opioid antagonists. Antagonize opioids carefully in patients with pain because the antagonist also reverses analgesia.
2. Antagonism of opioids with naloxone has been associated with catecholamine release, hypertension, dysrhythmias, and even fatal outcomes in people. Dilute naloxone with saline and give by slow intravenous titration to decrease the likelihood of untoward side effects.
3. Nalbuphine and butorphanol are associated with fewer reversal side effects than complete antagonism with naloxone.
   a. Titration of a 1:10 diluted solution of nalbuphine (5 mg/ml diluted to 0.5 mg/ml) appears to antagonize sedation and respiratory depression, maintain analgesia, and avoid the dangerous side effects associated with high-dose naloxone reversal.
   b. Butorphanol may be used for antagonism of mu opioids (e.g., oxymorphone) in veterinary patients.

III. Local Anesthesia

A. Epidurals

1. General considerations.
   a. Useful for intraoperative management of high-risk patients, perioperative analgesia, cesarean section, caudal anesthesia/analgesia, thoracotomies, and forelimb amputations (see Appendix E).
   b. Contraindications include hemorrhagic diathesis and sepsis. Epidural administration of local anesthetics, but not opioids, is contraindicated in hypovolemia; pretreatment with fluids may improve response.
   c. Decrease the dose of anesthetic in geriatric, pregnant, and obese patients plus those with space-occupying lesions. Also decrease the dose by 50% if CSF fluid is encountered when performing an epidural.
   d. Complications include infection, hemorrhage, and failure to produce analgesia or anesthesia.
2. Administration of local anesthetics epidurally.
   a. Results in sensory and motor blockade.
   b. Results in no or mild sedation, minimal nausea and vomiting, and occasionally urinary retention.
   c. May result in decreased heart rate, cardiac output, and blood pressure. Postural hypotension can be expected.
   d. Appropriate doses usually does not impair the respiratory system, but excessive doses can produce convulsions.
3. Epidural administration of opioids.
   a. Affects only sensory function.
   b. May cause marked sedation, nausea, vomiting, urinary retention, or pruritus.
   c. At appropriate dosages produces minimal change in heart rate, cardiac output, or blood pressure but may cause early and late respiratory depression. The respiratory depression can be antagonized.

B. Intercostal and Interpleural Neural Blocks

1. Intercostal nerve blocks.
   a. Postthoracotomy interpleural administration or intercostal bupivacaine hydrochloride nerve blocks have proven efficacious, especially when combined with systemic opioid administration.
   b. Block the intercostal nerves supplying the incision site, two nerves cranial to the site, and two nerves caudal to the thoracotomy incision.
2. Interpleural nerve blocks.
   a. Is an alternative to intercostal neural blockade and offers prolonged analgesia without multiple needle sticks.
   b. Dilute bupivacaine with saline and instill in the chest tube of the thoracotomy patient. Place the operated side down and allow sufficient time (20 minutes for bupivacaine) for absorption of the local anesthetic. If a chest tube is present additional bupivacaine can be placed postoperatively (e.g., after 6 hours).
   c. If intercostal and interpleural blocks are both employed, adjust the bupivacaine dose to stay below 2 mg/kg total dose.

IV. Regional Techniques

A. Wound Perfusion/Infiltration

1. The simplest technique for providing wound analgesia, but there is poor efficacy in infected wounds.
2. Brachial plexus anesthesia alleviates pain distal to the elbow. Infiltration of nerve stumps after amputation or brachial plexus block before amputation provides postsurgical pain relief.
3. When performing a splash block following an ear ablation, the local anesthetic should remain in contact with tissues for 15 to 20 minutes before being removed.

V. Nonsteroidal Antiinflammatory Drugs

A. Most nonsteroidal antiinflammatory drugs (NSAIDs) are marketed as oral preparations and have not been utilized in perioperative pain management. They can be associated with clotting problems, gastrointestinal ulceration, and potential renal damage, which limits their utility. Some NSAIDs are available as injectable preparations and may be effective analgesic adjuncts.

VI. Postoperative Patient Evaluation

A. Monitor heart rate, respiration, and mucous membrane color. They should normalize.

B. Appropriate analgesia causes the patient to be sedate but arousable. It is appropriate for the patient to sleep.

C. Monitor for normal behaviors such as eating, drinking, urinating, and grooming, which indicate that the patient is not in severe pain.

PART

II

Soft Tissue Surgery

13

Surgery of the Integumentary System (*SAS*, pp. 91-152)

Wound Management (SAS, pp. 91-132)

Surgical Anatomy

I. Skin Layers

A. Epidermis

1. Thickest on the nose and foot pads, where it is keratinized.
2. Avascular–receives nourishment from fluid that penetrates the deeper layers and from dermal capillaries.

B. Dermis

1. Thicker than the epidermis; composed of collagenous, reticular, and elastic fibers surrounded by a mucopolysaccharide ground substance.
2. Contains blood and lymph vessels, nerves, hair follicles, glands, ducts, and smooth muscle fibers.

C. Hypodermis or Subcutis, Lies below the Dermis

II. Vascular Supply of Skin

A. Direct Cutaneous Vessels

1. Supply the skin of dogs and cats.
2. Travel parallel to the skin and form terminal arteries and veins, which form the subdermal (deep), cutaneous (middle), and subpapillary (superficial) plexi.
   a. Subdermal plexus is of major importance to skin viability. In areas where there is a panniculus muscle, the subdermal plexus lies both superficial and deep to it. **Undermine in the fascial plane beneath the cutaneous musculature to preserve the integrity of the subdermal plexus. Where the panniculus is absent (i.e., extremities), the subdermal plexus runs in the deep surface of the dermis, necessitating that you undermine well below the dermal surface.**

b. The capillary loop system is poorly developed in dogs and cats compared with human beings and swine, which is why canine skin does not usually blister with superficial burns.

B. Musculocutaneous Vessels

1. Primary vessels supplying skin in human beings, apes, and swine; not present in dogs and other loose-skinned animals.
2. Run perpendicular to the skin surface.

Wound Healing

I. Stages of Wound Healing

A. Inflammatory Phase

1. Hemorrhage cleans and fills wounds immediately after injury.
2. Blood vessels initially constrict (for 5 to 10 minutes) to limit hemorrhage, but then dilate and leak fibrinogen and clotting elements into wounds.
3. Fibrin and plasma transudates fill wounds and plug lymphatics, localizing inflammation and "gluing" wound edges together.
4. Inflammatory mediators (i.e., histamine, serotonin) cause inflammation that begins immediately after injury and lasts approximately 5 days.

B. Debridement Phase

1. Neutrophils and monocytes appear (approximately 6 hours and 12 hours after injury, respectively) and initiate debridement.
2. Monocytes become macrophages within wounds at 24 to 48 hours. They remove necrotic tissue, bacteria, and foreign material and are chemotactic.
3. Lymphocytes appear later in this phase than neutrophils and macrophages.

C. Repair Phase

1. Usually begins 3 to 5 days after injury.
2. Fibroblasts and collagen.
   a. Migrate into wounds just ahead of new capillary buds as the inflammatory phase subsides (2 to 3 days).
   b. Invade wounds to synthesize and deposit collagen, elastin, and proteoglycans that mature into fibrous tissue.
   c. Orientation is initially haphazard, but after 5 days, tension on wounds causes fibroblasts, fibers, and capillaries to orient parallel to the incision or wound margin.
   d. Amount of collagen reaches a maximum within 2 to 3 weeks after wounding.
3. Granulation tissue.
   a. Fills defects and protects wounds.
   b. Provides a barrier to infection, a surface for epithelial migration, and a source of special fibroblasts called myofibroblasts.
   c. Healthy granulation tissue is highly vascular and inhibits wound infection.
4. Epithelialization.
   a. Begins almost immediately (24 to 48 hours) in sutured wounds with good edge-to-edge apposition.
   b. In open wounds, it begins when an adequate granulation bed has formed (usually 4 to 5 days).

c. Contact with other epithelial cells on all sides inhibits cell migration (contact inhibition) and thus stops epithelialization.
d. Initially, new epithelium is only one cell layer thick and is fragile, but it gradually thickens as additional cell layers form.
e. Epithelialization of suture tracts can be minimized by early removal of sutures.

5. Wound contraction.
   a. Reduces the size of wounds subsequent to myofibroblast contraction in granulation tissue.
   b. Occurs simultaneously with granulation and epithelialization but is independent of epithelialization. It progresses at a rate of approximately 0.6 to 0.7 mm/day.
   c. Is limited if skin around wounds is fixed, inelastic, or under tension, and it is inhibited if myofibroblast development or function is impaired.
   d. Can also be impaired by antiinflammatory steroids, antimicrotubular drugs, and local application of smooth muscle relaxants.
   e. Stops when wound edges meet, tension is excessive, or myofibroblasts are inadequate.

D. Maturation Phase

1. Begins once collagen has been adequately deposited in wounds (17 to 20 days postinjury) and may continue for several years.
2. Wound strength increases to its maximum level because of changes in the scar during this phase.

II. Host Factors That Delay Wound Healing

A. Old age (probably because of concurrent diseases or debilitation).

B. Malnourishment.

C. Serum protein concentrations less than 1.5 to 2 g/dl.

D. Hyperadrenocorticism.

E. Diabetes mellitus.

F. Uremia occurring within 5 days of injury.

III. Wound Characteristics That Delay Healing

A. Intense inflammatory reaction caused by some foreign materials (e.g., debris, sutures, surgical implants).

B. Exposure of the wound to antiseptics.

C. Wound infection (interferes with the repair phase of healing).

D. Impairment of blood supply by trauma, tight bandages, or wound movement.

E. Accumulation of fluid in dead space:
1. Hypoxic fluid environment of a seroma inhibits migration of reparative cells into wounds.
2. Fluid mechanically prevents adhesion of flaps or grafts to the wound bed.

IV. Wound Characteristics That Promote Healing

A. Warmth (30° C or 86° F).

B. Moisture (promotes recruitment of vital host defenses and cells).

V. External Factors That Delay Wound Healing

A. Corticosteroids depress all phases of wound healing and increase the chance of infection. Vitamin A and anabolic steroids may reverse the effects of corticosteroids on wound healing.

B. Antiinflammatory drugs suppress inflammation, but have little effect on wound strength.

C. Some chemotherapeutic drugs (e.g., cyclophosphamide, methotrexate, doxorubicin) significantly delay wound healing.

D. Radiation therapy may delay wound healing, depending on the dose and time of exposure relative to time of injury. It decreases the quantity of blood vessels and causes increasing dermal fibrosis.

Management of Open and Superficial Wounds

I. Covering Wounds

A. Use a clean, dry bandage immediately after injury or at presentation to prevent further contamination and hemorrhage.

II. The "Golden Period"

A. The first 6 to 8 hours between wound contamination at injury and bacterial multiplication greater than 10^5 organisms per gram of tissue.

B. A wound is classified as infected rather than contaminated when bacterial numbers exceed 10^5 organisms per gram of tissue.

C. Treat wounds less than 6 to 8 hours with minimal trauma and contamination by lavage, debridement, and primary closure.

D. Treat severely traumatized and contaminated wounds, wounds older than 6 to 8 hours, or infected wounds as open wounds to allow debridement and reduction of bacterial numbers.

III. Open Wound Care

A. Culture severely contaminated or infected wounds.

B. Clip and prep the area surrounding the wound. Protect the wound from clipped hair and detergents by applying a sterile water-soluble lubricant (K-Y Jelly) or placing saline-soaked sponges in the wound. Alternatively, close the wound temporarily with sutures, towel clamps, staples, or Michel clips.

C. Prepare the clipped skin with povidone-iodine or chlorhexidine gluconate. Do not use detergents or alcohol.

D. Lavage the wound with copious amounts of warm, sterile saline or tap water (500 to 1000 ml). Lavaging is preferred to scrubbing the wound with sponges. Bacteria are effectively removed from the wound surface by high-pressure lavage using a 35- or 60-ml syringe and 18-gauge needle, which generates approximately 7 to 8 psi of pressure.

E. Remove devitalized tissue by surgical excision, enzymes, or wet-dry bandages. The extent of devitalized tissue is usually obvious within 48 hours of injury.

F. After surgical debridement, leave the wound open and treat with medications and wet-dry bandages. Close the wound when it appears healthy or when a bed of healthy granulation tissue has formed or allow it to contract and epithelialize.

Antibiotics

I. General Considerations

A. Unnecessary for minimally or moderately contaminated wounds within the golden period.

B. Consider antibiotics for severely contaminated, crushed, or infected wounds or wounds older than 6 to 8 hours.

C. Culture contaminated wounds and those with established infection before initiating antibiotics, and base antibiotic selection on results of culture and sensitivity testing.

D. Give systemic antibiotics if there is a high risk of bacteremia or disseminated infections.

Topical Wound Medications

I. Topical Antibiotics

A. General Considerations

1. Mildly or moderately contaminated wounds typically do not benefit from combined topical and systemic antibiotic therapy; how-

ever, combined therapy is advantageous in heavily contaminated wounds.

2. Antibiotics used effectively as topical ointments or added to lavage solutions are penicillin, ampicillin, carbenicillin, tetracycline, kanamycin, neomycin, bacitracin, polymyxin, and the cephalosporins.
3. Advantages of topical antibiotics over antiseptics include selective bacterial toxicity, efficacy in the presence of organic material, and combined efficacy with systemic antibiotics.
4. Disadvantages of topical antibiotics include expense, reduced antimicrobial spectrum, potential for bacterial resistance, creation of superinfections, systemic or local toxicity, hypersensitivity, and increased nosocomial infections.
5. Use solutions rather than ointments and powders.

B. Triple Antibiotic Ointment

1. Broad spectrum; efficacy against *Pseudomonas* spp. is poor.
2. Poorly absorbed so systemic toxicosis (nephrotoxicity, ototoxicity, neurotoxicity) is rare.
3. More effective for preventing infections than treating them.

C. Silver Sulfadiazine (Silvadene)

1. Effective against most gram-positive and gram-negative bacteria and most fungi.
2. Penetrates necrotic tissue and enhances wound epithelialization.
3. Drug of choice to treat burn wounds.

D. Nitrofurazone

1. Broad-spectrum antibacterial and hydrophilic properties.
2. May delay wound epithelialization.

E. Gentamicin Sulfate

1. Available as a 1% ointment or powder.
2. Especially effective in controlling gram-negative bacterial growth (*Pseudomonas* spp., *Escherichia coli, Proteus* organisms).
3. Gentamicin in an oil-in-water cream base may initially inhibit wound contraction. Gentamicin in an isotonic solution promotes epithelialization.

II. Enzymatic Debriding Agents

A. Beneficial in patients that are poor anesthetic risks or when surgical debridement may damage healthy tissue needed for reconstruction.

B. Travase ointment contains bacillus subtilis protease as a debriding enzyme.

C. Preparation H is a hemorrhoid medication composed of a water-soluble extract of yeast (brewers' yeast, *Saccharomyces cerevisiae*) sometimes used on granulating wounds. It stimulates oxygen consumption, angiogenesis, epithelialization, and collagen synthesis in wounds and has been called the wound respiratory factor.

III. Other Topical Agents

A. Aloe Vera

1. Has been used on burns for its antibacterial activity against *Pseudomonas aeruginosa.*

2. Its antiprostaglandin and antithromboxane properties are beneficial in maintaining vascular patency and thus helping avert dermal ischemia.

IV. Lavage Solutions

A. Chlorhexidine Diacetate

1. Use a 0.05% solution for wound lavage and as a wetting solution.
2. Has a wide spectrum of antimicrobial activity and sustained residual activity.
3. Has antibacterial activity in the presence of blood and other organic debris, has minimal systemic absorption and toxicity, and promotes rapid healing.
4. **Make a 0.05% solution by diluting one part of stock solution with 40 parts of sterile water. Do not use saline for dilution because a precipitate will form.**

B. Povidone-Iodine

1. A 1% or 0.1% povidone-iodine solution (10% stock solution diluted 1:10 or 1:100, respectively) is frequently used as a wound lavage solution because of its wide spectrum of antimicrobial activity.
2. Iodine compounds are active against vegetative and sporulated bacteria, fungi, viruses, protozoa, and yeast.
3. Povidone-iodine is a water-soluble, strongly acidic (pH 3.2) iodophor produced by combining molecular iodine with polyvinylpyrrolidone.
4. Frequent reapplication (every 4 to 6 hours) is required when it is used as a wetting solution because residual activity lasts only 4 to 8 hours and organic matter (i.e., blood, serous exudate) inactivates the free iodine in povidone-iodine.
5. Contact hypersensitivities are common.

C. Tris-EDTA

1. When added to lavage solutions causes increased permeability of gram-negative bacteria to extracellular solutes and leakage of intracellular solutes.

D. Acetic Acid

1. Its antibacterial effect is achieved by lowering the wound pH.
2. Wound acidification is beneficial in wounds containing urea-splitting organisms such as *Pseudomonas* spp.; however, resistance may develop.

E. Lavage Solutions Not Recommended

1. Hydrogen peroxide damages tissues and is a poor antiseptic.
2. Dakin's solution (0.5% solution of sodium hypochlorite–1:10 dilution of laundry bleach) releases free chlorine and oxygen into tissues, killing bacteria and liquefying necrotic tissue. Even at half or quarter strength Dakin's solution is detrimental to neutrophils, fibroblasts, and endothelial cells; therefore it should not be used as a wound lavage solution.

Assessment of Skin Viability

I. Clinical Assessment

A. Nonviable skin is black, bluish-black, or white, and the area may be nonpliable, cool, and devoid of sensation.

B. Normal skin is warm, pliable, and pink with normal capillary refill (difficult to assess) and pain sensation.

C. Areas of questionable viability are often blue or purple and capillary refill and sensation are poor.

D. Other methods of assessing skin viability include dyes, transcutaneous oxygen or carbon dioxide, and laser-Doppler velocimetry. Intravenous injection of the vital stains fluorescein (10 mg/kg) or xylenol orange (90 mg/kg) have not been shown to be advantageous over visual observation.

Principles of Integumentary Surgery

I. Preservation of the Deep or Subdermal Plexus

A. The deep or subdermal plexus must be preserved during dissection and excision to ensure skin survival.

B. Undermine at the level of the subcutaneous fat to avoid transection of the subdermal plexus.

C. Dissect under the cutaneous trunci muscle, or in the distal extremities in the deep dermal layer, to avoid transecting the direct cutaneous arteries that supply the subdermal plexus.

D. Fundamental surgical principles for reconstructive surgery are listed in Table 13-1.

Drains

I. Passive Drains

A. Depend on gravity for fluid evacuation vs. active drains, which require a vacuum.

B. Penrose drains.

1. Secure to the skin at the dorsal aspect of the wound by direct visualization or blind suture placement.
2. Exit through a stab incision at least 1 cm from the primary incision. Do not exit from the primary incision.
3. Do not fenestrate.
4. Protect with a bandage that is changed before "strike-through" occurs.

II. Active Drains

A. May be open, with an air vent into the wound, or closed.

B. An effective closed-suction drain can be easily made using a butterfly

Table 13-1
Fundamental surgical principles

- Use strict asepsis in preparation of surgical team, room, and instruments, and during surgery.
- Handle tissues gently.
- Preserve vascularity.
- Remove necrotic tissue.
- Maintain hemostasis.
- Approximate tissues anatomically without tension.
- Obliterate dead space.
- Use appropriate suture materials and implants.

catheter and an evacuated tube or syringe. Remove the syringe adaptor from the plastic tubing and fenestrate the tube before placing the drain in the wound. After wound closure insert the needle into the evacuated tube (5 to 10 ml) to apply suction. Alternatively, remove the needle, fenestrate the tube, and attach the adaptor to a syringe with suction applied. Replace the vacuum tube when it loses negative pressure or fills with fluid.

Wound Closure

I. Definitions

A. **Primary wound closure**–immediate closure of the wound.

B. **Delayed primary wound closure**–closure of the wound within 1 to 3 days after injury when wound is free of infection but before granulation tissue has appeared.

C. **Secondary closure**–wound closure after the formation of granulation tissue.

D. **Second intention healing**–allowing the wound to contract and epithelialize.

II. Bandages

A. Layers

1. Contact or primary layer.
   a. Used to debride tissue, deliver medication, transmit wound exudate, or form an occlusive seal over the wound.
   b. Use an adherent contact layer when wound debridement is required; select a nonadherent contact layer when granulation tissue has formed.
   c. Semiocclusive bandages allow air to penetrate and exudate to escape from the wound surface.

   d. Occlusive bandages are impermeable to air; use on nonexudative wounds to keep tissues moist.
2. Intermediate or secondary layer.
   a. Absorbent layer that removes and stores deleterious agents (e.g., blood, serum, exudate, debris, bacteria, enzymes) away from the wound surface.
   b. Also serves to pad the wound from trauma, splint the wound to prevent movement, and hold the contact layer against the wound.
   c. Use absorbent cotton, combine roll, or cast padding (Specialist cast padding or Kerlix Rolls).
3. Outer or tertiary layer.
   a. Holds the other bandage layers in place and protects them from external contamination.
   b. Use roll gauze (Conform Stretch Bandages or Kling), stockinette (Specialist tubular stockinette), or surgical adhesive tape.
   c. Elastic adhesive tapes (Elastikon porous adhesive tape or Vetrap) apply pressure, conform to the area, and immobilize it. Support rods or splints may be incorporated into the outer layer of the bandage if additional immobilization is required.

B. Types of Bandages

1. Absorbent bandages.
   a. Indicated for open contaminated and infected wounds.
   b. Contact layer–an absorbent pad (Kerlix) followed by an absorbent intermediate layer (Kerlix Rolls) to hold the pad in place.
   c. Outer layer–an elastic contouring wrap (Conform Stretch Bandages or Kling); apply slight pressure. Adhesive tape is the final covering.
2. Adherent bandages.
   a. Wet-dry.
      i. Assist debridement by liquefying coagulum and absorbing necrotic debris while leaving viable tissue intact.
      ii. Advantages.
         (a) Antimicrobials can be used in the wetting solution.
         (b) A physiologic environment can be maintained.
         (c) Comfort is maintained.
         (d) Exudate is removed.
      iii. Place several layers of sterile gauze sponges over the wound and soak them with saline or a 0.05% to 0.1% chlorhexidine solution. Cover the wet sponges with an absorbent bandage. Change the bandage daily or more often if strike-through occurs. To remove the primary layers of the bandage (dry gauze sponges), moisten the sponges with saline and lift them from the wound.
   b. Wet-wet.
      i. Similar to a wet-dry bandage except the contact layer is not allowed to dry before bandage removal.
      ii. Used on wounds with large amounts of viscous exudate and little debris or necrotic tissue.
   c. Dry-dry.
      i. Used on wounds with loose necrotic tissue and debris or large quantities of low-viscosity exudate.
      ii. Apply a dry, wide-mesh gauze to the wound, followed by an absorbent intermediate layer and tape. Leave the bandage in place until absorbed fluid and debris have dried in the intermediate layer.
3. Nonadherent bandages.
   a. Use when drainage becomes serosanguineous and granulation tissue forms on the wound.
   b. Place an elastic contouring wrap (Conform Stretch Bandages or

Kling) over the absorbent wrap to conform the bandage and apply slight pressure. Place adhesive tape as the final covering. Change the bandage every 1 to 3 days, or as needed.

4. Tie-over bandages.
   a. Used to hold the contact and absorbent layers of a bandage in place when the wound is in an area inaccessible to standard bandaging techniques (e.g., hip, shoulder, axilla).
   b. Place several sutures (e.g., 2-0 or 0 nylon or polypropylene) in the skin surrounding the wound, tieing them with a loose loop. Apply an adherent or nonadherent contact layer and an intermediate bandage layer on the wound. Hold these layers in place by lacing sterile gauze or umbilical tape through the loose skin sutures. Cover the area with an outer bandage layer, if possible.
5. Pressure bandages.
   a. Used to facilitate control of minor hemorrhage, edema, and excess granulation tissue.
   b. Apply an absorbent nonadherent contact layer over the area of hemorrhage or excess granulation tissue. Use a thick absorbent intermediate layer and elastic adhesive tape for the outer bandage layer. Wrap the elastic tape carefully to avoid excess pressure, which can impair arterial, venous, and lymphatic circulation, and cause tissue necrosis or nerve damage. Observe for discomfort, swelling, hypothermia, dryness, or odor, which may indicate the area has been bandaged too tightly. Remove the bandage within 24 to 48 hours if it was applied to control hemorrhage.
6. Pressure relief bandages.
   a. Designed to prevent pressure over an area (usually a bony prominence); used to treat or prevent pressure sores.
   b. Create a doughnut-shaped bandage by rolling a towel or cloth into a tight cylinder, securely tape it to maintain the roll, and form it into an appropriately sized circle. Center the doughnut-shaped bandage over the lesion or bony prominence and secure it to the skin with tape so it will not slip. These bandages may be difficult to maintain in position. Taping directly to the skin may cause skin irritation.
   c. Pipe insulation bandages are usually used to protect the olecranon. Create bandages from foam rubber pipe insulation tubes by splitting the tube and cutting a hole where the bony prominence will lie. If necessary, use two or three thicknesses of pipe. Stack and tape the pieces of pipe together. When using over the olecranon, first pad the cranial surface of the radial-humeral joint with cast padding to prevent joint flexion and keep the dog from lying in sternal recumbency. Then, tape the cast padding and pipe insulation in place.

C. Bandaging Techniques

1. Thorax and abdomen.
   a. Apply an adherent or nonadherent contact layer over the incision or wound. Place several layers of sterile gauze sponges over the end of Penrose drains. Hold the contact layer in position with combine rolls, cast padding, or cotton. Use padding, gauze, and tape rolls 3 to 6 inches in width. Wrap the padding circumferentially around the torso with slight pressure. Overlap each wrap by approximately one half to one third the width of the roll.
   b. Reduce rostral or caudal slippage of the bandage by wrapping the intermediate and outer bandage layers between the legs and over the shoulders or hips in a criss-cross fashion. Encircle the torso with one wrap of bandage material, then direct the bandage from the right inguinal area (axillary area) to the left perineal area (shoulder

area). Encircle the torso again and continue across the right perineal area (shoulder area), through the left inguinal area (axillary area), to the left flank (thorax). Repeat the criss-cross pattern several times. Also reduce slippage by adhering 0.5 to 1 inch of tape to the hair. Do not wrap the bandage so tightly that thoracic expansion is inhibited.

   c. Hold the intermediate layer in place with elastic gauze (Kling) or stockinette. Cut a length of stockinette (3 inches for cats and small dogs; 4 to 6 inches for medium and large dogs) slightly longer than the length of the body from head to rump. Cut small holes in the stockinette to accommodate the legs. Place the stockinette over the head and pull the front legs through the leg holes before rolling the stockinette caudally. Pull the hind legs through the leg holes. Secure the bandage with tape. In male dogs cut a hole in the bandage to accommodate the prepuce or divert urine with a catheter to keep the bandage dry. During bandaging manipulate the ends of tube drains so they can be easily accessed for aspiration or infusion.

2. Head.
   a. Apply 1-inch porous tape directly to the edge of the pinna to form a stirrup, fold the ear over an absorbent pad or gauze sponges onto the dorsum of the head, and wrap the tape around the head to secure the ear in position. Using a similar technique pad and place the opposite pinna over the first pinna if indicated. Place a nonadherent contact layer over an incision or gauze sponges over the end of a passive drain. Hold the pinna and contact layers in position with 2-to 3-inch cast padding or cotton roll.
   b. Encircle the head, passing the rolls of bandage material cranial and caudal to the opposite ear unless both ears are being immobilized. Starting under the chin, wrap loosely and overlap each wrap by approximately one third the width of the roll. Cover this intermediate bandage layer with overlapping wraps of elastic gauze or a stockinette.
   c. To prevent slippage secure the bandage in position with elastic tape attached to the skin and hair at the cranial and caudal edges of the bandage. During bandaging manipulate the ends of tube drains so they can be easily accessed for aspiration or infusion. If necessary to medicate the ear, cut holes in the bandaging over the external acoustic meatus.
3. Extremities.
   a. Begin by applying a 1-inch porous tape stirrup to the dorsal and ventral or medial and lateral surfaces of the paw. Extend stirrups 3 to 8 inches beyond the digits to help prevent the bandage from slipping distally. If necessary, use a loose layer of elastic gauze to help secure the stirrups. Insert small pledgets of cotton or other absorbent material between the digits and the metatarsal/metacarpal pads and digital pads. Apply an appropriate contact layer over the wound. Snugly apply cast padding around the paw beginning at the level of the second and fifth digital pads. Wrap obliquely so the third and fourth digits protrude slightly beyond the bandage. Overlap the cast padding (2- to 3-inch width) one half to two thirds of its width as it is advanced up the leg. Continue the bandage to the proximal radius and ulna (tibia and fibula) or above the elbow (stifle), depending on the site of the injury. Use enough padding to create the bulkiness necessary for protection. Snugly wrap elastic gauze (2- to 3-inch width) over the cast padding to conform the padding to the limb, overlapping each turn by one half the width of the material. Separate the tape stirrups and attach them to their respective sides of the bandage. Apply an outer layer of elastic tape

(2- to 3-inch width), overlapping one half the width with each turn. Avoid overstretching the tape to prevent compromising limb circulation. Check exposed digits three and four frequently for swelling, coolness, and discomfort; remove the bandage and evaluate the limb if these signs are observed.

b. For onychectomy, digit amputation, or pad reconstruction apply stirrups laterally and cover the digits with gauze sponges or a nonadherent contact layer. Reflect layers of 2-inch cast padding from dorsal to ventral and then ventral to dorsal over the end of the paw. Extend the cast padding in a spiral pattern to the midradius and ulna (tibia and fibula). Leave the proximal ends of the tape stirrup exposed to aid bandage removal. Cover the cast padding with elastic gauze. Fold the tape stirrups to their respective sides. Cover the bandage with tape from the distal extremity to the proximal hair.

Suture Patterns

I. Walking Sutures

A. Walking sutures move skin across a defect, obliterate dead space, and distribute tension over the wound surface. They do not penetrate the skin surface.

B. Advance skin toward the center of the wound by placing rows of interrupted, subdermal sutures beginning at the depths of the wound.

II. External Tension Relieving Sutures

A. External tension relieving sutures help prevent sutures from cutting out, which occurs when pressure on skin within the suture loop exceeds the pressure that allows blood flow.

B. The standard tension-relieving suture is the vertical mattress suture.

Treatment of "Dog Ears"

I. Prevention

A. Prevent dog ears by placing sutures close together on the convex side of the defect and further apart on the concave side of the wound.

II. Correction

A. Correct dog ears by outlining with an elliptical incision, removing redundant skin, and apposing the skin edges in a linear or curvilinear fashion.

Relaxing Incisions

I. Simple Relaxing Incisions

A. Close the wound and make a relaxing incision at the point where undermining stopped or where tension lines are observed.

B. Begin the incision at the point of maximum skin tension and extend as necessary to relieve excess tension.

II. Multiple Punctate Relaxing Incisions

A. Make small, parallel, staggered incisions in skin adjacent to a wound to allow closure with reduced tension.

III. V-to-Y Plasty

A. A type of relaxing incision that provides an advancement flap to cover a wound. It is used to close chronic, inelastic wounds or wounds that would distort adjacent structures if closed under tension.

B. Make a V-shaped incision adjacent to the wound. Close the original wound after undermining skin. Close the V relief incision in the shape of a Y.

IV. Z Plasty

A. A technique that lengthens or relaxes an incision.

B. The Z may be incorporated into the wound or a separate Z made adjacent to the wound to facilitate closure with less tension.

C. The central limb of the Z is the wound or primary incision. The two arms of the Z are made the same length as the central limb. The angles of the Z can vary between 30 and 90 degrees, but 60 degrees is advised.

Pedicle Flaps

I. General Considerations

A. Are "tongues" of epidermis and dermis that are partially detached from donor sites and used to cover defects. The base or pedicle of the flap contains the blood supply essential for flap survival.

B. Most flaps are called *subdermal plexus flaps;* however, those with direct cutaneous vessels are termed *axial pattern flaps.*

C. The base of flaps should be slightly wider than the width of the flap body.

D. Delaying flap transfer 18 to 21 days after initial creation may improve circulation and survival in ischemic flaps (delay phenomenon).

II. Advancement Flaps

A. Are local subdermal plexus flaps.

B. Flaps are formed in adjacent, loose, elastic skin that can be slid over the defect.

III. Rotational Flaps

A. Local flaps that are pivoted over a defect with which they share a common border.

B. They are semicircular in shape and may be paired or single. A curved incision is created and undermined in a stepwise fashion until it covers the defect without tension.

IV. Transposition Flaps

A. Rectangular, local flaps that bring additional skin when rotated into defects.

B. The width of the flap equals the width of the defect.

V. Pouch and Hinge Flaps

A. Pouch flaps (bipedicle flaps) and hinge flaps (single pedicle flaps) are direct, distant flaps useful for reconstructing lower extremity skin defects.

B. Although this technique is successful in covering distal extremity skin defects, some animals may not tolerate the limb being positioned against the body wall; moreover, it causes temporary joint stiffness.

After granulation tissue has formed, prepare the skin on the limb and ipsilateral thoracoabdominal wall for aseptic surgery. Position the limb along the animal's side and make two parallel dorsoventral incisions at locations that allow complete coverage of the defect (if pad tissue is absent only a single cranial incision is necessary). Undermine the flap and place the foot within the pouch. Appose skin at the wound edges with the edges of the flap using interrupted approximating sutures (e.g., 3-0 or 4-0 polypropylene or nylon). Place three to four interrupted sutures through the skin of the flap into the granulation tissue to immobilize the flap over the defect. Bandage the limb against the body for 14 days and change the bandage every 3 to 4 days. Release the limb from the pouch by making two horizontal incisions (dorsal and ventral) an appropriate distance from the paw to allow coverage of the palmar aspect of

the defect. Lavage the medial aspect of the paw to remove exudate and debride if necessary. Trim the ends of the skin flap and suture in place. Lavage the donor site and close with interrupted approximating sutures (e.g., 3-0 to 4-0 polypropylene or nylon).

VI. Tubed Pedicle Flaps

A. Uses a multistaged procedure to "walk" an indirect, distant flap to a recipient site. The disadvantage of this technique is the number of stages and time required to accomplish wound closure.

Create the tube by making two parallel incisions through the skin in an area where remaining skin can be reapposed without excess tension. Undermine skin between the two incisions. Suture the incised edges of the flap together with approximating sutures creating a tube attached at both ends. Appose edges of the donor site with approximating sutures. After 18 to 21 days transect one end of the tube and transpose it to the recipient bed. Alternatively, transpose the end of the tube nearer the donor site and after an additional 18 to 21 days transect and transpose the other end of the tube over the defect. Incise the tube and unroll as needed to cover the defect and suture the edges of the tube to the edges of the defect. Appose skin edges at the tube's origin. Transect the remaining end of the tube after 18 to 21 days to complete coverage of the defect if necessary.

VII. Axial Pattern Flaps

A. Are pedicle flaps that include a direct cutaneous artery and vein at their base. They are elevated and transferred to cutaneous defects within their radius.

B. Specific axial pattern flaps are described in Table 13-2.

C. They require careful planning, measuring, and mapping on the skin surface to minimize errors.

Skin Grafts

I. General Considerations

A. Skin grafts are the transfer of a segment of free dermis and epidermis to a distant recipient site.

B. Autografts (same animal) are most useful; however, allografts (same species) and xenografts (different species) that are eventually rejected may be used to temporarily cover and protect large burned or denuded areas.

Table 13-2
Axial pattern flaps

Flap	Indications	Blood supply	Boundaries
Caudal auricular	head and neck defects	sternocleidomastoideus branch of the caudal auricular artery and vein	**base**—centered over lateral aspect of the wing of the atlas **caudal**—parallel to base, rostral to scapular spine **dorsal and ventral**—parallel, connecting caudal incision to base far enough to cover defect
Omocervical	face, head, ear, shoulder, neck, and axilla defects	superficial cervical branch of the omocervical artery and vein	**caudal**—scapular spine **center and ventral**—cranial shoulder depression at cranial edge of scapula **dorsal**—midline or contralateral scapulohumeral joint
Thoracodorsal	shoulder, forelimb, elbow, axilla, and thorax defects	cutaneous branch of the thoraco-dorsal artery and vein	**base**—ventral; caudal shoulder depression parallel to dorsal border of acromion **cranial**—scapular spine **caudal**—parallel scapular spine, twice the distance from the shoulder depression to acromion **dorsal**—dorsal midline or contralateral scapulohumeral joint
Superficial brachial	antebrachial and elbow defects	superficial brachial artery and vein	**base**—anterior one third of flexor surface of the elbow **medial and lateral**—parallel to the humeral shaft, converge at greater tubercle **dorsal**—below or at greater tubercle
Caudal superficial epigastric	caudal abdomen, flank, prepuce, perineum, thigh, and hindlimb defects	caudal superficial epigastric artery and vein	**base**—caudal inguinal ring **medial**—ventral abdominal midline **lateral**—equidistant from teats to midline **cranial**—between 1st and 2nd or 2nd and 3rd mammary glands

Deep circumflex iliac	**dorsal**—caudal thorax, lateral abdominal wall, ipsilateral flank, lateral lumbar area, medial or lateral thigh, greater trochanter, and pelvic defects	dorsal branch of the deep circumflex iliac artery and vein	**base**—cranioventral to wing of the ilium **caudal**—midway between cranial border of ileal wing and greater trochanter **cranial**—equal distance from ileal wing as caudal incision **dorsal**—midline
	ventral—lateral abdominal wall and pelvic and sacral defects	ventral branch of the deep circumflex iliac artery and vein	**base**—dorsal **caudal**—cranial border of femoral shaft **cranial**—parallel to caudal incision **ventral**—above patella
Genicular	lateral and medial tibial defects (possibly tibiotarsal joint defects)	genicular branch of the saphenous artery and medial saphenous vein	**base**—lateral stifle; 1 cm proximal to patella and 1.5 cm distal to tibial tuberosity **medial and lateral**—parallel to femoral shaft **dorsal**—base of greater trochanter
Reverse saphenous conduit	defects at or below the tarsus	cranial branch of the saphenous artery and vein	**base**—ventral **dorsal**—central one third of medial thigh or slightly above patella **medial and lateral**—0.5-1.0 cm cranial and caudal to branches off saphenous artery and medial saphenous vein
Lateral caudal	caudodorsal trunk and hindlimb defects	lateral caudal (coccygeal) artery and vein	dorsal defect **base**—ventral **incision**—dorsal midline ventral defect **base**—dorsal **incision**—ventral midline

C. Bone, cartilage, tendon, and nerve that are denuded of their overlying connective tissue do not support grafts. Chronic granulation tissue should be excised to allow new granulation tissue to form before grafting (approximately 4 to 5 days).

D. Plasmatic imbibition initially nourishes the graft and keeps the graft vessels dilated until the graft revascularizes. Vascular sprouts may be found within the lower layers of the graft in 48 to 72 hours.

E. Fluid accumulation within or under the graft and movement of the graft prevent good vascular connections from developing between the graft and the bed.

F. The most common causes of graft failure are separation from the graft bed, infection, and movement.

G. Donor site skin should have hair of the same color, texture, length, and thickness as hair surrounding the recipient site. The donor site should have enough skin to allow closure without tension after graft removal.

II. Full-Thickness Skin Grafts

A. Include the epidermis and entire dermis. Indicated to cover large defects on flexor surfaces thus preventing contracture and distal extremity defects.

B. Sheet grafts.
   1. Indicated to prevent contracture of defects on the distal aspect of the limbs and over flexor surfaces.
   2. Use over noninfected granulation beds and when minimal fluid production is expected because graft adhesion is prevented by fluid accumulation or drains.

Aseptically prepare the surgical sites. Debride, lavage, and control hemorrhage in the graft bed before placing the graft. Make a pattern of the defect using a sterile towel or paper template. Using the pattern of the defect as a guide, harvest a segment of skin from the donor site with the hair oriented in the proper direction. Excise all subcutaneous tissue from the graft with a scalpel blade during harvest or it will interfere with revascularization. Alternatively, excise the graft, stretch, and fix it to a piece of stiff cardboard and then remove subcutaneous tissues with scissors. Keep the donor site moist with saline-soaked sponges while the graft is being placed. Place the graft in the defect with the hair properly oriented. Tack the graft in position with interrupted sutures. Place a closed suction drain beneath the graft and appose the edges of the graft and wound with staples or simple interrupted or continuous sutures placed 3 to 4 mm apart. Close the donor site by undermining and apposing wound edges or using a pedicle flap. Bandage the graft site with a nonadherent, absorbable bandage. Change the evacuation tube as needed. Change the bandage and evaluate the graft 24 to 48 hours after surgery. Continue rebandaging as needed for 21 days.

C. Plug, punch, or seed grafts and strip grafts.
   1. Place in a prepared granulation tissue bed. Indicated for limb wounds and wounds with low-grade infection or irregular surfaces.

Prepare the graft bed by debriding and treating as an open wound for several days. Harvest plugs of skin from the donor site with a 5-mm biopsy punch or

tent the skin and resect a small piece of tissue. Harvest 5-mm-wide strips of skin free-hand for strip grafting. Remove subcutaneous tissues from the dermis. For plugs make small slitlike pockets (2 to 4 mm deep, 5 to 7 mm apart) in the granulation tissue, almost parallel to the wound surface. Insert a plug in each pocket, holding it in position with gentle pressure for 1 to 2 minutes. Alternatively, cut holes in the granulation tissue with a 4-mm skin biopsy punch and insert the skin plugs into these holes. Make grooves 2 mm wide and 3 to 5 mm apart for strip grafting. After hemorrhage has been controlled lay a skin strip in each groove and anchor it with an interrupted suture at each end. Bandage and splint the graft site with nonadherent, absorbent materials. Excise and reappose the donor site or treat as an open wound with bandages. Change the graft bandage 3 to 4 days after surgery, being careful to avoid dislodging any of the grafts. Rebandage the area as needed until healing is complete.

D. Mesh grafts.
   1. Mesh grafts may be either full-thickness or split-thickness grafts in which parallel rows of staggered slits have been cut. Meshing a sheet graft allows drainage, flexibility, conformity, and expansion.

III. Split-Thickness Skin Grafts

A. General Considerations

1. Composed of epidermis and a variable thickness of dermis. Feline skin is too thin for split-thickness grafting.
2. Graft take with split-thickness grafts is similar to that of full-thickness grafts. Split-thickness grafts are less durable and more subject to trauma than full-thickness grafts, and hair growth may be absent or sparse.
3. Skin of the lateral thoracic wall, back, shoulder, or another area with abundant skin may be used as the donor site.

Aseptically prepare the surgical sites. Debride, lavage, and control hemorrhage in the graft bed before placing the graft. Harvest the split-thickness graft with a dermatome or free-hand. Inject sterile saline subcutaneously under the donor site to elevate the skin. Lubricate the skin surface with sterile mineral oil or water-soluble gel if using a dermatome. Pull the skin in opposite directions over the donor site to make it taut. Harvest the graft. Using a scalpel, make a partial-thickness incision perpendicular to the skin surface. Then, holding a modified safety razor almost parallel to the skin surface, begin cutting. Place stay sutures in the cut edge of the graft to apply traction while cutting. Change blades as they become dull. Place the graft on the bed with hair growth oriented in the proper direction. Overlap the wound edges with the graft by 2 to 4 mm. Anchor the graft in place with interrupted sutures or skin staples. Irrigate under the graft with saline or thrombin. Apply a nonadherent absorbent bandage with a splint to immobilize the area. Use a tie-over bandage if necessary. Holes inadvertently perforating the graft will allow drainage and eventually heal. After harvest and grafting, excise the donor site and close it or manage it as an open wound with bandages. Increased pain is associated with the wound when it is managed as an open wound. Perform the first bandage change 24 to 48 hours after surgery. Drain the area if a seroma or hematoma has formed by making a small incision in the graft and aspirating. Expect the graft overlapping the skin to necrose. Rebandage the area and change the bandage only as needed because movement of the graft bed interferes with revascularization.

Surgical Management of Specific Skin Disorders (*SAS*, pp. 132-142)

Burns and Other Thermal Injuries (*SAS*, pp. 132-134)

I. Definitions

A. **Eschar**–residue of skin elements that have been coagulated by heat. It is composed almost entirely of tough denatured collagen fibers.

B. **Scabs**–contain dead cells and flimsy fibrin and are not a strong protective covering like an eschar.

C. **Superficial** or **first-degree burns.**
   1. Affect only epidermis.
   2. Painful, thickened, erythematous, and desquamated.
   3. Healing occurs rapidly (within 3 to 6 days) by epithelialization from the stratum germinativum or adnexal structures of the dermis.

D. **Superficial partial-thickness burns.**
   1. Are moist, blanch with pressure, and are sensitive to pain.
   2. Usually heal within 3 weeks because of epithelialization from deeper portions of the skin appendages.
   3. Healing is usually complete and occurs without grafting.

E. **Deep, partial-thickness** or **second-degree burns.**
   1. Cause marked destruction of the dermis.
   2. The only remaining adnexal epithelium is in the upper layers of the subcutaneous fat.
   3. Healing occurs by reepithelialization from deep adnexa and wound margins.

F. **Full-thickness** or **third-degree burns.**
   1. Form a dark brown, insensitive, leathery eschar.
   2. All skin structures are destroyed and hair epilates easily.
   3. Less painful than first- or second-degree burns because nerves have been destroyed.
   4. Healing occurs by contraction and reepithelialization unless the wound is reconstructed.

G. Estimating the size of the burn wound.
   1. Measure area of burned skin with a metric ruler; divide area by the total surface area of the animal (Table 13-3); multiply by 100.
   2. Rule-of-nine; each forelimb of the animal represents approximately 9% of the total body surface area (TBSA), each rear limb is 18% (two nines), and the dorsal and ventral thorax and abdomen are each 18%.

Table 13-3
Burns: calculation of total body surface area

Conversion chart
Body weight (kg) to total body surface area (m^2)

kg	m^2	kg	m^2
1.0	0.10	26.0	0.88
2.0	0.15	27.0	0.90
3.0	0.20	28.0	0.92
4.0	0.25	29.0	0.94
5.0	0.29	30.0	0.96
6.0	0.33	31.0	0.99
7.0	0.36	32.0	1.01
8.0	0.40	33.0	1.03
9.0	0.43	34.0	1.05
10.0	0.46	35.0	1.07
11.0	0.49	36.0	1.09
12.0	0.52	37.0	1.11
13.0	0.55	38.0	1.13
14.0	0.58	39.0	1.15
15.0	0.60	40.0	1.17
16.0	0.63	41.0	1.19
17.0	0.66	42.0	1.21
18.0	0.69	43.0	1.23
19.0	0.71	44.0	1.25
20.0	0.74	45.0	1.26
21.0	0.76	46.0	1.28
22.0	0.78	47.0	1.30
23.0	0.81	48.0	1.32
24.0	0.83	49.0	1.34
25.0	0.85	50.0	1.36

Total body surface area = $\text{weight}^{0.425} \times \text{height}^{0.725} \times 0.007184$ ($m^2 = kg^{0.425} \times cm^{0.725} \times 0.007184$)
or total body surface area = $0.1 \times \text{weight (kg)}^{2/3}$

From Swaim SF: *Surgery of traumatized skin: management and reconstruction in the dog and cat,* Philadelphia, 1980, WB Saunders.

II. Treatment

A. Minimize tissue loss by administering first aid and preventing shock.
1. Administer shock doses of lactated Ringer's solution or hypertonic saline solution to minimize and reverse signs of shock.
2. Hypertonic saline (4 ml/kg bolus) plus lactated Ringer's solution (1 ml/kg/percent of TBSA of burn) may be administered.

B. Prevent septic complications by good wound management.
1. Perform early wound debridement and reconstruction.

2. Immediately after thermal injury (within 2 hours), cool the affected areas to limit further extension of tissue destruction. Lavage the area with cold water or apply cold packs to the wound.

C. Provide analgesics as necessary to alleviate pain.

D. Monitor vital signs, mental status, hematocrit, total protein, urine output, central venous pressure, electrolytes, blood gases, and daily body weight.

E. Burn wound management.
1. Debride necrotic tissue from burn wounds with enzymes or dissection. Perform early burn excision to minimize secondary infections and systemic effects.

Estimate the burn depth and calculate the size of the burn in relationship to the TBSA obtained from a weight-conversion chart. Clip the wound and surrounding hair before gently lavaging with an antiseptic solution (e.g., 0.05% chlorhexidine diacetate). Cover the wound with a topical aloe vera compound or silver sulfadiazine. If treatment is begun soon after the burn, use aloe vera or dipyridamole (thromboxane synthetase blocker) to help preserve patency of the dermal vasculature. After the first 24 hours apply water-soluble, 1% silver sulfadiazine cream (Silvadene cream) to the wound once or twice daily. Silver sulfadiazine is bactericidal with activity against gram-positive and gram-negative bacteria and Candida spp. Bandage the wound and aseptically manage it during daily bandage changes. Remove the proteinaceous gel from the surface of the wound during bandage changes and before reapplication of silver sulfadiazine. Use gentle hydrotherapy to remove debris and clean the wound.

Electrical Injuries (*SAS*, pp. 134-135)

I. General Considerations

A. Chewing on electrical cords is the most common cause of electrical injury in small animals.

B. Tissue damage may be massive because of deep extension of the generated heat. Immediate death can result from respiratory paralysis or ventricular fibrillation. Animals are often found collapsed in a tonic state with an electrical cord in their mouth.

C. If the animal survives, the tonic state resolves when the cord is removed from the mouth, although the animal may be weak and ataxic for a short period. Burns primarily occur on the lips, gums, and palate.

II. Treatment

A. Pulmonary edema.
1. Diuretics (e.g., furosemide 2.5 to 5.0 mg/kg intramuscularly or intravenously, once or twice a day).

2. Aminophylline (10 mg/kg intravenously or intramuscularly three times a day).
3. Morphine (0.4 mg/kg intramuscularly or subcutaneously) may be given to dogs to reduce anxiety.
4. Ventilatory support is needed if there is no response to medication.

B. Repair of damaged tissue should be delayed until the full extent of the injury is known.

Frostbite (*SAS*, p. 135)

I. General Considerations

A. Extremities (e.g., ear, tail, scrotum, mammary glands) are most commonly affected because of sparse hair coat and poor peripheral circulation.

B. Frozen tissue is pale, hypoesthetic, and cool. Thawed viable tissue is hyperemic, painful, and scaly. Nonviable tissue undergoes dry gangrene or mummification and sloughs.

II. Treatment

A. Rapidly rewarm affected body parts in warm water (102° to 107.6° F or 39° to 42° C) for about 20 minutes to improve circulation.

B. Apply topical aloe vera or silver sulfadiazine to the affected areas.

C. Use bandages to prevent self-trauma.

D. Continue conservative therapy until viable tissue can be distinguished from nonviable tissue (3 to 6 weeks). Debride necrotic tissue and reconstruct the area if necessary.

Chemical Injuries (*SAS*, pp. 135-136)

I. General Considerations

A. Chemical burns from strong acids or alkalis destroy tissue by denaturing proteins or interfering with cell metabolism.

B. Corrosives (e.g., sodium-containing drain and oven cleaners, phenol disinfectants) cause protein denaturation resulting in erosion and ulceration.

C. Dehydrating chemicals (e.g., sulfuric and hydrochloric acid) desiccate tissues, whereas oxidizing agents (e.g., chromic acid, hypochlorite, potassium permanganate) coagulate protein.

D. Denaturizing agents (e.g., picric acid, tannic acid, acetic acid, formic acid, hydrofluoric acid) fix or stabilize tissue by the formation of salts.

E. Vesicants (e.g., dimethyl sulfoxide, cantharides, halogenated hydrocarbons, gasoline) liberate tissue amines (histamine, serotonin), causing blisters.

II. Treatment

A. Immediately after chemical exposure, flush resultant burns with large volumes of water to remove the chemical and prevent further injury.

B. Neutralize hydrofluoric acid to stop penetration.
   1. Apply aqueous benzalkonium chloride, which precipitates residual fluoride ion.
   2. Then inject 10% calcium gluconate into and around the lesion (0.5 ml/cm^2).

C. Prevent the animal from licking the wound to avoid chemical burns of the tongue, oropharynx, and esophagus.

D. Apply antimicrobials as described for thermal burns.

Snakebites (*SAS*, pp. 136-137)

I. Types of Venomous Snakes in the United States

A. Crotalidae (pit vipers): copperhead, cottonmouth water moccasin, rattlesnake.
   1. Identifiable characteristics.
      a. Triangular head with facial pits located between the nostrils and eyes.
      b. Vertically elliptical pupils.
   2. Crotalid snake venom.
      a. Venoms are primarily enzymatic in activity (i.e., hematotoxic, vasculotoxic, necrogenic). They alter the resistance and integrity of blood vessels causing hypotension and bleeding, affect cardiac dynamics and nervous system function, and produce respiratory depression and myonecrosis.
      b. Bites most commonly occur on the face and legs. Erythema, edema, and pain are immediate local effects. Envenomation has not occurred if these signs are not seen within 20 minutes of the bite.
      c. Progressive swelling and sometimes local hemorrhage occur with moderate to severe envenomation.
      d. Systemic signs of envenomation are usually lethargy, vomiting, diarrhea, hypotension, and shock. Other signs may include anorexia, salivation, thirst, lymph node pain, weakness, bradycardia or tachycardia, generalized tremors, coma, tachypnea, pulmonary edema, urinary and fecal incontinence, paralysis, convulsions, and hemorrhage. Venom-induced coagulation defects may be severe.

B. Elapidae subfamilies (coral snakes).
1. Identifiable characteristics.
   a. Round heads; no pits; round pupils.
   b. Small fangs in the cranial mandible allow them to hang from the animals they bite.
2. Coral snake venom.
   a. Primarily neurotoxic, causing moderate tissue reaction and pain at puncture sites. Neurotoxicity is characterized by central nervous system depression, vasomotor instability, and muscle paralysis.
   b. There is a delay of several hours before onset of systemic signs, which worsen gradually over 18 hours. Effects may last 7 to 10 days.
   c. Envenomation may cause lethargy, tremors, ptosis, dysphonia, incoordination, and hematuria. Larger doses may cause vomiting, salivation, defecation, and generalized parasympathetic stimulation followed by paralysis and death. The primary cause of death is respiratory paralysis.

II. Treatment

A. Immobilize the bite wound and avoid excitement or exertion. Lavage the wound and clean it with antiseptics or germicidal soaps.

B. Clip the site to facilitate examination for fang marks.

C. Hospitalize the patient and observe for systemic signs. Monitor results of hemograms, coagulation profiles, urinalysis, and serum biochemical analyses every 6 hours.

D. Monitor an electrocardiogram.

E. Measure the circumference of the edematous area around the bite and record it to monitor progression.

F. Administer antivenin (Antivenin Crotalidae Polyvalent or North American Coral Snake Antivenin) only if a snake bite is known to have occurred. Administer as soon as possible to limit tissue necrosis and prevent systemic reactions. Pretreat with antihistamines and skin test the animal with antivenin prior to intravenous administration to decrease anaphylactic reactions. Recommended doses range from 1 to 5 vials.

G. Give intravenous fluids. Corticosteroids may help reduce edema. Use broad-spectrum antibiotics to inhibit wound infection. Additional supportive care may include analgesics, sedatives, transfusions, and oxygen.

H. Treat necrotic tissue as an open, infected wound.

Pressure Sores (*SAS*, p. 137)

I. Susceptible Areas

A. The lateral humeral epicondyle, tuber calcanei, greater femoral trochanter, tuber coxae, and ischiatic tuberosity are most susceptible to pressure sores.

B. Pressure sores may also develop under improperly fitted or padded casts and bandages.

II. Treatment

A. Treat early pressure sores by using padded bedding and bandaging the limb to eliminate pressure over the bony prominence. Apply a well-padded doughnut-type bandage or pipe insulation bandage to prevent trauma.

B. Treat open wounds with topical antibiotics and wet-dry bandages to encourage debridement and granulation. Drain dead space and surgically debride infected tissues and bone when deep ulcers are present. Perform secondary closure after healthy granulation tissue has formed in large, deep wounds.

Elbow Hygroma (Elbow Seroma, Olecranon Bursitis) (*SAS*, pp. 137-138)

I. General Considerations

A. A fluid-filled cavity surrounded by dense fibrous connective tissue occurring over the lateral aspect of the olecranon.

B. Caused by chronic trauma and typically occur in young (6 to 18 months old), large-breed dogs before a protective callus forms over the bony prominence.

II. Treatment

A. Eliminate repeated elbow trauma (e.g., soft, padded bed and padded elbow bandage).

B. Aspiration of the hygroma is of little benefit and may introduce bacteria. Although surgery should be avoided if possible, development of a fibrous capsule or infection may necessitate it. Infection requires drainage and administration of appropriate antibiotics.

For nonulcerated (infected or sterile) hygromas, prepare the limb for aseptic surgery and make several dorsal and ventral stab wounds into the hygroma cavity. Probe the cavity, breaking down fibrous septa, and lavage it. Place multiple Penrose drains into the hygroma cavity and secure them. Apply a nonadherent absorbent bandage to absorb drainage and prevent trauma. Change the bandage daily. Remove drains when drainage becomes minimal and scar tissue adherence occurs (2 to 3 weeks). Continue to bandage the elbow for at least 1 week after drain removal or until healing is complete.

Lick Granulomas (*SAS*, pp. 138-139)

I. General Considerations

A. Are self-induced by continuous licking or chewing.

B. May occur anywhere, although the cranial aspect of the carpus/metacarpus and lateral aspect of the tarsus/metatarsus are most commonly affected.

C. The lesion is sparsely haired, thickened, firm, ulcerated, erythematous, and surrounded by a hyperpigmented halo.

II. Treatment

A. Initiate treatment before the lesion becomes chronic and nonresponsive. If an underlying cause is identified, treat or eliminate it. Numerous treatments have been tried with marginal success.

B. Surgical excision of a lick granuloma followed by reconstruction using direct apposition, flaps, or grafts is possible. The surgical site should be protected with a bandage until suture removal. However, the lesion usually recurs at the same or a different site unless the causative factor(s) is eliminated.

Dermoid Sinus (Pilonidal Sinus) (*SAS*, p. 139)

I. General Considerations

A. A tubular skin indentation that extends ventrally as a blind sac from the dorsal midline.

B. It is a neural tube defect caused by incomplete separation of skin and the neural tube during embryonic development.

C. Most common in Rhodesian ridgebacks, occurring along the dorsal midline cranial and caudal to their midline ridge.

D. Because the lesion is believed to be hereditary, affected animals should be neutered.

II. Treatment

A. Resect if they are associated with drainage or neurologic signs.

Clip and aseptically prepare a large area around the sinus. Position the dog in ventral recumbency and make an elliptical incision around the sinus opening. Carefully dissect the sinus to its origin and free its attachment. Divide or split the

nuchal ligament if necessary. Perform a laminectomy or hemilaminectomy if the sinus tract extends to the dura. Lavage thoroughly before closure. If the nuchal ligament has been transected, reappose it with a locking loop or modified Bunnel's suture pattern. Appose muscles and deep tissues with interrupted absorbable sutures to eliminate dead space (e.g., 3-0 or 4-0 polydioxanone or polyglyconate). If a large amount of dead space is still present, place a closed suction drain at the site. Appose subcutaneous tissues and skin routinely. Submit tissue samples for culture and sensitivity testing and histologic evaluation. Give analgesics and antibiotics, and bandage the site after surgery.

Interdigital Pyoderma (Granuloma, Acne, Furunculosis) (*SAS*, pp. 139-140)

I. General Considerations

A. A bacterial pododermatitis that may coexist with other conditions. It may be caused by parasites; allergies; mycoses; irritants; neoplasms; and metabolic, neurologic, or autoimmune disease.

B. Immunosuppression is suspected in some animals. The primary bacterial pathogen is *Staphylococcus intermedius.*

C. Varying degrees of pruritus, pain, paronychia, swelling, erythema, and hyperpigmentation are common.

D. Antibiotic and steroid therapy may cause remission, but recurrence is common. The underlying cause should be identified and treated.

II. Treatment

A. Medicate lesions with antibacterial agents (e.g., chlorhexidine, povidone-iodine, nitrofurazone) and bandage for 24 to 48 hours. Subsequently, soak with an antibacterial solution for 15 to 20 minutes twice daily.

B. Continue oral antibiotics (chosen based on sensitivity testing) for 6 to 8 weeks.

C. Consider fusion podoplasty for lesions failing to respond to this treatment.

Redundant Skin Folds (*SAS*, pp. 140-142)

I. General Considerations

A. Redundant skin is characteristic of some breeds and is exacerbated by obesity. Chronic skin overlap or apposition creates skin folds of varying depths.

B. Pyoderma occurs in the skin fold recesses (intertriginous dermatitis).

C. Affected areas become painful and foul smelling, causing the animal to further traumatize the area by scooting, rubbing, licking, or scratching.

D. Skin fold resection is the most effective treatment for skin fold pyoderma. First, medical therapy should reduce infection, inflammation, and secretions or exudates.

1. Clip hair from the folds and surrounding area.
2. Apply topical antibacterial solutions and medicated soaps (use antiseborrheic shampoos and astringents).
3. Give appropriate systemic antimicrobials.

II. Lip Folds

A. General Considerations

1. Breeds with excessive mandibular labial tissue (large pendulous lips) (e.g., spaniels, St. Bernards, Newfoundlands, Labrador retrievers, golden retrievers, Irish setters) most commonly have lip fold dermatitis. It may also occur following partial maxillectomy or mandibulectomy.
2. The fold usually occurs behind the mandibular canine tooth where food and saliva accumulate.
3. Affected dogs rub and paw their faces, and the skin becomes inflamed and thickened. Halitosis and pruritus are the most common presenting complaints.

B. Lip Fold Resection (Cheiloplasty)

Position the anesthetized animal in dorsal recumbency to allow access to both lips. Clip and aseptically prepare the mandibular area. Make an elliptical incision around the affected area, paralleling the horizontal ramus of the mandible. The incision may involve the mucocutaneous junction. Elevate and remove the outlined skin segment, preserving underlying muscles. Control hemorrhage with ligation, electrocoagulation, and pressure. Assess the adequacy of resection and excise additional skin if necessary. Lavage the site and appose subcutaneous and subcuticular tissues with continuous or interrupted approximating sutures (e.g., 3-0 or 4-0 polydioxanone or polyglyconate). Place interrupted appositional sutures in the skin (e.g., 3-0 or 4-0 polypropylene or nylon). Use an Elizabethan collar or bucket to prevent self-inflicted trauma to the surgical site. Keep the area clean and dry, removing food and saliva as needed.

C. Antidrool Cheiloplasty

Position the anesthetized patient in lateral recumbency. Clip the lateral face, lavage the oral cavity, and aseptically prepare the skin for surgery. Grasp the lower lip 2 to 3 cm rostral to the commissure and elevate it dorsally until the lip is taut when the dog's mouth is completely opened. The site of maximal tautness is usually near the level of the caudal root of the upper fourth premolar. Beginning near an imaginary line between the medial canthus of the eye and the commissure, make a 2.5- to 3-cm, horizontal, full-thickness incision through the maxillary skin at the site of tautness. Control hemorrhage with ligation or electrocoagulation. The dorsal labial vein lies just dorsal to the proposed incision site. Use scissors to remove a 2-mm strip of mucosa adjacent to the mucocutaneous junction of the lower lip, beginning 2 cm rostral to the commissure and extending 2.5 cm. Create 0.5- to 0.75-cm mucosal and skin

flaps by undermining on each side of the incision. Place stay sutures at the rostral and caudal aspects of the flaps. Evert the flaps through the cheek incision with the stay sutures. Secure and bury the flap edges in the cheek skin incision with 3 to 4 preplaced vertical mattress sutures (e.g., 2-0 or 3-0 polypropylene or nylon). Add additional approximating skin sutures if necessary to achieve good skin apposition. Reposition the patient and repeat the procedure on the other side. Lavage the oral cavity with water after meals. Fit the dog with an Elizabethan collar or bucket to prevent self-inflicted trauma if necessary. Remove sutures at 21 days. Delay suture removal because constant lip movement may interfere with healing.

III. Nasal Folds

A. General Considerations

1. Brachycephalic breeds (e.g., English bulldogs, French bulldogs, Pekingese, Boston terriers, pugs, Persian cats) characteristically have facial or nasal skin folds across the bridge of the nose. Prominent folds cause pyoderma and a foul odor.
2. Hair rubbing on the cornea is associated with keratitis, ulceration, epiphora, pain, and blepharospasm.

B. Nasal Skin Fold Resection

Position the patient in ventral recumbency. Protect the eyes with a petrolatum-based ophthalmic ointment. Clip and aseptically prepare the dorsum of the nose and lips. Estimate the amount of skin that must be resected to eliminate the skin folds without causing excessive tension or ectropion. Make an elliptical incision around or through the skin folds in nonmacerated tissue. Keep the caudal incision approximately 1 cm away from the medial canthus. Undermine and remove the outlined skin segment. Avoid traumatizing the nasolabialis muscle and facial vessels during dissection. Control hemorrhage with ligatures, electrocoagulation, and pressure. Lavage the area with sterile saline. Bury three or four interrupted sutures in the subcutaneous and subcuticular tissues to align and appose the skin edges and assess the adequacy of resection. Resect more skin if skin recesses remain. If necessary, undermine the skin edges to allow apposition without tension. Place additional interrupted, subcuticular sutures (e.g., 4-0 polydioxanone or polyglyconate) with buried knots. Use approximating skin sutures (e.g., 4-0 nylon or polypropylene) and cut the ends short to prevent further corneal irritation. Place an Elizabethan collar or bucket to prevent self-trauma. Keep the site free of exudates and ocular discharge. Continue to medicate the eyes.

IV. Vulvar Folds

A. Occur in obese females and those with infantile, recessed vulvas. Urine and vaginal secretions are trapped by the skin fold resulting in superficial perivulvar dermatitis.

B. Clinical signs include perineal pain, odor, and urinary tract infections.

C. Episioplasty is a vulvar reconstructive procedure that removes the skin fold. Skin fold pyoderma should be resolved medically before surgery.

V. Tail Folds

A. General Considerations

1. Redundant skin often overlaps deformed terminal caudal vertebrae ("screwtails," "corkscrew" tails, ingrown tails). Occurs most commonly in brachycephalic breeds.
2. To remove all skin recesses at the tailhead, complete caudectomy is necessary.

B. Tail Fold Resection

Give perioperative antibiotics based on skin fold culture and sensitivity results. Scrub the skin folds separate from the remainder of the surgical field. Resect the tail and skin folds en bloc, being careful during dissection to avoid penetrating the skin folds or traumatizing the rectum. Manipulate the tail with bone-holding forceps or towel clamps. Ankylosis or severe ventral deviation may make the vertebrae immobile. Transect the tail cranial to the deviated vertebrae with Gigli wire or a bone cutter if the intervertebral space cannot be located. Smooth sharp bone edges with rongeurs. Lavage thoroughly and insert Penrose drains before apposing the subcutaneous tissues with absorbable sutures (e.g., 3-0 or 4-0 polydioxanone or polyglyconate). Drains should exit ventral to the incision and lateral to the anus. Close skin with nonabsorbable sutures (e.g., 3-0 or 4-0 nylon or polypropylene). Keep the area clean and free of exudate and fecal contamination by applying warm moist compresses two to three times daily for 15 to 20 minutes. Remove drains in 3 to 5 days.

Surgery of the Tail (*SAS*, pp. 142-145)

I. Caudectomy in Puppies (Tail Docking)

A. Perform in puppies between 3 and 5 days of age when it does not require anesthesia. If performed after the first week of life, delay the procedure until the puppy is 8 to 12 weeks old and use a general anesthetic.

B. Determine the desired tail length by referring to breed standards and consulting with the owner (Table 13-4).

Have an assistant restrain the puppy. Clip and aseptically prepare the proposed site of resection. Retract the tail's skin toward the tailhead. Immobilize the tail between the thumb and index finger and apply pressure to help control hemorrhage. Palpate the desired transection site. Transect the tail between adjacent caudal vertebrae with Mayo scissors, nail trimmers, scalpel blade, or a tail docker/cutter (Tail Docker/Cutter). You may use scissors to assist with skin retraction. Place the ventral blade at the desired transection site. Position the dorsal blade more distally at an oblique angle. Rotate the blades into a perpendicular position while maintaining firm contact with the skin to push the skin cranially. Maintaining the scissors in this position, transect through an intervertebral space. Control hemorrhage with pressure or electrocautery. Extend the retracted skin over the remaining tail, assess the tail length, and resect more if necessary. Appose skin edges with two or three approximating sutures (e.g., 4-0 nylon or polypropylene).

Table 13-4
Tail docking guidelines

Breed	Length at less than 1 week
Sporting Breeds	
Brittany spaniel	Leave 1″
Clumber spaniel	Leave 1/4 to 1/3 of length
Cocker spaniel	Leave 1/3 of length (approximately 3/4″)
English cocker spaniel	Leave 1/3 of length
English springer spaniel	Leave 1/3 of length
Field spaniel	Leave 1/3 of length
German shorthaired pointer	Leave 2/5 of length
German wirehaired pointer	Leave 2/5 of length
Sussex spaniel	Leave 1/3 of length
Vizsla	Leave 2/3 of length
Weimaraner	Leave 3/5 of length (approximately 1 1/2″)
Welsh springer spaniel	Leave 1/3 to 1/2 of length
Wirehaired pointing griffon	Leave 1/3 of length
Working Breeds	
Bouvier des Flanders	Leave 1/2 to 3/4″
Boxer	Leave 1/2 to 3/4″ (two vertebrae)
Doberman pinscher	Leave 3/4″ (two vertebrae)
Giant schnauzer	Leave 1 1/4″ (three vertebrae)
Old English sheepdog	Leave one vertebrae (close to body)
Rottweiler	Leave one vertebrae (close to body)
Standard schnauzer	Leave 1″ (2 vertebrae)
Welsh corgi (Pembroke)	Leave one vertebrae (close to body)
Terrier Breeds	
Airedale terrier	Leave 2/3 to 3/4 of length*
Australian terrier	Leave 2/5 of length
Fox terrier	Leave 2/3 to 3/4 of length*
Irish terrier	Leave 3/4 of length
Kerry blue terrier	Leave 1/2 to 2/3 of length
Lakeland terrier	Leave 2/3 to 3/4 of length
Miniature schnauzer	Leave 3/4″ (less than 1″)
Norwich terrier	Leave 1/4 to 1/3 of length
Sealyham terrier	Leave 1/3 to 1/2 of length
Soft-coated wheaten terrier	Leave 1/2 to 3/4 of length
Welsh terrier	Leave 2/3 to 3/4 of length*

*Tip of docked tail should be approximately level with top of skull when puppy is in show position.

Table 13-4
Tail docking guidelines—cont'd

Breed	Length at less than 1 week
Toy Breeds	
Affenpinscher	Leave ⅓″ (close to body)
Brussels griffon	Leave ¼ to ⅓ of length (approximately ⅓″)
English toy spaniel	Leave ⅓ of length (approximately 1½″)
Miniature pinscher	Leave ½″ (two vertebrae)
Silky terrier	Leave ⅓ of length (approximately ½″)
Toy poodle	Leave ½ to ⅔ (approximately 1″)
Yorkshire terrier	Leave ⅓ of length (approximately ½″)
Nonsporting Breeds	
Miniature poodle	Leave ½ to ⅔ of length (approximately 1⅛″)
Schipperke	Close to body
Standard poodle	Leave ½ to ⅔ of length (approximately 1½″)
Miscellaneous Breeds	
Cavalier King Charles spaniel (optional)	Leave ⅔ of length with white tip
Spinoni Italiani	Leave ⅗ of length

II. Caudectomy in Adults

A. Partial Amputation

Anesthetize the patient and wrap the distal tail with gauze or insert it into an exam glove and secure the covering with tape. Clip a generous area near the amputation site and aseptically prepare it for surgery. Position the patient in a perineal position or lateral recumbency. Retract the skin toward the tailhead. Make a double V incision in the skin distal to the desired intervertebral transection site. Orient the V to create dorsal and ventral skin flaps that are longer than the desired tail length. Identify and ligate the medial and lateral caudal arteries and veins slightly cranial to the transection site. Incise soft tissues slightly distal to the desired intervertebral space and disarticulate the distal tail with a scalpel blade. If bleeding occurs place a circumferential ligature around the distal end of the remaining tail or religate the caudal vessels. Appose subcutaneous tissue and muscle over the exposed vertebrae with interrupted approximating sutures (e.g., 3-0 polydioxanone or polyglyconate). Fold the dorsal skin flap over the caudal vertebrae. Trim the ventral skin flap as needed to allow skin apposition without tension. Appose skin edges with approximating sutures (e.g., 3-0 or 4-0 nylon or polypropylene with a reverse cutting needle). Protect the surgical site with a bandage or by placing an Elizabethan collar or bucket over the animal's head.

B. Complete Caudectomy

Anesthetize the patient and clip and aseptically prepare the entire perineum and tailhead area. Position the animal in ventral recumbency. Make an elliptical

incision around the tail base. Incise subcutaneous tissues to expose the muscles. Separate the attachments of the levator ani, rectococcygeus, and coccygeus muscles to the caudal vertebra. Ligate the medial and lateral caudal arteries and veins before or after transection. Transect the tail by disarticulation with a scalpel blade at the second or third caudal vertebra. Lavage the site after hemostasis is controlled. Appose the levator ani muscles and subcutaneous tissues with simple interrupted or continuous suture patterns (e.g., 3-0 or 4-0 polydioxanone or polyglyconate). Excise redundant skin if necessary and appose skin edges with approximating, nonabsorbable sutures (e.g., 3-0 or 4-0 nylon or polypropylene).

Surgery of the Digits and Footpads (*SAS*, pp. 145-152)

I. Onychectomy (Declawing)

A. Removal of the third digital phalanx (P3) (usually of only the forelimbs)

B. Dissection onychectomy.
   1. In cats either a scalpel or guillotine-type nail clipper may be used. Use the dissection technique for canine onychectomy.

Anesthetize the patient and in dogs clip hair from the paw and around the toes. Aseptically scrub the paw, digits, and nails for surgery. Position the animal in lateral recumbency and apply a tourniquet below the elbow to minimize blood loss and improve visualization. Drape the feet. Extend the claw by grasping the tip with a towel clamp or by pushing up on the digital pad. Circumferentially incise the hairless, cuticle-like skin away from the claw near the articulation between the second and third phalanx. Transect the common digital extensor tendon and dorsal ligaments with a No. 11 or No. 12 scalpel blade. Follow the contour of the proximal end of P3 to transect the deep digital flexor tendon and dissect the phalanx from the digital pad and other soft tissue attachments (i.e., joint capsule, collateral ligaments, other tendons). Avoid cutting the digital pad. Remove all 10 claws from the front paws for elective onychectomy. Appose skin edges with a bandage, single interrupted cruciate sutures, or cyanoacrylate tissue adhesive (e.g., Vetbond Tissue Adhesive). Do not place sutures through the digital pads. Apply tissue adhesives over the apposed surface of the skin and not between the cut edges. Apply a bandage from the paw to the distal antebrachium and remove the tourniquet.

C. Nail clipper onychectomy.

Prepare the paws for surgery as described above. Trim the claws to facilitate positioning the nail trimmer in the interphalangeal space. Position a sharp guillotine-type nail clipper (Resco nail shears) around the claw. Extend the claw by grasping the tip with a towel clamp. Position the blade dorsally at the joint space and transect the extensor tendon(s). Rotate the blade ventrally with continuous contact with the skin. Lift the claw dorsally to close the joint space and deviate the flexor process ventrally. After ensuring that the digital pad is proximal to the line of transection and the instrument is in the joint space, close the instrument to amputate the phalanx. Inspect the articular surfaces for complete excision of P3. If a small portion of the palmar aspect of P3 remains,

Table 13-5
Breeds recommended for dewclaw removal

• Alaskan malamute	• Komondor
• Basset hound*	• Lakeland terrier
• Belgian Malinois	• Norwegian elkhound
• Belgian sheepdog	• Papillon
• Belgian Tervuren	• Puli*
• Bernese mountain dog	• Rottweiler
• Boxer	• Shetland sheepdog
• Cardigan Welsh corgi	• Siberian husky
• Chesapeake Bay retriever	• Silky terrier
• Dalmatian	• St. Bernard
• Dandie Dinmont terrier	• Vizsla
• Kerry blue terrier	• Weimaraner

*Optional removal.

grasp it with thumb forceps and carefully dissect it from the digital pad with a scalpel blade. Remove all 10 claws from the front paws for elective onychectomy. Appose skin edges with tissue adhesive. Apply a bandage from the paw to the distal antebrachium and remove the tourniquet. Expect mild bleeding when the bandage is removed after 12 to 24 hours; reapply the bandage. Use shredded paper, instead of litter, for 2 weeks while the nailbeds heal.

II. Dewclaw Removal

A. General Considerations

1. The dewclaw is the first digit of the canine rear paws. Refer to Table 13-5 for breed standards.
2. Remove dewclaws at 3 to 5 days of age, at the same time as caudectomy. After 5 days of age, hemorrhage is more excessive and anesthetics are necessary.

B. Puppy Dewclaw Removal

Aseptically prepare the medial aspect of the paw. Have an assistant cup the puppy in his or her hands and immobilize the paw. Abduct the digit and transect the web of skin attaching the dewclaw to the paw with Mayo scissors. Disarticulate the metatarsal (carpal)-phalangeal joint or transect the bone near the metatarsal or metacarpal bone with a scalpel blade or Mayo scissors. Control hemorrhage with pressure or electrocautery. Appose skin margins with a single approximating suture or allow second intention healing.

C. Adult Dewclaw Removal

1. If dewclaw removal is not performed within the first week of life, delay it until after 3 months of age and use a general anesthetic.

Position the patient in lateral recumbency. Clip and aseptically prepare the paws for surgery. Make an elliptical incision around the base of the digit where it articulates with the metatarsal or metacarpal bone. Abduct the digit and dissect subcutaneous tissues to the metacarpophalangeal or metatarsophalangeal joint. If the first and second phalanges are firmly attached, free them with a No. 11 blade. Ligate the dorsal common and axial palmar digital arteries.

Disarticulate the metacarpophalangeal or metatarsophalangeal joint with a scalpel blade. Results using bone cutters to transect the first phalanx near the metacarpophalangeal or metatarsophalangeal joint are less cosmetic. Appose subcutaneous tissues with 3-0 or 4-0 simple continuous or interrupted approximating sutures using absorbable suture material (e.g., polydioxanone, polyglyconate, polyglactin 910, or chromic catgut). Appose skin with interrupted approximating sutures (3-0 or 4-0 nylon or polypropylene). Apply a soft, padded bandage to protect the surgical site for 3 to 5 days. Remove sutures at 7 to 10 days.

III. Digit Amputation

A. Performed because of neoplasia, chronic bacterial or fungal infections, osteomyelitis, or severe trauma.

Clip and aseptically prepare the paw for surgery. Position the dog in ventral or lateral recumbency with the leg suspended. Place a tourniquet and drape the area. Release the aseptically prepared paw into the sterile field. Begin a dorsal skin incision at the distal end of the appropriate metacarpal (metatarsal) or proximal end of the first phalanx. Make a transverse encircling incision at the appropriate interphalangeal joint (inverse Y incision). Preserve the digital pad if only the third phalanx is removed. Transect the flexor and extensor tendons, ligaments, and joint capsule. Ligate the digital arteries and veins with 3-0 or 4-0 absorbable suture. Disarticulate with a scalpel blade or transect the phalanx with bone cutters. Include the sesamoid bones with the excision. Suture the extensor tendon to the dorsal surface of the pad when it is preserved. Appose subcutaneous tissues over the end of the bone with interrupted absorbable sutures (e.g., 3-0 or 4-0 polydioxanone or polyglyconate). Appose skin with approximating sutures (e.g., 3-0 or 4-0 nylon or polypropylene). Apply a padded bandage and if necessary an Elizabethan collar or bucket. Keep the bandage clean and dry. Change the bandage in 2 to 3 days or as needed to evaluate the wound. Remove the bandage and sutures after 7 to 10 days.

Footpad Injuries

I. Superficial Pad Loss

A. Allow to heal by second intention and treat with nonadherent absorbent or semiabsorbent bandages and a spoon splint.

B. Splint the paw to promote healing because wound contractile forces are antagonized by weight bearing, which pushes the wound edges apart.

C. Restrict exercise while the limb is bandaged.

II. Lacerations

Acute lacerations—*thoroughly lavage and minimally debride.*
Old, severely contaminated, or infected lacerations—*apply wet-dry bandages*

for several days. Debride the edges of chronic lacerations to remove necrotic tissue and provide a bleeding edge for apposition. Appose deep layers of the pad with buried simple interrupted absorbable sutures (e.g., 3-0 and 4-0 polydioxanone or polyglyconate). Appose epithelial edges with interrupted approximating sutures (e.g., 3-0 or 4-0 polypropylene or nylon), taking bites several millimeters from the cut edge. After closure protect the pad with a nonadherent, thick, absorbent bandage and a spoon splint. After suture removal, reapply the splint/bandage for 3-4 days. Alternatively, use a commercial boot after suture removal (Dog Bootie). Restrict exercise while the limb is bandaged.

14

Surgery of the Ear (*SAS*, pp. 153-178)

General Principles and Techniques (*SAS*, pp. 153-163)

I. Definitions

A. **Otitis externa** is inflammation of the vertical and/or horizontal ear canal(s).

B. **Otitis media** is inflammation of the tympanic cavity and membrane.

II. Preoperative Concerns

A. Determine the extent and severity of ear disease.
   1. Note the presence of a head tilt, circling, nystagmus, or vestibular dysfunction, which might indicate otitis media/interna.
   2. Assess facial nerve function (palpebral reflex, lip droop, facial spasms), which might suggest middle ear disease.
   3. Perform a Schirmer's tear test in animals with ocular discharge to differentiate preoperative abnormalities in tear production (i.e., "dry eye") from surgically induced facial nerve trauma.
   4. Perform an otoscopic examination to determine if the tympanic membrane is intact and define the severity of horizontal and vertical canal changes.
   5. Assess skull radiographs to determine if concurrent middle ear disease or neoplasia exists before cleaning the ear.
   6. Consider owner's expectations when determining which surgical procedure is most appropriate.

III. Anesthetic Considerations

A. Provide analgesics (see Appendix F). Ear surgery is painful.
   1. Oxymorphone appears to be a good analgesic for dogs undergoing ear surgery.
   2. Consider a splash block (bupivacaine hydrochloride; do not exceed 2 mg/kg) before closing the incision following resections or ablations. Do not flush the area for at least 20 minutes.

3. Use postoperative analgesic. If oxymorphone was used as a premedicant, readminister it 3 to 4 hours later (0.05 to 0.1 mg/kg intravenously, subcutaneously, or intramuscularly).
4. Use tranquilizers only in animals that have been given sufficient analgesics.
   a. Give acepromazine if there are no contraindications (i.e., hypotension, seizures).
   b. Acepromazine–0.025 to 0.05 mg/kg subcutaneously, intramuscularly, or intravenously; not to exceed 1 mg.
   c. See Appendix G-1 for selected anesthetic protocols for animals undergoing ear surgery.

IV. Antibiotics

A. Severe Otitis Externa

1. Perform bacterial cultures in animals with purulent discharge and initiate appropriate antibiotic therapy before surgery.
2. Treat for several weeks before surgery with systemic or topical antibiotics.

B. Moderate Otitis Externa

1. Give broad-spectrum antibiotics before the surgical procedure, or during surgery but after intraoperative cultures have been taken.
2. Culture deep tissues during surgery.
3. If possible, avoid ototoxic antibiotics (e.g., gentamicin, kanamycin, neomycin, streptomycin, tobramycin, amikacin, polymyxin B); however, careful systemic use of aminoglycosides is necessary in some patients (e.g., *Pseudomonas* spp.).

V. Surgical Anatomy

A. The ear is composed of three parts: (1) the inner ear, which consists of a membranous and a bony labyrinth and functions for hearing and balance; (2) the middle ear, which is formed by the tympanic cavity and connects to the pharynx via the auditory tube (eustachian tube); and (3) the external ear formed by the auditory meatus and a short canal (see *SAS,* Fig. 14-2).

B. The three auditory ossicles (stapes, malleus, and incus) connect the tympanic membrane to the inner ear.

C. The feline tympanic cavity is divided into two compartments by a thin, bony septum that arises along the cranial aspect of the bulla and curves to attach to the midpoint of the lateral wall.

D. The facial nerve exits the stylomastoid foramen caudal to the ear and courses ventral to the horizontal canal in close proximity to the middle ear.

VI. Surgical Techniques

A. Lateral Ear Canal Resection (*SAS,* pp. 156-158)

1. Indications.
   a. Use to increase drainage and improve ventilation of the ear canal

and to facilitate placement of topical agents into the horizontal canal.

b. Indicated in patients with minimal hyperplasia of the ear canal epithelium or small neoplastic lesions of the lateral aspect of the vertical canal.

2. Contraindications.
   a. Do not perform in animals with obstruction or stenosis of the horizontal ear canal, concurrent otitis media (unless performed in conjunction with ventral bulla osteotomy; see below), or in those with severe epithelial hyperplasia.
   b. Note that dogs with underlying disease (e.g., hypothyroidism or primary idiopathic seborrhea) often respond poorly to this surgery.
   c. Be sure that owners understand that lateral ear canal resection is not a curative procedure and that medical management of the ear may be necessary for the remainder of the animal's life.
3. Procedure.

Clip the entire side of the face and both sides of the pinna. Gently flush the ear and remove as much debris as possible. Position the animal in lateral recumbency with the head elevated on a towel and prepare the pinna and surrounding skin for aseptic surgery. Place quarter drapes around the ear with the entire pinna draped into the surgical site. Stand at the ventral aspect of the dog's head and position a forceps into the vertical ear canal to determine its ventral extent. Mark a site below the horizontal ear canal that is one half the length of the vertical ear canal. Make two parallel incisions in the skin lateral to the vertical ear canal that extend from the tragus ventrally to the marked site. These incisions should be one and one half times the length of the vertical ear canal. Connect the skin incisions ventrally and, using a combination of sharp and blunt dissection, reflect the skin flap dorsally, exposing the lateral cartilaginous wall of the vertical ear canal. During dissection stay as close as possible to the cartilage of the ear canal to avoid inadvertently damaging the facial nerve. Note the parotid gland at the ventral extent of the incision and avoid damaging it. While standing at the dorsal aspect of the animal's head, use Mayo scissors to cut the vertical canal. Place one blade of the scissors within the canal at the pretragic or tragohelicine incisure at the cranial (medial) aspect of the external auditory meatus and incise the canal ventrally to the level of the horizontal canal. Repeat the process beginning at the intertragic incisure (caudal or lateral aspect of the external auditory meatus). Angle the scissors 30 degrees while making the cuts. Do not allow the incision to converge toward the lateral aspect of the canal or the drainboard will be too narrow. Be sure to extend the incisions as far distally as the beginning of the horizontal canal or the drainboard will not lie flat against the skin. Reflect the cartilage flap distally, inspect the opening of the horizontal canal, and, if indicated, obtain cultures. Occasionally the opening can be widened by making two small cuts at the cranial and caudal aspect. Resect the distal one half of the cartilage flap to make the drainboard, and remove the skin flap. The ligament between the horizontal and vertical flaps usually acts as a hinge to allow the drainboard to lie flat, but in some cases scoring the cartilage on the ventral aspect of the drainboard will facilitate this. Place absorbable or nonabsorbable monofilament sutures (3-0 or 4-0) from the epithelial tissues to skin. Begin suturing at the opening of the horizontal canal first, then suture the drainboard. Last, suture the cranial and caudal aspects of the medial wall of the vertical ear canal to skin.

B. Vertical Ear Canal Ablation (*SAS,* pp. 158, 159)

1. Indications.
   a. Perform when the entire vertical canal is diseased but the horizontal canal is normal.

   b. Consider this procedure when neoplasia is confined to the vertical canal and in some animals with chronic otitis externa.
2. Contraindications.
   a. Do not perform this technique in animals with stenotic horizontal canals.
3. Procedure.

Position and prep the animal as for a lateral ear canal resection. Make a T-shaped incision with the horizontal component parallel and just below the upper edge of the tragus. From the midpoint of the horizontal incision make a vertical incision that extends to the level of the horizontal canal. Retract the skin flaps, reflect loose connective tissue, and expose the lateral aspect of the vertical canal. Continue the horizontal incision through the cartilage around the external auditory meatus with a scalpel blade. Remove as much of the diseased tissue on the medial surface of the pinna as possible, but avoid damaging the major branches of the great auricular artery. Use curved Mayo scissors to dissect around the proximal and medial aspect of the vertical canal. During dissection stay as close as possible to the cartilage of the ear canal to avoid inadvertently damaging the facial nerve. Free the entire vertical canal from all muscular and fascial attachments. Transect the vertical canal ventrally 1 to 2 cm dorsal to the horizontal canal and submit it for histologic examination. Incise the remnant of the vertical canal cranially and caudally to create dorsal and ventral flaps. Reflect the ventral flap downward and suture it to the skin for a drainboard using absorbable or nonabsorbable monofilament sutures (2-0 to 4-0). Suture the dorsal flap to the skin and close subcutaneous tissues with an absorbable suture material (2-0 or 3-0). Then close skin in a T shape.

C. Total Ear Canal Ablation (*SAS,* pp. 158-160)

1. Indications.
   a. Perform in animals with chronic otitis externa in which appropriate medical management has failed, when severe calcification/ossification of the ear cartilage is present, or when severe epithelial hyperplasia extends beyond the pinna or vertical ear canal.
   b. It is commonly performed in animals with lateral ear resections that have failed. Animals with severely stenotic ear canals may also benefit from this procedure.
   c. Occasionally, neoplasia of the horizontal canal can be treated by total ear canal ablation.
2. Contraindications.
   a. Do not perform in animals with mild disease because of the potential for serious complications.
   b. Do not perform if you are unfamiliar with the anatomy of the ear.
   c. Treat associated skin disease (e.g., seborrhea, atopy, food or contact allergy dermatitis) first or concurrently.
   d. Most animals with severe, chronic otitis externa have concurrent otitis media. Removing the avenue for exudative material to drain by performing a total ear canal ablation without treating the otitis media is disastrous. Therefore always perform a bulla osteotomy in conjunction with total ear canal ablation for otitis externa/media.
3. Procedure.

Position the animal in lateral recumbency with the head elevated with a towel and prepare the pinna and surrounding skin for aseptic surgery. Make a T-shaped incision with the horizontal component parallel and just below the upper edge of the tragus. From the midpoint of the horizontal incision make a vertical incision that extends to just past the level of the horizontal canal. Retract the skin flaps, reflect loose connective tissue, and expose the lateral aspect of the vertical canal. Continue the horizontal incision around the opening

of the vertical ear canal with a scalpel blade. Then use curved Mayo scissors to dissect around the proximal and medial aspect of the vertical canal. During dissection stay as close as possible to the cartilage of the ear canal to avoid inadvertently damaging the facial nerve. Avoid damaging the major branches of the great auricular artery at the medial aspect of the vertical canal. Identify the facial nerve as it courses caudoventrally to the horizontal canal (gently retract it if necessary). If the facial nerve is entrapped within thickened and calcified horizontal canal tissue, carefully dissect the nerve from the horizontal canal. Continue the dissection to the level of the external acoustic meatus. Excise the horizontal canal attachment to the external acoustic meatus with a scalpel blade, rongeur, or Mayo scissors, but be careful to avoid damaging the facial nerve. Remove the entire ear canal and obtain deep cultures around or just inside the external acoustic meatus. Submit the ear for histologic examination. Use a curette to carefully remove secretory tissue that is adherent to the rim of the external acoustic meatus. Be sure to remove all epithelial tissues in this region or chronic fistulation will occur. Perform a lateral bulla osteotomy (see below). Flush the area with sterile saline solution before closure. If obvious infection remains or extensive drainage is likely, place an ingress-egress drain to allow the area to be flushed postoperatively. Otherwise use blunt dissection to exit a Penrose drain (¼ to ½ inch wide) or soft rubber tubing ventral to the incision in a dependent area (through a separate stab incision), or use closed suction drainage (e.g., butterfly catheter and Vacutainer tube). The end of the drain near the tympanic cavity may be secured with a single suture of chromic catgut (4-0 or 5-0). Secure the drain to the skin at the exit site. If an ingress-egress system is used, place the tube via a separate stab incision proximal to the surgical incision at the dorsal aspect of the head and exit it ventrally through a separate incision. Close the subcutaneous tissues with an absorbable suture material (2-0 or 3-0) and close skin in a T shape.

D. Lateral Bulla Osteotomy (*SAS,* pp. 160-161)

1. Indications.
   a. Perform in conjunction with total ear canal ablation in animals with chronic otitis externa and middle ear disease.
2. Contraindications.
   a. Do not perform if you are unfamiliar with the anatomy of the middle ear because serious complications (i.e., vestibular dysfunction) may result.
3. Procedure.

Bluntly dissect the tissues from the lateral aspect of the bulla using a small periosteal elevator. Rongeur the lateral aspect of the bulla until the caudal aspect of the middle ear canal is exposed. Extend the bony excision as needed to fully visualize contents of the tympanic cavity. Use a curette to remove infected materials but avoid curetting in the dorsal or dorsomedial area of the tympanic cavity so as to not damage the auditory ossicles or inner ear structures. Gently irrigate the cavity with saline in order to remove all remaining debris.

E. Ventral Bulla Osteotomy (*SAS,* pp. 161, 162)

1. Indications.
   a. Provides better drainage of the bulla than does lateral bulla osteotomy and allows both bullae to be opened without repositioning the animal.
   b. It is the technique of choice for suspected middle ear neoplasia and nasopharyngeal polyps involving the feline middle ear.
   c. Can be performed alone or in conjunction with lateral ear resection.

2. Contraindications.
   a. Requires repositioning of the animal if done in conjunction with a vertical ear canal ablation; therefore lateral bullae osteotomies are more commonly performed in such animals.
3. Procedure.

Place the patient in dorsal recumbency and prepare a generous area surrounding the angle of the mandible for aseptic surgery. Palpate the bulla immediately caudal and medial to the vertical ramus of the mandible. Draw an imaginary line connecting the mandibular rami and a second imaginary line along the long axis of the ventral aspect of the head. Make a 7- to 10-cm incision parallel with the midline of the dog and centered 2 cm toward the affected side from where these imaginary lines intersect. Incise the platysma muscle, retract the linguofacial vein if necessary, and deepen the incision by bluntly dissecting the digastricus muscle (lateral) from the hyoglossus and styloglossus muscles (medial). Avoid damaging the hypoglossal nerve located on the lateral aspect of the hypoglossus muscle. Confirm the location of the bulla and use self-retaining retractors (e.g., Gelpi or Weitlander) to spread the digastricus and glossal muscles and retract them from the bulla. Palpate the bulla craniomedial to the cornu process of the hyoid bone and caudomedial to the angle of the mandible. Bluntly dissect tissues from the ventral surface of the bulla and use a Steinmann pin to make a hole in its ventral aspect. Enlarge the opening with small rongeurs (e.g., Lempert). Examine the interior of the bulla for inflammatory debris, neoplastic tissue, or foreign bodies, and obtain samples for culture, sensitivity, and histopathologic examination. Be sure to examine both compartments of the bulla in cats. Flush the cavity with warm saline, and if there is evidence of infection, or if continued drainage is anticipated, place a small fenestrated drain tube within the cavity and exit it through a separate stab incision. Suture the fenestrated portion of the drain tube to the bulla with small (4-0 to 6-0) chromic gut suture. Depending on the amount of exudation, remove the drain in 3 to 7 days.

VII. Suture Materials/Special Instruments

A. Necessary instruments.
   1. Rongeurs (to remove the lateral aspect of the bulla when performing a total ear canal resection).
   2. A Steinmann pin, hand chuck, and rongeurs are necessary for ventral bulla osteotomy (unless the bone has been eroded by infection or neoplasia).

B. Self-retaining retractors are useful when performing a ventral bulla osteotomy to allow retraction of the muscles that are superficial to the bulla.

C. Use monofilament suture (e.g., polydioxanone, polyglyconate, polypropylene, nylon) to suture the epithelial tissues of the canal to skin.

VIII. Postoperative Care and Assessment

A. Administer postoperative analgesics after ear canal resections or ablations and possibly tranquilizers if the animal appears dysphoric or anxious.

Table 14-1
Modified Tris-EDTA solution*

1 liter of distilled water
1.2 g EDTA
6.05 g Tris
1 ml glacial acetic acid

Note: pH of solution should be approximately 8.
Modified from Neer TM, Howard PE: Otitis media, *Compend Contin Educ Pract Vet* 4:410, 1982.
*Add 1-3 ml with gentamicin otic drops 2-3 times a day to affected ear.

B. Place a bandage over the ear(s) and use an Elizabethan collar or sidebar to prevent bandage removal and ear mutilation.

C. Hot pack the side of the face if swelling is excessive.

D. Monitor the animal after surgery because bandages and excessive swelling (particularly after bilateral total ear canal ablation and lateral bulla osteotomy) may impair respiration.

E. Continue antibiotics (based on culture results) for 3 to 4 weeks.

F. If ingress-egress drains have been placed, flush them with sterile saline, dilute chlorhexidine (0.05%), or a Tris-ethylenediaminetetraacetic acid (EDTA) solution (Table 14-1) 2 to 3 times a day until the infection appears to be resolving (i.e., decreased bacterial numbers, nondegenerative neutrophils).

G. Remove Penrose drains in 3 to 7 days and remove sutures in 10 to 14 days.

IX. Complications

A. Lateral and Vertical Ear Canal Ablation

1. Complications other than inadequate drainage and continued otitis externa are uncommon.
2. Relief of clinical signs associated with otitis externa may not occur in dogs with underlying dermatologic disease that cannot be effectively managed.
3. Making the opening of the horizontal canal insufficient for drainage and performing these techniques in animals with concurrent middle ear disease without treating the middle ear infection results in persistent or recurrent signs of otitis externa.

B. Total Ear Canal Ablation

1. Complications of total ear canal ablation include superficial wound infections, facial nerve paralysis, vestibular dysfunction, deafness, chronic fistulation or abscessation, and avascular necrosis of the skin of the pinna.
2. Facial nerve paralysis.
   a. Usually resolves within a few weeks of surgery and is caused by stretching or retraction of the nerve; however, permanent damage occurs if the nerve is transected or severely stretched.

b. May result in loss of the blink response and parasympathetic nerve innervation to the lacrimal glands.
c. Keep the eye moistened with artificial tears or an ophthalmic lubricant to prevent corneal ulceration.
d. Consider enucleaton if normal lid function does not return within 4 to 6 weeks or ulceration of the eye occurs because of chronic drying; however, this is seldom necessary.
e. If signs of middle and inner ear disease worsen acutely after surgery, suspect an abscess of the tympanic cavity.
f. Superficial wound infections are common and are attributed to surgical manipulation of infected tissues, inadequate closure of dead space, inadequate drainage, and resistance to antibiotics.
g. In cats surgical curettage of the tympanic cavity may cause a transient Horner's syndrome, which usually resolves in 2 to 3 weeks. Facial nerve paralysis has also been reported after ventral bulla osteotomy in cats.

Otitis Externa (*SAS*, pp. 163-168)

I. Definitions

A. **Otitis externa** is an inflammation of the epithelium of the horizontal and vertical ear canals and surrounding structures (i.e., external auditory meatus and pinna).

B. **Swimmer's ear** is a term used to describe otitis externa that occurs after swimming or bathing.

II. General Considerations and Clinically Relevant Pathophysiology

A. Otitis externa may be associated with other dermatologic diseases, particularly allergic or immune-mediated skin disease (food allergy dermatitis, atopy, contact dermatitis) or systemic diseases (endocrinopathies such as hypothyroidism or Sertoli cell tumors). Bacterial infections, foreign bodies (foxtails), parasites (*Otodectes cynotis, Demodex canis, Sarcoptes scabiei, Notoedres cati,* ticks), fungi, yeasts *(Mallassezia pachydermis),* or neoplasia may also be the cause.

B. *O. cynotis* is responsible for more than 50% of feline otitis externa.

C. Predisposing causes of otitis externa include excessive moisture or increased humidity in the canal, narrow ear canal conformation, or obstruction of the ear canal.

D. The most frequent bacteria isolated from ears of dogs with chronic otitis externa are *Corynebacterium* spp., *Escherichia coli, Proteus mirabilis, Pseudomonas aeruginosa,* and *Staphylococcus intermedius.* From the ears of cats: *Pasteurella multocida* and *Staphylococcus intermedius.*

III. Diagnosis

A. Clinical Presentation

1. Signalment.
   a. Dogs with long, pendulous ears (e.g., spaniels, basset hounds) and those with abundant hair in the ear canal (e.g., poodles) are commonly affected.
   b. Of the erect-eared dogs, German shepherds are most frequently affected.
   c. Spaniel breeds, particularly cocker spaniels, may have abnormal keratinization and increased sebaceous gland secretion of the pinna or ear canal, often leading to scarring and ear canal obstruction.
2. History.
   a. Animals with otitis externa may present for evaluation of acute or chronic signs. If a foreign body is lodged in the ear of an animal, head shaking and scratching at or near the ear are typical. Head shaking and ear scratching are also common among animals with parasitic infections and acute bacterial infections.
   b. A purulent, odoriferous discharge may be noted with chronic infections. The dog may constantly rub his head on objects and appear to be in pain when his head or ear is touched.

B. Physical Examination Findings

1. Palpate the ear and perform a thorough otoscopic examination. General anesthesia may be necessary to allow meticulous inspection. Determine the extent of involvement of the vertical and horizontal ear canals and the status of the tympanic membrane.
2. Perform a complete dermatologic examination unless an obvious cause such as a foreign body is found.

C. Radiography

1. Perform skull radiographs to determine if concurrent otitis media exists.
2. Note calcification of the external auditory canal or radiographic signs suggestive of neoplasia (i.e., bony lysis of the petrous temporal bone).

IV. Differential Diagnosis

A. Identify treatable underlying causes of otitis externa before considering surgical intervention; optimal results require underlying diseases to be appropriately treated.

B. Identify concurrent otitis media in animals with otitis externa.

V. Medical Management

A. Identifying underlying or perpetuating causes of otitis externa, clean and dry the ear, and use appropriate topical or systemic medications.

1. See Table 14-2 for topical agents available for treatment of otitis externa.
2. Thoroughly clean the ears before treating because ceruminous mate-

Table 14-2
Topical otic preparations

		Active ingredients					
Product	Company	Antibiotics	Antiinflammatory	Antiparasitic	Antiyeast	Other (e.g., anesthetics, astringents)	Vehicle
Adams ear desiccant	Adams		aloe vera			colloidal sulfur, dioctyl sodium sulfosuccinate, urea peroxide, EDTA	propylene glycol
Adams ear mite lotion	Adams		aloe vera	pyrethrins			
Cerumite	Evsco			pyrethrins			squalene
Clear$_x$ treatment dryer	DVM		hydrocortisone			acetic acid, colloidal sulfur, dioctyl sodium sulfosuccinate, urea peroxide	
Conofite 1% lotion	Pitmann Moore				micronazole nitrate		polyethylene glycol
Cort/Astrin	Vedco		hydrocortisone			Burow's solution	water
Epi-Otic	Allerderm					lactic acid, salicylic acid	propylene glycol
Forte topical	Upjohn	procaine penicillin, neomycin, polymyxin	hydrocortisone				mineral oil
Gentocin otic	Schering	gentamicin	betamethasone				alcohol, glycerin, propylene glycol

Continued

Table 14-2
Topical otic preparations—cont'd

		Active ingredients					
Product	Company	Antibiotics	Antiinflammatory	Antiparasitic	Antiyeast	Other (e.g., anesthetics, astringents)	Vehicle
Liquichlor	Evsco	chloramphenicol	prednisolone			tetracaine	mineral oil, squalene
Micropearls Coal Tar Spray	Evsco					coal tar	water
Mitiban	Upjohn			amitraz			water
Mitox	SmithKline-Beecham	neomycin		carbaryl		sulfactamide, tetracaine	mineral oil
Oti-Clens	SmithKline-Beecham					malic acid, benzoic acid, salicylic acid	propylene glycol
Otomax	Schering-Plough	gentamicin	betamethasone		clotrimazole		mineral oil
Otomite	Allerderm			0.05% pyrethrins			olive oil
Otomite Plus	Allerderm			0.15% pyrethrins			olive oil
Panalog ointment	Solvay	neomycin, thiostreptosin	triamcinolone acetonide		nystatin		polyethylene, mineral oil
Panodry	Solvay					boric acid, isopropyl alcohol	silicone fluid
Solvaprep	Solvay					surfactants	propylene glycol
Synotic	Syntex		fluocinolone, DMSO				propylene glycol
Tresaderm	MSD-Agvet	neomycin	dexamethasone	thiabendazole	thiabendazole	alcohol, glycerin	propylene glycol

rial decreases the ability of topical medications to reach the infection and may inactivate some drugs.

VI. Surgical Treatment

A. Indications

1. Consider surgical therapy of otitis externa when medical management fails, or in cases where there are proliferative growths or stenotic canals.
2. Surgical alternatives in animals with otitis externa that do not have middle ear involvement include a lateral ear canal resection, vertical ear canal ablation, or total ear canal resection. If otitis media exists, a lateral ear canal resection in conjunction with a ventral bulla osteotomy or an ear canal ablation with lateral bulla osteotomy can be performed.

B. Preoperative Management

1. Perform bacterial cultures if purulent discharge is present and initiate appropriate antibiotics before surgery or give β-lactamase–resistant penicillins or cephalosporins intravenously immediately before the surgical procedure or during surgery after intraoperative cultures have been obtained.
2. Surgical Technique.
   a. The choice of surgical technique depends on the severity of the disease and the owner's expectations.
   b. See surgical techniques detailed earlier in this chapter.

C. Prognosis

1. Less than half of dogs undergoing lateral ear resection for the treatment of chronic otitis externa have resolution of their clinical signs.
2. Total ear canal ablation combined with bulla osteotomy resolves clinical signs in the vast majority of surgically treated ears.
3. Partial or complete facial nerve paralysis has been reported to occur in 5% to 58% of cases treated with total ear canal ablation. Other complications include persistent infection (dissecting cellulitis, prolonged wound drainage, incisional dehiscence, periauricular abscess formation), nystagmus, head tilt, postural abnormalities, and loss of hearing.

Otitis Media/Interna (*SAS*, pp. 168-171)

I. Definitions

A. **Otitis media** is inflammation of the middle ear.

B. **Otitis interna** is inflammation of the inner ear.

C. **Myringotomy** is a surgical puncture of the tympanic membrane to relieve pressure or obtain samples for analysis.

Table 14-3
Clinical signs associated with otitis interna (vestibular dysfunction)

- Head tilt to affected side
- Circling to affected side
- Falling to affected side
- Rolling to affected side
- Nystagmus (horizontal or rotary), with fast component away from affected side
- Asymmetric ataxia with strength preserved
- Positional or vestibular strabismus with the eyeball ipsilateral to the lesion deviated ventrally
- Postural reactions (except for the righting reflex)

II. General Considerations and Clinically Relevant Pathophysiology

A. Infection

1. The most common cause of otitis media is bacterial infection; more than half of the animals with chronic end-stage otitis externa have documented evidence of otitis media at surgery.
2. Bilateral otitis media is usually indicative of bacterial infection. Otitis media may lead to otitis interna (Table 14-3).

B. Polyps

1. Inflammatory or nasopharyngeal polyps are benign masses that may be located in the nasopharynx, auditory tube, or tympanic cavity. Rarely, they may rupture the tympanic membrane and protrude into the external ear canal. They often cause signs of unilateral otitis media when located in the tympanic cavity.
2. Polyps may occur as a result of ascending infection from the pharynx or may arise as a result of chronic otitis media. Suspected congenital polyps have also been reported in kittens.

C. Neoplasia

1. Neoplasia originating in the middle ear is uncommon in both dogs and cats. Tumors originating in the external ear canal that secondarily extend into the tympanic cavity are more common than primary middle ear tumors in dogs.
2. Dogs: Benign tumors of the middle ear cavity (e.g., papillary adenomas, fibromas) have been more commonly reported than malignant tumors.
3. Cats: Squamous cell carcinoma is the most common tumor of the middle and inner ear. Other tumors found in the middle ear of cats have included fibrosarcomas, anaplastic carcinomas, lymphoblastic lymphosarcoma, and ceruminous gland adenocarcinoma.

III. Diagnosis

A. Clinical Presentation

1. Signalment.
   a. Most animals that develop otitis media secondary to otitis externa are middle-aged.

   b. Older animals more commonly develop neoplasia of the middle ear.
   c. Young cats are more apt to have nasopharyngeal polyps.
   d. There is no known breed or sex predisposition in cats with nasopharyngeal polyps or animals with neoplastic middle ear disease.
2. History.
   a. The history and clinical signs of animals with otitis media do not differ substantially from those with otitis externa alone.
   b. Some animals present for evaluation of vestibular signs caused by otitis interna (see Table 14-3).
   c. Pain during eating or when the mouth is opened may be noted, especially in cats with neoplastic middle ear disease.
   d. Ipsilateral facial nerve paralysis is common in animals with middle ear neoplasia.
   e. Neoplastic lesions of the middle ear rarely extend into the nasopharynx, causing gagging, retching, or dyspnea.
   f. Cats with nasopharyngeal polyps often have nasal discharge, sneezing, or stridor. If there is a concurrent pharyngeal polyp, dysphagia or dyspnea may be noted.
   g. Deafness may be reported with bilateral disease, but loss of hearing is seldom evident with unilateral lesions.

B. Physical Examination Findings

1. Discharge from the external auditory canal, hyperplasia, and ulceration of the aural epithelial tissues are often obvious in animals with otitis media and externa.
2. Neurologic abnormalities referable to the inner ear or facial nerve paralysis (Table 14-4) are not present in most animals with otitis media.
3. Horner's syndrome may occur as a result of damage of the sympathetic trunk as it courses through the middle ear. Clinical signs associated with the syndrome are ptosis, miosis, enophthalmus, and protrusion of the third eyelid.
4. Perform an otoscopic examination of these patients under general anesthesia.
   a. Inflammatory polyps usually appear as pedunculated, smooth, shiny, light-pink masses. The oral cavity of animals with inflammatory polyps or neoplastic masses should be carefully examined because extension into the pharynx may occur.
   b. Neoplastic lesions may be friable, but they are often difficult to differentiate grossly from chronically infected tissue.

C. Radiography

1. To view the tympanic bullae perform a frontal open-mouth view (also known as rostrocaudal open-mouth view). Place the animal on its back with his head flexed 80 to 90 degrees to the film. Hold the mouth open with gauze strips hooked on the upper and lower canine teeth and center the x-ray beam on the temporomandibular joints. Retract the tongue and endotracheal tube from the field of view, using gauze secured to the lower mandible.
2. To see individual bullae, perform lateral oblique views with the head tilted 10 to 15 degrees; use ventrodorsal or dorsoventral views to evaluate the external ear canals and architecture of the petrous temporal bones. Consider neoplasia if there is lysis or periosteal reaction of the bullae and petrous temporal bone.
3. The most common findings with middle ear disease are opacification of the air-filled tympanic cavities and thickening and sclerosis of the walls of the bullae.

Table 14-4
Clinical signs associated with facial nerve paralysis

- Diminished palpebral reflex
- Widened palpebral fissure
- Drooping of the ear and lip
- Excessive drooling
- Blepharospasm
- Elevation and wrinkling of the lip
- Caudal displacement of the labial commissure
- Elevation of the ear on the affected side

4. Remember that radiography is not sensitive for detecting middle ear disease; up to 25% of animals with middle ear disease do not have radiographic abnormalities.

IV. Medical Management

A. Medical management of animals with acute otitis media consists of myringotomy, cultures of middle ear contents, irrigation of the tympanic cavity, and topical (see Table 14-2) and systemic antibiotics.

B. If there is no improvement within 3 to 4 weeks, consider ventral bulla osteotomy.

V. Surgical Treatment

A. General Considerations

1. Surgical treatment of otitis media caused by infection includes bulla osteotomy, culture of affected tissues or exudate, drainage, and long-term antibiotics. If neurologic signs are present before surgery, warn the owner that they are likely to persist after surgery.
2. Benign neoplastic or inflammatory lesions can usually be removed via a bulla osteotomy; however, Horner's syndrome is a common, short-term complication of bulla osteotomy in cats. Neoplasia of the bulla warrants a poor prognosis.
3. Anesthesia.
   a. Do not use chamber or mask induction in dyspneic animals (e.g., some cats with nasopharyngeal polyps).
   b. Because nitrous oxide increases middle ear pressure, it may be wise to avoid its use in animals with middle ear disease.
4. Surgical technique.
   a. Approach the middle ear via a lateral bulla osteotomy in conjunction with a total ear canal ablation or via a ventral bulla osteotomy.

VI. Postoperative Care and Assessment

A. Cats with concurrent upper airway disease (e.g., nasopharyngeal polyps) may have respiratory distress after extubation and may require supplementary oxygen. Oxygen may be given by mask or nasal insufflation in these animals.

VII. Prognosis

A. Animals with bacterial otitis media may have persistent neurologic signs despite surgical treatment.

B. The prognosis for benign tumors is good; however, surgical cures are rare with malignant tumors (because of their extensive nature at the time of diagnosis).

C. Inflammatory polyps may recur if they are simply removed from the external ear using traction. Recurrence is less likely if traction plus bulla osteotomy is performed.

Aural Hematomas and Traumatic Lesions of the Pinna (*SAS*, pp. 171-176)

I. Definitions

A. An **aural hematoma** is a collection of blood within the cartilage plate of the ear.

II. General Considerations and Clinically Relevant Pathophysiology

A. Aural hematomas may occur in dogs or cats and are usually characterized as fluctuant, fluid-filled swellings on the concave surface of the pinna. The entire portion of the concave surface of the pinna may be involved, or only a portion.

B. The cause of aural hematomas is not well understood; however, it appears that head shaking or scratching at the ear caused by pain or irritation associated with otitis externa (usually bacterial otitis in dogs and *Otodectes cynotis* in cats) is responsible in many cases. Head shaking may cause sinusoidal wave motions to occur in the ear, resulting in cartilage fracture.

III. Diagnosis

A. Clinical Presentation

1. Signalment: dogs and cats with otitis externa are at increased risk to develop aural hematomas.
2. History: a history of violent head shaking or acute or chronic otitis externa may be noted; in some animals there may be no history of previous ear disease.

B. Physical Examination Findings

1. Hematomas initially appear fluid filled, soft, and fluctuant, but eventually may become firm and thickened as a result of fibrosis. The ear may then develop a "cauliflower" appearance.

C. Radiography

1. Skull radiographs may be indicated if underlying otitis externa/media has predisposed the animal to aural hematoma.

IV. Medical Management

A. Underlying ear disease should be appropriately treated.

B. Needle aspiration of aural hematomas has been attempted (with and without concurrent injection of corticosteroid); however, recurrence is common with this technique.

V. Surgical Treatment

A. Hemotomas

1. The goals of surgery are to remove the hematoma, prevent recurrence, and retain the natural appearance of the ear (i.e., minimize thickening and scarring).
2. To prevent enlargement or fibrosis, hematomas should be treated soon after they occur (i.e., within several days).

B. Linear Lacerations of the Pinna

1. If lacerations involve only one skin surface, leave them to heal by second intention or suture them. Clean the laceration and debride the edges if necrotic tissue is present. Appose the skin margins with simple interrupted sutures. If a flap of tissue has been elevated away from the cartilage, suture it. Place sutures through the skin at the margins of the wound; additionally, place sutures through the skin and cartilage at the center of the flap to obliterate any dead space where fluid might collect.
2. Suture full-thickness injuries through the ear margin. Suture the skin on both sides of the defect with simple interrupted sutures, or use a vertical mattress suture to appose the skin and cartilage on one side of the ear and simple interrupted sutures to appose the skin on the opposite side of the ear.

C. Preoperative Management

1. Treat concurrent otitis externa simultaneously.

D. Surgical Anatomy

1. Branches of the great auricular arteries and veins supply the pinna. These main vessels are located along the convex surface of the ear and small branches penetrate the scapha to supply the concave surface.
2. Sensory innervation to the ear is supplied by the second cervical nerve (convex surface) and the auriculotemporal branches of the trigeminal nerve (concave surface).

E. Surgical Techniques

1. Aural hematomas.

Make an S-shaped incision on the concave surface of the ear and expose the hematoma and its contents from end to end. Remove the fibrin clot and irrigate the cavity. Place ¾- to 1-cm-long sutures through the skin on the concave surface of the ear and underlying cartilage. Place the sutures parallel to the major vessels (vertical rather than horizontal). They may be placed through the cartilage without incorporating the skin on the convex surface of the ear or they may be full thickness. Place an ample number of sutures so that there are no pockets in which fluid can accumulate. Do not ligate the branches of the great auricular artery visible on the convex surface of the ear. Do not suture the incision closed; it should gap slightly to allow for continued drainage. Place a light protective bandage over the ear and support the ear over the animal's head. Remove the bandage and sutures in 10 to 14 days.

If there is minimal fibrin present, a teat cannula or drain can be placed in lieu of the above-described procedure. Trim half of the collar of the cannula to allow the tube to rest comfortably against the ear. Aspirate the contents of the hematoma using a large needle (14 or 16 gauge) inserted into the hematoma at its most distal margin. Insert the cannula through the needle hole and suture it to the ear. (The cannula is placed in the most distal aspect of the hematoma—even in erect-eared animals—to prevent drainage from entering the concha). Do not bandage or support the ear over the top of the head.

A ¼-inch fenestrated latex drain can be used instead of a teat cannula. Make a stab incision in the proximal and distal limits of the hematoma. Empty the hematoma of fluid and fibrin and use a mosquito or alligator forceps to bring the drain into the hematoma cavity. Suture the ends of the drain to the skin where they protrude from the cavity. Place a light bandage over the ear.

2. Avulsions of the ear margin.

Small avulsions of the ear margin may be treated by resecting surrounding tissue to restore a normal ear contour. The skin edges are sutured over the cartilage using a continuous suture pattern. Larger defects of the ear may be repaired using a pedicle flap obtained from the side of the neck in dogs with pendulous ears or the dorsum of the head in dogs with erect ears.

Prepare the ear and donor site for aseptic surgery. Debride the margins of the ear defect. Place the ear on the donor site and incise the skin, extending the limbs 0.5 to 1 cm longer than the defect. Suture the flap to the skin on the convex surface of the ear. Place a nonadherent dressing over the wound and leave the ear bandaged for 10 to 14 days. Then sever the flap from the donor site in the shape of the defect on the concave side of the ear. Gently fold the flap over the ear margin and suture it to the skin. Remove skin sutures in 10 to 14 days.

VI. Suture Materials/Special Instruments

A. Monofilament, nonabsorbable (e.g., polypropylene or nylon) or absorbable (e.g., polydioxanone or polyglyconate) suture material (3-0 or 4-0) should be used to suture the ear.

B. Other materials that may be used in animals with aural hematomas are Dr. Larson's plastic teat tubes and Silastic medical grade tubing.

VII. Postoperative Care and Assessment

A. A bandage can be used to protect the ear from contamination and self-inflicted trauma after hematoma repair.

B. Be sure to check head bandages periodically to ensure that they are not too tight and are not restricting breathing.

VIII. Prognosis

A. Aural hematomas seldom recur if they are properly treated and the underlying ear disease is appropriately treated.

Neoplasia of the Pinna and External Ear Canal (*SAS*, pp. 176-178)

I. General Considerations and Clinically Relevant Pathophysiology

A. Neoplasms of the external ear canal are relatively uncommon in dogs and cats; however, they may arise from any structure that lines or supports the ear canal. The most common tumors of the external ear canal arise from the ceruminous glands (ceruminous gland adenomas or adenocarcinomas). Squamous cell carcinomas, basal cell tumors, and mast cell tumors may also be found.

B. Although tumors of the external ear canal are more common than those arising within the internal or middle ear cavities, clinical signs of middle or inner ear disease may predominate if these tumors extend through the tympanic membrane.

C. Most canine ceruminous gland tumors are benign; such tumors are usually malignant in cats.

D. Any tumor that affects the skin may arise on the pinna, but the most frequent tumor of the pinna in cats is squamous cell carcinoma. These tumors are most commonly diagnosed in older cats, particularly white cats. The association between a lack of protective pigmentation and the occurrence of these tumors suggests that solar radiation may be a causative factor. Although these tumors are highly invasive, metastasis is uncommon. If metastasis does occur it is usually to the regional lymph nodes and lungs. Tumors may also be noted on the nares and eyelids.

E. Other tumors of the pinna of dogs and cats are melanoma, fibrosarcoma, basal cell tumor, fibroma, lymphoma, histiocytoma, papilloma, and mast cell tumor.

II. Diagnosis

A. Clinical Presentation

1. Signalment.

a. Most neoplastic lesions of the external ear are found in middle-aged to older animals.
   i. Older male cats may be at increased risk to develop ceruminous gland tumors of the ear canal.
   ii. Squamous cell carcinoma of the ear pinna occurs almost exclusively in older white-eared cats or multicolored cats with little pigmentation of their pinna.

2. History.
   a. The history of a patient with a tumor arising from the external ear canal usually differs minimally from those with primary bacterial otitis externa.
   b. The history of cats with squamous cell carcinoma is often insidious and begins with the owner intermittently noticing crusty eczematous lesions at the edge of the ear.

B. Physical Examination Findings

1. Small, pedunculated masses of the external ear canal suggest ceruminous gland hyperplasia or adenomas, papillomas, or inflammatory polyps.
2. Infiltrative masses suggest ceruminous gland adenocarcinoma.
3. Squamous cell carcinomas usually originate on the tips of the ears where there is little hair and may initially appear as hyperemic skin. As the lesions progress, erosion, ulceration, crusting, and thickening become noticeable. The ear may bleed with mild trauma.

C. Radiography

1. Radiographic signs of neoplasia (i.e., bony lysis of the petrous temporal bone) may be noted on skull radiographs of animals with neoplasia of the external ear canal.
2. Although metastasis usually occurs late in the course of disease, pulmonary metastasis may be noted with some ear tumors; therefore thoracic radiographs are recommended.

III. Medical Management

A. Squamous cell carcinoma may be prevented or reduced by applying sunscreens to nonpigmented areas of the ear and preventing physical exposure to ultraviolet radiation.

B. Cryotherapy and radiation are alternatives to surgical removal of the pinna. Cryotherapy may be curative in small, superficial tumors, but local recurrence is common.

C. Radiation therapy is less disfiguring than surgical removal of the lesions and is a viable alternative for small, superficial tumors and preneoplastic lesions.

IV. Surgical Treatment

A. General Considerations

1. For neoplasms of the external ear canal, vertical or total ear canal ablations are usually required.
2. The aim of surgical treatment of squamous cell carcinoma is to remove the neoplasm with a wide margin of normal surrounding skin. This may require pinnectomy alone, or a vertical ear canal ablation

plus removal of the pinna. Be sure to prepare the owner for the resulting cosmetic deformity.

B. Preoperative Management

1. If concurrent otitis externa is present, perioperative antibiotics based on culture results should be given.
2. Perform preoperative cytology to help determine the need for radical resection when neoplasia is suspected.

C. Surgical Technique

1. The most important aspect of surgery of ear neoplasms is to achieve wide margins to prevent local recurrence. This may require that the entire pinna and ear canal be removed. If aggressive surgical therapy cannot provide clean margins, adjunctive therapy (i.e., radiation) should be considered.
2. Pinnectomy.

For pinnectomy, remove the affected portion of the ear and suture the remaining skin over the exposed cartilage. For small tumors on the central portion of the convex surface of the pinna, resect the neoplasm and mobilize the skin around the defect by undermining between the cartilage and skin. Suture the skin margins, or, if necessary, leave the defect open to heal by second intention under a light bandage. For small tumors on the concave surface of the ear, repair the skin defect by elevating a flap from surrounding skin and rotating it into the defect. Suture the flap to the wound margins. After a delay of 10 to 14 days, transect the flap and suture the edge to the defect. Close the donor site primarily.

V. Postoperative Care and Assessment

A. Use an Elizabethan collar or sidebar to prevent the animal from mutilating the ear after surgery.

VI. Prognosis

A. For malignant ceruminous gland tumors of the external ear, ablation is seldom curative. Adjunctive therapy (radiation therapy) should be considered.

B. Local recurrence of squamous cell carcinomas is common if wide margins are not obtained at surgery. The prognosis is poor with squamous cell carcinoma of the middle and inner ear; however, amputation of the pinna for squamous cell carcinoma of the ear margin may be curative.

15

Surgery of the Abdominal Cavity (*SAS*, pp. 179-199)

General Principles and Techniques (*SAS*, pp. 179-184)

I. Definitions

A. **Celiotomy** is a surgical incision into the abdominal cavity.

B. **Laparotomy** is often used synonymously with celiotomy, although it technically refers to a flank incision.

C. An **acute abdomen** is the term used to describe a sudden onset of clinical signs referable to the abdominal cavity (e.g., abdominal distention, pain, vomiting).

D. The **cranial pubic ligament** (prepubic tendon) is a band of transverse fibers that connects the iliopectineal eminence and pectineal muscle origin of one side with those on the other side. This ligament attaches the rectus abdominis muscle to the pelvis.

E. The **inguinal canal** is a sagittal slit in the caudoventral abdominal wall through which the genital branch of the genitofemoral nerve, artery, and vein, the external pudendal vessel, and the spermatic cord (males) or round ligament (females) pass. The vascular structures are located in the caudomedial aspect of the canal. The inguinal canal is bounded by the internal and external inguinal rings.

F. The **internal inguinal ring** is formed by the caudal edge of the internal abdominal oblique muscle (cranial), rectus abdominis muscle (medial), and inguinal ligament (lateral and caudal).

G. The **external inguinal ring** is a longitudinal slit in the aponeurosis of the external abdominal oblique muscle.

H. **Abdominocentesis** is the percutaneous removal of fluid from the abdominal cavity, usually for diagnostic purposes, although it may occasionally be therapeutic.

II. Preoperative Concerns

A. Some conditions (e.g., gastric dilation-volvulus, colonic perforation, severe hemorrhage) are life threatening, and initiation of appropriate therapy must be prompt. Although obviously unnecessary surgery must be avoided, surgery cannot always be delayed until it is certain the patient will benefit from it.

B. Physical examination can be unreliable in predicting the severity of abdominal trauma.

1. Depressed or lethargic animals may not exhibit pain during abdominal palpation.
2. Clinical signs of hemorrhage often are not apparent immediately after trauma; delays of 3 to 4 hours between trauma and development of shock and collapse are common in patients with liver or spleen lacerations.
3. Animals with traumatic bile peritonitis often are without clinical signs for several weeks.
4. Traumatic mesenteric avulsion is seldom associated with clinical signs until subsequent peritonitis develops (usually days after trauma occurs).

C. Physical examination accurately predicts which traumatized animals require surgery in only about 50% of cases.

D. Preoperative management of most animals undergoing exploratory laparotomy is dictated by their underlying abdominal disease.

1. Perform serial examinations to detect trends or deterioration in patient status.
2. Determine at least hematocrit, serum total protein, serum glucose concentrations, complete blood count (CBC), platelet count, and blood urea nitrogen in an animal with an acute abdomen. Perform other laboratory tests (serum biochemistry profile, clotting parameters) depending on the animal's condition and suspected underlying disease.
3. Collect urine via cystocentesis or catheterization for urinalysis. Place an indwelling urinary catheter to quantitate urinary output if necessary.
4. Evaluate abdominal radiographs for peritoneal fluid (e.g., uroabdomen, peritonitis) or abnormal accumulations of air.
   a. Perform surgery if free air is present in the abdominal cavity because this usually indicates rupture or perforation of the gastrointestinal tract.
   b. Perform diagnostic peritoneal lavage in animals with acute abdominal signs of uncertain cause if radiographs are nondiagnostic.
5. Correct electrolyte and hydration abnormalities before surgery.

III. Anesthetic Considerations

A. Young, healthy animals can be premedicated with an anticholinergic and opioid (e.g., oxymorphone, butorphanol, buprenorphine) and induced with thiopental, propofol, or a combination of diazepam and ketamine given intravenously to effect (Appendix G-2).

B. Refer to subsequent chapters for the anesthetic management of sick or debilitated animals.

IV. Antibiotics

A. The appropriate use of antibiotics in patients undergoing abdominal surgery depends on the underlying disease, the animal's overall general health, and the length and type of surgical procedure being performed.

B. Surgeries of less than 1.5 to 2 hours in which a contaminated, hollow viscus is not opened do not usually warrant prophylactic antibiotics (see Chapter 10).

V. Surgical Techniques

A. Ventral Midline Celiotomy (*SAS,* pp. 180-181)

1. General considerations.
   a. Prepare the entire abdomen (including inguinal areas) and caudal thorax for aseptic surgery to allow extension of the incision into the thoracic or pelvic cavities if necessary. Prepping too small an area is a common mistake, particularly when abdominal exploration is performed in trauma patients.
   b. Count surgical sponges before surgery and before abdominal closure to help prevent inadvertently leaving them in the abdominal cavity.
   c. To adequately visualize all abdominal structures, extend the incision from the xiphoid process to the pubis.
      i. Make a caudal abdominal incision that extends from the umbilicus to the pubis for bladder exploration.
      ii. Make a cranial abdominal incision (i.e., umbilicus to xiphoid process) for evaluation of the liver and stomach.
      iii. Extend the incision laterally at the xiphoid process (1 cm caudal to the last rib) to facilitate exposure of the liver, biliary system, and diaphragm.
2. Surgical procedure.
   a. Ventral midline celiotomy in cats and female dogs.

With the patient in dorsal recumbency make a ventral midline skin incision beginning near the xiphoid process and extending caudally to the pubis. Sharply incise the subcutaneous tissues until the external fascia of the rectus abdominis muscle is exposed. Ligate or cauterize small subcutaneous bleeders and identify the linea alba. Tent the abdominal wall and make a sharp incision into the linea alba with a scalpel blade. Palpate the interior surface of the linea for adhesions. Use scissors to extend the incision cranially or caudally to near the extent of the skin incision. Digitally break down the attachments of one side of the falciform ligament to the body wall or excise it and remove it entirely if it interferes with visualization of cranial abdominal structures. Clamp the cranial end of the falciform ligament and ligate or cauterize bleeders before removing it.

   b. Ventral midline celiotomy in male dogs.

With the dog positioned in dorsal recumbency, place a towel clamp on the prepuce and clamp it to the skin on one side of the body. Drape the tip of the prepuce and clamp outside the surgical field. Make a ventral midline skin

incision beginning at the xiphoid process and continuing caudally to the prepuce. Curve the incision to the left or right (the opposite side from where the prepuce is clamped) of the penis and prepuce and extend it to the level of the pubis. Incise subcutaneous tissues and fibers of the preputialis muscle to the level of rectus fascia in the same plane as the skin incision. Ligate or cauterize large branches of the caudal superficial epigastric vein at the cranial aspect of the prepuce. Retract incised skin and subcutaneous tissues laterally and locate the linea alba and external fascia of the rectus abdominis muscle. Do not attempt to locate the caudal linea alba until subcutaneous tissues have been incised and abdominal musculature fascia identified. Tent the abdominal wall and make a sharp incision into the linea alba with a scalpel blade. Palpate the interior surface of the linea for adhesions. Use scissors to extend the incision cranially or caudally to near the extent of the skin incision.

B. Paracostal Celiotomy (*SAS,* p. 181)

1. General considerations.
   a. Use to expose the kidney and adrenal glands (it is most commonly used for unilateral adrenalectomy).
2. Surgical procedure.

Position the animal in lateral recumbency and place a rolled towel or sandbag between the animal and the operating table. Make a skin incision from the ventral vertebral column to near the ventral midline. Center the incision halfway between the wing of the ilium and the last rib. Extend the incision through the external abdominal oblique muscle with scissors. Separate internal abdominal oblique and transversus abdominis muscle fibers and expose peritoneal and transversalis fascia. Tent the peritoneum and sharply incise it with scissors.

C. Abdominal Exploration (*SAS,* pp. 181-182)

1. Systematically explore the entire abdomen (Table 15-1).
   a. Use moistened laparotomy sponges to protect tissues from drying during the procedure.
   b. If generalized infection is present or if diffuse intraoperative contamination has occurred, flush the abdomen with copious amounts of warmed, sterile saline solution.
      i. Do not use povidone-iodine; it has not shown a beneficial effect in repeated experimental and clinical trials and may be detrimental in animals with established peritonitis because the carrier, polyvinylpyrrolidone, inhibits macrophage chemotaxis.
      ii. There is no substantial evidence that adding antibiotics to lavage fluid benefits patients treated with appropriate systemic antibiotics.
      iii. Remove lavage fluid and blood and inspect the abdominal cavity before abdominal closure to ensure that all foreign material and surgical equipment have been removed.
   c. Perform a sponge count and compare it with the preoperative count to ensure that surgical sponges have not been left in the abdominal cavity.

D. Abdominal Wall Closure (*SAS,* pp. 182-183)

1. General considerations.
   a. Close the linea alba with simple interrupted sutures or a simple continuous suture pattern. A simple continuous suture pattern does not increase the risk of dehiscence when properly performed (i.e., secure knots, appropriate suture material), and it allows for rapid closure.

Table 15-1
Systematic exploration of the abdominal cavity

1) Explore the cranial quadrant
   - Examine the diaphragm (including esophageal hiatus) and entire liver (palpate the liver)
   - Inspect the gallbladder and biliary tree; express the gallbladder to determine patency
   - Examine the stomach, pylorus, proximal duodenum, and spleen
   - Examine both pancreatic limbs (palpate it gently!), portal vein, hepatic arteries, and caudal vena cava
2) Explore the caudal quadrant
   - Inspect the descending colon, urinary bladder, urethra, and prostate or uterine horns
   - Inspect the inguinal rings
3) Explore the intestinal tract
   - Palpate the intestinal tract from the duodenum to the descending colon and observe the mesenteric vasculature and nodes
4) Explore the gutters
   - Use the mesoduodenum to retract the intestine to the left and examine the right "gutter;" palpate the kidney and examine the adrenal gland, ureter, and ovary
   - Use the descending colon to retract the abdominal contents to the right; examine the left kidney, adrenal gland, ureter, and ovary

b. Use a strong, absorbable suture material (e.g., polydioxanone or polyglyconate) for continuous suture patterns and six to eight knots placed at each end of the incision line.

c. Avoid monofilament, nonabsorbable suture material (e.g., nylon, polypropylene) for continuous sutures because it has been associated with suture sinus formation in dogs.

d. Do not use surgical gut or stainless steel wire for continuous suture patterns.

2. Surgical procedure.

a. Ventral midline celiotomy closure.

On each side of the incision incorporate 4 to 10 mm of fascia in each suture. Place interrupted sutures 5 to 10 mm apart, depending on the animal's size. Tighten sutures sufficiently to appose, but not strangulate, tissue because the latter will adversely affect wound healing.

Incorporate full-thickness bites of the abdominal wall in the sutures if the incision is midline (i.e., through the linea alba). Do not incorporate the falciform ligament between the fascial edges. If the incision is lateral to the linea alba and muscular tissue is exposed (i.e., paramedian), close the external rectus sheath without including muscle in the sutures. Do not attempt to include peritoneum in the sutures. Close subcutaneous tissues with a simple continuous pattern of absorbable suture material and reappose preputialis muscle fibers. Use nonabsorbable (simple interrupted or continuous appositional patterns; see Chapter 9) sutures or stainless steel staples to close skin. Place skin sutures without tension.

b. Paracostal celiotomy closure.

Close individual muscle layers with synthetic absorbable or nonabsorbable suture material in a continuous or interrupted pattern. Attempt to eliminate dead space between muscle layers. Appose subcutaneous tissue with absorb-

able suture in a continuous or interrupted pattern and close skin with non-absorbable suture in a simple interrupted or continuous pattern.

VI. Healing of the Abdominal Wall

A. Be sure to include fascia in the suture line because it is the holding layer of abdominal incisions; dehiscence is common if rectus fascia is not incorporated in sutures.

B. Peritoneum heals rapidly across the incision and does not contribute to wound strength; therefore closure of this layer is not beneficial. Experimental and clinical studies in dogs suggest that suturing peritoneum may increase the incidence of postoperative intraabdominal adhesions.

C. Early signs of altered wound healing are inflammation and edema. Serosanguineous drainage from the incision and swelling are consistent signs of acute incisional dehiscence. Dehiscence usually occurs 3 to 5 days postoperatively when minimal healing has occurred and the sutures have weakened; however, it may occur earlier if knots were tied improperly or if fascia was not incorporated into the sutures. Evisceration usually results in sepsis and severe blood loss secondary to mutilation of exposed intestine and must be treated promptly.

D. Wound disruption after 10 to 21 days usually results in hernia formation rather than evisceration.

VII. Suture Materials/Special Instruments

A. Useful instruments for celiotomy include Balfour abdominal retractors, Poole or Yankauer suction tips, malleable retractors, and Mixter (right-angle) forceps.

B. Use laparotomy pads and 4 × 4 sponges that have radiopaque markers.

C. See the previous discussion on abdominal wall closure for choice of suture material.

VIII. Postoperative Care and Assessment

A. Check the abdominal incision twice daily for evidence of redness, swelling, or discharge.

B. If the animal licks or chews at the incision, use an Elizabethan collar or sidebar to prevent iatrogenic suture removal.

C. If dehiscence occurs bandage the abdomen, initiate fluid therapy, and administer broad-spectrum antibiotics while the animal is prepared for surgery.
   1. If technical failure is suspected (e.g., poor knot tieing, improper suturing), remove and replace the entire suture line. Do not debride the wound edges because it will delay wound healing.

2. Inspect the intestines for viability and resect damaged sections if appropriate.
3. Lavage the abdominal cavity with copious amounts of warmed, sterile saline.
4. Consider open abdominal drainage in animals with generalized peritonitis.

IX. Complications

A. Dehiscence (Incisional Hernias)

1. May occur if improper surgical technique is used (see the discussion above).
2. The most common causes of wound dehiscence in the early postoperative period are suture breakage, knot slippage or untieing, or sutures cutting through tissue.
3. An increased rate of dehiscence may occur in animals with wound infections, fluid or electrolyte imbalances, anemia, hypoproteinemia, metabolic disease, treatment with corticosteroids or chemotherapeutic agents or radiation, immunosuppression (i.e., feline immunodeficiency virus [FIV], feline leukemia virus), or abdominal distention.

Umbilical and Abdominal Hernias (*SAS*, pp. 184-187)

I. Definitions

A. **External abdominal hernias** are defects in the external wall of the abdomen that allow protrusion of abdominal contents.

B. **Internal abdominal hernias** are those that occur through a ring of tissue confined within the abdomen or thorax (e.g., diaphragmatic hernia, hiatal hernia).

C. **Umbilical hernias** occur through the umbilical ring.

D. **True hernias** are those in which the contents are enclosed within a peritoneal sac.

E. **False hernias** allow protrusion of organs outside of a normal abdominal opening; the contents are seldom contained within a peritoneal sac.

F. **Omphaloceles** are large midline umbilical and skin defects.

II. General Considerations and Clinically Relevant Pathophysiology

A. Abdominal hernias generally occur secondary to trauma (e.g., vehicular accidents, bite wounds); however, they have occasionally been reported as congenital lesions.

1. Abdominal hernias are false hernias because they do not contain a hernial sac. When associated with blunt trauma, they arise as a result of rupture of the wall from within because intraabdominal pressure is increased while abdominal muscles are contracted. The most common sites for traumatic abdominal hernias are the prepubic region and flank.
2. Congenital cranial abdominal hernias (i.e., cranial to the umbilicus) have been reported in association with peritoneopericardial diaphragmatic hernias in dogs and cats.

B. Cranial pubic ligament hernias often occur in association with pubic fractures.

C. Paracostal hernias may result in migration of abdominal contents along the thoracic wall.

D. Umbilical hernias.

1. Are usually congenital and caused by flawed embryogenesis.
2. Umbilical vessels, the vitelline duct, and the stalk of the allantois pass through the umbilical ring in the fetus, but this aperture closes at birth leaving an umbilical cicatrix. If the aperture fails to contract or it is too large or improperly formed, a hernia results.
3. The hernia is lined by a peritoneal sac, and these hernias are considered true hernias.
4. The cause of umbilical hernias is seldom known, but most are thought to be inherited.
5. Many male dogs with umbilical hernias are also cryptorchid.

E. Omphaloceles allow abdominal organs to protrude externally (eviscerate). The abdominal contents are initially covered by amniotic tissue, but this membrane covering is easily ruptured. Most affected neonates either die or are euthanized at birth.

III. Diagnosis

A. Clinical Presentation

1. Signalment.
   a. A majority of animals with umbilical or abdominal hernias are young.
   b. Umbilical hernias are believed to be heritable in some breeds (e.g., Airedale, basenji, Pekingese).
   c. Cranial ventral abdominal hernias associated with peritoneopericardial diaphragmatic hernias may be inherited in weimaraners.
2. History.
   a. A history of trauma is common with abdominal hernias. The hernia may initially be overlooked while more obvious or life-threatening injuries are treated.
   b. Small umbilical hernias often are not noticed until the animal is examined for neutering.
   c. If strangulation or intestinal obstruction occurs the animal may present for vomiting, abdominal pain, anorexia, or depression.

B. Physical Examination Findings

1. Abdominal structures (i.e., organs or omentum) in the subcutaneous space or between muscle layers usually cause asymmetry of the abdominal contour.

2. Carefully palpate the swelling to discern the contents of the hernia (e.g., intestine, bladder, spleen) and to locate the abdominal defect.
3. Umbilical hernias usually present as a soft ventral abdominal mass at the umbilical scar. Perform deep palpation of the swelling to determine umbilical ring size and help characterize contents.
   a. The hernial ring is not palpable in some animals because the ring closes subsequent to falciform fat or omental herniation.
   b. Occasionally, intestine or other abdominal structures can be palpated; they can generally be reduced into the abdominal cavity.
   c. If the umbilical sac is warm or painful and the contents are irreducible, intestinal strangulation or obstruction should be suspected.

C. Radiography/Ultrasonography

1. Radiographs should be taken in animals with abdominal hernias.
   a. Routine ventral dorsal and lateral views may show the presence of associated abdominal or thoracic injury (e.g., abdominal fluid, diaphragmatic hernia).
   b. Abdominal radiographs may help confirm the presence of a hernia (e.g., subcutaneous intestinal loops and loss of the ventral abdominal stripe) when the abdominal wall defect cannot be palpated because of swelling or pain.
2. Radiographs are generally not indicated in small umbilical hernias. Ultrasound may also help define the contents of hernias.

IV. Medical Management

A. Initial treatment of animals with abdominal hernias is directed toward diagnosing and treating shock and concurrent life-threatening internal injuries.

V. Surgical Treatment

A. Abdominal Hernias

1. General considerations.
   a. Most abdominal hernias can be repaired by suturing torn muscle edges or apposing the disrupted abdominal wall edge to pubis, ribs, or adjacent fascia. Rarely, synthetic mesh is needed to repair the defect.
   b. Some hernias (e.g., intestinal strangulation, urinary obstruction, concurrent organ trauma) require emergency surgical correction. However, the extent of devitalized muscle may not initially be apparent and delaying surgery until muscle damage can be accurately assessed will facilitate surgical correction in stable patients.
   c. Abdominal hernias secondary to bite wounds are usually contaminated; wound infection and dehiscence of skin or hernial repair are common. Mesh should not be placed in these hernias, and the wounds should be drained. Treatment of infected wounds includes cultures, drainage, antibiotics, and flushing.
   d. Abdominal exploration should be performed at herniorrhaphy to

diagnose concurrent abdominal organ injury (e.g., mesenteric avulsion, gastric or intestinal perforation, diaphragmatic herniation, bladder rupture).

2. Surgical procedure.

For most abdominal hernias perform a ventral midline abdominal incision to allow the entire abdomen to be explored. Assess the extent of visceral herniation. Reduce herniated contents and amputate or excise necrotic or devitalized tissue around the hernia. Close muscle layers of the hernia with simple interrupted or simple continuous sutures. If a large area of devitalized tissue is removed, use synthetic mesh such as Marlex or Prolene to close the defect (do not place in infected sites). Fold the edges of the mesh over and suture folded edges to viable tissue using simple interrupted sutures. Cranial pubic ligament injuries can be difficult to repair. If necessary, drill holes in the pubic bone to anchor sutures.

Paracostal hernias: Repair paracostal hernias via a midline incision or one made directly over the hernia. Explore the hernia and suture the torn edges of the transverse, internal, and external abdominal oblique muscles. Incorporate a rib in the suture if muscle has been avulsed from the costal arch.

Cranial pubic ligament hernias: With cranial pubic ligament injuries, make a ventral midline skin incision and identify the ruptured tendon and its pubic insertion. Evaluate inguinal rings and vascular lacuna; these hernias may extend into the femoral region as a result of inguinal ligament rupture. Reattach the free edge of the abdominal wall to the cranial pubic ligament with simple interrupted sutures. Alternatively, suture the tendon remnant to muscle fascia and periosteum, covering the pubis, or anchor it to the pubis by drilling holes in the pubic bone through which sutures can be placed. If the hernia extends into the femoral region, it may be necessary to suture body wall to the medial fascia of the adductor muscles. Take care when doing so to avoid damaging the femoral vessels or nerves.

B. Umbilical Hernias

1. General considerations.
   a. Many umbilical hernias resolve spontaneously in young animals or are small and are not corrected until the animal is neutered. Spontaneous closure may occur as late as 6 months of age.
   b. Intestinal strangulation is most likely when the hernial defect is about the size of intestine and the hernial sac is large. Strangulation is unlikely in very small or large defects. If abdominal viscera contained within the hernia cannot be reduced, surgery should be performed as soon as possible.
2. Surgical procedure.

For umbilical hernias palpate the hernial ring, reduce abdominal contents if possible, and incise skin over the umbilicus. If the hernia contains only fat or omentum, ligate the hernial neck and excise the sac and its contents. Alternatively, if adhesions are not present, invert the sac and its contents into the abdominal cavity. Do not debride wound margins. Suture edges of the defect with monofilament, synthetic, absorbable suture (e.g., polydioxanone or polyglyconate) in a simple interrupted pattern. If hernial contents cannot be reduced make an elliptical incision around the swelling to prevent damaging the contents. Incise the hernial sac and replace contents into the abdominal cavity. If the contents are irreducible or strangulation or intestinal obstruction is present, extend the abdominal defect on the midline. Explore the abdomen before closing the defect and inspect the intestines for viability. Umbilical hernia repair seldom requires mesh implantation.

VI. Suture Materials/Special Instruments

A. Use strong absorbable (polydioxanone or polyglyconate) or nonabsorbable (polypropylene or nylon) suture to repair abdominal or ventral hernias.

B. Consider synthetic mesh to repair some large defects (e.g., Marlex mesh, Prolene mesh).

Inguinal, Scrotal, and Femoral Hernias (*SAS*, pp. 187-193)

I. Definitions

A. **Inguinal hernias** are protrusions of organs or tissues through the inguinal canal adjacent to the vaginal process.

B. **Scrotal hernias** occur when inguinal ring defects allow abdominal contents to protrude into the vaginal process adjacent to the spermatic cord.

C. **Femoral hernias** occur through a defect in the femoral canal.

II. General Considerations and Clinically Relevant Pathophysiology

A. Inguinal Hernias

1. May arise as a result of a congenital inguinal ring abnormality or may occur following trauma. Congenital hernias may be associated with other abnormalities (e.g., umbilical hernias, perineal hernias, cryptorchidism).
2. Presumably arise in young male dogs because late testicular descent causes delayed inguinal ring closure. Older bitches may be predisposed to develop inguinal hernias because they have a relatively large diameter ring with a short canal.
3. The inguinal ring defect allows abdominal contents (e.g., intestine, bladder, uterus) to enter subcutaneous spaces.

B. Scrotal Hernias

1. Are rare, indirect hernias.
2. They are usually unilateral, and strangulation of abdominal contents is common.
3. An increased incidence of testicular tumors has been reported in conjunction with scrotal hernias.

C. Femoral Hernias

1. Are rare in dogs and cats.
2. They occur when abdominal contents or fat protrudes through the

femoral canal, caudomedial to the femoral vessels, and may be mistaken for inguinal hernias.

3. Femoral hernias may occur following trauma and avulsion of the cranial pubic ligaments, or they may be caused by transecting the origin of the pectineus muscle from the pubis during subtotal pectineal myectomy.

III. Diagnosis

A. Clinical Presentation

1. Signalment.
   a. Inguinal hernias.
      i. Nontraumatic inguinal hernias are most frequently reported in intact, middle-aged female dogs or young (less than 2 years of age) male dogs.
      ii. Breeds that are predisposed include Pekingese, cairn terrier, basset, basenji, and West Highland white terrier.
      iii. Rare in cats.
   b. Scrotal hernias.
      i. Have been reported most commonly in chondrodystrophic dogs, particularly shar-peis.
   c. Femoral hernias.
      i. No breed or sex predisposition has been reported for femoral hernias.
2. History.
   a. Inguinal hernias.
      i. Animals with inguinal hernias may present for evaluation of a nonpainful swelling in the inguinal region, or for vomiting, lethargy, pain, or depression if the hernial contents are incarcerated.
      ii. Omentum is the most common organ present in canine inguinal hernias.
      iii. Uterus is often located within the hernias of affected intact females. These hernias are often chronic and do not cause clinical signs until pregnancy or pyometra develops.
   b. Scrotal and femoral hernias.
      i. Affected animals usually present for evaluation of scrotal (scrotal hernias) or medial thigh swelling (femoral hernias), or for vomiting and pain if intestinal incarceration occurs.

B. Physical Examination Findings

1. Inguinal hernias.
   a. The physical characteristics of the swelling vary depending on the hernial contents and the degree of associated vascular obstruction. Often a soft, nonpainful, unilateral or bilateral swelling is noted in the inguinal region.
   b. If intestinal strangulation has occurred, or a gravid uterus or urinary bladder is contained within the hernia, the swelling may be large, fluctuant, and painful.
   c. Finding nonviable small intestine is more common in young (less than 2 years) male dogs with nontraumatic hernias than in older animals. Associated vascular or lymphatic obstruction may cause testicular and spermatic cord edema. Concurrent abnormalities (e.g., perineal hernia, cryptorchidism) may be noted.
   d. Unilateral inguinal hernias are more common than bilateral hernias. Bilateral hernias occur more commonly in young dogs, and careful palpation of the contralateral inguinal region for occult hernias is recommended in all dogs.

2. Scrotal hernias.
   a. Usually appear as a firm, cordlike mass extending into the caudal aspect of the scrotum. Pain and bluish-black tissue discoloration may be noted if intestinal strangulation has occurred.
3. Femoral hernias.
   a. Cause swelling on the medial aspect of the thigh that may extend into the inguinal region. The swelling is located caudal to the inguinal ligament and ventrolateral to the pelvic brim.

C. Radiography/Ultrasonography

1. Abdominal radiographs may help identify herniation of a gravid uterus, intestine, or bladder in an inguinal hernia.
2. Loss of the caudal abdominal stripe may be noted in affected animals.
3. Ultrasonography is useful with scrotal hernias to assess viability of testicular blood flow and whether spermatic cord torsion or hydrocele is present.

IV. Differential Diagnoses

A. Do not mistake the caudal abdominal fat pad in older obese cats for a hernia.

V. Surgical Treatment

A. Inguinal Hernias

1. General considerations.
   a. Correct these hernias promptly to prevent complications associated with intestinal strangulation or pregnancy.
   b. Remove nondescended testicles at inguinal hernia repair. Necrosis of ipsilateral descended testicles may occur secondary to vascular obstruction and necessitate orchiectomy.
   c. If a gravid uterus is contained within the inguinal hernia, spay the animal, or if the fetus is viable and pregnancy termination is not desired, reduce the uterus and close the inguinal ring. Warn owners that parturition or uterine enlargement may be associated with recurrence.
2. Surgical technique.

The goal of surgery is to reduce the abdominal contents and close the external inguinal ring so that herniation of abdominal contents cannot recur. The approach for inguinal hernias depends on whether the hernia is unilateral or bilateral, whether the contents can be reduced, and whether intestinal strangulation or concurrent abdominal trauma is present. Although an incision can be made parallel to the flank fold directly over the lateral aspect of the swelling, a midline incision is usually preferred in female dogs because it allows palpation and closure of both inguinal rings through a single skin incision. Inguinal hernias can usually be closed without the use of prosthetic materials. Occasionally repair of recurrent or large traumatic defects requires synthetic mesh placement or a cranial sartorius muscle flap.

Make a caudal abdominal midline skin incision in female dogs cranially from the brim of the pelvis. Deepen the incision through subcutaneous tissues to the ventral rectus sheath. Expose the hernial sac by bluntly dissecting beneath mammary tissue, and identify the hernial sac and ring. Reduce abdominal contents by twisting the sac and milking contents through the ring, or if necessary incise the hernial sac and make an incision in the craniomedial

aspect of the ring to enlarge it. After reducing abdominal contents amputate the base of the hernial sac and close it with horizontal mattress sutures, a simple continuous suture pattern, or an inverting suture pattern (i.e., Cushing plus Lembert). Close the inguinal ring with simple interrupted sutures of absorbable or nonabsorbable synthetic suture material. Avoid compromising the external pudendal vessels and genitofemoral nerve that exit from the caudomedial aspect of the ring (or the spermatic cord in intact male dogs). Palpate the contralateral ring and close it if necessary before skin closure.

If hernial contents cannot be reduced, perform a celiotomy and explore abdominal contents. Expose the inguinal ring as described above and reduce hernial contents (enlarge the inguinal ring if necessary). Resect nonviable intestine or perform an ovariohysterectomy and close the inguinal ring(s).

B. Scrotal Hernias

1. General considerations.
   a. Bilateral orchiectomy is recommended with scrotal hernias to lessen recurrence.
2. Surgical technique.

Expose the hernial sac and reduce abdominal contents (incise the hernial sac if necessary). If hernial repair is performed in conjunction with orchiectomy (preferred), open the hernial sac and ligate the contents of the spermatic cord. Remove the testicle after disrupting the ligament of the tail of the epididymis and ligate the hernial sac at the level of the internal inguinal ring. If castration is not being performed, make an incision into the hernial sac (parietal vaginal tunic) and evaluate the hernial contents. Reduce the herniated contents and place a transfixing ligature or several horizontal mattress sutures in the hernial sac to reduce the size of the vaginal orifice. Partially close the external inguinal ring with interrupted sutures. Do not compromise the spermatic cord or vascular structures at the caudomedial ring aspect.

If hernial contents cannot be reduced or if viscera are strangulated and necrotic, perform a midline celiotomy as described previously. After resecting intestine, expose the inguinal ring and repair the hernia. Perform a scrotal ablation if severe contamination of the vaginal process and scrotum has occurred.

C. Femoral Hernias

Incise skin parallel to the inguinal ligament and expose the hernial sac. Reduce sac contents and ligate the hernial sac as high in the femoral canal as possible. If the inguinal ligament is intact, close the femoral canal by placing sutures between the inguinal ligament and pectineal fascia. Do not damage or compromise neurovascular structures of the femoral canal. Close subcutaneous tissues and skin. If strangulation of abdominal organs is present, perform a midline celiotomy. Reduce abdominal contents, then invert and ligate the sac. Dissect laterally from the skin incision to the femoral canal and close the femoral canal defect as described above.

VI. Suture Materials/Special Instruments

A. Use monofilament absorbable (polydioxanone or polyglyconate) or nonabsorbable (polypropylene or nylon) suture material to close the hernial ring. Multifilament nonabsorbable suture may be associated with a higher incidence of wound infection.

B. Consider mesh as an overlay to reinforce the primary hernia repair.

VII. Postoperative Care and Assessment

A. Assess hernial sites postoperatively if evidence of infection or hematoma/seroma formation.

B. Remove skin sutures and initiate drainage and topical therapy if abscessation occurs to prevent dehiscence of the hernia repair.

C. Restrict exercise to leash walks for several weeks.

D. Use an Elizabethan collar to prevent the animal from licking at the surgical site.

E. Testicular swelling postoperatively may indicate compromise of testicular lymphatic or vascular drainage.

F. With femoral hernias, consider hobbles during healing to prevent limb abduction and assess femoral nerve function postoperatively. Nerve deficits or severe pain may indicate compromise of the femoral nerve during the repair; reoperation is warranted in such cases.

Peritonitis (*SAS*, pp. 193-199)

I. General Considerations and Clinically Relevant Pathophysiology

A. Secondary generalized peritonitis is the predominant form of peritonitis in dogs and is usually caused by bacteria.

B. Primary generalized peritonitis occurs in cats associated with feline infectious peritonitis.

C. Generalized peritonitis may result from intestinal or gallbladder perforation, rupture, or necrosis (e.g., gastric or intestinal foreign bodies, intussusception, mesenteric avulsion, gastric dilation-volvulus, necrotizing cholecystitis), pancreatic abscessation, prostatic abscesses, or foreign body penetration.

II. Diagnosis

A. Clinical Presentation

1. Signalment.
   a. Any age, sex, or breed of dog or cat may develop peritonitis. It is particularly common in young animals that have perforating foreign bodies and in those that receive abdominal trauma (e.g., vehicular trauma or bite wounds).
2. History.
   a. The history of peritonitis in a patient is often nonspecific. The animal may not show signs of illness for several days after the traumatic episode.

b. Most animals are presented for lethargy, anorexia, vomiting, diarrhea, or abdominal pain.

B. Physical Examination Findings

1. Affected animals are usually in pain during abdominal palpation. The pain may be localized but generalized pain is more common and the animal will often tense or "splint" the abdomen during palpation.
2. Abdominal distention may be noted if sufficient fluid has accumulated.
3. Pale mucous membranes, prolonged capillary refill times, and tachycardia may indicate that the animal is in shock. Dehydration and arrhythmias may also occur.

C. Radiography/Ultrasonography

1. The classic radiographic finding in animals with peritonitis is loss of abdominal detail with a focal or generalized "ground-glass" appearance
2. Free air in the abdomen may be noted with rupture of a hollow organ or sometimes occurs without gut rupture as a result of gas-producing anaerobes.
3. A more localized peritonitis may occur secondary to pancreatitis and can cause the duodenum to appear fixed and elevated.
4. Ultrasonography is useful to localize fluid accumulation and help determine etiology.

D. Laboratory Findings

1. The most common laboratory finding in animals with peritonitis is a marked leukocytosis. The predominant cell type is the neutrophil, and a left shift is often apparent.
2. Other abnormalities may include anemia, dehydration, and electrolyte and acid-base abnormalities.
3. Perform abdominocentesis and analyze fluid retrieved.
   a. Inflammatory fluids should have an elevated number of neutrophils, which may appear degenerative. Significant numbers of leukocytes accumulate in the peritoneal cavity within 2 to 3 hours of contamination with blood, bile, urine, feces, or gastric or pancreatic secretions.
      i. Leukocyte counts in abdominal fluid of normal dogs are usually less than 500 cells/ml.
      ii. Following peritoneal lavage in dogs, white blood cell (WBC) counts of 1000 to 2000 cells/ml are indicative of mild to moderate irritation, while counts of greater than 2000 cells/ml indicate marked peritonitis.
   b. The presence of degenerate leukocytes and bacteria in the lavage fluid suggests intraabdominal infection. However, always correlate the presence and number of WBCs with other clinical findings when considering abdominal exploration.
   c. Estimate the amount of blood in the abdominal cavity by observing the lavage sample.
      i. A red color reflects the presence of red blood cells (RBCs) and a deep red color usually indicates severe hemorrhage. If newsprint cannot be read through the plastic tubing, then hemorrhage is significant. If print can be seen through the tubing, only moderate or minimal hemorrhage is present.
      ii. Surgical intervention is indicated when there is a substantial increase in the packed cell volume (PCV) of lavage samples taken within 5 to 20 minutes of each other, or if an animal in shock does not respond to aggressive fluid therapy.

III. Medical Management

A. The goals of management of animals with peritonitis are to treat the cause of the contamination, resolve the infection, and restore normal fluid and electrolyte balances.

B. Withhold food if the animal is vomiting.

C. Initiate fluid replacement therapy as soon as possible, particularly if the animal is dehydrated or appears to be in shock (up to 90 ml/kg intravenously, based on the animal's condition).

D. Assess electrolytes and supplement potassium (Appendix H) if necessary.

E. If hypoglycemia is present (common if the animal has septic shock [systemic inflammatory response syndrome]), add glucose to the fluids (e.g., 2.5% to 5% dextrose).

F. Initiate standard shock therapy (i.e., fluid replacement, antibiotics, plus or minus soluble corticosteroids). If severe metabolic acidosis is present, consider administering bicarbonate (Appendix C).

G. Initiate broad-spectrum antibiotic therapy as soon as the diagnosis is made.
   1. Ampicillin plus enrofloxacin (Appendix I) is an effective combination against most bacteria responsible for peritonitis in dogs.
   2. Amikacin sulfate plus clindamycin or amikacin sulfate plus metronidazole may be necessary if anaerobic infection is present (Appendix I).
   3. A second-generation cephalosporin such as cefoxitin sodium (Appendix I) may also be used if gram-negative plus anaerobic infection is suspected.
   4. If renal compromise is present in an animal with a resistant bacterial infection, imipenem may be considered (Appendix I).
   5. Alter initial antibiotic therapy based on results of aerobic and anaerobic culture results of lavage fluid or cultures obtained at surgery.

H. Consider low-dose heparin (Appendix I) therapy to increase survival and reduce abscess formation in experimental peritonitis. Although the exact mechanism of its beneficial effect is still unknown, there does not appear to be any doubt that heparin is indicated in patients with severe peritonitis.

I. Heparin may also be incubated with plasma and given to animals with disseminated intravascular coagulation (DIC) (Appendix I).

IV. Surgical Treatment

A. General Considerations

1. Exploratory surgery is indicated when the cause of peritonitis cannot be determined or when bowel rupture, intestinal obstruction (e.g., bowel incarceration, neoplasia), or mesenteric avulsion is suspected.
2. The role that protein levels play in healing intestinal incisions is not well understood. However, most surgeons are concerned that

hypoproteinemic patients may not heal as quickly as patients with normal protein levels.

3. Lavage.
   a. Although the practice of lavaging the abdominal cavity of animals with peritonitis is controversial, lavage is generally indicated with diffuse peritonitis.
   b. Perform lavage with care in animals with localized peritonitis to prevent causing diffuse dissemination of infection.
   c. Remove as much of the fluid as possible because fluid inhibits the body's ability to fight off infection, probably by inhibiting neutrophil function.
   d. Warmed, sterile physiologic saline is the most appropriate lavage fluid.
4. Open abdominal drainage (OAD).
   a. OAD is a useful technique for managing animals with peritonitis.
   b. Reported advantages include improvement in the patient's metabolic condition secondary to improved drainage, reduced abdominal adhesion and abscess formation, and access for repeated inspection and exploration of the abdomen.

B. Preoperative Management

1. Stabilize animals with peritonitis before surgery if they are in shock (see Medical Management above).
2. If the animal is debilitated, vomiting, or not likely to resume eating for several days after surgery, consider enteral or parenteral hyperalimentation (see Chapter 11).

C. Anesthesia

1. Correct hypotension before surgery and prevent it during and after surgery in animals with peritonitis. Consider dobutamine (2 to 10 μg/kg/min IV) or dopamine (2 to 10 μg/kg/min IV) during surgery for inotropic support.
   a. Dobutamine is less arrhythmogenic and chronotropic than dopamine and is preferred if the patient is hypotensive and anuric.
   b. If the patient is anuric and normotensive, low-dose dopamine (0.5 to 1.5 μg/kg/min intravenously) plus furosemide (2.0 mg/kg intravenously) may be preferable.
   c. Monitor these patients for arrhythmias or tachycardia.
2. Animals with total protein less than 4.0 g/dl or albumin less than 1.5 g/dl may benefit from perioperative colloid administration.
   a. Colloids may be given preoperatively, intraoperatively, or postoperatively for a total dose of 20 ml/kg/day. If colloids are given during surgery (7 to 10 ml/kg), acute intraoperative hypotension should be treated with crystalloids.
3. Hepatic dysfunction.
   a. Do not use acepromazine in animals with peritonitis if severe hepatic dysfunction is suspected. Diazepam plus an opioid are useful premedicants in patients with hepatic disease. Diazepam used alone may disinhibit some behaviors. It should be used with caution in hypoalbuminemic patients.
   b. Most opioids have little or no adverse effect on the liver; however, intravenous morphine should be avoided in dogs with hepatic dysfunction because it may cause hepatic congestion as a result of histamine release and hepatic vein spasm. Although some opioid analgesics may have prolonged action when hepatic function is reduced, their effects can be antagonized.
   c. Barbiturates (e.g., thiopental) should be used cautiously or avoided in patients with significant hepatic dysfunction.
   d. Selected anesthetic protocols for use in animals with peritonitis are

provided in Appendix G-3. An anticholinergic (atropine or glycopyrollate) may be given if the animal is bradycardic.

D. Surgical Techniques

1. Abdominocentesis.

Insert an 18- or 20-gauge, 1.5-inch plastic over-the-needle catheter (with added side holes) into the abdominal cavity at the most dependent part of the abdomen. Do not attach a syringe; instead allow the fluid to drip from the needle and collect in a sterile tube. If sufficient fluid is obtained, place the fluid in a clot tube and an ethylenediaminetetraacetic acid (EDTA) tube, submit samples for aerobic and anaerobic culture, and make four to six smears for analysis. If fluid is not obtained, apply gentle suction using a 3-ml syringe. It is difficult to puncture bowel by this method because mobile loops of bowel move away from the tip of the needle as it strikes them. Perforations created by a needle this size usually heal without complications. The major disadvantage of needle paracentesis is that it is insensitive to the presence of the small volumes of intraperitoneal fluid and thus a negative result can be meaningless. At least 5 to 6 ml of fluid/kg body weight must be present in the abdominal cavity of dogs to obtain positive results in a majority of cases using this technique.

2. Diagnostic peritoneal lavage.

Make a 2-cm skin incision just caudal to the umbilicus and ligate any bleeders to avoid false-positive results. Spread loose subcutaneous tissues and make a small incision in the linea alba. Hold the edges of the incision with forceps while the peritoneal lavage catheter (Stylocath) (without the trocar) is inserted into the abdominal cavity. Direct the catheter caudally into the pelvis. With the catheter in place, apply gentle suction. If blood or fluid cannot be aspirated, connect the catheter to a bottle of warm sterile saline and infuse 20 ml/kg of fluid into the abdominal cavity. When the calculated volume of fluid has been delivered, roll the patient gently from side to side, place the bottle on the floor, vent it, and collect the fluid by gravity drainage. Do not be surprised if you do not retrieve all of the fluid, particularly in dehydrated animals.

3. Exploratory laparotomy.

Perform a ventral midline incision from the xiphoid process to the pubis (see SAS, pp. 180-181). Obtain a sample of fluid for culture and analysis. Explore and inspect the entire abdomen. Find the source of infection and correct it. Break down adhesions that may hinder drainage. Lavage the abdomen with copious amounts of warm sterile saline if the infection is generalized. Remove as much necrotic debris and fluid as possible. Close the abdomen routinely or perform open abdominal drainage.

4. Open abdominal drainage.

After completing the abdominal procedure, leave a portion of the abdominal incision (usually the most dependent portion) open to drain. Generally, make the opening just large enough to allow a gloved hand to be inserted. Close the cranial and caudal aspects of the incision with monofilament suture using a continuous suture pattern. Place a sterile laparotomy pad over the opening, then place a sterile wrap over the laparotomy pad. Change the wrap at least twice daily initially with the animal standing; sedation is seldom necessary (use sterile bandage materials and wear sterile gloves). The volume of drainage dictates the number of wrap changes needed. Break down adhesions to the incision that may interfere with drainage. Abdominal lavage may be attempted but is seldom necessary. Place a diaper over the wrap to decrease contamination from urine. Assess the fluid daily for bacterial numbers and cell

morphology. When bacterial numbers have decreased and normal neutrophil morphology is present (nondegenerative), close the incision (generally in 3 to 5 days). If the opening is small it may be left to heal by second intention.

V. Suture Materials/Special Instruments

A. Use monofilament synthetic nonabsorbable (polypropylene or nylon) or slowly absorbable (polydioxanone or polyglyconate) suture to close the abdomen in animals with peritonitis.

B. Do not use braided suture (Dacron, silk, braided nylon) or suture that may be rapidly degraded (chromic gut).

VI. Postoperative Care and Assessment

A. Continue fluid therapy postoperatively, particularly in those animals being managed with an open abdomen.

B. Assess electrolytes, acid-base, and serum protein in the postoperative period and correct as necessary.

C. Supplement nutrition to meet the increased need of animals with peritonitis (see Chapter 11).

D. If hypoproteinemia becomes severe, consider plasma transfusions.

16

Surgery of the Digestive System (*SAS*, pp. 200-366)

Surgery of the Oral Cavity and Oropharynx (*SAS*, pp. 200-232)

I. Definitions

A. **Maxillectomy** is removal of a portion of the maxilla.

B. **Mandibulectomy** is removal of a portion of the mandible.

C. **Tonsillectomy** is excision of one or both tonsils.

D. **Glossectomy** is excision of a portion of the tongue.

E. **Cheiloplasty** is performed to alter the shape of the lip, generally to reduce drooling.

F. **Mucoceles** are subcutaneous collections of saliva, mucus, or both.

G. **Ranulas** are collections of cystic fluid from the mandibular or sublingual salivary glands that occur beneath the tongue on either side of the frenulum.

II. Preoperative Concerns

A. Identifying Surgical Disease

1. Patients with oral cavity or oropharyngeal disease may present for drooling, dysphagia, anorexia, bleeding from the mouth, or fetid breath.
2. Others present because of a mass, oral hemorrhage, oral pain, difficulty eating, nasal regurgitation, chronic rhinitis, or dyspnea.
3. Some animals are asymptomatic until the lesions become large or are discovered on routine physical examination.

B. Preoperative Evaluation

1. Before performing major surgery, perform a thorough physical examination, complete blood cell count (CBC), serum biochemical profile, and urinalysis.

2. Cross-match the animal's blood before performing maxillectomy or mandibulectomy.
    a. Check the coagulation system of animals predisposed to coagulopathies.
    b. Evaluate Doberman pinschers for the presence of von Willebrand's disease.
3. Skull radiographs or CT scans will help determine the extent of the lesion.
4. Radiograph the thorax to evaluate for metastasis, cardiac size, and pulmonary disease.
5. Clean the teeth of animals with periodontal disease several days before major reconstructive surgery to improve tissue health and reduce oral bacterial numbers.
6. Maintain nutrition by tube feeding if necessary. Feed animals with oronasal fistulae via feeding tubes to decrease rhinitis and inhalation pneumonia before surgery.
7. Correct metabolic abnormalities and fast mature animals 12 to 18 hours (pediatric animals 4 to 8 hours) before anesthetic induction.
8. Flush the mouth after induction with dilute betadine or chlorhexidine solution to reduce bacterial numbers.

III. Anesthetic Considerations

A. Endotracheal Tubes

1. If an orally placed endotracheal tube hinders oral cavity and oropharyngeal surgery, perform endotracheal intubation through a pharyngotomy or tracheotomy incision.
2. Inflate the endotracheal tube cuff to prevent blood and fluid from entering the lower airways.
3. Place one or two gauze sponges in the oropharynx around the endotracheal tube to help absorb fluids.

B. Monitoring and Care

1. Minimize postoperative swelling by corticosteroid pretreatment (e.g., dexamethasone, 1 to 2 mg/kg SC or IM before anesthetic induction or IV at induction) to prevent potential obstruction of the glottis.
2. Have blood, hypertonic saline, or both available in the event that severe hemorrhage occurs. Place two cephalic catheters to allow simultaneous administration of blood and inotropes, if necessary.
3. Evaluate arterial blood pressure during surgery.
4. Avoid acepromazine.
5. See Appendix G-4 for selected anesthetic protocols for use in animals with oral disease.

IV. Antibiotics

A. The oral cavity and oropharynx are contaminated, but saliva is antimicrobial and the blood supply to this region is excellent; thus infections after oral surgery are rare.

B. One dose of prophylactic antibiotic effective against gram-positive aerobes and anaerobes (e.g., amoxicillin) may be given at induction. Therapeutic antibiotics (e.g., cefazolin plus metronidazole, amoxicillin, or clindamycin; see Appendix I) are indicated in debilitated and immunosuppressed patients and those with severe periodontal disease.

V. Surgical Anatomy

A. The blood supply to this region originates from branches of the common carotid arteries.
   1. Note the location of the paired major and minor palatine arteries when performing surgeries involving the hard palate.
   2. The mandible is mainly supplied by the mandibular alveolar artery, which enters the mandibular canal on the medial surface of the mandible. The mandibular canal also transmits the mandibular vein and mandibular alveolar nerve.

VI. Surgical Techniques

A. General Guidelines

1. Atraumatic surgical technique is important to reduce tissue damage and swelling and to encourage rapid healing.
2. Hemorrhage.
   a. Control hemorrhage with pressure and vessel ligation.
   b. Use electrosurgery sparingly because excessive use delays healing and may result in dehiscence. Apply electrocoagulation only to discrete, isolated areas.
3. Closure.
   a. During reconstructive procedures, create flaps that are approximately 2 to 4 mm larger than the defect and preserve major vessels entering these flaps.
   b. Minimize tension on these flaps by adequate mobilization.
   c. Manipulate flaps with skin hooks or stay sutures to minimize trauma.
   d. Place suture lines over connective tissue or bone, rather than the defect, to help support mucosal flaps.

B. Biopsy Techniques (*SAS,* pp. 202-203)

1. General guidelines.
   a. Obtain impression smears or aspirates from oral lesions before incisional or excisional biopsy.
   b. When obtaining biopsies, avoid areas of superficial necrosis; sample deeper, viable tissues.
   c. **Submit all specimens** for histologic evaluation.
2. Incisional biopsies.
   a. General considerations.
      i. Perform an incisional biopsy using a needle or wedge biopsy technique if the definitive diagnosis will change the course of therapy.
   b. Technique.

Use a Tru-Cut or Vim-Silverman needle to obtain small cores from several areas of the mass. Perform a wedge biopsy from nonnecrotic areas of the mass when larger pieces of tissue are needed. Use a loop or needle electrode of an electrosurgical unit in obtaining oral biopsies. The specimen will be nondiagnostic if too much current is applied, especially to a small sample. Prevent tissue coagulation by keeping the power setting on the electrosurgical unit as low as possible. Diseased tissue is often friable and difficult to appose with sutures after a biopsy; however, pressure over the cut area is usually sufficient to control hemorrhage. If necessary, use silver nitrate cautery.

3. Excisional biopsy.
   a. General considerations
      i. Perform an excisional biopsy and reconstruct the area if the definitive histologic diagnosis will not alter the course of therapy.

C. Temporary Carotid Artery Ligation (*SAS,* p. 203)

1. Indications
   a. Perform before maxillectomy to minimize blood loss.
   b. **This procedure may not be safe in cats.**
2. Procedure

Place the animal in dorsal recumbency and prepare the ventral cervical area for surgery. Expose the trachea through a 5- to 8-cm ventral cervical midline incision. Palpate the carotid pulse and exteriorize the carotid sheath. Separate the common carotid artery from the vagosympathetic trunk and internal jugular vein. Temporarily occlude the carotid artery with a vascular clamp or tie. Repeat the procedure on the opposite carotid artery. Temporarily appose skin with a continuous suture pattern or staples during the maxillectomy procedure. After maxillectomy, reopen the cervical wound and remove the vascular clamps or ties. Lavage the area thoroughly and appose the sternohyoid muscles, subcutaneous tissue, and skin in separate layers.

D. Partial Maxillectomy (*SAS,* pp. 203-204)

1. Indications.
   a. The most common reason for maxillectomy is to resect an oral neoplasm.
2. Procedure.

Clip and aseptically prepare the maxillary and nasal skin. Flush the mouth with antiseptic solution. Place the patient in dorsal recumbency for lesions of the premaxilla, and open the mouth to its maximum extent by placing a mouth speculum or taping the mouth open. Place the patient in lateral or dorsal recumbency for lesions caudal to the premaxilla. Determine the extent of resection based on the size of the soft tissue lesion and radiographic degree of bony involvement. Generally, excise the mass and a minimum of 1 to 2 cm of normal soft tissue and bone on all borders. Remove the mass en bloc by first making mucosal (buccal, gingival, and hard palate) incisions around the tissue to be resected. Avoid rectangular excision because the corners are susceptible to dehiscence. Then, using a periosteal elevator, undermine and reflect the gingival and palatal mucosa. Use an oscillating saw or an osteotome and mallet to cut the maxilla, incisive bone, and/or palate. Resect all premolar and molar teeth for lesions extending to the third premolar because of the outward turn of the dental arch. When performing a caudal maxillectomy, remove a portion of the zygomatic arch and orbit if necessary to obtain clean borders. Elevate the tissue block and sever any remaining soft tissue attachments to complete the resection. The nasal cavity is exposed. Remove involved nasal turbinates with ronguers and hemostats if disease extends into the nasal cavity. Control hemorrhage by ligating identifiable vessels and applying pressure to other areas. Isolate and ligate the major palatine and infraorbital artery and vein if included in the resection site. Use bone wax or electrofulguration to help control bone hemorrhage. Lavage and inspect the defect to ensure all grossly diseased tissue has been excised. Close the defect by elevating a buccal mucosal flap from the adjacent cheek or lip. Elevate enough buccal mucosa and submucosa to allow a tension-free approximation with the gingival and palatal mucosa. Place the first layer of simple interrupted sutures in the submucosa with the knot directed toward the nasal cavity. Place a second layer of interrupted approximating sutures (i.e., simple, cruciate, vertical) to accurately appose buccal mucosa to the palatal and gingival mucosa. A double-flap technique may be used to close premaxillectomy defects to provide mucosa on

both the nasal and oral surfaces. However, an epithelial surface on the nasal aspect of the flap is not necessary because the connective tissue surface of the flap is covered with respiratory epithelium within 1 to 2 weeks. If carotid artery occlusion was performed, release the occlusion after the defect is closed.

E. Partial Mandibulectomy (*SAS,* pp. 204-207)

1. Indications.
   a. Usually performed to resect an oral neoplasm.
   b. Occasionally mandibular fractures are also treated by partial mandibulectomy.
2. Procedure.

Position the patient in lateral, sternal, or dorsal recumbency with the neck extended. Clip and aseptically prepare the skin of the lateral face and ventral mandible. Flush the mouth with antiseptic solution. Determine the amount to be resected based on size of the soft tissue lesion and radiographic degree of bony involvement. Generally, excise the mass and a minimum of 1 to 2 cm of normal soft tissue and bone on all borders. Retract the commissure and lip to give maximal exposure. If necessary, improve visualization by incising the commissure to the level of the mandibular angle. Begin en bloc resection by first incising mucosa (buccal, gingival, and sublingual) around the diseased area. Using a periosteal elevator, undermine and reflect gingival mucosa to expose the lateral and ventral aspects of the ramus. Transect or elevate and retract muscles (mentalis, orbicularis oris, buccinator, mylohyoideus, geniohyoideus, genioglossus, masseter, digastricus, temporalis, and pterygoideus) attached to the portion of the mandible being resected. Use an oscillating saw or an osteotome and mallet to transect the ramus and separate the symphysis. Alternatively, use a Gigli wire to transect the ramus. Complete a total hemimandibulectomy by incising the joint capsule and disarticulating the temporomandibular joint. Locate the temporomandibular joint by rotating the mandible and palpating the articulation. Ligate or cauterize the mandibular artery. Sever any remaining soft tissue attachments to complete the resection. Avoid traumatizing the lingual frenulum or sublingual and mandibular salivary ducts. Contour the ostectomy sites with bone rongeurs, removing sharp bone and tapering the edges to facilitate closure. Stabilizing the remaining mandible is not necessary. During rostral mandibulectomies, redundant skin and mucosa may be eliminated by excising and apposing V-shaped wedges. The base of the V is along the mucocutaneous junction.

Close the defect by elevating a mucosal flap from the adjacent lip or cheek. Elevate enough mucosa and submucosa to allow a tension-free approximation with the gingival and sublingual mucosa. Place the first layer of simple interrupted sutures in the submucosa with the knots buried. Place a second layer of interrupted approximating sutures (simple, cruciate, or vertical) to accurately appose the labial, sublingual, and gingival mucosa.

Following mandibulectomy, perform cheiloplasty (commissuroplasty) to minimize excessive drooling and lateral protrusion of the tongue if necessary. ***Remove the mucocutaneous junction of the upper and lower lip to the level of the second premolar or canine tooth. Advance the commissure rostrally during closure. Appose the upper and lower lip margins in three layers (oral mucosa, muscle and connective tissue, and skin). Opening the mouth fully during the first 2 weeks may cause dehiscence. Use tension-relieving button sutures or a loose tape muzzle to help prevent this.***

F. Tonsillectomy (*SAS,* pp. 206, 208)

1. Indications.
   a. Neoplasia of the palatine tonsils; squamous cell carcinoma and lymphosarcoma are the most common tumors of the tonsils.

b. Airway obstruction or dysphagia caused by enlarged tonsils may require tonsillectomy.
c. To treat nonresponsive chronic tonsillitis.

2. Procedure.

Administer dexamethasone (1 to 2 mg/kg) at the time of induction to minimize postoperative swelling and edema. Position the animal in ventral recumbency with the maxilla suspended from an IV stand or similar device. Open the mouth maximally and secure it open with tape or gauze. Locate the tonsil in the tonsillar fossa or crypt on the dorsolateral wall of the oropharynx just caudal to the palatoglossal arch. Retract the edge of the tonsillar crypt caudodorsally to expose the tonsil. Grasp the tonsil at its base with an Allis tissue forceps or hemostat and retract it from the crypt. Transect the hilar mucosa at the base of the tonsil with Metzenbaum scissors or a tonsillectomy snare. Ligate the tonsillar artery as it enters the caudal aspect of the tonsil. (Some surgeons excise the tonsil using electrosurgery or laser surgery.) Appose the edges of the tonsillar crypt with a simple continuous suture pattern of 3-0 or 4-0 monofilament absorbable suture to minimize hemorrhage.

G. Glossectomy (*SAS,* pp. 208, 209)

1. Indications
   a. Neoplasia is the most common reason for tongue removal.
      i. Tumors usually occurs on the margin or base of the tongue.
      ii. The most common tongue tumor is squamous cell carcinoma; others include malignant melanoma, granular cell myeloblastoma, and mast cell tumor.
   b. Amputation of 40% to 60% of the rostral tongue is usually well tolerated.
   c. Amputation at the base of the tongue makes eating and drinking difficult; however, intake can be accomplished by learning to suck in food and water or by tossing chunks of food to the base of the tongue.
   d. Most lacerations of the tongue are amenable to repair with a one- or two-layer closure rather than amputation.
2. Procedure.

When performing partial glossectomy, resect the diseased portion of tongue and a minimum of 2 cm of normal tissue after placing a noncrushing clamp across the base of the tongue. Wedge the incision so slightly more tongue muscle than dorsal or ventral mucosa is excised. Control hemorrhage by ligation, pressure, or electrosurgery. Appose the epithelial edges with a simple continuous suture pattern using 3-0 or 4-0 monofilament absorbable suture.

H. Pharyngotomy (*SAS,* p. 209)

1. See Chapter 11.

VII. Suture Materials/Special Instruments

A. Although many suture materials may be used successfully in the oral cavity and oropharynx, 3-0 or 4-0 polydioxanone or polyglyconate (monofilament absorbable) and 3-0 or 4-0 polypropylene or nylon (monofilament nonabsorbable) are preferred.

VIII. Postoperative Care and Assessment

A. Recovery

1. Remove gauze sponges from the caudal pharynx, and suction the nasopharynx.
2. Delay extubation until a well-developed swallowing reflex is present. Recover patients in a slightly head-down position, and remove the tube with the cuff slightly inflated to encourage blood clots to be expelled through the mouth, rather than being aspirated or swallowed.
3. Monitor patients for signs of airway obstruction or pain, and provide analgesics as needed.
4. Use Elizabethan collars or similar restraining devices in some animals to prevent disruption of the surgical site.
5. Use an acrylic oral splint to protect the surgical site if warranted.

B. Oral Intake

1. Do not allow oral intake for the first 8 to 12 hours after surgery (except in pediatric patients who are at risk for hypoglycemia); maintain hydration with intravenous fluids. Offer water after 12 hours and observe the animal for signs of dysphagia, pain, and regurgitation.
2. If no serious problems are identified, offer soft food between 12 and 24 hours after surgery. Gruel is not necessary and may seep between sutures and inhibit healing. Feeding through a gastrostomy, pharyngostomy, or esophagostomy tube is occasionally necessary for animals with severe wounds or those unwilling to eat within 3 days after surgery.
3. Feed soft food until the wound is healed, and prevent the animal from chewing on sticks, toys, or other hard surfaces.

C. Postsurgical Sequelae

1. Maxillectomy.
   a. Consider cheiloplasty to decrease drooling and lateral tongue protrusion in animals after partial maxillectomies.
   b. After maxillectomy, expect epistaxis, serous to mucoid nasal discharge, and pain. Subcutaneous emphysema occasionally occurs when a large portion of the nasal cavity is exposed.
   c. Cosmesis is usually good with a slight facial concavity and lip elevation after lateral maxillectomy.
2. Mandibulectomy.
   a. Cosmesis and function after partial mandibulectomy are good.
   b. Mandibular "drift" and instability occur more often when the osteotomy is caudal to the second premolar. If erosion or ulceration develops, pull or shorten the involved canine tooth.
   c. Rostral mandibulectomy (bilateral) caudal to the third or fourth premolar may cause difficulty with prehension and is less cosmetic.

Congenital Oronasal Fistula (Cleft Palate) (*SAS*, pp. 211-216)

I. Definitions

A. A **congenital oronasal fistula** is an abnormal communication between the oral and nasal cavities involving the soft palate, hard palate, premaxilla, or lip.

B. Incomplete closure of the primary palate (lip and premaxilla) is a **primary cleft** or **cleft lip** (harelip).

C. Incomplete closure of the hard or soft palate is a **secondary cleft** or **cleft palate.**

II. General Considerations

A. Primary cleft palate alone is rare; however, secondary cleft palate may occur alone or in combination with primary clefts.

B. Secondary clefts are often undiagnosed at birth.

III. Diagnosis

A. Clinical Presentation

1. Signalment.
   a. Dogs, particularly brachycephalic breeds, are more commonly affected with cleft palate than cats.
   b. Purebred dogs have a higher incidence than mixed breeds.
   c. Breeds at high risk for cleft palate include Boston terrier, Pekingese, bulldog, miniature schnauzer, beagle, cocker spaniel, and dachshund.
   d. Siamese cats have a higher incidence than other cat breeds.
2. History.
   a. A history of difficulty nursing, nasal regurgitation, nasal discharge, and failure to thrive are common problems.
   b. Signs related to incomplete separation of the oral and nasal cavity include drainage of milk from the nares during or after nursing; gagging, coughing, or sneezing while eating; poor growth; and respiratory infection (e.g., rhinitis, aspiration pneumonia).

B. Physical Examination Findings

1. Check all puppies and kittens for evidence of a cleft palate on initial presentation.
2. A thorough oral exam is required to identify incomplete closure of the premaxilla, hard palate, or soft palate. Anesthesia may be necessary to thoroughly assess the soft palate.
3. A secondary cleft may occur without a primary cleft.
4. Patients may be thin and stunted.
5. Auscult for abnormal respiratory sounds, which will be present with aspiration pneumonia.
6. Carefully evaluate affected neonates for concurrent congenital anomalies.

IV. Medical Management

A. Tube feed affected patients to maintain an adequate nutritional status and to decrease the incidence of aspiration pneumonia until they are old enough for surgery.

B. Treat aspiration pneumonia with antibiotics, fluids, oxygen, bronchodilators, or expectorants. Perform a tracheal wash with culture and sensitivity if aspiration pneumonia is severe.

C. For severe aspiration or purulent rhinitis, administer broad-spectrum antibiotics with efficacy against anaerobes (e.g., trimethoprim-sulfadiazine, ampicillin, clindamycin).

V. Surgical Treatment

A. General Considerations

1. Most animals with defects of the primary and secondary palate are euthanized or die.
2. Delay surgical treatment until the patient is at least 8 to 12 weeks of age in order to allow growth and easier access to the palate.
3. Multiple procedures may be necessary before the entire cleft is permanently reconstructed.
4. Neuter affected patients.

B. Preoperative Management

1. Do not fast pediatric patients more than 4 to 8 hours.
2. Feed poorly nourished animals through a gastrostomy or esophagostomy tube for several days before surgery.
3. Flush the nasal and oral cavities with saline and a dilute antiseptic solution.
4. If the animal is not on antibiotics, give perioperative antibiotics intravenously at induction.

C. Anesthesia

1. Use guarded tracheostomy tubes to prevent kinking during the procedure.
2. Take care to prevent and recognize dislodgement of the anesthetic tubing from the endotracheal tube during oral manipulations.

D. Positioning

1. Place the animal in dorsal recumbency with the mouth maximally opened to facilitate repair of a secondary palate.
2. Position the animal in ventral or dorsal recumbency to repair a primary palate.

VI. Surgical Techniques

A. Closure of Hard Palate Defects

1. Sliding bipedical flap method.
   a. The disadvantage of this technique is that the repair is unsupported and directly over the defect.
   b. Procedure.

Incise the margins of the defect and make bilateral releasing incisions along the margins of the dental arcade, lateral to the palatine arteries. Elevate the mucoperiosteal layer on both sides of the defect with a periosteal elevator. Avoid damaging the major palatine arteries. Control hemorrhage with pressure and suction. Appose the nasal mucosal edges or periosteum at the margin of the defect with buried interrupted sutures (knots within the nasal cavity), if possible. Slide the elevated mucoperiosteal flaps across the defect and appose with simple interrupted sutures. Allow the denuded hard palate near the dental arcades to heal by second intention.

2. Overlapping flap method.
   a. This technique is advantageous because it does not place the repair over the palate defect.
   b. Procedure.

Incise one margin of the defect separating the oral and nasal mucosa. Elevate the mucoperiosteum at this edge approximately 5 mm. At the opposite side of the defect create a mucoperiosteal rotational flap large enough to cover the defect with its base hinged at the margin of the palatal defect. Begin the incision near and parallel to the dental arcade creating a flap 2 to 4 mm larger than the defect. Make perpendicular incisions at the rostral and caudal end of the incision extending to the cleft. Elevate this mucoperiosteal flap being careful not to disrupt the margin of the defect. Dissect carefully around the palatine artery to release it from fibrous tissue. Rotate the flap across the defect. Place the edge of the flap under the mucoperiosteal flap on the opposite side. Preplace and then tie a series of horizontal mattress sutures to secure the flaps in position.

B. Closure of Soft Palate Defects

1. An overlapping flap technique, rotational flaps from the hard or soft palate, or nasopharyngeal mucosal flaps can also be used to repair soft palate defects.
2. Procedure.

Close soft palate clefts by first incising the margins of the cleft to separate the oral and nasal mucosa. Continue incisions made in the margins of hard palate clefts caudally into the soft palate. Isolate the nasal mucosa, palatal muscles, and oral mucosa. Appose the palatal edges in three layers beginning caudally and working rostrally to a point adjacent to the caudal or midpoint of the tonsil. First appose the nasal mucosa using a series of simple interrupted sutures with nasally oriented knots or use a simple continuous pattern. Then appose the palatal muscle and connective tissue mucosa with a simple continuous suture pattern. Last, appose the oral mucosa with a simple continuous or interrupted suture pattern. Make tension-relieving incisions in the oral mucosa from the lingual aspect of the last molar to near the tip of the soft palate.

C. Closure of Primary Clefts

Create a mucosal flap to separate the nasal from the oral cavity. If the cleft extends into the premaxilla, evaluate the position of the deciduous incisors and pull them if necessary. Suture the buccal or gingival mucosal flap to the nasal mucosa. Use a free-hand modified Z-plasty for reconstruction of the lip defect (see Chapter 13). Close the lip defect so the distance from the ventral nostril to the free ventral edge of the lip is the same on both sides. Make multiple small flaps if necessary for a cosmetic closure. Place a layer of sutures in the fibromuscular layer (orbicularis oris muscle and connective tissue) before skin closure.

VII. Postoperative Care and Assessment

A. Feed soft food for a minimum of 2 weeks after surgery, and prevent chewing on hard objects (e.g., bones, sticks, chew toys).

B. Gastrostomy or esophagostomy feeding for 7 to 14 days may facilitate healing.

VIII. Prognosis

A. The prognosis is good for animals with successful cleft palate repair; however, multiple surgeries may be required.

B. Chronic rhinitis and aspiration pneumonia persist if large defects are not repaired.

C. Untreated patients with small clefts may have few clinical signs.

Acquired Oronasal Fistulae (*SAS*, pp. 216-222)

I. Definitions

A. **Acquired oronasal fistulae** are abnormal communications between the nasal and oral cavity caused by trauma or disease.

II. General Considerations and Clinically Relevant Pathophysiology

A. Acquired palatal defects are most frequently caused by dental disease.

B. An oronasal fistula may also result from trauma or be a complication of surgery, radiation, or hyperthermic treatment of oral lesions.

C. Foreign bodies lodged between the dental arcades may cause pressure necrosis of the hard palate and subsequent oronasal fistula.

D. Ingested food that passes through the fistula into the nasal cavity may be expelled from the nostril by sneezing. Chronic rhinitis is common.

III. Diagnosis

A. Clinical Presentation

1. Signalment.
   a. Any breed or sex may acquire an oronasal fistula.
   b. Oronasal fistulae secondary to dental disease or tumors are seen more often in middle-aged to older animals.
   c. Oronasal fistulae secondary to trauma may occur at any age.
2. History.
   a. Oronasal fistula should be suspected in patients with chronic rhinitis and a history of dental disease, trauma, or previously treated oral tumors.
   b. Common clinical signs are sneezing and chronic unilateral serous or mucopurulent nasal discharge.

B. Physical Examination Findings

1. Diagnosis can be made by identifying an abnormal communication between the oral and nasal cavities.
2. Small fistulae associated with periodontal disease are not easily identified unless the area around the involved tooth is explored with a narrow dental probe. If passing the probe into the gingival pocket causes epistaxis, a fistula is present.

C. Radiography/Ultrasonography

1. Skull radiographs may identify underlying causes of fistulae, such as periapical abscesses, advanced periodontal disease, maxillary neoplasia, or broken and retained tooth roots.

IV. Surgical Treatment

A. Surgical Options and Considerations

1. Most oronasal fistulae require surgical reconstruction, although small or traumatic fistulae occasionally heal spontaneously.
2. Extract teeth involved in the fistula several weeks before reconstruction of the defect (at least 5 mm from each margin), to allow removal of necrotic or diseased bone.
3. Traumatic oronasal fistulae may require stabilization of the maxilla and hard palate with small pins or wire.

B. Preoperative Management

1. Do not fast pediatric patients for longer than 4 to 8 hours.
2. After anesthetic induction, flush the nasal and oral cavities with saline-diluted antiseptic solution.
3. Aggressive medical management of rhinitis may decrease infection and improve suture-holding capability of tissues.

C. Positioning

1. Position the patient in lateral recumbency to repair oronasal fistulae associated with the dental arcade.
2. Use dorsal recumbency with the mouth opened maximally to facilitate the repair of more centrally located fistulae involving the secondary palate.

D. Surgical Technique

1. General considerations.
   a. Perform direct apposition of the fistula only if the fistula is very small.
   b. Consider a double-flap technique with large dental fistulae and fistulae located in more central areas of the palate.
2. Procedures.
   a. Direct apposition.

Debride the fistula to healthy, bleeding mucosal edges. Incise or debride the margin of the fistula and elevate the edges enough to allow approximation without excess tension. Appose mucosa with interrupted appositional sutures (i.e., simple, cruciate, or vertical mattress).

   b. Single-layer flap repair.

Debride the epithelial margin of the fistula. Incise the gingival and buccal mucosa to outline a flap 2 to 4 mm larger than the debrided fistula. Make these incisions perpendicular to the dental arcade. Elevate the gingival mucosa with

a periosteal elevator. Then undermine the buccal mucosa until the flap can be advanced across the defect without tension. Using a rongeur, remove infected alveolar and maxillary bone. Expose approximately 1 to 2 mm of the hard palate at the medial aspect of the fistula by excising 1 to 2 mm of mucoperiosteum. Lavage the surgical site with saline. Suture the gingival-buccal flap to the mucoperiosteum of the hard palate using interrupted approximating (i.e., simple, cruciate, or vertical mattress) monofilament, absorbable sutures.

c. Rotational flap repair.

A rotational or advancement flap may be created from the hard palate or soft palate, or an overlapping technique similar to that described for repair of congenital oronasal fistulae may be used. Do not debride the palatal epithelial margin during debridement of the fistula because this edge serves as the base of the mucoperiosteal flap and must remain continuous with the nasal mucosa to be effective. Create a flap in the mucoperiosteum 2 to 4 mm larger than the debrided fistula. Elevate the flap without disrupting the palatal margin of the fistula. Fold the flap over the defect and suture it to the gingival mucosa with interrupted, approximating, monofilament, absorbable sutures. Granulation tissue fills the defect over the hard palate, and the area reepithelializes within a few weeks.

d. Double-flap repair.

Allow the extraction sites to heal before reconstruction. Create one or two mucoperiosteal flaps, 2 to 4 mm larger than the defect. To ensure a good blood supply, incorporate the major palatine artery in palatal flaps. Transpose and suture the flap in place for the first layer of the closure. This flap provides "nasal" mucosa. Cover this layer with a mucosal flap (gingival and buccal) to provide the "oral" mucosal layer of the closure. Allow the denuded hard palate to heal by second intention.

V. Postoperative Care and Assessment

A. Provide intravenous fluids until the animal begins eating and drinking (usually within 24 hours of surgery).

B. Feed soft food for 2 to 3 weeks, and prevent chewing on hard objects (e.g., toys, sticks) to avoid dehiscence or perforation of the flap separating the oral and nasal cavities.

C. If the animal paws at the mouth, use an Elizabethan collar.

D. Treat severe rhinitis with antibiotics if not resolved preoperatively.

E. Evaluate healing 2 and 4 weeks postoperatively.

VI. Prognosis

A. Traumatic clefts may heal spontaneously in 2 to 4 weeks.

B. The long-term prognosis for most patients with nontraumatic fistulae is poor when surgical correction is not possible because these fistulae do not heal without surgical reconstruction.

Oral Tumors (*SAS*, pp. 222-227)

I. Definitions

A. Oral tumors encompass those neoplasms that arise from gingiva, buccal mucosa, labial mucosa, tongue, tonsil, or dental elements.

II. General Considerations and Clinically Relevant Pathophysiology

A. The most common malignant canine tumors are malignant melanoma, squamous cell carcinoma, and fibrosarcoma, whereas squamous cell carcinoma is the most common malignant oral feline tumor.
  1. Malignant melanomas (Table 16-1) are the most frequently occurring malignant oral tumor in dogs; they rarely occur in cats.
  2. Squamous cell carcinomas (SCC) (Table 16-2) are the most common malignant oral tumors of cats and the second most common malignant oral tumor in dogs. The masses are red, friable, vascular, and sometimes ulcerated.

Table 16-1
Characteristics of oral malignant melanomas

- Most common malignant oral tumor in dogs (~20%)
- Rare in cats
- Most common on gingiva
- More common in male dogs
- Mean age of affected animals is 9 to 11 years (10.3)
- Breeds with pigmented oral mucosa, cocker spaniels, and German shepherds may be predisposed
- Metastasis is common
- Prognosis is poor; median survival is 8 to 9 months

Table 16-2
Characteristics of oral squamous cell carcinomas

- Most common tumor in cats (~70%)
- Second most common tumor in dogs (with fibrosarcoma) (~15%)
- Occur on gingiva, lip, tongue, or tonsil
- Biological behavior varies with location and species; regional lymph node involvement common with tongue and tonsillar SCC

3. Fibrosarcomas (Table 16-3) are primarily found in dogs. They most commonly occur on the maxillary gingiva and hard palate and appear as pink-red, firm, smooth, multilobulated masses that are often attached to underlying tissue.
4. Osteosarcomas make up approximately 10% of canine mandibular and maxillary tumors.

B. Benign oral tumors are rare in cats. The most common benign oral neoplasms in dogs are epulides (Table 16-4).

1. Oral papillomas are benign tumors that are caused by a papillomavirus or papovavirus in young dogs. They occur primarily on the buccal and gingival mucosa, appearing as multiple gray-white pedunculated lesions.

III. Diagnosis

A. Clinical Presentation

1. Signalment.
   a. Breeds that appear to be predisposed to oral tumors include boxers, German shepherds, golden retrievers, cocker spaniels, German shorthaired pointers, collies, Old English sheepdogs, and weimaraners.
   b. Oral tumors are generally observed in middle-aged and older animals. Exceptions to this include oral papillomatosis, which occurs in dogs 1 year old or less, and fibrosarcoma, which has a mean age of occurrence of approximately 5 years.
   c. Melanomas are more common in males with an average onset age of 9 to 11 years. Breeds with pigmented oral mucosa and cocker spaniels and German shepherds appear to have an increased incidence.

Table 16-3
Characteristics of oral fibrosarcomas

- Second most common malignant oral tumor in dogs (with squamous cell carcinoma)
- Occur most commonly on gingiva and hard palate
- More common in large breeds (i.e., >20 kg), male dogs
- Younger dogs may be affected (mean age <7 years)
- Locally invasive; high metastatic potential in dogs <2 years of age

Table 16-4
Characteristics of epulides

- Most common oral tumor in dogs (~30%)
- Mean age ~8.2 years
- More common in large breed (i.e., >20 kg) dogs
- Do not metastasize
- Acanthomatous epulis most common form

d. Squamous cell carcinomas are common in cats of either sex that are older than 10 years. Nontonsillar squamous cell carcinomas are most common in small-breed dogs of either sex between 8 and 10 years of age.
e. Fibrosarcomas occur more commonly in large breed dogs, particularly Dobermans and golden retrievers. Males are affected more frequently than females (2:1).

2. History.
   a. Oral tumors are often large when recognized by an owner; however, some are found during yearly examinations or routine dentistry.
   b. Affected animals frequently present for evaluation of a visible mass, oral bleeding, difficulty eating, or halitosis.

B. Physical Examination Findings

1. General anesthesia is often necessary to define the extent of disease.
2. Evaluate regional lymph nodes for evidence of enlargement, nodularity, and adherence to surrounding tissue.

C. Radiography

1. Perform thoracic radiographs to look for pulmonary metastasis and concurrent pulmonary or cardiovascular disease.
2. Perform skull radiographs under general anesthesia and assess the extent of the lesion and bony involvement.

IV. Medical Management

A. Cytologic analysis of the tumor and draining lymph nodes is indicated before surgery.

B. Refer to a medicine text for nonsurgical treatment of oral neoplasia.

V. Surgical Treatment

A. General Considerations

1. Because most gingival tumors invade bone, mandibulectomy or maxillectomy is usually necessary.
2. Shaving the tumor down to bone will generally result in recurrence.

B. Preoperative Management

1. Perioperative antibiotics are indicated for oral tumors, which often have focal areas of necrosis and infection.
2. Debilitated animals require intravenous fluids and enteral or parenteral hyperalimentation before surgery.

C. Positioning

1. Resect mandibular lesions with the patient in lateral recumbency.
2. Resect maxillary lesions with the patient in lateral or ventral recumbency.

D. Surgical Technique

Identify the soft tissue or bone to be resected and remove it according to the techniques for maxillectomy, mandibulectomy, glossectomy, and tonsillectomy. After mandibulectomy or maxillectomy but before closure you may radiograph

the excised segment to help determine whether adequate bone was removed; however, tumor growth up the mandibular foramen may necessitate wider margins than radiographic evaluation of bone destruction might predict. If available, intraoperative cytology is often more beneficial in determining the adequacy of resection. Submit excised tissues for histologic analysis. If additional bone is excised mark the caudal border to allow determination of whether additional resection is needed (i.e., if this margin contains tumor).

VI. Postoperative Care and Assessment

A. Remove sponges from the caudal oropharynx, and suction the oral cavity and nasopharynx before anesthetic recovery.

B. Offer soft food and water the day after surgery.

C. Discontinue intravenous fluids when the animal maintains hydration by drinking.

VII. Prognosis

A. Dogs with tumors rostral to the maxillary canine or the first mandibular premolar teeth have a better prognosis. This may be because of earlier recognition, altered tumor behavior based on location, or prevalence of tumor type.

B. Squamous cell carcinomas respond best to surgery because they are localized and usually have not metastasized. Fibrosarcomas are localized but locally aggressive and are often difficult to completely resect. Melanomas have the poorest prognosis because they metastasize early. Tumors arising from the tongue have a poor prognosis.

Salivary Mucoceles (*SAS*, pp. 227-232)

I. Definitions

A. A **salivary mucocele** is a collection of saliva that has leaked from a damaged salivary gland or duct and is surrounded by granulation tissue.

B. A **cervical mucocele** is a collection of saliva in the deeper structures of the intermandibular space, the angle of the jaw, or the upper cervical region.

C. A **sublingual mucocele** or **ranula** is a collection of saliva in the sublingual tissue caudal to the openings of the sublingual and mandibular ducts.

D. A **pharyngeal mucocele** is a collection of saliva in the tissues adjacent to the pharynx.

E. A **zygomatic mucocele** is a collection of saliva ventral to the globe.

F. **Marsupialization** is the process of incising a mucocele and suturing the edges to the mucosa.

II. General Considerations and Clinically Relevant Pathophysiology

A. Tearing of a salivary gland or duct results in leakage of saliva into the surrounding tissue.

B. Salivary mucoceles are not cysts.

C. The sublingual salivary gland is most commonly involved.

III. Diagnosis

A. Clinical Presentation

1. Signalment.
   a. Dogs are more frequently affected than cats.
   b. All breeds are susceptible, but some reports indicate that poodles, German shepherds, dachshunds, and Australian silky terriers are more commonly affected.
   c. There is a slight predisposition for males to be affected.
2. History.
   a. Clinical signs depend on the location of the mucocele.
   b. Respiratory distress and dysphagia are common in patients with pharyngeal mucoceles.

B. Physical Examination Findings

1. Most mucoceles are soft and fluctuant, while tumors and abscesses are generally firm.
2. Mucoceles are nonpainful except during the acute phase of swelling.
3. Examining these animals in dorsal recumbency often allows the mucocele to gravitate to the affected side.
4. Blood-tinged saliva may occur in patients with sublingual mucoceles because teeth often traumatize the mucocele.

C. Radiography

1. Sialography, the injection of an iodinated water-soluble contrast agent into a salivary duct, is difficult and usually unnecessary to confirm the diagnosis or determine the site of origin.

D. Laboratory Findings

1. Aspiration of a clear, yellowish, or blood-tinged, ropey, mucoid fluid with a low cell count is consistent with saliva.

IV. Surgical Treatment

A. General Considerations

1. Medical management will not resolve the lesion.
2. Completely excise the involved gland-duct complex and drain the mucocele.

B. Preoperative Management

1. Animals with pharyngeal mucoceles may present in acute respiratory distress, and rapid intubation may be necessary. Intubation may not be possible through the mouth. A temporary tracheostomy may be required.

C. Surgical Anatomy

1. The parotid salivary gland is triangular and located just ventral to the ear canal; its duct opens in the labial mucosa at the level of the upper carnassial tooth.
2. The mandibular salivary gland is ovoid and located ventral to the parotid gland; its duct opens on a papilla lateral to the rostral border of the frenulum.
3. The sublingual salivary gland is located in several lobes along the mandibular salivary duct; its duct opens with the mandibular duct.
4. The zygomatic salivary gland is located ventral to the orbit and medial to the zygomatic arch; its duct opens lateral to the last upper molar tooth.

D. Positioning

1. Perform salivary gland excision with the animal in lateral recumbency.
2. Use ventral recumbency and maximal opening of the mouth to facilitate marsupialization of pharyngeal mucoceles and ranulas.

E. Surgical Technique

1. General considerations.
   a. The mandibular and sublingual salivary glands are excised together because the sublingual gland is intimately associated with the mandibular salivary gland duct; removal of one would traumatize the other.
2. Mandibular and sublingual salivary gland excision.

Position the patient in lateral recumbency. Place a pad under the neck to rotate the ventral aspect dorsally and fix the neck in an extended position. Locate the mandibular salivary gland between the linguofacial and maxillary veins as they join the external jugular vein. Incise skin, subcutaneous tissue, and platysma muscle from the angle of the mandible caudally to the external jugular vein to expose the fibrous capsule of the mandibular gland. Avoiding the branch of the second cervical nerve that crosses the capsule, incise the capsule and dissect it away from the mandibular and monostomatic sublingual salivary glands. Ligate the artery (branch of the great auricular artery) and vein as they are encountered on the dorsomedial aspect of the gland. Continue dissecting cranially, following the mandibular duct, sublingual duct, and polystomatic sublingual glands toward the mouth. Incise the fascia between the masseter and digastricus muscles. Expose the entire mandibular and sublingual salivary gland complex by retracting the digastricus muscle and applying caudal traction on the mandibular gland. If necessary, perform digastricus muscle myotomy or tunnel the caudal sublingual gland duct complex under the digastricus muscle to improve visualization. Dissect (digital and sharp) rostrally until the lingual branch of the trigeminal nerve is identified and only ducts remain in the complex. Avoid traumatizing the lingual or hypoglossal nerves. Try to identify the gland-duct defect causing the mucocele because failure to identify this defect may indicate that the mucocele originated from the contralateral gland-duct complex. Ligate and transect the mandibular sublingual gland-duct complex just caudal to the lingual nerve. Traction on the gland-duct complex may cause the ducts to tear. If this occurs near the point of proposed transection or on the oral aspect of the gland-duct defect, no further dissection is needed. However, if the tear occurs before the gland-duct defect, no further

dissection is needed. However, if the tear ocurs before the gland-duct defect or when the defect is not identified and glandular tissue is identified oral to the tear, further resection of glandular tissue is recommended to prevent recurrence. Lavage the surgical site before closure. Appose the digastric muscle if it has been incised with horizontal mattress or cruciate sutures. Close the dead space with a few sutures in the capsule and deep tissue. Routinely appose superficial muscles, subcutaneous tissue, and skin. Following excision, submit the glands and ducts to rule out neoplasia, and submit a portion of the mucocele wall to rule out congenital cysts.

3. Mucocele reduction.

Drain cervical mucoceles by making a stab incision at the most dependent point; place a Penrose drain if desired. Protect the drain with an absorbent bandage. Change the bandage and cleanse discharge from the neck as needed to prevent excoriation of the skin. Maintain the drain for 1 to 5 days, removing it when there is minimal discharge. Allow the stab incision to heal by second intention. Redundant skin resumes its normal appearance within several weeks. Drain sublingual mucoceles (ranula) by excising an elliptical full-thickness section of the mucocele wall. Suture the granulation tissue lining to the sublingual mucosa (marsupialization) to encourage drainage for several days. Drain pharyngeal mucoceles by aspiration or marsupialization. Excise redundant pharyngeal tissue to prevent airway obstruction after evacuation of the mucocele. **Marsupialized ranulas contract and heal quickly by second intention. After bilateral mandibular and sublingual salivary gland excision, dogs still have sufficient saliva to adequately moisten their food.**

4. Zygomatic gland excision.

Position the patient in lateral or ventral recumbency. Protect the animal's eye from irritants with ophthalmic ointment. Incise skin and subcutaneous tissues over the dorsal rim of the zygomatic arch. Incise the palpebral fascia, retractor anguli oculi muscle, and orbital ligament and elevate them dorsally with the skin and globe. Further expose the gland by partially removing the zygomatic arch via rongeurs or osteotomy. Retract the globe dorsally to expose the periorbital fat and underlying zygomatic gland. Remove the gland by blunt dissection (the gland is friable). Avoid the ventrally located anastomotic branch between the deep facial and external ophthalmic veins. Drain the mucocele if present. If possible, replace the zygomatic arch by securing the bone with suture placed through predrilled holes. Lavage the area and appose the palpebral fascia to the zygomatic periosteum with sutures. Close subcutaneous tissues and skin.

5. Parotid gland excision.

Position the patient in lateral recumbency. Incise skin from 1 to 2 cm ventral to the external acoustic meatus to a point midway between the ramus of the mandible and the bifurcation of the jugular vein. Incise the platysma muscle to expose the parotidoauricularis muscle, vertical ear canal, and parotid salivary gland. Sever and retract the parotidoauricularis muscle from its vertical ear canal attachment. Ligate and divide the caudal auricular vein. Begin dissection of the parotid gland at its dorsocaudal angle. Separate the parotid from the mandibular gland ventrally. Continue dissection between the gland and the vertical ear canal. Avoid traumatizing the facial nerve at the base of the horizontal ear canal. Ligate and divide the superficial temporal vein (a branch of the maxillary vein) coursing through the gland. Cauterize or ligate small vessels on the gland's medial surface. Ligate and transect the parotid duct as it leaves the

gland. Lavage the area. Reappose the parotidoauricularis muscle. Complete closure by apposing subcutaneous tissues and skin.

V. Postoperative Care and Assessment

A. Change bandages daily if a Penrose drain has been placed. Remove the drain 24 to 72 hours after surgery. Allow the drain site to heal by second intention.

B. Feed soft food for 3 to 5 days following ranula marsupialization or excision of pharyngeal mucoceles.

VI. Prognosis

A. Rarely, a mucocele will resolve without surgery.

B. The prognosis is excellent if the disease is accurately diagnosed and excision is complete.

Surgery of the Esophagus (*SAS*, pp. 232-261)

I. Definitions

A. **Esophagotomy** is an incision into the esophageal lumen; **esophagectomy** is partial resection of the esophagus.

B. **Regurgitation** is the passive expulsion of undigested food or fluid from the esophagus.

C. **Vomiting** is a centrally mediated reflex causing expulsion of food or fluid from the stomach, duodenum, or both.

II. General Considerations and Clinically Relevant Pathophysiology

A. The predominant clinical signs of esophageal pathology are regurgitation and dysphagia. The patient's appetite may be normal, ravenous, or depressed. Undigested food may be regurgitated with either partial or complete obstructions. Partial esophageal obstruction causes progressive emaciation.

B. Esophageal perforations may cause septic mediastinitis evidenced by fever, pleural effusion, respiratory distress, and eventual death.

III. Diagnosis

A. Assess plain radiographs of the esophagus extending from the caudal portion of the oral cavity to the stomach for radiopaque foreign bodies, esophageal size and location, periesophageal fluid or gas densities, and the presence or absence of aspiration pneumonia.

B. Flouroscopy. Use aqueous iodine or Iohexol, rather than barium, if esophageal perforation is suspected.

C. Esophagoscopy allows mucosal lesions to be biopsied and foreign bodies to be removed or advanced into the stomach.

IV. Preoperative Concerns

A. Treat aspiration pneumonia (Table 16-5) and esophagitis (Table 16-6) before surgery.

V. Anesthetic Considerations

A. Correct fluid, electrolyte, and acid-base imbalances before anesthetic induction.

B. If feasible, fast mature animals 12 to 18 hours before esophageal surgery; fast young puppies and kittens for shorter periods (4 to 8 hours) to prevent hypoglycemia.

C. See Appendix G-5 for anesthetic protocols for animals undergoing esophageal surgery.

VI. Antibiotics

A. Give perioperative antibiotics to prevent infection of periesophageal tissues (see Chapter 10).

B. Use broad-spectrum antibiotics effective against anaerobes (e.g., ampicillin, cephalosporins). Treat animals with preoperative perforation or severe esophageal trauma with therapeutic antibiotics.

VII. Surgical Anatomy

A. The cervical and proximal thoracic portions of the esophagus lie to the left of midline; however, the esophagus lies slightly to the right of midline from the tracheal bifurcation to the stomach.

B. Layers of the esophageal wall include mucosa, submucosa, muscularis, and adventitia. The esophagus has no serosa; therefore early fibrin sealing of esophagotomy sites may be slower than other areas of the gastrointestinal tract.

Table 16-5
Treatment of aspiration pneumonia

Aminophylline

Dogs—11 mg/kg PO, IM, IV, TID

Cats—5 mg/kg PO, BID

Oxtriphylline Elixir (Choledyl SA)

Dogs—14-15 mg/kg PO, TID

Cats—6-8 mg/kg PO, BID to TID

Terbutaline (Brethine, Bricanyl)

Dogs—1.25-5.0 mg/dog SC, PO, BID to TID

Cats—1.25 mg/cat SC, PO, BID

Ampicillin

22 mg/kg IV, IM, SC, PO, TID to QID

Cefazolin (Ancef, Kefzol)

20 mg/kg IV, IM, TID

Clindamycin (Antirobe, Cleocin)

11 mg/kg PO, IV, BID

Enrofloxacin (Baytril)

5-10 mg/kg PO, IV, BID

Amikacin (Amiglyde-V)

10 mg/kg IV, IM, SC, TID or 30 mg/kg SID

Trimethoprim-Sulfadiazine (Tribrissen)

Dogs—15 mg/kg IM, PO, BID

Cats—15 mg/kg PO, BID

Table 16-6
Treatment of esophagitis

Cimetidine (Tagamet)

10 mg/kg PO, IV, SC, TID to QID

Ranitidine (Zantac)

2 mg/kg PO, IV, IM, BID

Famotidine (Pepcid)

0.5 mg/kg PO, SID to BID

Omeprazole (Prilosec)

0.7-1.5 mg/kg PO, SID

Sucralfate (Carafate)*

0.5-1.0 g PO, TID to QID

Cisapride (Propulsid)

Dogs—0.25-0.5 mg/kg PO, BID to TID

Cats—2.5-5.0 mg/cat PO, BID to TID

*Carafate impairs absorption or reduces bioavailability of metidine; give at different intervals.

C. The submucosa is the holding layer of the esophagus; it must be incorporated with all sutures.

VIII. Surgical Techniques

A. Approach to the Cervical Esophagus

Position the patient in dorsal recumbency. Incise skin on the midline, beginning at the larynx and extending caudally to the manubrium. Incise and retract the platysma muscle and subcutaneous tissues. Separate the paired sternohyoid muscles along the midline to expose the underlying trachea. Retract the thyroidea ima vein with the sternohyoid muscle or ligate it. If access is needed to the caudal cervical esophagus, separate and retract the sternocephalicus muscles. Retract the trachea to the right to expose the adjacent anatomic structures, including the esophagus, the thyroid gland, cranial and caudal thyroid vessels, the recurrent laryngeal nerve, and the carotid sheath (vagosympathetic trunk, carotid artery, and internal jugular vein). Pass a stomach tube or esophageal stethoscope to facilitate identification of the esophagus and lesion. After completing the definitive procedure, lavage the surgical site with warmed sterile saline and return the trachea to its normal position. Close the incision by apposing the sternohyoid muscles using absorbable suture material (3-0 or 4-0) in a simple continuous suture pattern. Appose subcutaneous tissues with a simple continuous pattern (3-0 or 4-0) of absorbable suture material. Use nonabsorbable sutures (3-0 or 4-0 monofilament) and an appositional suture pattern to appose skin.

B. Approach to the Cranial Thoracic Esophagus via a Lateral Intercostal Thoracotomy

Position the patient in right lateral recumbency over a rolled towel placed perpendicular to the long axis of the body. Choose the appropriate intercostal space incision based on the radiographic location of the abnormality. Most abnormalities cranial to the heart base can be accessed through a left third or fourth intercostal space incision (see Chapter 26). Identify the esophagus in the mediastinum dorsal to the brachiocephalic trunk. Identification may be aided by passage of a stomach tube or by palpating the abnormality. Dissect the mediastinal pleura overlapping the esophagus to just above and below the proposed surgical site. Preserve the branch of the internal thoracic vein and the costocervical vein that crosses the cranial esophagus.

C. Approach to the Esophagus at the Heart Base via a Right Lateral Thoracotomy

Use the same approach as that for the cranial esophagus except make the incision through the right fourth or fifth intercostal space. Identify the esophagus located just dorsal to the trachea in the mediastinum. Dissect and retract the azygous vein from the esophagus to allow adequate exposure. Ligate the azygous vein if necessary to adequately expose the esophagus. Closure is the same as for cranial thoracotomy.

D. Approach to the Caudal Esophagus via a Caudal Lateral Thoracotomy

Position the patient in lateral recumbency as described above for cranial lateral thoracotomy. Perform a caudal lateral thoracotomy. Although the caudal

esophagus can be approached through either a left or right eighth or ninth intercostal space incision, the left ninth space is preferred. Expose the caudal esophagus by transecting the pulmonary ligament and packing the caudal lung lobes cranially. Identify the esophagus just ventral to the aorta. Identify the dorsal and ventral vagal nerve branches on the lateral aspect of the esophagus and protect them.

E. Esophagotomy

Pack off the esophagus from the remainder of the field with moistened laparotomy pads. Suction material from the cranial esophagus before making the esophagotomy incision to minimize contamination of the surgical site. If ingesta and secretions have not been completely suctioned, occlude the lumen cranial and caudal to the proposed esophagotomy site with fingers or noncrushing forceps. Place stay sutures adjacent to the proposed incision site to stabilize, aid manipulation, and avoid trauma to the esophageal edges. Make a stab incision into the lumen of the esophagus and extend the incision longitudinally as necessary to remove the foreign body or observe the lumen. Make the incision over the foreign body if the esophageal wall appears normal. If the wall appears compromised, make the incision caudal to the lesion or foreign body. Remove foreign bodies with forceps, taking care to avoid further esophageal trauma (tearing or perforation). Examine the esophageal lumen. Obtain culture specimens from necrotic and perforated areas. Debride and close perforations surrounded by healthy tissue that involve less than one fourth the circumference of the esophagus. Identify large necrotic areas or extensive perforations and perform a resection and anastomosis (see below).

Use either a one- or two-layer closure. A two-layer simple interrupted closure results in greater immediate wound strength, better tissue apposition, and improved healing after esophagotomy but takes longer to perform than single-layer techniques. *Place each suture approximately 2 mm from the edge and 2 mm apart. Incorporate the mucosa and submucosa in the first layer of a two-layer simple interrupted closure. Place sutures so that the knots are within the esophageal lumen. Incorporate adventitia, muscularis, and submucosa in the second layer of sutures with the knots tied extraluminally. When a one-layer closure is used, pass each suture through all layers of the esophageal wall and tie the knots on the extraluminal surface. Check closure integrity by occluding the lumen, injecting saline, applying pressure, and observing for leakage between sutures.*

F. Partial Esophagectomy

1. Although 20% to 50% of the esophagus has been resected and primarily anastomosed without tension-relieving techniques, resection of more than 3 to 5 cm risks anastomotic dehiscence.
2. Circumferential myotomy is a partial-thickness myotomy through the longitudinal muscle layers 2 to 3 cm cranial and caudal to the anastomosis. Do not incise the inner circular muscle layers to avoid damaging the submucosal blood supply.
3. Esophageal replacement may be necessary if segments of more than 3 to 5 cm are resected.
4. Esophectomy.

Occlude and stabilize the esophagus with fingers (scissor action of middle and index fingers) or noncrushing forceps. Resect the diseased portion of the esophagus. Suction debris from the lumen of the remaining esophagus. Place three equally spaced stay sutures at each end of the remaining esophagus to facilitate gentle handling of the esophagus and help maintain apposition and alignment of the transected ends. Bring the esophageal ends into apposition

with the stay sutures and suture it using a one- or two-layer closure as described for esophagotomy. Place sutures in the contralateral (far) wall first and then in the more accessible ipsilateral (near) wall. When using a two-layer closure, appose the esophagus in four steps. First, appose adventitia and muscularis of the contralateral wall around approximately one half of the esophageal circumference. Next, appose mucosa and submucosa of the contralateral wall. Then, appose mucosa and submucosa of the ipsilateral wall. Last, appose adventitia and muscularis of the ipsilateral wall. Check closure integrity by occluding the lumen, injecting saline, applying pressure, and observing for leakage between sutures.

IX. Postoperative Care and Assessment

A. After esophageal surgery, provide analgesics as described for thoracotomy patients in Chapter 26.

B. Withhold oral intake for 24 to 48 hours. Continue intravenous fluids until oral intake resumes. Offer water 24 hours postoperatively if the esophagus is in good condition and regurgitation or vomiting does not occur. Offer blenderized food (gruel) during the next 24 hours if no vomiting or regurgitation occurs after water consumption. Continue a diet of blenderized food for 5 to 7 days and then gradually return the animal to its normal diet over the next week. If oral intake is not anticipated or possible within 48 to 72 hours after surgery, perform feeding via a gastrostomy tube.

C. Treat esophagitis and aspiration pneumonia. Dysphagia and regurgitation occurring 3 to 6 weeks after surgery may indicate esophageal stricture formation.

Esophageal Foreign Bodies (*SAS*, pp. 243-245)

I. Definitions

A. **Foreign bodies** are inanimate objects that may cause obstruction or partial obstruction of the esophageal lumen.

II. General Considerations and Clinically Relevant Pathophysiology

A. The most common foreign bodies are bones, although sharp metal objects (e.g., needles, fish hooks), balls, string, and an assortment of other objects have lodged in canine and feline esophagi.

B. They are most commonly found at the thoracic inlet, heart base, or epiphrenic (diaphragm) area.

C. Sharp objects may abrade or lacerate the esophageal mucosa causing irritation and inflammation of the underlying tissues (esophagitis). Sharp objects may also perforate the esophageal wall and allow bacteria, ingesta, and secretions to contaminate the periesophageal tissues. Occasionally, sharp objects will perforate the esophageal wall and one of the great vessels at the heart base, causing severe hemorrhage.

III. Diagnosis

A. Clinical Presentation

1. Signalment.
   a. Indiscriminate eaters (dogs) are more commonly affected than more particular eaters (cats).
   b. Although any breed of dog or cat may have an esophageal foreign body, small-breed dogs are more frequently affected.
   c. Cats (having a tendency to play and hunt) more commonly present with string or needle foreign bodies than bones.
   d. Foreign bodies may occur in any age animal, but are most common during the first 3 years of life.
2. History.
   a. An acute onset of dysphagia or regurgitation is the initial clinical sign.
   b. Other signs may include gagging, excessive salivation, retching, inappetence, restlessness, depression, dehydration, and respiratory distress.

B. Physical Examination Findings

1. Most patients are normal to slightly depressed and dehydrated on physical examination.
2. Poor body condition may be present if the patient has been anorexic or regurgitating for several weeks.

C. Radiography/Ultrasonography/Endoscopy

1. Most foreign bodies are identified on good-quality plain radiographs.
2. Examine patients closely for signs of subcutaneous emphysema, pneumomediastinum, pleural effusion, or pneumothorax that suggest esophageal perforation.

IV. Differential Diagnosis

A. Differentiate vascular ring anomalies, extraluminal masses, esophageal neoplasia, strictures, esophagitis, gastroesophageal intussusception, esophageal diverticula, hiatal hernias, megaesophagus, and cricopharyngeal dysfunction from esophageal foreign bodies.

V. Surgical Treatment

A. General Considerations

1. Most esophageal foreign bodies can be successfully removed by nonsurgical means.
2. Forcing an object that is firmly embedded in the esophageal wall is contraindicated because doing so may cause perforation or enlargement of a preexisting perforation. Embedded fishhooks are an

exception to this policy; however, take care to avoid lacerating vessels during their removal.

B. Preoperative Management

1. Initiate therapy to correct dehydration and electrolyte and acid-base imbalances before surgery.
2. Give perioperative antibiotics to prevent infection of periesophageal tissues.
3. Treat animals with preoperative perforation or severe esophageal trauma with therapeutic antibiotics.

C. Anesthesia

1. See Appendix G-5.
2. Do not use nitrous oxide.

D. Surgical Technique

1. General considerations.
   a. Consider endoscopic removal only for foreign bodies with a relatively smooth contour. During endoscopic procedures, extend the neck and insufflate the esophagus carefully to avoid rupturing weakened areas or causing tension pneumothorax.
   b. After removal via endoscopy or gastrotomy, reevaluate the esophagus for evidence of perforation by careful endoscopic evaluation or radiography. Debride and close perforations surgically.
2. Technique.
   a. Endoscopic removal.

Pass a balloon catheter distal to the object. Dilate the esophageal lumen beyond its normal size by inflating the balloon, and disengage the object from the esophageal wall, by endoscopic manipulations if necessary, and remove it by pulling the catheter out through the mouth.

   b. Removal via a gastrotomy–use for distal esophageal foreign bodies.
   c. Removal via an esophagotomy or partial esophagectomy.
      i. Perform when foreign bodies are not successfully removed by other means; the risk of esophageal perforation or laceration is high; or evidence of mediastinitis, pleuritis, or esophageal necrosis exists.
      ii. Debride all esophageal disruptions if necessary and close in one or two layers as for esophagotomy.

VI. Postoperative Care and Assessment

A. Observe all patients carefully for 2 to 3 days for signs of esophageal leakage and infection.

B. Treat esophagitis and aspiration pneumonia.

C. Continue intravenous fluids until feeding resumes. To avoid delays in healing, withhold all oral intake (food, water, medications) for a minimum of 24 hours after foreign body removal. If no regurgitation has been observed, gradually introduce water and then a bland gruel.

D. Mild esophageal trauma.
   1. Offer water to animals with minimal esophageal trauma within 24 to 48 hours, followed by small meals of gruel. After 3 to 7 days of

feeding gruel, offer soft, moist food for 5 to 7 days, followed by a gradual return to a normal diet.

E. Moderate to severe esophageal trauma.
   1. Avoid oral intake in animals with moderate to severe esophageal trauma for 3 to 7 days. In debilitated patients or those requiring no oral intake for longer than 3 days, place a gastrostomy feeding tube.
   2. Continue antibiotics for several days if the esophageal mucosa is severely eroded or lacerated.
   3. Treat severe esophagitis with H_2 antagonists or proton pump inhibitors to reduce gastric acidity, sucralfate to protect denuded mucosa, and cisapride to empty the stomach. Administer antibiotics effective against oral anaerobes (ampicillin, amoxicillin, clindamycin). Corticosteroids may help prevent cicatrix formation.

VII. Prognosis

A. Foreign body removal is essential.

B. The prognosis is good if perforation has not occurred; however, it is guarded if perforation has resulted in mediastinitis or pyothorax.

Esophageal Strictures (*SAS*, pp. 245-247)

I. Definitions

A. **Esophageal strictures** are bands of intraluminal or intramural fibrous tissue that may cause obstruction or partial obstruction of the esophagus.

II. General Considerations and Clinically Relevant Pathophysiology

A. Esophageal strictures may occur as a result of esophageal foreign bodies, surgery, esophagitis, caustic agents, or circumferential esophageal trauma.

B. Gastroesophageal reflux may occur during general anesthesia and result in stricture 1 to 5 weeks after surgery.

III. Diagnosis

A. Clinical Presentation

1. Signalment.
   a. Any age, breed, or sex of dog or cat may be affected.
2. History.
   a. Regurgitation is the most common presenting sign, and stricture

should be suspected in animals experiencing frequent regurgitation with a history of previous esophageal trauma or surgery.

B. Physical Examination Findings

1. Although animals with esophageal strictures may be thin and depressed, physical examination is usually normal. Occasionally, the cervical esophagus is dilated.

C. Radiography/Ultrasonography/Endoscopy

1. Esophageal strictures can be difficult to identify. Positive contrast esophagrams facilitate diagnosis.
2. Partial strictures are more readily identified if barium is mixed with food.
3. Esophagoscopy allows visualization (plus biopsy usually) of the lesion.
4. Biopsy the stricture if neoplasia is suspected.

IV. Surgical Treatment

A. General Considerations

1. Treat strictures by correcting the cause and then reducing the narrowing with balloon catheter dilation or bouginage.
2. Balloon catheter dilation is the preferred method for dilation of esophageal strictures because there is less chance of perforation and fewer dilations are required.

B. Preoperative Management

1. Fast animals before esophageal dilation.
2. Initiate treatment for esophagitis and aspiration pneumonia before stricture treatment.

C. Surgical Technique

1. Bouginage involves the dilation of a stricture using blunt dilators that are graduated in size.

Perform balloon dilation of strictures with the aid of an endoscope. First, endoscopically place a guide wire through the stricture site. Use a wire that is stiff at one end and floppy at the other. Insert the floppy end of the wire through the scope's biopsy channel and through the stricture. Then withdraw the endoscope from the patient while continually feeding the wire into the patient, thus removing the endoscope from around the wire while the latter is kept in the stricture. Next place the balloon in the stricture by running the balloon catheter over the wire while observing it endoscopically. Once the balloon is positioned so that the middle of it is near the center of the stricture, inflate the balloon with fluid or air (depending on the type of balloon) and deflate it after a minute or so. The balloon must stay in the stricture during this process. If the balloon is not correctly positioned, it will migrate out of the stricture as it is inflated and the stricture will not be dilated. Progressively larger balloons may be used until the desired degree of dilation is achieved.

V. Postoperative Care and Assessment

A. Monitor patients closely for signs of perforation.

B. Repeat dilation is often necessary within 4 to 7 days.

C. Treat preexisting esophagitis and aspiration pneumonia.

D. Gastrostomy tube placement may be beneficial in these patients so that oral feeding can be avoided for 7 to 10 days.

VI. Prognosis

A. Most patients with esophageal strictures can be helped by dilation, but strictures may reform.

B. Patients with severe or long strictures often require multiple dilations.

Esophageal Neoplasia (*SAS*, pp. 249-250)

I. Definitions

A. **Esophageal neoplasia** is any abnormal, noninflammatory proliferation of cells in the esophagus.

II. General Considerations and Clinically Relevant Pathophysiology

A. Neoplasia of the esophagus is rare. The most common types of tumors include sarcomas, squamous cell carcinomas, and leiomyomas.

B. Primary esophageal carcinomas are of unknown etiology. Primary esophageal sarcomas (osteosarcoma, fibrosarcoma) are often located in the vicinity of parasitic granulomas caused by *Spirocerca lupi.*

C. Most esophageal tumors are locally invasive and metastasize to draining lymph nodes.

III. Diagnosis

A. Clinical Presentation

1. Signalment.
   a. In cats, squamous cell carcinomas are usually seen in females in the middle third of the esophagus just caudal to the thoracic inlet.
   b. Most esophageal tumors occur in dogs and cats over 6 to 8 years of age.
2. History.
   a. Suspect neoplasia with chronic progressive signs of obstructive esophageal disease in middle-aged to older animals.

B. Physical Examination Findings

1. Physical examination is usually normal.

2. Hypertrophic osteopathy and spondylosis deformans may be noted, especially with *S. lupi*–induced sarcomas.

C. Radiography/Ultrasonography/Esophagoscopy

1. Aerophagia, displacement of the esophagus, and megaesophagus are signs of esophageal neoplasia.
2. Evaluate the lungs for metastatic lesions.
3. Contrast esophagrams may demonstrate an intraluminal mass (mucosal irregularities, filling defects, or stricture) with primary tumors, or an impinging extraluminal mass with secondary tumors.
4. Esophagoscopy allows direct visualization of intraluminal masses and biopsy for definitive diagnosis.

IV. Surgical Treatment

A. General Considerations

1. It is important to make an early diagnosis before metastasis or extensive esophageal involvement has occurred.
2. Partial esophagectomy with end-to-end anastomosis is indicated when approximation can be accomplished without excess tension.

B. Preoperative Management

1. Medical treatment (anthelmentics; fenbendazole, 50 mg/kg PO; ivermectin, 50 to 200 μg/kg PO; disophenol, 10 mg/kg SC; or diethylcarbamazine, 20 to 500 mg/kg PO) can be attempted for *S. lupi,* but if a sarcoma is already present, treatment is not recommended.

V. Prognosis

A. Most esophageal tumors are advanced at the time of diagnosis and do not respond well to radiation therapy or chemotherapy.

B. With surgery the prognosis is guarded for cure or palliation because resection is difficult as a result of the advanced nature of most tumors at the time of detection.

Hiatal Hernias (*SAS*, pp. 250-254)

I. Definitions

A. **Hiatal hernias** are protrusions of the abdominal esophagus, gastroesophageal junction, and sometimes a portion of the gastric fundus through the esophageal hiatus into the caudal mediastinum cranial to the diaphragm.

II. General Considerations and Clinically Relevant Pathophysiology

A. Hiatal hernias are usually caused by congenital abnormalities of the hiatus that allow cranial movement of the abdominal esophagus and stomach.

B. Gastroesophageal reflux and subsequent esophagitis and megaesophagus are responsible for most of the clinical signs.

C. Hiatal hernia is occasionally secondary to trauma and has occurred concurrently with respiratory distress.

D. The stomach commonly slides in and out of the thorax. Other abdominal viscera may also be cranially displaced. Various types of hiatal abnormalities have been described.

III. Diagnosis

A. Clinical Presentation

1. Signalment.
   a. Hiatal hernias may occur in a variety of dog and cat breeds; however, males and Chinese shar-pei dogs appear to be predisposed to this condition.
   b. Most symptomatic animals have signs relating to congenital hiatal hernia before reaching 1 year of age, although diagnosis may occur later.
2. History.
   a. Regurgitation is the primary clinical sign in symptomatic individuals, but many patients are asymptomatic.
   b. Other signs may include vomiting, hypersalivation, dysphagia, respiratory distress, hematemesis, anorexia, and weight loss.

B. Radiography/Ultrasonography

1. Hiatal hernias usually appear as a mass near the esophageal hiatus in the caudodorsal thoracic region on survey radiographs. With sliding hernias, several radiographs may be necessary to identify the herniation because herniation may be intermittent.
2. Fluoroscopy.
   a. Fluoroscopy may demonstrate hypomotility, delayed clearing of the distal esophagus, or gastroesophageal reflux.
   b. Compressing the abdomen while observing fluoroscopy may help identify hernias.

IV. Surgical Treatment

A. General Considerations

1. Medical treatment for gastroesophageal reflux or esophagitis may be beneficial; however, surgery is generally recommended in symptomatic animals with congenital disease.
2. Perform diaphragmatic hiatal reduction and plication, esophagopexy, and left-sided fundic gastropexy. Gastropexy is probably the most important step in the repair.

B. Preoperative Management

1. Treat reflux esophagitis and aspiration pneumonia before anesthetic induction.
2. Feed frequent, small meals of high-protein/low-fat foods.
3. If megaesophagus is present, feed affected animals in a standing, upright position.

C. Anesthesia

1. Utilize positive pressure ventilation if pneumothorax is created during hiatal manipulations.
2. Do not use nitrous oxide.

D. Surgical Anatomy

1. The esophageal hiatus is more centrally located than the caval foramen (located ventrally) or aortic hiatus (located dorsally).
2. The esophageal hiatus is surrounded by the phrenicoesophageal ligament, the thickened collagen fibers of which are weakened, stretched, or in some way defective in hiatal hernias.

E. Positioning

1. Position patients in dorsal recumbency, and prepare the caudal thorax and ventral abdomen for aseptic surgery.

F. Surgical Technique

Make a cranial ventral midline incision extending caudal to the umbilicus to expose the diaphragm and stomach. Retract the left lobes of the liver medially to expose the esophageal hiatus. Pass a stomach tube (28 to 32 French) to help identify and manipulate the esophagus. Grasp the stomach and reduce the hernia with gentle traction. Examine the hiatus. Dissect the phrenicoesophageal membrane, freeing the esophagus from the diaphragm ventrally. Preserve the vagal trunks and esophageal vessels during dissection. Place an umbilical tape sling around the abdominal esophagus to displace it caudally and facilitate manipulations. Perform a diaphragmatic hiatal plication/reduction, esophagopexy, and left-sided fundic gastropexy. Accomplish diaphragmatic hiatal plication/reduction by excoriating or debriding the margins of the hiatus and then place three to five sutures (2-0 polydioxanone or polypropylene) to appose the edges and narrow the hiatus. Plication should occur around a large stomach tube (28 to 32 French). The hiatus is reduced to 1 to 2 cm, a size that allows passage of one finger. Esophagopexy is accomplished by placing sutures (3-0 or 2-0 polydioxanone or polypropylene) from the remaining margin of the hiatus through the adventitia and muscular layers of the abdominal esophagus. Either a left-sided tube gastropexy or incisional gastropexy completes the repair. The fundus is fixed with slight to moderate caudal traction to prevent cranial movement of the gastroesophageal junction into the thorax. Evacuate air from the chest via thoracentesis or tube thoracostomy and lavage and close the abdomen.

V. Postoperative Care and Assessment

A. Monitor patients postoperatively for dyspnea resulting from pneumothorax, and evacuate air from the thorax as necessary.

B. Continue treatment of esophagitis and aspiration pneumonia postoperatively.

VI. Prognosis

A. The prognosis is good with the described surgical repair; however, aspiration pneumonia must be controlled for a favorable outcome.

Gastroesophageal Intussusception (*SAS*, pp. 254-255)

I. Definitions

A. **Gastroesophageal intussusception** is the invagination of the gastric cardia into the distal esophagus with or without the spleen, duodenum, pancreas, and omentum.

II. General Considerations and Clinically Relevant Pathophysiology

A. Gastroesophageal intussusception can be confused with esophageal hiatal hernia. However, the gastroesophageal junction does not move cranially into the thorax as with sliding hiatal hernia, and the cardia is within the esophageal lumen rather than external to the esophagus as with paraesophageal hiatal hernia.

III. Diagnosis

A. Clinical Presentation

1. Signalment.
   a. Although several breeds have been reported with gastroesophageal intussusception, German shepherds and other large-breed dogs seem to be at increased risk.
   b. Gastroesophageal intussusception has not been reported in cats.
   c. It is most common in young dogs, usually less than 3 months of age.
2. History.
   a. In most cases the onset of clinical signs is acute, with rapid deterioration and death within 1 to 3 days if the condition is not treated immediately.
   b. Signs may mimic those of aspiration pneumonia, making diagnosis difficult.
   c. Affected animals often have a history of esophageal disease.
   d. An acute onset of clinical signs (i.e., regurgitation, vomiting, dyspnea, hematemesis, abdominal discomfort, rapid deterioration, death) is common.

B. Radiography/Esophagoscopy

1. Radiographs show a dilated distal esophagus with a luminal soft tissue mass.

2. Esophagoscopy reveals a dilated esophagus with gastric rugal folds within the distal esophageal lumen. Esophagitis may be apparent. It may not be possible to advance the endoscope into the distal esophagus or stomach.

IV. Surgical Treatment

A. Perform surgical intervention as soon as possible after diagnosis.

B. Preoperative management.
   1. Initiate shock treatment (i.e., fluid therapy, broad-spectrum antibiotics, plus or minus steroids) and correct electrolyte and acid-base abnormalities before anesthetic induction.

C. Surgical Technique.

Make a ventral midline abdominal incision from the xiphoid process to several centimeters caudal to the umbilicus. Explore the abdomen and locate the duodenum and stomach. Apply gentle traction on the duodenum and stomach to reduce the intussusception. If necessary, digitally dilate or enlarge the esophageal hiatus to allow complete reduction of the intussusception. Examine the distal esophagus, stomach, and any other involved viscera for evidence of vascular thrombosis, avulsion, ischemia, or necrosis. Resect devitalized tissue. Reduce the size of the esophageal hiatus to 1 to 2 cm if it is too large or lax. Perform an incisional gastropexy at the gastric fundus to prevent recurrence. Lavage and close the abdomen.

V. Postoperative Care and Assessment

A. Withhold oral intake to encourage resolution of esophagitis and gastritis. Offer water after 24 to 48 hours. If vomiting or regurgitation does not occur, offer small amounts of a low-fat gruel several times a day. If megaesophagus is present, feed the animal in an upright position.

B. Esophageal weakness may not resolve. Gastrostomy tube feeding may be helpful.

C. Devitalization of a portion of the esophagus or stomach may occur as a result of preoperative vascular compromise.

D. Dysphagia is common for several days after surgery; however, persistent dysphagia may occur if the hiatus is overly narrowed by surgery. Such patients require reoperation.

VI. Prognosis

A. Antemortem diagnosis is rare (mortality approaches 95%); thus few cases of gastroesophageal intussusception have been diagnosed and treated successfully.

Cricopharyngeal Achalasia (*SAS*, pp. 255-258)

I. Definitions

A. **Cricopharyngeal achalasia** is one type of pharyngeal dysphagia where there is a failure of the sphincter to open correctly.

II. General Considerations and Clinically Relevant Pathophysiology

A. Differentiate cricopharyngeal achalasia from other forms of oropharyngeal dysphagia, because it is treatable.

B. Cricopharyngeal achalasia is characterized by inadequate relaxation of the cricopharyngeal muscle in coordination with pharyngeal muscle contractions during swallowing.

III. Diagnosis

A. Clinical Presentation

1. Signalment.
   a. The condition seems to be more common in springer and cocker spaniels, but has been seen in a variety of breeds.
2. History.
   a. Most dogs appear normal until they begin eating solid food. At that time repeated unsuccessful attempts to swallow, with gagging, retching, and expulsion of saliva-covered food is noted.
   b. Regurgitation occurs immediately after swallowing.

B. Physical Examination Findings

1. Observe the animal eating and drinking to confirm dysphagia and to characterize it as oral or pharyngeal.
   a. Patients with oral dysphagia have difficulty with prehension and bolus formation.
   b. Those with pharyngeal dysphagia have difficulty transporting the bolus into the esophagus.
2. Patients with cricopharyngeal dysphagia usually have more difficulty with food, whereas those with other types of pharyngeal dysphagias may have more difficulty (i.e., may aspirate more readily) when swallowing liquids.

C. Radiography/Ultrasonography

1. Evaluate survey thoracic radiographs for aspiration pneumonia and esophageal size.
2. Definitive diagnosis requires fluoroscopic or cinefluoroscopic evaluation during a barium swallow.

3. Patients with cricopharyngeal achalasia have adequate pharyngeal strength to push the food bolus into the esophagus, but the cricopharyngeal sphincter stays shut or opens at the wrong time during the swallowing reflex.

IV. Surgical Treatment

A. Cricopharyngeal myectomy is curative for cricopharyngeal achalasia.

B. Preoperative management.
   1. Provide preoperative nutritional support with a gastrostomy tube if necessary.
   2. Treat aspiration pneumonia with fluids, appropriate antibiotics, and expectorants.

C. Surgical anatomy.
   1. The cricopharyngeal muscle lies on the larynx and pharynx immediately caudal to the thyropharyngeal muscle.
   2. It can be identified as a bundle of transverse muscle fibers converging on the dorsal midline and blending into the longitudinal muscle fibers of the cranial esophagus.

D. Positioning.
   1. Position the animal in dorsal recumbency with the legs positioned lateral to the thorax.
   2. Prepare the ventral neck (from the angle of the mandible to the manubrium) for aseptic surgery.

E. Surgical technique.

Make a ventral midline cervical incision beginning cranial to the larynx and extending caudally to the midcervical area. Separate and retract the sternohyoid muscles laterally to expose the trachea. Rotate the larynx and trachea laterally via traction on the sternothyroid muscle to expose the cricopharyngeal musculature. Place a suture through the lamina of the thyroid cartilage to maintain laryngeal rotation and exposure of the cricopharyngeal muscle and dorsal esophagus. Pass a gastric tube into the esophagus to aid identification of the esophageal wall. Identify the cricopharyngeal muscles. Incise the cricopharyngeal muscle on its midline. Elevate the muscle fibers from the underlying esophageal submucosa with care to avoid perforating the esophageal wall. Resect the lateral portion of each cricopharyngeus muscle. Inspect the esophageal wall for damage and lavage the area. Allow the larynx and trachea to return to their normal position. Appose the sternohyoid muscles with a continuous suture pattern. Close subcutaneous tissues and skin routinely.

V. Postoperative Care

A. Feed a gruel or canned food for the first 1 to 2 days postoperatively, then gradually return to normal food consistency over the next 3 to 4 days.

VI. Prognosis

A. The prognosis is good if the only abnormality present is cricopharyngeal achalasia and guarded if other dysphagias are present.

Vascular Ring Anomalies (*SAS*, pp. 258-261)

I. Definitions

A. **Vascular ring anomalies** are congenital malformations of the great vessels and their branches that cause constriction of the esophagus and signs of esophageal obstruction.

II. General Considerations and Clinically Relevant Pathophysiology

A. The most common type of vascular ring anomaly is a persistent fourth right aortic arch (PRAA).

B. The left pulmonary artery and the descending aorta are connected by the ligamentum arteriosum.

III. Diagnosis

A. Clinical Presentation

1. Signalment.
   a. Vascular ring anomalies occur in both dogs and cats, but are more common in dogs.
   b. German shepherds, Irish setters, and Boston terriers are the most commonly affected dog breeds. Siamese and Persian cats have been diagnosed more often than other cat breeds.
2. History.
   a. The classic history is acute onset of regurgitation when solid or semisolid food is first fed.
   b. Coughing with respiratory distress may be a result of aspiration pneumonia or tracheal stenosis secondary to a double aortic arch.

B. Physical Examination Findings

1. Affected animals are often thin and small.
2. An enlarged esophagus may sometimes be palpated at the thoracic inlet and neck.

C. Radiography/Ultrasonography/Endoscopy

1. Thoracic radiographs may reveal a dilated esophagus cranial to the heart containing air, water, or food.

2. Positive contrast radiography using a barium suspension or barium with food will demonstrate esophageal constriction at the base of the heart with varying degrees of esophageal dilatation extending cranially.
3. Endoscopic examination of the esophagus helps rule out other causes of esophageal stricture or obstruction and may reveal esophageal ulceration.

IV. Medical Management

A. Perform surgery as soon after onset of clinical signs as possible to reduce damage to the esophageal muscles and nerves.

B. Treat aspiration pneumonia and improve the animal's nutritional status.

V. Surgical Treatment

A. Preoperative Management

1. Correct hydration, electrolyte, and acid-base abnormalities before surgery if possible.

B. Positioning

1. Most patients with vascular ring anomalies should be positioned in right lateral recumbency for a left lateral thoracotomy; however, those with persistent right ligamentum arteriosum are positioned in left lateral recumbency.
2. Positioning of animals with double aortic arches varies depending on the dominant arch.

C. Surgical Technique

Perform a lateral thoracotomy at the left fourth (fifth) intercostal space for patients with PRAA. Pack the cranial lung caudally to expose the mediastinum dorsal to the heart. Identify the aorta, pulmonary artery, ligamentum arteriosum, vagus, and phrenic nerves. Identify the anomalous structure(s). If a persistent left cranial cava is present, dissect and retract the vena cava to improve visualization. If a prominent hemiazygous vein is also present, dissect, ligate, and divide it. If a constricting subclavian artery is identified, isolate, ligate, and transect it. Incise the mediastinum, dissect, and elevate the ligamentum arteriosum. Double ligate the ligamentum arteriosum and then transect it. Pass a ballooned catheter or large orogastric tube through the constricted esophagus to aid identification of constricting fibrous bands and to dilate the site. Dissect and transect these fibrous bands from the esophageal wall. Lavage the area, reposition the lung lobes, place a thoracostomy tube if necessary, and close the thorax routinely.

VI. Postoperative Care and Assessment

A. Monitor closely for dyspnea and tap the chest if necessary.

B. Monitor pediatric patients closely for hypoglycemia in the postoperative period.

C. Resume oral intake within 12 to 24 hours of surgery. Initially, feed a canned food gruel with the animal in an upright posture. Maintain this stance for 10 to 20 minutes after eating to help prevent distention of the dilated esophagus and help reestablish esophageal muscle tone and esophageal size. Owners may gradually reduce the amount of water in the food 2 to 4 weeks after surgery if minimal regurgitation has occurred with gruel feeding.

VII. Prognosis

A. Most patients surviving surgery improve.

B. The prognosis is poor if there is esophageal dilatation caudal to the constriction because this area is often hypomotile and frequently does not regain normal size.

C. Without surgery, regurgitation usually continues and worsens as the esophagus continues to dilate.

Surgery of the Stomach (*SAS*, pp. 261-292)

I. Definitions

A. **Gastrotomy** is an incision through the stomach wall into the lumen.

B. **Partial gastrectomy** is a resection of a portion of the stomach.

C. **Gastrostomy** is creation of an artificial opening into the gastric lumen.

D. **Gastropexy** permanently adheres the stomach to the body wall.

II. Preoperative Concerns

A. Gastric disease may cause vomiting (intermittent or profuse and continuous) or just anorexia.

B. Dehydration and hypokalemia are common in vomiting animals and should be corrected before anesthetic induction.

C. Alkalosis may occur as a result of gastric fluid loss; however, metabolic acidosis may also be seen.

D. Esophagitis.
  1. Mild esophagitis can generally be treated by withholding food for 24 to 48 hours and need not delay gastric surgery.
  2. Severe esophagitis may necessitate withholding oral food for 7 to 10 days.

E. When possible, withhold food for 8 to 12 hours before surgery to ensure that the stomach is empty.

III. Anesthetic Considerations

A. See anesthetic protocols for animals with gastric disorders (Appendixes G-6 and G-7).

B. Avoid nitrous oxide whenever gastric or intestinal distention is present (e.g., gastric dilatation-volvulus, intestinal volvulus/torsion), because it rapidly diffuses into gas-filled areas, causing additional organ distention.

C. Rapid induction and immediate intubation are essential if vomiting is a concern; however, mask induction is acceptable if vomiting is not a concern.

IV. Antibiotics

A. Consider using perioperative antibiotics (see Chapter 10) if the gastric lumen will be entered; however, they are not necessary with a simple gastrotomy.

V. Surgical Anatomy

A. The stomach can be divided into the cardia, fundus, body, pyloric antrum, pyloric canal, and pyloric ostium.

B. Blood supply.
   1. The gastric (lesser curvature) and gastroepiploic (greater curvature) arteries supply the stomach and are derived from the celiac artery.
   2. The short gastric arteries arise from the splenic artery and supply the greater curvature.

VI. Surgical Techniques

A. Gastrotomy

Make a ventral midline abdominal incision from the xiphoid to the pubis. Use Balfour retractors to retract the abdominal wall and provide adequate exposure to the gastrointestinal tract. Inspect the entire abdominal contents before incising the stomach. To decrease contamination, isolate the stomach from remaining abdominal contents with moistened laparotomy sponges. Place stay sutures to assist in manipulation of the stomach and help prevent spillage of gastric contents. Make the gastric incision in a hypovascular area of the ventral aspect of the stomach, between the greater and lesser curvatures. Be sure that the incision is not near the pylorus, lest closure of the incision cause excessive tissue to be infolded into the gastric lumen, producing outflow obstruction. Make a stab incision into the gastric lumen with a scalpel, and enlarge the incision with Metzenbaum scissors. Use suction to aspirate gastric contents and decrease spillage. Close the stomach with 2-0 or 3-0 suture material in a two-layer inverting seromuscular pattern, using an absorbable suture material such as polydioxanone or polyglyconate suture. Include serosa, muscularis, and submucosa in the first layer, using a Cushing or simple continuous pattern, then follow it with a Lembert or Cushing pattern that incorporates the serosal and muscularis layers. Alternatively, close the mucosa with a simple continuous

suture pattern as a separate layer, to decrease postoperative bleeding. Substitute sterile instruments and gloves for ones contaminated by gastric contents before closing the abdominal incision. Whenever you remove a gastric foreign body, be sure to check the entire intestinal tract for additional material that could cause an intestinal obstruction.

B. Partial Gastrectomy and Invagination of Gastric Tissue

1. General considerations.
   a. Partial gastrectomy is indicated when necrosis, ulceration, or neoplasia involves the greater curvature, or middle portion, of the stomach.
   b. Invagination does not require opening of the gastric lumen; however, obstruction from excessive intraluminal tissue is possible.
   c. Assess the extent of necrosis by observing serosal color, gastric wall texture, vascular patency, and bleeding on incision; however, it is difficult to determine tissue viability in many cases with these techniques.
2. Procedure.

To remove the greater curvature of the stomach, ligate branches of the left gastroepiploic vessels or short gastric vessels along the section of the stomach to be removed. Excise the necrotic tissue, leaving a margin of normal, actively bleeding tissue to suture. Close the stomach with a two-layer inverting suture pattern, using an absorbable suture (e.g., polydioxanone or polyglyconate suture; 2-0 or 3-0). Incorporate submucosa, muscularis, and serosal layers in a Cushing or simple continuous pattern in the first layer. Then use a Cushing or Lembert pattern to invert the serosa and muscularis over the first layer. Alternatively, you may use a thoracoabdominal (TA) stapling device to close the incision. To invaginate necrotic tissue, use a simple continuous suture pattern followed by an inverting suture pattern. Place sutures in healthy gastric tissue on both sides of the tissue that is to be invaginated, bringing the healthy tissue over the top of the necrotic tissue. Be sure that sutures are placed in healthy tissues to prevent dehiscence.

If removing neoplasia or ulcerated tissue, ligate branches of the right and left gastric artery and vein (lesser curvature) and left gastroepiploic artery and vein (greater curvature), and remove omental attachments. Following removal of the suspect tissues, perform a two-layer end-to-end anastomosis of the stomach. If the luminal circumferences are of disparate size, the larger circumference can be partially closed using a two-layer suture pattern. Close the mucosa and submucosa of the dorsal surface of the stomach with a simple continuous pattern, using an absorbable suture material (2-0 or 3-0), then close the ventral aspect. Suture the serosa and muscularis layers with an inverting suture pattern (e.g., Cushing or Lembert).

C. Temporary Gastrostomy

1. General considerations.
   a. Temporary gastrostomy is recommended only if surgery for GDV must be delayed and alternative techniques fail to keep the stomach decompressed.
   b. It can usually be performed with local anesthesia (e.g., 2% lidocaine), using a reverse-7 local block or direct infiltration over the proposed incision. Tranquilization or sedation may be necessary if the dog is fractious.
2. Procedure.

Make a 6- to 10-cm full-thickness incision in the right paracostal body wall, and identify the stomach. Before incising into the gastric lumen, suture the

stomach to skin using a simple continuous suture pattern. Then make an incision in the stomach. Be sure that the stomach is securely sutured to the skin to prevent leakage of gastric contents subcutaneously. Place Vaseline on the skin to prevent scalding from gastric contents.

D. Pylorectomy with Gastroduodenostomy (Billroth I)

1. Indicated for neoplasia, outflow obstruction due to pyloric muscular hypertrophy, or ulceration of the gastric outflow tract.
2. Procedure.

Identify the common bile duct and pancreatic ducts, then place stay sutures in the proximal duodenum and pyloric antrum. If increased caudoventral retraction of the pylorus is desired, identify and transect a portion of the hepatogastric ligament. Ligate branches of the right gastric and right gastroepiploic artery and vein to the affected tissues, and remove the omental and mesenteric attachments. Use noncrushing forceps (Doyen) or fingers to occlude the stomach and duodenum proximal and distal to the area to be resected. Excise the area of pylorus to be removed, using Metzenbaum scissors or a scalpel blade, and inspect the remaining edges to ensure that all abnormal tissue has been excised. If there is marked disparity in the size of the gastric and duodenal lumens, incise the duodenum at an angle, or partially close the antrum. Perform a one- or two-layer end-to-end anastomosis of the pyloric antrum to the duodenum, using 2-0 or 3-0 absorbable suture material in a simple continuous, crushing, or simple interrupted pattern. In one study no difference was noted in the prevalence of postoperative leakage and incisional dehiscence between a one-layer and two-layer closure. Close the far (dorsal) aspect of the incision first, followed by the near (ventral) aspect. Avoid inverting excessive tissue, which might decrease the diameter of the gastric outflow tract.

E. Partial Gastrectomy with Gastrojejunostomy (Billroth II)

1. Perform if the extent of the lesion precludes an end-to-end anastomosis of the pyloric antrum to the duodenum.
2. Procedure.

Resect the pylorus, antrum, and proximal duodenum as described above, ligating appropriate branches of the right and left gastric and gastroepiploic vessels. Close the duodenal and pyloric antral stumps with a two-layer suture pattern. For the first layer, incorporate the mucosa and submucosa in a simple interrupted or simple continuous suture pattern of 2-0 or 3-0 absorbable suture material. Then place an inverting suture pattern (e.g., Lembert) in the seromuscular layer. Identify an avascular area between the gastric incision and greater curvature. Bring a loop of proximal jejunum to the selected site, and attach it to the stomach with stay sutures. Suture the seromuscular layers of the stomach and intestine together, using a simple continuous suture pattern. Make full-thickness, longitudinal incisions into the stomach and intestinal lumens, near the suture line. Suture mucosa and submucosa of the stomach to the intestine with a continuous suture pattern of absorbable suture material (3-0 or 4-0). Next place a continuous suture pattern in the serosa and muscularis.

F. Pyloromyotomy and Pyloroplasty

1. General considerations.
   a. Pyloromyotomy and pyloroplasty increase the diameter of the pylorus and are used to correct gastric outflow obstruction (i.e.,

chronic antral mucosal hypertrophy or pyloric stenosis). However, do not perform these procedures routinely in dogs without evidence of pyloric dysfunction (e.g., most dogs with GDV), because they can slow gastric emptying.

2. Fredet-Ramstedt pyloromyotomy.

Hold the pylorus between the index finger and thumb in the nondominant hand. Select a hypovascular area of the ventral pylorus, and make a longitudinal incision through the serosa and muscularis, but not through the mucosa. Make sure that the muscularis layer is completely incised, to allow the mucosa to bulge into the incision site. If the mucosa is inadvertently penetrated, suture it with interrupted sutures of 2-0 or 3-0 absorbable suture material.

3. Heineke-Mikulicz pyloroplasty.

Make a full-thickness, longitudinal incision in the ventral surface of the pylorus. Place traction sutures at the center of the incision, and orient the incision transversely. Suture the transverse incision with a one-layer suture pattern (simple interrupted or crushing) of 2-0 or 3-0 absorbable suture material. Place the sutures carefully, so that the incision edges are properly aligned and tissue inversion avoided.

4. Y-U pyloroplasty.

Make a longitudinal incision (limb) in the serosa overlying the ventral pylorus, and extend it into the stomach by making two incisions (arms) that run parallel to the lesser and greater curvature of the stomach (creating a Y-shaped incision). Be sure that the angle of the Y is not overly narrow or necrosis may result. The limbs and arms of the Y-shaped incision should be approximately the same length. Make a full-thickness incision. Inspect the mucosa, and if necessary, resect it. If mucosa is resected, appose the remaining mucosal edges with a continuous suture pattern of absorbable suture material before closing the Y incision. Suture the base of the antral flap to the distal end of the duodenal incision with a simple interrupted suture (absorbable 2-0 or 3-0 suture material), creating a U-shaped closure. Close the remainder of the incision (the limbs) with simple interrupted sutures. Be sure that tissue approximation is adequate to prevent leakage and that minimal tissue has been infolded into the pyloric lumen.

G. Gastropexy

1. General considerations.
   a. Gastropexy techniques are designed to permanently adhere the stomach to the body wall. The most common indications are GDV (pyloric antrum to right body wall) and hiatal herniation (fundus to left body wall).
   b. To create a permanent adhesion, the gastric muscle must be in contact with the muscle of the body wall; intact gastric serosa will not form permanent adhesions to an intact peritoneal surface.
2. Tube gastropexy.

Make a stab incision into the right abdominal wall, caudal to the last rib and 4 to 10 cm lateral to the midline. Place a Foley catheter (18 to 30 French) through the stab incision. Select a site in a hypovascular region of the seromuscular layer of the ventral surface of the pyloric antrum where the balloon of the catheter will not obstruct gastric outflow. Place a purse-string suture of 2-0 absorbable suture (e.g., polydioxanone or polyglyconate suture) at this site. Make a stab incision through the purse-string suture and insert the Foley catheter tip into the gastric lumen. (Note: The Foley catheter can be

placed through the omentum before entry into the stomach so that the omentum is secured between the stomach and body wall, or the omentum can be wrapped around the site after the stomach has been secured to the body wall.) Inflate the bulb of the Foley catheter with saline (not air), and secure the purse-string suture around the tube. Preplace three to four absorbable sutures between the pyloric antrum and the body wall, where the tube exits. Avoid penetrating the catheter or balloon when placing the sutures. Draw the stomach to the body wall by placing traction on the catheter, and tie the preplaced sutures. Secure the tube to skin with a Roman sandal suture pattern, but avoid penetrating it with a suture. Place a bandage around the dog's abdomen and over the tube to prevent its premature removal (and use an Elizabethan collar if necessary). Leave the tube in place 7 to 10 days, then deflate the balloon and remove it. Leave the skin incision open to facilitate drainage. Place a light bandage over the open wound if desired.

3. Circumcostal gastropexy.

Make either a one- or two-layer hinged flap (approximately 5 to 6 cm long in large dogs) by incising through the seromuscular layer of the pyloric antrum. Do not incise the gastric mucosa or enter the lumen (if this occurs, suture the mucosa with 3-0 absorbable suture material). Elevate the flap by dissecting under the muscularis. If a one-hinged flap is made, place the hinge toward the lesser curvature. Make a 5- to 6-cm incision over the eleventh or twelfth rib at the level of the costochondral junction. Be sure that the incision does not penetrate the diaphragmatic attachments to the body wall, causing pneumothorax. Form a tunnel under the rib using a Carmalt clamp or hemostat. Place stay sutures on the flap (if using a two-flap technique, place the sutures on the flap nearest the lesser curvature). Pass the gastric antral flap craniodorsal under the rib and suture it with 2-0 absorbable suture material to the original gastric margin (one-flap technique) or the other flap (two-flap technique).

4. Muscular flap (incisional) gastropexy.

Make two hinged flaps in the seromuscular layer of the gastric antrum (similar to that for a circumcostal gastropexy). Then make similar flaps in the right ventrolateral abdominal wall by incising the peritoneum and internal fascia of the rectus abdominis or transverse abdominis muscles. Elevate flaps by dissecting ventral to the muscle layer. Invert the flaps, and suture the edge of the abdominal flaps to the gastric flaps, using a simple continuous suture pattern of 2-0 absorbable or nonabsorbable suture. Ensure that the muscularis layer of the stomach is in contact with the abdominal wall muscle. Suture the cranial margin first, followed by the caudal margin. Be sure to place sufficient sutures so that a loop of bowel cannot become incarcerated between the flaps.

5. Belt-loop gastropexy.

Elevate a seromuscular flap in the gastric antrum. Make two transverse incisions in the ventrolateral abdominal wall by incising the peritoneum and abdominal musculature. The incisions should be 2.5 to 4 cm apart and 3 to 5 cm long. Create a tunnel under the abdominal musculature with forceps. Place stay sutures in the edge of the antral flap, and use them to pass the flap from cranial to caudal under the muscular flap. Suture the flap to its original gastric margin, using a simple continuous suture pattern of 2-0 absorbable or nonabsorbable suture material. You may wish to place additional sutures between the body wall and the stomach to decrease tension on the gastropexy.

VII. Gastric Wound Healing

A. The extraordinarily rich blood supply, reduced bacterial numbers (as a result of gastric acidity), rapidly regenerating epithelium, and defense mechanisms provided by the omentum allow gastric incisions to heal quickly.

VIII. Suture Materials

A. Use monofilament absorbable suture material (e.g., polydioxanone [PDS] or polyglyconate [Maxon]) for gastrointestinal surgery.

IX. Postoperative Care and Assessment

A. Monitor electrolytes (especially potassium) postoperatively.

B. If prolonged vomiting or anorexia is anticipated, provide enteral hyperalimentation via a gastrostomy or enterostomy (if the animal is vomiting) tube.

Gastric Foreign Bodies (*SAS*, pp. 275-277)

I. Definitions

A. **Gastric foreign bodies** are anything ingested by an animal that cannot be digested (e.g., plastic) or is slowly digested (e.g., bones).

B. **Linear foreign bodies** are usually pieces of string, yarn, thread, cloth, or dental floss.

II. General Considerations and Clinically Relevant Pathophysiology

A. Foreign bodies may occur in the stomach and small intestine concurrently; therefore perform a complete exploration of the entire intestinal tract whenever you do surgery to remove a gastric foreign body.

B. **Repeat the radiographs immediately before surgery to ensure that the object has not moved** (even if they were just taken the day before).

III. Diagnosis

A. Clinical Presentation

1. Signalment.
   a. Young animals more commonly ingest foreign bodies than do older animals, and gastric or intestinal foreign bodies should be suspected in any puppy or kitten presenting for acute or persistent vomiting.
2. History.
   a. Most animals with gastric foreign bodies present for vomiting, anorexia, or depression.
   b. The vomiting may be intermittent, and some animals may continue to eat and remain active.
   c. Vomiting is often absent if the foreign body is in the gastric fundus and does not obstruct the pylorus.

B. Physical Examination Findings

1. Physical examination is often unremarkable.
2. Plicated intestines may be felt if there is a linear foreign object, and pain may be evident if gastric perforation has caused peritonitis.
3. Thorough examination of the mouth, including ventral to the tongue, is mandatory in all animals with suspected linear foreign objects.

C. Radiography/Endoscopy

1. Radiopaque foreign bodies can be diagnosed with plain films; however, many foreign bodies are radiolucent.
2. Contrast studies may be necessary to delineate radiolucent foreign bodies.

IV. Medical Management

A. If the object is small and has rounded edges, vomiting can be induced using apomorphine in the dog or xylazine in the cat. However, this should only be attempted when the clinician is certain it will be expelled without causing harm.

V. Surgical Treatment

A. Preoperative Management

1. If possible, identify and correct metabolic and acid-base abnormalities, and withhold food for 12 hours.
2. Take radiographs immediately before surgery to verify the position of the object in the digestive tract.
3. Perioperative antibiotics may be given at induction and continued for up to 12 hours postoperatively (see Chapter 10).

B. Positioning

1. Place the animal in dorsal recumbency and prepare the abdomen for a ventral midline incision.
2. Prep an area from midthorax to the pubis to allow the entire digestive system to be explored for foreign objects.

C. Surgical Technique

Inspect the entire digestive system for material that could cause obstruction or perforation. If a linear foreign body is found in the pylorus and extends into the intestinal tract, do not try to pull it into the stomach unless it moves easily. Instead, make several incisions into the stomach and intestines to avoid causing further damage to the intestinal tract. Inspect the stomach for perforation or necrosis, and remove or patch abnormal tissue, depending on the location. Close the gastric incision as described for gastrotomy.

VI. Postoperative Care and Assessment

A. Monitor the patient's fluid status and maintain hydration with intravenous fluids postoperatively until the animal is drinking.

B. Correct electrolyte abnormalities.

C. Feed a bland diet for 12 to 24 hours after surgery if the patient is not vomiting. If vomiting continues, use centrally acting antiemetics such as chlorpromazine, metoclopramide, or ondansetron, and withhold oral intake.

Gastric Dilatation-Volvulus (*SAS*, pp. 277-283)

I. Definitions

A. **Gastric dilatation-volvulus** (GDV) is an enlargement of the stomach associated with rotation on its mesenteric axis.

B. **Simple dilatation** refers to a stomach that is engorged with air or froth, but not malpositioned.

II. General Considerations and Clinically Relevant Pathophysiology

A. Classically, the GDV syndrome is an acute condition with a mortality rate of 30% to 45% in treated animals.

B. The cause of GDV is unknown, but exercise after ingestion of large meals of highly processed foods or water has been suggested to contribute. Recommendations for clients of animals at high risk are provided in Table 16-7.

C. Generally, the stomach rotates in a clockwise direction when viewed from the surgeon's perspective (with the dog on its back and the clinician standing at the dog's side, facing cranially).

Table 16-7
Recommendations for clients

• Feed several small meals a day, rather than one large meal
• Avoid stress during feeding (if necessary, separate dogs in multiple-dog households during feeding)
• Restrict exercise before and after meals
• For high-risk dogs, consider prophylactic gastropexy
• Seek veterinary care as soon as signs of bloat are noted

D. Partial or chronic GDV may occur in dogs and is usually a progressive but non–life-threatening syndrome that may be associated with vomiting, anorexia, or weight loss. These dogs may have chronic, intermittent signs and appear normal between episodes.

III. Diagnosis

A. Clinical Presentation

1. Signalment.
   a. GDV primarily occurs in large, deep-chested breeds (e.g., Great Dane, weimaraner, Saint Bernard, German shepherd, Irish and Gordon setters, Doberman pinscher), but has been reported in cats and small-breed dogs, including shar-peis and basset hounds.
   b. Large breed size, degree of purity of breed, and increase of weight are significant risk factors for development of this disease.
   c. GDV may occur in any age dog, but is most common in middle-aged to older animals.
2. History.
   a. A dog with GDV may present with a history of a progressively distending and tympanic abdomen, or the owner may simply find the animal recumbent and depressed, with a distended abdomen.
   b. Nonproductive retching, hypersalivation, and restlessness are common.

B. Physical Examination Findings

1. Abdominal palpation often reveals various degrees of abdominal tympany or enlargement; however, it may be difficult to feel gastric distention in heavily muscled, large-breed, or very obese dogs.
2. Clinical signs associated with shock, including weak peripheral pulses, tachycardia, prolonged capillary refill time, pale mucous membranes, or dyspnea, may be present.

C. Radiography

1. Radiographic evaluation is necessary to differentiate simple dilatation from dilatation plus volvulus.
2. Decompress affected animals before taking radiographs. Take right lateral and dorsoventral radiographic views.
   a. In normal dogs, the pylorus is located ventral to the fundus on the lateral view, and on the right side of the abdomen on the dorsoventral view.
   b. On a right lateral view of a dog with GDV, the pylorus lies cranial to the body of the stomach and is separated from the rest of the stomach by soft tissue (reverse C sign).

c. On the dorsoventral view, the pylorus appears as a gas-filled structure to the left of midline.
d. Free abdominal air suggests gastric rupture and warrants immediate surgery.

D. Laboratory Findings

1. Although normal or increased potassium concentrations may occur, hypokalemia is more common.
2. Vascular stasis may cause increased lactic acid production, resulting in a metabolic acidosis. However, metabolic alkalosis caused by sequestration of hydrogen ions in the gastric lumen can offset the metabolic acidosis, causing the pH to be normal (i.e., a mixed acid-base disorder). Respiratory acidosis may be caused by hypoventilation secondary to gastric impingement on the diaphragm and decreased ventilatory compliance. **Hence, routine use of sodium bicarbonate is inappropriate.**

IV. Medical Management

A. Stabilization

1. Place a large-bore intravenous catheter(s) in either a jugular or both cephalic veins. Give either isotonic fluids (90 ml/kg/hr), hypertonic 7% saline (4 to 5 ml/kg over 5 to 15 min), or hetastarch (5 to 10 ml/kg over 10 to 15 min). If hypertonic saline or hetastarch is given, adjust the rate of subsequent crystalloid administration.
2. Draw blood for blood gas analyses, a CBC, and a biochemical panel.
3. Give broad-spectrum antibiotics (e.g., cefazolin, ampicillin plus enrofloxacin) and possibly flunixin meglumine (for septic shock).

B. Gastric Decompression

1. General considerations.
   a. Perform gastric decompression while initiating shock therapy.
   b. Decompress the stomach by passing a stomach tube, or percutaneously with several large-bore intravenous catheters or a small trocar.
2. Technique.

Measure the stomach tube from the point of the nose to the xiphoid process and mark the correct length with a piece of tape. Place a roll of tape between the incisors and pass the tube through the center hole. Attempt to pass the tube to the measured point, but do not perforate the esophagus with overly rigorous attempts. Placing the animal in different positions (e.g., sitting, reclining on a tilt-table) may help if it is difficult to advance the tube into the stomach. If these attempts fail, attempt percutaneous decompression of the stomach. This may relieve pressure on the cardia and allow the tube to enter the stomach. Once the air has been removed, flush the stomach with warm water. If blood is seen in the fluid from the stomach, prompt surgical intervention is warranted because this may indicate gastric necrosis. If immediate surgery is not possible in an animal in which a stomach tube was passed but that dilates rapidly after decompression, the stomach tube can be exteriorized through a pharyngostomy approach. This will prevent the animal from chewing on the tube, until definitive surgery can be performed.

3. Temporary gastrostomy. If the stomach tube still cannot be passed, and immediate surgical correction is not possible, consider a temporary gastrostomy. Do not place a Foley catheter into the stomach percutaneously.

V. Surgical Treatment

A. General Considerations

1. Perform surgery as soon as the animal has been stabilized, even if the stomach has been decompressed.
2. Rotation of a nondistended stomach interferes with gastric blood flow and may potentiate gastric necrosis.

B. Preoperative Management

1. See Medical Management, previous page.

C. Anesthesia

1. If the animal has been decompressed and stabilized and cardiac arrhythmias are not present, the animal may be given oxymorphone (0.1 mg/kg IV) and diazepam (0.2 mg/kg IV) in incremental doses as necessary for intubation (Appendix G-8).
2. If necessary for intubation, administer etomidate or reduced dosages of thiobarbiturates or propofol (in addition to oxymorphone and diazepam).
3. Etomidate (0.5 to 1.5 mg/kg IV) is a good choice for induction if the animal has not been well stabilized because it maintains cardiac output and is not arrhythmogenic.
4. Alternatively, a combination of lidocaine and thiobarbiturate may be used if arrhythmias are present. For the latter, 9 mg/kg of each is drawn up and half is given initially, intravenously. Additional drug is given to effect to allow the dog to be intubated. Generally, no more than 6 mg/kg of lidocaine is given intravenously to prevent toxicity. If bradycardia occurs, give anticholinergics (e.g., atropine or glycopyrrolate).
5. Maintenance.
   a. Do not use nitrous oxide in dogs with GDV.
   b. Use isoflurane because it is less arrhythmogenic than halothane.

D. Surgical Anatomy

1. Rupture of the short gastrics in dogs with GDV is common and may contribute to blood loss and gastric infarction or necrosis.
2. Eighty percent of the arterial flow is to the mucosa and the remainder is to the muscularis and serosa; therefore observation of mucosal color is not a reliable indicator of gastric wall viability. The mucosa often appears darkened because of vascular compromise, even when full-thickness necrosis is not present.

E. Positioning

1. Place the dog in dorsal recumbency and prepare the abdomen for a midline abdominal incision.
2. Extend the prepped area from midthorax to the pubis. If performing a tube gastropexy, extend the prepped area cranially and dorsally to allow the tube to be exteriorized behind the caudal right rib.

F. Surgical Technique

Decompress the stomach before repositioning, by using a large-bore needle (i.e., 14 or 16 gauge) attached to suction. If the needle becomes occluded with ingesta, have an assistant pass an orogastric stomach tube and perform gastric lavage. Intraoperative manipulation of the cardia will usually allow the tube to be passed into the stomach without difficulty. If adequate decompression is still not achieved, or an assistant is not available, perform a small gastrotomy incision to remove the gastric contents, although this should be avoided if

possible. For a clockwise rotation, once the stomach has been decompressed, rotate it counterclockwise by grasping the pylorus (usually found below the esophagus) with the right hand and the greater curvature with the left. Push the greater curvature, or fundus, of the stomach toward the table while simultaneously elevating the pylorus (toward the incision). Check to make sure that the spleen is normally positioned in the left abdominal quadrant. If there is splenic necrosis or significant infarction, perform a partial or complete splenectomy (see Chapter 20). Remove or invaginate necrotic gastric tissues. Avoid entering the gastric lumen if possible. If you are uncertain whether gastric tissue will remain viable, invaginate the abnormal tissue. Verify that the gastrosplenic ligament is not torsed, and before closure, palpate the intra-abdominal esophagus to ensure that the stomach is derotated.

VI. Postoperative Care and Assessment

A. Closely monitor electrolyte, fluid, and acid-basis status postoperatively. Many dogs with GDV are hypokalemic postoperatively and require potassium supplementation.

B. Offer small amounts of water and soft, low-fat food 12 to 24 hours after surgery, and observe patients for vomiting.

C. If vomiting is severe or continuous, give a centrally acting antiemetic.

D. Secondary gastric ulcers may occur and require treatment. H_2 receptor blockers (e.g., cimetidine, ranitidine, or famotidine) decrease gastric acidity and may be beneficial.

E. Ventricular arrhythmias are common in dogs with GDV and usually begin 12 to 36 hours postoperatively.
   1. Treatment of cardiac arrhythmias includes maintenance of normal hydration and correction of electrolyte imbalances. Some antiarrhythmic drugs (e.g., lidocaine) are ineffective when the animal is hypokalemic.
      a. Try a test bolus (2 mg/kg) of lidocaine first. Use a constant rate of infusion if the arrhythmias are controlled (Table 16-8).
      b. If arrhythmias are not controlled, try procainamide or sotolol.

Table 16-8
Antiarrhythmic therapy

Lidocaine (Xylocaine)
IV bolus (2 mg/kg increments up to total dose of 8 mg/kg) then IV drip at 50 µg/kg/min (500 mg in 500 ml of fluid administered at maintenance rate [66 ml/kg/day])
Procainamide (Pronestyl)
10-15 mg/kg slow IV bolus or 25-60 µg/kg/min as a continuous IV infusion or 15 mg/kg IM, PO, BID to QID
Sotolol (Betapace)
1.0-2.0 mg/kg PO, BID

VII. Prognosis

A. With timely surgery, the prognosis is fair; however, mortality rates as high as 45% and greater have been reported.

B. Tube gastropexy has the highest reported recurrence rate, varying from 5% to 29%.

C. The reported recurrence rates of dogs operated on for GDV in which the stomach has been repositioned but gastropexy not performed approaches 80%.

Benign Gastric Outflow Obstruction (*SAS*, pp. 283-286)

I. Definitions

A. **Pyloric stenosis** refers to benign muscular hypertrophy of the pylorus.

B. **Chronic antral mucosal hypertrophy** refers to benign hypertrophy of the pyloric mucosa causing outflow obstruction.

C. **Chronic hypertrophic pyloric gastropathy** (CHPG) is a term that denotes pyloric hypertrophy, without specifying whether the mucosa or muscularis is involved.

II. Synonyms

A. Pyloric stenosis synonyms: benign antral muscular hypertrophy, congenital hypertrophic stenosis, congenital pyloric muscle hypertrophy.

B. Chronic antral mucosal hypertrophy synonyms: pyloric or gastric mucosal hypertrophy, chronic hypertrophic gastritis, multiple polyps of the gastric mucosa, acquired hypertrophy.

III. General Considerations and Clinically Relevant Pathophysiology

A. Gastric outlet obstruction may be caused by pyloric abnormalities, disorders of gastric motility, or extrinsic lesions compressing the outflow tract (e.g., pancreatic, duodenal, or hepatic neoplasia).

B. The cause of pyloric stenosis is unknown, but excessive gastrin production has been implicated.

IV. Diagnosis

A. Clinical Presentation

1. Signalment.
   a. In dogs, pyloric stenosis is most commonly seen in brachycephalic (e.g., boxer, bulldog, and Boston terrier) breeds. Siamese cats have also been reported with this condition.
   b. Chronic antral mucosal hypertrophy occurs most commonly in small-breed dogs, particularly Lhasa apso, shih tzu, and Maltese breeds. Some dogs reported with chronic antral mucosal hypertrophy have been considered particularly excitable or vicious.
   c. Males may be more commonly affected than females.
   d. Pyloric stenosis is more common in young animals; however, animals of any age may be affected.
   e. Chronic antral mucosal hypertrophy is more common in middle-aged to older dogs and may mimic neoplasia.
2. History.
   a. Vomiting is the most common sign; however, vomiting may be intermittent or delayed hours after feeding.
   b. Cats commonly have regurgitation and vomiting.
   c. The frequency of vomiting varies from several times daily to once or twice a week.

B. Physical Examination Findings

1. Findings are generally nonspecific; they may include weight loss, anorexia, depression, or dehydration.

C. Radiography/Ultrasonography/Endoscopy

1. Survey abdominal radiographs may reveal gastric distention.
2. If gastric outlet obstruction is suspected, endoscopy is usually recommended because it is diagnostic and allows biopsy.
3. Contrast radiographs may show delayed emptying, pyloric wall thickening, or a filling defect in the pylorus. However, normal elimination of liquid barium does not rule out gastric outflow obstruction.
4. Ultrasonography usually reveals pyloric wall thickening and often detects neoplastic metastases. Ultrasonography also detects extrinsic lesions (e.g., abscess or neoplasia) that may cause gastric outflow obstruction.

V. Medical Management

A. Correct dehydration and electrolyte and acid-base abnormalities before surgery or endoscopy.

VI. Surgical Treatment

A. General Considerations

1. Surgery is recommended for benign pyloric obstruction. The goal is to remove the obstruction and reestablish normal gastric emptying.
2. Submit a full-thickness biopsy to ensure that the thickening is benign.

B. Preoperative Management

1. Withhold food for 24 hours before surgery.

C. Positioning

1. Place the animal in dorsal recumbency and prepare the abdomen for a ventral midline incision.
2. Extend the prepped area from midthorax to near the pubis.

D. Surgical Technique

1. Surgical procedures to correct outlet obstruction due to mucosal or muscular hypertrophy include pyloroplasty and Billroth I procedures. Pyloromyotomy is often ineffective and is not recommended.
2. When mucosal hypertrophy is present, perform either a Y-U pyloroplasty or Billroth I.

VII. Postoperative Care and Assessment

A. Give small amounts of water the day following surgery and observe the patient for vomiting. If vomiting does not occur, give small amounts of moist food 24 hours postoperatively. Discontinue fluid therapy when the animal is eating and drinking normally.

B. Monitor electrolyte abnormalities postoperatively and correct as necessary.

VIII. Prognosis

A. The prognosis with surgical correction of these conditions is good.

B. A poor outcome is generally the result of technical failures (e.g., dehiscence or leakage) or choosing an inappropriate surgical technique for the lesion.

Gastric Ulceration/Erosion (*SAS*, pp. 286-289)

I. Definitions

A. **Ulcers** are mucosal defects extending through the muscularis mucosae into the submucosa or deeper layers of the stomach.

B. **Erosions** do not penetrate the muscularis mucosae.

II. General Considerations and Clinically Relevant Pathophysiology

A. Gastric ulceration in small animals is often iatrogenic (i.e., caused by nonsteroidal antiinflammatory drugs [NSAIDs]) or occurs secondary to an underlying disease process (e.g., mast cell disease, shock, tumor, hepatic failure). **Avoid the concurrent use of steroids and NSAIDs.**

B. The most common sites for gastric ulcers are in the non–acid-producing parts (i.e., fundus and pyloric antrum).

C. Zollinger-Ellison syndrome can cause severe duodenal ulceration, and removal of the pancreatic mass may be necessary to alleviate clinical signs.

D. Thrombosis associated with disseminated intravascular coagulation (DIC) may decrease gastric blood flow and enhance ulcer formation.

E. Both acute and chronic liver disease may be associated with gastrointestinal bleeding and ulcer formation.

F. Circulatory shock and the resultant poor gastric perfusion may cause "stress ulcers."

G. Ulcers may also form secondary to septic shock and commonly occur in dogs with intervertebral disc disease (IVDD).

H. Other conditions associated with gastrointestinal ulceration in small animals include inflammatory bowel disease, gastric or duodenal neoplasia, reflux of bile acid into the stomach, major surgery, uremia, pythiosis, recurrent pancreatitis, and possibly psychologic stress.

III. Diagnosis

A. Clinical Presentation

1. Signalment.
   a. Gastric ulceration or erosion occurs more commonly in dogs than cats.
   b. Most noniatrogenic gastric ulcers in dogs occur in middle-aged or older dogs.
   c. There is no breed predisposition.
2. History.
   a. Although vomiting is a common clinical sign of gastrointestinal ulceration, some dogs present for anorexia or anemia, without vomiting. Vomitus may or may not contain digested blood, fresh blood, or blood clots. Digested blood looks like coffee grounds.
   b. Owners may or may not report that the stools of dogs with ulcers are black (melena) and that the dog has a poor appetite.

B. Physical Examination Findings

1. Abdominal pain may be present on abdominal palpation; however, many dogs with nonperforating gastric ulcers are not obviously in pain.
2. Other signs of ulcer disease include anemia, edema (caused by hypoproteinemia), melena, nausea, and weight loss.

C. Radiography/Ultrasonography/Endoscopy

1. If gastroduodenal ulceration is suspected, the most sensitive and specific test is gastroduodenoscopy.

D. Laboratory Findings

1. Animals with gastric ulcers may be anemic, hypoproteinemic, or both.

2. Gastrinomas are uncommon, but if no other underlying cause is identified, measure serum gastrin levels.

IV. Medical Management

A. Consider symptomatic therapy (e.g., fluids, antibiotics, blood, antiemetics). Identify and treat underlying diseases (e.g., discontinue ulcerogenic drugs, remove mast cell tumors or gastrinomas, treat renal or hepatic disease).

B. Initially, control bleeding medically if perforation seems unlikely.

C. Agents used for treating ulcers include those that lessen gastric acidity and those that protect the gastric mucosa from damage, such as sucralfate (Carafate), cimetidine (Tagamet), ranitidine (Zantac), famotidine (Pepcid), omeprazole (Prilosec), and misoprostol (Cytotec).

V. Surgical Treatment

A. General Considerations

1. Consider surgery if medical therapy is not successful in alleviating clinical signs within 5 to 7 days, bleeding is profuse and life-threatening, or perforation is believed imminent.

B. Preoperative Management

1. If possible, stabilize the animal before surgery.
2. Give whole blood if the animal is severely anemic (i.e., PCV less than 20%).
3. Correct electrolyte and acid-base abnormalities and initiate fluid therapy.

C. Positioning

1. Place the animal in dorsal recumbency and prepare the abdomen for a ventral midline incision.
2. Extend the prepped area from midthorax to the pubis.

D. Surgical Technique

If possible, remove the ulcer with a full-thickness gastric resection, and submit tissue for histopathologic examination. Assess the regional lymph nodes and liver for evidence of metastatic neoplasia or pythiosis, and biopsy them if they appear abnormal. Check both limbs of the pancreas for masses. Occasionally, the location of the ulcer near the pylorus makes full-thickness resection difficult. If the ulcer is located at the pylorus and perforation is present or imminent, perform a serosal patch over the site to help prevent leakage and promote ulcer healing. A serosal patch is simpler to perform than a pylorectomy and gastroduodenostomy (Billroth I). Occasionally, a localized abscess will be noted where an ulcer has perforated, but the omentum or other abdominal structures have walled the site off. If this is the case, carefully drain the abscess, and resect or patch the ulcer. Preoperative or intraoperative endoscopy is helpful in locating ulcers; some are difficult to discern from the serosal surface. If there is extensive disease secondary to something that may not resolve quickly (e.g., inflammatory bowel disease, hepatic failure) place an enterostomy feeding tube.

VI. Postoperative Care and Assessment

A. Give small amounts of water the day following surgery and observe the patient for vomiting.

B. If vomiting does not occur, give small amounts of food 24 hours postoperatively.

C. Feed a low-fat diet with moderate amounts of protein and carbohydrates to aid gastric emptying.

VII. Prognosis

A. The prognosis is good if the ulcer is the result of treatable disease and perforation has not occurred.

Gastric Neoplasia and Infiltrative Disease (*SAS*, pp. 289-292)

I. Definitions

A. **Pythiosis** is a fungal infection caused by *Pythiosis insidiosum* that may cause a severe inflammatory and infiltrative lesion in the stomach.

B. **Phycomycosis** is a more general term for mycoses caused by fungi of the group *Phycomycetes.*

II. General Considerations and Clinically Relevant Pathophysiology

A. Benign gastric tumors are more commonly found in dogs than in cats; however, most gastric neoplasms are malignant.

B. Adenocarcinoma is the most common canine stomach tumor, usually occurring in the pyloric antrum or lesser curvature.

C. Lymphoma is the most common gastric tumor in cats; adenocarcinomas are rare. Most affected cats are feline leukemia virus (FeLV) negative.

D. Leiomyomas are the most common benign canine gastric tumor. They tend to be slow growing, submucosal, and expansile.

E. Pythiosis is a fungal infection caused by *P. insidiosum* that affects any part of the alimentary tract (as well as skin).

III. Diagnosis

A. Clinical Presentation

1. Signalment.
   a. Belgian sheepdogs (adenocarcinomas) and beagles (leiomyoma) may have an increased incidence of gastric neoplasia.
   b. Males appear to be more commonly affected than females.
2. History.
   a. Animals with gastric neoplasia or other infiltrative disease usually present with a history of anorexia. Chronic vomiting, hematemesis, melena, lethargy, weight loss, or edema may also occur.
   b. Many animals are asymptomatic until the tumor becomes large enough to cause gastric outlet obstruction.

B. Physical Examination

1. Findings in animals with gastric neoplasia or pythiosis are often nonspecific (e.g., weight loss, anemia, or edema).

C. Radiography/Ultrasonography/Endoscopy

1. Noncontrast radiographs are generally nondiagnostic.
2. Contrast radiographs may reveal filling defects, delayed gastric emptying, ulceration, loss of normal rugal folds, mucosal thickening, or loss of gastric wall compliance.
3. If a gastric neoplasm is suspected, perform endoscopy because it allows mucosal biopsy of the stomach and duodenum.
   a. Tumors may be difficult to diagnose with endoscopy if they are scirrhous or completely submucosal.
   b. Pythiosis is particularly difficult to diagnose by flexible endoscopic biopsy because the organisms are found in the submucosa.
4. Take thoracic radiographs to rule out pulmonary metastasis.

IV. Surgical Treatment

A. Preoperative Management

1. Withhold food for 12 hours before surgery.
2. Give perioperative antibiotics at anesthetic induction and continue for up to 12 hours postoperatively.

B. Positioning

1. Place the animal in dorsal recumbency and prepare the abdomen for a ventral midline incision.
2. Extend the prepped area from midthorax to the pubis.

C. Surgical Technique

1. Gastric neoplasia.
   a. With the exception of lymphoma, surgery is the only viable treatment for gastric neoplasia.
   b. Palpate the regional lymph nodes for evidence of metastasis. Inspect the liver and other abdominal structures for metastasis or thickening, and biopsy suspicious lesions.
   c. If the lesion appears localized to the stomach, gastric resection might be curative.
2. Pythiosis.
   a. Wide surgical excision is currently the only potentially curative therapy available for pythiosis; however, obtaining wide surgical

margins is difficult because of the extensive nature of the disease at diagnosis. Gastric drainage procedures, such as Billroth II procedures, may be warranted in some cases.

b. Itraconazole therapy is being investigated and may help some patients.

V. Postoperative Care and Assessment

A. Monitor the electrolyte and fluid status of the patient postoperatively, and correct deficiencies.

B. Feed the animal a low-fat, bland diet beginning 24 hours after surgery if vomiting does not occur. If vomiting continues, give a centrally acting antiemetic such as chlorpromazine, metoclopramide, or ondansetron. Consider using an enterostomy feeding tube to help provide nutrition in the postoperative period.

VI. Prognosis

A. The prognosis is guarded for most gastric neoplasms because of their malignant characteristics and size at the time of diagnosis.

B. Pythiosis may be difficult to treat surgically because of its rapid growth rate and extensive nature, but surgical cures have been achieved.

Surgery of the Small Intestine (*SAS*, pp. 292-319)

I. Definitions

A. **Enterotomy** is an incision into the intestine.

B. **Enterectomy** is removal of a segment of intestine.

C. **Intestinal resection and anastomosis** is an enterectomy with reestablishment of continuity between the divided ends.

D. **Enteroenteropexy** or **intestinal plication** is surgical fixation of one intestinal segment to another.

E. **Enteropexy** is fixation of an intestinal segment to the body wall or another loop of intestine.

F. **Serosal patching** is placement of an antimesenteric border of the small intestine over a suture line or organ defect and securing it with sutures.

II. Preoperative Concerns

A. Ascertain diet, medications, stressful events, and response to previous therapy from the owners.

B. Clinical signs of small intestinal disease are variable and nonspecific; vomiting, diarrhea, anorexia, depression, and weight loss are common (Table 16-9).
   1. Severe vomiting, shock, or an acute abdomen suggests intestinal malposition, ischemia, perforation, or upper intestinal obstruction.
   2. Chronic disease is more typical of lower intestinal tract disease or partial obstruction.

C. Perform hematologic and biochemical profiles on animals with suspected small intestinal abnormalities to help identify concurrent systemic disease and to direct preoperative therapy.

D. Radiographs.
   1. Plain radiographs may demonstrate abnormal gas-fluid patterns, masses, foreign bodies, abdominal fluid, or displaced viscera. Take right-lateral recumbent and ventrodorsal views.
   2. Contrast studies are useful for demonstrating foreign bodies, obstructions, abnormal displacements, abnormal bowel wall thickness, irregular mucosal patterns, and distortion of the bowel wall.

Table 16-9
Clinical signs of chronic intestinal disease

Clinical sign	Small intestine	Large intestine
Weight loss	Consistent	Infrequent
Appetite	Variable	Usually normal; variable
Vomiting	Occasional	Rare
Belching	Occasional	Rare
Flatulence and borborygmus	Occasional	Rare
Distended abdomen	Variable	Rare
Defecation quantity	Normal to large	Small to normal
Defecation frequency	Normal to slightly increased	Normal to very frequent
Blood in feces	If present, usually dark, black (melena)	If present, usually fresh, red (hematochezia)
Mucus in feces	Absent	Present or absent
Steatorrhea	Occasional	Absent
Fecalith	Absent	Sometimes
Urgency or tenesmus	Absent	Sometimes present
Dyschezia	Absent	Present with rectal disease
Rectal exam	Normal	May be normal or abnormal (blood, mucus, pain, mass)
Abdominal pain	Variable	Variable
Poor hair coat	Variable	Uncommon
Depression	Variable	Uncommon

a. When intestinal perforation is suspected, use iodinated contrast or iohexol. **Do not use barium!**

E. Use ultrasonography to define intestinal and other abdominal masses and provide information about the intestine.

F. Gastrointestinal endoscopy allows visualization and biopsy of the duodenum (and sometimes the upper jejunum and ileum) for detection of inflammation, ulcers, masses, and changes in wall thickness or texture.

III. Anesthetic Considerations

A. Fast mature animals 12 to 18 hours before surgery, but only fast pediatric patients for 4 to 8 hours.

B. Special anesthetic considerations are needed when dealing with patients having bowel obstruction, ischemia, or perforation.
   1. Do not use nitrous oxide in patients with intestinal obstruction.
   2. Visceral manipulation may induce bradycardia; have atropine or glycopyrrolate available.

C. See Appendix G-9 for anesthetic protocols for animals undergoing intestinal surgery.

IV. Antibiotics

A. Use antibiotics in animals with severe mucosal damage or acute gastrointestinal disease associated with bloody diarrhea, fever, leukocytosis, leukopenia, or shock.

B. Use prophylactic antibiotics in animals with intestinal obstruction because there is an increased risk of contamination associated with bacterial overgrowth.

C. Antibiotics are also indicated when devascularized and traumatized tissue are present and when surgical times are expected to be greater than 2 to 3 hours.

D. Administer first-generation cephalosporins (e.g., cefazolin; Appendix I) before surgery on the upper and middle small intestine. Use second-generation cephalosporins (e.g., cefmetazole or cefoxitin; Appendix I) for procedures involving the distal small intestine and large intestine.

E. Redose antibiotics 2 hours after the initial dose.

V. Surgical Anatomy

A. The common bile duct and pancreatic duct open in the first few centimeters of the duodenum at the major duodenal papilla in dogs. The accessory pancreatic duct enters caudal to this at the minor duodenal papilla.

B. Submucosa is the intestinal layer that provides mechanical strength; thus engage it when suturing intestine to provide a secure closure.

VI. Surgical Techniques

A. General Considerations

1. Perform surgical correction of mechanical obstructions within 12 hours of diagnosis, if possible.
   a. Weigh the benefits of stabilizing the patient against the risk of ischemic necrosis caused by vascular disruption, which increases with time.
   b. Perform surgery for penetrating abdominal wounds, intestinal perforation, volvulus, or peritonitis as soon as the diagnosis is made.
2. Routine criteria to assess bowel viability include observation of intestinal color (pink to red rather than blue to black), wall texture, peristalsis, pulsation of arteries, and bleeding when incised.
   a. Resect bowel of questionable viability.

B. Intestinal Biopsy

1. General considerations.
   a. Perform laparotomy and enterotomy if endoscopic or ultrasound biopsy is not possible or is nondiagnostic.
   b. Obtain multiple biopsies and be sure that the samples are reasonably large (4 to 5 mm) and contain adequate amounts of mucosa.
   c. Explore the entire abdomen thoroughly before biopsies are performed.
2. Technique.

Exteriorize and isolate the diseased or desired intestine from the abdomen by packing with towels or laparotomy sponges. Gently milk chyme (intestinal contents) from the lumen of the identified intestinal segment. To minimize spillage of chyme, occlude the lumen at both ends of the isolated segment by having an assistant use a scissorlike grip with the index and middle fingers, 4 to 6 cm on each side of the proposed enterotomy site. If an assistant is not available, noncrushing intestinal forceps (Doyen) or a Penrose drain tourniquet can also be used to occlude the intestinal lumen. Make a full-thickness stab incision into the intestinal lumen on the antimesenteric border with a No. 11 scalpel blade. Obtain full-thickness biopsies 2 to 3 mm wide by either making a second longitudinal incision parallel to the first with the scalpel blade or by removing an ellipse of intestinal wall at one margin of the first incision with Metzenbaum scissors. Transverse enterotomy incisions can also be made to obtain biopsies. Place the biopsy serosal side down on a heavy piece of sterile paper to help prevent curling of the specimen. Close the incision as described below with simple interrupted sutures. Simple continuous or crushing sutures may also be used to close the enterotomy. If a foreign body is present, make the incision in healthy-appearing tissue distal to the foreign body. Lengthen the incision along the intestine's long axis with Metzenbaum scissors or scalpel as necessary to allow foreign body removal without tearing the intestine. After biopsy or foreign body removal, prepare the incision for closure by trimming everted mucosa so that its edge is even with the serosal edge (if necessary). Suction the isolated lumen. Close the incision with gentle appositional force in a longitudinal or transverse direction using simple interrupted sutures. Place sutures through all layers of the intestinal wall, 2 mm from the edge and 2 to 3 mm apart, with extraluminal knots. Angle the needle so the serosa is engaged slightly further from the edge than the mucosa to help reposition everting

mucosa within the lumen. Tie each suture carefully without cutting through layers of the intestinal wall so as to gently appose all intestinal layers without crushing the tissue. Use a monofilament absorbable suture material (4-0 or 3-0 polydioxanone or polyglyconate) with a swaged-on taper or tapercut point needle. Consider a monofilament nonabsorbable suture (4-0 or 3-0 polypropylene or nylon) if the patient has an albumin level less than or equal to 2.0 g/dl. While maintaining luminal occlusion near the enterotomy site, moderately distend the lumen with sterile saline, apply gentle digital pressure, and observe for leakage between sutures or through needle holes. Place additional sutures if leakage occurs between sutures. Lavage the isolated intestine and the entire abdomen if contamination has occurred. Place omentum over the suture line before abdominal closure. Use a serosal patch rather than omentum if intestinal integrity is questionable or if leakage occurs from needle holes. Replace contaminated instruments and gloves before abdominal closure.

C. Intestinal Resection and Anastomosis

Make an abdominal incision long enough to allow exploration of the abdomen. Thoroughly explore the abdomen and collect any nonintestinal specimens, then exteriorize and isolate the diseased intestine from the abdomen by packing with towels or laparotomy sponges. Assess intestinal viability and determine the amount of intestine needing resection. Double ligate and transect the arcadial mesenteric vessels from the cranial mesenteric artery that supplies this segment of intestine. Double ligate the terminal arcade vessels and vasa recta vessels within the mesenteric fat at the points of proposed intestinal transection. Gently milk chyme (intestinal contents) from the lumen of the identified intestinal segment. Occlude the lumen at both ends of the segment to minimize spillage of chyme (see above). Place forceps across each end of the diseased bowel segment (these forceps may be either crushing or noncrushing because this segment of the intestine will be excised). Transect the intestine with either a scalpel blade or Metzenbaum scissors along the outside of the forceps. Make the incision either perpendicular or oblique to the long axis. Use a perpendicular incision (75- to 90-degree angle) at each end if the luminal diameters are the same. When luminal sizes of the intestinal ends are expected to be unequal, use a perpendicular incision across the intestine with the larger luminal diameter and an oblique incision (45- to 60-degree angle) across the intestine with the smaller luminal diameter to help correct size disparity. Make the oblique incision such that the antimesenteric border is shorter than the mesenteric border. Suction the intestinal ends and remove any debris clinging to the cut edges with a moistened gauze sponge. Trim everting mucosa with Metzenbaum scissors just before beginning the end-to-end anastomosis.

Use 3-0 or 4-0 monofilament, absorbable suture (polydioxanone or polyglyconate) with a swaged-on taper or tapercut point needle. In peritonitis cases monofilament nonabsorbable suture (3-0 or 4-0 polypropylene or nylon) is sometimes used. Place simple interrupted sutures through all layers of the intestinal wall. Angle the needle so the serosa is engaged slightly further from the edge than the mucosa. This helps reposition everting mucosa within the lumen. Tie each suture carefully so as to gently appose the edges of the intestine with the knots extraluminally. Tying sutures roughly or with too much tension causes the suture to cut through the serosa, muscularis, and mucosa and creates a crushing suture. Some surgeons prefer this suture, and others use a simple continuous pattern. Pulling continuous sutures too tight will have a purse-string effect, and significant stenosis may occur. A continuous pattern around the intestine may limit dilation at the anastomotic site and cause a partial obstruction. Appose intestinal ends by first placing a simple interrupted suture at the mesenteric border and then placing a second suture at the antimesenteric border approximately 180 degrees from the first (this divides the suture line into equal halves and allows determination of whether the ends are of approximately equal diameter). The mesenteric suture is the most difficult suture to place in the anastomosis because of mesenteric fat. It is also the most common site of leakage. If the ends are of equal diameter, space additional sutures between the first two sutures approximately 2 mm from the edge and 2 to 3 mm apart. If minor disparity still exists between lumen sizes, space the sutures around the larger lumen slightly further apart than the sutures in the intestine with the smaller lumen. To correct luminal disparity that cannot be accommodated by the angle of the incisions or by suture spacing, resect a small wedge (1 to 2 cm long and 1 to 3 mm wide) from the antimesenteric border of the intestine with the smaller lumen. This enlarges the perimeter of the stoma, giving it an oval shape. Do not suture together the edges of the intestine with the larger lumen in an attempt to reduce luminal size to that of the smaller intestine. Narrowing the larger lumen is not recommended because there is greater tendency for stricture at the anastomotic site when the dilated intestine contracts to a normal size. After suture placement inspect the anastomosis and check for leakage. While maintaining luminal occlusion adjacent to the anastomotic site, moderately distend the lumen with sterile saline, apply gentle digital pressure, and observe for leakage between sutures or through needle holes. This is a subjective test because all anastomoses can be made to leak if enough pressure is applied. Place additional sutures if leakage occurs between sutures. Close the mesenteric defect with a simple continuous or interrupted suture pattern (4-0 polydioxanone or polyglyconate), being careful not to penetrate or traumatize arcadial vessels near the defect. Lavage the isolated intestine and the entire abdomen if abdominal contamination has occurred. Wrap the anastomotic site with omentum before abdominal closure or use a serosal patch if intestinal integrity is questionable and leakage is likely.

D. Serosal Patching

Use one or more loops of intestine to form the patch. Use gentle loops to avoid stretching, twisting, or kinking the intestine and mesenteric vessels. If using more than one loop of intestine, suture these loops together before securing the patch to the damaged area. All sutures used to create or secure the patch engage the submucosa, muscularis, and serosa; they should not penetrate the intestinal lumen. Place interrupted or continuous sutures in healthy tissue to secure the patch and isolate the damaged area.

E. Bowel Plication

Place small intestinal loops side by side to form a series of gentle loops from the distal duodenum to the distal ileum. Secure the loops by placing sutures that engage the submucosa, muscularis, and serosa 6 to 10 cm. Use 3-0 or 4-0 monofilament absorbable or nonabsorbable sutures with a swaged-on taper point needle. Avoid positioning the intestinal loops at acute angles lest intestinal obstruction occur.

VII. Healing of the Small Intestine

A. Approximating suture patterns facilitate rapid healing. Everting and inverting suture patterns retard intestinal healing and may result in greater stricture formation.

B. Systemic factors such as hypovolemia, shock, hypoproteinemia, debilitation, and concurrent infections may delay healing and increase the risk of incisional breakdown.

C. Tension on the repair caused by accumulated ingesta, fluid, gas, or poor mobilization of the bowel increases the potential for intestinal suture breakdown.

D. Dehiscence most commonly occurs between 3 and 5 days after intestinal surgery.

VIII. Suture Materials/Special Instruments

A. Consider long-lasting monofilament absorbable (polydioxanone or polyglyconate) or nonabsorbable (nylon or polypropylene) sutures for patients with low albumin levels.

IX. Postoperative Care and Assessment

A. Monitor the animal closely for vomiting during recovery. Provide analgesics (e.g., oxymorphone, butorphanol, or buprenorphine) as needed.

B. Maintain hydration with intravenous fluids; monitor and correct electrolyte and acid-base abnormalities. Offer small amounts of water 8 to 12 hours after surgery.

C. If no vomiting occurs, offer small amounts of food 12 to 24 hours after surgery.

1. Feed animals a bland, low-fat food three to four times daily.
2. Reintroduce the normal diet gradually, beginning 48 to 72 hours after surgery.
3. Monitor clinical signs and response to abdominal palpation for evidence of leakage and subsequent peritonitis or abscess formation.

D. Provide nutritional support via an enterostomy tube if the patient is debilitated, is vomiting, or remains anorexic.

Intestinal Foreign Bodies (*SAS*, pp. 305-309)

I. Definitions

A. **Intestinal foreign bodies** are ingested objects that may cause complete or partial intraluminal obstruction.

II. General Considerations and Clinically Relevant Pathophysiology

A. Foreign bodies that traverse the esophagus and stomach may become lodged in the smaller-diameter intestine.

B. The clinical course and signs are more severe in animals with complete intraluminal obstructions than in those with partial obstructions.
   1. With complete intraluminal obstruction, the intestine oral to the lesion distends with gas and fluid.
   2. Clinical signs of distal and incomplete obstructions may be insidious, with vague, intermittent anorexia, lethargy, and occasional vomiting spanning several days or weeks.

C. Proximal or high obstructions (i.e., duodenum or proximal jejunum) cause persistent vomiting, loss of gastric secretions, electrolyte imbalances, and dehydration. The major cause of death from upper small intestinal obstruction is severe, rapid hypovolemia.

III. Diagnosis

A. Clinical Presentation

1. Signalment.
   a. There is no breed or sex predisposition; however, cats more commonly ingest linear foreign bodies than dogs.
2. History.
   a. An acute onset of vomiting, anorexia, and depression are the most common presenting complaints.

B. Physical Examination Findings

1. Physical examination may reveal abdominal distention, diarrhea, abdominal pain, abnormal posture, or shock.
2. Animals with high obstruction may be severely dehydrated; those with low obstructions may be thin as a result of severe weight loss.

C. Radiography/Ultrasonography/Endoscopy

1. Radiography will often diagnose complete or near-complete obstructions and may identify the cause.
2. Obstructed intestinal loops become distended with air, fluid, or ingesta.
3. Linear foreign bodies cause the intestines to appear bunched or pleated together with small gas bubbles in the lumen and without gas-distended intestinal loops.
4. Ultrasonography may identify foreign objects with a hyperechoic margin plus or minus fluid accumulation. It also allows motility to be assessed.
5. Linear foreign bodies lodged at the pylorus that prevent scope passage into the duodenum may be recognized endoscopically.

IV. Medical Management

A. Foreign body advancement may be monitored radiographically unless vomiting is severe, debilitation occurs, or there is evidence of peritonitis.

B. **Always repeat radiographs before surgery** (even if they were taken the previous evening) because the foreign body may have moved into the colon or passed in the feces.

V. Surgical Treatment

A. General Considerations

1. In cases of partial obstruction, failure to radiographically demonstrate foreign body movement within the intestine over an 8-hour period, or failure to pass the object within approximately 36 hours, indicates the need for surgery.
2. Do not delay surgery to observe for passage of the object through the intestinal tract if abdominal pain, fever, vomiting, or lethargy is apparent.
3. Most foreign bodies can be removed by enterotomy rather than resection and anastomosis unless intestinal necrosis or perforation is present.
4. Multiple enterotomies (two to four) are often necessary to remove linear foreign bodies.

B. Preoperative Management

1. Correct fluid, electrolyte, and acid-base deficits before surgery, if possible.

C. Surgical Technique

Make an incision through the linea alba that is sufficient to allow complete exploration of the abdomen. Explore the entire abdomen and gastrointestinal tract to avoid overlooking concurrent abnormalities or multiple foreign bodies. Once the foreign body has been located, isolate this loop of intestine from the remainder of the abdominal cavity with laparotomy pads or sterile towels. Complete obstructions may cause the bowel to be severely distended and appear cyanotic; however, reserve determination of intestinal viability until the bowel has been decompressed and the foreign body has been removed by enterotomy. Bathe the intestine in warm saline for a few minutes to help improve its color and peristalsis. Normally the appearance of the intestine improves rapidly after decompression. If the intestinal segment is determined to be viable, close the enterotomy with simple interrupted sutures as described on pp. 201-202. Resect nonviable or questionable intestine and reestablish bowel continuity by end-to-end anastomosis. After foreign body removal, carefully examine the intestine for evidence of perforation that might necessitate resection of the involved segment(s).

Intestinal Neoplasia (*SAS*, pp. 309-311)

I. Definitions

A. **Intestinal neoplasia** includes those tumors that arise from one of the layers of the intestinal wall, its glands, or associated cells or lymphatics.

II. General Considerations and Clinically Relevant Pathophysiology

A. Intestinal tumors occur most commonly in the canine rectum and colon and the feline small intestine.

B. Most intestinal tumors are malignant.
   1. They most commonly invade the muscular layer of the intestinal wall, where they compromise the lumen diameter and reduce distensibility.
   2. At the time of diagnosis the disease is usually advanced, and most malignant tumors have metastasized.

C. In dogs adenocarcinoma is the most common intestinal tumor, and leiomyosarcoma is the most common sarcoma.

D. In cats lymphosarcoma is most common, followed by adenocarcinoma and mast cell tumor.

E. Adenocarcinomas.
   1. Adenocarcinomas are locally invasive and slow growing.
   2. They most commonly arise in the duodenum and colon in dogs and distal jejunum and ileum in cats.

F. Lymphosarcoma.
   1. Lymphosarcoma may be caused by FeLV or feline immunodeficiency virus (FIV). In dogs the etiology is unknown.
   2. It may be diffuse or nodular.

G. Adenomatous polyps are found in the feline duodenum and canine rectum.

H. Intestinal leiomyosarcomas are malignant smooth-muscle tumors of older dogs and most commonly occur in the cecum and jejunum.

III. Diagnosis

A. Clinical Presentation

1. Signalment.
   a. Older animals are most commonly affected.
2. History.
   a. Patients initially have vague clinical signs of depression, anorexia, and lethargy, which may progress to diarrhea or vomiting.
   b. Weight loss is progressive.

B. Physical Examination Findings

1. Abdominal palpation may reveal a firm abdominal mass, thickened intestinal loops, or mesenteric lymphadenopathy.
2. Weight loss may be evident.

C. Radiography/Ultrasonography

1. Take thoracic and abdominal radiographs if neoplasia is suspected.
2. Abdominal ultrasonography often delineates the mass and may facilitate percutaneous biopsy.

IV. Medical Management

A. Lymphosarcoma may respond to chemotherapy.

B. Refer to a medicine text for additional information and chemotherapeutic protocols.

V. Surgical Treatment

A. General Considerations

1. Surgical resection is the treatment of choice for intestinal tumors; however, many tumors are too advanced to allow complete resection by the time they are diagnosed.

B. Preoperative Management

1. Correct fluid, electrolyte, and acid-base deficits before surgery if possible.

C. Surgical Technique

Make an incision through the linea alba from the xiphoid process to the pubis to allow complete abdominal exploration. Explore the entire abdomen and gastrointestinal tract to avoid overlooking concurrent abnormalities. Biopsy mesenteric lymph nodes and other organs as needed before incising intestine. Resect the mass with 4- to 8-cm margins of grossly normal tissue and perform an end-to-end anastomosis. Pay special attention to surgical technique because these patients are frequently debilitated. Submit tissues for histopathologic evaluation and tumor staging.

VI. Postoperative Care and Assessment

A. Provide postoperative care as described in the section on surgery of the small intestine.

Intussusception (*SAS*, pp. 311-314)

I. Definitions

A. **Intussusception** is the telescoping or invagination of one intestinal segment **(intussusceptum)** into the lumen of an adjacent segment **(intussuscipiens).**

II. General Considerations and Clinically Relevant Pathophysiology

A. Gastrointestinal tract intussusceptions may occur anywhere; however, ileocolic and jejuno-jejunal intussusceptions are most common.

B. The cause of most intussusceptions is unknown. They may be associated with enteritis or systemic illness, or occur after surgery.

III. Diagnosis

A. Clinical Presentation

1. Signalment.
   a. Intussusceptions occur more commonly in dogs than cats.
   b. Suspect parasitism or enteritis as a cause for intussusception in young dogs. Suspect intestinal thickening or masses in adults.
2. History.
   a. The severity and type of clinical signs depend on the location, completeness, vascular integrity, and duration of intestinal obstruction.
   b. Consider acute intussusceptions in puppies with parvoviral enteritis that suddenly become worse.
   c. Patients with chronic intussusception often have intractable, intermittent diarrhea and hypoalbuminemia.

B. Physical Examination Findings

1. A presumptive diagnosis of intussusception can be made when an elongated, thickened intestinal loop (sausage-shaped mass) is palpated.
2. Jejuno-jejunal intussusceptions are easier to palpate than ileocolic intussusceptions because they are usually more caudal and ventral in the abdomen.

C. Radiography/Ultrasonography

1. On radiographs, jejunal intussusceptions more often result in obstructive patterns than ileocolic intussusception.
2. Ultrasonography is useful in detecting intussusceptions.

IV. Medical Management

A. Most intussusceptions require surgical reduction and ancillary procedures to prevent recurrence.

V. Surgical Treatment

A. General Considerations

1. Because recurrence is common, treat intussusceptions surgically even if they can be manually reduced.

B. Preoperative Management

1. Correct fluid, electrolyte, and acid-base deficits before surgery if possible.

C. Surgical Technique

Explore the abdomen, collect specimens, and isolate the involved intestine with laparotomy pads. Reduce intussusceptions manually if possible by gently applying traction on the neck of the intussusceptum while milking its apex (leading edge) out of the intussuscipiens. Avoid excessive traction because this may tear the compromised intestine. Manual reduction is successful only if fibrin has not formed firm serosal adhesions. Evaluate the reduced intestine for viability and perforation. Carefully palpate the leading edge of the intussusceptum to detect mass lesions. Perform a resection and anastomosis if manual reduction is impossible, tissue is devitalized, or mesenteric vessels have been avulsed from a portion of the involved intestine. Submit biopsies of the involved intestine to identify the cause of the intussusception. Perform an enteroenteropexy to prevent recurrence.

VI. Postoperative Care and Assessment

A. Provide postoperative care as described on p. 203.

VII. Prognosis

A. Recurrence is expected in 20% to 30% of affected animals without enteropexy.

Intestinal Volvulus/Torsion (*SAS*, pp. 316-319)

I. Definitions

A. **Intestinal volvulus** is defined as twisting of the intestine, which causes obstruction.

B. **Intestinal torsion** is twisting of the intestines about the root of the mesentery.

II. General Considerations and Clinically Relevant Pathophysiology

A. Intestinal volvulus/torsion is uncommon in small animals because they have short mesenteric attachments. When it does occur the jejunum is most commonly involved.

B. Intestinal volvulus is a medical and surgical emergency.

III. Diagnosis

A. Clinical Presentation

1. Signalment.
   a. Male, medium-to-large, sporting or working breeds are most commonly diagnosed with intestinal volvulus/torsion.
   b. German shepherds (with pancreatic insufficiency) and English pointers appear predisposed to intestinal volvulus/torsion.
   c. Young adult dogs (2 to 3 years) are most commonly affected.
2. History.
   a. Vigorous activity, dietary indiscretion, or trauma often precedes volvulus.
   b. Signs are typically acute.

B. Physical Examination Findings

1. Affected animals usually present in shock with an acute abdomen.
2. Pain and dilated loops of intestine may be detected by abdominal palpation.

C. Radiography

1. Plain radiographs are often diagnostic with the entire intestinal tract uniformly distended with gas.

IV. Medical Management

A. Shock therapy (fluids, antibiotics, plus or minus corticosteroids; see below) is essential but not curative. Immediate diagnosis and surgery are necessary if the patient is to survive.

V. Surgical Treatment

A. Preoperative Management

1. Initial treatment consists of aggressive shock therapy and correction of electrolyte and acid-base abnormalities. Rapidly administer shock doses of fluids (e.g., 90 ml/kg/hr) and monitor central venous pressure to avoid volume overload. Alternatively, give hypertonic saline or hetastarch (Appendix B).
2. Administer broad-spectrum antibiotic therapy and possibly a nonsteroidal antiinflammatory drug.

B. Anesthesia

1. These patients are extreme anesthetic risks. Use a balanced anesthetic protocol (e.g., opioids plus isoflurane) (Appendix G-10).
2. Preoxygenate before surgery.
3. Placing two venous catheters (e.g., two cephalic or a cephalic and jugular catheter) before surgery is recommended to allow fluids, blood, pressors, or other agents to be given simultaneously if needed.
4. Correct hypotension before and prevent during and after surgery. If the total protein is less than 4.0 g/dl or albumin is less than 1.5 g/dl, give perioperative colloids.
5. Consider giving dobutamine (2 to 10 μg/kg/min, IV) or dopamine (2 to 10 μg/kg/min, IV) during surgery for inotropic support.
6. Monitor these patients for arrhythmias or tachycardia. Monitor an

ECG, pulse oximeter, and direct and indirect blood pressure measurements throughout surgery.

7. Do not use nitrous oxide.

C. Surgical Technique

Quickly explore the abdomen to confirm the diagnosis and determine the direction of twisting. The intestine will appear dilated, edematous, and discolored with the serosal surfaces ranging from red to black in color. Decompress the intestine if necessary to allow derotation and reposition the intestines. Allow the intestine to reperfuse and stabilize while the abdomen is more thoroughly explored. Evaluate intestinal viability and resect devitalized tissue. Thoroughly lavage the abdomen with warm physiologic saline or balanced electrolyte solution. Perform open peritoneal drainage if intestinal necrosis and peritonitis are identified.

VI. Postoperative Care and Assessment

A. Provide postoperative care as described on p. 203.

VII. Prognosis

A. Mortality rates approach 100%. Most animals who have survived have been incidentally diagnosed during celiotomy for another problem, had rotation limited to 180 degrees, and were operated on within a few hours of occurrence.

Surgery of the Large Intestine (*SAS*, pp. 319-335)

I. Definitions

A. **Colopexy** is surgical fixation of the colon.

B. **Colectomy** is partial or complete resection of the colon.

C. **Typhlectomy** is resection of the cecum.

D. **Tenesmus** is straining to defecate.

E. **Dyschezia** is pain or discomfort on defecation.

F. **Hematochezia** is the passage of stools that contain red blood.

G. **Melena** is passage of tarry stools (i.e., digested blood).

II. Preoperative Concerns

A. Differentiation of large bowel disease from small intestinal disorders is usually based on history and physical examination; however, in some cases (e.g., fungal, infectious, neoplastic), radiographs, ultrasonography, endoscopy, or biopsy may be necessary.

B. Physical examination findings vary depending on the disease and its location in the large bowel.

C. The colon contains more bacteria than the rest of the gastrointestinal tract. Mechanical emptying and cleansing are indicated to reduce bacterial numbers unless the colon is perforated or obstructed.
   1. Feed an elemental diet that requires no digestion (composed of glucose, amino acids, etc.) to reduce colonic bacterial numbers.
   2. Withhold food 24 hours before surgery, but allow free access to water.
   3. Give laxatives, cathartics, and warm-water enemas 24 hours before surgery. Colon electrolyte solutions (Colyte or GoLytely) more effectively cleanse the colon than enemas; the only contraindication to their use is obstruction.

III. Anesthetic Considerations

A. Avoid nitrous oxide in patients with intestinal obstruction, because it increases the volume of air trapped in hollow viscera.

IV. Antibiotics

A. There is a high risk of infection after colorectal surgery. Although controversial, the use of antibiotics in colorectal surgery reduces morbidity and mortality associated with infection.

B. Give systemic perioperative antibiotics effective against gram-negative aerobes and anaerobes.
   1. Recommended drugs include second-generation cephalosporins (e.g., cefmetazole, cefoxitin, cefotetan) given at the time of induction.
   2. Gentamicin plus cefazolin can be given intravenously at induction.
   3. Aminoglycosides (e.g., neomycin, kanamycin) in combination with metronidazole can be given orally beginning 24 hours before surgery.

V. Surgical Anatomy

A. Note the different conformation of the vessels supplying the large and small intestine before performing a colectomy.

VI. Surgical Techniques

A. Colopexy

1. General considerations.
   a. Colopexy is done to create permanent adhesions between the

serosal surfaces of the colon and abdominal wall so as to prevent caudal movement of the colon and rectum.

b. The most common indication is to prevent recurring rectal prolapse.

2. Technique.

Expose and explore the abdomen. Locate and isolate the descending colon from the remainder of the abdomen. Pull the descending colon cranially to reduce the prolapse. Verify prolapse reduction by having a nonsterile assistant inspect the anus visually and perform a rectal examination. Make a 3- to 5-cm longitudinal incision along the antimesenteric border of the distal descending colon through only the serosal and muscularis layers. Create a similar incision on the left abdominal wall several centimeters lateral (2.5 cm or more) to the linea alba through the peritoneum and underlying muscle. Appose each edge of the colonic and abdominal wall incisions with two simple continuous or simple interrupted rows of sutures using 2-0 or 3-0 monofilament absorbable (e.g., polydioxanone or polyglyconate) or nonabsorbable (nylon, polypropylene) suture material. Engage the submucosa as each suture is placed. Lavage the surgical site and surround it with omentum before abdominal closure. Alternatively, scarify an 8- to 10-cm antimesenteric segment of the descending colon by scraping the serosa with a scalpel blade or rubbing it with a gauze sponge. On the left abdominal wall opposite the prepared colon, scarify the peritoneum in the same manner. Preplace, then tie, six to eight horizontal mattress sutures between the two scarified surfaces. Roll the colon toward the midline and place a second row of six to eight sutures. Use 2-0 to 3-0 monofilament absorbable or nonabsorbable sutures that engage the submucosa, but do not penetrate the colonic mucosa. Tie the sutures apposing the scarified surfaces.

B. Resection

1. During subtotal colectomy, 90% to 95% of the colon is resected; the primary adverse effect is frequent and soft stools.
2. Technique.

Explore the entire abdomen through a ventral midline celiotomy. Collect nonintestinal specimens before entering the bowel lumen. Carefully isolate the diseased bowel with laparotomy pads or sterile towels. Assess intestinal viability and determine resection sites. Double ligate all the vasa recta vessels to the diseased segment, but do not ligate the major colic vessels running parallel to the mesenteric border of the bowel unless performing a colectomy. Gently milk fecal material from the lumen of the isolated bowel. Occlude the lumen at both ends to minimize fecal contamination by having an assistant use a scissorlike grip with the index and middle fingers positioned 4 to 6 cm from the diseased tissue on the colonic wall. Noncrushing intestinal forceps (Doyen) or a Penrose drain tourniquet can also be used to occlude the intestinal lumen. Place another pair of forceps (either crushing [Carmalt] or noncrushing [Doyen]) across each end of the diseased bowel segment. Transect through healthy colon using a scalpel blade or Metzenbaum scissors along the outside of the crushing forceps. Make the incision perpendicular to the long axis if the lumen sizes are about equal. Use an oblique (45- to 60-degree angle) incision across the smaller intestinal segment when lumen sizes are expected to be unequal. Angle the incision so the antimesenteric border is shorter than the mesenteric border. Suction the intestinal ends and remove any debris clinging to the cut edges with a moistened gauze sponge. Trim everting mucosa with Metzenbaum scissors just before beginning the anastomosis.

C. Anastomoses

1. General considerations.

   a. Luminal disparity that cannot be accommodated by the angle of the incisions or suture spacing is usually correctable by resecting a small wedge (1 to 2 cm long, 1 to 3 mm wide) from the antimesenteric border of the intestine with the smaller lumen. This enlarges the stomal perimeter and gives it an oval shape.

2. Sutured anastomoses.

Reappose intestinal ends with a one- or two-layer suture closure or with staples. Use 3-0 or 4-0 monofilament absorbable (polydioxanone, polyglyconate) or nonabsorbable (nylon, polypropylene) suture with a taper or tapercut, swaged-on needle. Place simple interrupted sutures through all layers of the wall and position knots extraluminally when a one-layer closure is used. Angle the needle so slightly more serosa than mucosa is engaged with each bite to help prevent mucosa from protruding between sutures. Begin by placing one suture at the mesenteric border and one at the antimesenteric border. If the intestinal ends are of equal diameter, space additional sutures between the first two sutures approximately 2 mm from the edge and 2 to 3 mm apart. Gently appose the tissue edges when tying knots to prevent tissue strangulation and disruption of blood supply. If minor disparity still exists between lumen sizes, space sutures around the larger lumen slightly further apart than the sutures in the intestinal segment with the smaller lumen. After completing the anastomosis, check for leakage by moderately distending the lumen with saline and applying gentle digital pressure. Look for leakage between sutures or through suture holes. Place additional sutures if leakage occurs between sutures. Close the mesenteric defect. Lavage the isolated intestine thoroughly without allowing the fluid to seep into the abdominal cavity. Remove the laparotomy pads and change gloves and instruments. Lavage the abdomen with sterile, warm saline, then use suction to remove the fluid. Wrap the anastomotic site with omentum or create a serosal patch.

3. Stapled anastomoses.

For an end-to-side technique first insert the end-to-end stapling instrument (without anvil) through the open transected end of the colon. Advance the center rod through an antimesenteric stab wound surrounded by a purse-string suture. Tie the suture and place the anvil on the center rod. Introduce the anvil into the lumen of the ileum. Tie the ileal purse-string suture, close the instrument, and fire the staples. Gently rotate and remove the instrument. Inspect the anastomotic site for hemostasis and integrity. Close the transected colon with a transverse stapler. Lavage the surgical sites and place an omental or serosal patch.

D. Typhlectomy

Begin typhlectomy for a noninverted cecum by ligating cecal branches of the ileocecal artery within the ileocecal mesenteric attachment (ileocecal fold). Dissect the ileocecal fold, freeing the cecum from the ileum and colon. Place a clamp across the base of the cecum. Milk intestinal contents from the ascending colon and ileum adjacent to the cecocolic orifice and occlude the lumen. Transect the cecum where it joins the ascending colon. Close the defect with simple interrupted sutures. Alternatively, place a transverse or linear cutting stapling instrument across the base of the cecum. Activate the stapler. Transect the cecum before removing the transverse stapling instrument. Lavage, then cover the surgical site with an omental or serosal patch. If the cecum is inverted, manually reduce it, if possible, before resection. Perform an antimesenteric colotomy and exteriorize the cecum if it cannot be manually reduced. Resect the cecum and close the cecocolic orifice with sutures or staples as described above.

VII. Healing of the Large Intestine

A. Colonic healing is similar to that in the small intestine, but delayed.
   1. Collateral circulation to the large intestine is poor compared with the small intestine.
   2. There are large numbers of anaerobic and aerobic intraluminal bacteria with more anaerobes than aerobes.
   3. High intraluminal pressure develops during passage of a solid fecal bolus.

B. Risk of dehiscence during the first 3 to 4 days is high because collagen lysis exceeds synthesis.

VIII. Postoperative Care and Assessment

A. Monitor animals closely for vomiting or regurgitation during recovery to prevent aspiration pneumonia.

B. Provide postoperative care as described in the section on surgery of the small intestine, p. 203.

Large Intestinal Neoplasia (*SAS*, pp. 327-330)

I. Definitions

A. **Colorectal neoplasia** includes any tumor occurring in the colon or rectum.

B. **Polyps** are grossly visible protrusions from the mucosal surface of either neoplastic or nonneoplastic cells.

II. General Considerations and Clinically Relevant Pathophysiology

A. Adenomatous polyps and adenocarcinomas are the most common colorectal neoplasms.

B. Clinical signs of tenesmus, dyschezia, and hematochezia can be attributed to the presence of a friable luminal mass that bleeds when abraded by the passage of feces.

C. Adenocarcinomas of the colon and rectum are rare in dogs and cats. Most adenocarcinomas of the large intestine are located in the canine and feline rectum (more than 50% are midrectum).

D. Leiomyomas are benign neoplasms of smooth muscle occurring sporadically in the large intestine.

III. Diagnosis

A. Clinical Presentation

1. Signalment.
   a. Colorectal tumors are more frequent in dogs than cats.
   b. The incidence of polyps is equal in males and females; however, colonic carcinomas are two to three times more common in males than females.
   c. Mixed-breed dogs, poodles, German shepherds, collies, West Highland white terriers, Airedale terriers, and Lhasa apsos appear to be most commonly affected.
2. History.
   a. Most dogs present because owners have noticed blood and mucus in feces.
   b. Common clinical signs include straining to defecate, passage of blood and mucus with feces, painful defecation, and passage of ribbonlike feces.

B. Physical Examination

1. Abdominal or rectal palpation often identifies colorectal masses.
2. Blood may be noted on rectal exam.

C. Radiography/Ultrasonography/Endoscopy

1. Take thoracic and abdominal radiographs to evaluate the extent of disease.
   a. Evaluate sublumbar lymph node size because enlargement is often indicative of metastasis.
2. Perform proctoscopy/colonoscopy to identify diffuse or multiple lesions and to localize lesions to the distal colon and rectum.
3. **Biopsy all lesions** and include submucosa in biopsies with obvious, deep infiltrating disease.

IV. Surgical Treatment

A. General Considerations

1. Surgical resection is the treatment of choice for intestinal tumors.
   a. Unfortunately many tumors are too far advanced for successful resection when diagnosed.
   b. Incontinence may occur after resection.

B. Preoperative Management

1. Correct hydration, electrolyte, and acid-base abnormalities before surgery.
2. If the animal has no obstruction, bacterial numbers may be reduced by evacuating the colon with oral cathartics, enemas, and fasting.
3. Give antibiotics effective against aerobic and anaerobic intestinal bacteria flora.

C. Positioning

1. Approach tumors of the cecum and colon via a ventral celiotomy with the patient in dorsal recumbency.
2. Approach rectal tumors using either a ventral midline celiotomy with pelvic osteotomy, anal eversion, or perineal dissection.
3. Approach tumors of the cranial to middle rectum with the patient in dorsal recumbency using a ventral celiotomy and pelvic osteotomy.
4. Approach tumors of the caudal rectum and anal canal with the

patient in ventral recumbency using the DePage position and anal eversion, or a dorsal or lateral perineal approach.

D. Surgical Technique

1. General considerations.
   a. Surgical resection is the most common treatment for large intestinal neoplasia. Margins of 4 to 8 cm are recommended during partial colectomy for malignant tumors.
   b. Noninvasive anal or rectal masses are often everted through the anus and excised with limited normal tissue margins.
2. Procedure.

Dilate and retract the anus to allow visualization of the mass. Place stay sutures in the rectal mucosa near the mass to facilitate eversion through the anus. Use an electrosurgical electrode, laser, or scalpel blade to incise mucosa and submucosa surrounding the mass. Remove the mass and appose mucosa and submucosa with simple interrupted 4-0 absorbable (e.g., polydioxanone, polyglyconate, or polyglactin 910) sutures.

V. Suture Materials/Special Instruments

A. Absorbable (e.g., polydioxanone, polyglyconate, polyglactin 910) sutures are preferred when removing masses from the rectum.

B. Absorbable or nonabsorbable sutures may be used for colectomy, but the former is preferred.

VI. Postoperative Care and Assessment

A. Provide postoperative care as described in the section on surgery of the small intestine, p. 203.

VII. Prognosis

A. Give a guarded prognosis to animals with nonresectable tumors because other modes of therapy are ineffective, of questionable value, or non-applicable because of severe side effects.

B. The prognosis for patients with benign masses is generally good to excellent if excision is complete; however, recurrence and malignant transformation are possible when polyp excision is incomplete.

Megacolon (*SAS*, pp. 332-335)

I. Definitions

A. **Megacolon** is a descriptive term for persistent increased large intestinal diameter and hypomotility associated with severe constipation or obstipation (no feces may be passed).

II. General Considerations and Clinically Relevant Pathophysiology

A. Megacolon is most frequently diagnosed in cats.
  1. It is not a specific disease but a clinical sign associated with failure to normally void feces.
  2. It may be congenital or acquired and occurs secondary to colonic inertia and outlet obstruction.

B. Feces that are retained in the colon for prolonged periods dehydrate and solidify because of continued water absorption.
  1. The fecal mass may become so large and hard that passage through the pelvic canal is impossible.
  2. Prolonged severe colonic distention eventually causes irreversible changes in colonic smooth muscles and nerves, causing inertia.

III. Diagnosis

A. Clinical Presentation

1. Signalment.
   a. Idiopathic megacolon is primarily seen in cats but rarely occurs in dogs.
   b. Megacolon secondary to neurologic, obstructive, or medical disease may occur in any animal.
2. History.
   a. Affected animals present for evaluation of constipation or obstipation.
   b. They may be depressed or anorexic or have tenesmus, weakness, lethargy, poor hair coat, vomiting, weight loss, and occasionally watery, mucoid, or bloody diarrhea.

B. Physical Examination Findings

1. A lean body condition and poor hair coat may be evident on physical examination. Some animals are depressed and dehydrated.
2. Abdominal palpation reveals a distended colon.

C. Radiography

1. Abdominal radiographs demonstrate a distended colon impacted with fecal material.
2. Perform radiographs to rule out obstructive diseases (e.g., pelvic fracture malunions, sacrocaudal spinal trauma or deformities, and intramural or mural colonic or rectoanal obstructive lesions).

IV. Medical Management

A. Constipation is difficult to treat once megacolon develops; however, medical management should be attempted before colectomy.
  1. Initial management includes correction of hydration, electrolyte, and acid-base abnormalities in severely affected animals.
  2. Evacuate the colon with stool softeners, enemas, or digital evacuation.
  3. To control constipation, use long-term high-fiber diets, stool softeners, bulk laxatives, and enemas. Osmotic laxatives (e.g., lactulose or ice

cream or milk in some cats) and prokinetic drugs (e.g., cisapride) may help prevent recurrence once the colon is evacuated by enemas.

V. Surgical Treatment

A. General Considerations

1. Surgery for megacolon entails removing all of the colon except a short distal segment needed to reestablish intestinal continuity.

B. Preoperative Management

1. Preoperative intestinal preparation using multiple enemas to evacuate the large colon is ineffective and unnecessary.
2. Give prophylactic antibiotics effective against aerobic and anaerobic colonic bacteria.

C. Subtotal Colectomy

Explore the abdomen and biopsy abnormal tissues. Isolate the distal small intestine, cecum, and colon from the remainder of the abdomen with several moistened laparotomy pads. Identify resection sites at the distal jejunum or proximal ileum and distal 1 to 2 cm of colon. Choose sites that will allow apposition without tension. Ligate and transect branches of the ileal artery and vein, ileocolic artery and vein, caudal mesenteric artery and vein, and cranial rectal artery and vein. An alternative procedure is to preserve the ileocolic sphincter; however, it is more difficult to achieve a tension-free apposition if the ileocolic sphincter is preserved. Ileocolic anastomosis is technically easier and allows removal of more colon. If the ileocolic valve is preserved, ligate the right colic, middle colic, and caudal mesenteric vessels. If the ileum is partially or completely removed, also ligate the ileocolic and terminal ileal arcadial vessels. Milk feces into the dilated colon, which will be resected. Place intestinal forceps proximal and distal to the planned resection site. Resect the dilated colon at its junction with the small intestine or just distal to the cecum. Perform an end-to-end anastomosis with either a circular stapler or sutures. Correct for luminal size disparity when performing a suture anastomosis by altering the angle of transection (oblique angles on small lumens and perpendicular angles on large lumens) using unequal suture spacing (further apart on the large lumen) or resecting an antimesenteric wedge from the intestine. If a staple technique is used, place purse-string sutures at each colonic end before resection. Insert the stapler into the colon transanally or through an antimesenteric incision in the cecum or colon. Transanal introduction of the stapler may not be possible in all cats because of their small anus and narrow pelvic canal. Lavage the anastomotic site and close the mesenteric defect. Remove laparotomy pads, lavage the abdomen, and place omentum over the surgical site.

VI. Suture Materials/Special Instruments

A. Polydioxanone and polyglyconate (3-0 or 4-0) are preferred sutures for colectomy.

B. Nonabsorbable (e.g., nylon or polypropylene) sutures may be used in debilitated or hypoalbuminemic animals.

VII. Postoperative Care and Assessment

A. Maintain hydration with intravenous or subcutaneous fluids for 1 to 3 days after surgery, and give analgesics as necessary.

B. Offer food within 24 hours of surgery, although anorexia may persist for 5 or more days.
   1. Use diazepam (0.5 mg/day IV) or cyproheptadine (2.0 mg/dose PO, BID) to stimulate eating in some cats.
   2. It may be necessary to keep animals on a low-volume, high-caloric diet for 10 to 14 days.

C. Expect liquid, tarry feces and tenesmus immediately after surgery. The character of the feces changes gradually from diarrhea to soft, formed stool in 80% of cats by 6 weeks after surgery.

D. Keep the litter pan clean to encourage defecation.

VIII. Prognosis

A. Long-term results of subtotal colectomy for idiopathic megacolon in cats are usually good to excellent.

B. Semiformed stools and, rarely, diarrhea persist in some cats.

C. The frequency of defecation is usually increased (30% to 50%) compared with normal cats; however, most cats are continent.

Surgery of the Perineum, Rectum, and Anus (*SAS*, pp. 335-366)

I. Definitions

A. **Rectal resection** is removal of a portion of the terminal large intestine.

B. **Rectal pull-through** is resection of the terminal colon, midrectum, or both using an anal approach, with or without an abdominal approach.

C. **Anal sacculectomy** is removal of the anal sac(s).

II. Diagnosis

A. Clinical Presentation

1. Scooting, anal licking, constipation, tenesmus, and dyschezia are typical presenting complaints associated with perineal and rectal disease.
2. Many conditions can be diagnosed on physical examination, and a thorough rectal examination is crucial.

3. Anesthesia may be required for adequate rectal examination of animals with pain.
4. Visual inspection of the perineum may reveal unilateral or bilateral swelling, perianal masses, ulceration, fistulae, fecal soiling, or prolapsed mucosa.

B. Laboratory Findings

1. Laboratory findings of hypercalcemia, anemia, and other paraneoplastic syndromes may be associated with neoplastic masses.

C. Radiography/Endoscopy

1. If possible, evacuate the colon and rectum with enemas, laxatives, or cathartics before radiographic studies.
   a. Enlarged sublumbar lymph nodes suggest metastasis.
2. Proctoscopy helps define rectal disease, but it should be combined with colonoscopy because tumors and inflammatory disease may also affect the colon.
3. Collect samples for culture, cytology, and biopsy.
   a. Biopsy normal tissue in addition to thickened folds, masses, strictures, or ulcers.

III. Preoperative Concerns

A. Preoperative patient preparation methods (for mechanical emptying and cleansing) are similar to those used before colon surgery (p. 212). Minimally, digitally evacuate the terminal rectum of all patients while under anesthesia, just before surgery.

B. Although these colonic lavage solutions work well, enemas facilitate complete cleansing. Give a warm-water enema the day before surgery and a 10% povidone-iodine enema 3 hours before surgery.

C. After anesthetic induction, place a urinary catheter to aid intraoperative identification of the urethra, manually clean the rectum (if necessary), and express the anal sacs.

IV. Anesthetic Considerations

A. Avoid nitrous oxide in patients with intestinal obstruction.

B. If there are no contraindications (e.g., sepsis, bleeding diatheses, hypovolemia [for epidurals using local anesthetics]), epidurals may be used in dogs to supplement general anesthesia. Because local anesthetics in epidurals may cause hypotension, correct dehydration before performing the procedure.

C. See Appendix G-11 for selected anesthetic protocols for animals undergoing perineal, rectal, or anal surgery.

V. Antibiotics

A. There is a high risk of infection after colorectal surgery. Although controversial, the use of antibiotics in colorectal surgery reduces morbidity and mortality associated with infection.

B. Give systemic perioperative antibiotics effective against gram-negative aerobes and anaerobes.

1. Recommended drugs include second-generation cephalosporins (e.g., cefmetazole, cefoxitin, cefotetan) given at the time of induction.
2. Third-generation cephalosporins effective against gram-positive and gram-negative aerobes and some anaerobes are available, albeit expensive.
3. Gentamicin plus cefazolin can be given intravenously at induction.
4. Aminoglycosides (e.g., neomycin, kanamycin) and metronidazole can be given orally in combination beginning 24 hours before surgery.

VI. Surgical Anatomy

A. The cranial rectal artery is a branch of the caudal mesenteric artery and is the major blood supply to the rectum. To ensure adequate anastomotic blood supply, preserve the cranial rectal artery in dogs unless the intrapelvic rectum is resected.

B. The internal and external sphincter muscles surround the terminal rectum and anal canal to control defecation. The internal anal sphincter is a caudal thickening of the circular smooth muscle lining the anal canal.

1. Note the location of the perineal nerves.
2. The blood supply to the external anal sphincter is from the perineal arteries.

VII. Surgical Techniques

A. General Considerations

1. For optimal healing, use a monofilament, synthetic absorbable suture (e.g., polydioxanone, polyglyconate) and approximating suture patterns (simple interrupted, Gambee, crushing, or simple continuous) for rectoanal surgery.
2. Fecal incontinence usually occurs if more than 4 cm or the final 1.5 cm of the terminal rectum is resected, if the perineal nerves are damaged, or if more than half the external anal sphincter is damaged.

B. Techniques for Rectal Resection

1. Ventral approach.

For pubic symphysiotomy, incise the entire length of the adductor aponeurosis. Divide the pubis and ischium on the midline with an osteotome and mallet or an oscillating saw. Separate the pubis and ischium with a self-retaining retractor (e.g., pediatric Finochietto).

2. Anal approach.

With the patient in ventral recumbency, dilate the anus with three or four stay sutures placed through the mucocutaneous junction. Evert the rectal wall by placing stay sutures (e.g., 3-0 nylon or other monofilament suture) in the rectal mucosa cranial or caudal to the mass/lesion and applying caudal traction. Place additional stay sutures to further retract the mass/lesion if necessary. Use electrosurgery, laser, or scalpel incisions to remove masses. Make a partial or full-thickness incision, depending on malignancy and need for wide borders. Appose cut edges with simple interrupted sutures (e.g., 3-0 or 4-0 polydiox-

anone or polyglyconate). Remove the stay sutures and allow the surgical site to retract within the pelvic canal.

3. Rectal pull-through approach.

Position the animal in ventral recumbency with the hindquarters elevated. Evert the rectum with stay sutures placed cranial to the mucocutaneous junction (1.5 cm or more if possible). Using the stay sutures, apply caudal traction to the cranial rectum. Begin a full-thickness 360-degree incision through the rectum, leaving a 1.5-cm cuff of nondiseased rectal wall attached to the anus if possible. Place three or four stay sutures in the rectal cuff. Mobilize the rectum by bluntly dissecting along the external wall. Continue dissection as far cranially as the cranial rectal artery if necessary. Ligate or coagulate rectal vessels as they are encountered. Split the rectum longitudinally until normal tissue is identified if the lesion is diffuse. Transect the diseased rectum in stages with 1 to 2 cm of normal tissue at each end. Transect one fourth to one third of the circumference and then appose the cranial end of the rectum to the caudal rectal cuff with simple interrupted sutures (e.g., 3-0 or 4-0 polydioxanone or polyglyconate). Continue transecting and apposing until all diseased tissue has been excised. Some surgeons prefer a two-layer closure: first appose the seromuscular layer and then the mucosa/submucosal layer.

4. Swenson's pull-through approach.

For this procedure, position the patient in dorsal recumbency so both a ventral abdominal and anal approach may be used. Transect the colon proximal to the mass. Oversew the ends of the colon and rectum. Use linear cutting or transverse stapling instruments to reappose the colon and rectum. Ligate vessels supplying the distal colon and rectum. Place stay sutures through the end of the remaining colon or ileum and rectum. Grasp the sutures with transanally placed forceps and evert the rectum through the anus. Advance colon or ileum through the pelvic canal with stay sutures. Resect the lesion and anastomose the end of the colon or ileum to the terminal rectum as described above. Gently replace the intestine into the pelvic canal.

5. Dorsal approach.

Position the patient in ventral recumbency with the pelvis elevated and the tail fixed over the back. Pad the cranial aspect of the hindlimbs to prevent pressure on the femoral nerves. Make a curvilinear incision from one ischiatic tuberosity to the other curving dorsal to the anus. Incise subcutaneous fat and perineal fascia. Locate the rectum, external anal sphincter, levator ani, and coccygeus muscles laterally and the rectococcygeus muscles dorsally. Transect the paired rectococcygeus muscles near their origin on the rectal wall or insertion on the caudal vertebrae. Elevate the external anal sphincter and caudal edge of the levator ani to the level of the caudal rectal nerve. Partially transect the levator ani muscles for more cranial rectal resections if necessary. Position a self-retaining retractor (e.g., Gelpi or Weitlaner) to improve visualization if necessary. Gently retract the rectum caudally and mobilize the rectum cranially to normal bowel. Repair the lacerated rectum or resect the diseased bowel. Ligate or cauterize vessels to the diseased bowel. Place stay sutures in the cranial bowel before transection. Appose the bowel ends with interrupted appositional sutures (e.g., 3-0 or 4-0 polydioxanone or polyglyconate) or an end-to-end stapling device. Reappose transected levator ani muscle with appositional cruciate or mattress sutures. Some surgeons reattach the rectococcygeus muscles and external anal sphincter to the rectus muscle. Thoroughly lavage the area and place drains if significant contamination has occurred. Placement of a drain against the anastomotic site may cause

dehiscence. Separately appose the subcutaneous tissue and skin with continuous or interrupted sutures of 3-0 or 4-0 polydioxanone and 3-0 or 4-0 nylon or polypropylene, respectively.

6. Lateral approach.

Make a curvilinear incision 2 to 3 cm lateral to the anus, beginning dorsal to the tail head and extending ventral to the anus. Incise subcutaneous tissues to expose the pelvic diaphragm. Separate the fascia between the external anal sphincter and the levator ani muscle. Preserve the caudal rectal nerve to the external anal sphincter. Repair the laceration with a one- or two-layer closure using simple interrupted sutures (e.g., 3-0 or 4-0 polydioxanone or polyglyconate). Thoroughly lavage the area and place a Penrose or closed-suction drain if soft tissues were contaminated with feces. Resect diverticula with a linear stapling device. Reappose the external anal sphincter and levator ani muscles with interrupted appositional sutures. Place additional sutures between the external anal sphincter and internal obturator muscle if this fascial plane is disrupted. Close subcutaneous tissues and skin routinely.

VIII. Healing of the Rectum

A. Rectal healing is affected by the same factors that affect colonic healing.

IX. Postoperative Care and Assessment

A. Provide postoperative care as described for surgery of the small intestine.

B. General considerations.
   1. Use an Elizabethan collar, bucket, or side-bars to protect the surgical site.
   2. Give a stool softener when oral intake begins and continue for 2 weeks, or as needed.
   3. Ileus may be minimized by encouraging early ambulation and eating.

C. Increased frequency of defecation may occur after major colorectal resections.

D. Perineal surgery.
   1. Patients having perineal surgery may resume their normal diet with the first feeding.
   2. Apply warm compresses two to three times daily for 15 to 20 minutes to minimize postoperative swelling after perianal or perineal surgery.
   3. Perianal and perineal area surgeries are predisposed to infection because of high bacterial numbers in these areas.
   4. Assessment.
      a. Assess anal sphincter function, continence, perineal swelling, and draining daily.
      b. Remove purse-string sutures immediately or within 2 to 3 days postoperatively.

Anal Neoplasia (*SAS*, pp. 344-348)

I. Definition

A. **Perianal glands** are modified sebaceous glands.

II. General Considerations and Clinically Relevant Pathophysiology

A. The most common perianal tumors are adenomas and carcinomas of the perianal and apocrine glands. Apocrine gland tumors usually involve the anal sacs. The most common malignant tumors are perianal gland adenocarcinomas and apocrine gland adenocarcinomas.

B. Perianal adenomas are the most common canine perianal tumors.
   1. They are the third most frequent tumor in male dogs.
   2. They occur 12 times more often in intact males than in intact females and are more common in ovariohysterectomized females than in intact females.
   3. They are hormone dependent and usually decrease in size after castration.

C. Perianal gland adenocarcinomas cannot be grossly differentiated from adenomas. These tumors are not hormone responsive.

D. Anal sac apocrine gland adenocarcinomas (anal sac adenocarcinoma, apocrine gland adenocarcinoma) arise in the anal sac. These tumors can release parathyroid hormone–like activity, causing hypercalcemia, polyuria, and polydipsia.

E. Anal squamous cell carcinomas arise from the anocutaneous line. They are typically malignant and metastasize quickly.

III. Diagnosis

A. Clinical Presentation

1. Signalment.
   a. Perianal tumors are common in middle-aged and older male dogs, but rare in females.
   b. Adenomas are more prevalent in cocker spaniels, beagles, bulldogs, and Samoyeds.
   c. Apocrine gland adenocarcinomas usually occur in dogs, especially old, ovariohysterectomized females.
2. History.
   a. Tumors in the perianal region cause irritation with subsequent licking, scooting, and tenesmus.
   b. Constipation, obstipation, and dyschezia may occur with large, invasive tumors.
   c. Some tumors are asymptomatic and found incidentally on physical examination.
   d. In castrated males, consider perianal tumors malignant until proven otherwise.

e. Paraneoplastic hypercalcemia is common with anal sac adenocarcinomas.

B. Physical Examination Findings

1. Multiple perianal masses are often identified around the circumference of the anus in the hairless area. They may be of variable size, covered with epithelium or ulcerated, friable, and broad based.
2. Most adenomas are well circumscribed, whereas carcinomas are invasive.

C. Radiography/Ultrasonography

1. Radiographs of the abdomen and thorax help stage the disease. Enlarged sublumbar lymph nodes suggest metastasis.
2. Abdominal ultrasonography allows lymph node evaluation.

D. Laboratory Findings

1. Cytology helps, but histology is necessary to differentiate perianal adenomas from carcinomas.
2. Anal sac tumors often cause hypercalcemia and renal dysfunction.

IV. Differential Diagnosis

A. Differential diagnoses of anal and perianal irritation include anal sacculitis, dermatitis, endoparasites, perianal fistula, and tumors.

B. Differential diagnoses for perianal swelling include perineal hernia, perianal neoplasia, perianal gland hyperplasia, anal sacculitis, anal sac neoplasia, atresia ani, rectal pythiosis, and vaginal tumors.

C. Differential diagnoses for dyschezia include rectal foreign body, perineal hernia, perianal fistula, anal stricture, rectal stricture, anal sac abscess, rectal or anal neoplasia, anal trauma, anal dermatitis, anorectal prolapse, inflammatory bowel disease, histoplasmosis, and pythiosis.

V. Medical Treatment

A. Some perianal tumors respond to chemotherapy or radiation therapy, but reports documenting effectiveness are lacking.

B. Perianal gland adenomas may shrink after a short course of diethylstilbestrol (0.5 to 1.0 mg/day for 2 to 3 weeks).

C. Radiation therapy or chemotherapy is recommended for nonresectable malignancies.

VI. Surgical Treatment

A. General Considerations

1. Surgical excision is the treatment of choice for perianal tumors.
   a. Castrate the animal and resect small masses, or biopsy multiple or large masses.
2. Generally, perianal masses not involving the anal sacs are perianal adenomas.
3. Reevaluate patients in 4 to 6 weeks. Adenomas will be smaller at this

time and can generally be resected with less trauma to the external anal sphincter. Some adenomas regress completely after castration.

4. If malignancy is identified histologically, promptly perform a wide resection.

B. Preoperative Management

1. Correct fluid, electrolyte, and acid-base abnormalities before surgery.
2. Perioperative antibiotics are indicated in old or debilitated patients.
3. Do not administer enemas on the day of surgery because they may increase contamination of the surgical site.
4. Hypercalcemia.
   a. Rehydrate mildly to moderately hypercalcemic animals with physiologic saline solution.
   b. If they are urinating, give furosemide and prednisone.
   c. Severely affected animals may also be treated with alkalinizing agents (e.g., sodium bicarbonate) and bone resorption inhibitors (etidronate disodium or salmon calcitonin).

C. Anesthesia

1. Patients with perianal tumors may be old, debilitated, and have other serious medical problems, requiring special care during anesthesia.
2. Anesthetic recommendations for animals undergoing perianal surgery are listed in Appendix G-11.

D. Surgical Technique

Begin by performing a prescrotal or caudal castration on intact male dogs with perianal adenomas. Incise perianal skin surrounding perianal adenomas with minimal margins of normal tissue. Dissect the tumor from subcutaneous tissues and the external anal sphincter with minimal trauma. Thoroughly lavage the area. Close dead space with monofilament absorbable sutures (e.g., 3-0 to 4-0 polydioxanone or polyglyconate), and skin with interrupted appositional sutures (e.g., monofilament, 3-0 to 4-0 nylon or polypropylene). Submit the excised masses and testicles for histologic evaluation. Resect malignant tumors with a minimum of 1 cm of normal tissue on all borders. This includes partial resection of the external anal sphincter, anal canal, and anal sacs in some cases. Appose the epithelial edges to avoid anal stricture.

VII. Postoperative Care and Assessment

A. Treat hypercalcemia until serum calcium is normal. Most animals are normocalcemic within 24 hours of primary tumor resection.

B. Keep the perianal area clean, and use an Elizabethan collar or similar restraint device to keep the patient from licking at surgical sites.

C. If not vomiting, offer water and food within 8 to 12 hours. A stool softener may be added to the food for 2 to 3 weeks.

VIII. Prognosis

A. The prognosis after surgery is good for benign perianal tumors but guarded to poor for malignant tumors, although some malignant tumors may be slow growing and late to metastasize.

B. Adenomas occasionally recur (less than 10%) and should be rebiopsied.

C. Early, complete excision of perianal gland adenocarcinomas can be curative, but most carcinomas are invasive or metastasize to lymph nodes.

D. Anal sac adenocarcinomas in female dogs warrant a poor prognosis because they frequently spread locally and to lymph nodes by the time of diagnosis.

Anal Sac Infection/Impaction (*SAS*, pp. 348-352)

I. Definitions

A. **Anal sac impaction** is an abnormal accumulation of anal sac secretions secondary to inflammation, infection, or duct obstruction.

II. General Considerations and Clinically Relevant Pathophysiology

A. Anal sacculitis is common, affecting approximately 10% of dogs, and is usually caused by infection or duct obstruction.

B. Anal sacculitis also occurs without duct obstruction. In these cases hypersecretion occurs and the sac is easy to express. Secretions are more liquid than normal with yellowish-white granules.

III. Diagnosis

A. Clinical Presentation

1. Signalment.
   a. Anal sacculitis may occur in any age, breed, or sex of animal; however, it is most common in small and toy breed dogs and rare in cats.
   b. Anal sacculitis may be associated with seborrheic dermatitis or other dermatoses in some animals.
2. History.
   a. Many animals have a history of recent (1 to 3 weeks) diarrhea or soft stools or estrus.
   b. They usually evidence anal irritation (e.g., scooting, licking, and biting at the tailhead or anus).

B. Physical Examination Findings

1. The anal sac region may appear swollen and inflamed. Abscesses or impaction may cause the anal sac to rupture and create a draining lesion at the 4 o'clock or 7 o'clock position.
2. Impaction is diagnosed when the sac is distended, mildly painful, and not readily expressed.

C. Radiography

1. Plain radiographs are recommended if neoplasia is suspected.
2. A fistulogram may help determine whether a draining tract is associated with the anal sac region or some other perineal location.

IV. Differential Diagnosis

A. The primary differentials for anal sacculitis are flea allergy (from licking and biting), perianal tumor (caused by swelling and ulceration), perianal fistulae, or tail fold pyoderma (the result of abscessation and draining tracts).

B. Differential diagnoses for anal or perianal irritation include anal sacculitis, dermatitis, endoparasites, perianal fistulae, and tumors.

C. Differential diagnoses for perianal swelling include perianal hernia, perianal neoplasia, perianal gland hyperplasia, anal sacculitis, anal sac neoplasia, atresia ani, rectal pythiosis, and vaginal tumors.

V. Medical Treatment

A. Most anal sac problems can be medically managed by manual expression, lavage, antibiotics, and dietary change.

VI. Surgical Treatment

A. General Considerations

1. Failure of medical therapy and suspicion of neoplasia are indications for anal sacculectomy.
2. If a draining tract persists after anal sac rupture, surgery should be delayed until inflammation is controlled.
3. Both anal sacs should be removed, even if only one is obviously involved, to avoid a second surgery.

B. Preoperative Management

1. Treat anal sacculitis, abscessation, or fistulation for several days as described above to reduce inflammation before surgery.

C. Surgical Anatomy

1. One anal sac lies on each side of the anus between the internal and external anal sphincters.
2. The ducts of the anal sacs open in the cutaneous zone at approximately the 4 o'clock to 5 o'clock and 7 o'clock to 8 o'clock positions.
3. The duct opening in cats is more lateral to the anocutaneous line than in dogs.

D. Surgical Technique

1. Closed technique.

Manually evacuate feces from the rectum if present. Prepare the perineal area for surgery. Insert a small probe or hemostat into the orifice of the anal sac duct. Advance the instrument until the lateral extent of the sac is identified.

Alternatively, wax or synthetic resin may be infused to distend the sac before resection. Make a curvilinear incision over the anal sac. Dissecting directly against the anal sac, separate the internal and external anal sphincter muscle fibers from the sac's exterior with small Metzenbaum or iris scissors. Avoid excising or traumatizing the muscles or the caudal rectal artery medial to the duct. Continue dissecting to free the sac and duct to its mucocutaneous junction at the anal canal. Perforation of the sac may occur during dissection, and tissues may be contaminated with secretions. Place a ligature around the duct at the mucocutaneous junction (e.g., 4-0 polydioxanone or polyglyconate). Excise the anal sac and duct, then inspect for completeness of removal. Control hemorrhage with ligatures, electrocoagulation, or pressure. Lavage the tissues thoroughly. Appose subcutaneous tissues with interrupted sutures of 4-0 polydioxanone or polyglyconate and skin with 3-0 or 4-0 nylon or polypropylene.

2. Open technique.

Prepare as described above. Place a scissors blade or groove director into the duct of the anal sac. Apply medial traction on the duct while incising through skin, subcutaneous tissue, external anal sphincter, duct, and sac. Continue the incision to the lateral extent of the anal sac. Elevate the cut edge of the sac and use small Metzenbaum or iris scissors to dissect the sac free of its attachments to muscle and surrounding tissue. The lining of the anal sac is grayish and glistening and is easily distinguished from surrounding tissue. Complete the procedure as for closed sacculectomy.

VII. Postoperative Care and Assessment

A. Keep the perianal area clean, and use an Elizabethan collar or similar restraint device to keep the patient from licking the sites.

B. Offer food and water within 8 to 12 hours if no vomiting has been noted.

C. A stool softener may be added to the food for 2 to 3 weeks.

D. Monitor the surgical site for signs of infection or drainage, and palpate the rectum and perianal area for evidence of stricture when sutures are removed at 7 to 10 days.

VIII. Prognosis

A. The prognosis for nonneoplastic anal sac disease is good if it is not associated with perianal fistulae.

Perineal Hernia (*SAS*, pp. 352-356)

I. Definitions

A. **Perineal hernias** occur when the perineal muscles separate, allowing rectum, pelvic, or abdominal contents to displace perineal skin.

II. General Considerations and Clinically Relevant Pathophysiology

A. Perineal hernia occurs when pelvic diaphragm muscles fail to support the rectal wall, allowing persistent rectal distention and impaired defecation.

B. The cause of pelvic diaphragm weakening is poorly understood but is believed to be associated with male hormones, straining, and congenital or acquired muscle weakness or atrophy.

C. Herniation may be unilateral or bilateral. Most occur between the levator ani, external anal sphincter, and internal obturator muscles (caudal hernia).

III. Diagnosis

A. Clinical Presentation

1. Signalment.
   a. Perineal hernias are common in dogs and rare in cats. They occur almost exclusively in intact male dogs.
   b. Breeds most commonly affected are Boston terriers, boxers, Welsh corgis, Pekingese, collies, poodles, and mongrels.
   c. Most perineal hernias occur in dogs older than 5 years.
2. History.
   a. Affected animals usually present because of difficulty defecating.
   b. Some owners notice a swelling lateral to the anus.
   c. Occasionally animals present as emergencies because of postrenal uremia associated with bladder entrapment or shock associated with intestinal strangulation.
   d. Clinical signs may include perineal swelling, constipation, obstipation, dyschezia, tenesmus, rectal prolapse, stranguria, anuria, vomiting, flatulence, and fecal incontinence.

B. Physical Examination Findings

1. Diagnosis is based on finding a perineal swelling lateral to the anus and a weakened pelvic diaphragm.
2. Cats typically have bilateral hernias, which seldom cause obvious perineal swelling.
3. Rectal palpation of the pelvic diaphragm reveals a weakness or separation of the muscles.

C. Radiography

1. Radiographs are seldom needed; however, they may reveal the position of the urinary bladder and prostate and asymmetry or enlargement.

IV. Medical Treatment

A. The goals of treatment are to relieve and prevent constipation and dysuria and to prevent organ strangulation.

B. Normal defecation can sometimes be maintained using laxatives, stool softeners, dietary changes, periodic enemas, or manual rectal evacuation.

V. Surgical Treatment

A. General Considerations

1. Herniorrhaphy should always be recommended.
2. Retroflexion of the urinary bladder and visceral entrapment are emergencies requiring immediate surgery.
3. Castration, although controversial, is recommended during herniorrhaphy because it has been reported to reduce recurrence.

B. Preoperative Management

1. Give stool softeners 2 to 3 days before surgery.
2. Evacuate the large intestine with laxatives, cathartics, enemas, and manual extraction.
3. Give prophylactic antibiotics effective against gram-negative and anaerobic organisms intravenously after anesthetic induction.
4. If the urinary bladder is retroflexed into the hernia, place a urinary catheter or perform cystocentesis via the perineum to relieve distress and prevent further physiologic deterioration.

C. Surgical Anatomy

1. The pelvic diaphragm is composed of the paired medial coccygeal and levator ani muscles.
2. The sacrotuberous ligament in the dog is a fibrous band running from the transverse process of the last sacral and first caudal vertebrae to the lateral angle of the ischiatic tuberosity rostral to the pelvic diaphragm. Cats do not have a sacrotuberous ligament. The sciatic nerve lies just cranial and lateral to the sacrotuberous ligament.
3. The internal obturator muscle is a fan-shaped muscle covering the dorsal surface of the ischium.
4. The internal pudendal artery and vein and the pudendal nerve run caudomedially through the pelvic canal on the dorsal surface of the internal obturator muscle, lateral to the coccygeus and levator ani muscles. The pudendal nerve is dorsal to the vessels and divides into the caudal rectal and perineal nerves.

D. Positioning

1. Clip and aseptically prepare the perineum for surgery. The prepared area should extend 10 to 15 cm cranial to the tail base, laterally beyond the ischial tuberosity, and ventrally to include the scrotum.
2. Position the animal in ventral recumbency with the tail fixed over the back, the pelvis elevated, and the hindlegs padded. Alternatively, use a well-padded perineal stand.

E. Surgical Technique

1. Approach.

Make a curvilinear incision beginning cranial to the coccygeus muscles, curving over the hernial bulge 1 to 2 cm lateral to the anus, and extending 2 to 3 cm ventral to the pelvic floor. Incise subcutaneous tissue and hernial sac. Identify and reduce hernial contents by dissecting subcutaneous and fibrous attachments. Biopsy any abnormal structures within the hernia (e.g., prostate, masses). Maintain hernial reduction by packing the defect with a moistened, tagged sponge. Identify the muscles involved in the hernia, internal pudendal artery and vein, pudendal nerve, caudal rectal vessels and nerve, and sacrotuberous ligament. Repair the hernia with one of the described techniques. After herniorrhaphy perform a caudal castration through a median perineal incision.

2. Traditional or anatomic herniorrhaphy.

Preplace simple interrupted 0 or 2-0 monofilament sutures using a large, curved needle. Begin suture placement between the external anal sphincter and levator ani, coccygeus, or both muscles. Space sutures less than 1 cm apart. As placement progresses ventrally and laterally, incorporate the sacrotuberous ligament for a secure repair if necessary. Place sutures through rather than around the sacrotuberous ligament to avoid sciatic nerve entrapment. Direct ventral sutures between the external anal sphincter and the internal obturator muscle. Be cognizant of the pudendal vessels and nerves at all times to prevent traumatizing these structures. Tie sutures beginning dorsally and progressing ventrally. Remove the sponge used to maintain reduction before tying the last few sutures. Evaluate the repair; place additional sutures if weaknesses or defects persist. Lavage the area. Close subcutaneous tissues with an interrupted or continuous appositional pattern (e.g., 3-0 or 4-0 polydioxanone or polyglyconate), and skin with an appositional interrupted pattern (e.g., 3-0 or 4-0 nylon).

3. Internal obturator transposition herniorrhaphy.

Incise fascia and periosteum along the caudal border of the ischium and origin of the internal obturator muscle. Using a periosteal elevator, elevate the periosteum and internal obturator muscle from the ischium. Transpose dorsomedially or roll up the muscle into the defect to allow apposition between the coccygeus, levator ani, and external anal sphincter. Transect the internal obturator tendon of insertion if necessary to get adequate coverage of the defect. The internal obturator tendon is often difficult to visualize, making transection difficult. Use care to avoid transection of the caudal gluteal vessels and perineal nerve. Preplace simple interrupted sutures as with the traditional technique. Begin by apposing the combined levator ani and coccygeus muscles with the external anal sphincter muscle dorsally. Then place sutures between the internal obturator and external anal sphincter medially and the levator ani and coccygeus muscles laterally.

VI. Postoperative Care and Assessment

A. If rectal prolapse occurs, place a purse-string suture.

B. After herniorrhaphy, monitor patients for signs of wound infection (e.g., redness, pain, swelling, discharge).

C. Continue stool softeners for 1 to 2 months.

VII. Prognosis

A. The prognosis is fair to good when surgery is performed by an experienced surgeon.

B. Patients with bladder retroflexion have the poorest prognosis.

C. Preexisting neurologic abnormalities (e.g., anal sphincter incompetence or compromised urinary bladder innervation) will not be corrected by the herniorrhaphy.

Perianal Fistulae (*SAS*, pp. 356-360)

I. Definition

A. **Perianal fistulae** are suppurative, progressive, deep, ulcerating tracts in the perianal tissues.

II. General Considerations and Clinically Relevant Pathophysiology

A. The etiology of perianal fistulae is unknown.
   1. The combination of infection and abscessation of glands around the anus; the moist, contaminated anal environment; and a broad-based, low-set tail conformation are believed to contribute to perianal fistula formation.
   2. German shepherds have a greater density of apocrine glands in the cutaneous zone of the anal canal, which may predispose them to perianal fistulae.

III. Diagnosis

A. Clinical Presentation

1. Signalment.
   a. Perianal fistulae occur most commonly in German shepherds, but Irish setters also are predisposed.
   b. The disease appears to be more common in males than females, with a predominance in intact animals.
2. History.
   a. Dogs with perianal fistulae usually exhibit anal discomfort, constipation, diarrhea, odor, licking, scooting, tenesmus, dyschezia, ulceration, or purulent perianal discharge.

B. Physical Examination Findings

1. The perineum is often painful, and affected dogs may snap, bite, or cry when the tail is lifted, necessitating sedation or general anesthesia for thorough perineal examination.
2. Perform a rectal exam to determine the depth of involvement, degree of fibrosis, and relationship of anal sacs to fistulae.

IV. Medical Treatment

A. Cyclosporine therapy is reportedly effective for the treatment of perianal fistulae. This therapy has reduced the need for surgery in many animals.

V. Surgical Treatment

A. General Considerations

1. The goals of surgery are to eliminate necrotic or unhealthy tissue and stimulate second intention healing without causing fecal incontinence or anal stenosis.
2. Radical resection is the excision of all diseased skin, subcutaneous tissue, muscle, and fascia. The rectum is apposed to remaining skin with widely spaced interrupted sutures. The remainder of the defect is allowed to heal by second intention. Fecal incontinence is a common postoperative problem.
3. Debridement and fulguration of fistulae have less potential for causing fecal incontinence than extensive resection but tend to be ineffective in severe cases.
4. Debridement and chemical cauterization (resection of epithelium overlying coalescing fistulous tracts, followed by the application of an irritant chemical to the underlying granulation tissue) may be performed using a strong (7%) iodine solution.

Rectal Prolapse (*SAS*, pp. 360-363)

I. Definitions

A. **Rectal prolapse** is a protrusion of rectal mucosa from the anus.

II. General Considerations and Clinically Relevant Pathophysiology

A. Rectal prolapse is principally associated with endoparasitism or enteritis in young animals, and tumors or perineal hernias in middle-aged to older animals.

B. However, any condition causing tenesmus may result in rectal prolapse.

III. Diagnosis

A. Clinical Presentation

1. Signalment.
   a. Rectal prolapse occurs in dogs and cats, with no documented breed predispositions.
   b. It may occur more often in Manx cats because of their anal laxity.
2. History.
   a. Straining or recent perineal surgery are common.
   b. Constipation, diarrhea, prostatitis, urinary tract infections, dyspnea, and dystocia may produce tenesmus.
   c. Perineal or perianal irritation from trauma or surgery may also cause straining and rectal prolapse.

B. Physical Examination

1. The protrusion of anorectal mucosa is usually obvious.

IV. Differential Diagnosis

A. The primary differential diagnosis for rectal prolapse is intussusception.

B. Insertion of a probe (e.g., thermometer or smooth tube) alongside the prolapsed mass is possible with an intussusception but not with a rectal prolapse.

V. Medical Treatment

A. Acute rectal prolapse is easily treated, but chronic disease may require resection.

B. Manual reduction and placement of a purse-string suture around the anus are recommended for acute prolapses with minimal tissue damage and edema.
   1. Apply warm saline lavages, massage, and lubrication (e.g., with a water-soluble gel) to the everted tissue before digital reduction.
   2. Place a purse-string suture tight enough to maintain prolapse reduction without interfering with passage of soft stool.

VI. Surgical Treatment

A. General Considerations

1. Nonreducible or severely traumatized prolapses necessitate amputation.
2. Perform colopexy when rectal prolapse repeatedly recurs after manual reduction or amputation.

B. Preoperative Management

1. Give prophylactic antibiotics effective against gram-negative and anaerobic bacteria at the time of anesthetic induction.
2. Lavage the exposed tissue with warm sterile saline and lubricate with a water-soluble gel.

C. Positioning

1. After the perianal area has been clipped and aseptically prepared for surgery, lavage and lubricate the everted tissue again.
2. Position the patient in ventral recumbency with the hind legs over the end of the table. Elevate the pelvis with padding, and secure the tail over the back. Pad the end of the table to avoid pressure on the femoral nerves.

D. Surgical Technique

Place a sterile test tube or syringe case into the rectal lumen to serve as a guide. Place three horizontal mattress stay sutures (at the 12 o'clock, 5 o'clock, and 8 o'clock positions) through all layers of the prolapse just cranial to the proposed transection site. These sutures should enter the rectal lumen with the needle being deflected by the probe before being passed through the rectal

tissues again. Transect the traumatized tissue in stages caudal to the stay sutures. Anatomically appose the transected edges with simple interrupted sutures (e.g., 3-0 or 4-0 polydioxanone or polyglyconate) after each stage of the resection. Space sutures approximately 2 mm apart and 2 mm from the cut edge. Inspect the anastomosis for gaps between sutures. Remove the stay sutures and gently replace the anastomotic site within the pelvic or anal canal. Place a purse-string suture around the anus if postoperative tenesmus is anticipated.

VII. Postoperative Care and Assessment

A. The cause of the prolapse must be treated to prevent recurrence.

B. Feed a low-fiber diet while the purse-string suture is in place.

C. Give stool softeners for 2 to 3 weeks after resection.

D. Remove the purse-string suture 3 to 5 days after manual reduction and 1 to 2 days after resection.

VIII. Prognosis

A. The prognosis for most animals treated surgically is good, provided the primary cause of tenesmus or irritation is appropriately treated.

17

Surgery of the Liver (*SAS*, pp. 367-388)

General Principles and Techniques (*SAS*, pp. 367-373)

I. Definitions

A. **Hepatectomy** is removal of either the entire liver (total hepatectomy) or a portion (partial hepatectomy).

II. Preoperative Concerns

A. Clinical signs of hepatic disease may not be apparent until the disease is advanced.

B. Hepatic failure may affect other organ systems (e.g., CNS, kidney, intestines, and heart).

C. Severe or chronic hepatic disease may cause coagulopathy because of decreased synthesis of clotting factors. Evaluate clotting parameters before surgery.

D. Hypoalbuminemia is common with advanced hepatic disease. Fluid therapy may further dilute albumin. Serum albumin less than 2.0 g/dl may delay wound healing.

E. Electrolyte abnormalities are uncommon, but always measure serum potassium.

F. Anemia occurs because of nutritional deficiencies, coagulation abnormalities, or gastrointestinal hemorrhage. Give blood transfusions if the hematocrit is less than 20% (see Appendix A).

G. Hypoglycemia may occur with severe hepatic insufficiency.

H. Massive ascites may cause diaphragmatic displacement and restriction of lung expansion.

I. Treat hepatic encephalopathy with dietary therapy, appropriate antibiotics, enemas, fluids, and other medications to decrease or eliminate clinical signs before surgery.

III. Anesthetic Considerations

A. Hepatic dysfunction impairs ability to metabolize and inactivate some drugs. Prolonged duration of action or altered function of drugs may result.

B. Acetylpromazine lowers the seizure threshold, lowers systemic vascular resistance and blood pressure, and alters the metabolism of some drugs (i.e., procaine, succinylcholine). Avoid it.

C. Diazepam is a useful premedicant (see Appendix G-12) that causes mild, dose-related CNS depression, does not depress the cardiopulmonary system, raises the seizure threshold, and can be antagonized with flumazenil. Consider using diazepam in conjunction with an opioid. Use it with caution in hypoalbuminemic patients.

D. Intravenous morphine may cause hepatic congestion because of histamine release and hepatic vein spasm. Some opioid analgesics have prolonged action when hepatic function is reduced, but their effects can be antagonized.

E. Barbiturates (e.g., thiopental) may have a prolonged duration of action in patients with significant hepatic disease.

F. Ketamine is metabolized in the liver of dogs (it is excreted largely unchanged in the urine of cats). It may precipitate seizures in encephalopathic patients; administer it at reduced dosages to dogs with mild hepatic dysfunction and avoid it in patients with severe dysfunction.

G. Use inhalation anesthetics.

1. Avoid hyperventilating these patients, because it may decrease portal blood flow.
2. Halothane and isoflurane decrease portal blood flow, but hepatic arterial blood flow tends to increase during isoflurane anesthesia, preserving hepatic oxygenation. Isoflurane, unlike halothane, has not been associated with postoperative hepatic dysfunction.
3. Isoflurane is the inhalation agent of choice for patients with severe hepatic disease.

IV. Antibiotics

A. Anaerobic bacteria residing in the liver may proliferate if there is hepatic ischemia or hypoxia. Use prophylactic antibiotics in most patients undergoing hepatic surgery.

B. Broad-spectrum antibiotics (i.e., penicillin derivatives, metronidazole, clindamycin) are indicated in the treatment of hepatic encephalopathy, bacterial hepatitis, and hepatic abscesses.

1. Metronidazole can cause neurologic signs (e.g., ataxia, nystagmus, head tilt, and seizures) when administered at greater than 60 mg/kg of body weight.
2. Avoid potentially hepatotoxic antibiotics (e.g., chloramphenicol, chlortetracycline, or erythromycin).

V. Surgical Anatomy

A. The diaphragmatic (i.e., parietal) surface of the liver is convex and lies mainly in touch with the diaphragm. The visceral surface faces caudoventrally and to the left and contacts the stomach, duodenum, pancreas, and right kidney.
   1. There are six hepatic lobes.
   2. The liver borders are normally sharp, but they appear more rounded in young animals and in those with infiltrated, congested, or scarred livers.

B. The liver has two afferent blood supplies: a low-pressure portal system and a high-pressure arterial system. The portal vein drains the stomach, intestines, pancreas, and spleen and supplies four fifths of the blood that enters the liver.
   1. The efferent drainage of the liver is through the hepatic veins.
   2. In the fetal pup, the ductus venosus shunts blood from the umbilical vein to the hepatic venous system.

C. Bile, formed in the liver, is discharged into bile canaliculi that unite to form interlobular ducts that ultimately merge to form lobar or bile ducts.

D. The portal vein, bile ducts, hepatic artery, lymphatics, and nerves are contained in the lacelike and nonsupporting portion of the lesser omentum known as the hepatoduodenal ligament.

VI. Surgical Techniques

A. Hepatic Biopsy (*SAS,* p. 369)

1. General considerations.
   a. Hepatic tissue is friable, making sharp dissection difficult. Retraction of blood vessels and bile ducts within the friable stroma occurs, and ligation of blood vessels and bile ducts after they have been cut is difficult. Packing the liver firmly enough to obtain hemostasis may cause ischemia and necrosis.
   b. Maintaining hepatic blood supply is important because the liver normally harbors pathogenic anaerobes.
   c. Hepatic biopsies are commonly indicated and may be obtained percutaneously, with laparoscopy or at surgery. Partial hepatectomies may be indicated for focal neoplasms or trauma.
   d. The standard approach for hepatic surgery is a cranial ventral midline abdominal incision. Split the caudal aspect of the sternum if additional exposure is needed.
2. Percutaneous liver biopsy (*SAS*, pp. 369-370).
   a. General considerations.
      i. Patient selection.
         (a) Percutaneous core biopsies or fine-needle aspirations are most successful in patients with diffuse hepatic disease; however, ultrasound guidance allows some focal lesions to be biopsied.
         (b) Do not perform percutaneous core biopsies in patients with clinical bleeding, severe thrombocytopenia (i.e.,

<20,000 platelets/μl), cavitary lesions, or highly vascular lesions (determined with ultrasound).

(c) Percutaneous biopsies may be obtained under tranquilization or heavy sedation using a transthoracic or transabdominal approach.

ii. Tissue core biopsies.

(a) Use a Tru-cut biopsy or an automated biopsy device (e.g., Bard Biopty Instrument).

(b) Obtain two or three (2-cm long) samples.

iii. Fine-needle aspirate (FNA).

(a) Obtain with a hand-held syringe or an aspiration gun with syringe attached to a 20- to 25-gauge, 1- to 3-inch needle.

(b) For histopathology, remove the needle from the syringe or gun and placed it in formalin. Once the sample has been fixed, remove it from the needle for processing.

(c) FNA is most likely to be diagnostic for diffuse hepatic neoplasia (e.g., lymphosarcoma), fungal disease, and idiopathic hepatic lipidosis. Inability to diagnose these conditions on an FNA does not preclude disease.

b. Transabdominal approach.

i. Surgical technique.

With the animal in dorsal recumbency, clip the hair from the area surrounding the xiphoid process and prepare it for aseptic surgery. Make a small incision in the skin on the left side between the costal arch and xiphoid process. Insert the biopsy needle through the skin incision in a craniodorsal direction, angling it slightly toward the left of midline. Advance the needle until resistance is met or ultrasound guidance shows the needle to be positioned at the surface of the liver. Advance the biopsy needle into the hepatic tissue and obtain the biopsy.

3. Surgical liver biopsy (*SAS,* p. 370).

a. General considerations.

i. Surgical biopsy allows the entire liver to be thoroughly inspected and palpated, and focal lesions to be biopsied. Hemorrhage can be identified and controlled.

ii. The biopsy can be taken from the most accessible site (marginal biopsy samples) in generalized disease.

iii. With focal disease, the entire liver should be palpated for the presence of intraparenchymal nodules or cavities and representative samples obtained.

b. The "guillotine" method.

i. Surgical technique.

Place a loop of suture around the protruding margin of a liver lobe. Pull the ligature tight and allow it to crush through the hepatic parenchyma before tying it. As the suture tears through the soft hepatic tissue, vessels and biliary ducts are ligated. Hold the liver gently between the fingers and, using a sharp blade, cut the hepatic tissue approximately 5 mm distal to the ligature (allowing the stump of crushed tissue to remain with the ligature). To avoid crushing the biopsy sample and causing artifacts, do not handle it with tissue forceps. Place a portion of the sample in formalin for histologic examination; reserve the remainder for culture and cytologic examination. Check the biopsy site for hemorrhage. If hemorrhage continues, place a pledget of absorbable gelatin foam over the site. Alternatively, if a focal (nonmarginal) area of the liver is to be biopsied, use a punch biopsy or Tru-cut biopsy or place several overlapping guillotine sutures around the margin of the lesion and excise it. Use caution with a punch biopsy to avoid penetrating more than half the thickness of the liver with each biopsy. Apply

pressure to the site until bleeding stops. If hemorrhage continues, place a pledget of absorbable gelatin foam over the site.

B. Partial Lobectomy (*SAS*, pp. 370-371)

1. General considerations.
   a. Sometimes indicated when disease involves only a portion of a liver lobe (e.g., peripheral hepatic arteriovenous fistulae, focal neoplasia, hepatic abscesses, or trauma).
   b. May be challenging because of difficulty in obtaining hemostasis. Should be done cautiously in animals with bleeding disorders.
   c. Stapling instruments may allow hemorrhage if the staples do not adequately compress hepatic tissue.
2. Surgical procedure.

Determine the line of separation between normal hepatic parenchyma and that to be removed and sharply incise the liver capsule along the selected site. Bluntly fracture the liver with fingers or the blunt end of a Bard Parker scalpel handle and expose parenchymal vessels. Ligate large vessels (hemoclips may be used) and electrocoagulate small bleeders that are encountered during the dissection. Alternately, place a stapling device (Autosuture TA 90, 55, or 30) across the base of the lobe and deploy the staples. Excise the hepatic parenchyma distal to the ligatures or staples. Before closing the abdomen, ensure that the raw surface of the liver is dry and free of hemorrhage. In small dogs and cats, you may place several overlapping guillotine sutures (as described above) along the entire line of demarcation. Be sure the entire width of the hepatic parenchyma is included in the sutures. After tightening the sutures securely, use a sharp blade to cut the hepatic tissue distal to the ligature, allowing a stump of crushed tissue to remain with the ligature.

C. Complete Lobectomy (*SAS*, pp. 371-372)

1. General considerations.
   a. Indicated in some focal lesions involving one or two hepatic lobes (e.g., traumatic lacerations of the liver or hepatic arteriovenous fistulae).
   b. The left lobes (i.e., left lateral and left medial lobes) maintain their separation near the hilus more than do the other lobes; therefore these lobes can often be removed in small dogs and cats by placing a single encircling ligature around the base of the lobe.
   c. For the right lateral and caudate lobes, careful dissection around the hepatic caudal vena cava is usually necessary.
2. Surgical procedure.

For the left lobes in small dogs and cats, crush the parenchyma near the hilus with fingers or forceps. Place an encircling ligature around the crushed area and tie. For the left lobes in larger dogs and right and caudate lobes, carefully dissect, if necessary, the lobe from the caudal vena cava. Isolate the blood vessels and biliary ducts near the hilus and ligate them. Double ligate or oversew the ends of large vessels. Resect the parenchymal tissue, leaving a stump of tissue distal to the ligatures to prevent retraction of the hepatic tissue from the ligatures and subsequent hemorrhage. Before performing the dissection, umbilical tape can be passed around the portal vein, celiac artery, cranial mesenteric arteries, and the caudal vena cava in front of and behind the liver. The umbilical tape is passed through rubber tubing, which can be used to occlude the hepatic blood supply if uncontrollable hemorrhage occurs.

VII. Healing of the Liver

A. Liver has a relative absence of connective tissue stroma, is highly susceptible to small changes in blood flow, and has an enormous regenerative capacity (adequate liver function is possible after 80% of the organ has been removed).

B. Close lacerations only when bleeding is profuse. If lacerations are sutured, do not create an internal pocket of bile or blood or cause ischemia of the surrounding cells.

C. In an emergency, ligate the proper hepatic artery to control hemorrhage from extensive liver lacerations.

D. Treat complex fractures or severe contusions by hepatic lobectomy if ligation of the hepatic artery does not stop hemorrhage.

VIII. Suture Materials/Special Instruments

A. Perform guillotine biopsies with large (0 or 2-0) chromic gut suture or polyglactin 910.

B. Suture with good knot security (e.g., silk suture) facilitates partial hepatectomy. Do not use braided, nonabsorbable suture if infection is present.

C. Use polydioxanone or polyglyconate suture for vessel ligation in complete and partial lobectomies.

IX. Postoperative Care and Assessment

A. Keep in mind that increased half-life of some drugs in patients with hepatic dysfunction may prolong recovery.

B. Monitor glucose concentrations; transient hypoglycemia is common after removal of large portions of the liver.

C. Maintain albumin levels (i.e., 2.0 g/dl) by administering plasma or whole blood.

D. Assess clotting factors if hemorrhage or petechiation occurs.

E. Continue antibiotics for 2 to 3 days if partial hepatectomy has been performed.

X. Special Age Considerations

A. Young animals undergoing portosystemic shunt ligation are prone to hypoglycemia.

B. Hypothermia, common in young patients, decreases the minimum alveolar concentration (MAC) of inhalants used for anesthetic maintenance.

Portosystemic Vascular Anomalies (*SAS*, pp. 374-384)

I. Definitions

A. **Portosystemic vascular anomalies (PSVA)** or **portosystemic shunts (PSS)** are anomalous vessels that allow portal blood draining the stomach, intestines, pancreas, and spleen to pass directly into the systemic circulation without first passing through the liver.

B. **Extrahepatic shunts** are located outside the hepatic parenchyma and may be congenital or acquired; intrahepatic shunts are within the liver.

C. The term **"portocaval shunt"** technically refers to a specific type of vascular anomaly (i.e., portal vein to caudal cava).

II. General Considerations and Clinically Relevant Pathophysiology

A. Problems arise when portal blood bypasses the liver.
   1. Hepatotrophic substances from the pancreas and intestines do not reach the liver, resulting in hepatic atrophy or failure of the liver to obtain normal size.
   2. Hepatic encephalopathy is a clinical syndrome of altered CNS function resulting from hepatic insufficiency. "Toxins" that are normally deactivated in the liver enter the systemic circulation.

B. Types.
   1. Extrahepatic shunts.
      a. Account for nearly 63% of single shunts in dogs; they also occur in cats.
      b. Congenital.
         i. Usually single anomalous vessels connecting the portal vein to the systemic circulation.
         ii. Different PSS have been described in dogs and cats.
            (a) Portal vein to caudal vena cava.
            (b) Portal vein to azygous.
            (c) Left gastric vein to caudal vena cava.
            (d) Splenic vein to caudal vena cava.
            (e) Left gastric, cranial mesenteric, caudal mesenteric, or gastroduodenal vein to the caudal vena cava.
            (f) Combinations of the above.
      c. Acquired.
         i. Typically multiple and represent about 20% of all canine PSS.
         ii. They arise because of increased resistance to portal blood flow and subsequent portal hypertension.
         iii. Multiple shunts are most commonly associated with chronic, severe hepatic disease (i.e., cirrhosis), but have been reported secondary to hepatoportal fibrosis in young dogs.

iv. Venoocclusive hepatic disease is a cause of multiple PSS in young cocker spaniels.
v. Multiple shunts most commonly occur in the left renal area and root of the mesentery, and connections to the caudal vena cava or azygous veins are usually observed.

2. Intrahepatic shunts.
   a. Are usually congenital, singular shunts that occur because of a failure of the ductus venosus to close following birth, or they may arise when other portal to hepatic vein or caudal vena cava anastomoses exist.
   b. Congenital intrahepatic PSS constitute about 35% of single shunts in dogs.
3. Arteriovenous (A-V) fistulae.
   a. Account for about 2% of single shunts and may be congenital or acquired.
   b. Acquired A-V fistulae occur secondary to trauma, tumors, surgical procedures, or degenerative processes that cause arteries to rupture into adjacent veins.
   c. Congenital A-V fistula develop as a result of failure of the common embryologic capillary plexus to differentiate into an artery or a vein.
   d. Affected animals develop portal hypertension and multiple collateral shunting vessels and frequently have ascites.

III. Diagnosis

A. Clinical Presentation

1. Signalment.
   a. Single PSS are usually congenital and are most commonly diagnosed in animals less than 1 year of age.
   b. Extrahepatic shunts have been most frequently diagnosed in miniature and toy-breed dogs (e.g., miniature schnauzers, Yorkshire terriers, poodles, Lhaso apsos, and Pekingese).
   c. Intrahepatic PSS are more commonly diagnosed in large-breed dogs (e.g., German shepherds, golden retrievers, Doberman pinschers, Labrador retrievers, Irish setters, Samoyeds, and Irish wolfhounds).
   d. Congenital extrahepatic and intrahepatic shunts have been reported in cats.
   e. Multiple shunts are commonly diagnosed in animals between 1 and 7 years of age; however, multiple acquired PSS secondary to hepatoportal fibrosis have been reported in dogs as young as 4 months of age. Breeds most commonly affected include the German shepherd, Doberman pinscher, and cocker spaniel.
   f. Most dogs with hepatic A-V fistulae are young (i.e., younger than 1.5 years) at the time of diagnosis.
2. History.
   a. The history is variable.
   b. Affected animals usually have failure to grow, small body stature, or weight loss.
   c. Intermittent anorexia, depression, vomiting, polydipsia or polyuria, ptyalism (especially in cats), pica, amaurosis, and behavioral changes are common.
   d. Urinary dysfunction (i.e., hematuria, dysuria, pollakiuria, stranguria, urethral obstruction) associated with urate urolithiasis may occur.

e. Occasionally, the first abnormality noted is prolonged response to anesthetic agents or tranquilizers.

f. Hepatic encephalopathy (i.e., ataxia, weakness, stupor, head pressing, circling, amaurosis, pacing, seizures, or coma) may be intermittent and is usually worse after eating a high-protein diet.
   i. Signs vary and some patients appear overly quiet.
   ii. Hepatic encephalopathy may worsen after gastrointestinal hemorrhage (e.g., parasites or ulceration).

g. The most common presenting signs caused by hepatic A-V fistula are sudden onsets of depression, ascites, and vomiting.
   i. The ascites is typically a pure transudate despite a serum albumin greater than 1.8 g/dl.
   ii. Many animals have concurrent gastrointestinal foreign bodies.

B. Physical Examination Findings

1. Most animals with PSS have microhepatia.
2. Kidneys may feel prominent or "plump."
3. A golden or copper color to the iris has been observed in many cats with PSS.
4. Neurologic abnormalities may be noted.
5. Ptyalism is common in cats, but rare in dogs.
6. Animals with hepatic A-V fistulae may have a palpably enlarged liver (rare) or ascites. An audible bruit can sometimes be auscultated in the cranial abdomen of affected animals.

C. Radiography, Ultrasonography, Nuclear Imaging

1. Definitive diagnosis of PSS is made via surgical identification of the shunt, intraoperative positive contrast portography, ultrasound, or nuclear hepatic scintigraphy.
   a. Positive contrast techniques include splenoportography, cranial mesenteric arterial portography, celiac arteriography, transsplenic portal catheterization, and jejunal vein portography.
   b. Jejunal vein portography is the simplest and most effective portographic technique.
   c. The most consistent finding on plain abdominal radiographs is microhepatia.
2. Intrahepatic and extrahepatic shunts have been identified with ultrasound.
   a. Assess the bladder and renal pelves for calculi; urate stones are usually radiolucent and difficult to see on plain abdominal radiographs.
   b. Ultrasound is also useful to identify the anechoic, tortuous vessels seen with hepatic A-V fistulae.
3. Nuclear scintigraphy is a rapid, noninvasive method of documenting abnormal hepatic blood flow.
   a. After colonic administration of ^{99m}Tc, the time when activity in the region of the liver is first noted is compared with the time when activity appears in the region of the heart. Animals with liver-to-heart time intervals greater than 2 seconds are considered normal.
   b. False negative results may occur if a small shunt involves only a peripheral portion of the portal system or if the animal has microvascular hepatic dysplasia.

D. Laboratory Findings

1. Hematologic abnormalities include microcytosis with normochromic erythrocytes, mild nonregenerative anemia, target cell formation, or poikilocytosis.

2. Biochemical tests.
   a. Low plasma albumin is common in dogs; however, some dogs (and most cats) with PSS have normal albumin levels.
   b. Low BUN results from reduced conversion of ammonia to urea.
   c. Mild increases in serum alanine aminotransferase, aspartate aminotransferase, and alkaline phosphatase occasionally occur.
   d. Serum bilirubin concentration is usually normal.
   e. Hypocholesterolemia and fasting hypoglycemia may occur.
   f. Prothrombin time, activated partial thromboplastin time, and activated coagulation time are usually normal.
3. Urinalysis may disclose dilute urine or ammonium biurate crystals. Hematuria, pyuria, and proteinuria may occur if urate calculi form.
4. The hematologic and biochemical profiles of canine hepatic A-V fistulae can be similar to those of dogs with single or multiple PSS.
5. Liver function tests (e.g., fasting and postprandial serum bile acids and the ammonia tolerance test [ATT]).
   a. In animals with PSS the abnormal blood flow results in abnormal hepatic clearance of bile acids and elevated postprandial concentrations. Fasting samples often have normal bile acid concentrations. *Obtain fasting and postprandial bile acids.*
      i. The animal should be fasted for 12 hours.
      ii. Collect a serum sample.
      iii. Feed 1 to 2 tbsp p/d (dogs) or c/d (cats).
      iv. Collect a serum sample 2 hours after feeding.
   b. Abnormalities in serum bile acids occur with other diseases, but young dogs with elevated (e.g., ≥100 μmol/L) postprandial serum bile acids in conjunction with microhepatia often have PSS.
   c. Ammonia is generated by RBCs; therefore blood samples have to be refrigerated immediately and transported on ice, and the plasma and blood cells separated promptly in a refrigerated centrifuge.

IV. Differential Diagnosis

A. PSS must be differentiated from other diseases causing hepatic insufficiency (e.g., cirrhosis) or neurologic abnormalities (e.g., hydrocephalus, epilepsy) in dogs and cats.

V. Medical Management

A. Surgery is the treatment of choice for animals with PSS. Continued deterioration of hepatic function is expected as long as the majority of blood is shunted away from the liver.

B. Life expectancy of medically managed animals is generally 2 months to 2 years.

C. Medical management should be initiated before surgical intervention in animals with signs of hepatic encephalopathy.

1. Precipitating factors for hepatic encephalopathy include high-protein meals, bacterial infections, gastrointestinal bleeding, blood transfusions, inappropriate drug therapy, and electrolyte/acid-base abnormalities.
2. General supportive care includes fluid therapy (0.9% NaCl or 0.45%

NaCl and 2.5% dextrose), normalization of acid-base disturbances, and supplementation of potassium.

3. Feed the highest-protein diet the animal will tolerate. Consider moderately protein-restricted diets (i.e., k/d or in some animals u/d; Hill's Pet Products) that contain high levels of branched-chain amino acids and arginine.
4. Antibiotics reduce enteric flora responsible for the production of many of the toxins (i.e., ammonia) thought to cause hepatic encephalopathy see Appendix I.
   a. Oral neomycin is used, but avoid it in azotemic animals.
   b. Metronidazole or ampicillin, given either orally or parenterally, also reduces intestinal ammonia concentrations.
5. Lactulose (see Appendix I) is a synthetic disaccharide that acidifies colonic contents and traps ammonium ions in the lumen.
   a. It is also an osmotic cathartic that reduces intestinal transit time and decreases production and absorption of ammonia.
   b. Give it orally or as a retention enema.
   c. Side effects include diarrhea, vomiting, anorexia, and increased gastrointestinal loss of potassium and water.
6. Treatment of hepatic coma.
   a. Cleansing enemas (warm water) and retention enemas with neomycin and/or lactulose.
   b. Identify and correct acid-base and electrolyte abnormalities and hypoglycemia.

VI. Surgical Treatment

A. General Considerations

1. The goal is to identify and ligate or attenuate the abnormal vessel. It is often not possible to totally occlude shunts without producing life-threatening portal hypertension; these shunts should only be attenuated.
2. When total ligation is not possible, a second surgery several months after the first operation to totally occlude the shunt may be necessary; however, in some animals the shunts will thrombose.
3. If the shunt(s) is identified during abdominal exploration, positive contrast portography examination is not necessary. However, if a shunt is not identified visually, intraoperative portography is necessary.

B. Preoperative Management

1. Stabilize encephalopathic patients before surgery.
2. Use perioperative antibiotics (e.g., cephalosporins) in patients with PSS.
3. Correct fluid and electrolyte imbalances.

C. Anesthesia

1. Reduced liver function and abnormal hepatic blood flow markedly reduce drug absorption, metabolism, and clearance (see Appendix G-13).
   a. Highly protein-bound drugs are affected by the low albumin concentrations that may accompany PSS (i.e., increased levels of circulating unbound drug).
   b. Avoid drugs metabolized by the liver (e.g., barbiturates and phenothiazine tranquilizers) and those that are highly protein bound (e.g., diazepam).

c. Benzodiazepines may negatively affect neurologic function in hepatoencephalopathic patients.
d. Reversible opioids may be administered with an anticholinergic, followed by mask or chamber induction with isoflurane and oxygen and endotracheal intubation.
e. Monitor blood glucose levels because patients with PSS may have reduced hepatic glycogen stores.
f. Prevent hypothermia.
g. Inotropic support (i.e., dobutamine [2-10 mg/kg/min; IV] or dopamine [2-10 mg/kg/min; IV]) may be necessary. Monitor these patients for arrhythmias or tachycardia.

D. Surgical Anatomy

1. The canine portal vein varies from 3 to 8 cm long and usually originates at the level of the first lumbar vertebra.
   a. It is formed by confluence of the cranial and caudal mesenteric veins and splenic vein.
   b. The splenic vein enters the portal vein at the level of the thoracolumbar junction.
   c. The phrenicoabdominal veins terminate in the caudal vena cava about 1 cm cranial to the renal veins.
2. Any vein entering the caudal vena cava cranial to the phrenicoabdominal veins (before the hepatic veins) may be considered an anomalous structure.

E. Positioning

1. Perform a standard ventral midline celiotomy from the xiphoid cartilage caudally.
2. For intrahepatic shunts and A-V fistulae, extend the incision cranially through the xiphoid process and caudal sternebrae, as needed.

VII. Surgical Technique

A. Portosytemic Shunt Ligation/Attenuation

1. General considerations.
   a. Ligate or attenuate single extrahepatic and intrahepatic shunts.
   b. Treat arteriovenous fistulae by removing the affected liver lobe.
   c. Measure portal pressures when occluding intrahepatic or extrahepatic shunts.
      i. Normal portal pressure in dogs is 8 to 13 cm H_2O, which is 7 to 8 cm H_2O higher than systemic venous pressure.
      ii. Animals with single PSS often have resting portal pressures closer to systemic venous pressures.
      iii. Excessive portal venous pressures can cause splanchnic congestion, portal hypertension, and death.
2. Surgical procedures.
   a. Ligation of single extrahepatic shunts.
      i. General considerations.
         (a) Shunt occlusion should cause a rapid increase in portal pressure, which aids in confirmation of the anomalous vessel.
         (b) Check portal pressures carefully before and during shunt ligation.
         (c) If you are unsure whether complete ligation should be attempted, only attenuate the shunt.

(d) If you are uncertain whether the vessel you have occluded is the shunt, perform jejunal portography.

ii. Surgical technique.

Perform a midline abdominal incision. Identify the portal vein by retracting the duodenum to the left and ventrally. Locate the caudal vena cava, renal veins, phrenicoabdominal veins, and portal vein (ventral to the caudal vena cava at the most dorsal aspect of the mesoduodenum). Note any veins entering the caudal vena cava proximal to the phrenicoabdominal veins. If the shunt has not been identified, open the omental bursa and retract the stomach cranially, the duodenum to the right and ventrally, and the left lobe of the pancreas caudally. Identify shunts that communicate with the caudal vena cava through the epiploic foramen by observing abnormal tributaries of the portal vein, left gastric vein, or splenic vein. Once the anomalous vessel is identified, isolate it and pass 2-0 silk suture around the vessel. If jejunal portography was not performed (see below), exteriorize a segment of jejunum and insert a 20- to 22-gauge over-the-needle catheter (Angiocath, Abbocath) into a jejunal vein. Do not damage the corresponding jejunal artery. Obtain baseline portal pressures. Temporarily occlude the shunt and observe portal pressures during this manipulation. If there is any doubt as to whether a vessel is a shunt, perform portography.

Once you have positively identified the shunt, slowly tighten the ligature while monitoring portal pressures. If possible, completely occlude the shunting vessel but do not allow postligation portal pressures to exceed 10 cm H_2O (8 mm Hg) above baseline pressures or 20 to 23 cm H_2O (15 to 18 mm Hg). You may be able to only attenuate the vessel. Observe the viscera for evidence of splanchnic congestion for 5 to 10 minutes. If excessive splanchnic congestion is noted, loosen the suture. Remove the jejunal vein catheter and ligate the vein. Examine the kidneys and bladder for the presence of calculi. If cystic calculi are present and the patient is stable, remove the calculi during the shunt ligation surgery. If operative time has been lengthy or renal calculi are present, it may be best to schedule a second surgery. Obtain a liver biopsy before closing the abdomen.

b. Jejunal portography.

i. General considerations.

(a) Perform to determine if the shunt is extrahepatic or intrahepatic. If the caudal extent of the PSS is cranial to T_{13}, the shunt is probably intrahepatic. If the caudal extent of the shunt is caudal to T_{13}, it is probably extrahepatic.

(b) With multiple hepatic shunts, radiographic confirmation of the shunts is rarely necessary. The technique is the same as for single PSS, except that exposures should be delayed approximately 3 or 4 seconds after the start of injection of the contrast material, to enable adequate filling of the shunting vessels.

ii. Surgical technique.

Exteriorize a loop of jejunum. Identify a jejunal vein near the mesenteric border of the intestine and place two sutures around the vessel. Insert a 20- to 22-gauge over-the-needle catheter into the vessel and use the preplaced sutures to secure it to the vessel. Attach a heparinized extension set and three-way stop-cock to the catheter. Close the abdominal incision temporarily. Inject a water-soluble contrast agent (e.g., Renovist) (2 ml/kg body weight) as a bolus into the catheter and make an exposure when the last milliliter is being injected. Making a lateral and ventrodorsal projection will help more fully define the location of the shunt. The catheter can also be used for pressure measurement.

c. Ligation of intrahepatic shunts.
   i. General considerations.
      (a) Intravascular and extravascular methods exist.
      (b) The vessel is often difficult to locate. Occasionally, the shunt can be identified as a palpable depression or soft spot in a liver lobe, or it may be seen entering into the caudal vena cava if it is not completely encircled by hepatic parenchymal tissue.
      (c) Intraoperative ultrasound can identify the shunt in hepatic tissue, but this technique is not always successful.
      (d) Intravascular technique involving temporary hepatic vascular occlusion (see below, under A-V fistula) in conjunction with caudal caval venotomy: the shunting vessel is identified entering the lumen of the caudal cava cranial to the liver. The vessel is completely occluded or attenuated by suturing the ostium.
      (e) Direct isolation of shunts involving the left medial or lateral liver lobes that are not completely surrounded by hepatic tissue may be possible.
   ii. Surgical technique.

Extend the abdominal incision proximally into the caudal sternebrae. Incise the left triangular ligament and free the left lateral liver lobe so that it can be retracted to the right. Use a combination of sharp and blunt dissection to isolate the anomalous vessel at its junction with the hepatic vein. Place a single silk ligature around the vessel and attenuate flow while measuring portal pressures.

d. Caudal vena cava banding for multiple shunts.
   i. General considerations.
      (a) Surgical management of multiple PSS involves suture attenuation (or banding) of the abdominal vena cava, just caudal to the hepatic hilus. The intent is to raise the systemic venous pressure within the abdomen to, or slightly above, that of the portal venous system.
      (b) Potential negative results of vena caval banding include accentuation of ascitic fluid formation and subcutaneous edema in the rear quarters.
      (c) Two venous catheters are needed to simultaneously monitor both the portal venous and the abdominal caudal vena caval pressures. The mesenteric catheter previously described is used to monitor portal venous pressure. A second catheter placed either through a purse-string suture in the abdominal vena cava, caudal to the banding ligature, or percutaneously into the lateral or medial saphenous vein and extending into the caudal vena cava, is used to monitor systemic venous pressure.
      (d) Multiple extrahepatic PSS in the area of the left kidney are usually evident at exploratory laparotomy. Take care when incising the abdominal wall in patients with suspected multiple PSS because large, dilated vessels may be present in the falciform ligament and/or the greater omentum.
   ii. Surgical technique.

Explore the abdominal cavity and observe the mesenteric circulation. Examine the portal system as described above for single PSS. Examine the left renal area by temporarily exteriorizing the spleen and using the descending colon and associated mesocolon to retract the remaining intestines to the right. Evaluate the left paravertebral area and note vascular connections between the

portal system and the azygous vein. Use right-angled forceps to isolate the abdominal vena cava as close to the liver as possible. Place silk suture (0 or 1) around the vena cava and constrict it. Monitor vena cava and portal venous pressures using a two-channel pressure transducer or two water manometers (Note: Fine modulations in ligature tension are more difficult with the latter technique because the water manometers respond more slowly to changing pressures). Partially attenuate the caudal vena cava until systemic venous pressures caudal to the ligation equal or just exceed (by 1 to 2 mm Hg) portal venous pressures. Pressures should be closely monitored at the time of knot-tying because the vena caval pressure often drops rapidly for a time after suture attenuation. Following banding, closely observe the mesenteric circulation for up to 20 minutes for signs of excessive congestion. Within a few minutes of occlusion, vena caval pressures transiently drop to less than those recorded at the time of banding. Do not attempt to individually or collectively ligate the anomalous vessels. Remove the venous catheters and obtain a liver biopsy.

e. Partial hepatectomy for removal of hepatic A-V fistula.
  i. General considerations.
    (a) Treatment of hepatic A-V fistulae involves removal of the affected lobes and abnormal vascular structures with or without temporary hepatic vascular occlusion.
    (b) If temporary vascular occlusion is used, the vascular clamps and occlusive ligatures should be released within 15 minutes.
  ii. Surgical technique.

Extend the abdominal incision cranially through the caudal sternebrae and incise the diaphragm down to and partially around the hiatus of the caudal vena cava. Place moistened umbilical tapes around the thoracic portion of the caudal vena cava, abdominal portion of the caudal vena cava (between the liver and renal veins), and the portal vein (just proximal to the first hepatic branch). Pass the umbilical tapes through a piece of rubber tubing (Rumel tourniquet). Identify, isolate, and ligate the phrenicoabdominal veins and isolate the celiac and cranial mesenteric arteries. Place a purse-string suture in the portal vein or a splenic tributary and pass a 3.5- or 5-French catheter into the vessel to monitor portal pressures. Monitor blood pressure carefully during surgery; manipulation and ligation of the fistula may cause sudden, severe fluctuations. Isolate the affected lobes by dissection of the triangular, coronary, and hepatorenal ligaments and ligaments of the lesser omentum. Identify the hepatic arterial branch supplying the affected lobe and temporarily occlude it to see if pressure within the fistula diminishes. Double ligate the arterial supply of the fistula with nonabsorbable suture (e.g., 2-0 silk). Isolate the portal branch and biliary ducts to the affected lobe and double ligate them. Temporarily occlude the vasculature by tightening the preplaced umbilical tape ligatures and by placing vascular clamps on the celiac and cranial mesenteric arteries. Sharply dissect the liver parenchyma to resect the affected lobe. Ligate any vascular structures not already occluded and control hemorrhage by packing the area for several minutes. Sometimes the affected portion of the liver can be removed by partial hepatectomy without performing vascular occlusion as described here.

VIII. Suture Materials/Special Instruments

A. Blunt-tipped, right-angled, or Mixter forceps are useful for dissecting around venous structures.

B. Shunt ligation is usually performed with silk suture because of the knot security this suture affords.

C. Delayed wound healing may be a problem if the patient is hypoproteinemic.

D. A long-lasting absorbable suture material such as polydioxanone or a nonabsorbable suture material should be used to close the linea alba.

IX. Postoperative Care and Assessment

A. Portal hypertension can develop several hours postoperatively and may not be evident immediately after shunt ligation or attenuation.
1. Hypertension and splanchnic congestion may cause a painful abdomen, hemorrhagic diarrhea, endotoxic shock, and death.
2. Many shunt patients experience painful abdomens during the early postoperative period, and recognition of life-threatening portal hypertension may be difficult.
3. If signs of endotoxic shock or hemorrhagic diarrhea or other signs of a deteriorating condition occur, perform emergency surgery to remove or loosen the ligature around the shunting vessel.
4. Portal vein thrombosis is a potentially life-threatening complication. If a shunt is only partially ligated, consider a single anticoagulant dose of heparin at the time of shunt attenuation.
5. Self-limiting ascites may occur following single shunt ligation.
   a. Use diuretics if drainage from the surgical incision site is present or if the animal experiences discomfort secondary to the abdominal distention.

B. Status epilepticus may occur 2 to 3 days after PSS ligation.
1. Long-term anticonvulsant therapy may be needed.
2. Permanent neurologic abnormalities may occur (e.g., blindness).

C. Medical management of hepatic encephalopathy should be continued postoperatively until the hepatic parenchyma regenerate.

D. If there is no improvement in clinical signs within 2 to 3 months, nuclear scintigraphy or jejunal portography should be repeated.

E. Postoperative management of the patient with multiple PSS is often less demanding.
1. Ascites is a commonly observed postoperative problem.
   a. Modulate by the intermittent use of diuretics.
   b. Perform abdominocentesis only if absolutely necessary.
   c. Dietary management (low-salt diet) may also be helpful.
   d. Ascites formation often decreases as hepatic function improves.
2. Less common problems are subcutaneous edema and peripheral venous congestion, particularly in the rear quarters or ventral abdomen.

X. Prognosis

A. Surgical mortality associated with the treatment of single PSS is 14% to 21%.

B. Complete occlusion of the PSS usually allows an excellent quality of life and normal life span.

C. Clinical signs may continue postoperatively in patients that tolerate only partial occlusion and require dietary and medical management. Reoperation and total shunt occlusion are recommended in such animals.

D. Hemorrhage, hypotension, and acute hepatic congestion are common complications during surgical correction of intrahepatic PSS in dogs. A 25% mortality rate associated with surgery has been reported in these dogs.

E. The prognosis following venal caval banding in patients with multiple PSS depends on the reversibility of the primary inciting cause and the degree of portal hypertension present at surgery.
1. If shunts are secondary to primary hepatocellular disease, caudal vena cava banding is of questionable benefit.

F. The long-term prognosis is good for dogs with hepatic A-V fistulae that survive surgery.

Cavitary Hepatic Lesions (*SAS*, pp. 384-386)

I. Definitions

A. **Cavitary hepatic lesions** are usually cysts or abscesses; however, large neoplastic lesions (i.e., hemangiomas, adenomas) occasionally cavitate.

B. **Hepatic abscesses** are localized collections of pus in the hepatic parenchyma.

C. **Hepatic cysts** are closed, fluid-filled sacs lined by secretory epithelium.

II. General Considerations and Clinically Relevant Pathophysiology

A. Hepatic abscesses are rare.

B. They are usually associated with extrahepatic infection (i.e., ascending biliary tract infections, hematogenous infection via the portal vein or hepatic artery, or direct extension from areas adjacent to the liver), hepatic trauma (i.e., surgical biopsy, penetrating wounds, or blunt trauma), or neoplasia.
1. Hepatic abscesses are frequently a complication of omphalophlebitis in puppies.
2. Diabetes mellitus has been associated with hepatic abscesses.
3. Small abscesses may not be associated with clinical signs and may resorb without therapy.

C. Hepatic cysts are usually incidental findings, but rarely become so large that they interfere with normal function of adjacent organs.
   1. A single hepatic cyst may be noted, or several cysts may be present in the same or different lobes.
   2. Concurrent polycystic renal disease has been reported in cats.
   3. If there is clinical evidence of hepatic dysfunction, liver biopsy is often warranted to determine the cause.

III. Diagnosis

A. Clinical Presentation

1. Signalment.
   a. There is no reported sex or breed predisposition for hepatic abscesses or cysts.
2. History.
   a. Clinical signs of hepatic abscesses may include anorexia, lethargy, weight loss, and intermittent abdominal pain.
   b. Most animals with hepatic cysts are asymptomatic; however, some cysts cause abdominal distention.

B. Physical Examination Findings

1. Hepatic abscesses may cause persistent fever, hepatomegaly, and abdominal enlargement.
2. A firm abdominal mass and marked abdominal distention may be noted in animals with hepatic cysts.

C. Radiography/Ultrasonography

1. Hepatic cysts.
   a. Small ones are often incidental findings on abdominal radiographs or ultrasonography.
   b. Large cysts are usually well-defined radiopaque structures located in the cranial abdomen.
2. Hepatic abscesses.
   a. Radiographs may demonstrate hepatomegaly, but a well-defined hepatic mass is seldom evident.
   b. Gas within the hepatic parenchyma can be noted, which strongly suggests abscesses caused by gas-forming bacteria.
   c. Ultrasonography is the most useful diagnostic test for abscesses and cysts.
      i. Hepatic abscesses appear as hypoechoic or anechoic structures that may contain mixed echo densities, depending on cellularity.
      ii. Scintigraphy and computed tomography are also highly sensitive, but less commonly used.
      iii. Ultrasound-guided FNAs of hepatic abscesses can be performed before surgery; however, there is a risk that the abscess will rupture or drain into the abdomen and cause diffuse peritonitis.
      iv. Fluid removed from cysts during FNA is usually transudative in nature.

D. Laboratory Findings

1. Laboratory abnormalities are seldom present with hepatic cysts.
2. Abnormalities with hepatic abscesses.
   a. Inflammatory leukogram and nonregenerative anemia.
   b. Hypoalbuminemia, hypokalemia, hyperglycemia, and elevated

hepatic enzymes; however, elevation of alanine transaminase activity is not a consistent finding.

IV. Differential Diagnosis

A. Hepatic cysts, abscesses, neoplasms, and parasitic lesions must be differentiated.

B. Hepatic abscesses produce nonspecific signs that may be masked by associated disease processes.

C. Large neoplastic hepatic lesions may necrose and become secondarily infected.

D. Hepatic cysts may become infected.

E. Histologic evaluation of surgically resected tissue is important.

V. Medical Management

A. Medical management of hepatic abscesses entails fluid therapy, correcting electrolyte and acid-base abnormalities, and initiating appropriate antibiotics.

B. Resect hepatic abscesses as soon as the animal has been stabilized.

C. Base preoperative parenteral antibiotic therapy on culture and sensitivity results, or use antibiotics with bactericidal activity against anaerobes and gram-negative bacteria (e.g., amoxicillin plus clavulanic acid, cefoxitin, cefazolin plus metronidazole; see Appendix I).

VI. Surgical Treatment

A. General Considerations

1. Whether hepatic cysts should be removed when diagnosed in asymptomatic animals is not clear.
2. Promptly resect hepatic cysts associated with clinical signs and hepatic abscesses.

B. Preoperative Management

1. Stabilize symptomatic animals before surgery.
2. Initiate antibiotics before surgery.

C. Positioning

1. Place in dorsal recumbency and prep from midthorax to the pubis.

VII. Surgical Technique

A. Abscess/Cyst

1. General considerations.
   a. Hepatic abscesses and cysts are generally treated by partial hepatectomy.

b. Try to remove the cyst without entering the lumen.
c. Culturing hepatic cysts may be optional if the fluid does not appear infected cytologically; however, some cysts can develop secondary bacterial infections.

2. Surgical technique.

Pack the area surrounding the liver with moistened laparotomy sponges to decrease intraoperative contamination if the lumen of the abscess or cyst is entered. If possible, resect the affected portion of the liver without entering the lesion. Culture the lesion and submit it for histologic examination. Palpate the remainder of the liver parenchyma for other nodules and explore the abdominal cavity for associated infections or disease.

VIII. Postoperative Care and Assessment

A. Continue fluid therapy in animals with hepatic abscesses until the animal is drinking normally.

B. Continue antibiotic therapy for 7 to 10 days.

C. Monitor the animal for leukocytosis, fever, abdominal fluid, and abdominal pain if abdominal contamination occurred.

D. Minimal postoperative care is needed for most animals with hepatic cysts.

IX. Prognosis

A. The prognosis for hepatic abscesses depends on the rapidity with which the abscess is diagnosed, whether concurrent peritonitis is present, and the overall health of the animal.

B. The prognosis for hepatic cysts (with or without surgery) is good unless there is concurrent hepatic or renal disease.

Hepatobiliary Neoplasia (*SAS*, pp. 386-388)

I. Definitions

A. **Hepatocellular tumors** arise from hepatocytes.

B. **Cholangiocellular neoplasms** arise from intrahepatic or extrahepatic bile duct epithelium.

C. **Hepatoma** refers to both hepatocellular carcinomas and hepatocellular adenomas.

D. **Cholangiocellular carcinomas** are also known as bile duct carcinomas.

II. General Considerations and Clinically Relevant Pathophysiology

A. Primary hepatic neoplasms are uncommon and may be of epithelial or mesenchymal origin.

B. Hepatocellular carcinomas and cholangiocellular carcinomas are the most commonly diagnosed primary hepatic malignancies in dogs.
   1. Hepatocellular carcinomas may involve a single liver lobe or may be nodular or diffuse and involve multiple lobes.

C. In cats, cholangiocellular adenomas are the most common primary tumor.

D. Hepatic carcinoids are rare tumors that arise from neuroectodermal cells in the liver.

E. Benign hepatic masses (i.e., adenomas or cysts) are often incidental findings at necropsy.

F. Cholangiocellular carcinomas arise primarily from intrahepatic bile duct epithelium.

G. Neoplasms of the extrahepatic bile duct and gallbladder are rare.

H. Most malignant primary hepatic tumors are highly metastatic.
   1. The most common sites for epithelial tumors to metastasize are the regional lymph nodes and lungs.
   2. Mesenchymal tumors most often metastasize to the spleen.

I. Metastatic neoplasia is more common in the liver than are primary tumors.

J. Lymphosarcoma is the most common secondary hepatic tumor.

III. Diagnosis

A. Clinical Presentation

1. Signalment.
   a. Primary hepatic neoplasia is usually a disease of aged dogs and cats.
   b. Hepatocellular carcinomas may be more common in male dogs, whereas cholangiocellular carcinomas may be more common in cats and female dogs.
2. History.
   a. Animals with primary hepatic neoplasia usually present with signs associated with hepatic failure (i.e., lethargic, weak, anorexic, losing weight, or vomiting, and/or have polyuria/polydipsia).
   b. The clinical signs associated with metastatic hepatic neoplasia are highly variable.

B. Physical Examination Findings

1. Hepatomegaly is common in animals with primary hepatic tumors.
2. Hepatic carcinoids may not cause significant hepatomegaly.
3. Additional findings may include jaundice and ascites.

4. Hepatocellular adenomas may rupture and cause hemoperitoneum.
5. Marked hepatomegaly is less common with metastatic neoplasia; however, lymphosarcoma often causes diffuse hepatic enlargement.

C. Radiography/Ultrasonography

1. Radiographs help localize the mass to the liver and may reveal extrahepatic metastasis.
2. Radiographs may be useless if ascites is present.
3. Take thoracic radiographs whenever hepatic neoplasia is suspected, because pulmonary metastasis is common.
4. Ultrasonography localizes and defines the extent of disease. It is particularly useful in animals with ascites.
5. Ultrasound-guided biopsies may allow presurgical diagnosis.

D. Laboratory Findings

1. Neutrophilia and biochemical abnormalities compatible with hepatic disease (increased serum alanine transaminase, aspartate transaminase, serum alkaline phosphate) are common but inconsistent.
2. Serum bilirubin concentrations may be increased, particularly if extrahepatic biliary obstruction occurs.
3. Hypoglycemia occasionally causes clinical signs.
4. Albumin levels are usually normal in patients with primary hepatic neoplasia.

IV. Differential Diagnosis

A. Primary hepatobiliary tumors must be differentiated from nodular hyperplasia, abscesses, hematomas, or cysts.

B. Do not perform percutaneous biopsies in animals with clinical bleeding disorders, or if the lesions appear cavitary or highly vascular.

C. Cytologic evaluation of abdominal fluid is seldom helpful in differentiating between these lesions.

V. Medical Management

A. Surgical excision of primary malignant hepatic tumors is the treatment of choice.

B. They are usually diagnosed in older animals, and concurrent cardiac, renal, or other metabolic problems are common.

C. Medical therapy should aim at correcting fluid and electrolyte imbalances and providing nutrition to improve chances of surviving surgery.

VI. Surgical Treatment

A. General Considerations

1. If the tumor is localized to a single lobe or confined to the gallbladder, surgical resection may be curative.
   a. Perform surgical biopsies on all animals with hepatomegaly or nodularity because differentiation requires histopathology.

b. Multiple hepatic masses do not indicate metastatic disease because primary hepatic tumors may spread to other portions of the liver.
c. If neoplasia is suspected, assess the draining lymph nodes and surrounding organs for metastasis.
d. Hepatocellular tumors are most commonly found in the left medial and left lateral liver lobes.

B. Preoperative Management

1. Stabilize the animal with fluid and electrolyte therapy before surgery.
2. Give blood transfusions to animals that are severely anemic (i.e., PCV less than 20%), especially if bleeding tendencies are present (i.e., petechiation, ecchymosis, or hemorrhage).
3. Consider plasma or whole blood transfusions if the animal has clinical evidence of coagulopathy or is severely thrombocytopenic (i.e., less than 20,000 platelets/μl).
4. If the patient has massive ascites, slowly remove some fluid before anesthetic induction to help prevent hypoventilation associated with positioning the patient while it is being prepared for surgery.

C. Anesthesia

1. Ventilation of patients with ascites may require intermittent positive-pressure ventilation.
2. Compression of the caudal vena cava in patients with large hepatic masses or massive ascites may cause decreased venous return and reduced cardiac output.

D. Positioning

1. Perform a cranial ventral midline abdominal incision.
2. Extend the incision paracostally to allow enhanced visualization and manipulation of large tumors.
3. Extend the prepped area from midthorax to the pubis.

VII. Surgical Technique

A. See partial hepatectomy and cholecystectomy.

VIII. Suture Material/Special Instruments

A. Absorbable suture material is used for hepatic biopsy.

B. Ligation of the cystic duct for cholecystectomy is generally done with nonabsorbable suture material.

IX. Postoperative Care and Assessment

A. Postoperative nutritional support of patients with hepatic neoplasia is often necessary.

B. Nonresectable primary hepatic tumors seldom respond to chemotherapy or radiation therapy, but chemotherapy may palliate hepatic lymphosarcoma.

X. Prognosis

A. The prognosis for dogs and cats with primary hepatobiliary malignancies is often poor.

B. The high rate of metastasis and degree of invasion make surgical resection unlikely to be curative in most patients.

C. Benign tumors may be surgically resected, and long-term survival of patients with benign hepatic tumors has been reported.

18

Surgery of the Extrahepatic Biliary System (*SAS*, pp. 389-399)

General Principles and Techniques (*SAS*, pp. 389-395)

I. Definitions

A. **Cholecystotomy** is the creation of an opening into the gallbladder for drainage.

B. **Cholecystectomy** is removal of the gallbladder.

C. **Choledochotomy** is incision of the common bile duct for exploration or removal of a calculus.

D. **Choledochoduodenostomy** is a rarely indicated procedure in dogs and cats that involves surgical anastomosis of the common bile duct to the duodenum.

E. **Cholecystoduodenostomy** and **cholecystojejunostomy** are surgical anastomoses of the gallbladder to the duodenum or jejunum, respectively.

F. Calculi may form in the gallbladder **(cholelithiasis)** or the common bile duct **(choledocholithiasis).**

II. Preoperative Concerns

A. Biliary disease may be due to obstruction of the extrahepatic biliary system, neoplasia, infection, or trauma.

B. Lesions that cause obstruction of the extrahepatic biliary system may be extraluminal or intraluminal.
   1. Extraluminal obstruction may be caused by pancreatic neoplasia, duodenal or pyloric neoplasia, hepatic or biliary neoplasia, pancreatitis, or pancreatic abscessation.
   2. Intraluminal obstruction is less common but may occur in association with cholelithiasis, choledocholithiasis, or inspissated bile.

3. Pancreatic disease is the most common cause of extrahepatic biliary obstruction in dogs.

C. Correct electrolyte and fluid abnormalities preoperatively.

D. Prolonged biliary obstruction may cause vitamin K malabsorption, resulting in deficiencies of factors VII, IX, and X.
1. If there is clinical evidence of bleeding, give vitamin K_1 (Aqua-Mephyton, Mephyton) 0.1 to 0.2 mg/kg SC, SID.

E. Partial or complete biliary obstruction may allow ascending aerobic and anaerobic infection and subsequent bacteremia. Perioperative antibiotic therapy is indicated.

F. Extrahepatic biliary injury may occur because of blunt or penetrating trauma.
1. Common bile duct, gallbladder, cystic duct, or hepatic duct lacerations may cause bile peritonitis, or (if the infection is "walled-off") a localized inflammatory process with adherence to surrounding organs.
2. Necrotizing cholecystitis occurs when bacteria damage the gallbladder wall, often resulting in peritoneal spillage of bile.

III. Anesthetic Considerations

A. Anesthetic requirements and concerns for biliary disease are similar to those for hepatic disease.

B. An additional concern in patients with obstructive biliary disease relates to the effect of mu-agonists (e.g., oxymorphone, morphine) on smooth muscle tone. These drugs increase sphincter tone and enhance pain.
1. Mixed agonist antagonists (e.g., butorphanol) may be preferable as premedicants and analgesics in these patients.
   a. Butorphanol.
      i. 0.2 to 0.4 mg/kg IV, IM, or SC as a premedicant.
      ii. Repeat dose q 2 to 4 hours as needed for analgesia.

IV. Antibiotics

A. Use prophylactic antibiotics in patients undergoing biliary surgery.

B. The most common organisms isolated from biliary infections are *E. coli*, *Klebsiella* spp., *Enterobacter* spp., *Proteus* spp., and *Pseudomonas* spp.

C. Antibiotics that are excreted in active form in the bile include amoxicillin, cefazolin, and enrofloxacin (see Appendix I).

D. Chloramphenicol is dependent on hepatic metabolism; avoid using it in patients with severe hepatic dysfunction.

V. Surgical Anatomy

A. The hepatic and cystic ducts and the common bile duct plus the gallbladder constitute the extrahepatic biliary system.

1. Bile drains from the hepatic ducts into the bile duct and is stored and concentrated in the gallbladder.
2. The gallbladder lies between the quadrate lobe of the liver medially and the right medial lobe laterally.
3. Between the neck of the gallbladder (i.e., the tapering end leading into the cystic duct) and the fundus is the body, or middle portion, of the gallbladder.
4. The cystic duct extends from the neck of the gallbladder to the junction with the first tributary from the liver. From this point to the opening of the biliary system into the duodenum, the duct is termed the bile duct.

B. The bile duct runs through the lesser omentum for approximately 5 cm and enters the mesenteric wall of the duodenum.

1. The canine bile duct terminates in the duodenum near the opening of the minor pancreatic duct. This combined opening of the minor pancreatic duct and bile duct is the major duodenal papilla.
2. The feline bile duct usually joins the major pancreatic duct before entering the duodenum.

VI. Surgical Techniques

A. General Considerations

1. Perform exploratory laparotomy when leakage of bile into the abdomen is suspected; when obstruction of bile flow is not clearly due to pancreatitis; and when neoplasia (biliary tract, intestinal, or pancreatic), parasitic disease, or biliary calculi is suspected.
2. Ensure patency of the common bile duct by manually expressing the gallbladder, or by retrograde (i.e., from the duodenum) or normograde (i.e., from the gallbladder) catheterization of the duct.
3. Initially treat animals with biliary obstruction secondary to benign pancreatic disease medically for pancreatitis.
   a. If clinical or laboratory improvement is not seen within 7 to 10 days of initiating appropriate therapy, or if clinical deterioration occurs despite appropriate medical therapy, consider cholecystoduodenostomy or cholecystojejunostomy.
4. In extremely ill patients with biliary obstruction who cannot undergo surgical exploration, temporary decompression of the gallbladder using ultrasound-guided aspiration, or a Foley or self-retaining accordion catheter, may be warranted.

B. Cholecystotomy

1. General considerations.
   a. It is rarely performed.
   b. It is indicated to remove some choleliths or when the gallbladder contents are inspissated and cannot be aspirated into a syringe.
2. Surgical procedure.

Pack the area surrounding the gallbladder with sterile, moistened laparotomy sponges. Place stay sutures in the gallbladder to facilitate manipulation and decrease spillage. Make an incision in the fundus of the gallbladder. Remove the gallbladder contents and submit for culture. Lavage the gallbladder with warmed, sterile saline. Catheterize the common bile duct via the cystic duct with a 3.5- or 5-French soft catheter and flush it to ensure patency. Close the incision with a one- or two-layer inverting suture pattern using absorbable suture material (3-0 to 5-0).

C. Cholecystectomy

1. General considerations.
   a. Cholecystitis and cholelithiasis are best treated by cholecystectomy.
   b. Cholecystectomy may also be indicated for primary neoplasia or traumatic rupture of the gallbladder.
   c. Always determine the patency of the common bile duct before performing this technique.
2. Surgical procedure.

Expose the gallbladder and incise the visceral peritoneum along the junction of the gallbladder and liver with Metzenbaum scissors. Apply gentle traction to the gallbladder and, using blunt dissection, free it from the liver. Free the cystic duct to its junction with the common bile duct. Be sure to identify the common bile duct and avoid damaging it during the procedure. If necessary, identify the common bile duct by placing a 3.5- or 5-French soft catheter into the duct via the duodenal papilla. Make a small enterotomy in the proximal duodenum, locate the duodenal papilla, and place a small red rubber tube into the common bile duct. Flush the duct to ensure its patency. Clamp and double ligate the cystic duct and cystic artery with nonabsorbable suture material (2-0 to 4-0). Sever the duct distal to the ligatures and remove the gallbladder. Submit a portion of the wall, plus bile, for culture if infection is suspected. Submit the remainder of the gallbladder for histologic analysis if indicated (for cholecystitis or neoplasia). Close the duodenal incision with simple interrupted sutures of absorbable suture material.

D. Choledochotomy

1. General considerations.
   a. Only perform direct incision of the bile duct in animals in which the duct is markedly dilated (e.g., chronic obstruction), and when the obstruction can be removed (i.e., choledocholithiasis, biliary sludge).
   b. First try to remove the obstruction by flushing the common bile duct, using a catheter placed via an enterotomy or cholecystotomy.
   c. Extraluminal obstruction or stricture of the duct is best treated with biliary diversion techniques.
2. Surgical procedure.

Pack the area surrounding the common bile duct with sterile, moistened laparotomy sponges. Place traction sutures into the distended duct. Make a small incision into the duct and remove the obstruction. Flush the duct with copious amounts of warmed, sterile saline and pass a 3.5- to 5-French soft catheter into the gallbladder and duodenum to ensure patency. Close the incision with a simple continuous or simple interrupted suture pattern of absorbable suture material (4-0 or 5-0). If leakage is a concern, pass a catheter into the duct via an incision in the proximal duodenum (see above). Small leaks may be treated by stenting the incision with a 3.5- to 5-French soft catheter (see discussion on repairing common bile duct injuries).

E. Bile Flow Diversion

1. General considerations.
   a. Bile flow diversion is indicated when common bile duct obstruction is present or the duct is severely traumatized, and the gallbladder is not directly involved in the disease process.
   b. Cholecystojejunostomy or cholecystoduodenostomy is preferred over choledochoduodenostomy.
      i. If cholecystojejunostomy is performed, the proximal jejunum

should be used to decrease the incidence of postoperative maldigestion of lipids.

ii. Duodenal ulceration may occur more commonly as a sequela to cholecystojejunostomy than as a sequela to cholecystoduodenostomy.

iii. In dogs, make the stoma between the bowel and the gallbladder at least 2.5 cm long to minimize the potential for obstruction of bile flow or retention of bowel contents in the gallbladder.

(a) Making the stoma too small is more likely to result in ascending or chronic cholecystitis than is making the stoma too large.

2. Surgical procedure.

Mobilize the gallbladder from the liver as described for cholecystectomy. Place stay sutures approximately 3 cm apart in the gallbladder. Bring the gallbladder into apposition with the antimesenteric surface of the descending duodenum so that there is little or no tension on the gallbladder or intestine. Pack the area surrounding the gallbladder and duodenum with sterile, moistened laparotomy sponges. Place a continuous suture of absorbable suture material between the serosa of the gallbladder and the serosa of the duodenum, near the mesentery (referred to as original suture line). Make the suture line 3 to 4 cm in length. Leave the ends of the suture long and use them to manipulate the intestine and gallbladder. Drain the gallbladder and make a 2.5- to 3-cm incision into it, parallel to the preplaced suture line. Have an assistant occlude the duodenum proximal and distal to the proposed incision site. Make a similar parallel incision in the antimesenteric surface of the duodenum. Place a continuous suture line of absorbable suture material (2-0 to 4-0) from the mucosa of the gallbladder to the mucosa of the duodenum, beginning with the edges closest to the original suture line. Then use the same suture material to suture the mucosal edges of the stoma farthest from the original suture line. Complete the stoma by suturing the serosal edges of the gallbladder and intestine over the near side of the stoma (i.e., the side farthest from the original suture line).

F. Repair of Common Bile Duct Injuries

1. General considerations.

a. The surgical technique that should be used to repair lacerations of the common bile duct depends on the location and severity of the lesion.

i. Severely damaged ducts, particularly if there has been bile leakage or adhesion formation, are difficult to repair primarily.

ii. If the injury is distal to the entrance of the hepatic ducts, ligate the common bile duct proximal and perform distal to the injury and biliary diversion (i.e., cholecystoduodenostomy or cholecystojejunostomy; see above).

b. Primary suturing and anastomosis.

i. Consider for cases in which the duct has been cleanly severed and the luminal diameter is greater than 4 to 5 mm. Proximal lacerations or perforations may also be treated with primary suturing.

ii. Accurately reappose the mucosa of the bile duct.

iii. Use small sutures and avoid tension on the suture line.

c. Stenting catheters.

i. Their use in the common bile duct is controversial, but temporary bile diversion may allow bile duct injuries to heal that would otherwise dehisce, leak, or stricture.

ii. Disadvantages include an increased potential for stricture because of the presence of a foreign body at the injured site, obstruction of the tube, and ascending infection.

iii. If you stent the bile duct, use a soft, straight catheter that is smaller than the diameter of the duct to minimize irritation to the duct wall.

2. Surgical procedure.

Identify the common bile duct. This may be facilitated by passing a catheter into the duct from the duodenum (see above discussion of cholecystectomy). Be careful not to interfere with the blood supply to the duct during manipulation. Carefully debride the transected ends of the duct, but be sure to leave adequate duct length to avoid having tension on the suture line when the ends are reapposed. Reappose the ends of the duct with absorbable suture material using simple interrupted sutures (4-0 to 6-0). Place a 3.5- to 5-French soft catheter in the duct from the duodenum to stent the suture line. Suture the distal end of the catheter to the duodenal lumen with a small chromic gut suture (3-0 or 4-0). As the suture dissolves, peristalsis causes the catheter to enter the intestinal lumen, where it will pass in the feces.

VII. Healing of the Biliary Tract

A. If a small strip of the common bile duct wall remains intact, the duct will regenerate.

B. Longitudinal tension on the suture line of a repaired biliary duct causes severe stenosis.

C. Intraluminal tubes may interfere with normal biliary drainage, thus promoting cholangitis.

D. Cholecystojejunostomies are performed over direct repair of the common bile duct.

VIII. Suture Materials/Special Instruments

A. Use absorbable suture material in the biliary tree. Nonabsorbable suture may act as a nidus for stone formation.

B. Empty the gallbladder with a syringe and needle or a needle attached to suction before surgical manipulations to decrease spillage of bile during biliary diversion surgery.

IX. Postoperative Care and Assessment

A. Continue fluid therapy until the animal is able to maintain hydration with oral fluids. Monitor and correct electrolytes and acid-base status.

B. Many patients with bile peritonitis are debilitated before surgery, and nutritional supplementation may be beneficial.

C. Continue antibiotic therapy for 7 to 10 days if cholecystitis was present or bile leakage occurred before or during surgery. Consider open abdominal drainage in patients with generalized bile peritonitis.

X. Special Age Considerations

A. Trauma should be suspected in young animals presenting with bile peritonitis.

B. Obstruction secondary to pancreatitis or neoplasia is more common in middle-aged or older animals.

Cholelithiasis (*SAS*, pp. 395-397)

I. Definitions

A. Calculi (i.e., gallstones) in the gallbladder are **choleliths,** and those found in the common bile duct are **choledocholiths.**

II. General Considerations and Clinically Relevant Pathophysiology

A. Choleliths are often fortuitous findings at necropsy or during imaging with radiographs or ultrasound.

B. Stones may cause cholecystitis, vomiting, anorexia, icterus, fever, or abdominal pain.

C. Cholesterol, bilirubin, and mixed stones have been reported.

III. Diagnosis

A. Clinical Presentation

1. Signalment.
   a. Aged female small-breed dogs appear to be at increased risk for development of choleliths.
2. History.
   a. Most animals are asymptomatic.
   b. Fever, vomiting, icterus, or abdominal pain may occur if cholecystitis or biliary obstruction occurs. Clinical signs may be mild and intermittent in some animals.

B. Physical Examination Findings

1. Icterus may occur if the calculus causes biliary obstruction or ascending cholangitis.

2. Abdominal pain and vomiting may also occur.
3. Choleliths rarely cause perforation of the gallbladder or common bile duct.

C. Radiography/Ultrasonography

1. Gallstones are seldom radiodense, but they are readily identified by ultrasound.
2. If obstruction is present, dilation of the common bile duct or hepatic ducts may be seen.

D. Laboratory Findings

1. Abnormalities are uncommon.
2. Symptomatic animals may show abnormalities compatible with extrahepatic biliary obstruction (i.e., increased serum alkaline phosphatase, usually with hyperbilirubinemia), or ascending cholangitis.
3. Hypercholesterolemia may be found secondary to biliary tract obstruction.
4. Bilirubinuria usually occurs before hyperbilirubinemia.

IV. Differential Diagnosis

A. Evidence of concurrent cholecystitis should be sought in symptomatic animals with choleliths.

B. Sludge and true concretions may be difficult to differentiate in some animals before surgery.

V. Medical Management

A. Treat concurrent cholecystitis with appropriate antibiotics.

VI. Surgical Treatment

A. General Considerations

1. Remove choleliths if they are found in a patient with biliary tract disease.

B. Preoperative Management

1. See preoperative management of patients with biliary obstruction.

C. Positioning

1. Place the patient in dorsal recumbency.
2. Prepare the abdomen from the xiphoid to the pubis.

VII. Surgical Technique

A. Cholecystectomy is the surgical treatment of choice for cholelithiasis causing clinical signs.

1. If stones are also present in the common bile duct, catheterize the duct via the duodenum and flush the stones into the gallbladder.
2. If the bile duct is enlarged, incise the duct (choledochotomy) and remove the stones.

B. There is a greatly increased mortality in human patients with cholelithiasis when choledochotomy is performed versus cholecystectomy.

C. Culture the bile.

VIII. Suture Materials/Special Instruments

A. Suture the gallbladder and common bile duct with absorbable suture material to decrease the likelihood of suture serving as a nidus for calculi formation.

IX. Postoperative Care and Assessment

A. See postoperative management of patients with obstructive biliary disorders.

B. The prognosis is excellent with proper surgical technique.

Bile Peritonitis (*SAS*, pp. 397-399)

I. Definitions

A. **Bile peritonitis** (i.e., bilious ascites) is inflammation of the peritoneum caused by bile leakage into the abdomen.

II. General Considerations and Clinically Relevant Pathophysiology

A. An acute condition in the abdomen (i.e., shock and/or pain caused by severe abdominal disease) may be caused by leakage of bile into the abdominal cavity, particularly if there is concurrent septic peritonitis.

B. Leakage of bile into the abdominal cavity may occur with traumatic rupture of any portion of the extrahepatic biliary tree or may be secondary to necrotizing cholecystitis or chronic obstruction (rare).

C. Untreated bile peritonitis is often lethal. Clinical signs of bile peritonitis usually develop quickly if rupture is associated with biliary tract infection.

D. Dogs with sterile bile peritonitis (i.e., rupture caused by trauma) may not have clinical signs other than ascites and icterus for weeks.
1. Changes in intestinal mucosal permeability may lead to secondary bacterial infection of the effusion.
2. If diagnosis of a ruptured biliary tract is delayed, repair of the biliary tract will be complicated by necrotic tissues and adhesions.

E. Diagnostic peritoneal lavage assists in the early diagnosis of bile peritonitis (before onset of clinical signs) in animals sustaining abdominal trauma.

F. Rupture of the extrahepatic biliary ducts or gallbladder may be due to blunt abdominal trauma; cholecystitis; or obstruction secondary to calculi, neoplasia, or parasites.
1. Trauma usually causes rupture of the common bile duct rather than the gallbladder.
2. The most common site of ductal rupture appears to be the common bile duct just distal to the entrance of the last hepatic duct; however, rupture may occur in the distal common bile duct, cystic duct (rare), or hepatic ducts.
3. Gallbladder rupture is principally due to necrotizing cholecystitis or cholelithiasis.

III. Diagnosis

A. Clinical Presentation

1. Signalment.
   a. Traumatic rupture of the common bile duct or gallbladder may occur in animals of any age.
   b. Necrotizing cholecystitis is more common in middle-aged or older animals.
2. History.
   a. The animal may have sustained trauma several weeks before presentation.
   b. Clinical signs may be slowly progressive or acute if the bile becomes infected.

B. Physical Examination Findings

1. Animals with infected bile peritonitis generally present in shock with acute abdominal pain, fever, vomiting, and anorexia.
2. Animals with localized peritonitis secondary to inspissated bile tend not to be as sick as those with diffuse peritonitis.
3. Some animals are diagnosed before a diseased gallbladder ruptures, in which case signs are similar to those with localized peritonitis.

C. Radiography/Ultrasonography

1. Radiographs can show a generalized loss of abdominal detail if the peritonitis is diffuse, or a soft-tissue density in the cranial abdomen if the infection is localized.
2. Plain radiographs may reveal radiodense gallstones or air in the gallbladder wall or lumen.

3. Ultrasonography can delineate the location of mass lesions.
4. Exploratory laparotomy is indicated in any patient with bile peritonitis and negates the need for extensive diagnostic workups.

D. Laboratory Findings

1. Bilious effusions have bilirubin concentrations greater than those found in serum.
2. Neutrophilia is expected if peritonitis is generalized; however, the white blood cell count may be normal in localized infections.
3. *E. coli* is a common bacterial isolate from animals with bilious effusions.

IV. Differential Diagnosis

A. Bilious effusion is obvious because the fluid looks like bile. If there is any doubt as to whether the fluid is bilious or bile stained, compare simultaneous bilirubin concentrations in the serum and effusion.

V. Medical Management

A. Animals with bile peritonitis may be anemic, hypoproteinemic, dehydrated, or have electrolyte imbalances.

B. Bile causes peritoneal inflammation and fluid transudation into the abdominal cavity, and the animal may present in hypovolemic and/or septic shock.

C. Administer broad-spectrum antibiotics before, during, and after surgery.

D. Consider vitamin K_1 administration (or fresh whole blood), because disruption of bile flow occasionally causes vitamin K malabsorption and coagulation disturbances.

VI. Surgical Treatment

A. General Considerations

1. Surgical treatments for common bile duct rupture include ductal repair or biliary diversion.
2. Repair is possible if the rupture is diagnosed early but becomes difficult once adhesions develop. Cholecystoduodenostomy or cholecystojejunostomy is usually easier and safer.
3. Rupture of a hepatic duct can be treated by ligation of the leaking duct. Gallbladder rupture secondary to infective processes should be treated by cholecystectomy.
4. Treatment of necrotizing cholecystitis includes cholecystectomy, antibiotics, and appropriate therapy for peritonitis.
   a. Attempts to salvage the gallbladder by closing the defect are inappropriate because the wall is usually necrotic.
   b. Be sure that the common bile duct is not ligated when the gallbladder is removed.

B. Preoperative Management

1. Perform surgery as soon as the animal has been stabilized.

C. Anesthesia

1. Induce hypovolemic or septic dogs or dogs in shock with oxymorphone plus diazepam (Appendix G-14).
2. If intubation is not possible, give etomidate or mask induce with isoflurane if the patient is not vomiting.
3. For stable patients, see anesthetic management of patients with hepatobiliary disease, p. 263.

D. Positioning

1. Prepare the caudal thorax and entire abdomen for aseptic surgery.
2. Expose the gallbladder via a cranial midline abdominal incision.

VII. Surgical Technique

A. Treat lacerations or transections of the bile ducts by primary repair or biliary diversion.

B. Ligate damaged hepatic duct because alternative routes for biliary drainage from a single liver lobe will develop.

C. Culture the abdominal fluid and/or site of rupture or perforation during surgery. Once the site of leakage has been identified and corrected, flush the abdomen with copious amounts of warmed, sterile fluids.

D. Consider open abdominal drainage if generalized peritonitis is present.

VIII. Suture Materials/Special Instruments

A. A Poole suction tip is useful to remove abdominal fluid and help identify the site of leakage. Use it also to remove fluid instilled in the abdomen during lavage.

IX. Postoperative Care and Assessment

A. Many patients with bile peritonitis are extremely debilitated before surgery.

B. Continue fluid therapy and monitor electrolytes and acid-base status.

C. Bile peritonitis is painful; provide postoperative analgesia with oxymorphone. Butorphanol is effective but of shorter duration.

D. Nutritional supplementation via jejunostomy or parenterally is beneficial.

E. Continue antibiotic therapy based on culture of bile for at least 7 to 14 days postoperatively.

X. Prognosis

A. The prognosis for patients with diffuse, septic bile peritonitis is guarded. Without aggressive surgical management, most of these patients will die.

B. The prognosis is better if the condition is diagnosed and treated early and is better in animals with nonseptic biliary effusions.

19

Surgery of the Endocrine System (*SAS*, pp. 401-441)

Surgery of the Adrenal and Pituitary Glands (*SAS*, pp. 401-414)

I. Definitions

A. **Adrenalectomy** is the removal of one or both adrenal glands.

B. **Hypophysectomy** is removal of the pituitary gland (hypophysis).

C. **Hyperadrenocorticism** is a multisystemic disorder that results from excessive glucocorticoids.

D. **Cushing's disease** refers to hyperadrenocorticism caused by a pituitary adenoma.

E. **Addison's disease** is due to deficiency of glucocorticoids and/or mineralocorticoids.

II. Preoperative Concerns

A. Adrenocortical insufficiency may be naturally occurring or iatrogenic because of administration of glucocorticoids, progestins, or adreno-corticolytic drugs.
   1. Severely suppressed glucocorticoid secretion may cause collapse and weakness without evidence of electrolyte abnormalities.
   2. Suppression of mineralocorticoids causes electrolyte abnormalities (i.e., hyponatremia, hyperkalemia) and azotemia.
      a. Reduced ability to retain sodium causes volume depletion, decreased cardiac output, reduced vascular tone, and acute vascular collapse.
      b. Correct electrolyte concentrations before surgery.
   3. Some dogs with hypoadrenocorticism are hypoalbuminemic.
   4. Animals with hypoadrenocorticism may be unable to respond to surgical stress and often require glucocorticoid supplementation before and during surgery.
      a. When minor elective surgery is performed in animals with

Table 19-1
Protocol for glucocorticoid administration in animals with adrenocortical insufficiency undergoing minor elective procedures

1. 1 hr before surgery give *one* of the following IV:
Prednisolone Sodium Succinate
1.0-2.0 mg/kg, or
Dexamethasone
0.1-0.2 mg/kg, or
Soluble Hydrocortisone
4-5 mg/kg
2. Repeat dose at recovery IV or IM
3. Resume maintenance glucocorticoid therapy on first postoperative day, if needed

Modified from Short CE: *Principles and practice of veterinary anesthesia,* Los Angeles, 1987, Williams & Wilkins.

adrenocortical insufficiency, give glucocorticoid therapy intravenously before induction of anesthesia (Table 19-1). The same dose can be given intravenously or intramuscularly after recovery from anesthesia, and then the animal returned to its oral maintenance glucocorticoid therapy the day following surgery.

b. For major surgery, use a similar protocol but continue glucocorticoid therapy at approximately five times the maintenance dose for 2 to 3 days (Table 19-2). Normal maintenance doses are then reinstituted. Once the animal is eating, medications can be given orally rather than by injection.

5. Iatrogenic hyperadrenocorticism is the most common form.

B. Spontaneous hyperadrenocorticism.

1. Usually caused by excessive pituitary secretion of adrenocorticotropic hormone (ACTH) resulting in bilateral adrenocortical hyperplasia.
2. Functional adrenocortical tumors are less common.
3. Muscle wasting, weakness, and thin, fragile skin are common.
4. Electrolyte and/or acid-base abnormalities, hyperglycemia, and hypertension may be present.
5. Intraabdominal fat deposition, combined with muscular weakness, sometimes causes ventilatory abnormalities.
6. Cardiovascular abnormalities may occur secondary to hypertension.
7. Animals with hyperadrenocorticism are at increased risk for postoperative pulmonary thromboembolism. If hypercoagulopathies are suspected preoperatively, consider preventative measures (e.g., low-dose heparin therapy).
8. Most animals with hyperadrenocorticism have urinary tract infection, even when the urinalysis shows no evidence of it.

III. Anesthetic Considerations

A. Maintenance of electrolyte and glucose levels is important.

B. Glucocorticoid supplementation is often necessary in animals with adrenocortical insufficiency undergoing surgery.

Table 19-2
Protocol for glucocorticoid administration in animals with adrenocortical insufficiency undergoing major elective procedures

1. Administer preoperative steroids as described in Table 19-1
2. Repeat dose at recovery IV or IM
3. Days 1 and 2 postoperatively—administer one of the following IV or IM:

Prednisolone

0.5 mg/kg BID, or

Dexamethasone

0.1 mg/kg SID, or

Prednisone

0.5 mg/kg BID, or

Cortisone Acetate

2.5 mg/kg BID

4. Resume maintenance glucocorticoid therapy on third postoperative day, unless complications arise

Modified from Short CE: *Principles and practice of veterinary anesthesia,* Los Angeles, 1987, Williams & Wilkins.

C. Begin glucocorticoid therapy preoperatively in patients with hyperadrenocorticism that are undergoing adrenalectomy.

D. Retraction of the caudal cava is often necessary for adrenalectomy. Monitor vascular pressures closely during surgery, and retract carefully to prevent obstructing venous return.

E. Animals with pheochromocytomas require special anesthetic considerations to avoid complications associated with excessive catecholamine secretion.

IV. Antibiotics

A. Animals with hyperadrenocorticism are at increased risk for developing postoperative infections. Perioperative prophylactic antibiotics are recommended.

V. Surgical Anatomy

A. Location.
   1. The adrenal glands are located near the craniomedial pole of the kidneys.
   2. The left adrenal is slightly larger than the right. The left gland lies beneath the lateral process of the second lumbar vertebra, whereas the right adrenal is more cranial, lying beneath the lateral process of the last thoracic vertebra.
   3. The phrenicoabdominal vessels cross the ventral surface of the adrenal.

B. Adrenal glands are composed of two functionally and structurally different regions.

1. The outer cortex produces mineralocorticoids, glucocorticoids, and small amounts of androgenic hormones.
   a. Mineralocorticoids regulate sodium and potassium concentrations.
2. The adrenal medulla secretes epinephrine and norepinephrine in response to sympathetic stimulation.
   a. Epinephrine and norepinephrine have almost the same effects as direct sympathetic stimulation.
   b. Their effects last significantly longer because they are slowly removed from circulation.

VI. Surgical Techniques

A. Adrenalectomy (*SAS,* pp. 403-404)

1. General considerations.
   a. Usually performed for adrenal tumors.
   b. Bilateral adrenalectomy for treatment of Cushing's disease is controversial and not commonly performed.
      i. A ventral midline approach allows the entire abdomen to be explored for metastasis and bilateral adrenalectomy to be performed with a single surgical incision.
         (a) Exposure and dissection of the adrenal may be difficult with this approach, particularly in large dogs.
      ii. A paracostal incision provides improved access to the adrenal gland but does not allow evaluation of the liver or other organs for metastasis.
         (a) Consider this for animals with unilateral lesions, without evidence of metastasis on ultrasound, computed tomography, or magnetic resonance imaging.
   c. Adrenalectomy is not advised if extensive tumor metastasis is present, or if invasion of the caudal cava and surrounding organs makes complete removal of neoplastic tissue unlikely.
   d. Concurrent diabetes mellitus might be a contraindication to bilateral adrenalectomy because lack of endogenous catecholamines may make it difficult to regulate the diabetes.
2. Adrenalectomy via a midline abdominal approach (*SAS,* p. 403).
   a. Surgical procedure.

Prepare the entire ventral abdomen and caudal thorax for aseptic surgery. Perform a ventral midline abdominal incision that extends from the xiphoid cartilage to near the pubis. Identify the enlarged adrenal, and carefully inspect the entire abdomen (including the other adrenal) for abnormalities or evidence of metastasis. Palpate the liver for evidence of nodularity, and biopsy if indicated. Palpate the caudal vena cava near the adrenals for evidence of tumor invasion or thrombosis. If additional exposure is needed for adrenalectomy, extend the incision paracostally on the side of the affected gland by incising the fascia of the rectus abdominis muscle and fibers of the external abdominal oblique, internal abdominal oblique, and transversus abdominis muscles, respectively. Use self-retaining retractors to improve visualization of the abdominal cavity. Retract liver, spleen, and stomach cranially, kidney caudally, and vena cava medially, to expose the entire gland. Identify the blood supply and ureter to the ipsilateral kidney, and avoid these structures during dissection. Ligate the phrenicoabdominal vein, and divide it between sutures. Carefully dissect the adrenal gland from surrounding tissues, using a combination of sharp and blunt dissection. Numerous vessels may be

Adrenal Neoplasia (*SAS*, pp. 405-410)

I. Definitions

A. **Adrenal carcinomas** are autonomously functioning malignant tumors of the adrenal cortex.

B. **Adrenal adenomas** are benign adrenocortical tumors.

C. **Pheochromocytomas** (i.e., paraganglioma) are catecholamine-secreting tumors that usually arise in adrenal medullary tissue.

II. General Considerations and Clinically Relevant Pathophysiology

A. The most common tumors of the canine adrenal glands are adrenal adenomas, carcinomas, and pheochromocytomas.

B. Most adrenal tumors are not functional, and clinical signs are caused by local invasion of the tumor into surrounding tissue and/or distant metastases.

C. Spontaneous hyperadrenocorticism may be caused by adrenocortical tumors.
   1. Pituitary-dependent hyperadrenocorticism is more common than adrenal neoplasia.
   2. Adrenocortical adenomas and carcinomas appear to occur with equal frequency.
      a. They are usually unilateral.
      b. Ultrasonographic evaluation of the adrenals often identifies adrenomegaly and localizes the tumor to one side of the body.
   3. Colonic perforation is a rare sequel of excessive glucocorticoid secretion.

D. Pheochromocytomas secrete excessive amounts of catecholamines and other vasoactive peptides.
   1. Excessive catecholamine and vasoactive peptide levels may manifest as cardiovascular, respiratory, or CNS disease.
   2. Regional invasion and distant metastases (liver, regional lymph nodes, lungs, spleen, ovary, diaphragm, vertebrae) occur in 50% of affected dogs.
      a. Invasion of the caudal vena cava, phrenicoabdominal artery or vein, renal artery or vein, or hepatic vein may cause ascites, edema, or venous distention.
      b. Pheochromocytomas are usually unilateral.
   3. Occasionally, pheochromocytomas are associated with neoplastic transformation of multiple endocrine tissues of neuroectoderm origin.
   4. Extraadrenal pheochromocytomas have been reported in dogs and cats.

E. Other tumors that arise from the adrenal medulla are neuroblastomas and ganglioneuromas; however, they are rare.

III. Diagnosis

A. Clinical Presentation

1. Signalment.
   a. Usually occur in older, large-breed dogs.
   b. Diagnosed more commonly in females.
   c. Pheochromocytomas usually occur in older dogs but have been reported in dogs as young as 1 year of age.
      i. Boxers may be predisposed to this tumor.
      ii. Adrenal tumors are rarely diagnosed in cats.
2. History.
   a. Functional adrenocortical tumors commonly cause hyperadrenocorticism (i.e., polyuria, polydipsia, polyphagia, abdominal enlargement, endocrine alopecia, muscle wasting, weakness, lethargy, panting, and/or hyperpigmentation).
   b. Nonfunctional adrenocortical tumors often cause anorexia, abdominal enlargement, abdominal pain, diarrhea, vomiting, and lethargy.
   c. Occasionally dogs are asymptomatic, and the adrenal mass is a fortuitous finding at surgery or necropsy.

B. Physical Examination Findings

1. Depend on whether the tumors are functional.
2. Clinical findings of hyperadrenocorticism are usually present in those with functional tumors.
3. Ascites, abdominal pain, edema, diarrhea, and vomiting are common with nonfunctional tumors.
4. Clinical findings in animals with pheochromocytomas may include tachycardia/cardiac arrhythmias, acute collapse, polypnea, panting, cough, lethargy, anorexia, dyspnea, weakness, abdominal distention, congestive heart failure, ataxia, incoordination, polyuria/polydipsia, and alopecia.
   a. Hypertension (paroxysmal or sustained) is frequently present.

C. Radiography/Ultrasonography

1. Adrenal tumors are difficult to detect radiographically unless they cause significant adrenal enlargement (≥20 mm) or calcification.
   a. Withhold food for 24 hours before radiography.
   b. Mineralization of tissue cranial to the kidney may be seen on plain radiographs and may or may not be associated with obvious adrenal enlargement. This finding is suggestive of adrenocortical neoplasia (adenoma or carcinoma).
      i. Nonneoplastic mineralization of adrenal glands is uncommon; however, bilateral adrenal calcification may occur with pituitary-dependent hyperadrenocorticism.
2. Ultrasonography is useful to assess adrenal gland size, echogenicity, and shape.
   a. The normal canine adrenal gland (in mature dogs) is 2 to 3 cm long, 1 cm wide, and 0.5 cm thick.
   b. Pheochromocytomas have been reported to have mixed echo patterns and cannot be definitively differentiated from adrenocortical tumors.
   c. Bilateral adrenal enlargement is suggestive of pituitary-dependent

Table 19-4
ACTH-stimulation test in dogs

1. Obtain serum for pre-ACTH.
2. Administer 0.25 mg synthetic ACTH (Cortosyn)/dog IV.
3. Obtain serum 1 hr post-ACTH administration.

hyperadrenocorticism while functional adrenocortical tumors typically cause atrophy of the contralateral gland.

d. Adrenal metastasis may be diagnosed with ultrasound.

3. X-ray computed tomography (CT) and magnetic resonance imaging enable accurate localization of adrenal neoplasia; but do not differentiate adrenal adenomas, carcinomas, and pheochromocytomas.
   a. Masses that are poorly demarcated, have irregular shape, and are nonhomogeneous with mineralization are usually carcinomas.
   b. Determination of caudal vena cava invasion is not usually possible with CT.
   c. Perform caudal vena caval angiography preoperatively if caudal caval thrombosis is suspected.
   d. Excretory urography may help identify tumor invasion necessitating nephrectomy (i.e., ureteral obstruction or renal invasion).

D. Laboratory Findings

1. Laboratory abnormalities are inconsistent and nonspecific with pheochromocytomas.
2. Common (not invariable) laboratory abnormalities with hyperadrenocorticism include increased serum alkaline phosphatase, neutrophilic leukocytosis, lymphopenia, eosinopenia, mild polycythemia, increased alanine aminotransferase, and hypercholesterolemia.
3. Urinary tract abnormalities may include hyposthenuria or isosthenuria, and urinary tract infections are common (even when bacteria and inflammatory cells are absent on urinalysis).
4. Spontaneous hyperadrenocorticism is diagnosed by an ACTH-stimulation test (Table 19-4) and/or low-dose dexamethasone suppression (LDDS) test. These tests should be performed after exogenous steroid administration has been stopped (Table 19-5).
   a. Approximately 85% of hyperadrenal dogs have increased post-ACTH plasma cortisol concentrations.
   b. False-positive tests may occur in dogs that are chronically stressed or ill.
   c. If plasma cortisol concentrations are normal on the ACTH-stimulation test, but clinical signs suggest hyperadrenocorticism, an LDDS test should be performed.
5. After making a definitive diagnosis of hyperadrenocorticism, differentiate adrenal-dependent and pituitary-dependent causes by LDDS, high-dose dexamethasone suppression test, ultrasonography, or measurement of endogenous ACTH.

IV. Differential Diagnosis

A. Pheochromocytomas and adrenocortical tumors must be differentiated because of different operative management.

Table 19-5
Patterns of ACTH-stimulation tests (post-ACTH cortisol)*

>24 µg/dl—strongly suggestive of hyperadrenocorticism
19-24 µg/dl—suggestive of hyperadrenocorticism
8-18 µg/dl—normal
<8 µg/dl—suggestive of iatrogenic Cushing's disease

*There may be substantial variation between laboratories.
To convert µg/dl to nmol/L, multiply µg/dl × 27.59.

B. Pheochromocytomas may be identified grossly by application of Zenker's solution (potassium dichromate or iodate), which results in oxidation of catecholamines, forming a dark brown pigment within 10 to 20 minutes after application to the surface of a freshly sectioned tumor.

C. Differentiation of adenomas and carcinomas is impossible without histopathology.
1. Apparent metastatic lesions in the liver or draining lymph nodes may suggest malignancy, but care should be used to differentiate benign hepatic nodules from neoplastic disease.

V. Medical Management

A. Adrenergic blockade (i.e., phenoxybenzamine, phentolamine, prazosin) is used in patients with pheochromocytomas to control blood pressure.
1. If tachycardia or cardiac arrhythmias are present, use β-adrenergic blockade; however, unopposed β-blockade may result in severe hypertension.

B. Mitotane (o,p′-DDD) (Lysodren).
1. May control clinical signs in animals with adrenocortical tumors.
2. Larger doses are required to obtain and maintain control in these dogs than in those with pituitary-dependent hyperadrenocorticism, and greater side effects (i.e., gastric irritation, vomiting) can be expected.
   a. Administer 50 to 75 mg/kg/day for 14 days.
   b. If needed, increase the dose by another 50 mg/kg for another 14 days.
   c. Repeat this increment every 14 days until the disease is controlled or the animal does not tolerate this drug.

C. Ketoconazole is an alternative to mitotane (Table 19-6).
1. It is less toxic, causes reversible inhibition of adrenal steroid production, and has little effect on mineralocorticoid production.
2. It may be used in animals with malignant adrenocortical tumors who are not surgical candidates because of metastasis.
3. Ketoconazole used preoperatively reduces the risk of anesthesia and surgery in animals with uncontrolled hyperadrenocorticism.
4. It can be used as a diagnostic trial in dogs in whom equivocal test results make the diagnosis of hyperadrenocorticism difficult. Give it for a minimum of 4 to 8 weeks for this purpose.
   a. It must be given for the duration of the animal's life if it is used to control clinical signs.

Table 19-6
Ketoconazole treatment for adrenal tumors

1. Administer 5 mg/kg with food BID for 7 days.
2. Increase dose to 10 mg/kg BID for 7-14 days.
3. Perform ACTH-stimulation test 2 to 4 hr after giving ketoconazole dose.
4. If there is a lack of adrenocortical response to ACTH and clinical improvement without causing illness, continue same dosage.
5. If there is a response to ACTH or no clinical improvement, increase the dosage to 15 mg/kg BID.

b. Anorexia, depression, vomiting, diarrhea, or icterus may necessitate stopping the drug or reducing the dosage.

D. Rechecks (including ACTH-stimulation) are recommended every 3 to 6 months.

VI. Surgical Treatment

A. General Considerations

1. The overall health, presence of unresectable metastases and apparent invasiveness of the tumor should be considered.
   a. Prolonged survival has occurred in dogs with invasive, malignant tumors that required caudal caval venotomy.
   b. Survival greater than 1 year may be possible, even in dogs with widespread metastatic lesions.
   c. If the tumor appears invasive, a midline abdominal approach is preferred to allow evaluation of the caudal cava and other abdominal structures.
   d. Thrombus removal may require that the midline incision be extended into the caudal thorax via a caudal median sternotomy approach.
   e. Small tumors, or those that do not appear invasive, may be removed from a paralumbar approach.

B. Preoperative Management

1. Determine renal function before surgery, in case ipsilateral nephrectomy is necessary.
2. Correct electrolyte or acid-base abnormalities, hyperglycemia, and hypertension before surgery.
3. Initiate fluid therapy before anesthetic induction.
4. Animals with hyperadrenocorticism are at increased risk to develop pulmonary thromboembolism postoperatively. If hypercoagulability is suspected, consider preventative low-dose heparin therapy (see Appendix I).
5. Administer perioperative antibiotics and continue them postoperatively in hyperadrenal animals.
6. Examine the cardiovascular system for evidence of arrhythmias or congestive heart failure in animals with pheochromocytomas.

C. Anesthesia

1. Complications are common during adrenalectomy for pheochromocytomas, and wide fluctuations in heart rate and blood pressure are frequent.
2. Monitor cardiac rhythm, arterial blood pressure, and pulse oximetry.

3. Treatment for several days before surgery with an α-adrenergic blocker (i.e., phenoxybenzamine; 0.2-0.4 mg/kg PO, BID) is recommended. Increase the dose of phenoxybenzamine until blood pressure is within the normal range.
4. Control heart rate, if necessary, with a β-blocker (i.e., propranolol, esmolol; see Appendix I); however, do not initiate it until adequate α-blockade is established (i.e., normal blood pressure). Intraoperative β-blockade with esmolol is preferred because of its short half-life.
5. Treat cardiac arrhythmias with lidocaine (see Table 16-8).
6. Hypertension.
   a. May result from tumor manipulation and can be minimized by isolating the tumor's blood supply before manipulating the tumor.
   b. Treat with phentolamine given as an IV bolus.
   c. Sodium nitroprusside may also be infused for maintenance of blood pressure.
7. Hypotension.
   a. Frequently occurs after tumor removal.
   b. High doses of crystalloids may be necessary to maintain perfusion.
   c. If hypotension persists, give dobutamine.
8. Significant intraoperative hemorrhage may require blood transfusions.
9. Avoid atropine, xylazine, and ketamine with suspected pheochromocytomas.
10. Isoflurane is the inhalation agent of choice because it does not sensitize the myocardium to epinephrine-induced arrhythmias.

D. Positioning

1. Position the animal in either dorsal recumbency or lateral recumbency with the affected side up.
2. Clip and prepare a generous area to allow a caudal thoracotomy to be performed if necessary.

VII. Surgical Technique

A. General Considerations

1. Perform an adrenalectomy via either a midline abdominal or a paralumbar approach.
2. Concurrent nephrectomy may be necessary with invasive tumors.
3. Ensure complete tumor removal. Perform an en bloc resection, if possible, to avoid leaving small fragments of neoplastic tissue.
4. Isolate the vascular supply to pheochromocytomas before tumor manipulation, to decrease catecholamine release or to help prevent shedding of tumor cells.
5. Explore the entire abdomen with special attention paid to the bladder, pelvic canal, kidney, aorta, and near the junction of the caudal mesenteric artery, where extraadrenal neoplasia is reported to occur.

VIII. Suture Materials/Special Instruments

A. Delayed wound healing may occur.

B. Self-retaining retractors (e.g., Balfour abdominal retractors) and malleable retractors help improve visualization of the adrenal glands.

C. Electrocautery and hemoclips allow hemostasis to be obtained more easily with vascular tumors than does suture ligation of vessels.

IX. Postoperative Care and Assessment

A. Hypoadrenocorticism often develops postoperatively in hyperadrenal dogs because of atrophy of the contralateral gland. These animals require glucocorticoid therapy postoperatively.

B. If hyperadrenocorticism continues postoperatively, consider therapy with mitotane.

C. Continue fluid therapy until the animal is able to maintain hydration.

D. Monitor blood pressure and heart rate and rhythm. Blood transfusions may be required intraoperatively or postoperatively in some patients.

X. Prognosis

A. Prolonged survival (1 to 2 years) can occur in dogs with invasive, metastatic pheochromocytomas after aggressive surgical resection.

B. Prognosis for dogs with adrenocortical carcinomas depends on the tumor's size and invasiveness, but generally the prognosis is poor.

Pituitary Neoplasia (*SAS*, pp. 410-414)

I. Definitions

A. **Pituitary tumors** arise from the hypophysis in the sella turcica.

II. General Considerations and Clinically Relevant Pathophysiology

A. Pituitary tumors may be functional (60%) or nonfunctional (40%).

B. Functional pituitary tumors are the most common cause of canine hyperadrenocorticism.

C. Large tumors often grow dorsally into the brain because the diaphragm of the sella is incomplete.
   1. Nonfunctional tumors may cause clinical signs by impinging on adjacent brain tissue (i.e., optic chiasm, hypothalamus, thalamus, infundibular recess, and third ventricle).
   2. Tumor size and development of neurologic signs do not always correlate.

D. Adenomas are classified as microadenomas (less than 1 cm in diameter) or macroadenomas (greater than 1 cm in diameter).

E. Microadenomas account for nearly 70% of pituitary tumors.

III. Diagnosis

A. Clinical Presentation

1. Signalment.
   a. Poodles, dachshunds, and boxers may be predisposed to pituitary-dependent hyperadrenocorticism.
   b. Middle-aged and older dogs are most commonly affected.
2. History.
   a. Most dogs present with signs of hyperadrenocorticism (i.e., polyuria, polydipsia, polyphagia, abdominal enlargement, endocrine alopecia, muscle wasting, weakness, lethargy, panting, and/or hyperpigmentation).
   b. Concurrent neurologic signs (seizures, visual deficits, ataxia, incoordination, facial hemiplegia, head tilt, somnolence, compulsive walking, depression) may also be noted.
   c. Mental depression and stupor were reported as the most common abnormalities in two studies.
   d. Nonfunctional macroadenomas or carcinomas may only cause neurologic signs.

B. Physical Examination Findings

1. Typical signs of hyperadrenocorticism are expected with functional pituitary tumors.
2. Papillary edema, ataxia, and incoordination occasionally occur.

C. Radiography/Imaging

1. Diagnosis is best made with CT or magnetic resonance imaging.
2. Adenomas and carcinomas cannot be differentiated with CT; however, differentiation of animals with microadenomas, which might benefit from hypophysectomy, and those with macroadenomas (in which surgical therapy is seldom indicated) is possible.
3. Bilateral adrenal enlargement, diagnosed by ultrasonography, is usually indicative of pituitary-dependent hyperadrenocorticism.

D. Laboratory Findings

1. Laboratory abnormalities are generally consistent with hyperadrenocorticism.
2. Small, nonfunctional pituitary tumors seldom cause laboratory abnormalities.
3. Large tumors may increase intracranial pressure.

IV. Differential Diagnosis

A. Cushing's syndrome must be differentiated from iatrogenic hyperadrenocorticism or adrenocortical neoplasms.

B. After pituitary dysfunction has been diagnosed, pituitary neoplasms must be differentiated from other pituitary lesions (i.e., cysts, abscesses, craniopharyngiomas).

V. Medical Management

A. Hyperadrenocorticism may be treated with mitotane, ketoconazole, or deprenyl.

B. External-beam radiation therapy can be effective treatment for large pituitary tumors, when combined with concurrent adrenal-suppressive treatment (mitotane or ketoconazole).

VI. Surgical Treatment

A. General Considerations

1. Hypophysectomy is rarely performed in animals with pituitary microadenomas and functional adenohypophyseal hyperplasia.
   a. Advocates of this procedure suggest that the majority of dogs with pituitary-dependent hyperadrenocorticism tumors are surgical candidates for hypophysectomy and that this technique is preferable to long-term medical management.
   b. If concurrent neurologic signs are present, or tumor has extended intracranially or transsphenoidally, hypophysectomy is not indicated.
   c. Hypophysectomy renders animals infertile.
   d. There are no data suggesting that hypophysectomy is safe and effective in cats.
   e. Radiographic markers, combined with a cranial sinus venogram, are necessary to identify the pituitary location in some animals.
   f. Placement of the endotracheal tube via a tracheotomy and use of an operating microscope are recommended.

B. Preoperative Management

1. Extensive preoperative workup is indicated to confirm and localize the lesion and define landmarks for surgery.
2. Catheterization of the angularis oculi vein preoperatively has been recommended to help identify landmarks.
3. Radiographic markers are placed on the sphenoid bone in conjunction with venous sinus angiography.
4. Animals with hyperadrenocorticism are at increased risk to develop postoperative infections.

C. Anesthesia

1. Most animals with pituitary tumors do not require special anesthetic consideration; however, patients that have large masses increasing intracranial pressures need special precautions.
   a. Restrict fluid therapy to the volume required to maintain adequate circulation.
   b. Use isoflurane.
   c. Avoid ketamine in patients with intracranial masses and other conditions in which increased intracranial pressures may occur as a result of surgery.
   d. Hyperventilate patients with increased intracranial pressures.

D. Surgical Anatomy

1. The pituitary occupies a shallow, oval recess in the basisphenoid bone, called the sella turcica.

2. Pituitary size varies, but is usually approximately 1 cm in length.
3. The pituitary is composed of the adenohypophysis (subdivided into the pars proximalis, pars intermedia, and pars distalis) and neurohypophysis.
4. The arterial supply of the pituitary arises from the internal carotid arteries and caudal communicating arteries.

E. Positioning

1. Position the animal in dorsal recumbency, with the neck flexed and the hard palate at 30 degrees to the horizontal surface of the table.
2. Open the mouth maximally and secure the jaw with tape. The lower jaw should be approximately 80 degrees to the table surface.
3. Retract the tongue against the lower jaw with tongue forceps.
4. Flush the oral cavity and wipe it with a sterile surgical sponge impregnated with 0.05% dilute chlorhexidine solution.

VII. Surgical Technique

A. Transsphenoidal Approach

1. General considerations.
   a. Bleeding can be excessive; have bone wax handy to fill the burr hole.
2. Surgical technique.

Make a midline incision along the rostral two thirds of the soft palate, and retract the palate with Gelpi retractors. Use electrocautery to control hemorrhage. Make a midline incision in the nasopharyngeal mucoperiosteum, and subperiosteally elevate the mucoperiosteum to expose the caudal aspect of the presphenoid and rostral aspect of the basisphenoid bones. Identify a small vascular foramen on the midline of the rostral portion of the basisphenoid bone, 2 to 6 mm caudal to the suture line between the presphenoid and basisphenoid bones. Use a 2- to 4-mm diameter egg-shaped drill to burr a hole centered on the vascular foramen. With the drill positioned 45 degrees to the horizontal plane, remove the outer cortex of bone. Control bleeding with continuous suction, and occlude larger bleeders with bone wax. Partially remove the inner cortex with the drill; use a curette to excise the remaining portion of the cortex and expose the dura mater. Make a cruciate incision in the dura mater, but avoid the cavernous venous sinuses that lie lateral to the hypophysis. Break or loosen the dural attachments with a fine, blunt instrument. Apply traction to the hypophysis, using a 2- to 4-mm diameter suction tip. To prevent small tissue fragments from being lost in the suction, place a tissue filter as an interphase between the suction tip and tubing. Excise any visible remnant of the pituitary stalk. Fill the burr hole with bone wax or a muscle graft harvested from the soft palate incision. Appose the nasopharyngeal mucoperiosteum over the hole (do not suture). Close the soft palate incision with a two-layer simple interrupted pattern.

VIII. Suture Materials/Special Instruments

A. Delayed wound healing may occur; close incisions with strong, slowly absorbed or nonabsorbable suture material (e.g., polydioxanone, polyglyconate, polypropylene, or nylon).

B. A drill with a 2- to 4-mm egg-shaped burr is required for hypophysectomy.

C. Bone wax, a suction device, a tissue filter (approximately 150 mm), and a fine, blunt instrument (e.g., Steven's tenotomy hook) are recommended.

IX. Postoperative Care and Assessment

A. Continue fluid therapy until the animal is able to maintain its hydration.

B. Give desmopressin acetate (DDAVP) for up to 2 weeks (2 μg/dog [2-4 drops of 100 μg/ml] intranasally or in conjunctiva SID to BID).

C. Begin corticosteroid therapy before surgery and continue it postoperatively (prednisone or prednisolone; 0.2 mg/kg SID).

D. Begin thyroid hormone supplementation (Soloxine, Thyrotabs, Synthroid; 22 μg/kg PO, BID) after surgery and continue it for life.

E. If bone wax was used to control hemorrhage, continue antibiotic therapy for 7 to 10 days.

F. Nasal discharge and impaired swallowing may be observed for the first few days postoperatively. Persistence of these signs may indicate palate dehiscence.

X. Prognosis

A. Long-term survival is possible following hypophysectomy, radiation therapy plus chemotherapy, or chemotherapy alone in dogs with pituitary-dependent hyperadrenocorticism caused by microadenomas.

B. Long-term survival has also been reported in dogs with large, functional tumors, following radiation therapy.

Surgery of the Pancreas (*SAS*, pp. 414-428)

I. Definitions

A. **Pancreatectomy** is surgical removal of all or part of the pancreas.

B. **Insulinoma** is a functional tumor of pancreatic β-islet cells.

C. **Zollinger-Ellison** syndrome is a condition caused by non–β-islet cell tumors, in which excess gastrin is secreted.

II. Preoperative Concerns

A. Pancreatic inflammation often causes vomiting and may also be accompanied by weight loss and debilitation; however, cats with pancreatitis do not show vomiting as reliably as do dogs.
   1. Vomiting animals require fluid therapy and correction of electrolyte and acid-base abnormalities before surgery.

B. Evaluate diabetic animals carefully for overall metabolic status before surgery (i.e., CBC, serum biochemical panel and urinalysis).
   1. Correct severe hyperglycemia (>300 mg/dl) or ketoacidosis with insulin administration, intravenous fluids, and electrolytes before surgery.

III. Anesthetic Considerations

A. Blood glucose concentrations ideally should be maintained between 100 and 300 mg/dl during surgery.
   1. Hypoglycemia may occur if animals are given their regular insulin dose and food is withheld before surgery; however, the stress of surgery usually results in hyperglycemia.
   2. Feed animals their normal diet the day before surgery, and administer their regular dose of insulin. Withhold food 12 hours before surgery or give a small meal after the morning insulin.
   3. Perform surgery in the morning.
   4. Measure blood glucose concentrations the morning of surgery. If the blood glucose concentration is between 150 and 300 mg/dl 1 to 2 hours before surgery, give the animal one half of its usual morning dose of insulin subcutaneously.
   5. Check blood glucose at induction and hourly thereafter. If the blood glucose level is low, administer 0.45% saline and 2.5% dextrose (5 ml/kg for the first hour and then 2.5 ml/kg thereafter). If blood glucose is normal, administer lactated Ringer's solution (at the same rate). Change fluids to 5% dextrose and give an additional small dose of regular insulin if the blood glucose concentration is greater than 300 mg/dl.

B. Premedicate these animals with an anticholinergic and opioid, induce with thiobarbiturates or propofol, and maintain on either halothane or isoflurane inhalants (see Appendixes G-14 and G-15).

C. Animals that are not vomiting may be induced with a mask or placed in a chamber, or they may be given thiopental or propofol at reduced dosages.

D. Use reduced dosages of diazepam and ketamine in cats.

IV. Antibiotics

A. Use prophylactic antibiotics in animals undergoing pancreatic biopsy or partial pancreatectomy.

B. Pancreatic infections may be polymicrobial; use broad-spectrum antimicrobial therapy (e.g., cefazolin).

V. Surgical Anatomy

A. The pancreas of dogs and cats is composed of a right and left limb and a small central body.
   1. The right limb of the pancreas lies within the mesoduodenum and is closely associated with the duodenum, particularly at its cranial aspect.
   2. The dorsal aspect of the right pancreatic lobe is visualized by retracting the duodenum ventrally and toward the midline; the ventral aspect of the right pancreatic lobe is examined by retracting the duodenum laterally.
   3. The pancreatic body (angle) lies in the bend formed by the pylorus and duodenum.
   4. The left pancreatic lobe is viewed within the deep leaf of the greater omentum by retracting the stomach cranially and the transverse colon caudally.

B. The main blood supply to the left pancreatic lobe is via branches of the splenic artery; however, branches from the common hepatic and gastroduodenal arteries also supply portions of it.
   1. The main vessels of the right lobe of the pancreas are the pancreatic branches of the cranial and caudal pancreaticoduodenal arteries that anastomose in the gland.
   2. The cranial pancreaticoduodenal artery is a terminal branch of the hepatic artery; the caudal pancreaticoduodenal arises from the cranial mesenteric vessel. Use care to avoid damaging these branches of this vessel during pancreatic surgery, or devitalization of the duodenum may occur.

C. Digestive secretions enter the duodenum via one of two ducts.
   1. These ducts may communicate within the gland or may cross each other.
   2. When the two ducts do not communicate, the pancreatic duct drains the right lobe and the accessory pancreatic duct drains the left lobe.
   3. The accessory pancreatic duct is the largest excretory pancreatic duct in dogs. It opens into the duodenum at the minor duodenal papilla.
   4. The pancreatic duct is the principal, and often only, duct in cats.

VI. Surgical Techniques

A. General Considerations

1. Perform a ventral midline abdominal incision extending from the xiphoid cartilage to caudal to the umbilicus.
   a. Gently examine the pancreas using a combination of gentle palpation and visual examination to avoid causing pancreatitis.
   b. Retract the free portion of the greater omentum cranially and cover it with moist sponges.
   c. Bluntly separate the omental leaf overlying the pancreas to allow direct visualization of the left pancreas.
   d. When neoplasia is suspected, examine lymph nodes that lie along the splenic vessels and portal vein and those at the hilus of the liver and head of the pancreas.
2. It is difficult to diagnose feline pancreatitis; biopsy may be more commonly indicated than presently used.
   a. Laparoscopic biopsy is well tolerated in cats.

3. Partial pancreatectomy is indicated in animals with insulin- or gastrin-secreting tumors and for pancreatic adenocarcinoma.
4. Total pancreatectomy is usually performed in conjunction with resection and anastomosis of the proximal duodenum, common bile duct ligation, and cholecystojejunostomy. It is associated with high morbidity and mortality.
5. Pancreatic drainage is indicated in some conditions (e.g., large abscesses or cysts) in which pancreatectomy is not feasible. A Penrose drain or double-lumen sump drain is sutured to the surrounding tissues with chromic gut suture and exteriorized lateral to the abdominal incision.

B. Pancreatic Biopsy (*SAS,* p. 417)

1. General considerations.
   a. If diffuse pancreatic disease is present, obtain a biopsy by removing a small portion of the caudal aspect of the right pancreatic limb.
   b. Remove focal lesions near the extremity of the pancreas similarly.
2. Surgical technique.

For focal lesions within the pancreatic parenchyma, use a Tru-Cut or Vim-Silverman needle, or shave off a portion of the lesion with a scalpel to obtain a small sample of pancreatic tissue. Use care to avoid damaging adjacent blood vessels or pancreatic ducts.

C. Partial Pancreatectomy (*SAS,* pp. 417-418)

1. General considerations.
   a. Remove focal lesions near the extremity of the pancreas by the suture fracture technique.
2. Surgical technique.

Incise the mesoduodenum or omentum on each side of the pancreas to be removed. Pass nonabsorbable suture material from one side of the pancreas to the other, through the incisions, so that the suture is just proximal to the lesion being excised. Tighten the suture and allow it to crush through the parenchyma, which ligates vessels and ducts. Excise the specimen distal to the ligature. Close any holes in the mesoduodenum with absorbable suture material. Blunt separation of pancreatic lobules and ligation of ducts can be performed for lesions anywhere within the pancreas. With small lesions it may be possible to identify and preserve the pancreatic ducts. Identify the lesion to be removed, and gently incise the mesoduodenum or omentum overlying it. For lesions involving the pancreatic body or proximal aspect of the right lobe, bluntly dissect pancreatic tissue from the pancreaticoduodenal vessels using gauze sponges. Ligate or cauterize small pancreatic vessels, but avoid damaging the pancreaticoduodenal vessels. Separate the affected lobules from adjoining tissue by blunt dissection, using sterile Q-tips or Halsted mosquito hemostats. Identify blood vessels and ducts supplying the portion of pancreas to be removed and ligate them. Excise the affected pancreatic tissue, and close any holes in the mesoduodenum.

VII. Healing of the Pancreas

A. Pancreatic duct obstruction is seldom caused by wound contraction; rather, parenchymal edema or obstruction at the duodenal papilla is usually responsible.

B. The main concern associated with pancreatic healing following surgery is the effect of healing on the flow and drainage of pancreatic secretions.

C. As much as 80% of the pancreas can be removed without causing deleterious decreases in exocrine or endocrine function, if the duct to the remaining portion is left intact.

VIII. Suture Material/Special Instruments

A. Ligate the duct with nonabsorbable suture material (i.e., polypropylene, nylon) in animals with inflammatory, aseptic, or neoplastic conditions.

B. In septic conditions of the pancreas, use monofilament absorbable suture material (e.g., polydioxanone, polyglyconate); avoid braided suture material. Chromic gut suture is rapidly digested by pancreatic enzymes.

IX. Postoperative Care and Assessment

A. Delay oral feedings for 2 to 5 days after extensive pancreatic surgery and hydration, and maintain electrolytes with intravenous fluid therapy.

B. First feed water to observe whether vomiting occurs. If the animal does not vomit, give small amounts of low-fat (less than 2% fat on a dry-matter basis), bland food (e.g., rice and defatted chicken).

C. Animals with diffuse pancreatic disease or those that develop pancreatitis postoperatively may require total parenteral nutrition postoperatively.

D. With septic conditions, use broad-spectrum antibiotic therapy for 10 to 14 days postoperatively.

X. Special Age Considerations

A. Pancreatic disease is usually found in middle-aged or older animals.

B. Parenteral hyperalimentation may be necessary before and after surgery in these patients.

Pancreatic Abscesses and Pseudocysts (*SAS*, pp. 419-421)

I. Definitions

A. **Pancreatic abscesses** are a collection of purulent material and necrotic tissue within, and extending from, the pancreatic parenchyma.

B. **Pancreatic pseudocysts** are collections of pancreatic fluid enclosed within a wall of granulation tissue.

II. General Considerations and Clinically Relevant Pathophysiology

A. Pancreatic abscesses usually occur as a consequence of acute pancreatitis.

B. Pancreatic pseudocysts are rarely diagnosed in small animals. They may be incidental findings or may be associated with nonspecific abdominal signs (e.g., pain, vomiting).
   1. The fluid contained within the cysts is a combination of blood and pancreatic fluids and enzymes.

III. Diagnosis

A. Clinical Presentation

1. Signalment.
   a. Pancreatic abscesses generally arise following acute bouts of pancreatitis.
   b. Most animals are middle-aged to older, and dogs are more commonly affected than cats.
2. History.
   a. Most animals with pancreatic abscesses have a previous history of acute onset of anorexia, depression, diarrhea, or vomiting, and most have previously been treated for gastroenteritis that was probably pancreatitis.
   b. Animals with pancreatic cysts may be asymptomatic or show vague signs of abdominal discomfort.

B. Physical Examination Findings

1. Pancreatic abscesses may cause pain during abdominal palpation, depression, icterus, pyrexia, palpable cranial abdominal mass, or abdominal distention; however, the animal may have none of these findings. Pyrexia is inconsistent.

C. Radiography/Ultrasonography

1. The most consistent finding with pancreatic abscesses on survey abdominal radiographs is an ill-defined increase in soft tissue density in the right cranial abdominal quadrant.
2. A generalized increase in soft tissue density and loss of visceral contrast throughout the abdomen may be observed if peritonitis is present.
3. Abdominal ultrasonography is more sensitive and usually reveals a mass in the area of the pancreas. Gallbladder and bile duct distention may also be noted.
4. Gastric outflow obstruction is occasionally observed on contrast studies of the upper gastrointestinal tract.
5. Ultrasound examination is the best tool to identify pancreatic pseudocysts; however, differentiation of pseudocysts from other fluid-filled masses is not possible without fluid evaluation.
   a. Percutaneous fine-needle aspiration (FNA) of masses can be considered; however, the risk of abdominal contamination usually outweighs any advantages.

D. Laboratory Findings

1. Hematology may reveal leukocytosis, neutrophilia with or without a left shift, lymphopenia, or monocytosis.
2. Serum biochemical abnormalities may include hyperbilirubinemia, high serum alkaline phosphatase, high alanine aminotransferase, hypocholesterolemia, hyponatremia, hypochloremia, and hypokalemia.
3. Blood work in animals with pseudocysts may be consistent with pancreatitis or may be normal.

IV. Differential Diagnosis

A. Pancreatic abscesses must be differentiated from pancreatitis, gastric foreign bodies, intestinal foreign bodies, gastritis, cholecystitis, pancreatic neoplasia, and gastrointestinal neoplasia.

B. Ultrasound is the most useful test to differentiate these abnormalities preoperatively; however, exploratory surgery may be required to make a definitive diagnosis.

C. Pancreatic pseudocysts must be differentiated from pancreatic abscesses or neoplasia, based on gross appearance, culture results, and histopathologic examination.

V. Medical Management

A. Pancreatic abscesses are surgical diseases.

B. Small pancreatic pseudocysts may resolve spontaneously without therapy.

VI. Surgical Treatment

A. General Considerations

1. Generalized peritonitis is present in some dogs with pancreatic abscesses.
   a. A mass is usually observed originating from the pancreas in the cranial portion of the abdomen. The mass may be firm and fibrotic or friable.
   b. Multiple adhesions to omentum and adjacent loops of small or large intestine are frequently present. Adhesions may be present with pseudocysts if the cyst has ruptured and reformed; however, fewer adhesions are expected than with pancreatic abscesses.
   c. Pseudocysts may be drained at surgery or by FNA. The former is associated with a lower rate of recurrence.

B. Preoperative Management

1. With pancreatic abscesses, initiate medical management before surgery.
2. Begin fluid therapy based on the serum biochemical analyses.
3. Administer broad-spectrum antibiotics intravenously before surgery and continue for at least 10 to 14 days postoperatively.

C. Positioning

1. Position the animal in dorsal recumbency, and prepare the caudal thorax and entire abdomen.

VII. Surgical Technique

A. Pancreatic Abscesses

1. Surgical technique.

Perform a midline abdominal laparotomy that extends from the xiphoid cartilage caudally to distal to the umbilicus. Gently explore the abdomen. Locate the pancreatic mass and obtain cultures of infected tissues. Gently break down adhesions to the intestine and omentum. Try to preserve the pancreatic ducts, common bile ducts, and adjacent vascular structures during dissection. Debride necrotic or purulent areas of the pancreas using a combination of sharp and blunt dissection. Resect as much of the infected and necrotic pancreas as possible. If the mass is not resectable, debride it and place a Penrose drain(s) into the mass, and exteriorize it lateral to the abdominal incision. Determine common bile duct patency by gently expressing the gallbladder. If the common bile duct is not patent, catheterize the duct and try to obtain flow, or perform a cholecystoenterostomy. Make sure you do not ligate the common bile duct. If generalized peritonitis is present, lavage the abdomen thoroughly with warmed, sterile saline or lactated Ringer's solution. The abdomen may be closed or left open for drainage.

B. Pancreatic Pseudocysts

1. Surgical technique.

Explore the abdominal cavity as described above. Locate the pancreatic mass and obtain cultures of the cystic fluid. Gently break down adhesions, if present. Resect as much of the fibrous wall surrounding the pseudocyst as possible. If the mass is not resectable, aspirate the fluid. A Penrose drain can be placed; however, this increases the risk of iatrogenic infection. Close the abdomen routinely.

VIII. Suture Materials/Special Instruments

A. Use absorbable suture material for partial pancreatectomy in animals with pancreatic abscesses.

B. Have aerobic and anaerobic culture swabs available.

C. Use copious amounts of warmed fluids for abdominal flushing; suction allows complete removal of instilled fluid and facilitates dilution of infected fluids in the abdominal cavity.

IX. Postoperative Care and Assessment

A. Continue antibiotic therapy based on results of culture and sensitivity of abdominal fluid or infected pancreatic tissues.

B. Continue fluid therapy until the animal is eating and drinking normally.

C. Initiate needle-catheter jejunostomy or parenteral feeding postoperatively, if needed.

D. Monitor animals postoperatively for continued infection (continued pyrexia, worsening or lack of improvement in CBC, or sudden deterioration). Repeat surgeries may be necessary in such animals.
   1. Blood cultures are warranted if bacteremia is suspected.

E. Hypoproteinemia and hypoalbuminemia may be severe (particularly if open abdominal drainage is performed) and warrant plasma transfusions.

X. Prognosis

A. The prognosis in animals with pancreatic abscesses is guarded.
   1. Early recognition and aggressive therapy may improve survival.

B. The prognosis for pancreatic pseudocysts is good. Many resolve spontaneously.

Insulinoma (*SAS*, pp. 421-425)

I. Definitions

A. **Insulinomas** (i.e., pancreatic β-cell tumors, adenomas, or adenocarcinomas of the pancreatic islets) are functional tumors of the β-cells of the islands of Langerhans that autonomously secrete insulin, even in the presence of hypoglycemia.

II. General Considerations and Clinically Relevant Pathophysiology

A. Insulinomas secrete excessive amounts of insulin, causing hypoglycemia.

B. They are more commonly recognized in dogs than in cats.

C. Malignant tumors predominate in dogs.

D. Insulinomas are slow growing tumors that compress adjacent pancreatic parenchyma.

E. Insulinomas are usually sharply delineated and encapsulated, and although most are malignant, surgical excision is often palliative.

III. Diagnosis

A. Clinical Presentation

1. Signalment.

a. Tumors generally occur in middle-aged to older dogs, with no sex predisposition.
b. Medium- to large-breed dogs (e.g., Irish setters, German shepherds, Labrador retrievers, standard poodles, and boxers) appear to be more commonly affected.

2. History.
   a. Clinical signs are attributable to hypoglycemia and include muscle tremors, muscle weakness, ataxia, mental dullness, disorientation, collapse, and/or convulsions.
   b. Dogs may be easily agitated and may have intermittent periods of excitability and restlessness.
   c. Clinical signs are often intermittent initially, but occur more commonly as the disease progresses.
   d. Clinical signs often diminish or resolve with feeding.
   e. Many animals are treated with anticonvulsants before the diagnosis is made.

B. Physical Examination Findings

1. Physical examination findings may reveal a normal or ataxic animal, muscle weakness, mental dullness, or disorientation.
2. Affected dogs do not usually have physical examination abnormalities between hypoglycemic episodes.
3. Withholding food before and during the evaluation may precipitate seizures.
4. Neuronal demyelination and axonal degeneration may occur from chronic hypoglycemia.

C. Radiography/Ultrasonography

1. Location of the tumor within the pancreas can sometimes be determined with ultrasound.
2. Ultrasonography may indicate metastasis to the liver and regional lymph nodes in some affected animals.
3. Radiographs are indicated, but pulmonary metastasis is rare.

D. Laboratory Findings

1. Tentative diagnosis of insulinoma is based on demonstration of Whipple's triad.
   a. Clinical signs associated with hypoglycemia (usually neurologic).
   b. Fasting blood glucose concentrations less than or equal to 40 mg/dl.
   c. Relief of neurologic signs with feeding or glucose administration.
2. Fasting or nonfasting blood glucose concentrations are often less than 70 mg/dl.
3. Most affected dogs can be made hypoglycemic by fasting for 12 to 24 hours. Measure blood glucose every 2 to 3 hours when fasting animals, until hypoglycemia is detected.
4. Once hypoglycemia has been confirmed, measure serum insulin levels. Normal fasting serum immunoreactive insulin concentrations range from 5 to 26 μU/ml, whereas insulin levels in affected animals often exceed 70 μU/ml. If insulin levels fall within the normal range, an amended insulin:glucose ratio can be determined; however, false-positive results are possible.
   a. $$\frac{\text{Serum insulin } (\mu\text{U/ml} \times 100)}{\text{Plasma glucose (mg/dl)} - 30}$$
5. Definitive diagnosis of insulinoma may require exploratory surgery.

IV. Differential Diagnosis

A. Insulinoma is a differential diagnosis in any dog with persistent and progressive seizures.

B. Once hypoglycemia has been verified, these tumors must be differentiated from extrapancreatic neoplasms, hunting dog or puppy hypoglycemia, sepsis, hepatic failure, hypoadrenocorticism, and hypopituitarism.

C. Consider laboratory error in "hypoglycemic" animals that do not have clinical signs of hypoglycemia.

V. Medical Management

A. Feed dogs with insulinomas 3 to 6 small meals per day of a diet that is high in protein and complex carbohydrates, but low in refined sugar.

B. Restrict exercise to help alleviate clinical signs.

C. Glucocorticoid therapy may also help prevent hypoglycemia.
   1. Prednisone or prednisolone–0.25 to 2 mg/kg BID
   2. If clinical signs of hyperadrenocorticism occur, decrease glucocorticoid therapy and use alternate drugs; however, hyperadrenocorticism may be preferable to hypoglycemia.

D. Diazoxide is an oral hyperglycemic agent that inhibits pancreatic insulin secretion and glucose uptake by tissues.
   1. Start with 10 mg/kg divided BID with meals. The dosage may gradually be increased to 60 mg/kg divided BID. Concurrent administration of hydrochlorothiazide may enhance effects.
   2. Side effects (e.g., anorexia, vomiting, aplastic anemia, cataracts, bone marrow suppression, thrombocytopenia, anorexia, diarrhea, tachycardia, and fluid retention) may occur.

E. If hypoglycemia is severe and unresponsive, intravenous 5% or 10% dextrose may be necessary to maintain blood glucose concentrations until surgery can be performed.

F. Streptozocin is nephrotoxic in dogs. Alloxan and a somatostatin analog (octreotide; 1-2 μg/kg SC before surgery) have been used in a few dogs with insulinomas; however, data are too scarce to recommend their use at this time.

VI. Surgical Treatment

A. Preoperative Management

1. Initiate fluid therapy with 5% glucose 12 to 24 hours before surgery.
2. Withhold food 12 hours before surgery.
3. Measure blood glucose concentrations immediately before surgery and administer additional glucose if the concentration is less than 75 to 100 mg/dl.

B. Anesthesia

1. Maintain blood glucose concentrations greater than 75 to 100 mg/dl.
2. Use thiobarbiturates or etomidate because either decreases cerebral glucose metabolism.
3. Maintain anesthesia with isoflurane or halothane.
4. Monitor blood glucose concentrations every 20 to 40 minutes during surgery to avoid intraoperative hypoglycemia.

C. Positioning

1. Position the animal in dorsal recumbency and prepare the caudoventral thorax and entire abdomen.

VII. Surgical Technique

A. General Considerations

1. Explore the cranial abdominal cavity thoroughly for evidence of neoplasia. Carefully and gently palpate the entire pancreas for evidence of tumor nodules.
   a. Most dogs have solitary nodules. Tumors are located with equal frequency in the left and right lobes of the pancreas and in the body.
   b. Metastasis is noted in approximately 50% of cases at the time of surgery. Metastasis usually occurs to the regional lymph nodes and liver.

B. Surgical Technique

1. Administer methylene blue intravenously if the tumor cannot be identified to help differentiate it from surrounding normal tissue. Maximal staining occurs within 30 minutes. A common side effect of methylene blue administration is hemolytic anemia caused by Heinz body formation.
   a. Dilute 3 mg/kg of 1% methylene blue in 250 ml of 0.9% sterile saline and give IV over 30 to 40 minutes.

Perform a partial pancreatectomy, removing tumor nodules with as wide a margin of normal tissue as possible. Submit excised lesions for histopathologic examination. Excise metastatic nodules, if possible.

VIII. Suture Materials/Special Instruments

A. Balfour abdominal retractors are useful for abdominal exploration.

B. Sterile Q-tips or fine hemostats are useful for separating pancreatic tissues during partial pancreatectomy.

C. Duct ligation is performed using 3-0 or 4-0 nonabsorbable suture material.

IX. Postoperative Care and Assessment

A. Measure blood glucose concentrations frequently during the first 24 hours postoperatively.

B. Pancreatitis may result from surgical manipulation of the pancreas.

C. Administer small amounts of water the day following surgery, and if vomiting does not occur, feed small, frequent meals.

D. Once the blood glucose concentration stabilizes at 75 to 100 mg/dl or greater, stop the glucose infusion.
   1. If persistent hypoglycemia continues, initiate medical therapy (glucocorticoids, diazoxide).

E. Neurologic signs (i.e., ataxia, bizarre behavior, coma, seizures) may persist despite normoglycemia.

F. Transient hyperglycemia occasionally persists for years after surgery.
   1. Insulin therapy may be indicated if blood glucose concentrations greater than 180 mg/dl persist for more than 3 to 5 days.

X. Prognosis

A. Nearly 50% of dogs without evidence of metastasis at the time of surgery will be normoglycemic for at least 1 year after partial pancreatectomy.

B. Long-term disease-free periods can be obtained in some dogs with multiple surgeries to remove hepatic nodules as clinical signs occur.

C. Young dogs may have a poorer prognosis than older dogs.

Gastrinomas (*SAS*, pp. 425-427)

I. Definitions

A. **Gastrinomas** (i.e., non–β-cell tumors, gastrin-secreting tumors) are tumors that secrete excessive gastrin.

B. **Zollinger-Ellison syndrome** is a term used to describe a syndrome of gastric acid hypersecretion, gastrointestinal ulceration, and non–β-cell pancreatic tumors.

II. General Considerations and Clinically Relevant Pathophysiology

A. Gastrinomas are rare.

B. Excess gastrin causes hyperacidity, which can cause multiple ulcerations in the duodenal mucosa.

C. Pancreatic gastrin-secreting tumors are usually locally invasive into adjacent parenchyma and frequently metastasize to regional lymph nodes and/or liver.

III. Diagnosis

A. Clinical Presentation

1. Signalment.
   a. Dogs and cats may be affected.
2. History.
   a. Most animals present with clinical signs of anorexia, vomiting (which is occasionally blood-tinged), regurgitation, intermittent diarrhea, weight loss, and/or dehydration.
   b. Clinical signs may be present for several days or months before diagnosis.

B. Physical Examination Findings

1. Clinical findings may include dehydration, diarrhea, melena, hematemesis (coffee-ground appearance), steatorrhea, and/or weight loss.
2. Abdominal pain is inconsistent. Perforation of a gastric ulcer may cause generalized peritonitis.

C. Radiography/Ultrasonography/Endoscopy

1. Radiographs and ultrasonography are nondiagnostic because pancreatic masses are generally too small to be visualized.
2. Endoscopy is the most useful technique for diagnosing esophagitis, gastric mucosal hypertrophy, and/or duodenal ulceration.
3. Ulcers are most commonly located in the proximal duodenum.

D. Laboratory Findings

1. Nonspecific laboratory abnormalities include anemia, hypoproteinemia, and/or leukocytosis.
2. Hypochloremic, hypokalemic, metabolic alkalosis, or metabolic acidosis may occur if vomiting has been severe.
3. Preoperative diagnosis of gastrinoma is based on demonstration of hypergastrinemia.
4. Blood samples for serum gastrin analysis should be obtained after a 12-hour fast.
   a. Basal serum gastrin levels in normal dogs and cats
      i. Dogs–less than 190 pg/ml
      ii. Cats–less than 135 pg/ml
   b. These values may vary between laboratories.

IV. Differential Diagnosis

A. Gastrinomas must be differentiated from other causes of ulceration, including nonsteroidal antiinflammatory drugs (NSAIDs), corticosteroids, gastric neoplasia, infiltrative disease, mast cell tumors, disseminated intravascular coagulation, hepatic disease, circulatory shock, and septic shock.

B. Other causes of hypergastrinemia include renal failure, gastric outflow obstruction, and current H_2-blocker therapy.

V. Medical Management

A. The prognosis for long-term cure is poor; however, aggressive medical management may be helpful.

1. Proton-pump inhibitors (e.g., omeprazole) are the most potent inhibitors of gastric-acid secretion known (see Appendix I).
2. H_2 receptor blockers decrease acid secretion; however, they tend to be much less effective for this disease than omeprazole.

B. Sucralfate can be used to treat ulcers that develop in spite of antacid therapy (see Appendix I).

VI. Surgical Treatment

A. General Considerations

1. Surgical resection of the pancreatic mass may provide a cure if metastasis is not present.
   a. If metastasis is present, surgical debulking of the mass and removal of operable metastatic lesions may improve efficacy of medical therapy and prolong survival.
2. Inspect the gastrointestinal tract during surgery for ulcers that may perforate. Remove such lesions or perform serosal patching over them.

B. Preoperative Management

1. Give whole blood if the PCV is less than 20%. Oxygenate anemic animals before induction.
2. Correct electrolyte and acid-base abnormalities.

C. Positioning

1. Place the animal in dorsal recumbency and prepare the caudal thorax and entire ventral abdomen.

VII. Surgical Technique

Perform a thorough abdominal exploration. Inspect the draining lymph nodes, liver, duodenum, and mesentery for evidence of metastasis. Inspect the entire pancreas for a mass lesion. Perform a partial pancreatectomy and resect metastatic lesions that are accessible. Submit excised tissues for histopathologic examination.

VIII. Suture Materials/Special Instruments

A. If the animal is severely hypoproteinemic or anemic, wound healing may be delayed.

1. Use polydioxanone or polyglyconate suture (2-0 or 3-0) to close gastrotomy and abdominal incisions.
2. These sutures may also be used to perform a serosal patch.

B. Postoperative care and assessment.

1. Give small amounts of water the day following surgery and observe for vomiting. If vomiting does not occur, give small amounts of food 24 hours postoperatively.
2. The diet should be low-fat and contain moderate amounts of protein and carbohydrates to aid gastric emptying.
3. Continue medical therapy for ulcers until clinical signs resolve.

IX. Prognosis

A. The long-term prognosis is guarded.

Exocrine Pancreatic Neoplasia (*SAS*, pp. 427-428)

I. Definitions

A. **Exocrine pancreatic carcinomas** (i.e., pancreatic carcinomas) are malignant tumors that arise from either acinar or ductular epithelial cells.

II. General Considerations and Clinically Relevant Pathophysiology

A. Most pancreatic tumors are aggressive, malignant adenocarcinomas that invade locally and metastasize readily.

B. The most common sites for metastasis are liver, lungs, peritoneum, and regional lymph nodes.

C. Benign pancreatic tumors (i.e., adenomas) are rare.

III. Diagnosis

A. Clinical Presentation

1. Signalment.
   a. Pancreatic adenocarcinomas may be slightly more common in cats than in dogs.
   b. They occur more commonly in older animals, and Airedale terriers and boxers have been reported to have higher risk for this tumor.
2. History.
   a. Vomiting, abdominal pain, anorexia, weight loss, lethargy, abdominal distention, and/or diarrhea may be seen.
   b. The history may be acute or chronic.

B. Physical Examination Findings

1. Physical examination findings may include abdominal pain on palpation and/or ascites (secondary to compression of the portal vein or other vessels or resulting from widespread abdominal metastasis).
2. The first clinical sign may be icterus resulting from common bile duct obstruction.

C. Radiography/Ultrasonography

1. An ill-defined increase in soft tissue density in the right cranial abdominal quadrant may be noted on survey abdominal radiographs.
   a. Ascites causes loss of visceral contrast.

2. Abdominal ultrasonography often reveals a mass in the area of the pancreas.
   a. Distention of the gallbladder and bile ducts may be noted if there is extrahepatic biliary tract obstruction.

D. Laboratory Findings

1. Abnormalities consistent with extrahepatic cholestasis (i.e., elevated alkaline phosphatase and hyperbilirubinemia) are often present.

IV. Differential Diagnosis

A. Nodular pancreatic hyperplasia, a condition seen in older animals, is characterized by multiple small, white lesions that protrude minimally from the pancreatic surface.

B. Adenomas are usually small masses that may contain cysts.

C. Pancreatic carcinomas are usually well advanced at the time of diagnosis.

V. Medical Management

A. Only patients with resectable lesions at the time of laparotomy have a fair prognosis.

B. Chemotherapeutic agents have not prolonged the life of people or animals with this tumor.

VI. Surgical Treatment

A. General Considerations

1. Surgical resection is the treatment of choice; however, most animals are presented with advanced disease, and surgical resection is not possible.

B. Preoperative Management

1. Stabilize the animal before surgery with intravenous fluids and correction of acid-base and electrolyte abnormalities.

C. Positioning

1. Position the animal in dorsal recumbency and prepare the entire abdomen and caudal thorax.

VII. Surgical Technique

Make an abdominal incision that extends from the xiphoid cartilage as far caudally as necessary to allow complete exploration of the abdominal cavity. After identifying the pancreatic mass, explore abdominal organs, peritoneum, and regional nodes for evidence of metastasis. Euthanasia should be considered in animals with widespread metastasis. Perform a partial pancreatectomy, if possible. Confirm the patency of the common bile duct before abdominal closure.

VIII. Suture Materials/Special Instruments

A. A standard soft-tissue pack or general surgery pack is generally all that is required.

IX. Postoperative Care and Assessment

A. Debilitated animals may need enteral or parenteral hyperalimentation.

X. Prognosis

A. The prognosis is extremely poor for animals with pancreatic carcinomas.

Surgery of the Thyroid and Parathyroid Glands (*SAS*, pp. 428-441)

I. Definitions

A. **Thyroidectomy** is removal of a thyroid gland.

B. **Hypothyroidism** is deficient secretion of thyroxine.
   1. **Goitrous hypothyroidism** is caused by an abnormal iodine uptake or by defects in iodine uptake, organification, or thyroglobulin formation.
   2. **Nongoitrous hypothyroidism** is spontaneous hypothyroidism that may be immune-mediated (i.e., lymphocytic thyroiditis) or a result of idiopathic atrophy.

C. **Hyperthyroidism** is excessive secretion of thyroxine.

D. **Primary hyperparathyroidism** is excessive secretion of parathyroid hormone (PTH) by one or more abnormal parathyroid glands.

II. Preoperative Concerns

A. Hypothyroidism is usually due to thyroid dysfunction (primary hypothyroidism).

B. Primary hypothyroidism is usually caused by idiopathic follicular atrophy or lymphocytic thyroiditis.
   1. Dogs with lymphocytic thyroiditis have circulating thyroglobulin antibodies that form antigen-antibody complexes within the gland, causing functional glandular tissue to be replaced by fibrous tissue.

Table 19-7
Treatment of canine hypothyroidism

Maintenance
Thyroxine (Soloxine) 22 μg/kg PO, BID
Before Surgery (If not on Maintenance Therapy)
Oral—Levothyroxine (T_3; Cytobin or Cytomel) 4-6 μg/kg PO, TID or QID, or
IV—L-thyroxine; 20-40 μg/kg (1 dose)

2. Hypothyroidism in cats is usually caused by surgical removal of the thyroid glands or damage to their blood supply during thyroidectomy.

C. Hypothyroidism may be manifested as lethargy, exercise intolerance, weight gain, constipation, nonpruritic symmetric alopecia, peripheral neuropathies (i.e., laryngeal paralysis, vestibular deficits, megaesophagus), reproductive problems, cardiovascular changes (i.e., bradycardia, weak apex beat), and/or coagulopathies.

D. Hypothyroidism may cause decreased activity of factor VIII or factor VIII–related antigen, which may predispose to spontaneous bleeding or serious hemorrhage during surgery in animals with von Willebrand's disease.
1. Give animals with untreated hypothyroidism undergoing emergency procedures oral 1-triiodothyronine three to four times a day or a single intravenous dose of 1-thyroxine (Table 19-7).
2. Postpone elective procedures until replacement therapy has been maintained for a minimum of 2 weeks.
3. If excessive bleeding is noted despite thyroid supplementation, give whole blood or plasma (see Appendix A).

E. Functional parathyroid neoplasms cause hypercalcemia through excessive secretion of PTH, which results in increased renal calcium reabsorption and increased renal phosphorus excretion, increased calcium and phosphorus release from bone, and increased intestinal absorption of calcium and phosphorus.

F. Primary hypoparathyroidism is a rare cause of hypocalcemia in dogs and cats, affecting primarily middle-aged female dogs, secondary to lymphocytic parathyroiditis.

III. Anesthetic Considerations

A. Hypothyroidism may prolong anesthetic recovery.

B. Dosages of premedications and anesthetics may need to be decreased in moderately or severely affected animals.

C. Monitor blood pressure, cardiac function, and hematocrit during anesthesia and in the early postoperative period.

D. Hypothermia may be of greater concern in these patients.

IV. Antibiotics

A. Guidelines for appropriate perioperative antibiotic use should be followed in hypothyroid patients.

B. Consider prophylactic antibiotic therapy in animals that are debilitated, obese, and/or have concurrent hyperadrenocorticism.

V. Surgical Anatomy

A. The thyroid glands (or lobes) are dark red, elongated structures attached to the outer surface of the proximal portion of the trachea.

1. They are usually positioned laterally and slightly ventral to the fifth to eighth cartilage rings.
2. The left lobe is usually located one to three tracheal rings caudal to the right lobe. In adult dogs they are approximately 5 cm in length and 1.5 cm wide; in cats they are 2.0 cm long and 0.3 cm wide.
3. Functional accessory thyroid tissue is common along the trachea, thoracic inlet, mediastinum, and thoracic portion of the descending aorta.

B. The cranial and caudal thyroid arteries are the thyroid's principal blood supply.

1. The cranial thyroid artery arises from the common carotid artery; the caudal thyroid artery typically arises from the brachiocephalic artery.
2. The cranial and caudal thyroid arteries anastomose on the dorsal surface of the gland, where they send numerous vessels that supply the gland.
3. The cranial thyroid artery in dogs usually sends a branch that supplies the external parathyroid gland before entering the thyroid parenchyma.
4. In cats the branch that supplies the external parathyroid gland may arise from the cranial thyroid artery after it has perforated the capsule.
5. Caudal thyroid arteries may not be present in cats.

C. The parathyroid glands are small ellipsoid disks, usually occurring as four structurally independent glands in close association with the thyroid glands.

1. The external parathyroid glands are normally found on the cranial dorsolateral surface of the thyroid.
2. The internal parathyroid glands are embedded within the thyroid parenchyma, usually at the caudomedial pole.

VI. Surgical Techniques

A. General Considerations

1. Thyroidectomy may be performed via an intracapsular or extracapsular approach.
    a. The extracapsular approach is used in dogs with malignant thyroid tumors, and no attempt is made to spare the ipsilateral parathyroid glands.

b. Intracapsular and modified extracapsular approaches have been described for thyroidectomy in cats.
  i. These techniques spare the external parathyroid glands.
  ii. Modification of the original intracapsular approach involves excising the majority of the thyroid capsule once the thyroid tissue has been removed.
  iii. Recurrence of hyperthyroidism in cats following thyroidectomy is thought to be the result of hypertrophy of small nests of functional thyroid tissue attached to the capsule.

VII. Healing of the Thyroid and Parathyroid Glands

A. Abnormal thyroid tissue appears to regenerate and hypertrophy following incomplete feline thyroidectomy.

B. Parathyroid tissue may be able to revascularize and regain function, even if it has been totally separated from its blood supply.
  1. Many surgeons recommend implanting an inadvertently excised parathyroid gland into surrounding muscle, rather than discarding it.

VIII. Suture Materials/Special Instruments

A. Delayed wound healing may occur in animals with hypothyroidism.

Feline Hyperthyroidism (*SAS*, pp. 431-436)

I. Definitions

A. **Hyperthyroidism** is a multisystemic disease resulting from excessive production and secretion of thyroxine (T_4).

B. **Goiter** is an enlargement of the thyroid gland.

C. **Graves' disease** describes an autoimmune disorder of human beings in which circulating autoantibodies stimulate thyroid tissue.

II. General Considerations and Clinically Relevant Pathophysiology

A. Hyperthyroidism is much more common in cats.

B. Most affected cats have bilateral adenomatous hyperplasia of one or both thyroid glands.
  1. Approximately 5% of cats have an ectopic thyroid mass at the thoracic inlet or in the cranial mediastinum.

C. Excessive circulating thyroxine causes multisystemic organ dysfunction.
   1. Up to 80% of affected cats have thyrotoxic heart disease, and approximately 20% of these may have congestive heart failure.
   2. Abnormalities of the CNS may include hyperexcitability, irritability, aggression, seizures, confusion, and stupor.

III. Diagnosis

A. Clinical Presentation

1. Signalment.
   a. Hyperthyroidism generally affects cats older than 8 years of age.
2. History.
   a. Most affected cats are presented because of weight loss despite a normal or voracious appetite, restlessness, and/or hyperactivity.
   b. Vomiting, diarrhea, polyuria, polydipsia, aggression, and/or a rough hair coat may also occur.
   c. Body temperature may be slightly elevated.
   d. Approximately 10% of hyperthyroid cats are depressed, lethargic, inappetent, and/or weak (i.e., "apathetic" hyperthyroidism).

B. Physical Examination Findings

1. A palpable cervical mass is present in most affected cats.
   a. Occasionally, the gland may descend into the thoracic inlet, where it can no longer be palpated.
2. Additional physical examination findings may include emaciation, a thin and/or roughened hair coat, and cardiac abnormalities (e.g., tachycardia, gallop rhythms, murmurs, left anterior fascicular block, and/or atrial and ventricular tachyarrhythmias).
3. Electrocardiographic abnormalities may include tachycardia, prolonged QRS duration, increased R-wave amplitudes in lead II, and ventricular preexcitation.

C. Radiography/Ultrasonography/Thyroid Imaging

1. An enlarged heart, consistent with hypertrophic cardiomyopathy, is often found on thoracic radiographs and echocardiography.
   a. Congestive heart failure may cause pleural effusion and/or pulmonary edema.
2. Thyroid imaging can detect functional ectopic thyroid tissue.

D. Laboratory Findings

1. Most affected cats have high serum free T_4 concentrations; however, hyperthyroidism cannot be excluded on the basis of normal thyroxine concentrations.
2. Other abnormalities may include increased PCV, neutrophilic leukocytosis, eosinopenia, lymphopenia, elevated alanine aminotransferase, and elevated alkaline phosphatase.
3. If baseline serum thyroxine concentrations are normal in a cat with appropriate clinical signs and a palpable ventral cervical mass, serum free T_4 concentration should be remeasured in 3 to 4 weeks.
   a. Alternatively, a T_3 suppression test or a thyrotropin-releasing hormone (TRH) stimulation test may be performed.
      i. Day 1–Obtain morning baseline serum T_4 and T_3 concentrations
      ii. Days 1 and 2–Give sodium liothyronine, 25 μg/cat PO, TID for 2 days
      iii. Morning of day 3–Administer sodium liothyronine, wait 2 to 4 hours, then measure serum T_4 and T_3.

4. Alternatively, response to oral antithyroid drugs or results of a sodium pertechnetate scan may be used to help confirm the diagnosis.

IV. Differential Diagnosis

A. Weight loss of vomiting caused by hyperthyroidism must be differentiated from that caused by intestinal lymphoma or inflammatory bowel disease.

B. Cats with neurologic signs must be differentiated from cats with primary CNS abnormalities.

C. Cardiac dysfunction secondary to hyperthyroidism should be differentiated from that resulting from other acquired or congenital causes.

V. Medical Management

A. Treatment of feline hyperthyroidism may include long-term administration of antithyroid drugs, iodine-131 (^{131}I), or surgical removal of the affected glands.

B. The choice of treatment for an individual cat depends on the age and condition of the cat and the treatment modalities available to the practitioner.

C. Administration of methimazole can cause remission; however, clinical signs return once the drug is discontinued.
   1. Rarely, drug-induced hepatopathy, thrombocytopenia, and agranulocytosis occur with chronic therapy.
   2. If thyroid carcinoma is suspected, medical therapy with antithyroid drugs may palliate clinical signs while allowing tumor growth.

D. Iodine-131 is a safe and effective method of treating hyperthyroidism.
   1. The cat must be confined for several weeks, during which it is a human health hazard.
   2. It is important to eliminate other diseases before treating with ^{131}I, so that minimal contact with the cat is required during treatment.
   3. The efficacy of radioactive iodine therapy is reduced by recent administration of antithyroid drugs because these drugs reduce incorporation of the radioactive iodine into the thyroid gland.

VI. Surgical Treatment

A. General Considerations

1. Surgical treatment of hyperthyroidism involves thyroidectomy.
2. The major complication of thyroidectomy is hypoparathyroidism secondary to removal or damage of the parathyroid glands.

B. Preoperative Management

1. Make cats euthyroid preoperatively by administering methimazole (5 mg/cat PO, BID or TID, followed by 2.5 to 5.0 mg/cat PO, BID, or TID). Generally, administration for 1 to 3 weeks before surgery is sufficient; however, repeat the T_4 concentration to ensure that it is within the normal range before surgery.

2. If preoperative therapy with methimazole is not tolerated, give propranolol for 1 to 2 weeks before surgery to decrease the heart rate (2.5 to 5 mg/cat PO, BID or TID).
   a. Discontinue propranolol 24 to 48 hours before surgery because of its β-blocking effects, which may interfere with treatment of hypotension.
3. Perform electrocardiogram, chest radiograph, and echocardiogram before surgery.
4. Many hyperthyroid cats have concurrent renal disease, hypokalemia and/or azotemia. Give these cats fluids before, during, and after surgery, and ensure that further deterioration of renal function does not occur during or after surgery, when cardiac output drops because the cat becomes euthyroid.

C. Anesthesia

1. Avoid inhalants that sensitize the heart to arrhythmias (e.g., halothane).
2. Premedicate cats with cardiomyopathy with butorphanol (0.2 mg/kg IM or SC) and induce with diazepam (0.2 mg/kg IV) followed by etomidate (1 to 3 mg/kg IV). Maintenance on isoflurane in oxygen should be used.
3. If the cat does not have cardiomyopathy, a variety of anesthetic protocols can be used (e.g., premedicate similarly and chamber induce with isoflurane in oxygen).
4. If arrhythmias occur during surgery that are not due to hypoxemia or the anesthetic, give esmolol as an intravenous bolus.

D. Positioning

1. Place the animal in dorsal recumbency, with the neck slightly hyperextended and forelimbs pulled caudally.
2. Prepare the entire ventral neck and cranioventral thorax.

VII. Surgical Technique

A. Intracapsular Thyroidectomy

1. Surgical technique.

Make a skin incision from the larynx to a point cranial to the manubrium. Bluntly separate the sternohyoid and sternothyroid muscles. Use a self-retaining retractor (i.e., Gelpi) to maintain exposure. Identify the enlarged thyroid gland and external parathyroid gland. Make an incision on the caudoventral surface of the gland in an avascular area, and extend it cranially with small scissors (i.e., iris scissors). Carefully remove the thyroid tissue from the capsule, using a combination of blunt and sharp dissection. Perform the dissection carefully to avoid damaging the parathyroid gland or its blood supply. Use bipolar cautery to achieve hemostasis but avoid damaging the gland's blood supply. After the thyroid parenchyma has been removed, excise the majority of the thyroid capsule; however, do not excise capsule that is intimately associated with the external parathyroid gland. Close subcutaneous tissue with a simple continuous suture pattern. Close skin with either a simple continuous or a simple interrupted suture pattern.

B. Modified Extracapsular Approach for Thyroidectomy

1. Surgical technique.

Position the animal as described above. Locate the thyroid gland as described above, and ligate or cauterize the caudal thyroid vein. Cauterize the

thyroid capsule approximately 2 mm from the external parathyroid gland, using fine-tipped bipolar-cautery forceps. With small, fine scissors cut the gland at the cauterized area, and remove the gland by sharp and blunt dissection from the parathyroid gland. Carefully dissect all thyroid gland from the surrounding tissues and parathyroid gland. Do not damage the cranial thyroid artery or its branches to the external parathyroid gland. Close as described above.

VIII. Suture Materials/Special Instruments

A. Small, fine instruments, such as iris scissors and Bishop-Harmon thumb forceps, facilitate removal of the thyroid glands.

B. Bipolar cautery forceps are advantageous for providing hemostasis because they allow finer control of coagulation than do unipolar forceps.

C. Sterile Q-tips are useful for dissecting the thyroid glands from the parathyroid glands.

IX. Postoperative Care and Assessment

A. Complications may include hypocalcemia, hypothyroidism, recurrence of hyperthyroidism, Horner's syndrome, and/or laryngeal paralysis.

B. Hypocalcemia (serum calcium levels <9 mg/dl in adult dogs and <8.5 mg/dl in adult cats) is the most important, acute, life-threatening complication of thyroidectomy.

1. Hypocalcemia may be permanent if all four parathyroid glands are removed or their blood supply is irreversibly damaged.
2. Temporary hypocalcemia is usually caused by disruption of the parathyroid blood supply.
3. Hypocalcemia should not occur after unilateral thyroidectomy.
4. Observe animals closely for signs of hypocalcemia (i.e., panting, nervousness, facial rubbing, muscle twitching, ataxia, seizures) for 2 to 4 days.
5. In cats, early signs may include lethargy, anorexia, panting, and facial rubbing.
   a. Clinical signs are usually noted within 24 to 96 hours, although delayed signs have been reported up to 5 to 6 days later.
6. Acute hypocalcemia may be treated with intravenous 10% calcium gluconate (Table 19-8). Give calcium slowly intravenously and monitor cardiac rate and rhythm during administration.
   a. It should be discontinued if bradycardia develops.
   b. Calcium gluconate can be added to the fluids, or the intravenous dose can be diluted in an equal volume of saline and given subcutaneously every 6 to 8 hours, until the animal is eating and able to be given oral medications.
      i. Discontinue subcutaneous or intravenous calcium when the serum calcium level is greater than 8 mg/dl.
   c. Maintenance therapy consists of oral calcium and vitamin D administration. The form of vitamin D most commonly used is dihydrotachysterol.

Table 19-8
Treatment of hypocalcemia following thyroidectomy

Management of Acute Signs
Give 0.5-1.5 ml/kg (5-15 mg Ca/kg) of 10% calcium gluconate slowly IV (over 10-20 min) and monitor the heart, then add 10 ml of 10% calcium gluconate into 250 ml of lactated Ringer's solution and drip at maintenance rate, or give IV dose diluted in equal volume of saline SC (in multiple sites). Monitor serum calcium frequently (2-3 times a day, if necessary).
Maintenance Therapy
Give calcium lactate 0.2-0.5 g/cat/day in divided doses PO and give vitamin D (dihydrotachysterol) PO 0.02-0.03 mg/kg/day for 5-7 days, then 0.01 mg/kg/day for 5-7 days, then 0.005 mg/kg/day for 1-4 mo.

i. Monitor serum calcium levels weekly and adjust the dosage of calcium accordingly.
ii. Discontinue vitamin D supplementation once the parathyroid gland revascularizes. Some animals require lifelong therapy.

C. Recurrent hyperthyroidism may result from hypertrophy if adenomatous tissue is not removed during thyroidectomy, or from adenomatous changes in ectopic thyroid tissue.

Hyperparathyroidism (*SAS*, pp. 436-438)

I. Definitions

A. **Primary hyperparathyroidism** results from excessive secretion of parathyroid hormone (PTH) by the parathyroid gland(s).

II. General Considerations and Clinically Relevant Pathophysiology

A. Primary hyperparathyroidism is uncommon.

B. It is usually caused by parathyroid adenomas.

C. Parathyroid adenomas are typically small, well-encapsulated tumors that appear brown or red and are located near the thyroid glands; however, ectopic adenomas may be located near the thoracic inlet or in the cranial mediastinum.

D. Clinical signs are caused by increased serum calcium levels and include dystrophic calcification, impaired renal tubular concentrating ability, nephrolithiasis, and calcium oxalate urolithiasis.

III. Diagnosis

A. Clinical Presentation

1. Signalment.
   a. Parathyroid tumors usually occur in older dogs.
   b. Keeshonden (and possibly German shepherds and Norwegian elkhounds) may be predisposed.
2. History.
   a. Dogs may be asymptomatic or may present for nonspecific signs (e.g., polyuria, polydipsia, vomiting, weakness, constipation, lethargy, and/or inappetence).
   b. The most common clinical signs in cats with primary hyperparathyroidism are anorexia, lethargy, vomiting, weakness, and weight loss.
   c. Occasionally bone and joint pain and pathologic fractures may occur secondary to skeletal demineralization.
   d. Cystic calculi may occur secondary to hypercalcemia.

B. Physical Examination Findings

1. Usually nonspecific, an enlarged parathyroid gland can seldom be palpated in dogs.
2. A cervical mass may be palpated in some cats.

C. Radiography/Ultrasonography

1. Cervical radiographs seldom identify the neoplasm.
2. Ultrasonographic evaluation of the cervical region occasionally reveals a parathyroid mass.
3. Marked demineralization of the skeleton, nephrolithiasis, and/or nephrocalcinosis may be noted radiographically.

D. Laboratory Findings

1. Serum biochemical abnormalities in dogs with primary hyperparathyroidism include hypercalcemia and hypophosphatemia. Hypercalcemia is the most consistent finding in affected cats.
2. Measurement of PTH in animals with normal renal function helps confirm hyperparathyroidism. Other causes of hypercalcemia are usually associated with low or low-normal levels of PTH.
   a. Renal dysfunction (which may occur secondary to hypercalcemia or be a primary disorder) may also elevate serum concentrations of PTH.
3. Definitive diagnosis of primary hyperparathyroidism requires surgical exploration of the parathyroid glands.

IV. Differential Diagnosis

A. Thoracic and abdominal radiographs, abdominal ultrasonography, routine blood work, and lymph node aspirations should be performed in hypercalcemic animals to look for other causes of hypercalcemia such as lymphosarcoma, apocrine gland adenocarcinoma, granulomatous disease, renal failure, hypoadrenocorticism, and hypervitaminosis D.

B. Thyroglossal cysts (formed when the embryonic thyroglossal duct fills with fluid) may be confused with parathyroid masses on palpation.

V. Medical Management

A. Hypercalcemia may be treated by diuresis.

B. Surgical removal of the neoplastic parathyroid tissue is the definitive treatment for primary hyperparathyroidism.

VI. Surgical Treatment

A. General Considerations

1. Parathyroidectomy is the treatment of choice for hyperparathyroidism caused by parathyroid neoplasia and primary hyperplasia.
   a. If the parathyroid glands are uniformly enlarged, secondary hyperparathyroidism should be suspected and other diagnostic tests performed to identify the cause.
   b. Enlargement of all four glands may occur with primary hyperplasia.
   c. Most dogs with primary hyperparathyroidism have a single parathyroid adenoma.
   d. If the parathyroid glands appear normal, ectopic parathyroid tissue may be located near the base of the heart.

B. Preoperative Management

1. Institute diuresis with physiologic saline solution before anesthetic induction to help lower serum calcium levels.
2. Once the animal has been appropriately hydrated, furosemide administration may promote further calciuresis.
3. Monitor electrolytes to avoid iatrogenic hypokalemia.

C. Anesthesia

1. Theoretically, marked hypercalcemia may cause bradycardia, peripheral vasoconstriction, and hypertension.
2. Hypotension may occur during anesthesia associated with relaxation of peripheral vascular tone.
3. Hypercalcemia may predispose to cardiac arrhythmias. Anesthetic agents that potentiate arrhythmias (i.e., thiobarbiturates, halothane) should be avoided.

D. Positioning

1. Place the animal in dorsal recumbency, with the neck slightly hyperextended and forelimbs pulled caudally.
2. Clip and prepare the entire ventral neck and cranioventral thorax.

VII. Surgical Technique

A. General Considerations

1. Inspect all four parathyroid glands.
2. If the external parathyroid gland is involved, the gland can be removed without removing the thyroid gland; however, removal of the internal parathyroid gland requires that thyroidectomy be performed.
3. Spare the external parathyroid gland when the internal parathyroid gland is neoplastic.

4. Facilitate visualization of the abnormal parathyroid gland with infusion of intravenous methylene blue in saline solution, if necessary.
   a. Abnormal parathyroid tissue may stain dark blue with this procedure.
   b. A common side effect of methylene blue administration is hemolytic anemia because of Heinz body formation.
5. If carcinoma is suspected, based on apparent invasiveness of the tumor, complete thyroidectomy and removal of draining lymph nodes are indicated.

VIII. Suture Materials/Special Instruments

A. Small, fine instruments, such as iris scissors and Bishop-Harmon thumb forceps, facilitate removal of the parathyroid glands.

B. Bipolar cautery forceps are advantageous for providing hemostasis because they allow finer control of coagulation than do unipolar forceps.

C. Sterile Q-tips are useful for dissecting the parathyroid glands from the thyroid glands.

IX. Postoperative Care and Assessment

A. Hypocalcemia is the most frequent postoperative complication in dogs; it may be less common in cats.
   1. Hypocalcemia may occur after removal of a single parathyroid adenoma because negative feedback from high circulating levels of PTH suppresses function in the other normal glands.
   2. Hypocalcemia may be most pronounced in animals with higher preoperative serum calcium levels and those with marked skeletal demineralization.
   3. Prolonged treatment of hypocalcemia should not be necessary.
   4. The prognosis for long-term survival following parathyroidectomy for hyperparathyroidism secondary to adenomas or hyperplasia is excellent if there is not severe renal damage.

Thyroid Carcinoma in Dogs (*SAS*, pp. 438-441)

I. Definitions

A. **Thyroid neoplasms** may be carcinomas (malignant) or adenomas (benign).

B. **Carcinomas** may arise from follicular cells and be classified as follicular, compact, papillary, or mixed, or they may arise from parafollicular or C-cells (medullary thyroid carcinomas).

II. General Considerations and Clinically Relevant Pathophysiology

A. Thyroid neoplasms make up 1% to 4% of all tumors in dogs.

B. Canine thyroid carcinomas are more common than adenomas, whereas functional adenomas prevail in cats.

C. Adenocarcinomas are generally rapidly growing, highly invasive tumors that frequently metastasize to the draining lymph nodes and lungs.

D. Large tumors (i.e., those >100 cm^3) are always associated with pulmonary metastasis.

E. Ectopic thyroid tumors have been reported at the heart base, caudal mediastinum, and tongue.

F. Tumors arising in cystic remnants of the thyroglossal duct are rarely reported in dogs.
   1. They are usually well-circumscribed, fluctuant, moveable enlargements in the ventral midline cervical region.

III. Diagnosis

A. Clinical Presentation

1. Signalment.
   a. Thyroid neoplasia is most common in medium- to large-breed dogs; boxers, beagles, and golden retrievers may be predisposed.
   b. Most affected dogs are middle-aged or older.
2. History.
   a. Affected animals often present for evaluation of a palpable cervical enlargement, dysphagia, dyspnea, coughing, voice change, and/or exercise intolerance.
   b. Respiratory abnormalities may be the result of tracheal compression or pulmonary metastasis.
   c. Hyperthyroidism (i.e., polydipsia, polyuria, weakness, restlessness, and a propensity to seek cool places) is rarely associated with canine thyroid carcinomas.

B. Physical Examination Findings

1. A ventral cervical mass is often palpable.
   a. Carcinomas usually appear firm and poorly encapsulated.
   b. Adenomas are typically small and freely moveable.
   c. Bilateral ptosis and prolapse of the nictitating membrane can be associated with paralysis of the extraocular and intraocular muscles secondary to thyroid adenocarcinoma invasion of the cavernous sinuses in dogs.

C. Radiography/Ultrasonography/Thyroid Imaging

1. Cervical radiographs or ultrasonography usually reveals diffuse cervical edema and soft-tissue swelling caudal to the mandible and surrounding the trachea. The mass may be partially mineralized.
2. Take thoracic radiographs to identify pulmonary metastasis.
3. Thyroid imaging may reveal abnormal thyroid gland uptake (heterog-

enous uptake with "hot" and "cold" regions, compared with normal thyroids or salivary gland uptake) and focal accumulations of the radiopharmaceutical in the lungs.

D. Laboratory Findings

1. Cytologic evaluation of an FNA of the cervical mass may reveal bizarre, pleomorphic cells, consistent with neoplasia.
2. Nondiagnostic samples may be obtained if the sample is contaminated with blood or is hypocellular.
3. Neoplastic follicular epithelial cells are fragile and are often broken during sample preparation.
4. Hyperthyroidism and hypothyroidism are occasionally associated with thyroid carcinomas; therefore measuring serum T_4 and T_3 concentrations is warranted.

IV. Differential Diagnosis

A. Cervical swelling because of thyroid neoplasia must be differentiated from abscesses, lymphadenopathy, or sialoadenopathy. This can usually be done by cytologic evaluation of fine-needle aspirates.

V. Medical Management

A. Dogs with thyroid carcinomas may be palliated with radioactive iodine (^{131}I); however, much larger doses of ^{131}I appear to be necessary in dogs than in cats with thyroid adenomas.

B. Chemotherapy with doxorubicin may benefit animals for whom complete excision is not possible.

C. External-beam (cobalt) irradiation appears beneficial in reducing tumor volume in animals, after debulking procedures; however, large doses are required.

VI. Surgical Treatment

A. General Considerations

1. Surgical excision of thyroid adenomas is the treatment of choice.
   a. Surgical removal of thyroid carcinomas is often difficult because of their invasive nature and pronounced vascularity but should be considered if metastasis is not evident, and the lesion is localized.
   b. Marginal excision (i.e., just outside the tumor pseudocapsule) in tumors that are freely moveable results in fewer complications than more extensive resection and does not appear to affect the local recurrence rate.
   c. Adjunctive radiation therapy or chemotherapy may be warranted if complete surgical excision is not possible.
   d. Have blood for transfusion available during surgery because hemorrhage is often excessive.

B. Preoperative Management

1. Correct electrolyte and acid-base abnormalities before surgery.
2. Initiate fluid therapy before surgery in geriatric patients with reduced renal function and in those that are dehydrated.

C. Anesthesia

1. Tachycardia or arrhythmias may occur because of catecholamine release; treatment should be anticipated.
2. Avoid drugs that are arrhythmogenic (e.g., barbiturates and halothane).

D. Surgical Anatomy

1. See surgical anatomy of the thyroid glands, p. 310.
2. The carotid artery, internal jugular vein, recurrent laryngeal nerve, and esophagus may adhere to or surround the tumor.

E. Positioning

1. Place the animal in dorsal recumbency, with the neck slightly hyperextended.
2. Tie the front limbs back away from the neck.
3. Clip and prepare the entire neck, cranial thorax, and caudal intermandibular space.

VII. Surgical Technique

Make a ventral midline incision over the thyroid glands. Identify the neoplastic mass and adjacent structures. If necessary, ligate the carotid artery and jugular vein. Remove the mass (thyroid and parathyroid glands) by a combination of sharp and blunt dissection. Identify and remove abnormal cervical lymph nodes. Use electrocautery and ligation to provide hemostasis. Inspect the contralateral thyroid, and biopsy or remove if indicated. Close the incision routinely. Submit tissue for histologic evaluation.

VIII. Suture Materials/Special Instruments

A. These tumors are frequently very vascular, and electrocautery is useful for obtaining hemostasis.

IX. Postoperative Care and Assessment

A. Use a light pressure wrap to decrease hemorrhage and swelling; place it with care to avoid causing airway obstruction.

B. Monitor the hematocrit postoperatively and transfuse as needed.

C. If unilateral thyroparathyroidectomy is performed, observe the animal for hypocalcemia or hypothyroidism, but supplementation is usually not necessary.

D. If bilateral thyroparathyroidectomy is performed, initiate vitamin D, calcium, and thyroid supplementation postoperatively.

X. Prognosis

A. The prognosis is guarded for thyroid carcinomas and depends on tumor size, resectability, and presence of metastasis.

B. Prognosis for thyroid adenomas is excellent.

20

Surgery of the Hemolymphatic System (*SAS*, pp. 443-459)

General Principles and Techniques (*SAS*, pp. 443-445)

I. Definitions

A. Tissue for histopathologic examination of lymph nodes may be obtained by removing the entire node **(lymphadenectomy)** or by excising a portion of it.

B. **Lymphangiomas** are benign tumors of peripheral lymphatics.

C. **Lymphangiosarcomas** are malignant tumors of lymphatic capillaries.

II. Preoperative Concerns

A. Lymphadenopathy is a common lymphatic abnormality.
   1. It may be due to focal infection, inflammation, neoplasia (metastic or primary), or systemic disease.
   2. Determine whether the enlargement is generalized or localized (regional).
      a. With localized lymphadenopathy, examine areas drained by the node for infection, inflammation, or neoplasia.
      b. Do fine-needle aspirates (FNAs) before lymph node biopsy because occasionally neoplastic cells or fungal elements are noted.
      c. Nondiagnostic aspirates may be obtained in animals with well-differentiated tumors and in those with focal infection or neoplasia.

B. The mandibular, superficial cervical, superficial inguinal, and popliteal lymph nodes are usually palpable.

C. The tonsils may be visualized within the oral cavity.

D. The axillary, accessory axillary, cervical, femoral, and retropharyngeal lymph nodes are usually only palpable when enlarged in dogs; however, the axillary node may be readily located in cats, even when only moderately enlarged.

E. Unless the animal is extremely thin or cachectic, sublumbar and mesenteric lymph nodes must be enlarged to be detected on rectal or abdominal palpation.

F. Acute enlargement (i.e., suppurative lymphadenitis) can be associated with pain, but lymphoid neoplasia usually causes painless enlargement.

1. Metastic neoplasia and fungal infections sometimes cause nodes to become fixed to surrounding tissues.
2. Clinical signs may result from lymphadenopathy.

G. Survey radiographs may detect internal lymphadenopathy.

1. Examine thoracic films for mediastinal, hilar, or sternal lymphadenopathy.
2. Abdominal radiographs may reveal ventral deviation of the colon resulting from sublumbar lymphadenopathy.

H. Lymphangiomas are rare, benign neoplasms originating from lymphatic capillaries.

1. They typically present as large, fluctuant swellings that are noticed incidentally or because of interference with normal structures.
2. Affected dogs are usually middle-aged or older.
3. Treatment for lymphangioma is complete surgical excision or marsupialization.

I. Lymphangiosarcomas are malignant tumors that arise from lymphatic capillaries.

1. The local invasiveness of this tumor often necessitates euthanasia. Surgical cures are unlikely.

III. Anesthetic Considerations

A. Excise superficial nodes (e.g., popliteal) under local anesthesia and sedation if possible.

B. Short-duration general anesthesia usually facilitates extirpation.

IV. Antibiotics

A. Perioperative antibiotics are seldom indicated in animals undergoing lymph node biopsy or removal.

V. Surgical Anatomy

A. Lymph nodes are bean-shaped with a convex surface and a small flat or concave hilus.

B. They are usually encased in fat at flexor angles or joints, in the mediastinum and mesentery, and in the angle formed by the origin of larger blood vessels.

VI. Surgical Techniques

A. Lymph Node Biopsy (*SAS,* pp. 444-445)

1. General considerations.
   a. There are no absolute contraindications to lymph node biopsy.
   b. Correct significant hemostatic disorders preoperatively, if possible, and properly ligate blood vessels.
   c. With generalized lymphadenopathy, the popliteal, inguinal, and prescapular lymph nodes are preferred biopsy sites.
      i. Biopsy at least two nodes.
      ii. Do not biopsy the mandibular lymph node and nodes draining the gastrointestinal tract because their morphologic appearance is often distorted by reactive hyperplasia caused by constant antigenic exposure.
   d. Incisional (wedge) biopsy of lymph nodes is indicated when lymphadenectomy may be difficult because of a node's size or location (i.e., nodes that are located close to major vessels or nerves).
2. Incisional biopsy (*SAS,* pp. 444-445).
   a. Surgical procedure.

Use a No. 15 scalpel blade to remove a wedge-shaped section of the parenchyma, and place the sample in a buffered formalin solution. In order to provide hemostasis, place a horizontal mattress suture of absorbable suture material (i.e., 3-0 chromic catgut) to close the incision.

3. Lymphadenectomy (*SAS,* p. 445).
   a. Surgical procedure.

Prepare the skin overlying the lymph node for aseptic surgery. Immobilize the lymph node firmly in one hand, and make an incision in the overlying skin. Bluntly dissect the node from surrounding tissue. Generally, a vessel near the hilus of the node requires ligation to prevent postoperative hemorrhage. Handle the node gently to prevent damage and distortion of the lymph node tissue. Section the node to provide samples for aerobic and anaerobic cultures, fungal cultures, histopathology, and cytology. Make impression smears by lightly blotting the cut edge of the node with absorbent paper and touching the sample lightly to a glass slide before placing it in formalin. Close dead space and suture skin routinely.

VII. Healing of the Lymphatic System

A. Healing of lymphatics is usually rapid.

B. Lymphedema rarely occurs following lymphadenectomy, and if it does occur, it is usually transient and seldom requires specific therapy.

VIII. Suture Materials/Special Instruments

A. Special instruments are not required for lymph node biopsy or removal.

B. Use absorbable suture in the lymph node parenchyma.

IX. Postoperative Care and Assessment

A. Observe for swelling at the surgical site.

B. Swelling is usually associated with hematoma formation caused by inadequate hemostasis or with seroma formation, if dead space was not obliterated.

X. Special Age Considerations

A. Increased lymph node size is expected in young animals as a part of an appropriate immunologic response.

B. As the animal ages, lymph node size usually decreases, making nodes difficult to palpate.

C. Loss of fat that normally surrounds the nodes in cachectic patients may make the nodes prominent.

Lymphedema (*SAS*, pp. 445-449)

I. Definitions

A. **Lymphedema** is an accumulation of fluid in the interstitial space.

B. **Primary lymphedema** is caused by an abnormality or disease of lymph vessels or lymph nodes.

C. **Secondary lymphedema** occurs because of lymphatic obstruction of the nodes or vessels by neoplasia, filariasis, lymphoproliferative disorders, or surgery.

II. General Considerations and Clinically Relevant Pathophysiology

A. Lymphedema results from a disturbance of the equilibrium between the amount of fluid in the interstitial space that needs to be cleared (capillary filtrate) and the capacity of the lymphatic and venous systems to remove this fluid.

1. Possible etiologies include overload of the lymphatic system, inadequate collection by the lymphatic terminal buds, abnormal lymphatic contractility, insufficient lymphatics, lymph node obstruction, and central vessel (i.e., thoracic duct) defects.
2. This edema is relatively protein-rich (2-5 g/dl).
3. Although the early stages are reversible, chronic edema is associated with thickening and fibrosis of tissues, making treatment difficult.
4. The dog is most commonly reported to have lymphedema.

B. Distinguishing between primary and secondary lymphedema is often difficult.

1. Lymph node obstruction, although more commonly associated with secondary lymphedema, has been associated with primary lymphedema.
2. Many of the dogs reported with primary lymphedema have had small or absent lymph nodes.
3. Secondary lymphedema may be caused by trauma, heat, irradiation, infection, or venous congestion (i.e., because of heart failure).

III. Diagnosis

A. Clinical Presentation

1. Signalment.
   a. Primary lymphedema is usually noted at birth or shortly thereafter; however, older animals may develop lymphedema associated with congenital abnormalities.
   b. The lymphatic system may function normally until a precipitating cause (e.g., infection or trauma) overwhelms the marginal lymphatic system.
   c. Congenital, hereditary lymphedema has been reported in bulldogs and poodles.
2. History.
   a. Lymphedema typically presents as a spontaneous, painless swelling of the extremities, with pitting edema.
   b. The rear limbs are more commonly affected, and unilateral swelling may be present.
   c. Lymphedema usually begins in the distal extremity and progresses proximally.
   d. Lameness and pain are uncommon without massive enlargement or cellulitis.

B. Physical Examination Findings

1. Lymphedema is diagnosed on the basis of clinical signs.
2. The limb is generally not excessively warm or cool.
3. Although frequently bilateral, the degree of swelling is often greater in one limb.
4. Occasionally, the swelling may be precipitated by minor trauma and/or superficial skin infections.
5. As the edema becomes chronic, fibrosis occurs, and the edema will tend to progressively pit less, until pitting is absent.

C. Lymphography/Lymphoscintigraphy

1. The classic diagnostic tool has been direct lymphography.
2. Oil-based contrast media are contraindicated.
3. Lymphoscintigraphy is an alternative approach for imaging peripheral lymphatics.

D. Laboratory Findings

1. Specific laboratory abnormalities are not found.

IV. Differential Diagnosis

A. The key differential diagnosis is abnormality of the venous system, such as venous stasis or arteriovenous fistula.

B. Typical changes in venous obstruction include varices, stasis hyperpigmentation, and cutaneous ulceration.

C. Typical changes in arteriovenous fistulae vary, depending on location; however, palpation of strong pulsatile vessels, often with a fremitus or "thrill," and auscultation of a machinery murmur, or bruit, are classic.
1. Angiography is necessary to confirm the diagnosis and determine the size, extent, and location of the fistula.

D. Physical examination should eliminate systemic causes of bilateral edema, including heart failure, renal failure, cirrhosis, and hypoproteinemia.

V. Medical Management

A. In the early stages of lymphedema, before the development of fibrosis, nonsurgical therapy may decrease the swelling.
1. Nonsurgical therapy consists of heavy bandages or splints that exert pressure on the limb, meticulous care of the skin to avoid infection, weight control, and appropriate use of antibiotics to treat and prevent cellulitis and lymphangitis.
2. Drugs include steroids, diuretics, anticoagulants, and fibrinolysin inhibitors. The proposed benefits of these pharmaceuticals have not been substantiated.
3. Do not use diurectics long-term.
4. The benzopyrones can be used to successfully treat experimental lymphedema in dogs.
   a. They seem to stimulate macrophages, which promotes proteolysis.
   b. Coumarin, O-(B-hydroxy-ethyl)-rutosides, diosmin, and rutin are such drugs.
      i. Rutin–50 to 100 mg/kg PO, TID.

VI. Surgical Treatment

A. General Considerations

1. With the exception of amputation, no current surgical treatment offers a cure for lymphedema.
2. Lymphangiography rarely provides information that helps manage animals with spontaneous lymphedema.
3. Biopsies of affected tissues should be submitted because lymphangiosarcoma, a highly malignant neoplasm, has been reported to occur in human beings with long-standing lymphedema.

B. Preoperative Management

1. Use perioperative antibiotics in patients undergoing lymphangiography because there is a high risk of subsequent lymphangitis.
   a. Inject 1 ml of 3% Evans Blue dye between the second and third or between the third and fourth digits before other preoperative procedures, to aid in the visualization and cannulation of lymphatics.

C. Anesthesia

1. General anesthesia is required for direct lymphangiography.

D. Surgical Anatomy

1. The lymphatic system of the extremities are divided into the superficial lymphatics and the deep, muscular lymphatics.

2. The superficial system appears to be the one most commonly involved in lymphedema.
   a. These lymphatics empty into a valved group of vessels that are found at the junction of the dermis and subcutaneous tissue. Lymph then drains into afferent lymphatics located in the subcutaneous fat.
   b. The superficial lymphatics of the pelvic limb consist of a larger medial group and a smaller lateral group.
   c. Lymphatics follow the branches of the medial saphenous vein and drain into the superficial inguinal lymph nodes.
   d. Deeper lymphatics drain the fascial planes surrounding skeletal muscles, joints, and synovium.

E. Positioning

1. Position the animal on the radiology table in lateral recumbency, with the affected limb down and the opposite limb retracted from the x-ray field.
2. Prepare and drape the dorsomedial aspect of the metatarsus for aseptic surgery.

F. Direct Lymphangiography

1. Surgical technique.

Make a 5-cm skin incision over the middorsomedial metatarsal region. Use sharp and blunt dissection until a blue-stained superficial metatarsal lymphatic vessel is identified. Meticulously dissect the lymphatic free from surrounding tissue with fine, blunt dissection probes, and cannulate the lymphatic, using a lymph duct cannulator or a 27- or 30-gauge over-the-needle catheter. Inject a small amount of sterile saline into the catheter or cannulator to verify patency. Then manually infuse an aqueous-based radiographic contrast agent into the lymphatic vessel. Take radiographs immediately following the injection; additional radiographs may be made, depending on the rate of lymphatic transport of the contrast agent, which varies from patient to patient. Upon completion of the lymphangiogram, withdraw the cannulator, ligate the lymphatic vessel, and close the incision in a routine fashion.

VII. Suture Materials/Special Instruments

A. A commercial lymphatic duct cannulator, such as a Tegtmeyer lymph duct cannulator, may facilitate cannulation of the lymphatic vessel.

VIII. Postoperative Care and Assessment

A. If the lymphatics appear abnormal in character or quantity, or if an obvious obstruction is not noted on the lymphangiogram, consider medical therapy or amputation.

IX. Prognosis

A. Primary lymphedema seldom resolves spontaneously.

B. Neoplastic alteration of chronic lymphedematous tissue may be a concern in animals.

Surgery of the Spleen (*SAS*, pp. 449-454)

I. Definitions

A. **Splenomegaly** is enlargement of the spleen from any cause.

B. **Splenectomy** is surgical removal of the spleen.

C. **Splenosis** is the congenital or traumatic presence of multiple nodules of normal splenic tissue in the abdomen.

D. **Siderotic plaques** are brown or rust-colored deposits of iron and calcium that may be found on the splenic surface.

II. Preoperative Concerns

A. Diffuse (symmetric) splenomegaly may be attributed to congestion (e.g., splenic torsion, right-sided heart failure, gastric dilatation-volvulus, or drugs) or infiltration as a result of infection (e.g., fungal, bacteria, or viral), immune-mediated disease (e.g., immune-mediated thrombocytopenia), or neoplasia (e.g., lymphosarcoma or feline mastocytosis).

B. Focal (asymmetric) splenomegaly may be caused by benign (e.g., nodular regeneration, hematoma, or trauma) or neoplastic processes (e.g., hemangiosarcoma).

C. Infiltrative splenomegaly resulting from neoplasia is one of the most common causes of spontaneous splenomegaly.

D. Anemia may be present because of acute hemorrhage associated with splenic trauma or hematoma rupture or associated with the underlying disease.
   1. Perform coagulation profiles in animals with evidence of bleeding not thought to be the result of trauma.
   2. Consider preoperative blood transfusions in normally hydrated animals with a PCV less than 20% or hemoglobin less than 5 to 7 g/dl.
   3. If disseminated intravascular hemolysis is suspected, consider heparin therapy (see Appendix I).

III. Anesthetic Considerations

A. Give anemic patients oxygen before induction and during recovery.

B. Use anticholinergic drugs to prevent bradycardia.

C. Avoid barbiturates that cause splenic congestion.

D. Avoid acetylpromazine in these patients because of potential red blood cell sequestration, hypotension, and impact on platelet function.

E. Monitor arterial blood pressure during surgery.

IV. Antibiotics

A. Perioperative antibiotics in healthy animals are usually unnecessary, but may be given at induction and discontinued within 24 hours.

B. Longer-term antibiotic therapy may be warranted in animals that are immunosuppressed or severely debilitated.

V. Surgical Anatomy

A. The spleen is in the left cranial abdominal quadrant.
   1. It usually lies parallel to the greater curvature of the stomach; however, its exact location is dependent on its size and on the position of other abdominal organs.
      a. When the stomach is contracted, the spleen usually lies within the rib cage, but with massive gastric enlargement it may be in the caudal abdomen.

B. The splenic capsule is composed of elastic and smooth muscle fibers.
   1. The parenchyma consists of a white pulp (i.e., lymphoid tissue) and red pulp (i.e., venous sinuses and cellular tissue filling the intravascular spaces).
   2. Large numbers of α-adrenergic receptors are responsible for splenic contraction.
   3. The spleen is normally red in color, but siderotic plaques or fibrin deposits may alter its appearance.

C. The arterial supply of the spleen is usually the splenic artery, a branch of the celiac artery.
   1. The splenic artery is generally over 2 mm in diameter and gives off three to five long primary branches as it courses in the greater omentum toward the ventral third of the spleen.
   2. The first branch is usually to the pancreas and is the main supply of the left limb of that organ.
   3. The two remaining branches run toward the proximal half of the spleen, where they send 20 to 30 splenic branches that enter the parenchyma.
   4. The branches then continue in the gastrosplenic ligament to the great curvature of the stomach, where they form the short gastric arteries (supplies fundus) and left gastroepiploic artery (supplies greater curvature of the stomach).
   5. Venous drainage is via the splenic vein into the gastrosplenic vein, which empties into the portal vein.

VI. Surgical Techniques

A. General Considerations

1. Approach the spleen via a ventral midline abdominal incision that extends from the xiphoid to a point caudal to the umbilicus.

B. Splenic Biopsy

1. General considerations.
   a. Splenic biopsies are indicated to ascertain the cause of clinically

significant splenomegaly or suspected metastatic lesions to the spleen.

i. They may be obtained percutaneously, by FNA, or at surgery.
ii. Ultrasound-guided biopsies improve the likelihood of obtaining diagnostic samples percutaneously.
iii. Percutaneous biopsies are often diagnostic for diffuse lesions (e.g., mastocytosis or lymphosarcoma); however, focal or nodular lesions may be missed.
iv. Differentiation of hemangiosarcoma and hematoma with cytologic analysis of samples obtained by FNA is rarely possible.
v. When cavitary lesions are identified with ultrasound, FNA should be performed with care, or not at all. Rupture of cavitary lesions may occur during aspiration and be fatal, especially in animals with coagulopathies.

b. Special preservatives are required for special staining techniques (e.g., for identification of viral inclusions, Bouin's fixative is preferred).
   i. Score (cut into) samples that are larger than 5 cm before placement in formalin, to allow the sample to fix properly.
   ii. Score large splenic masses at multiple sites, but leave the mass intact to allow identification of the entire lesion and its relationships. If this is not possible, submit multiple representative samples from diverse sites, including the margin of the abnormal and normal-appearing tissues.
   iii. If the lesion is cavitary, rupture it before placing in formalin.

2. Splenic aspiration
   a. Surgical technique.

Place the animal in right lateral or dorsal recumbency, using manual restraint or mild sedation. Avoid using phenothiazine tranquilizers or barbiturates because the resultant splenic congestion may cause a nondiagnostic sample as a result of blood dilution. Surgically prep a small area on the left side of the abdomen, and isolate the spleen. Using a plastic syringe attached to a small needle (23 or 25 gauge, 1 to 1.5 in), penetrate the abdominal wall and advance the needle into the spleen. Apply suction on the syringe several times. Before removing the needle from the abdomen, relieve suction on the syringe to prevent aspirating the contents of the needle into the syringe. Remove the needle from the abdomen, and place the specimen on a slide for evaluation.

3. Surgical biopsy.
   a. General considerations.
      i. During celiotomy, focal lesions may be biopsied by FNA or with a Tru-cut, Jamshidi, modified Franklin-Silverman, or punch biopsy.
   b. Surgical technique.

To remove focal lesions near the center of the spleen, make a rectangular or oval incision through the capsule and into the parenchyma, to sufficient depth to remove the lesion. Close the defect by placing simple interrupted or mattress sutures of absorbable material (3-0 or 4-0) in the splenic capsule.

C. Repair of Lacerations

1. General considerations.
   a. Splenorrhaphy is indicated to provide hemostasis in superficial traumatic lesions of the splenic capsule.

2. Surgical technique.

Explore the lesion and ligate any large traumatized vessels. Place simple interrupted or mattress sutures of absorbable material (3-0 or 4-0) in the splenic capsule. Apply gentle pressure to the area for several minutes. If bleeding continues, ligate the splenic branches supplying the lesion as close to the hilus of the spleen as possible. Small areas of ischemia will revascularize as a result of collateralization.

D. Partial Splenectomy

1. General considerations.
   a. May be performed if more diffuse lesions are present.
   b. Partial splenectomy is indicated in animals with traumatic or focal lesions of the spleen, to preserve splenic function.
2. Surgical technique.

Define the area of the spleen to be removed, and double ligate and incise hilar vessels supplying the area. Note the extent of ischemia that develops, and use this as a guideline for the resection. Squeeze the splenic tissue at this line between a thumb and forefinger, and milk the splenic pulp toward the ischemic area. Place forceps on the flattened portion, and divide the spleen between the forceps. Close the cut surface of the spleen adjacent to the forceps with a continuous suture pattern of absorbable suture material (3-0 or 4-0). Alternatively, place two rows of mattress sutures in a continuous overlapping fashion at the line of demarcation. If hemorrhage continues, oversew the end of the spleen with a continuous suture of absorbable suture material.

   a. Automated stapling devices (e.g., TA staplers) may also be used for partial splenectomy.
   b. If the staples are not secured in sufficient tissue, they will loosen and allow hemorrhage to occur from the splenic stump.
   c. Either 3.5- or 4.8-sized stainless steel staples are recommended.

E. Total Splenectomy

1. General considerations.
   a. Total splenectomy is most commonly performed in animals with splenic neoplasia, torsion (stomach or spleen), or severe trauma.
   b. Splenectomy has been advocated for immune-mediated hematologic disorders refractory to medical therapy.
   c. Life-threatening sepsis has been associated with complete splenectomy in humans, but has not been recognized in dogs.
   d. Partial splenectomy is preferred over total splenectomy, when possible.
   e. The major disadvantages of total splenectomy are loss of its reservoir, immune-defense, and hematopoiesis and filtration functions.
   f. Splenectomy is contraindicated in patients with bone marrow hypoplasia in which the spleen is a main site of hematopoiesis.
2. Surgical technique.

After exploring the abdomen, exteriorize the spleen, and place moistened abdominal sponges or laparotomy pads around the incision under the spleen. Double ligate and transect all vessels at the splenic hilus with absorbable (preferred) or nonabsorbable suture material. Preserve the short gastric branches supplying the gastric fundus, if possible. Alternatively, open the omental bursa, and isolate the splenic artery. Identify the branch(es) supplying the left limb of the pancreas. Double ligate and transect the splenic artery distal to this vessel(s).

a. Interference with blood flow through the pancreatic branch of the splenic artery may result in ischemic pancreatitis and peritonitis.

VII. Suture Materials/Special Instruments

A. Have a large number of clamps available.

B. Use absorbable suture material.

C. If generalized peritonitis is present, use monofilament synthetic absorbable suture material for vessel ligation (e.g., polydioxanone or polyglyconate).

VIII. Postoperative Care and Assessment

A. Following splenic biopsy or splenectomy, closely observe the animal for 24 hours for evidence of hemorrhage.

B. Evaluate the hematocrit every few hours until the animal is stable.

C. Administer nasal oxygen to anemic patients and give analgesics, if necessary.

D. Hemorrhage may be indicative of technical failures or disseminated intravascular coagulation.

E. Mild postoperative leukocytosis may occur following splenectomy in dogs because the spleen influences bone-marrow leukocyte production; however, large or prolonged elevations may indicate infection (i.e., splenic abscess or peritonitis).

F. Increased numbers of Howell-Jolly bodies, nucleated erythrocytes, target cells, or platelets may also be found postsplenectomy.

Splenic Torsion (*SAS*, pp. 454-456)

I. Definitions

A. **Splenic torsion** occurs when the spleen twists on its vascular pedicle.

II. General Considerations and Clinically Relevant Pathophysiology

A. Splenic torsion most commonly occurs in association with gastric dilatation-volvulus.

B. Isolated splenic torsion is rare.

1. Typically, the thin-walled splenic vein is occluded, although the splenic artery remains partially patent, resulting in congestive splenomegaly.
2. Vascular thrombosis (particularly of the splenic vein) may occur.
3. In some dogs, clinical signs are acute, although in others the torsion is presumably intermittent, and abnormalities are first noted weeks before diagnosis.

C. Splenic infarction may be associated with liver disease, renal disease, hyperadrenocorticism, neoplasia, or thrombosis associated with cardiovascular disease.

1. Splenic infarction in these dogs appears to be a sign of altered blood flow and coagulation, rather than of the primary disease.
2. Splenectomy should be reserved for those animals that have life-threatening complications, such as hemoabdomen or sepsis.

III. Diagnosis

A. Clinical Presentation

1. Signalment.
   a. Splenic torsion usually occurs in large-breed dogs (e.g., Great Danes), with no age or sex predilection.
2. History.
   a. Most animals present because of some combination of vomiting, weakness or depression, icterus, hematuria or hemoglobinuria, abdominal pain, and/or diarrhea.
   b. Clinical signs may be acute or chronic.
   c. Acute torsion may cause signs of cardiovascular collapse and shock.

B. Physical Examination Findings

1. The most prominent physical examination finding is splenic enlargement or a midabdominal mass.
2. Abdominal pain, fever, dehydration, pale mucous membranes, and/or icterus are sometimes found.

C. Radiography/Ultrasonography

1. The most common radiographic findings are decreased visceral detail associated with peritoneal effusion and small intestine displacement.
2. Occasionally, gas bubbles within the spleen may be identified, presumably formed by gas-producing bacteria.
3. Ultrasonography may reveal a markedly enlarged spleen that is diffusely hypoechoic, with linear echoes separating large, anechoic areas.

D. Laboratory Findings

1. Laboratory analysis may reveal anemia, leukocytosis, hemoglobinuria, elevated serum alkaline phosphatase activity, and/or elevated alanine transaminase activity.

IV. Differential Diagnosis

A. Differentials include other causes of splenomegaly (i.e., neoplasia, trauma, hematoma, abscess, or immune-mediated disease), peritoneal effusion (i.e., peritonitis or ascites), other midabdominal masses (e.g., gastrointestinal, pancreatic, renal, or lymph node enlargement), and gastric dilatation-volvulus.

V. Medical Management

A. Splenic torsion is a surgical disease; medical management is limited to stabilizing the animal for surgery.

B. If the animal is shocky, initiate intravenous fluids and antibiotic therapy.

VI. Surgical Treatment

A. General Considerations

1. Animals exhibiting shock should be operated on as quickly as possible after they have been stabilized.
2. Gastric dilation-volvulus may occur in dogs following splenic torsion and stretching of the gastric ligaments; prophylactic gastropexy may be warranted at the time of splenectomy.

B. Preoperative Management

1. Correct fluid deficits and electrolyte and acid-base abnormalities before surgery, if possible.
2. Give whole blood to animals with hematocrits less than 20%.
3. Perioperative antibiotic therapy is recommended.
4. Electrocardiograms are warranted to determine if cardiac arrhythmias are present that may require therapy before anesthetic induction or during surgery.
5. The enlarged and congested spleen may rupture with handling, causing abdominal hemorrhage; therefore have blood transfusion products available.

C. Anesthesia

1. See recommendations for gastric dilatation-volvulus, Appendix G-8.
2. Avoid barbiturates or other drugs that cause splenic congestion.

D. Positioning

1. Position the animal in dorsal recumbency, and prepare the entire ventral abdomen.
2. Extend the ventral incision from the xiphoid and make it long enough to allow the enlarged spleen to be manipulated and exteriorized.

VII. Surgical Technique

A. The treatment of splenic torsion is somewhat controversial.

B. Some authors recommend that in animals with acute torsion, the splenic pedicle be untwisted and the spleen repositioned. If vascular patency is present, restoration of blood flow will cause the spleen to decrease to near-normal size within a few minutes.

C. Splenectomy may be safer, because there is no good way to secure the spleen in its normal position, and torsion may recur.

1. Splenectomy is the only viable option in animals in whom the

vascular pedicle cannot be untwisted because of fibrosis, splenic rupture, or vascular thrombosis.

VIII. Postoperative Care and Assessment

A. Vomiting may occur postoperatively, associated with pancreatic ischemia and pancreatitis.

IX. Prognosis

A. The prognosis is generally good following surgical management of splenic torsion.

B. Delayed diagnosis may result in splenic necrosis, sepsis, peritonitis, and/or disseminated intravascular coagulation.

Splenic Neoplasia (*SAS*, pp. 456-459)

I. Definitions

A. **Hemangiosarcomas** (i.e., hemangiosarcoma-angiosarcoma, hemangioendothelioma) are malignant neoplasms that arise from blood vessels.

B. **Hemangiomas** are benign tumors of dilated blood vessels.

C. A **hematoma** is a swelling, or mass of blood (usually clotted), confined to an organ, tissue, or space, and caused by seepage as a result of coagulopathy.

II. General Considerations and Clinically Relevant Pathophysiology

A. The most common tumor in dogs is hemangiosarcoma. Other malignant and benign neoplasms may also occur.

B. The most frequently recognized nonneoplastic lesions of the spleen are nodular hyperplasia and hematomas.

C. Canine splenic hemangiosarcoma is more common than all other types of malignant splenic tumors combined.
   1. Between 24% and 45% of dogs with splenic hemangiosarcoma have concurrent right atrial hemangiosarcoma.
   2. Splenic hemangiosarcomas frequently metastasize to liver, omentum, and mesentery.
   3. Lung metastases may be more common in dogs with right atrial tumors than in those without.

D. Splenic hematomas are variably sized, encapsulated, blood and fibrin-filled masses that are often grossly indistinguishable from hemangiosarcomas.

1. They may result from trauma, occur spontaneously, or may be secondary to other diseases.

E. Hemangiomas and hemangiosarcomas may be difficult to distinguish histologically, but because the prognosis for these lesions is very different (see below), it is important that they be accurately differentiated.

1. Multiple sections of a malignant mass may be studied without seeing obvious malignancy.

F. Mastocytoma, lymphosarcoma, myeloproliferative disease, and hemangiosarcoma are the most common neoplasms of the feline spleen.

1. Splenic involvement is a consistent finding in cats with noncutaneous systemic mastocytosis.

III. Diagnosis

A. Clinical Presentation

1. Signalment.
   a. Splenic tumors (including hematomas) usually occur in medium-to-large sized dogs.
   b. German shepherd dogs are at increased risk for hemangiosarcoma and hemangioma.
2. History.
   a. Dogs with hemangiosarcoma may present for abdominal enlargement, anorexia, lethargy, depression, and/or vomiting or may have acute signs of weakness, depression, anorexia, and hypovolemic shock caused by splenic rupture and hemorrhage.
   b. Clinical signs with splenic hematoma are similar, except that rupture leading to collapse and anorexia are less common because large masses frequently become apparent before rupture occurs.
   c. Splenic rupture and hemorrhage are uncommon in dogs with nonangiogenic and nonlymphomatous splenic tumors.

B. Physical Examination Findings

1. Physical examination findings include lethargy, weakness, abdominal distention, and possibly splenomegaly or a splenic mass.
2. If rupture occurs, the animal may present with signs of hypovolemic shock (tachycardia, pale mucous membranes, and weak peripheral pulses).

C. Radiography/Ultrasonography

1. Abdominal masses are usually detected radiographically in dogs with hemangiosarcoma and nonangiogenic and nonlymphomatous sarcomas; however, peritoneal fluid may make locating the lesion in the spleen difficult.
2. Ultrasonography is more definitive in locating lesions in the spleen and detecting abdominal metastases.
3. Before surgery, echo the heart to look for right atrial involvement.
4. Take thoracic radiographs to detect pulmonary or thoracic neoplasia.

D. Laboratory Findings

1. Neutrophilic leukocytosis may be present.
2. Mild or moderate anemia associated with chronic disease and/or hemoperitoneum is common.

3. Numerous nucleated blood cells, Howell-Jolly bodies, poikilocytosis, acanthocytosis, schistocytosis, and/or thrombocytopenia may be found.
4. Thrombocytopenia caused by disseminated intravascular coagulation is common in dogs with splenic tumors.
5. Cytologic analysis of abdominal fluid rarely reveals tumor cells.

IV. Differential Diagnosis

A. Splenic hematoma and hemangioma must be differentiated from hemangiosarcoma and other neoplastic diseases.

B. When cavitary lesions are identified with ultrasound, perform FNA cautiously, or not at all.
1. Diagnosis of hemangiosarcoma is difficult with FNA.
2. Rupture of cavitary lesions may occur during aspiration and be fatal.
3. The presence of hepatic nodules may indicate metastasis and malignancy in dogs with splenic masses, but the hepatic nodules may also represent extramedullary hematopoiesis or nodular hyperplasia.

V. Medical Management

A. Surgical resection is the mainstay of therapy for splenic hemangiosarcoma.

VI. Surgical Treatment

A. General Considerations

1. Splenectomy is the treatment of choice for animals with splenic hematoma, hemangioma, hemangiosarcoma (if extensive metastasis or other organ failure does not preclude the short-term benefits of removing the enlarged and/or ruptured spleen).
2. Splenectomy may not be warranted in dogs with concurrent right atrial tumors.
3. Dogs with splenic lymphoma and clinical signs associated with massive splenomegaly, splenic rupture, and hemoperitoneum may benefit from splenectomy.

B. Preoperative Management

1. Anemic animals may require blood transfusions before surgery and should be preoxygenated.
2. Perform an ECG to determine if ventricular arrhythmias are present. Perioperative antibiotics may be indicated in some animals undergoing splenectomy.

C. Anesthesia

1. See recommendations for gastric dilatation-volvulus, Appendix G-8.
2. Avoid barbiturates or other drugs that cause splenic congestion.

D. Positioning

1. Place the animal in dorsal recumbency for a ventral midline celiotomy.

VII. Surgical Technique

A. Total splenectomy, rather than partial splenectomy, is warranted in animals with malignant tumors or large benign masses.

VIII. Suture Materials/Special Instruments

A. Strong, monofilament absorbable or nonabsorbable suture should be used in closing the abdominal incision.

IX. Postoperative Care and Assessment

A. Observe animals with splenic hemangiosarcoma for disseminated intravascular coagulation following splenectomy.

B. Monitor the hematocrit and give blood transfusions if the PCV is less than 20%.

C. Antibiotic therapy can be discontinued within 24 hours in most animals.

X. Prognosis

A. The prognosis for animals with hemangiosarcoma depends on whether clinical signs are apparent at the time of surgery.

B. Most dogs with splenic hemangioma live 1 year or more after surgery.

21

Surgery of the Kidney and Ureter (*SAS*, pp. 461-480)

General Principles and Techniques (*SAS*, pp. 461-470)

I. Definitions

A. **Nephrectomy** is excision of the kidney.

B. **Nephrotomy** is a surgical incision into the kidney.

C. **Nephrostomy** is the creation of a permanent fistula leading into the pelvis of the kidney; temporary nephrostomy tubes (nephropyelostomy) are occasionally used to divert urine when obstructive uropathy occurs or when the proximal ureter has been avulsed from the kidney.

D. **Pyelolithotomy** is an incision into the renal pelvis and proximal ureter.

E. **Ureterotomy** is an incision into the ureter.

F. **Neoureterostomy** is a surgical procedure performed to correct intramural ectopic ureters.

G. **Ureteroneocystostomy** involves implantation of a resected ureter into the bladder.

II. Preoperative Concerns

A. The minimum database for urinary dysfunction includes BUN, creatinine, urinalysis, hematocrit, total protein, albumin, electrolytes (especially potassium), total CO_2, and an ECG, if electrolytes are not readily available.

B. Acute renal disease usually causes moderate or severe dehydration.

C. Most oliguric animals have acute renal failure; however, many animals with nonobstructive acute renal failure are not oliguric.

D. Preoperative intravenous fluid therapy is needed to restore circulating blood volume and urine production; however, fluids must be administered judiciously to avoid overloading these patients.

E. Diuretics may also be helpful to enhance urine production in animals that are adequately hydrated.

F. Urine production of hydrated animals on maintenance fluids that do not have abnormal extrarenal losses should be at least 50 ml/kg/day or greater than 2 ml/kg/hr.

G. Electrolyte and acid–base abnormalities may occur.
1. Hyperkalemia is often present in acute obstructive renal disorders and some acute renal parenchymal disorders.
2. Hypokalemia may occur with acute or chronic renal disease and diuretic therapy.
3. Clinically important hypocalcemia is occasionally associated with acute renal disease.
4. Metabolic acidosis may be present in animals with acute or chronic renal disease.

H. Animals with chronic renal failure may be anemic.
1. Gastric ulceration, bleeding, or increased red cell fragility may occur in uremic patients.

III. Anesthetic Considerations

A. Give anemic patients oxygen before induction and during recovery.

B. Use anticholinergic drugs to prevent bradycardia.

C. Monitor systemic arterial blood pressure and urine output during surgery.
1. Avoid hypotensive drugs (e.g., acetylpromazine) in animals with renal impairment.
2. If the animal is oliguric but normotensive, use low-dose dopamine (1-2 μg/kg/min intravenously), with or without furosemide (0.2 mg/kg intravenously). Alternatively, mannitol (0.25-0.5 g/kg intravenously) may be used in cats.
3. If oliguria and hypotension coexist, administer dopamine (2-10 μg/kg/min intravenously) or dobutamine (2-10 μg/kg/min intravenously).

D. Avoid thiobarbiturates if arrhythmias are present.

E. Isoflurane is the inhalation agent of choice in arrhythmic patients.

F. Premedicate with an anticholinergic (i.e., atropine or glycopyrrolate) and oxymorphone, butorphanol, or buprenorphine (see Appendixes G-17 and G-18).

G. If the animal has minimal renal compromise, use a thiobarbiturate, propofol, or a mask for induction.

H. Avoid ketamine in cats with renal compromise.

I. If the dog is severely depressed, oxymorphone plus diazepam may allow intubation.

J. If additional drugs are needed, administer etomidate or a reduced dose of thiobarbiturate or propofol intravenously, or use mask induction if the animal is not vomiting.

K. Monitor urine output during and after surgery.

IV. Antibiotics

A. Animals with renal calculi or ectopic ureters may have concurrent infections. Use appropriate antibiotics, based on urine culture and susceptibility. Alternatively, withhold antibiotics until appropriate intra-operative cultures have been taken.
   1. Avoid potentially nephrotoxic antibiotics (i.e., aminoglycosides, tetracycline [except doxycycline], and sulfonamides).
   2. Penicillin drugs (i.e., penicillin G, ampicillin, amoxicillin, and combinations of clavulanic acid and amoxicillin) are highly concentrated in urine.
   3. Cephalosporins (e.g., cefazolin, 20 mg/kg intravenously at induction) have an enhanced gram-negative spectrum, are excreted in the urine, and are often used for perioperative antibiotic therapy.
   4. Fluoroquinolones (e.g., enrofloxacin) have a broad activity against aerobic gram-negative bacteria.

V. Surgical Anatomy

A. The kidneys lie in the retroperitoneal space lateral to the aorta and caudal vena cava.
   1. The cranial pole of the right kidney lies at the level of the thirteenth rib.

B. The renal pelvis is the funnel-shaped structure that receives urine and directs it into the ureter.
   1. There are generally five to six diverticula that curve outward from the renal pelvis.

C. The renal artery normally bifurcates into dorsal and ventral branches.

D. The ureter begins at the renal pelvis and enters the dorsal surface of the bladder obliquely, by means of two slitlike orifices.
   1. The blood supply to the ureter is from the cranial ureteral artery (from the renal artery) and the caudal ureteral artery (from the prostatic or vaginal artery).

VI. Surgical Techniques

A. Perform a ventral midline abdominal incision from the xiphoid to caudal to the umbilicus.
   1. If the distal ureter must be transected (i.e., for nephrectomy) or a cystotomy is necessary, extend the incision to the pubis.
   2. Use Balfour retractors to retract the abdominal wall and expose the kidney.
      a. Expose the right kidney by elevating the duodenum and displacing the other loops of intestine toward the animal's left side.
      b. Expose the left kidney by elevating the mesocolon so that the small intestine is retracted to the animal's right side.

B. Renal biopsy (*SAS*, p. 463).

1. General considerations.
    a. Renal biopsy may be indicated to diagnose the cause of renal insufficiency (especially acute renal failure), hematuria (rare), or proteinuria.
    b. It may be performed at surgery, or percutaneously, with the aid of ultrasound, laparoscopy, a keyhole abdominal incision, or blindly.
    c. Of the percutaneous techniques, ultrasound-guided biopsy is preferable.
        i. Avoid percutaneous biopsy in patients with bleeding disorders, large intrarenal cysts, perirenal abscesses, or obstructive uropathy.
        ii. Give fluids before, during, and shortly after biopsy to initiate and maintain a mild diuresis, which may decrease the formation of blood clots within the renal pelvis.
    d. Surgical biopsies may be performed using a biopsy instrument (e.g., Vim Tru-Cut or Franklin modified Vim-Silverman biopsy needles) or a wedge resection.
2. Needle biopsy.
    a. Surgical technique.

Perform a needle biopsy with a Tru-Cut instrument by placing the tip of the instrument on the kidney capsule, with the obturator specimen rod fully retracted within the outer cannula. Push the specimen rod into the lesion by advancing the plastic handle. Then advance the outer sheath of the needle into the tissue to sever the biopsy sample. Withdraw the needle, with the outer sheath over the specimen rod. Apply digital pressure to the site to control hemorrhage. Be sure that the sample is primarily cortical tissue.

3. Wedge biopsy.
    a. Surgical technique.

For a wedge biopsy, make an incision into the renal parenchyma with a No. 15 scalpel blade. Make another incision at an angle to the first incision to remove a wedged-shaped piece of parenchyma. Be sure to include cortex in the sample. Close the incision with a mattress suture of 3-0 absorbable suture material.

C. Nephrectomy (*SAS*, pp. 463-464).

1. General considerations.
    a. Nephrectomy is indicated for renal neoplasia, severe trauma resulting in uncontrollable hemorrhage or urine leakage, pyelonephritis that is resistant to medical therapy, hydronephrosis, and ureteral abnormalities (i.e., avulsion, stricture, rupture, or calculi) that defy surgical repair.
    b. Before nephrectomy, assess renal function in the opposite kidney by determining its glomerular filtration rate (GFR).
    c. Excretory urograms can produce anuric/oliguric renal failure in animals with previously mild or moderate renal disease.
    d. If renal neoplasia is suspected, perform radiography (thoracic and abdominal) and ultrasonography to help rule out metastasis (including to the opposite kidney).
    e. To avoid unintentional transection, always identify the opposite ureter.
2. Surgical technique.

Grasp the peritoneum over the kidney and incise it. Free the kidney from its sublumbar attachments, using a combination of blunt and sharp dissection. Elevate the kidney and retract it medially to locate the renal artery and vein on

the dorsal surface of the renal hilus. Identify any branches of the renal artery. Double ligate the renal artery with absorbable (e.g., polydioxanone or polyglyconate) or nonabsorbable (e.g., cardiovascular silk) suture close to the abdominal aorta, to ensure that all branches have been ligated. Identify the renal vein and ligate it similarly. The left ovarian and testicular veins drain into the renal vein and should not be ligated in intact dogs. Avoid ligating the renal artery and vein together to prevent an arteriovenous fistula from forming. Ligate the ureter near the bladder with absorbable suture material. Remove the kidney and ureter, and after procuring appropriate culture specimens, submit them for histologic examination.

D. Partial nephrectomy (*SAS*, p. 464-465).

1. General considerations.
    a. Partial nephrectomy is occasionally warranted for focal renal lesions, particularly if optimal preservation of renal function is necessary because of bilateral renal dysfunction.
        i. Avoid electrocoagulation of bleeding vessels because this causes excessive parenchymal damage.
        ii. Avoid partial nephrectomy in animals with clinically significant coagulopathies.
    b. Total nephrectomy is easier and has less risk of postoperative hemorrhage.
2. Surgical technique.

If possible, strip the renal capsule from the area of the kidney to be excised. Use absorbable suture (No. 0 or 1) with two long, straight needles attached. Thread the needles into the kidney at the proposed resection site. Tie the thread into three separate ligatures, but avoid damaging the renal vessels or ureter. Excise the renal tissue distal to these ligatures. Ligate any bleeders and suture the exposed diverticula with absorbable suture material (2-0 or 3-0). Approximate the capsule over the end of the kidney, and anchor it to the sublumbar tissues to prevent rotation of the kidney. Alternatively, clamp the renal vessels with vascular forceps, and excise the kidney parenchyma. Ligate parenchymal vessels, and close the renal pelvis and diverticula. Suture the capsule as described above, and remove the clamps from the renal vessels.

E. Nephrotomy (*SAS*, pp. 464-465, 466).

1. General considerations.
    a. Nephrotomy is usually performed to remove calculi lodged within the renal pelvis, but it may also be performed to explore the renal pelvis for neoplasia or hematuria.
    b. Avoid nephrotomy in patients with severe hydronephrosis.
    c. Nephrotomy may temporarily decrease renal function by 25% to 50%.
    d. Closure of nephrotomy incisions may be accomplished without sutures or with transparenchymal horizontal mattress sutures. The latter may cause increased vascular strangulation, pressure necrosis, infarction, and postoperative hemorrhage.
        i. Cyanoacrylate adhesive provides rapid hemostasis; however, if the adhesive enters the renal diverticula, calculus formation may occur.
2. Surgical technique.

Locate the renal vessels, and temporarily occlude them with vascular forceps, a tourniquet, or an assistant's fingers. Mobilize the kidney to expose the convex lateral surface. Make a sharp incision along the midline of the convex border of the kidney sufficient to allow removal of the calculi and

inspection of the entire renal pelvis. Extend the incision from the capsule to the pelvic diverticula. Alternatively, make a sharp incision through the capsule, and bluntly separate the renal parenchyma with forceps. Obtain a culture of the renal pelvis. Remove the calculi and flush the kidney with warm saline or lactated Ringer's solution. Assess the ureter for patency by placing a 3.5 French soft rubber catheter down the ureter and flushing it with warm fluids. Close the nephrotomy by apposing the cut tissues and applying digital pressure (for approximately 5 minutes), while restoring blood flow through the renal vessels (sutureless technique). Alternatively, appose the capsule with a continuous pattern of absorbable suture material. If adequate hemostasis is not achieved or urine leakage is a concern, place absorbable sutures through the cortex in a horizontal mattress fashion. Then suture the capsule with a continuous pattern of absorbable suture material. Replace the kidney in its original location. Sutures may be placed in the peritoneum where the kidney was elevated to help stabilize it.

F. Pyelolithotomy (*SAS,* pp. 465-466).
   1. General considerations.
      a. Pyelolithotomy may be performed to remove renal calculi if the proximal ureter and renal pelvis are sufficiently dilated.
      b. Pyelolithotomy is extremely difficult if the ureter is not dilated.
   2. Surgical technique.

Dissect the kidney from its sublumbar attachments, and expose the dorsal surface. Identify the ureter and renal vessels. Make an incision over the dilated pelvis and proximal ureter, and remove the calculi. Flush the renal pelvis and diverticula with warm saline to remove small debris. Next flush the ureter to ensure its patency. Close the incision with a continuous suture of 4-0 or 5-0 absorbable suture material.

G. Ureterotomy (*SAS,* pp. 466-467).
   1. General considerations.
      a. Ureterotomy is occasionally performed to remove obstructive calculi.
      b. There is a risk of postoperative leakage and stricture formation.
      c. If obstruction is not present, dietary dissolution of struvite calculi may be attempted. However, removal of calculi is indicated if obstruction occurs or seems likely (e.g., hydroureter or hydronephrosis).
      d. Some stones located in the distal ureter may be flushed or pulled into the bladder through a cystotomy, making a ureterotomy unnecessary.
      e. Use of stenting catheters is controversial because they may promote stricture formation and infection.
      f. Transverse or longitudinal incisions may be made in the ureter; however, there may be less tension on transverse ureterotomies, and thus they may heal more readily.
   2. Surgical technique.

Make a transverse or longitudinal incision in the dilated ureter proximal to the calculi and remove them. Place a small, soft rubber catheter into the ureter proximal and distal to the incision, and flush the ureter with warm fluid. Be certain that all calculi have been removed and that the ureter is patent. Close the incision with simple interrupted sutures of 5-0 to 7-0 absorbable suture material. Alternatively, if the ureter is not dilated and stricture formation seems likely, make a longitudinal incision over the calculi, and close the incision in a transverse fashion. If the ureter has been damaged, perform a resection and anastomosis or proximal urinary diversion.

H. Ureteral anastomosis (*SAS*, pp. 467-469).

1. General considerations.
   a. Ureteral anastomosis is difficult in small patients and has a high rate of postoperative obstruction.
   b. If the ureter is transected or damaged near the bladder, ureteroneocystostomy may be performed (explained later in this chapter).
   c. If the ureter is avulsed from the renal pelvis, urinary drainage can be performed by placing a catheter through the renal parenchyma into the ureter.
      i. If function is adequate in the opposite kidney, consider nephrectomy.
   d. Do minimal dissection around the ureter to avoid compromising its blood supply.
   e. To avoid damaging the ureter, use stay sutures for manipulation and avoid traumatic forceps.
   f. Avoid tension across the anastomotic site.
   g. A bladder-flap ureteroplasty has been described for ureteral trauma near the bladder.
2. Surgical technique.

For ureteral anastomosis, suture the ureter directly, or spatulate it by making a longitudinal incision on opposite sides of each end of the ureter. Preplace absorbable sutures (5-0 or 6-0) at the apex of the spatulated incisions and align the ureteral ends. Appose the ureteral ends with simple interrupted sutures, using the preplaced sutures. Close the remainder of the ureter with simple interrupted sutures. Ensure that the ends of the ureter are not twisted and that sufficient sutures have been placed to prevent leakage.

I. Neoureterostomy (*SAS*, p. 467).

1. General considerations.
   a. Neoureterostomy is performed for intramural ectopic ureters.

J. Ureteroneocystostomy (*SAS*, p. 467).

1. General considerations.
   a. Ureteroneocystostomy is performed for extraluminal ectopic ureters and to repair ureters that are damaged near the bladder.
   b. The ureter is resected or debrided and reimplanted into the bladder lumen.

VII. Healing of the Kidney and Ureter

A. Scar production occurs and may obliterate some functional nephrons, but wound contraction is usually minimal.

B. Renal pelvis and collecting ducts experience wound contraction and scar tissue formation, resulting in strictures.

C. Uroepithelium may seal a damaged area within 48 hours. If at least 50% of the ureteral circumference remains, the ureter will heal by epithelization, fibrous connective tissue synthesis, and longitudinal versus circumferential wound contraction.

D. Peristalsis is absent in the distal segment of a transected ureter for at least 10 days after repair.

1. Immobilizing the ureter to surrounding structures will also inhibit peristalsis and diminish urine flow.

VIII. Suture Materials/Special Instruments

A. Use absorbable suture material such as polyglactin 910 (Vicryl), polyglycolic acid (Dexon), polydioxanone (PDS), or polyglyconate (Maxon).

B. PDS and Maxon maintain tensile strength and are more slowly absorbed than is desirable for most urinary surgery, but they have less tissue drag than Dexon or Vicryl.

C. The use of pediatric or ophthalmic instruments will facilitate surgery of the ureter.

IX. Postoperative Care and Assessment

A. Perform abdominocentesis if hemorrhage or leakage is suspected.

B. Monitor central venous pressure and urine output. Indwelling urinary catheters allow urine output measurement.

C. Monitor animals for urethral obstruction following repair of ectopic ureters.
   1. This will typically go undetected unless the surgery was bilateral or abdominal radiographs or ultrasonography documents significant hydroureter or hydronephrosis.

D. Diagnose urinary leakage by abdominocentesis and measurement of fluid creatinine levels (not BUN). With uroperitoneum, creatinine levels in the abdominal fluid will be greater than serum creatinine levels.

X. Special Age Considerations

A. Older animals often have some degree of renal compromise and require careful monitoring during any surgical procedure.

B. Avoid hypotension during surgery and the postoperative period to prevent further renal damage.

C. If cardiac disease is also present, use fluids judiciously to prevent overhydration while maintaining renal blood flow.

Ectopic Ureter (*SAS*, pp. 470-475)

I. Definitions

A. **Ectopic ureter** (i.e., ureteral ectopia) is a congenital anomaly in which one or both ureters empty outside the bladder.

B. **Extraluminal ectopic ureters** are those that completely bypass the bladder.

C. **Intraluminal ectopic ureters** course submucosally in the bladder to open in the urethra or vagina.

II. General Considerations and Clinically Relevant Pathophysiology

A. The ureter normally enters the dorsolateral, caudal surface of the bladder and empties into the trigone after a short intramural course.

B. Associated abnormalities (i.e., urethral sphincter incompetence, bladder hypoplasia, vestibulovaginal abnormalities, or ureteroceles) may occur concurrently with ectopic ureters.

C. Surgical correction of ureteral ectopia is recommended; however, the presence of other abnormalities increases the likelihood of postoperative incontinence.

D. Approximately 70% to 80% of affected dogs have unilateral intramural or extramural ectopia.
   1. Intramural lesions are more common.

E. Ureteral ectopia is less common in cats, but bilateral ectopia may occur more frequently in cats than in dogs.

F. Pyelonephritis and cystitis are common in dogs with ureteral ectopia.
   1. Hydroureter is the most frequent urogenital abnormality in dogs with ureteral ectopia and may be caused by chronic infection, obstructed urine outflow, or a primary lack of ureteral peristalsis.
   2. With unilateral ectopia, hydroureter and hydronephrosis may occur in the contralateral ureter as a result of chronic ascending urinary tract infections (UTIs).

G. Hypoplastic bladders or intrapelvic bladders may be congenital or secondary to lack of normal filling of the bladder.

III. Diagnosis

A. Clinical Presentation

1. Signalment.
   a. Ectopic ureters are usually seen in female dogs.
   b. Siberian huskies have an increased incidence of ureteral ectopia; golden retrievers, Labrador retrievers, miniature poodles, and some terrier breeds may also have a higher-than-expected incidence.
   c. Ureteral ectopia should be suspected in any young animal that presents with a history of incontinence since birth; however, this condition should also be included as a differential in older animals with lifelong urinary incontinence.
2. History.
   a. Urinary incontinence is usually constant, but may be intermittent.
   b. Many affected animals are able to urinate normally.

B. Physical Examination Findings

1. Physical examination findings include wetness of perivulvar hair, odor, and irritation or urine-scalding of surrounding skin.

C. Radiography/Ultrasonography

1. The size and shape of the kidneys, bladder, and prostate should be assessed with survey abdominal radiographs.
2. Excretory urography is the most commonly used method for confirming ectopic ureters and defining associated urogenital abnormalities (i.e., hydronephrosis, hydroureter, hypoplastic bladder, and ureteroceles).
   a. Extramural ectopia is best identified before the bladder completely fills with contrast.
   b. Contrast radiography does not accurately identify all ectopic ureters and often fails to differentiate between intramural and extramural lesions.
3. Retrograde cystography, pneumocystography (with animal in dorsoventral position to allow gas contrast to rise adjacent to ureters), and vaginoscopy may help correctly define ectopic ureter morphology.
4. Cystoscopy may be the most reliable method for diagnosing ectopic ureters in females.

D. Laboratory Findings

1. Concomitant urinary tract infection is common.
2. Renal failure may be present because of chronic pyelonephritis, obstructive uropathy, or concurrent congenital abnormalities.

IV. Differential Diagnosis

A. Ureteral ectopia should be considered likely in any young animal presenting for incontinence.

B. Other causes of incontinence include, behavioral incontinence, urge incontinence (associated with inflammation or infection), neurogenic disorders (i.e., lower and upper motor neuron disorders or reflex dyssynergia), anatomic outflow obstruction (i.e., paradoxical incontinence), and urethral sphincter incontinence (i.e., hormone-responsive incontinence).

C. Eliminate behavioral, urge, neurogenic, and hormone-responsive incontinence before considering tests for ectopia in older animals.

V. Medical Management

A. Incontinence may persist after surgical correction if there is concomitant urethral sphincter incompetence.

B. α-Adrenergic agonists (i.e., phenylpropanolamine or ephedrine) or diethylstilbestrol may be used to increase urethral sphincter tone.

1. Phenylpropanolamine.
   a. Dogs–1.5 to 2.0 mg/kg PO, BID
   b. Cats–1.5 mg/kg PO, TID

VI. Surgical Treatment

A. Surgical correction is the treatment of choice for ectopic ureters, even if marginal improvement occurs with medical management.
1. Perform surgery as soon as possible to prevent secondary abnormalities resulting from ascending urinary tract infections or outflow obstruction.
2. Perform neoureterostomy for intramural ectopic ureters.
3. If the ureter is extraluminal, resect the ureter and reimplant it into the bladder lumen.

B. Preoperative management.
1. Use appropriate antibiotics, as indicated by urine culture and susceptibility testing. If antibiotic therapy has not been initiated before surgery, administer antibiotics (e.g., cefazolin) after intraoperative cultures have been taken.
2. Determine renal function before surgery if there is hydronephrosis or renal fibrosis.
3. Remove nonfunctional kidneys.

C. Anesthesia.
1. If renal impairment is not present, many different anesthetic regimens can be used safely (see Appendixes G-17 and G-18).

D. Positioning.
1. Place the animal in dorsal recumbency and prepare the abdomen from above the xiphoid to below the pubis.

VII. Surgical Technique

A. General Considerations

1. Explore the entire urinary system before repairing the ureter.
2. Remove nonfunctional kidneys and their ureter, but first consider bilateral ectopia.
3. Ligate the end of the ectopic ureter as close to its termination as possible.

B. Neoureterostomy

1. General considerations.
   a. Handle the bladder tissues with extreme care, and use stay sutures whenever possible.
   b. Once the bladder has been emptied of urine, use sterile Q-tips to absorb urine (rather than a sponge) to avoid abrading the mucosal surface.
   c. Use pediatric instruments to help decrease tissue trauma.
2. Surgical technique.

Make an incision into the ventral bladder, near the urethra. Place stay sutures to facilitate retraction of the bladder wall edges. Inspect the trigone for ureteral openings. Identify a submucosal swelling or ridge within the bladder wall; this may be facilitated by digitally occluding the urethra to cause ureteral dilation. Use a No. 15 scalpel blade to make a 3- to 5-mm longitudinal incision through the bladder mucosa into the ureteral lumen. Use simple interrupted sutures to suture the ureteral mucosa to the bladder with a 5-0 to 7-0 absorbable suture material. Place a 3.5- or 5-French catheter into the distal

ureter. Just distal to the new stoma, pass one or two nonabsorbable sutures (3-0 or 4-0) from the serosal surface circumferentially around the tube, staying beneath the mucosa. Be sure that the suture does not penetrate the bladder lumen. Use this suture to ligate the distal ureter after removing the catheter. Close the proximal urethra with simple interrupted or simple continuous sutures (single or double layer), but ensure that the urethral diameter is not compromised. Close the bladder in such a manner as to ensure a water-tight seal (i.e., simple continuous or inverting suture pattern, depending on the bladder wall thickness).

C. Ureteroneocystostomy

1. General considerations.
   a. If the ureter is extraluminal, resect and reimplant it into the bladder lumen.
   b. In dogs, implant the ureter into the bladder using a simple transverse pull-through or an intramural tunnel (3 : 1 tunnel length to ureteral orifice diameter) technique.
   c. Microsurgical techniques may be necessary to prevent ureteral obstruction in cats.
2. Surgical technique.

Perform a ventral cystotomy as described above for neoureterostomy. Ligate the ureter and transect it, preserving as much length as possible. Place a stay suture on the proximal end of the transected ureter. Incise the bladder mucosa, and create a short oblique submucosal tunnel in the bladder wall. Use the stay suture to draw the ureter into the bladder lumen to avoid damaging the ureter. Make a 1- to 2-mm longitudinal incision in the ureter end (i.e., spatulate it) and suture it to the bladder mucosa with absorbable suture (e.g., polyglycolic acid or polyglactin 910).

VIII. Suture Materials/Special Instruments

A. Use absorbable suture material such as polyglactin 910 (Vicryl), polyglycolic acid (Dexon), polydioxanone (PDS), or polyglyconate (Maxon).

B. Small suture (i.e., 4-0 or 5-0) is preferred to suture the ureter to the bladder mucosa.

C. Ligate the distal ureter with nonabsorbable suture because incontinence may recur as a result of recanalization of the distal ureter following the use of absorbable suture material.

IX. Postoperative Care and Assessment

A. Closely observe the animal after surgery for signs of urinary obstruction or leakage.

B. If urethral obstruction occurs because of postoperative swelling, place an indwelling urinary catheter for 3 to 4 days.

C. If bilateral ectopia is corrected during the same surgery (or significant renal impairment exists in the contralateral kidney with unilateral surgery), monitor the animal for signs of renal failure as a result of ureteral swelling and subsequent obstruction.

D. If incontinence continues for longer than 2 to 3 months postoperatively, perform an excretory urogram or cystoscopy to evaluate the ureters.

X. Prognosis

A. Thirty to 55% of patients continue to show some degree of incontinence following surgery.

B. Obtaining urethral pressure measurements before surgery and after phenylpropanolamine therapy is instituted may help predict the likelihood of continence after surgery.

C. Siberian huskies are particularly prone to postoperative incontinence because of a high incidence of urethral sphincter incompetence. These dogs may respond to α-adrenergic agonists.

D. If bladder hypoplasia is present, incontinence may continue until the bladder enlarges and properly functions as a reservoir.

E. Dogs with ureteral troughs may have a poorer prognosis than dogs with nondistended intramural ectopic ureters.

Renal and Ureteral Calculi (*SAS*, pp. 475-478)

I. Definitions

A. **Urolithiasis** refers to having urinary calculi or uroliths (kidney, ureter, bladder, or urethra).

B. Having renal or ureteral calculi (i.e., nephroliths or ureteroliths) is **nephrolithiasis** or **ureterolithiasis,** respectively.

C. **Nephrolithotomy** (i.e., lithonephrotomy) is performed to remove renal calculi from the renal pelvis by incising through kidney parenchyma.

D. **Pyelolithotomy** is an incision into the renal pelvis and proximal ureter.

E. **Ureterolithotomy** is removal of calculi from the ureter by incision.

F. A **staghorn calculus** is one that occurs in the renal pelvis and extends into the diverticula.

II. General Considerations and Clinically Relevant Pathophysiology

A. Only 5% to 10% of canine uroliths are in the kidney and ureter; calculi are found even less commonly at these sites in cats.

B. Uroliths are named according to their mineral content.
1. Struvite (magnesium ammonium phosphate) uroliths are most common. (This is discussed in Chapter 22; see Table 22-1 in particular.)

C. Some disease processes (i.e., portosystemic shunts or hepatic cirrhosis) are associated with a high rate of urolithiasis.

D. Certain breeds (i.e., dalmatians and dachshunds) also have a high incidence of urolithiasis because of metabolic abnormalities.

E. Whether all renal or ureteral stones should be removed is controversial.
1. If they are associated with infection, they should be removed; however, removal of noninfected stones from the renal pelvis may produce more renal damage than the stone caused.
2. Ureteral calculi frequently cause obstruction and often require prompt surgical removal.

F. Any stone that is surgically removed should be submitted for analysis.

G. Microbial cultures of urine (and possible calculi) are mandatory for patients with uroliths.

H. It is difficult to eliminate urinary tract infections if calculi are present.

III. Diagnosis

A. Clinical Presentation

1. Signalment.
   a. Siamese cats may have an increased incidence of nephrolithiasis.
   b. Middle-aged to older animals have a higher rate of urolithiasis than young animals.
   c. Some calculi occur in young animals (i.e., urate calculi associated with portosystemic shunts, struvite calculi in schnauzers).
2. History.
   a. The history varies, depending on whether or not the stone has caused obstruction or there is concurrent infection.
   b. Clinical signs may be intermittent, particularly if the animal has been treated with antibiotics.
   c. A previous history of urolithiasis is common if stone analysis was not performed or appropriate therapy was not instituted following previous surgery.

B. Physical Examination Findings

1. Renal calculi may be asymptomatic or associated with hematuria, flank pain, or renomegaly.
2. Hematuria is often the clinical sign noted in cats with nephrolithiasis.
3. Animals with pyelonephritis may be polyuric or polydipsic, lethargic,

depressed, febrile, anorexic, or uremic (i.e., anorexic, depressed, dehydrated, and vomiting).

4. Dysuria or stranguria may occur if there is concurrent cystitis.

C. Radiography/Ultrasonography

1. Renal calculi may be incidental findings on abdominal radiographs or with ultrasonography.
2. Most renal and ureteral calculi are radiopaque and thus appear as increased densities in the renal pelvis or ureter.
3. Whenever renal calculi are diagnosed, the ureters, bladder, and urethra should also be examined carefully for the presence of calculi.
4. Associated abnormalities (i.e., hydronephrosis or hydroureter) may be assessed by ultrasonography (preferred) or excretory urography.

D. Laboratory Findings

1. Concomitant urinary tract infection is common.
2. Renal failure may be present as a result of chronic pyelonephritis or obstructive uropathy.
3. Findings associated with hepatic disease (low BUN or hypoproteinemia) may be present in some animals with urate calculi.

IV. Differential Diagnosis

A. Uroliths should be considered in any animal presenting for chronic urinary tract infection, hematuria, stranguria, pollakiuria, or acute obstructive uropathy.

V. Medical Management

A. Identify and treat potential underlying causes of renal or ureteral calculi (i.e., infection, portosystemic shunts, or metabolic abnormalities).

B. Some stones can be managed with dietary therapy or pharmacologic agents (see Table 22-1 in Chapter 22).

1. If dietary therapy is used to dissolve renal calculi, there is a risk that the stones will become small enough to enter the ureter and cause obstruction. Therefore monitor these animals carefully for evidence of ureteral obstruction.

VI. Surgical Treatment

A. General Considerations

1. Consider surgical removal of renal and ureteral calculi when they are infected or cause obstruction. Perform surgery as soon as possible once the animal has been stabilized, to prevent irreversible renal damage.

B. Preoperative Management

1. Administer appropriate antibiotics, as indicated by urine culture and susceptibility testing. If antibiotic therapy has not been initiated before surgery, administer antibiotics (e.g., cefazolin) after intraoperative cultures have been taken.
2. Determine renal function before surgery.

3. Nephrectomy, rather than stone removal, is indicated in nonfunctional kidneys; otherwise the kidney and ureter should be preserved.

C. Anesthesia

1. If renal impairment is not present, many anesthetic regimens can be used safely (see Appendixes G-17 and G-18).

D. Positioning

1. Place the animal in dorsal recumbency and prepare the abdomen from above the xiphoid to caudal to the pubis.
2. If nephrectomy is performed, the incision will need to extend caudally, to allow the ureter to be ligated near the bladder.

VII. Surgical Technique

A. Explore the entire urinary system before removing the calculi.

B. Remove renal calculi via a nephrotomy or pyelolithotomy.
   1. If the renal pelvis and proximal ureter are sufficiently dilated, a pyelolithotomy is preferred.
   2. If the stone is large and involves the diverticula plus pelvis, nephrotomy is usually necessary.
   3. Occasionally, soft stones can be crushed and removed through the renal pelvis, but care is necessary to prevent ureteral damage.

C. Bilateral nephrotomy can be performed; however, there is risk that renal failure will occur postoperatively. Staged procedures are preferred.

D. Submit cultures of the renal pelvis or ureter.

E. Submit the stones for analysis and possibly microbial culture.

VIII. Suture Materials/Special Instruments

A. Use absorbable suture material such as polyglactin 910 (Vicryl), polyglycolic acid (Dexon), polydioxanone (PDS), or polyglyconate (Maxon) in the kidney and ureter.

IX. Postoperative Care and Assessment

A. Observe the animal closely after surgery for signs of urinary obstruction or leakage.

B. Renal failure may occur if bilateral nephrotomy was performed or if significant renal impairment was present in the contralateral kidney preoperatively.

X. Special Age Considerations

A. Older animals often have some degree of renal compromise and require careful monitoring during any surgical procedure.

B. Avoid hypotension during surgery and the postoperative period to avoid further renal damage.

C. If cardiac disease is also present, use fluids judiciously to prevent overhydration while maintaining renal blood flow.

XI. Prognosis

A. If the underlying disease, infection, or metabolic abnormality is not treated, most uroliths will recur.

Renal and Ureteral Neoplasia (*SAS*, pp. 478-480)

I. Definition

A. **Nephroblastomas** (i.e., embryonal adenomyosarcoma, nephroma, Wilms' tumor) are rapidly developing malignant mixed tumors that arise from embryonal elements of the kidney.

II. General Considerations and Clinically Relevant Pathophysiology

A. Primary renal tumors are uncommon and are usually malignant.
   1. In dogs, carcinomas are most common.
   2. Lymphoma is the most common renal neoplasm in cats and may be primary or metastatic.

B. Bilateral renal involvement occurs in nearly 30% of dogs with primary renal neoplasia.
   1. Metastasis to liver, adrenal glands, lung, lymph nodes, bone, and brain is common with renal tumors.
   2. Renal metastasis of other primary abdominal tumors is common.

C. Renal neoplasia may cause local signs or systemic manifestations of renal failure.

D. Tumors arising from the renal pelvis are more likely to cause hematuria or hydronephrosis than signs of renal failure.

E. Unilateral renal damage may not be associated with systemic clinical signs, even if the kidney becomes nonfunctional.

F. Large renal neoplasms may compress or invade the caudal vena cava, causing vascular obstruction.

III. Diagnosis

A. Clinical Presentation

1. Signalment.
   a. In German shepherd dogs, renal cystadenocarcinomas have been associated with generalized nodular dermatofibrosis.
   b. Renal neoplasia most commonly occurs in middle-aged to older animals.
   c. Nephroblastomas and undifferentiated renal sarcomas occur most commonly in young dogs and cats; however, they may also occur in older animals.
2. History.
   a. The history of animals with primary renal tumors is often vague and nonspecific.
   b. The most common signs are anorexia, depression, and weight loss.
   c. Occasionally, the only abnormality noted is abdominal enlargement associated with a renal mass.
   d. Renal failure is primarily seen with bilateral involvement (e.g., lymphoma in cats).
   e. Some benign neoplasms (i.e., hemangioma) cause intermittent or constant hematuria.

B. Physical Examination Findings

1. An abdominal mass is often palpated in dogs and cats with renal neoplasia.
2. Weight loss, anorexia, depression, anemia, dyspnea, and pyrexia may be seen.
3. Lameness has been associated with bony metastasis and hypertrophic osteopathy.

C. Radiography/Ultrasonography

1. Renal enlargement may be identified on survey abdominal radiographs; however, ultrasonography is more sensitive and specific.
2. Excretory urography may allow localization of renal neoplasia and assessment of parenchymal involvement.
3. If vascular involvement is suspected, selective angiography can be used to detect intravascular or extravascular (compressive) lesions.
4. Thoracic radiographs should be taken to detect pulmonary metastasis.

D. Laboratory Findings

1. Anemia and azotemia are common.
2. Gross hematuria may occur with mesenchymal (i.e., anaplastic sarcomas fibromas, hemangiosarcomas, and lymphosarcoma) and transitional cell tumors; however, microscopic hematuria is more common.

IV. Differential Diagnosis

A. Renal neoplasia must be differentiated from hydronephrosis; polycystic disease; and abscess and neoplasia of the adrenal glands, spleen, liver, or lymph nodes.

B. Abdominal ultrasonography is the most useful diagnostic tool.

1. Ultrasound-guided biopsy can be performed if the kidney does not appear fluid filled; however, the biopsy may cause peritonitis,

uncontrollable hemorrhage, or may seed the abdomen with tumor cells.

V. Medical Management

A. Preoperative medical management of animals with renal neoplasia is necessary if renal failure is present or anemia is severe (i.e., a PCV of less than 20%).

VI. Surgical Treatment

A. General Considerations

1. Nephrectomy is indicated for malignant renal tumors if they are unilateral and there is no evidence of metastasis.
2. Cats with renal lymphoma may respond to chemotherapy for variable time periods.

B. Preoperative Management

1. Perioperative antibiotic therapy is indicated in some patients (i.e., large neoplasms that may be secondarily infected or immunosuppressed or chronically debilitated patients). Treat animals with preexisting urinary tract infections before surgery.
2. Consider preoperative blood transfusions in moderately to severely anemic patients (see Appendix A).
3. Have blood available for intraoperative and postoperative transfusions.

C. Anesthesia

1. If renal impairment is not present, many anesthetic regimens can be used safely (see Appendixes G-17 and G-18).

D. Positioning

1. Place the animal in dorsal recumbency and prepare the abdomen from above the xiphoid to below the pubis.

VII. Surgical Technique

A. Explore the entire abdomen for metastasis before performing a nephrectomy.

B. Palpate the other kidney and biopsy it if bilateral involvement is suspected.

C. Locate the adjacent ureter to ensure that it is not inadvertently ligated.

D. Remove the entire ureter with the kidney.

E. Handle neoplastic kidney carefully and ligate the renal vein to help prevent seeding of neoplastic cells via the vasculature or directly into adjacent tissues.

VIII. Suture Materials/Special Instruments

A. Use absorbable suture material such as polyglactin 910 (Vicryl), polyglycolic acid (Dexon), polydioxanone (PDS), or polyglyconate (Maxon), or nonabsorbable cardiovascular silk to ligate the renal vessels and ureter.

IX. Postoperative Care and Assessment

A. See postoperative care of patients with renal disease.

B. The major complications of nephrectomy are hemorrhage and urinary leakage if the vessels or ureter are not adequately ligated.

C. If the animal had preexisting renal dysfunction, renal failure may occur postoperatively.

D. With large renal tumors, ligation of the opposite ureter is possible if care is not taken to determine its location intraoperatively.

X. Special Age Considerations

A. Older animals may have some degree of renal dysfunction in the contralateral kidney and require careful monitoring during the surgical procedure.

B. Many animals have bilateral renal neoplasia.

XI. Prognosis

A. The prognosis is typically poor; however, if nephrectomy is performed before metastasis, long-term survival is possible.

22

Surgery of the Urinary Bladder and Urethra (*SAS*, pp. 481-515)

General Principles and Techniques (*SAS*, pp. 481-495)

I. Definitions

A. **Cystotomy** is surgical incision into the urinary bladder.

B. **Cystectomy** is removal of a portion of the urinary bladder.

C. **Urethrotomy** is an incision into the urethra.

D. **Urethrostomy** is the creation of a permanent fistula into the urethra.

E. **Cystolithiasis** and **cystolithectomy** refer to the development of urinary bladder calculi and their removal, respectively.

F. **Uroabdomen** is the condition of having urinary leakage into the abdominal cavity.

II. Preoperative Concerns

A. General Considerations

1. Urinary obstruction.
   a. May occur if calculi become lodged in the urethra or a tumor obstructs the proximal urethra or trigone.
   b. Male cats with sterile cystitis may develop penile urethral obstruction.
   c. Obstruction to urinary flow may result in a distended urinary bladder, postrenal uremia, and hyperkalemia.
2. Bladder rupture.
   a. Common after motor vehicular trauma.
   b. Urine leakage may also occur from necrotic bladders (i.e., following damage to its blood supply) or as a complication of bladder surgery.
   c. Urinary leakage into the abdominal cavity results in uremia, dehydration, hypovolemia, hyperkalemia, and death if undiagnosed or untreated.

3. Urinary obstruction and uroperitoneum are *medical* emergencies, not surgical emergencies.
4. Hyperkalemia associated with these conditions makes the animal prone to cardiac arrhythmias; therefore correct fluid and electrolyte abnormalities before induction of anesthesia (see Appendix J).
   a. Treat mild or moderate hyperkalemia with IV fluids (i.e., 0.9% saline for dilution).
   b. If the animal has concurrent hyponatremia, avoid 5% dextrose solutions (i.e., D_5W) and half-strength saline.
   c. If the hyperkalemia appears immediately life-threatening, give 10% calcium gluconate slowly intravenously until other therapy lowers the plasma potassium concentration.
5. In animals with uroperitoneum, treat hyperkalemia and azotemia with fluids (dilution) and abdominal drainage.
   a. Penrose drains can be used for short-term management in patients with uroabdomen.
   b. Abdominal drainage for 6 to 12 hours is often adequate.
   c. Alternately, accomplish peritoneal drainage by placement of a peritoneal dialysis catheter.
6. Subcutaneous urine leakage causes bruising and/or swelling of the tissues
   a. The skin and subcutaneous tissues can necrose if left untreated.
   b. Management of patients with urethral rupture before surgery may necessitate placement of an indwelling urinary catheter and/or cutaneous urinary diversion (tube cystostomy).

III. Anesthetic Considerations

A. Correct electrolyte (e.g., hyperkalemia) and acid–base abnormalities (see Appendixes C and J) in patients with urinary obstruction or leakage before anesthetic induction.

B. Give intravenous fluids to restore normal hydration and combat postobstruction diuresis.

C. Monitor an ECG before, during, and after surgery for cardiac arrhythmias. If the animal is hyperkalemic, use 0.9% saline for fluid therapy. If the serum potassium is normal, use a balanced electrolyte solution.

D. Do not use anticholinergics for trauma patients because they may increase heart rate and oxygen consumption and cause a predisposition to cardiac arrhythmias.

E. Dogs.
1. If analgesia is needed, give butorphanol, oxymorphone, or buprenorphine in small, incremental doses (see Appendix F).
2. Only use acetylpromazine if volume replacement has been adequate and shock or severe blood loss is unlikely.
3. Use thiobarbiturates cautiously in animals with preexisting arrhythmias (see Appendixes G-19 and G-20).
4. Use combinations of opioids and benzodiazepines (diazepam), which do not cause severe vasodilation or myocardial depression, for inducing anesthesia despite hypovolemia or dehydration.
5. Consider etomidate for induction, because it maintains cardiovascular stability and is not arrhythmogenic.

6. If the patient is not vomiting, consider mask or chamber induction, or administer thiopental or propofol at reduced dosages.

F. Cats.
   1. Premedicate cats using low dosages of butorphanol, buprenorphine, or oxymorphone and induce with etomidate.
   2. Because cats excrete in their urine the active form of ketamine, use it very cautiously (if at all) if urinary obstruction or renal dysfunction is present.

G. Use isoflurane, because it is the least cardiodepressant inhalation anesthetic.

IV. Antibiotics

A. Consider perioperative antibiotic therapy in animals with urinary obstruction or leakage because infection prolongs healing and may promote stricture formation.

B. Place animals with cystic or urethral calculi on appropriate antibiotics based on urine culture and susceptibility, because they often have concurrent infections.

C. Alternatively, withhold antibiotics until appropriate intraoperative cultures have been taken.

D. Avoid potentially nephrotoxic antibiotics (i.e., aminoglycosides, tetracycline) in patients with obstructions.

V. Surgical Techniques

A. Cystotomy (*SAS,* pp. 483-485).
   1. General considerations.
      a. Make an incision on the dorsal or ventral surface of the bladder, away from the urethra.
      b. Perform ventral exposure if identification and/or catheterization of the ureteral openings is necessary.
      c. For closure, use a single- or double-layer appositional pattern or invert suture patterns using absorbable suture material.
         i. If the bladder wall is thick, use a single-layer appositional closure and do not penetrate the bladder lumen with the sutures.
         ii. In normal bladders, use of a double-layer inverting suture pattern with luminal penetration is common.
   2. Surgical technique.

Isolate the bladder from the rest of the abdominal cavity by placing moistened laparotomy pads beneath it. Place stay sutures on the bladder apex to facilitate manipulation. Make the incision in the dorsal or ventral aspect of the bladder, away from the ureters and urethra and between major blood vessels. Remove urine by suction (perform intraoperative cystocentesis before cystotomy if suction is not available). Excise a small section of the bladder wall

adjacent to the incision and submit it for culture. Check the bladder apex for a diverticulum and remove it if necessary. Examine the mucosa for defects and pass a catheter down the urethra to check for patency. Close the bladder in two or three layers with absorbable suture material. For a two-layer closure, suture the seromuscular layers with two continuous inverting suture lines (i.e., Cushing, followed by Lembert). If a three-layer closure is used, suture the mucosa as a separate layer with a simple continuous suture pattern.

B. See *SAS,* pp. 484-485 for cystostomy (prepubic catheterization), including Foley catheter placement and Stamey catheter placement.

C. Intrapelvic urethral anastomosis (*SAS,* pp. 486-487).

1. General considerations.
   a. For small lacerations or partial ruptures, divert urine through a urethral catheter or tube cystostomy for 7 to 21 days, and allow to heal by second intention.
   b. Perform primary suture repair of a completely transected urethra whenever possible.
2. Surgical technique.

Incise the caudal ventral midline of the abdomen and, if necessary, perform a pubic symphysiotomy or bilateral pubic and ischial osteotomy (explained later in this chapter). Locate the transected ends of the urethra and debride them. Minimize dissection around the urethra and bladder to avoid damaging the vascular or nerve supply to these structures. Suture the ends with six to eight absorbable interrupted sutures over a transurethral catheter (preferably a Foley catheter or other soft catheter). Leave the catheter in place for 7 to 10 days.

If the urethral tissues do not hold suture because of prolonged urine extravasation and subsequent tissue devitalization, perform delayed repair. Place a transurethral catheter to divert urine flow for 5 to 7 days. If a catheter cannot be placed from the penile orifice into the bladder, pass a catheter from the bladder into the traumatized tissue, tie it to a catheter placed from the penile urethral orifice, and use it to pull the penile catheter into the bladder. If the urethra does not heal completely in 7 to 10 days or stricture occurs, resect the urethral ends and suture them over a catheter as described for primary repair. Tube cystostomy can also be used to provide urinary diversion while the urethra is healing, but take care to ensure that the bladder is not allowed to distend or urethral flow of urine will occur.

Obtain adequate urethral exposure by splitting the symphysis on the midline. If necessary, remove the cranial aspect of the pubis. Bilateral pubic and ischial osteotomy allows exposure of the entire urogenital tract in female dogs.

Make a ventral midline incision from the umbilicus to the vulva. Perform a celiotomy from the umbilicus to the pubis, then sharply separate the adductor muscles on the midline of the pubis and ischium. Subperiostally elevate the adductor muscles until the obturator nerves and half of the obturator foramen are exposed. Transect the prepubic tendon along the left pubis to the proposed pubic osteotomy site. Predrill holes in the pubis and ischium on both sides of the four proposed osteotomy sites and craniocaudally along the left pubis. Osteotomize the pubis and elevate the internal obturator muscle from the left pubis and ischium, allowing reflection of the entire central bony plate to the right. To close the osteotomy sites, preplace orthopedic wire through the previously drilled holes on the right side. Then, before replacing the bone plate, place sutures through the lines of holes in the left pubis and ischium, through the left internal obturator muscle, and back through the adjacent holes in the pubis or ischium. Place orthopedic wire through the left osteotomy sites, then secure the preplaced wires and sutures. Reappose the adductor muscles and prepubic tendon before closing the linea alba.

D. Urethrotomy (*SAS,* pp. 487-490).

1. Prescrotal urethrotomy.

With the dog in dorsal recumbency, place a sterile catheter into the penile urethra to the scrotum or to the obstruction. Make a ventral midline incision through the skin and subcutaneous tissues, between the caudal aspect of the os penis and scrotum. Identify, mobilize, and retract the retractor penis muscle laterally to expose the urethra. Using a No. 15 scalpel blade, make an incision into the urethral lumen over the catheter. Iris scissors can be used to extend the incision, if necessary. Remove calculi with forceps and gently flush the urethra with warm saline. The incision may be left to heal by second intention or the urethra may be closed with simple interrupted absorbable sutures (4-0 or 5-0). Place the first layer in the urethral mucosa and corpus spongiosum, then appose subcutaneous tissues and skin with simple interrupted sutures or a continuous subcuticular suture pattern. Some surgeons prefer a continuous suture pattern in the urethra to promote hemostasis. Remove the urinary catheter following surgery, regardless of whether the urethra is sutured or not.

2. Perineal urethrotomy.

Place a purse-string suture in the anus. Place a sterile catheter into the urethra to the level of the bladder or the site of the obstruction. With the dog in sternal recumbency and the rear limbs hanging over the edge of the table, make a midline incision over the urethra, midway between the scrotum and anus. Identify the retractor penis muscle, elevate, and retract it. Separate the paired bulbospongiosus muscles at their raphe to expose the corpus spongiosum, then incise the corpus spongiosum to enter the urethral lumen. Close the incision as described above for prescrotal urethrotomy.

E. Urethrostomy (*SAS,* pp. 489-492).

Make a 3- to 4-cm incision in the urethral mucosa as described above. Make the length of the urethral incision 6 to 8 times its luminal diameter. Place periurethral sutures to the subcutaneous tissues using a simple continuous suture pattern of absorbable suture material. Place simple interrupted absorbable sutures (3-0 to 5-0) from the urethral mucosa to the skin beginning at the caudal aspect of the incision. Suture the remainder of the urethral mucosa to the skin with simple interrupted sutures (see SAS, Fig. 22-15). Suture skin at either end of the incision with simple interrupted sutures.

1. Scrotal urethrostomy.

If the dog is intact, castrate him and excise the scrotum; otherwise, perform scrotal ablation. Place a sterile catheter into the urethra to the level of the ischial arch or beyond. Make a midline incision over the urethra through the subcutaneous tissues. Identify the retractor penis muscle, mobilize, and retract it laterally to expose the urethra. Using a No. 15 scalpel blade, make a 3- to 4-cm incision into the urethral lumen over the catheter. Suture the urethra as described above for prescrotal urethrostomy.

2. Canine perineal urethrostomy.

Make a 4- to 6-cm incision in skin and overlying tissues and incise the perineal urethra as described above for perineal urethrotomy. The urethral incision should be 1.5 to 2.0 cm in length. Suture the urethral mucosa to the skin as described above for prescrotal urethrostomy.

3. Prepubic urethrostomy.

Make a ventral midline incision from the umbilicus to the pubis. Free the intrapelvic urethra from the pelvic floor using blunt dissection. Be sure to preserve the urethral artery and its branches. Sever the distal aspect of the intrapelvic urethra. It may be necessary to carefully dissect the prostate from the urethra to ensure that there is ample urethra to exteriorize in some male dogs. Preserve the blood supply to the neck of the bladder. In male dogs, exteriorize the urethra through a small stab incision 2 to 3 cm lateral to the prepuce or within the prepuce. In females, exteriorize the urethra through the ventral midline incision or 2 to 3 cm lateral to the linea alba. Spatulate the distal end of the urethra to increase the luminal diameter, then suture the urethral mucosa to skin with interrupted sutures of absorbable (e.g., polyglyconate or polydioxanone suture) or nonabsorbable (e.g., nylon or polypropylene) suture. Be sure that there is little tension on the urethrostomy site and that the urethra is not bent sharply. A Foley catheter can be placed into the bladder through the urethrostomy to divert urine during initial healing (i.e., 24-48 hours).

4. Subpubic urethrostomy.

Perform this procedure similarly to the one described above, but retract the skin caudally past the brim of the pubis. Expose the medial boundary of the obturator foramen by elevating the adductor muscle and cranial portion of the gracilis muscle from the periosteum of the pubis. Partially incise the prepubic tendon and reflect it laterally to expose the pubic rami. Osteotomize the pubic rami 1.5 cm lateral to the pubic symphysis. Make a transverse incision through the body of the pubic bone and across the pubic symphysis. Rotate the pubic flap ventrally to visualize the intrapelvic urethra. Transect the urethra cranial to the lesion (i.e., stricture) and replace the pubic flap. Reappose the muscular aponeuroses of the gracilis and adductor muscles with interrupted or horizontal mattress sutures. Make a 1-cm stab incision 3 cm distal to the caudal extent of the abdominal incision. Tunnel through the subcutaneous tissues and exteriorize the urethra. Spatulate the urethral end and suture it to the skin with 4-0 suture material. Close the abdominal incision but leave the caudal 1 cm of the linea alba open to avoid crimping the urethra as it passes over the pubic flap. Resect the tissues at the perineal urethrostomy site and either close them or leave them open to heal by second intention.

F. Urinary diversion is described in *SAS*, pp. 492-493.

VI. Healing of the Bladder and Urethra

A. Compared with other organs, the urinary bladder heals quickly, regaining 100% of normal tissue strength in 14 to 21 days.

B. If urethral continuity is not completely disrupted, the urethra can heal by regeneration of urethral mucosa in as little as 7 days.

C. Urine extravasation (particularly if infected) delays wound healing and promotes periurethral fibrosis and stricture formation. Urinary diversion via a urethral catheter or tube cystostomy is therefore indicated for small urethral lacerations.

D. When complete transection of the urethra occurs, fibrous tissue often leads to stricture and urinary obstruction. Perform primary anastomosis over an indwelling catheter (or proximal urinary diversion) to decrease the likelihood of stricture formation. Leave the catheter in place for 3 to 5 days.

VII. Suture Materials/Special Instruments

A. Use absorbable suture material (e.g., polydioxanone [PDS], polyglyconate [Maxon], polyglycolic acid [Dexon] or polyglactin-910 [Vicryl]) for bladder and urethral surgery.

B. Avoid nonabsorbable sutures because of their potential to promote calculi formation.

VIII. Postoperative Care and Assessment

A. Monitor urination closely in patients after urethral surgery to detect obstruction caused by tissue swelling, fibrosis, or necrosis.

B. Following removal of the urinary obstruction, maintain intravenous fluid therapy until postobstructive diuresis ceases.

C. Monitor electrolytes (particularly potassium) because hypokalemia may occur secondary to diuresis or medical therapy of hyperkalemia.

D. Monitor patients for pain postoperatively and provide analgesics.

E. Use Elizabethan collars in patients with indwelling urinary catheters, urethrotomies, or urethrostomies to prevent early catheter removal or self-mutilation.

F. With urethrotomy, observe the patient for postoperative hemorrhage. If necessary, use digital pressure on the surgical site to stop bleeding immediately after surgery or after urination (for 3 to 5 days).

G. Bladder atony may occur in as little as 12 hours if the animal is sedated or given narcotic analgesics postoperatively, or does not void because of pain.

H. Keep the bladder decompressed by manually expressing it until the patient is urinating normally.

I. In cats with urethrostomies, use paper instead of gravel litter until the wound is healed and perform urinary cultures routinely to check for UTI.

J. Do not use an indwelling catheter, which may promote stricture formation and UTI in cats following surgery.

IX. Special Age Considerations

A. Monitor older animals closely because they may have preexisting cardiac or renal dysfunction.

B. Young animals may have very small urethras, making surgical repair of complete transections difficult.

Uroabdomen (*SAS,* pp. 496-499)

I. Definition

A. **Uroabdomen** is an accumulation of urine in the peritoneal cavity. Urine may leak from the kidney, ureter, bladder, and/or proximal urethra.

II. General Considerations and Clinically Relevant Pathophysiology

A. Bladder rupture is the most common cause of uroabdomen in dogs and cats.
   1. It may occur spontaneously (associated with tumor, severe cystitis, or urethral obstruction), be due to blunt or penetrating abdominal trauma, or be iatrogenic following cystocentesis or bladder catheterization.
   2. Urinary tract leakage may also be a complication of surgery.

B. Assess any animal presenting after vehicular trauma for possible urinary tract trauma.

C. Immediate surgery is contraindicated in animals with uroabdomen that are hyperkalemic or uremic.
   1. For the correction of hyperkalcemia, see Preoperative Concerns, pp. 362-363, and Appendix J.

III. Diagnosis

A. Clinical Presentation

1. Signalment.
   a. There is no age, sex, or breed disposition associated with most causes of urinary tract leakages.
   b. Male dogs and cats with obstruction caused by calculi or sterile cystitis (FUS) have a high risk of bladder rupture if the obstruction is not alleviated promptly.
2. History.
   a. Clinical signs of urinary tract trauma are often vague and may be masked by other signs of trauma.
   b. The animal may present for azotemia (i.e., vomiting, anorexia, depression, lethargy), or hematuria, dysuria, abdominal pain, and/or abdominal swelling or herniation may be noted.
   c. Abdominal and perineal bruising are common with vehicular trauma, particularly if there are pelvic fractures, and may indicate subcutaneous urine leakage.
   d. In female dogs, there may be a history of previous catheterization using a rigid catheter.
   e. Rupture of the urethra is most frequently associated with pelvic fractures in male dogs.
   f. Remember that animals with ruptured bladders or unilateral ureteral trauma may urinate normal volumes, without evidence of hematuria. Similarly the ability to retrieve fluid while performing bladder catheterization does not preclude the diagnosis of a ruptured bladder.

B. Physical Examination Findings

1. Perform abdominal palpation to determine the size and shape of the bladder.
2. Examine the animal closely for abdominal swelling or fluid accumulation.
3. Monitor urine quantity and character (i.e., hematuria, dysuria) and bruising on the ventral abdomen or perineum.

C. Radiography/Fluoroscopy

1. Survey radiographs may show reduced size or absence of the urinary bladder, lack of contrast and increased size of the retroperitoneal space, and/or lack of normal intraabdominal contrast.
2. If a ruptured bladder is suspected, perform a positive contrast cystourethrogram.
   a. Free contrast agent in the abdominal cavity will coat and highlight abdominal organs.
3. During excretory urogram contrast leakage into the retroperitoneal space (for proximal lesions) or abdomen (for distal lesions) occurs with ureteral rupture or laceration.

D. Laboratory Findings

1. Perform a CBC and serum biochemical profile with electrolytes. Hyperkalemia and azotemia may be noted.
2. Perform analysis of abdominal fluid if urinary tract rupture is suspected.
   a. Measure creatinine (not BUN).
   b. With uroabdomen, expect creatinine levels of the abdominal fluid to be greater than those in the blood.
3. Renal failure may be present if obstruction preceded the rupture.
4. Bladder rupture secondary to UTI may result in septic peritonitis.

IV. Medical Management

A. If the animal is not hyperkalemic or azotemic, rehydrate it with 0.9% saline and perform immediate surgical repair.

B. If concurrent trauma delays surgery, perform abdominal drainage and/or urinary diversion (i.e., urethral catheter and/or tube cystostomy) until the animal is stable.

C. With delayed diagnosis, correct electrolytes, hydration, and acid–base balance before surgery.

D. Administer antibiotics based on culture results if infection is present, or prophylactically if abdominal drains are placed.

V. Surgical Treatment

A. General Considerations

1. Repair urethral trauma primary anastomosis (immediate or delayed), or allow the urethra to heal over a urinary catheter if it is not completely transected.
2. Repair ureteral rupture by anastomosis or reimplantation into the bladder, depending on location of the damage.

3. Bladder rupture generally occurs near the apex.
   a. Perform surgical exploration and repair the rupture, or if it is very small, keep the bladder decompressed and allow to heal.
   b. Explore the entire abdomen to determine the reason for rupture and/or identify concurrent trauma.
4. If bladder rupture is secondary to severe cystitis, tumor, or obstruction, the bladder may be extremely friable or large areas may be necrotic, making excision and primary closure of the rent difficult. In such cases, perform prolonged urinary diversion.
5. If cystitis or tumor is present, submit a biopsy of the bladder mucosa for culture and histologic examination.
6. In animals with rupture caused by obstruction from calculi, carefully check the urethra for calculi and verify its patency before repairing the bladder defect.

B. Preoperative Management

1. Evaluate an ECG for arrhythmias.
2. If possible, correct hydration, acid–base, and electrolyte abnormalities before surgery.
3. If antibiotic therapy has not been initiated before surgery, give perioperative antibiotics (e.g., cefazolin) at induction.

C. Anesthesia

1. See Appendix G-19 for anesthetic protocols for bladder surgery.
2. See Appendix G-20 for anesthetic recommendation for patients in renal failure.
3. If the animal is vomiting, avoid mask or chamber induction.

D. Positioning

1. Place the animal in dorsal recumbency and prepare the abdomen for a ventral midline incision.
2. For bladder rupture, prep the entire ventral abdomen to allow complete exploration of the abdomen.

E. Surgical Technique

1. See the description of cystotomy, p. 364.

Excise devitalized or necrotic bladder tissue and suture the rent with a one- or two-layer continuous suture pattern. If the bladder is markedly thickened, perform a single-layer anastomosing pattern; otherwise, use a two-layer inverting pattern. If tissues are friable and a water-tight seal is not achieved, perform a serosal patch over the incision line.

VI. Postoperative Care and Assessment

A. Give intravenous fluids until the animal is able to drink adequate fluids to maintain hydration.

B. Closely observe the patient after surgery for signs of urinary obstruction or peritonitis.

C. Urinary tract infection is common with indwelling or repeated catheterization.

D. If bladder atony is present, keep the bladder decompressed by intermittent urinary catheterization or by manual expression.

1. Use an α-blocker (e.g., phenoxybenzamine) and/or a somatic muscle relaxant (e.g., diazepam) to decrease urethral sphincter tone.
2. Bethanechol is a cholinergic that increases detrusor contractility and may aid voiding.
3. Manually express the bladder with care following surgery (particularly in patients with friable bladders secondary to infection or obstruction) to avoid disrupting the suture line.

VII. Prognosis

A. The prognosis is excellent for animals with traumatic bladder rupture. Occasionally rupture secondary to obstruction may have a guarded prognosis if the majority of the bladder is necrotic.

Bladder and Urethral Calculi (*SAS*, pp. 499-503)

I. Definitions

A. **Urolithiasis** is a term that refers to having urinary calculi or uroliths (kidney, ureter, bladder, or urethra).

B. **Cystolithiasis** and **cystolithectomy** refer to the development of urinary bladder calculi, and their removal, respectively.

II. General Considerations and Clinically Relevant Pathophysiology

A. The large majority of canine uroliths are found in the bladder or urethra.

B. Struvite (i.e., magnesium ammonium phosphate) calculi are the most common canine uroliths, followed by calcium oxalate, urate, silicate, cystine, and mixed types.

C. UTIs are an important predisposing cause for the formation of struvite calculi in dogs. Feline struvite formation usually occurs despite absence of UTI.

D. Although dissolution of some stones is possible, surgical removal is often necessary initially to allow a diagnosis of stone type.

E. Appropriate medical management may help decrease the recurrence of canine uroliths (Table 22-1).

Table 22-1
Treatment and prevention of canine urolithiasis

Urolith type	Treatment options	Prevention
Struvite	Surgical removal or dissolution Hill's s/d diet Control infection Urease inhibitor? Keep urine pH <6.5, BUN <10 mg/dl, and urine specific gravity <1.020	Hill's c/d diet Monitor urine pH and urine sediment; treat any infections quickly and appropriately
Calcium oxalate	Surgical removal	Hill's u/d diet? Potassium citrate?
Urate	Surgical removal or dissolution Hill's u/d diet Allopurinol Control infection	Hill's u/d diet Allopurinol if necessary Correct congenital portosystemic shunts
Silicate	Surgical removal	Hill's u/d diet Prevent consumption of dirt
Cystine	Surgical removal or dissolution Hill's u/d diet D-penicillamine *N*-(2-Mercaptopropionyl)-glycine (MPG)	Hill's u/d diet Thiol-containing drugs if necessary

Modified from Nelson R, Couto G: *Essentials of small animal internal medicine,* St Louis, 1995, Mosby.

III. Diagnosis

A. Clinical Presentation

1. Signalment.
   a. Uroliths may occur in dogs of any age, but they are most frequently observed in middle-aged dogs.
   b. Struvite uroliths.
      i. Are more common in female dogs than males because females more commonly have UTI; however, urethral obstruction from stones is more common in males.
      ii. Calculi in dogs less than 1 year of age are often struvite because of UTI.
   c. Calcium oxalate uroliths.
      i. Are more common in male dogs, particularly miniature schnauzers, miniature poodles, Yorkshire terriers, Lhasa apsos, and shih tzus.
      ii. Middle-aged to older dogs are most commonly affected.
   d. Urate uroliths.
      i. Sixty percent occur in dalmatians—most of the remainder are seen in breeds that commonly have portosystemic shunts (i.e., Yorkshire terriers, Pekingese, Lhasa apsos).
   e. Silicate uroliths.
      i. Middle-aged, male German shepherds seem to be at increased risk.
   f. Cystine uroliths.
      i. Frequently occur in middle-aged, male dachshunds.
2. History.
   a. Clinical signs of UTI (i.e., hematuria, pollakiuria, stranguria) are common.

b. Small stones may lodge in the urethra of male dogs and cause partial or complete urinary obstruction.
c. Bladder distention, abdominal pain, stranguria, paradoxical incontinence, and/or signs of postrenal azotemia (i.e., anorexia, vomiting, depression) may develop.
d. Occasionally bladder rupture will occur and result in uroabdomen.

B. Physical Examination Findings

1. The bladder wall is often thickened and the stones themselves are occasionally palpable.
2. Signs consistent with UTI may be noted.
3. Abdominal pain, anorexia, vomiting, and/or depression may be noted if urinary tract obstruction occurs.

C. Radiography/Ultrasonography

1. Radiograph and/or ultrasound any animal with urolithiasis. In addition to defining the number and location of bladder and urethral calculi, the procedures may indicate the presence of calculi in the kidney and/or ureter.
2. Calcium-containing uroliths (i.e., calcium phosphate and calcium oxalate) are the most radiodense, whereas cystine and urate uroliths are the least radiopaque.
3. Struvite calculi are normally radiodense and are usually observed with plain radiography.
4. Use retrograde cystourethrography to help identify radiolucent stones in the bladder or urethra.

D. Laboratory Findings

1. Concomitant UTI is common (i.e., pyuria, hematuria, proteinuria, and/or bacteriuria).
2. Renal failure may be present because of chronic pyelonephritis or obstructive uropathy.
3. Findings associated with hepatic insufficiency (low BUN, hypoalbuminemia) may be present in some animals with urate calculi.

IV. Medical Management

A. Relieve urethral obstruction and/or decompress bladder if necessary.
1. Insert a finger in the rectum and massage a urethral urolith toward the vagina to dislodge uroliths in female dogs.
2. Use urohydropropulsion to propel urethral stones back into the bladder in both male and female dogs (see *SAS*, pp. 501-502, Fig. 22-28).

V. Surgical Treatment

A. General Considerations

1. When the urolith has not been typed, consider surgery if there are concurrent or predisposing anatomic abnormalities (e.g., urachal diverticula), if medical dissolution is not possible, or if a bladder mucosal culture is required.
2. Although medical dissolution of struvite, urate, and cystine calculi is possible, surgical removal of calcium oxalate, calcium phosphate, and silicate stones is necessary.
3. Perform cystotomy preferentially over urethrotomy if the stones can be flushed into the bladder either preoperatively or intraoperatively.

4. Submit calculi for stone analysis (and possibly culture) to guide postoperative management and help prevent recurrence, particularly if stone type was not determined based on identification of urine crystals.

B. Preoperative Management

1. Treat postrenal azotemia and hyperkalemia before surgery (see Preoperative Concerns of Surgery of the Urinary Bladder and Urethra).
2. Initiate fluid therapy to promote diuresis.
3. Evaluate an ECG for arrythmias.
4. Eradicate UTI before surgery.
5. Consider perioperative antibiotics if the animal is not already receiving antibiotics. Withhold prophylactic antibiotics until after bladder mucosa has been excised for culture in animals with negative urine cultures.

C. Surgical Technique

Perform a cystotomy and incise a small piece of bladder at the incision and submit it for culture and possibly histologic examination. Remove the bladder stones and carefully check the urethra for additional calculi. In male dogs, place a catheter into the urethra from the penile orifice and occlude the vesicourethral opening with a finger from within the bladder lumen. Have an assistant gently occlude the penile urethra around the catheter with fingers to minimize fluid leakage. Flush the catheter with sterile saline to maximally dilate the urethra (i.e., when additional saline cannot be flushed into the catheter). While fluid is still being flushed into the catheter, remove the finger at the vesicourethral opening. Repeat this procedure until it is certain that no stones remain in the urethral lumen. Check the bladder for urachal diverticula and excise if necessary. Submit the stones for mineral analysis and possibly for microbial culture.

VI. Postoperative Care and Assessment

A. Monitor the animal closely for urinary obstruction or leakage following surgery.

B. Monitor urine sediment and pH regularly and treat UTI promptly.

C. Implement preventive treatment specific to the stone type to help prevent recurrence of urolithiasis.

D. Do not initiate D-penicillamine earlier than 2 weeks after surgery because it may inhibit wound healing.

E. Refer to other sources for specific recommendations regarding medical treatment and prevention of urolithiasis.

VII. Prognosis

A. Recurrence is more common in dogs with cystine and urate stones than in those with oxalate or phosphate stones.

B. Appropriate medical management (i.e., prevention of UTI) is necessary to decrease the recurrence of struvite calculi.

Urethral Prolapse (*SAS*, pp. 503-505) Bladder and Urethral Neoplasia (*SAS*, pp. 505-508)

I. General Considerations and Clinically Relevant Pathophysiology

A. Bladder neoplasia occurs more frequently than neoplasia of the remainder of the urinary system in dogs.

B. In cats, renal lymphosarcoma is more common than bladder neoplasia.

C. Most bladder tumors are malignant; metastasis to the sublumbar lymph nodes and lungs is common. Local extension to the ureters and/or urethra is also common.

D. Transitional cell carcinoma is the most common tumor type in canine and feline bladders.

E. Fibromas, other benign tumors, and inflammatory polyps may also be found.

F. Metastasis of other tumors to the bladder is uncommon although extension of prostatic or urethral tumors may occur.

G. Transitional cell carcinomas are the most common canine urethral neoplasm; urethral tumors are exceedingly rare in cats.

H. Granulomatous inflammation of the urethra in female dogs may cause clinical signs similar to urethral neoplasia and may be differentiated by cytologic evaluation of urethral aspirates or surgical biopsies. The cause is unknown.

II. Diagnosis

A. Clinical Presentation

1. Signalment.
   a. Bladder tumors are more common in dogs than cats.
   b. Older, neutered dogs weighing more than 10 kg are most commonly affected; however, botryoid rhabdomyosarcoma often occurs in young large-breed dogs.
   c. In feline bladder tumors, males are more commonly affected than females. Bladder tumors usually occur in older cats.
   d. Urethral tumors are more common in older female dogs.
2. History.
   a. Most dogs with bladder or urethral tumors are examined because of hematuria, pollakiuria, stranguria, and/or dysuria.
   b. The most common clinical sign in cats is intermittent or persistent hematuria.
   c. If the tumor causes urethral or bladder obstruction, signs of uremia (i.e., vomiting, anorexia, depression) may occur.

B. Physical Examination Findings

1. The physical examination findings are often normal, but may include

a urethral or caudal abdominal mass, prostatomegaly, bladder distention, abdominal pain, weakness, lymphadenopathy, cough or dyspnea, and/or lameness.

2. Urethral masses in females may be palpated rectally or by digital examination of the vagina.

C. Radiography/Ultrasonography

1. Survey abdominal radiographs are rarely diagnostic, but may exclude prostatic disease or urolithiasis.
   a. Examine the sublumbar lymph nodes, pelvis, and vertebrae for metastasis.
   b. Diffuse thickening or calcification of the bladder wall is occasionally noted.
   c. Take thoracic radiographs to identify pulmonary metastasis.
2. Positive-contrast urography and ultrasonography are the most useful tools for diagnosing urethral or bladder neoplasia.
3. Perform retrograde urethrography in dogs with suspected urethral neoplasia to determine the length of the urethra affected and to check for evidence of trigonal involvement.

D. Laboratory Findings

1. Perform a CBC, serum biochemical profile, and urinalysis in animals with bladder tumors. Hematuria, pyuria, proteinuria, and/or bacteriuria are common.
2. Although malignant cells may be found in the urine sediment of some dogs with bladder or urethral tumors, they are not detected in most cats with bladder neoplasia.
3. Take care to avoid confusing neoplastic cells from those that are merely dysplastic; atypical transitional cells are common in animals with cystitis.
4. Empty the bladder and perform cytologic evaluation of a saline wash because prolonged exposure to urine may make interpretation of abnormal cells difficult.

III. Medical Management

A. If partial or complete urinary obstruction is present, stabilize the animal before surgery with fluids and cutaneous urinary diversion (urethral catheter or tube cystostomy).

B. Correct electrolyte and acid–base abnormalities.

C. Treat concurrent UTI with appropriate antibiotics.

D. Evaluate an ECG for arrhythmias.

E. Piroxicam (0.3 mg/kg PO, EOD to SID) has been used to treat nonresectable transitional cell carcinoma of the urinary bladder in dogs. Concurrent use of misoprostol (1-5 μg/kg PO, TID) may be beneficial in these cases.

IV. Surgical Treatment

A. General Considerations

1. Surgical therapy is difficult because the most common site for urinary bladder neoplasia is the trigone.

a. Although the ureters can be transected and implanted into the apex of the bladder following partial cystectomy, incontinence typically occurs if the trigone is removed.
b. Similarly, implantation of the ureters at a distant site (i.e., the colon) following complete cystectomy typically causes pyelonephritis and/or incontinence.
2. Surgical excision of neoplastic lesions may be curative if the tumor is benign.
3. Resection of focal lesions of the urethra is possible with a transpubic surgical approach and urethral resection and anastomosis.
4. Perform prepubic urethrostomy with resection of neoplastic tissues if the distal urethra is involved.
5. Urethral tumors that involve the entire length of the urethra or the bladder trigone are generally inoperable.

B. Preoperative Management

1. See discussion on medical management.

C. Anesthesia

1. See Appendix G-19 for suggested anesthetic protocols.
2. For animals with impaired renal function, see Appendix G-20.

D. Positioning

1. Place the animal in dorsal recumbency, and prepare the abdomen for a ventral midline incision.
2. For bladder neoplasia, extend the incision from above the umbilicus to the brim of the pelvis.
3. With urethral neoplasia, extend the incision caudally to allow a pubic osteotomy to be performed.

E. Surgical Technique

1. Bladder neoplasia.

Examine the sublumbar lymph nodes, ureters, and other abdominal organs for evidence of tumor extension or metastasis. Locate the entrance of the ureters into the trigone and excise the tumor, removing at least 1 cm of normal tissue. Be sure to avoid damaging the ureters. If a large portion of the bladder has been removed, place a urinary catheter and suture the bladder with a continuous appositional suture pattern. Otherwise, a two-layer inverting pattern can be used. If the bladder trigone is involved, consider ureterocolonic urinary diversion, chemotherapy, or euthanasia.

2. Urethral neoplasia.

Check the trigone, ureters, sublumbar lymph nodes, and other abdominal tissues for evidence of neoplasia. Perform a pelvic osteotomy and carefully examine the entire urethra. If the tumor does not involve the entire urethra or trigone, perform a urethral resection and anastomosis. If only the distal urethra is involved and neoplastic tissues can be resected, consider a prepubic urethrostomy. Rarely a benign, pedunculated urethral tumor may be removed through a urethrotomy incision.

V. Postoperative Care and Assessment

A. Observe the animal for urinary leakage or obstruction following surgery.

B. Postoperative care for animals undergoing ureterocolonicanastomosis is described in *SAS,* p. 507.

VI. Prognosis

A. Because of the malignant nature of most lower urinary tract tumors, the prognosis is guarded.

B. Many tumors have already metastasized at diagnosis.

C. With aggressive surgery, urethral tumors may have a better prognosis than bladder tumors.

D. Chemotherapy may allow dogs with bladder tumors to survive for significantly longer periods than if they undergo surgery.

Urinary Incontinence (*SAS,* pp. 508-511)

I. Definitions

A. **Urinary incontinence** is due to failure of voluntary control of the vesical and urethral sphincters with constant or frequent involuntary passage of urine.

II. General Considerations and Clinically Relevant Pathophysiology

A. Poor urethral tone, marked urethral hypoplasia, "pelvic" bladders, ovariohysterectomy, obesity, and congenital abnormalities have all been implicated as potential causes of urinary sphincter mechanism incontinence in female dogs.

B. Congenital urethral sphincter mechanism incontinence has also been described in cats.

C. Some animals respond to estrogen supplementation or drugs that act on the autonomic nervous system.

D. Sympathomimetic drugs, particularly α-adrenergic stimulants (e.g., ephedrine, phenylpropanolamine, and imipramine) have been used to increase urethral sphincter tone.

E. Surgical alternatives to improve urethral resistance include urethral slings, artificial sphincters, urethral lengthening procedures, periurethral injections of polytetrafluoroethylene, colposuspension, and cystourethropexy (see *SAS,* pp. 508).

F. Because these techniques are not uniformly successful, or because success has not been well documented, reserve surgical treatment (other than for congenital abnormalities such as ectopic ureters) for animals that do not respond to medical management (explained later in this chapter), or when the owners refuse to consider long-term drug therapy.

III. Diagnosis

A. Clinical Presentation

1. Signalment.
   a. Medium-sized and large-breed dogs seem to be at increased risk, particularly Doberman pinschers, Old English sheepdogs, and springer spaniels.
   b. Among small-breed dogs, miniature poodles may be at increased risk.
   c. Incontinence may be first noted at any age, depending on the cause.
2. History.
   a. Animals may have a lifelong history of urinary incontinence, or it may occur after ovariohysterectomy.
   b. The incontinence may be continuous, intermittent, or occur only during excitement or when asleep.

B. Radiography

1. Perform excretory urography to identify the termination of the ureters into the bladder.
2. The vesicourethral junction may appear blunted and abnormally dilated, or the urethra may seem abnormally short.
3. In cats with vaginal aplasia, radiographic evidence of a communication between the lumen of the uterus and the bladder may be noted.

C. Laboratory Findings

1. Perform urine cultures in all animals with incontinence, even if the urinalysis is not suggestive of a UTI.

IV. Medical Management

A. Treat dogs with suspected urethral sphincter mechanism incompetence with estrogens and/or sympathomimetic drugs initially.

1. Use diethylstilbestrol (DES) and/or α-adrenergic agonists (i.e., phenylpropanolamine or ephedrine) to increase urethral sphincter tone.
2. If the animal responds to DES, decrease the frequency of administration to the lowest effective dose.
3. High doses of DES may cause estruslike signs, bone marrow toxicity, and/or alopecia; therefore use dosages greater than 1 mg daily with caution.
4. Use of α-adrenergic agonists with DES may allow lower dosages to be used.
5. Phenylpropanolamine is used more frequently than ephedrine because it has fewer side effects (i.e., hyperexcitability, panting, and/or anorexia) and greater efficacy over time.

B. Some male dogs with testosterone-responsive urinary incontinence may be managed by parenteral testosterone.

1. Repositol forms (i.e., testosterone cypionate) are most commonly used.
2. If prostatic enlargement or perianal adenomas are present (or occur during therapy), use phenylpropanolamine or ephedrine rather than testosterone.

V. Surgical Treatment

A. There is presently no single surgical procedure that will cure incontinence in all female dogs with urethral sphincter mechanism incontinence (see *SAS,* pp. 504-510).

B. Preoperative management.
   1. Treat concurrent UTIs before surgery.

C. Positioning.
   1. Place the animal in dorsal recumbency and prepare the abdomen for a ventral midline incision.
   2. Extend the prepped area from the pubis proximally to the umbilicus.

D. Surgical technique.
   1. Bladder flap reconstruction of a hypoplastic urethra.

Perform a ventral cystotomy that extends into the proximal aspect of the hypoplastic urethra. Identify the ureteral openings. Make two stab incisions into the bladder wall caudal and lateral to the ureteral stoma, with the distance between the stab incisions representing the desired circumference of the new urethral tube, in addition to an allowance for suturing. A 4-French (cats) or 8-French (dogs) catheter should pass easily into the newly created urethral tube. Use scissors to extend the incision towards the urethra, creating two full-thickness flaps. Reflect the flaps cranially. Suture the defect from the urethral end cranially to form the urethral tube with a two-layer simple continuous suture pattern or a simple continuous suture pattern and a Cushing's pattern. Use absorbable suture material (2-0 to 4-0). If the urethral lumen is compromised by placing two layers of sutures, suture the urethral tube with a single-layer appositional pattern using care to ensure sufficient apposition of sutures such that urine leakage will not occur. Suture the flaps together. Perform ovariohysterectomy in intact cats in which the uterine horns empty into the bladder.

   2. Colposuspension.

Place a Foley catheter into the bladder and empty it of urine. Make a caudal midline abdominal skin incision extending onto the pubis. Undermine subcutaneous fascia and fat and expose the prepubic tendon bilaterally. Extend the abdominal incision through the linea alba and expose the bladder. Place traction on the bladder and identify the bladder neck by inflating the bulb of the Foley catheter. Bluntly dissect the tissues between the urethra and the pelvic floor. Have an assistant displace the vagina cranially by placing a finger in the vulva. Separate the fat and fascia around the ventral bladder neck and proximal urethra and expose the vaginal wall dorsolateral to the urethra. While maintaining cranial traction on the vagina, place two sutures (0 or 1 monofilament nonabsorbable suture) on each side from the vagina to the prepubic tendon. Place sutures full-thickness through the vaginal wall taking care to ensure that the urethra is not compressed or displaced by the sutures.

VI. Postoperative Care and Assessment

A. See discussion of postoperative care, p. 368.

VII. Prognosis

A. Urinary continence or decreased frequency and volume of urine dribbling appear to occur in most animals with urethral hypoplasia following bladder flap reconstruction.

Feline Urologic Syndrome (Sterile Cystitis) (*SAS,* pp. 512-515)

I. Definition

A. **Feline urologic syndrome** (FUS) is a term used to describe an idiopathic inflammatory process of the feline lower urinary tract that sometimes results in partial or complete urethral obstruction. The current accepted terminology is **sterile cystitis.**

II. General Considerations and Clinically Relevant Pathophysiology

A. Affected cats may or may not have struvite crystals or calculi, and struvite crystalluria may be found without evidence of associated signs of sterile cystitis.

B. UTI is uncommon in cats with obstruction.

C. Dietary factors, obesity, urine alkalinity, UTI, decreased urine volume and decreased frequency of urination, viruses, and vesicourachal diverticula have all been implicated as causes of sterile cystitis in cats; however, the etiology is not defined and is probably multifactorial.

III. Diagnosis

A. Clinical Presentation

1. Signalment.
   a. Overweight cats may be predisposed to sterile cystitis.
   b. Males and females are equally affected; however, male cats are more likely to have obstruction because of the small diameter of their urethras.
   c. Middle-aged cats are more commonly affected and indoor cats may be at increased risk.
2. History.

a. Cats without obstruction usually present for evaluation of pollakiuria, stranguria, hematuria, and/or inappropriate urination.
b. Cats with obstruction may appear uncomfortable or anxious, restless, may attempt to urinate frequently, lick their genitalia, and may have abdominal pain.
c. If obstruction has been present for greater than 36 to 48 hours, anorexia, dehydration, vomiting, collapse, stupor, hypothermia, and/or bradycardia may be noted.

B. Physical Examination Findings

1. If the cat is obstructed, the bladder will feel distended and firm (unless it has ruptured) and cannot be expressed.
2. Abdominal palpation may elicit signs of pain.
3. Take care when palpating the bladder of cats with obstruction to prevent iatrogenic rupture.

IV. Medical Management

A. For cats with obstruction, begin fluid therapy before laboratory data are returned.
1. Give intravenous fluids to restore normal hydration and treat hyperkalemia.
2. Use 0.9% saline in case the cat is hyperkalemic; however, if serum potassium is later found to be normal, administer a balanced electrolyte solution.

B. Promptly relieve obstruction by urethral catheterization or gentle penile massage, if possible.
1. Anesthesia may be required unless the cat is severely depressed.
2. Use sterile isotonic fluid to flush plugs or calculi into the bladder.
3. Use nonmetal, smooth, well-lubricated catheters to minimize urethral trauma.
4. If the catheter cannot be advanced, cystocentesis may be helpful.

C. If a normal stream is not present following catheterization, or detrusor atony is present, an indwelling, soft urinary catheter may be sewn in place; however, this often promotes UTI.

D. Stabilize the cat before performing a perineal urethrostomy.

V. Surgical Treatment

A. General Considerations

1. There is a high incidence of postoperative bacterial UTI after urethrostomy because of anatomic alterations of the urethral meatus, compromised intrinsic defense mechanisms, and the underlying uropathy.
2. Many cats have a permanent loss of striated urethral sphincter function after this procedure, although incontinence is rare.

B. Preoperative Management

1. Correct electrolyte (i.e., hyperkalemia) and acid–base abnormalities before anesthetic induction (see Appendix J).
2. Give intravenous fluids to restore normal hydration and combat postobstruction diuresis.

a. Cats that were initially severely uremic will often have a marked postobstruction diuresis, during which time they require large volumes of intravenous fluids to prevent severe hypovolemia.
3. Monitor serum potassium concentrations to avoid hypokalemia.

C. Anesthesia

1. Monitor an ECG before, during, and after surgery for cardiac arrhythmias.
2. If the cat has been adequately stabilized (i.e., hydration and potassium are normal), use diazepam followed by ultra–short-acting thiobarbiturates (thiamylal sodium, thiopental sodium) or propofol, or mask induction (after premedicating with an opioid).
3. Use thiobarbiturates cautiously in animals with preexisting arrhythmias, as they are arrhythmogenic.
4. Use isoflurane for maintenance because it is the least cardiodepressant inhalation anesthetic.
5. Induce dehydrated or hypovolemic patients or patients in shock with diazepam followed by etomidate, after premedicating with an opioid.
6. Because ketamine is excreted in the urine in its active form, use it very cautiously (if at all) and at low dosages in cats with urinary obstruction.
7. Do not use mask induction if the cat is vomiting.

D. Positioning

1. Place the cat in sternal recumbency with the perineal region elevated slightly.
2. Ventilate, if necessary, when the cat is positioned in this manner.

E. Surgical Technique

1. Perineal urethrostomy.

Place a purse-string suture in the anus and catheterize the penis if possible. Make an elliptical incision around the scrotum and prepuce and excise them. Place an Allis tissue forceps on the end of the prepuce or around the catheter to help manipulate the penis. Reflect the penis dorsolaterally and sharply dissect the surrounding loose tissue on either side. Extend the dissection ventrally and laterally toward the penile attachments at the ischial arch. Elevate the penis dorsally and sharply sever the ventral penile ligament. Then, transect the ischiocavernosus muscles and ischiourethralis muscles at their insertion on the ischium to avoid damaging branches of the pudendal nerves and to minimize hemorrhage. Reflect the penis ventrally to expose the dorsal surface. Expose the bulbourethral glands proximal and dorsal to the bulbospongiosus muscle and cranial to the severed ischiocavernosus and ischiourethralis muscles. Avoid excessive dorsal dissection to prevent damaging the nerves and vessels supplying the urethral muscle. Elevate and remove the retractor penis muscle over the urethra and longitudinally incise the penile urethra using a No. 11 blade or sharp tenotomy scissors. Continue the urethra incision proximal to the pelvic urethra approximately 1 cm beyond the level of the bulbourethral glands. Pass a closed Halsted mosquito hemostat up the urethra to ensure that the urethral width is adequate. The hemostat should be able to be passed to the level of the box-locks without resistance. Suture the urethral mucosa to the skin using 4-0 absorbable (polydioxanone or polyglyconate) or nonabsorbable (nylon or polypropylene) suture on a taper-cut, swaged-on needle. Be sure to suture the urethral mucosa to skin (it is sometimes difficult to identify mucosa). Place the most proximal sutures at a 45-degree angle to the skin first, then place the remainder. Suture the proximal two thirds of the penile urethra to the skin and amputate the distal end by placing a horizontal mattress suture through the skin and penile tissues and severing the penis distal to this ligature. Close the remaining skin with simple interrupted sutures.

VI. Suture Materials/Special Instruments

A. Place a urinary catheter in the urethra to help locate it during the operation.

B. Use monofilament absorbable (polydioxanone or polyglyconate) or nonabsorbable (polypropylene or nylon) suture.

C. Tenotomy scissors and small, atraumatic forceps are useful.

VII. Postoperative Care and Assessment

A. Use paper instead of gravel litter until the wound is healed.

B. Remove the sutures 10 to 14 days after the surgery.

C. Perform urinary cultures periodically to check for UTI.

D. Do not routinely use indwelling catheters following surgery because they may promote stricture formation and/or UTI.

VIII. Prognosis

A. The mortality rate of obstructed cats may exceed 35%. This high rate is often due to the financial constraints of owners reluctant to finance multiple or prolonged hospitalizations.

B. Recurrence of obstruction is uncommon if perineal urethrostomy is performed properly; however, the cat should be monitored periodically for UTI for the remainder of its life.

23

Surgery of the Reproductive and Genital Systems (*SAS*, pp. 517-574)

General Principles and Techniques (*SAS*, pp. 517-538)

I. Definitions

A. **Ovariohysterectomy** (OHE) is the surgical removal of the ovaries and uterus.

B. **Orchiectomy** is the surgical removal of the testicles.

C. **Episiotomy** is an incision of the vulvar orifice to allow access to the vestibule and vagina.

D. **Episioplasty** is a reconstructive procedure most commonly performed to excise excess skin folds around the vulva that cause perivulvar dermatitis.

II. Preoperative Concerns

A. Females

1. Perform abdominal palpation to detect uterine enlargement, a mass, or pain.
2. Evaluate abnormal vulvar skin folds, conformation, discharge, or enlargement.
   a. During estrus and proestrus, expect the vulva to be swollen to 2 or 3 times normal size, and have a hemorrhagic to straw-colored discharge.
   b. Perform a digital and visual examination when vaginal discharge or enlargement is detected. Use an otoscope or vaginal speculum to view the vestibule and caudal vagina, and an endoscope for the cranial vagina and cervix. Consider positive contrast vaginography if vaginoscopy fails to define the problem.
   c. Obtain vaginal, uterine, or mammary gland cultures if infection is suspected, and perform Brucellosis testing if there is persistent vaginal discharge.
   d. Evaluate vaginal cytology, which should be consistent with the estrus cycle.
3. Inspect mammary glands for symmetry, size, mobility, and discharge.
4. Radiographaphy and ultrasonography.

a. The normal nongravid uterus usually is not identified by plain radiographs or ultrasonography.
b. Radiographs.
   i. Identify an enlarged gravid uterus within 31 to 38 days.
   ii. Observe fetal skeletal mineralization by 45 days after the luteinizing hormone peak.
c. Ultrasound.
   i. Detect pregnancy and fetal viability as early as 20 to 28 days into gestation.
   ii. Use it to identify ovarian masses and follicular changes, as well as uterine cysts, masses or fluid, premature placental separation, and a thickened uterine wall.

B. Males

1. Perform abdominal and rectal palpation to evaluate prostatic size, symmetry, texture and mobility, and sublumbar lymph node size.
   a. An abnormal prostate may be asymmetric, irregular, painful on palpation, and/or displace adjacent viscera.
2. Use abdominal radiographs to define prostatic size, shape, and location, and to evaluate sublumbar lymph nodes, lumbar vertebrae, and the bony pelvis for evidence of metastases.
   a. Consider a positive contrast cystourethrogram to evaluate prostatic position in relation to the bladder, urethral size, mucosal contour, and prostatic reflux.
3. Use ultrasonography to define parenchymal homogeneity, contour, disease distribution, and urethral diameter.
   a. Collect cytology and biopsy specimens with ultrasound guidance.
4. Perform cytologic evaluation of prostatic fluid obtained by ejaculation, prostatic washes, or fine-needle aspiration (FNA).
   a. Prostatic massage or ejaculation fluid in normal dogs has few transitional cells, rare neutrophils, and a varying number of erythrocytes.
   b. Obtain cultures of urine and prostatic fluid to detect bacterial infections.
5. Examine the scrotum for size, symmetry, thickening, masses, sensitivity, and scrotal adhesions.
6. Palpate the testicles for size, consistency, contour, symmetry, and sensitivity.
7. Use ultrasonography to evaluate scrotal swelling and testicular abnormalities.
8. Observe the prepuce and penis for signs of trauma, wounds, masses, irritation, and congenital abnormalities.
   a. Extrude the penis completely from the prepuce for thorough examination.
   b. Consider radiographs to help evaluate os penis fractures and urethral extension of disease.
   c. Perform cytologic evaluation on all accessible masses. A biopsy is necessary for definitive diagnosis.
9. Measurement of serum hormone (LH and FSH) concentrations may aid in determining whether a male dog has been neutered or has a hormone-producing tumor.

III. Anesthetic Considerations

A. General Considerations

1. See Appendix G-21 for suggested anesthetic protocols.
   a. Premedicate with atropine or glycopyrrolate to help prevent bradycardia induced by visceral manipulation.

b. Use opioids for preoperative and postoperative analgesia.
c. Do not use ketamine alone for procedures because it gives poor visceral analgesia.
2. Use fluids administration to compensate for evaporation during abdominal surgery.
3. Maintain body temperature.

B. Early Neutering

1. When performing early neutering (i.e., at 6 to 16 weeks of age) take additional precautions.
   a. Take extra care to prevent hypoglycemia, hypothermia, and hemorrhage.
   b. Avoid the use of acepromazine.
   c. Premedicate with an anticholinergic.
   d. Use isoflurane for maintenance of anesthesia.

C. Epidurals

1. Consider using an epidural in addition to general anesthesia or heavy sedation (Table 23-1).
   a. For epidurals using local anesthetics, assess for contraindications (e.g., sepsis, bleeding diatheses, hypovolemia).
   b. Reduce epidural doses if a spinal has been inadvertently performed, the patient is pregnant or obese, or there are space-occupying vertebral canal lesions.
   c. Opioids may be superior to local anesthetic drugs in epidurals because opioids cause sensory loss without motor block, and they do not promote hypotension.

IV. Antibiotics

A. When selecting antibiotics, base the choice on culture and susceptibility results or on expected pathogens in patients with pyometra, metritis, or bacterial prostatitis.

Table 23-1
Epidural anesthesia in dogs

Drug	Dose	Onset of action	Duration of action
Lidocaine 2%*	1 ml/3.4 kg (T_5) 1 ml/4.5 kg (T_{13}-L_1)†	10 min	1-1.5 hr
Bupivacaine 0.25% or 0.5%* (preservative free)	1 ml/4.5 kg	20-30 min	4.5-6 hr
Fentanyl	0.001 mg/kg	4-10 min	6 hr
Oxymorphone	0.1 mg/kg	15 min?	10 hr
Morphine (preservative free)	0.1 mg/kg‡	23 min	20 hr
Buprenorphine	0.005 mg/kg	30 min?	12-18 hr

*Avoid head-down position after epidural.
†A block to T_1 leads to intercostal nerve paralysis; a block to C_7-C_5 leads to phrenic nerve paralysis.
‡The dose for epidural morphine in cats is 0.03 mg/kg.

V. Surgical Anatomy

A. Female Reproductive Tract

1. Ovaries.
   a. The ovaries are located just caudal to the pole of each kidney, with the right ovary further cranial than the left.
   b. Each ovary is attached by the proper ligament to the uterine horn and via the suspensory ligament to the transversalis fascia medial to the last one or two ribs.
2. The ovarian pedicle (mesovarium) includes the suspensory ligament with its artery and vein, ovarian artery and vein, fat, and connective tissue.
3. The broad ligament (mesometrium) is the peritoneal fold that suspends the uterus.
4. The round ligament travels in the free edge of the broad ligament from the ovary through the inguinal canal with the vaginal process.

B. Male Reproductive Tract

1. Prostate gland.
   a. The prostate gland completely surrounds the neck of the bladder and beginning of the urethra.
   b. The blood and nerve supply (pelvic and hypogastric nerves) enter the prostate at the 10 o'clock and 2 o'clock positions when viewed in a transverse plane.
   c. The ductus deferens enter the craniodorsal surface of the prostate and course caudoventrally to enter the urethra.
   d. In cats, bulbourethral glands are found caudal to the prostate.
2. Penis.
3. Testicles.
   a. The spermatic cord begins at the inguinal ring where the testicular artery, testicular veins (pampiniform plexus), lymphatics, testicular autonomic nerve plexus, ductus deferens and its artery and vein, smooth muscle, and visceral layer of the vaginal tunic come together.

VI. Surgical Techniques

A. Elective Surgery

1. Withhold food from adults for 12 to 18 hours and from pediatric patients for 4 to 8 hours before surgery.
2. When preparing for a celiotomy, express the urinary bladder before aseptically preparing the skin.
3. In male dogs, clip and aseptically prepare the prescrotal area for castration. Do not clip the hair or allow soap on the sensitive scrotum.
4. In cats, pluck hair from the scrotum.

B. Pediatric Surgery

1. Handle the fragile pediatric tissue gently and use 3-0 to 5-0 ligatures.
2. Developmental effects of early neutering.
   a. Delays growth plate closure resulting in increased bone length in male and female dogs.
   b. Infantile vulva and mammary glands or penis, prepuce, and os penis persist.
   c. No effect on weight gain or activity level.

C. Ovariohysterectomy (OHE) (*SAS*, pp. 523-525)

1. General considerations.
   a. Many techniques are used for ovariohysterectomy; they all should accomplish the same goals: removal of the ovaries and uterine horns and body.
   b. In dogs, make the incision immediately caudal to the umbilicus, but in cats make the incision more caudal to allow ligation of the uterine body.
2. Technique.

Clip and surgically prepare the ventral abdomen from the xiphoid to the pubis. Identify the umbilicus and visually divide the caudal abdomen into thirds. In dogs, make the incision just caudal to the umbilicus in the cranial third of the caudal abdomen. More caudal incisions make it difficult to exteriorize canine ovaries. In deep-chested dogs or those with an enlarged uterus, extend the incision cranially or caudally to allow exteriorization of the tract without excessive traction. In cats, the body of the uterus is more caudal and difficult to exteriorize; therefore make the incision in the middle third of the caudal abdomen. Make a 4- to 8-cm incision through skin and subcutaneous tissues to expose the linea alba. Grasp the linea alba or ventral rectus sheath, tent it outward, and make a stab incision into the abdominal cavity. Extend the linea incision cranial and caudal to the stab with Mayo scissors. Elevate the left abdominal wall by grasping the linea or external rectus sheath with thumb forceps. Slide the ovariectomy hook (e.g., Covault, Snook), with the hook against the abdominal wall, 2- to 3-cm caudal to the kidney. Turn the hook medially to ensnare the uterine horn, broad ligament, or round ligament and gently elevate it from the abdomen. Anatomically confirm the identification of the uterine horn by following it to either the uterine bifurcation or ovary. If the uterine horn cannot be located with the hook, retroflex the bladder through the incision and locate the uterine body and horns between the colon and bladder. With caudal and medial traction on the uterine horn, identify the suspensory ligament by palpation as the taut fibrous band at the proximal edge of the ovarian pedicle. Stretch or break the suspensory ligament near the kidney, without tearing the ovarian vessels, to allow exteriorization of the ovary. Use the index finger to apply caudolateral traction on the suspensory ligament while maintaining caudomedial traction on the uterine horn.

Make a hole in the broad ligament caudal to the ovarian pedicle. Place one or two Rochester Carmalt forceps across the ovarian pedicle proximal (deep) to the ovary and one across the proper ligament of the ovary. The proximal (deep) clamp serves as a groove for the ligature, the middle clamp holds the pedicle for ligation and the distal clamp prevents backflow of blood after transection. When using two clamps, the ovarian pedicle clamp serves both to hold the pedicle and make a groove for the ligature. Place a figure-8 ligature proximal to (below) the ovarian pedicle clamps. Choose an absorbable suture material for ligatures (i.e., 2-0 or 3-0 chromic catgut, polydioxanone, polyglyconate, or polyglactin 910). Begin by directing the blunt end of the needle through the middle of the pedicle, loop the suture around one side of the pedicle, then redirect the needle through the original hole from the same direction and loop the ligature around the other half of the pedicle. Securely tie the ligature. Remove one clamp or "flash" a single clamp while tightening the ligature to allow pedicle compression. Place a second circumferential ligature proximal to (below) the first to control hemorrhage, which may occur from puncturing a vessel as the needle is passed through the pedicle. Place a mosquito hemostat on the suspensory ligament near the ovary. Transect the ovarian pedicle between the Carmalt and ovary. Open the ovarian bursa and examine the ovary to be certain that it has been removed in its entirety. Remove the Carmalt from the ovarian pedicle and observe for hemorrhage. Replace the Carmalt and religate the pedicle if hemorrhage is noted.

Trace the uterine horn to the uterine body. Grasp the other uterine horn and

follow it to the opposite ovary. Place clamps and ligatures as described above. Make a window in the broad ligament adjacent to the uterine body and uterine artery and vein. Place a Carmalt across the broad ligament on each side and transect. Apply a ligature around the broad ligament if the patient is in estrus, is pregnant, or the broad ligament is heavily infiltrated with vessels or fat. Apply cranial traction on the uterus and ligate the uterine body cranial to the cervix. Place a figure-8 suture through the body using the point of the needle and encircling the uterine vessels on each side. Place a circumferential ligature nearer the cervix. Place a Carmalt across the uterine body cranial to the ligatures. Grasp the uterine wall with forceps or mosquito hemostats cranial to the ligatures. Transect the uterine body and observe for hemorrhage. Religate if hemorrhage is observed. Some surgeons place one to three Carmalts across the uterine body before ligation. In cats, clamps may cut rather than crush a friable or engorged uterus and cause transection before ligature placement. Replace the uterine stump into the abdomen before releasing the hemostats or forceps. Close the abdominal wall in three layers (fascia/linea alba, subcutaneous tissue, and skin).

D. Orchiectomy (*SAS,* pp. 524-527)

1. General considerations.
   a. The risk of ligature slippage and loosening may be greater with closed than with open techniques; however, removal of the tunics may reduce postoperative swelling.
   b. Use either a prescrotal or perineal approach.
      i. A prescrotal approach is easier and more commonly performed.
      ii. Use a perineal approach to avoid repositioning for another surgery (e.g., perineal hernia repair).
2. Open, prescrotal castration.

Position the patient in dorsal recumbency. Verify the presence of both testicles in the scrotum. Clip and aseptically prepare the caudal abdomen and medial thighs. Avoid irritating the scrotum with clippers or antiseptics. Drape the surgical area to exclude the scrotum from the field. Apply pressure on the scrotum to advance one testicle as far as possible into the prescrotal area. Incise skin and subcutaneous tissues along the median raphe over the displaced testicle. Continue the incision through spermatic fascia to exteriorize the testicle. Incise the parietal vaginal tunic over the testicle. Do not incise the tunica albuginea, which would expose the testicular parenchyma. Place a hemostat across the vaginal tunic where it attaches to the epididymis. Digitally separate the ligament of the tail of the epididymis from the tunic while applying traction with the hemostat on the tunic. Further exteriorize the testicle by applying caudal and outward traction. Identify the structures of the spermatic cord. Individually ligate the vascular cord and ductus deferens, then place an encircling ligature around both. Many surgeons ligate the ductus deferens and pampiniform plexus together. Use 2-0 or 3-0 absorbable suture (e.g., chromic catgut, polyglactin 910, polydioxanone or polyglyconate) for ligatures. Alternatively, use hemostatic staples. Place a hemostat across the cord near the testicle. Grasp the ductus deferens with thumb forceps above the ligature and transect both the ductus deferens and vascular cord between the hemostat and ligatures. Inspect the cord for hemorrhage and replace the cord within the tunic. Encircle the cremaster muscle and tunic with a ligature. Advance the second testicle into the incision, incise the fascial covering, and remove the testicle as described. Appose the incised dense fascia on either side of the penis with interrupted or continuous sutures. Close subcutaneous tissues with a continuous pattern. Appose skin with an intradermal, subcuticular, or simple interrupted suture pattern.

3. Closed, prescrotal castration.
   a. Perform a "closed" castration similarly to the "open" technique, except do not incise the parietal vaginal tunic.

Maximally exteriorize the spermatic cord by reflecting fat and fascia from the parietal tunic with a gauze sponge. Place traction on the testicle while the fibrous attachments between the spermatic cord tunic and scrotum are torn. Place mass ligatures (e.g., 2-0 or 3-0 absorbable) around the entire spermatic cord and tunics. Pass the needle through the cremaster muscle if a transfixation ligature is desired. Hemostatic staples may also be used.

4. Perineal castration.
   a. Use the same technique as for an open, prescrotal castration, except displace the testicles into a caudal incision.
   b. An "open" technique must be used.

Make a midline skin and subcutaneous tissue incision dorsal to the scrotum in the perineum ventral to the anus. Advance one testicle to the incision and incise the spermatic fascia and tunic. Exteriorize the testicle and ligate the spermatic cord as described for an open, prescrotal castration.

5. Scrotal ablation (*SAS*, p. 527).
   a. Perform a scrotal ablation for neoplastic scrotal diseases and for castration performed in conjunction with scrotal urethrostomy in dogs and perineal urethrostomy in cats.
   b. Also perform because of severe scrotal trauma, abscesses, or ischemia.

Elevate the scrotum and testicles from the body wall. Make an elliptical skin incision at the base of the scrotum, being careful not to excise too much skin. Control hemorrhage with electrocoagulation, ligation, or pressure. Incise the vaginal tunics and remove the testicles as described for open castration. Remove the scrotum after incising its median septum. Appose subcutaneous tissues with a simple continuous suture pattern (e.g., 3-0 absorbable suture). Appose skin edges with approximating interrupted sutures (e.g., 3-0 or 4-0 nonabsorbable suture).

6. Feline castration.

Pluck hair from the scrotum rather than clipping. In kittens less than 16 to 20 weeks of age, plucking scrotal hair may be difficult. Use clippers to gently remove scrotal hair. Position the cat in dorsal or lateral recumbency with the hindlegs pulled cranially. Mobilize a testicle in the scrotum by applying pressure with the thumb and index finger at the base of the scrotum. Make a 1-cm incision over each testicle at the end of the scrotum from cranial to caudal. Incise the parietal vaginal tunic over the testicle. Digitally separate the attachment of the ligament of the tail of the epididymis to the vaginal tunic. Double ligate the spermatic cord with absorbable suture (e.g., 3-0 chromic catgut) or hemoclips or remove the ductus deferens from the testicle and tie it with the vessels (explained later in this chapter). Alternatively, use a figure-8 knot (explained later in this chapter). Transect the cord, inspect for bleeding, and replace it within the tunic. Excise the second testicle in a similar fashion. Resect any tags of tissue protruding from the scrotum. Allow the scrotal incision to heal by second intention.

To ligate the ductus deferens with the vessels, separate the ductus deferens from the testicle. Using the remainder of the spermatic cord (testicular vessels and testicle) as one strand and the ductus deferens as the other, tie two to three square knots (five to six throws). Sever the vessels with attached testicle and ductus deferens distal to the knot. Inspect for hemorrhage.

For an overhand or figure-8 knot, the spermatic cord is tied on itself with the aid of a curved mosquito hemostat. Place the hemostat on top of the cord. Wrap the distal (testicle) end of the cord over the hemostat once. Direct the wrapped hemostat ventral to the cord while holding the testicle in the opposite hand. Open the tips of the hemostat and grasp the distal end of the cord. Transect the spermatic cord near the testicle and manipulate the severed end of the cord through the loops around the hemostat. Make the knot snug, resect excess cord, inspect for bleeding, and replace the cord within the tunic before releasing.

E. Cryptorchid Castration (*SAS,* p. 527).

1. General considerations.
   a. Cryptorchidism is a congenital failure of one or both testicles to descend into the scrotum. Unilateral cryptorchidism is more common.
   b. There is little hope of further testicular descent after 2 months of age.
   c. Testicular agenesis is rare.
   d. Cryptorchidism testes are typically small and soft and may be located in the inguinal area or abdominal cavity. Testicles located in the inguinal region are often easier to locate when the animal is under anesthesia.
   e. Recommend bilateral castration to owners because retained canine testes are predisposed to neoplasia and the condition is believed to be inherited.
2. Inguinal testicles.

Advance unilateral, mobile inguinal testicles to the prescrotal incision and remove. Remove nonmobile testicles by making an incision over the inguinal ring. Dissect through subcutaneous fat and mobilize and remove the testicle. Submit the testicles for histologic examination to verify removal of testicular tissue and to rule out neoplasia.

3. Intraabdominal testicles.

Nonpalpable testes must be located via exploratory laparotomy. Make a ventral midline incision from the umbilicus to the pubis or a paramedian incision adjacent to the prepuce. Find the testicle(s) by retroflexing the bladder, locating the ductus deferens dorsal to the neck of the bladder, and following the ductus deferens to the testicle. If the ductus deferens travels into the inguinal ring and the testicle cannot be manipulated into the abdomen, perform an inguinal incision. Avulse the ligament of the tail of the epididymis. Double ligate the testicular artery and vein and ductus deferens separately. Transect and remove the testicle. Inspect for hemorrhage and close the abdomen in three layers.

F. Vasectomy (*SAS,* pp. 528, 530)

1. General considerations.
   a. This procedure is rarely recommended because although with it fertility is inhibited, male behavioral patterns such as roaming, aggression, and urine marking are maintained.
   b. Spermatozoa persist in canine ejaculates for 3 weeks and feline ejaculates for 7 weeks after vasectomy.
2. Technique.

Make a 1- to 2-cm incision over the spermatic cord between the scrotum and inguinal ring. Locate the spermatic cord, incise the vaginal tunic, and isolate the

ductus deferens by blunt dissection. Double ligate the ductus deferens and resect a 0.5-cm section of ductus between ligatures. Repeat the procedure on the contralateral spermatic cord. Appose subcutaneous tissues and skin.

G. Cesarean Section (*SAS,* pp. 528-531)

1. Indications.
   a. Use a cesarean section to remove fetuses from a uterus as quickly as possible because of dystocia or fetal putrefaction.
   b. Elective cesareans are often scheduled for brachycephalic breeds and other animals with a history of dystocia, or animals with pelvic fracture malunion.
   c. A cesarean may be performed in conjunction with an OHE, either as described and followed by OHE, or as an en bloc resection.
      i. Advantages of en bloc ovariohysterectomy of the gravid uterus include minimal anesthetic time, and minimal potential for abdominal contamination.
      ii. The disadvantage of this technique is that a second team is required to resuscitate the neonates.
      iii. Mothering and lactation are normal following OHE.
2. Preoperative management.
   a. Correct fluid and electrolyte abnormalities and hypocalcemia, if present.
   b. Administer antibiotics (e.g., cefazolin, 20 mg/kg IV) if fetal death or uterine infection is suspected.
   c. Be aware of the potential for greater anesthetic risk because of hypovolemia, hypoglycemia, hypocalcemia, and/or toxemia. In addition, a distended uterus may decrease tidal volume.
   d. Recognize that drugs that depress the mother also depress the fetus (see Appendix G-21 for suggested anesthetic protocols). Minimize anesthesia time and consider using an epidural or a lidocaine line block on the skin.
3. Cesarean without ovariohysterectomy.

Clip and perform a preliminary abdominal prep before anesthetic induction to minimize time from induction to delivery. Preoxygenate the bitch/queen if possible before induction. Anesthetize the patient using a general or regional protocol that is appropriate for the bitch/queen and minimizes neonatal depression (Appendix G-21). Position the patient in dorsal recumbency. Apply a final aseptic scrub to the ventral abdomen. Make a ventral midline incision from just cranial to the umbilicus to near the pubis. Elevate the external rectus sheath before making a stab incision through the linea alba to avoid inadvertent laceration of the uterus. Exteriorize the gravid uterine horns by carefully lifting rather than pulling them out of the abdomen, because uterine vessels are easily avulsed and the uterine wall readily tears. Isolate the uterus from the remainder of the abdomen with sterile towels or laparotomy pads. Tent and then incise the uterine body to avoid lacerating the neonate. Extend the incision with Metzenbaum scissors. The incision should be long enough to prevent tearing during extraction of the fetus. Empty each horn by gently squeezing (milking) cranial to each fetus to move it toward the incision, then grasping and gently pulling it from the uterus. Rupture the amniotic sac and clamp the umbilical cord as each neonate is presented. Avoid contaminating the abdomen and surgical field with amniotic fluids. Aseptically pass each neonate to an assistant (see following text for neonatal care). At term the placenta is often expelled with the neonate; however, if the placenta has not separated, gently pull it from the endometrium. Do not forcibly separate the placenta from the uterine wall or severe hemorrhage may occur. Palpate the pelvic canal and remove any fetus from this location.

Uterine contraction usually begins when the fetuses are removed. Administer oxytocin (1-5 units IM or IV for dogs; 0.5 units IM or IV with a maximum of 3 units for cats) or ergonovine maleate (0.02-0.1 mg/kg IM) if contraction has not occurred. Give oxytocin and compress the uterine walls if endometrial hemorrhage is severe. Lavage the external uterus to remove debris. Close the uterine incision with 3-0 or 4-0 absorbable sutures using an appositional pattern in a single-layer simple continuous pattern, a double-layer appositional closure (mucosa and submucosa followed by muscularis and serosa), or an appositional closure followed by a second layer inverting pattern (Cushing or Lembert). Lavage the surgical site and replace contaminated towels, sponges, instruments, and gloves. Inspect for uterine vessel avulsion and control hemorrhage. Lavage the abdomen if contamination or spillage of uterine contents has occurred. Cover the uterine incision with omentum. Appose the abdominal wall in three layers (rectus fascia, subcutaneous tissue, and skin). Use subcuticular or intradermal skin closure to eliminate suture ends that may irritate neonates. Lavage all antiseptics, blood, and debris from the ventral abdomen and mammae.

4. En bloc resection.

Perform en bloc ovariohysterectomy of the gravid uterus by first exteriorizing and isolating the ovarian pedicles and separating the broad ligament from the uterus to the point of the cervix. Manipulate fetuses in the vagina or cervix into the uterine body. Then, double- or triple clamp the ovarian pedicles and uterus just cranial to the cervix. Quickly transect between clamps and remove the ovaries and uterus. Give the uterus to a team of assistants to open and resuscitate the neonates. The time from clamping the uterus to removal of the neonates should be 30 to 60 seconds. Double ligate ovarian and uterine pedicles. Inspect for hemorrhage and close the abdomen.

5. Neonatal care.

Firmly cradle the neonate and gently swing downward to help clear fluid from the upper airways. Gently suction the nares and nasopharynx. Briskly rub and dry each neonate to stimulate the respiratory drive. If necessary, antagonize opioids (place a drop of naloxone under the tongue) and give doxapram (place a drop under the tongue) to stimulate respiration. Ligate, transect, and disinfect the umbilical cord. Inspect each neonate for congenital or developmental anomalies (i.e., cleft palate, limb deformity, hernia, imperforate anus). Place neonates in a warm environment (32° C, 90° F) until their mother is able to care for them. Allow nursing as soon as possible to ensure colostrum intake. Closely observe the mother and her behavior toward the neonates during the first few hours; some mothers will reject or kill their neonates. Discharge the bitch/queen and neonates from the hospital as soon as possible to reduce stress and exposure to potential pathogens.

H. Mastectomy (*SAS,* p. 531)

1. General considerations.
   a. One gland (simple mastectomy), several glands (regional mastectomy), or an entire chain (complete unilateral mastectomy) may be excised; however simultaneous removal of both chains causes significant suture line tension and is not recommended.
2. See Mammary Neoplasia for the surgical technique.

I. Episiotomy (*SAS,* pp. 531-532)

1. General considerations.
   a. Place an Elizabethan collar after surgery to prevent self-trauma.

b. To reduce inflammation and edema, apply cold compresses immediately after surgery and warm compresses the following day.

2. Technique.

With the animal in a perineal position, place a noncrushing clamp (i.e., Doyen) with one shaft in the vagina on each side of the perineal midline. Make a midline skin incision through the dorsal commissure of the vulvar lips to just distal of the external anal sphincter muscle with a scalpel blade. Continue the incision through the muscle and vaginal wall with Mayo scissors. Control hemorrhage with hemostats, electrocoagulation, and ligatures. Place two or three horizontal mattress stay sutures full-thickness through the skin and vaginal mucosa on each side of the incision to facilitate retraction and hemostasis. Then remove the Doyen clamps and position a self-retaining retractor (e.g., Gelpi) to improve exposure, if necessary. Evaluate the vagina and vestibule and perform any needed procedures. Close the episiotomy incision in three layers. Preplace an interrupted suture to realign and reappose the dorsal vulvar commissure. First reappose the vaginal mucosa with simple interrupted or continuous sutures (e.g., 3-0 or 4-0 polydioxanone or polyglyconate), tying the knots in the lumen. Then reappose muscles and subcutaneous tissues in a continuous pattern. Lastly, reappose skin with interrupted appositional sutures (e.g., 3-0 or 4-0 nylon or polypropylene).

J. Episioplasty (*SAS*, pp. 532-533)

With the patient in a perineal position, assess the amount of skin to be excised by elevating the skin fold and evaluating expected tension. Beginning near the ventral vulvar commissure, make a crescent-shaped incision encircling the vulva at the proposed lateral and dorsal borders of the resection. Make a second crescent shaped incision medial and parallel to the first to outline the ellipse of skin to be removed. Excise the outlined segment of skin and excess subcutaneous tissue. Place interrupted sutures at the 3 o'clock, 9 o'clock, and 12 o'clock positions to assess the effectiveness of the resection. Resect more skin along the outer margin if the vulva is still recessed or skin folds persist. Bring the skin edges into approximation by first apposing the subcutaneous tissues using interrupted sutures with buried knots (e.g., 3-0 or 4-0 polydioxanone or polyglyconate). Place the first sutures at the 12, 3, and 9 o'clock positions to symmetrically align the edges. Appose skin edges with simple interrupted sutures (e.g., 3-0 or 4-0 nylon or polypropylene). Place an Elizabethan collar or bucket over the head to prevent licking and chewing at the surgical site. Continue antibiotics if necessary to control the pyoderma.

K. Testicular Biopsy (*SAS*, pp. 532-533)

1. General considerations.

a. Use a testicular biopsy in a valuable breeding animal to help determine the etiology of infertility or reduced fertility.

b. Perform either a needle biopsy through the scrotal skin or a wedge resection through a prescrotal incision.

2. Technique.

Make a 1-cm incision through the tunica albuginea of one testicle with a sterile, thin razor blade or No. 11 scalpel blade. Excise a wedge of testicular parenchyma with the razor blade. Appose the tunica albuginea with 4-0 to 6-0 absorbable suture (i.e., polydioxanone or polyglyconate). Appose skin edges with intradermal (subcuticular) or simple interrupted sutures. Better preservation of architectural detail is obtained by placing the sample in Bouin's, Zenker's, or Stieve's fixative, rather than formalin.

L. Prostatic Biopsy (*SAS*, pp. 533-534)

1. General considerations.
   a. Percutaneous techniques are less invasive, but operative techniques allow collection of larger samples.
   b. Do not damage the prostatic urethra and do not perform a biopsy if an abscess or cyst is suspected.
   c. Perform percutaneous biopsies using a Tru-Cut or a Franklin-Silverman biopsy needle.
      i. Ultrasound-guided biopsy.

Position the patient in dorsal or lateral recumbency and ultrasonographically evaluate the prostate. Aseptically prepare the abdominal wall in the area the biopsy needle will be inserted. Nick the skin (3- to 5-mm incision) with a scalpel blade at the needle insertion site. Identify the desired biopsy site with ultrasound and visualize needle placement into the prostate. Collect two to three biopsies with a biopsy needle/instrument. Observe the prostate for hemorrhage or fluid leakage with ultrasound.

      ii. Palpation-guided biopsy.

Position the patient in a perineal position with the tail fixed over the back. Aseptically prepare the perineum around the anus. Mobilize and reposition the prostate in a more caudal position by having an assistant apply gentle pressure on the caudal abdomen. Make a nick incision (3 to 5 mm) slightly lateral to the midline, midway between the anus and ischial tuberosity. Confirm the location of the prostate by rectal examination. Insert the needle through the soft tissues ventral to the rectum. Guide the needle to the prostate digitally via rectal palpation. Penetrate the capsule at the caudal margin of the prostate with the needle in the closed position, then fully insert the inner cannula into the prostatic parenchyma. Quickly advance the outer cannula over the stationary inner cannula, or fire the trigger when using an automatic instrument, to cut the specimen. Remove the needle from the prostate in the closed position. Evaluate the specimen size and collect additional samples, if necessary.

      iii. Open biopsy.

Collect prostatic biopsies during exploratory laparotomy with a biopsy needle or wedge excision. Via a caudal midline abdominal incision, retract the urinary bladder cranially using stay sutures. Isolate the prostate from the remainder of the abdomen with sterile laparotomy pads. Palpate the prostate and select a biopsy site. Dissect periprostatic fat from the desired site. Excise a wedge of prostatic tissue using a No. 11 scalpel blade. Appose edges of the defect by placing cruciate or simple continuous absorbable sutures (e.g., 3-0 or 4-0 polydioxanone or polyglyconate) in the prostatic capsule. Lavage the surgical site(s) and replace periprostatic fat. Close the abdomen in three layers.

M. Prostatectomy (*SAS*, pp. 534-535)

1. Total prostatectomy.
   a. Consider a total prostatectomy for patients with tumors that have not metastasized; however, recognize that this procedure is infrequently performed because urinary incontinence commonly results.

Expose the prostate through a caudal ventral midline celiotomy and pubic osteotomy (SAS, p. 534). Place a urethral catheter. Retract the urinary bladder cranially with stay sutures. Dissect the lateral pedicles and periprostatic

fat directly from the capsule without damaging the dorsal plexus of vessels and nerves. Control hemostasis by ligation and electrocoagulation. Ligate and divide the prostatic vessels and ductus deferens as close to the prostate as possible. Dissect the prostate from the urinary bladder and extrapelvic urethra. Transect the urethra on both ends as close to the prostate as possible. Avoid the trigone and neck of the bladder. Remove the prostate. Advance the urethral catheter into the urinary bladder. Approximate the urethral ends with simple interrupted sutures using 4-0 to 6-0 synthetic absorbable suture (i.e., polydioxanone, polyglyconate) on a taper point swaged-on needle. Place the first two sutures at the 12 o'clock and 6 o'clock positions, leaving the ends long to aid rotation of the urethra during suturing. Place the dorsal suture first. Space sutures approximately 2 mm apart and 1.5 to 2.0 mm from the edge. Place a cystostomy tube or transurethral Foley catheter to divert urine for 5 to 7 days. Biopsy an iliac or sublumbar lymph node to evaluate for metastasis. Replace contaminated instruments and gloves. Lavage the surgical site and abdomen. Place omentum around the anastomosis. Wire the pubic segment into place. Perform a 3-layer abdominal wall closure.

2. Subtotal prostatectomy.
   a. General considerations.
      i. Consider a subtotal prostatectomy for recurrent abscessation or cysts that have not responded to drainage procedures.
      ii. Place a urinary catheter to aid urethral identification.
      iii. Approach and expose the prostate as for total prostatectomy.
   b. Subtotal prostatectomy with capsulectomy.

Isolate and ligate or cauterize all vessels as they enter the prostatic capsule. Excise the prostate within 5 mm of the urethra using scissors, an electrosurgical unit, or laser. Place a cystostomy tube if the urethral catheter is to be removed. Assess hemostasis and lavage the surgical site. Surround the prostatic urethra with omentum or prostatic fat. Close the abdomen routinely.

   c. Intracapsular subtotal prostatectomy.

Incise the ventral median septum with an electroscalpel. Continue the incision through the parenchyma into the ventral urethra. Using the electroscalpel, resect all parenchyma except a 2- to 3-mm shell attached to the capsule. Resect all the urethra except a 3- to 5-mm dorsal strip. Lavage the prostatic shell and close the capsule over a urethral catheter positioned in the urinary bladder. Use an approximating pattern for the first layer and an inverting pattern for the second layer of closure (e.g., 3-0 or 4-0 polydioxanone or polyglyconate). Maintain the catheter for 10 days. Alternatively, use an ultrasonic surgical aspirator to remove parenchyma and preserve the urethra.

VII. Healing of the Reproductive and Genital Systems

A. Reproductive organs heal like other visceral tissues. Additional considerations include the following.
   1. Incisions into testicular parenchyma may cause an immunologic response and subsequent sperm granuloma.
   2. Scarring of the uterus may inhibit placentation.

VIII. Postoperative Care and Assessment

A. Assess the incision site twice daily for redness, swelling, or discharge.

B. Limit activity to leash walks until sutures are removed (generally 10 to 14 days).

C. Provide analgesics and continue antibiotics as necessary.

D. Protect surgical sites by using an Elizabethan collar, bucket, sidebars, or bandage.

E. Administer stool softeners after prostatic or perineal surgery to minimize discomfort during defecation (Table 23-2).

F. After perineal surgery, apply warm compresses to the surgical site two to three times daily.

Surgery of the Female Reproduction Tract: Specific Diseases

Uterine Neoplasia (*SAS*, pp. 538-539)

I. General Considerations

A. Uterine neoplasia is rare in dogs and cats.

B. Tumors that may occur in the uterus are leiomyoma, leiomyosarcoma, adenocarcinoma, lipoma, fibroma, adenoma, and fibrosarcoma.

1. Leiomyomas.
   a. Leiomyomas are the most common uterine tumors.
   b. They are benign and generally noninvasive and slow growing.
   c. They may protrude into the uterine lumen on a stalk or cause the wall to bulge externally.
   d. German shepherd dogs have a syndrome characterized by multiple uterine leiomyomas, bilateral renal cystadenocarcinomas, and nodular dermatofibrosis.
2. Leiomyosarcomas.
   a. Leimyosarcomas are the most common malignant tumors of bitches.
   b. They are difficult to distinguish grossly from leiomyomas.
   c. They are invasive tumors that are usually slow to metastasize.
3. Adenocarcinomas.
   a. Adenocarcinomas are the most common malignant tumors of queens.

Table 23-2
Stool softeners

Dioctyl Sodium Sulfosuccinate or Docusate Sodium (Colace)
Dogs
50-200 mg PO, BID to TID
Cats
50 mg PO, SID to BID
Lactulose (Chronulac)
Dogs
1 ml/4.5 kg PO, TID to effect
Cats
5 ml/cat PO, TID
Psyllium (Metamucil)
Dogs
2-10 g PO, SID to BID or 1 tsp per 10 kg; twice daily in food
Cats
1-4 g PO, SID to BID or 1 tsp per 10 kg; twice daily in food

b. Adenocarcinomas cause the endometrium to become thickened and nodular.
c. Metastasis is usually present at the time of diagnosis and may occur to multiple sites.

II. Diagnosis

A. Clinical Presentation

1. Signalment.
   a. Middle-aged or older animals are typically affected.
2. History.
   a. Uterine tumors are typically asymptomatic unless they are large and compress the gastrointestinal or urinary tracts.
   b. Suspect uterine tumors with animals that have a history of abnormal estrus cycles and/or a mucoid or hemorrhagic vaginal discharge as a result of tumor irritation and vascular erosion.
   c. If uterine tumors obstruct the cervix, pyometra may result.

B. Physical Examination

1. Typically physical and digital vaginal examination are normal, but large masses may be palpated.
2. Observe for a hemorrhagic vaginal discharge and enlarged, asymmetric sublumbar lymph nodes if the tumor has metastasized.

C. Radiography/Ultrasonography/Endoscopy

1. Use abdominal radiography and ultrasonography to delineate a mass in the uterine area, lymph node enlargement or visceral metastasis. An ultrasound-guided biopsy may indicate tumor type.

2. Take thoracic radiographs to evaluate for metastasis.
3. Vaginoscopy may reveal abnormal discharge.

D. Laboratory Findings

1. Neoplastic cells are rarely identified on vaginal cytology.

III. Medical Management

A. The effectiveness of chemotherapy and radiation therapy on uterine masses is unknown.

IV. Surgical Treatment

A. Perform an OHE.

B. Preoperative management.

1. If pyometra is present, correct hydration and electrolyte and acid–base abnormalities, and initiate antibiotic therapy before surgery.

C. Positioning.

1. Position animals in dorsal recumbency.

D. Surgical technique.

Perform a ventral midline celiotomy. Explore the abdomen for evidence of metastasis or other abnormalities. Biopsy or excise abnormal structures. Perform an OHE, removing the cervix if it is within 1 to 2 cm of the tumor. Culture the uterus if metritis or pyometra is suspected.

V. Postoperative Care and Assessment

A. Antibiotics are not necessary unless a uterine infection is identified.

B. Evaluate thoracic and abdominal radiographs periodically if a malignant tumor was present.

VI. Prognosis

A. Inform owners that the prognosis for asymptomatic benign tumors without surgery is good unless the mass impinges on the gastrointestinal or urinary tracts, and prognosis is excellent following OHE.

B. Inform owners that the prognosis following OHE is good for malignant tumors if there is no evidence of metastasis or local infiltration. The prognosis for uterine adenocarcinomas is guarded because of its propensity to metastasize before diagnosis.

Mammary Neoplasia (*SAS*, pp. 539-544)

I. Definitions

A. **Lumpectomy** is removal of a mass or part of a mammae.

B. **Simple mastectomy** is excision of an entire gland.

C. **Regional mastectomy** is excision of the involved gland and adjacent glands.

D. **Unilateral mastectomy** is the removal of all mammary glands, subcutaneous tissues, and associated lymphatics on one side of the midline.

E. **Bilateral mastectomy** is the simultaneous removal of both mammary chains.

II. General Considerations

A. Canine Tumors

1. Mammary tumors are uncommon in male dogs but the most common tumor in female dogs.
2. Tumor types are benign mixed tumors, carcinomas, adenomas, malignant mixed tumors, sarcomas, and myeloepitheliomas.
3. Approximately 35% to 50% of canine mammary tumors and 90% of feline mammary tumors are malignant.
4. Malignant mammary tumors generally spread to the regional lymph nodes and lungs. Some "malignant" mammary tumors do not recur or spread after surgery.

B. Feline Tumors

1. Mammary tumors are less common in cats than dogs.
2. Adenocarcinomas are most common.
3. Expect feline mammary tumors to grow rapidly and metastasize to local lymph nodes and lungs early in the course of the disease.
4. Differentiate feline mammary tumors from lobular hyperplasia and fibroepithelial hyperplasia. Also be aware that mammary hypertrophy results from endogenous or exogenous progesterone stimulation and commonly occurs in young intact female cats 2 to 4 weeks after estrus.
5. Perform a unilateral mastectomy to remove feline mammary tumors because local recurrence is common with less radical procedures.
6. Survival for cats with malignant mammary tumors is generally less than 1 year.

C. Hormone Receptors

1. Recognize that many mammary gland neoplasias are hormone dependent, and most can be prevented if OHE is performed before 1 year of age.
2. Dogs with tumors containing estrogen or progesterone receptors live longer than those without. Progesterone administration may be

associated with the development of malignant mammary tumors in cats and benign tumors in dogs.

III. Diagnosis

A. Clinical Presentation

1. Signalment.
   a. Middle-aged or older female dogs and cats are commonly affected.
   b. Almost all feline mammary tumors (99%) occur in intact females.
2. History.
   a. Typically mammary tumors are discovered during routine physical examination, or the owner has noticed a lump and/or abnormal discharge from the mammae.
   b. Occasionally an animal presents because of dyspnea or lameness secondary to pulmonary or bone metastasis, respectively.

B. Physical Examination

1. Canine mammary tumors most commonly occur in the caudal glands. Multiple masses may be found in one or both mammary chains. Masses may be sessile or pedunculated, solid or cystic, and ulcerated or covered with skin and hair.
2. Suspect inflammatory carcinoma or mastitis if the glands are diffusely swollen.
   a. These tumors grow rapidly, invading cutaneous lymphatics and causing marked edema and inflammation. They are often ulcerated.
3. Palpate for axillary, inguinal, or sublumbar lymph node enlargement.
4. Lameness or limb edema is suggestive of metastasis.

C. Radiography/Ultrasonography

1. Take thoracic radiographs to evaluate for pulmonary metastasis.
2. Pleural fluid may occur in cats with metastatic pulmonary disease.
3. Abdominal radiographs may detect iliac lymph node enlargement with caudal tumors. Abdominal ultrasonography may detect abdominal metastasis.

D. Laboratory Findings

1. Obtain a definitive diagnosis by histopathology of each mass because different tumor types may occur in the same individual.
2. Perform lymph node aspiration to help stage the disease.
3. Evaluate pleural fluid cytologically, if present.
4. Consider a bone scan to help confirm bone metastasis.

IV. Medical Management

A. Neither chemotherapy, radiation therapy, nor hormonal therapy is routinely recommended as an adjunct to surgery.

V. Surgical Treatment

A. General Considerations

1. Perform surgical excision for all mammary tumors except inflammatory carcinomas. Excision allows histologic diagnosis and can be curative.

a. Inflammatory carcinomas are extremely aggressive and surgery is of no value in controlling or palliating the disease.
b. If complete excision is not possible with a single surgery, a second procedure should be delayed 3 to 4 weeks to allow healing and relaxation of stretched skin.

2. If performing an OHE at the time of tumor removal, complete it before mastectomy to prevent seeding the abdominal cavity with tumor cells.
3. Select the surgical technique based on tumor size and location.
   a. Perform a lumpectomy when the mass is small (less than 5 mm), encapsulated, noninvasive, and at the periphery of the gland.
      i. Milk and lymph leakage may cause postoperative inflammation and discomfort.
      ii. Local recurrence is decreased in cats when unilateral mastectomy is performed rather than a lumpectomy.
   b. Perform a simple mastectomy when the tumor involves the central area of the gland or the majority of the gland.
   c. Perform a regional mastectomy when multiple tumors occur in adjacent glands in the chain or when the mass occurs between two glands.
   d. Perform a unilateral mastectomy when numerous tumors occur throughout the chain.
   e. Perform a bilateral mastectomy when numerous masses occur in both chains; however, skin closure can be extremely difficult or impossible. Staged unilateral mastectomies are preferred.

B. Preoperative Management

1. Treat ulcerated, infected masses with warm compresses and antibiotics for several days before surgery to reduce inflammation and allow more accurate assessment of the gross tumor margins.

C. Surgical Anatomy

1. Dogs usually have five pairs of mammary glands and cats four pairs.
2. Lymph nodes.
   a. The axillary lymph node drains the three cranial glands and the inguinal lymph node drains the two caudal glands; however, there are lymphatic connections between glands and across the midline.

D. Positioning

1. Position the animal in dorsal recumbency.

E. Surgical Technique

Make an elliptical incision around the involved mammary gland(s), a minimum of 1 cm from the tumor. Continue the incision through subcutaneous tissues to the fascia of the external abdominal wall. Avoid incising mammary tissue; however, this is often impossible because mammary tissue may be confluent between adjacent glands. The midline separation between mammary chains is distinct. Control superficial hemorrhage with electrocoagulation, hemostats, and/or ligation. Perform an en bloc excision by elevating one edge of the incision and dissecting subcutaneous tissue from the pectoral and rectus fascia using a smooth gliding motion of the scissors. Use traction on the elevated skin segment to facilitate dissection. Abdominal and inguinal glands are loosely attached by fat and connective tissue and easily separated from rectus fascia. Thoracic glands adhere to the underlying pectoral muscles with little intervening fat or connective tissue. Resect the inguinal fat pad and lymph node(s) with the inguinal mammary gland. The axillary lymph node is not included with en bloc resection of the thoracic glands. Excise fascia if the tumor has invaded subcutaneous tissues. Some neoplastic lesions will invade the

abdominal musculature and excision must include a portion of the abdominal wall. Continue gliding scissor dissection until major vessels (i.e., cranial superficial epigastric and caudal superficial epigastrics) to the gland are encountered. Isolate and ligate these vessels. Ligate the cranial superficial epigastric vessel where it penetrates the rectus abdominis between the caudal thoracic and cranial abdominal (third) mammary glands. Ligate the caudal superficial epigastric vessel adjacent to the inguinal fat pad near the inguinal ring. Ligate branches supplying the first and second thoracic mammary glands as they are encountered penetrating the pectoral muscles. Lavage the wound and evaluate for abnormal tissue. Undermine the wound edges and advance skin toward the center of the defect with walking sutures. If deadspace is extensive, place a Penrose drain to help prevent fluid accumulation. Appose skin edges with a subcutaneous or subcuticular suture pattern. Use 3-0 or 4-0 absorbable suture (polydioxanone or polyglyconate) on a swaged-on taper point needle in either an interrupted or continuous pattern. Skin apposition is most difficult in the thoracic region because the ribs make the area less compressible than the abdomen and the skin is less mobile. Use appositional skin sutures (e.g., 3-0 or 4-0 nylon or polypropylene) or staples. Place a padded circumferential bandage to compress deadspace, mobilize tissue, and support the wound.

VI. Postoperative Care and Assessment

A. Provide analgesics.

B. Place an abdominal bandage to support the wound, compress deadspace, and absorb fluid for 5 to 7 days. Change bandages daily for the first 2 to 3 days, or as needed to keep it dry.

C. Remove Penrose drains, if used, when drainage diminishes to a minimal amount (usually within 3-5 days).

D. Reevaluate patients with malignant tumors every 3 to 4 months for local recurrence and metastasis.

VII. Prognosis

A. Canine

1. The prognosis with benign tumors is good with surgery.
2. The prognosis for dogs with malignant tumors depends on several factors, including tumor type and stage.
   a. Most dogs with malignant tumors, but without obvious metastasis at the time of surgery, die or are euthanized for tumor-related problems within 1 to 2 years.
   b. Tumors smaller than 3 cm have a better prognosis than tumors larger than 3 cm in diameter.
   c. The presence of multiple tumors does not affect the prognosis.

B. Feline

1. Tumors smaller than 2 cm have less local recurrence than those larger than 2 to 3 cm.
2. The presence of multiple tumors may decrease survival in cats.

C. Adenocarcinomas

1. When confined to the duct epithelium, adenocarcinomas have a good prognosis after surgery.
2. The prognosis worsens when neoplastic cells extend beyond the duct system.

D. Sarcoma and Inflammatory Carcinoma

1. Both tumor types have a very poor prognosis.

Pyometra (*SAS*, pp. 544-549)

I. Definition

A. **Pyometra** is an accumulation of purulent material within the uterus.

II. General Considerations

A. Pathophysiology

1. Pyometra is associated with cystic endometrial hyperplasia. Both of these conditions develop during diestrus or following exogenously administered progesterone.
2. Progesterone stimulates the growth and secretory activity of the endometrial glands and reduces myometrial activity. Excessive progesterone influence or an exaggerated progesterone response causes the uterine glandular tissue to become cystic, edematous, thickened, and infiltrated by lymphocytes and plasma cells.
3. Fluid accumulates in endometrial glands and the uterine lumen with cystic endometrial hyperplasia. This abnormal uterine environment allows bacterial colonization and pyometra.
4. Cats have a decreased incidence of pyometra because they are induced ovulators.

B. Infection

1. *E. coli* is the most common organism identified in canine and feline pyometra.
2. If the cervix is open, vaginal discharge occurs.
3. If the cervix is closed, discharge is prevented and more serious disease results.
4. Septicemia and endotoxemia can develop if pyometra is untreated.

C. Concurrent Abnormalities

1. Concurrent abnormalities may include hypoglycemia, renal and hepatic dysfunction, anemia, and cardiac arrhythmias, and coagulation abnormalities.

III. Diagnosis

A. Clinical Presentation

1. Signalment.
   a. Older (7 to 8 years) intact bitches and queens are typically affected, with bitches more often affected than queens.
   b. Younger animals given exogenous estrogen or progestins may be affected.

2. History.
   a. There is typically a history of estrus, mismating injections, or exogenous administration of estrogens or progestins several weeks before (i.e., in cats 1-4 weeks, in dogs 4-8 weeks) symptoms appear.
   b. The animal may present because of a purulent, sometimes bloody, vaginal discharge. Others have obvious abdominal distention, fever, partial-to-complete anorexia, lethargy, polyuria, polydipsia, vomiting, diarrhea, and/or weight loss.

B. Physical Examination

1. There is typically a purulent blood-tinged vaginal discharge if the cervix is open.
2. Dehydration is frequently present. Animals with endotoxemia or septicemia may be in shock, hypothermic, and moribund. Fever is infrequently present.

C. Radiography/Ultrasonography

1. Use abdominal radiographs or ultrasonography to detect a fluid-filled uterus.
2. Recognize that occasionally, with open pyometra or uterine rupture, enough drainage occurs so that the uterus is not radiographically detected. Note signs of uterine rupture and peritonitis (i.e., poor serosal contrast).
3. Rule out pregnancy.
   a. Radiographically, identify fetal calcification after 45 days of gestation.
   b. Ultrasonographically, identify fetal structures 21 days after onset of diestrus, and assess fetal viability at 24 to 30 days of gestation.

D. Laboratory Findings

1. Complete blood count.
   a. Evaluate the CBC for a neutrophilia with a left shift, monocytosis, and evidence of WBC toxicity. Do not rule out pyometra in animals with normal numbers of WBCs or leukopenia. Sequestration of neutrophils in the enlarged uterus may cause neutropenia despite severe infection.
   b. Assess for a mild normocytic, normochromic, nonregenerative anemia.
   c. Clotting abnormalities and disseminated intravascular coagulation may occur in severely affected patients.
2. Serum biochemistry.
   a. Evaluate the biochemistry profile for common biochemical abnormalities, including hyperproteinemia, hyperglobulinemia, and azotemia. Less common abnormalities include electrolyte abnormalities, increased alanine aminotransferase and alkaline phosphatase activities, hyperglycemia, or hypoglycemia.
3. Urinalysis.
   a. Perform a urinalysis to assess for isosthenuria, proteinuria, and bacteriuria.
   b. Do not perform a cystocentesis if pyometra is suspected.
4. Vaginal cytology.
   a. Use vaginal cytology to confirm a septic exudate with open pyometra.

IV. Medical Management

A. Consider medical therapy with antibiotics for 2 to 3 weeks and $PGF_{2\alpha}$ (0.1-0.25 mg/kg SC, SID or BID for 3-5 days) only for metabolically stable, valuable, breeding animals.

1. More than one series of prostaglandin injections may be necessary.
2. Inform owners that $PGF_{2\alpha}$ therapy is not approved for use in dogs and cats and that serious complications (e.g., uterine rupture and sepsis) are possible.
3. Be aware of the short-term side effects (30-60 minutes), including panting, salivation, emesis, defecation, urination, mydriasis, nesting, tenesmus, lordosis, vocalization, and intensive grooming.
4. $PGF_{2\alpha}$ therapy may cause reduced fertility.

V. Surgical Treatment

A. General Considerations

1. Do not delay OHE.
2. Surgical drainage of the uterus without OHE is not recommended, but has been successful in a few cases. The corpus lutea are removed and each horn lavaged and suctioned. Indwelling drains are placed through the cervix to allow daily lavage with dilute antiseptics.

B. Preoperative Management

1. Monitor urine output, glucose, and arrhythmias.
2. Correct hydration, electrolyte, and acid–base imbalances if possible.
3. Administer a broad-spectrum antibiotic (e.g., cefazolin) effective against *E. coli.*
4. In addition to fluid volume replacement, consider giving corticosteroids or flunixin meglumine (not both) to endotoxic or septicemic patients.

C. Anesthesia (see Appendix G-23)

1. For arrhythmic dogs, consider premedicating with oxymorphone and inducing with thiopental and lidocaine. For the latter, draw up 9 mg/kg of each and give half initially IV. Give additional drug to allow the dog to be intubated, but generally give no more than 6 mg/kg of lidocaine to prevent toxicity.
2. Correct hypotension before and during surgery.
   a. Colloids may be given (7-10 mg/kg) for a total dose of 20 ml/kg/day.
   b. Treat acute intraoperative hypotension with crystalloids.
   c. Dobutamine (2-10 μg/kg/min IV) or dopamine (2-10 μg/kg/min IV) may be given during surgery for inotropic support.

D. Positioning

1. Position the animal in dorsal recumbency.

E. Surgical Technique

Expose the abdomen through a ventral midline incision beginning 2 to 3 cm caudal to the xiphoid and extending to the pubis. Explore the abdomen and locate the distended uterus. Observe for evidence of peritonitis (i.e., serosal inflammation, increased abdominal fluid, petechiation). Obtain abdominal fluid for culture, evacuate the urinary bladder by cystocentesis, and collect a urine specimen for culture and analysis if not previously submitted. Carefully exteriorize the uterus without applying pressure or excessive traction. A fluid-filled uterus is often friable; therefore lift rather than pull the uterus out of the abdomen. Do not use a spay hook to locate and exteriorize the uterus because the uterus may tear. Do not correct uterine torsion because this will release bacteria and toxins. Isolate the uterus from the abdomen with laparotomy pads or sterile towels. Place clamps and ligatures as previously described for OHE except that the cervix may be resected in addition to ovaries,

uterine horns, and uterine body. Ligate the pedicles with absorbable monofilament suture material (i.e., 2-0 or 3-0 polydioxanone or polyglyconate) and transect at the junction of the cervix and vagina. Thoroughly lavage the vaginal stump. Culture the contents of the uterus without contaminating the surgical field. Remove laparotomy pads and replace contaminated instruments, gloves, and drapes. Lavage the abdomen and close the incision routinely. Submit the tract for pathologic evaluation.

VI. Postoperative Care and Assessment

A. Provide analgesics, fluid therapy, and antibiotics.

B. Closely monitor the patient for 24 to 48 hours for sepsis and shock, dehydration, and electrolyte or acid–base imbalances.

C. Low-dose dopamine or diuretics (see Appendix I) may be given postoperatively if urine production is reduced.

VII. Complications

A. In addition to complications associated with elective OHE, septicemia, endotoxemia, peritonitis, and cervical or stump pyometra may occur.

B. Advise owners that death occurs in 5% to 8% of patients despite appropriate therapy and is common after uterine rupture.

VIII. Prognosis

A. Inform owners that without surgical or medical therapy death usually occurs.

B. Make owners aware that pymetra commonly persists or recurs after prostaglandin therapy in dogs.

C. Inform owners that the prognosis following surgery is good if abdominal contamination is avoided, shock and sepsis are controlled, and renal damage is reversed by fluid therapy.

Vaginal Prolapse/Hyperplasia (*SAS*, pp. 549-551)

I. General Considerations

A. Normal estrogenic stimulation causes vaginal mucosa to become edematous.

B. The edematous mucosa may prolapse with hyperestrogenism or weakness of the vaginal connective tissue during proestrus and estrus, and occasionally, at the end of diestrus or parturition.

C. Although edema resolves spontaneously when ovarian production of estrogen has elapsed, prolapse may recur with each succeeding estrus cycle.

D. Do not breed these animals because vaginal prolapse/hyperplasia appears to be familial.

II. Diagnosis

A. Clinical Presentation

1. Signalment.
   a. Young (2 years or younger), large-breed dogs are most commonly affected.
   b. Vaginal prolapse/hyperplasia is extremely rare in cats.
2. History.
   a. There is typically a history of a protrusion of a mass from the vulva, vulvar discharge, or bleeding.
   b. Bitches may present because they refuse to allow intromission during breeding.

B. Physical Examination

1. Most commonly, a mass will be seen protruding between the vulvar lips, or the perineum will bulge.
   a. Acute prolapse and nonprotruding prolapses are characterized by a glistening, edematous, pale pink mucosal surface.
   b. Chronic prolapses appear leathery, corrugated, and sometimes ulcerated or fissured.
2. Assess the mass to determine origin, size at the base, locations of the vaginal lumen and urethral opening, and extent of tissue damage. The mass should arise from the ventral vaginal floor, and areas other than just cranial to the urethral orifice should feel normal.

C. Laboratory Findings

1. Perform vaginal cytology to confirm estrogen stimulation (i.e., RBCs in the absence of cornified vaginal epithelial cells).

III. Medical Management

A. If protrusion is not circumferential, vaginal prolapse will spontaneously resolve when estrogen influence diminishes.

B. Treat transmissible venereal tumors (TVT) with vincristine (0.025 mg/kg up to 1 mg or 0.5 mg/m^2 IV, weekly for 3-6 weeks) or combination chemotherapy. TVT also respond to local excision, radiation therapy, and immunotherapy. In addition, TVT sometimes regress spontaneously.

IV. Surgical Treatment

A. General Considerations

1. Perform an OHE to prevent recurrence and injury to the everted mucosa.

   a. Large, protruding masses may require manual reduction via an episiotomy and vulvar sutures to prevent recurrence until the edematous tissue shrinks.
   b. Resection of the protruding tissue without OHE is not recommended.
2. Resect the protruding tissue when the tissue is severely damaged or necrotic.
3. Perform an OHE and mass excision or biopsy for all vaginal tumors except TVT. Many vaginal tumors are under hormonal influence and regress after OHE.

B. Preoperative Management

1. Lavage the protruding mucosa with warm saline to remove debris and necrotic tissue, apply an antibiotic or antibiotic/steroid ointment, and replace the mass within the vagina or vestibule, if possible.
2. Place an Elizabethan collar to prevent self-trauma before surgery.

C. Positioning

1. Position the patient in dorsal recumbency for OHE.
2. Reposition the patient in perineal position for an episiotomy.

D. Surgical Technique

Perform an OHE and biopsy the mass to rule out neoplasia. Perform an episiotomy, if necessary, to allow biopsy. Replace the protruding mass into the vagina or vestibule. Lavage, lubricate, and reduce the prolapsed tissue by digital manipulation. Maintain reduction by placing two to three horizontal mattress sutures (e.g., 2-0 nylon or polypropylene) between the vulvar lips.

If resection of necrotic or severely traumatized tissue is necessary, position the patient in a perineal position and perform an episiotomy to expose the mass. Place and maintain a urethral catheter during the procedure. In stages, incise the base of the edematous tissue. Control hemorrhage with pressure, ligatures, and electrocoagulation. Appose adjacent mucosal edges with interrupted or continuous approximating sutures (e.g., 3-0 or 4-0 polydioxanone or polyglyconate). Edema should resolve within 5 to 7 days of OHE.

V. Postoperative Care and Assessment

A. Provide analgesics.

B. Apply cold compresses immediately after episiotomy and warm compresses the following day to reduce inflammation and swelling.

C. Place an Elizabethan collar after surgery to prevent self-trauma.

D. Recheck in 5 to 7 days, and remove the vulvar sutures if tissue eversion has regressed with minimal threat of reprotrusion.

VI. Prognosis

A. Inform owners that the prognosis following OHE is excellent.

B. Without OHE, recurrence during subsequent estrus and difficult conception are common.

Uterine Prolapse (*SAS*, pp. 551-552)

I. Definition

A. **Uterine prolapse** is an eversion and protrusion of a portion of the uterus through the cervix into the vagina during or near parturition.

II. General Considerations

A. Uterine prolapse is rare. It is associated with parturition (the cervix must be dilated) and involves the entire vaginal circumference.

B. The everted tissue is doughnut-shaped and discolored from venous congestion, trauma, and debris.

C. Uterine prolapse may result in tearing of the broad ligament and uterine artery hemorrhage, which must be repaired quickly.

III. Diagnosis

A. Clinical Presentation

1. Signalment.
   a. Any age animal near or at parturition may be affected.
2. History.
   a. There is typically a history of excessive straining during parturition.
   b. A mucosal mass is generally noticed protruding from the vulva.
   c. There may be signs of abdominal distress and tenesmus, or signs of hemorrhagic shock if the ovarian or uterine vessels have ruptured.

B. Physical Examination

1. Diagnose uterine prolapse by identifying everted mucosa protruding through the vulva or by digital examination of the vagina.
2. A fornix will be identified by inserting a probe or finger along the protruding mass if it is a vaginal mass or prolapse, but not if it is a uterine prolapse.

IV. Medical Management

A. Medical treatment is rarely successful.
   1. Lavage the protruding mass with warm saline and gently massage to reduce edema. Lavaging with hypertonic dextrose solution may reduce swelling.
   2. Lubricate the mass with a water-soluble gel and replace manually.

V. Surgical Treatment

A. General Considerations

1. Select from treatment options that include manual reduction, manual reduction with immediate OHE, reduction during celiotomy, and amputation of the mass.
2. Perform an OHE if the uterus is devitalized, irreducible, or vessels in the broad ligament have ruptured.
3. If uterine amputation is necessary to allow reduction, perform it similarly to amputation for vaginal prolapse/hyperplasia, ligating the arteries, then follow with an OHE.
   a. Catheterize the urethra during uterine amputation to prevent traumatizing it.
4. Consider performing a vaginapexy during cesarean section, celiotomy, or when the patient is stable.

B. Preoperative Management

1. Stabilize the animal with fluids and start antibiotics if necessary.
2. If the prolapsed tissue appears healthy, lavage and replace.

C. Anesthesia

1. Consider epidural anesthesia to facilitate prolapse reduction and reduce postoperative straining (see Appendix E).

D. Positioning

1. Position the animal in ventral, dorsal, or lateral recumbency for manual reduction.
2. Position the animal in a perineal position for episiotomy, and dorsal recumbency for celiotomy.

E. Surgical Technique

Reduce acute prolapses manually. Lavage the protruding tissue with warm saline or water and diluted antiseptic. Hypertonic agents (e.g., sugar) may help reduce edema and facilitate reduction. Gently compress the mass to reduce edema while attempting to reduce the prolapse. If necessary, perform an episiotomy to assist reduction. Insert a urethral catheter. Place horizontal mattress sutures between the vulvar lips to maintain reduction and prevent recurrence. If necessary, perform celiotomy to facilitate reduction by cranial uterine traction, ensure proper alignment of the uterine horns, and assess integrity of the vasculature.

VI. Postoperative Care and Assessment

A. Provide analgesics as necessary.

B. Monitor urination because swelling and pain may cause urethral obstruction.

VII. Prognosis

A. Complete uterine prolapse will not regress spontaneously.

B. Inform owners that survival following successful manual reduction of uterine prolapses is common, but infertility and dystocia may occur with subsequent breeding.

C. The prognosis following OHE is excellent if shock and hemorrhage are treated appropriately.

Surgery of the Male Reproduction Tract—Specific Diseases

Prostatic Hyperplasia (*SAS*, pp. 552-553)

I. Definition

A. **Prostatic hyperplasia** is a benign enlargement of the prostate secondary to androgenic hormone stimulation.

II. General Considerations

A. Benign prostatic hyperplasia (BPH) is the most common canine prostatic disorder.

B. BPH may potentially be caused by an abnormal ratio of androgens to estrogens, increased number of androgen receptors, or increased tissue sensitivity to androgens.

III. Diagnosis

A. Clinical Presentation

1. Signalment.
   a. Sexually intact male dogs are affected.
   b. Most intact dogs over 6 years of age have some degree of BPH.
2. History.
   a. There is typically a history of tenesmus, hematuria, and/or urethral bleeding.

B. Physical Examination

1. Most dogs are asymptomatic, but tenesmus, hematuria, or urethral bleeding may occur.
2. Perform rectal palpation to reveal symmetric, nonpainful prostatic enlargement.

C. Radiography/Ultrasonography

1. Assess radiographically for symmetrical enlargement of the prostate.

2. Ultrasonography shows diffuse, symmetric prostatic involvement and commonly small, multiple, diffuse cysts.

D. Laboratory Findings

1. Cytology typically reveals hemorrhage and mild inflammation without sepsis.
2. Perform histopathology for a definitive diagnosis.

IV. Medical Management

A. Estrogen therapy has been used to reduce prostatic size, but is not recommended because it causes infertility, squamous metaplasia, abscessation, and aplastic anemia.

B. Medroxyprogesterone acetate (3 mg/kg [minimum dose of 50 mg] SC; repeat in 4 to 6 weeks if signs persist) alleviated signs of hyperplasia within 4 to 6 weeks in more than half of the dogs treated in one study; however, most had recurrence.

1. Potential progestin side effects include increased appetite, weight gain, mammary neoplasia and dysplasia, and diabetes mellitus.

C. Ketoconazole may be safer but requires lifelong therapy.

V. Surgical Treatment

A. General Considerations

1. Do not treat asymptomatic animals.
2. Castration is the best treatment for dogs with clinical disease.

B. Preoperative Management

1. Treat constipation, tenesmus, and urine retention symptomatically.

C. Positioning

1. Position the animal in dorsal recumbency for prescrotal castration and in perineal position for perineal castration.

D. Surgical Technique

1. Perform castration.

VI. Postoperative Care and Assessment

A. Provide analgesics.

B. Evaluate prostatic involution ultrasonographically.

VII. Prognosis

A. Inform owners that the prognosis following castration is excellent.

B. Clinical signs recur or worsen without castration.

Prostatic Abscesses (*SAS,* pp. 553-558)

I. General Considerations

A. The source of bacteria is usually the urethra, although a hematogenous infection is possible.
   1. Microabscesses form and coalesce, causing large abscesses if not treated promptly.

B. Enlargement of the prostate compresses the colon (and rarely the urethra), causing obstruction.

C. Abscess rupture may cause septicemia, peritonitis, and cardiovascular collapse.

D. The prostatic epithelium creates a blood/prostate barrier because of its lipid bilayer.

II. Diagnosis

A. Clinical Presentation

1. Signalment.
   a. Older, sexually intact males with prostatitis, squamous metaplasia, or cysts are typically affected.
   b. Prostatic abscesses are rare in cats.
2. History.
   a. There is typically a history of recurrent or nonresponsive UTIs.
   b. Animals are usually presented because of an acute onset of depression/lethargy, straining to urinate or defecate, hematuria, vomiting, discomfort or pain, and polyuria/polydipsia.

B. Physical Examination

1. Abscessed prostates are generally enlarged, painful, and asymmetric with fluctuant areas (Table 23-3).
2. Palpate the scrotum and testicles for evidence of masses, enlargement, or increased sensitivity. Some animals have perineal hernias, subcutaneous edema, and/or feminization.
3. Depression, fever, anorexia, vomiting, diarrhea, and dehydration are associated with severe infections.

C. Radiography/Ultrasonography

1. Evaluate radiographs for changes, including prostatomegaly, indistinct borders, and occasional mineralization. Loss of abdominal detail suggests peritonitis.
2. Perform contrast procedures, which may show reflux into the prostatic parenchyma and alteration in urethral diameter.
3. Use ultrasound to identify hyperechoic, intraparenchymal, fluid-filled spaces.

D. Laboratory Findings

1. Complete blood count.

Table 23-3
Clinical signs of prostatic disease

Signs	Diagnosis			
	Hyperplasia	Infection abscess	Cyst	Neoplasia
Prostatomegaly	+	+	+	±
Symmetric prostatic enlargement	+	±	±	±
Pain on prostatic palpation	–	±	–	±
Fluctuant prostate	–	±	+	–
Lymph node enlargement	–	±	–	±
Ultrasound	Normal to ↑ echogenicity	Hypoechoic cavities	Anechoic cavities	Hyperechoic or heterogenous irregular urethra
Cytology	Hemorrhage	Inflammation, bacteria	Hemorrhage	Atypical cells ± inflammation and bacteria
Peripheral leukocytosis	–	+	–	±
Pyuria	Rare	+	Rare	±
Systemic signs	±	+	±	±

+, present; –, absent; ±, variable.

  a. Typically there is a neutrophilic leukocytosis with a left shift, toxic neutrophils, and monocytosis.
2. Serum chemistry.
   a. Alkaline phosphatase and alanine transaminase activities and creatinine concentrations may be elevated, along with hyperglobulinemia, hypoglycemia, and hypokalemia.
3. Urinalysis.
   a. Urinalysis commonly reveals hematuria, pyuria, and bacteriuria.
4. Prostatic wash or FNA cytology.
   a. Typically cytology yields highly cellular smears with large numbers of neutrophils and smaller numbers of macrophages and epithelial cells.
5. Bacterial culture.
   a. Culture most commonly isolates *E. coli*, *Pseudomonas* spp., *Staphylococcus* spp., *Streptococcus* spp., and *Proteus* spp.
   b. Occasionally, anaerobic organisms or *Mycoplasma* spp. are isolated.

III. Medical Management

A. Treat prostatitis and small prostatic abscesses with antibiotics, fluid therapy, and nutritional support.

Table 23-4
Shock treatment

Lactated Ringer's Solution or Physiologic Saline Solution
Dogs
Up to 90 ml/kg/hr (to effect)
Cats
Up to 60 ml/kg/hr (to effect)
OR
Hetastarch
5-10 ml/kg (up to 20 ml/kg/day)
OR
7% Hypertonic Saline
4-5 ml/kg (up to 10 ml/kg/day), then isotonic crystalloids at 10-20 ml/kg/hr (to effect)
OR
7% Saline and Dextran 70
3-5 ml/kg (up to 10 ml/kg/day), then isotonic crystalloids at 10-20 ml/kg/hr (to effect)
Flunixin Meglumine (Banamine)
1 mg/kg IV, once or twice if in septic shock
50% Dextrose
1-2 ml/kg IV

B. Treat for septic shock if necessary (Tables 23-4 and 23-5).

C. Monitor urine output (normal urine output is more than 1-2 ml/kg/hr).

IV. Surgical Treatment

A. General Considerations

1. When the patient is stable, drain large abscesses and perform castration.
2. Perform a prostatic biopsy during drainage or resection.
3. Select a subtotal prostatectomy for stable patients with recurrent abscessation or cysts that have not responded to drainage procedures. Rarely, a total prostatectomy is performed for recurrent prostatic infections.

B. Preoperative Management

1. Stabilize the animal before surgery.
2. Place a urinary catheter to facilitate intraoperative identification of the urethra.

C. Positioning

1. Position the animal in dorsal recumbency.
2. Flush the prepuce with a 0.1% povidone iodine or a 1:40 dilution of 2% chlorhexidine solution.

D. Surgical Technique

1. General considerations.
   a. Choose a procedure, based on the size and location of the abscess/cyst.

Table 23-5
Antibiotic therapy in animals with septic shock

Ampicillin
22 mg/kg IV, TID
Enrofloxacin (Baytril)
5-10 mg/kg IV, BID
Amikacin (Amiglyde-V)
30 mg/kg IV, SID
Clindamycin (Cleocin)
11 mg/kg IV, TID
Metronidazole (Flagyl)
10 mg/kg IV, TID
Cefoxitin (Mefoxin)
15-30 mg/kg IV, TID to QID
Imipenem (Primaxin)
3-10 mg/kg IV, TID to QID

i. Marsupialization is an option if the abscess/cyst can be mobilized to the ventral abdominal wall and the capsule is capable of holding sutures. It is more commonly used for cysts than for abscesses.
ii. Prostatic omentalization is a recently described technique that may decrease postoperative care.

b. Perform castration before performing the abdominal exploration.

2. Multiple drain technique.

Place a urethral catheter. Expose the prostate through a ventral midline celiotomy from umbilicus to the pubis. Extend the incision caudally and perform a pubic osteotomy, if necessary, to adequately expose the prostate. Place Balfour retractors to facilitate exposure. Explore the abdomen and isolate the bladder and prostate with laparotomy sponges. Place traction sutures through the bladder wall to retract the prostate cranially. Dissect the ventral fat pad from the prostatic capsule. Insert a large gauge needle into the abscess/cyst, collect a sample for culture and susceptibility testing, and suction its contents. Avoiding vessels and nerves, incise the ventral aspect of the prostate over the abscess/cyst cavity. Digitally break down all trabecula and fibrous bands to connect adjacent abscesses/cysts, creating a common cavity. Suction and lavage the cavity to remove fluid accumulations. Debride necrotic tissue. Place two to four Penrose drains (½ inch) transversely across the ventrolateral aspect of both lobes of the prostate. Periprostatic drains may also be placed. Alternatively, place a tube drain into the abscess/cyst cavity for continuous suction drainage. Exteriorize the end of the drain(s) 2 to 3 cm lateral to the abdominal incision and prepuce. Biopsy the prostatic parenchyma. Secure the drains to the skin with cruciate sutures (e.g., 3-0 nylon). Lavage the surgical site and entire abdomen if contamination has occurred. Surround the surgical site with omentum and periprostatic fat. Close the abdomen routinely. Remove drains in 1 to 3 weeks.

3. Omentalization.

Expose, isolate, and culture the prostate as described above for drain insertion. Make stab incisions bilaterally in the lateral aspects of the prostate gland and remove the purulent material by suction. Explore and digitally break

down any loculated abscesses within the parenchyma. Identify the prostatic urethra by palpation of the previously placed urethral catheter. Place a Penrose drain around the prostatic urethra within the parenchyma to elevate the gland and facilitate irrigation of the abscess cavities with warm saline. Enlarge the stab incisions by resection of the lateral capsular tissue. Submit excised tissue for histopathologic examination. Introduce omentum through one capsulotomy wound with forceps introduced through the contralateral wound. Pass the omentum around the prostatic urethra, exit it through the same incision, and anchor it to itself with absorbable mattress sutures. Close the abdomen routinely.

V. Postoperative Care and Assessment

A. Provide analgesics.

B. Monitor for sepsis, shock, and anemia, while providing fluid and nutritional support.

C. Administer appropriate antibiotics for 2 to 3 weeks.

D. Bandage the abdomen to protect drains or suction apparatus, and use an Elizabethan collar to prevent self-trauma and drain removal. Change bandages daily.

E. Remove drains when the discharge becomes serosanguineous and diminished in volume (1-3 weeks).

F. Identify recurring or persistent infection by culturing prostatic fluid and performing ultrasonography every 3 to 4 months for 1 year.

VI. Prognosis

A. With antibiotics and supportive therapy, small abscesses may resolve.

B. Large, untreated abscesses will eventually cause septicemia, toxemia, and death.

C. Fair to excellent results are expected if the patient survives 2 weeks after surgery.

D. The prognosis after omentalization appears good if sufficient omentum is placed within the prostate.

Prostatic Cysts (*SAS*, pp. 558-560)

I. General Considerations

A. Parenchymal prostatic cysts occur within or have a physical communication with the prostatic parenchyma.

1. They are common in dogs and may be associated with BPH.
2. Their etiology is unknown, but some are congenital.

B. Periprostatic cysts are adjacent and attached to the prostate, but seldom communicate with the parenchyma.
1. They are rare compared to other types of prostatic disease.
2. These cysts are often large, extending into the perineal fossa or abdomen.

C. Prostatic cysts may become infected and abscess.

II. Diagnosis

A. Clinical Presentation

1. Signalment.
   a. Older, intact male, large-breed dogs are most commonly affected.
2. History.
   a. Typically, dogs are asymptomatic until the cysts become large enough to cause rectal, bladder, or urethral obstruction.
   b. Animals are commonly presented for depression, inappetence, stranguria, tenesmus, and/or bloody penile discharge.

B. Physical Examination

1. Examination findings are generally similar to those caused by prostatic hyperplasia (see Table 23-3); however, periprostatic cysts are asymmetric, fluctuant, and sometimes cause abdominal distention.

C. Radiography/Ultrasonography

1. Evaluate plain radiographs for prostate or cyst wall calcification.
2. Use a cystourethrogram to differentiate prostatic cysts and periprostatic cysts from the urinary bladder.
3. On ultrasound, periprostatic cysts are usually large anechoic structures with internal septa.

D. Laboratory Findings

1. Perform aspiration to obtain a sterile, yellow to serosanguineous fluid with minimal inflammation.
2. Perform cytologic evaluation to reveal prostatic epithelial cells and few leukocytes, but more erythrocytes and hemosiderophages than with prostatic hyperplasia.

III. Medical Management

A. Treat constipation with stool softeners (see Table 23-2).

B. Treat urine retention by catheterization.

IV. Surgical Treatment

A. General Considerations

1. With small parenchymal cysts, treat by castration.
2. With large cysts, castrate the dog and either drain, resect, or debulk the cyst.

a. Culture the cystic fluid and obtain a prostatic biopsy.
b. Drain nonresectable cysts by marsupialization or multiple drains.
c. A subtotal prostatectomy may be appropriate for recurring cysts.

B. Positioning

1. Position the animal in dorsal recumbency.

C. Surgical Technique

1. Marsupialization.

Expose and isolate the prostate as described under Prostatic Abscesses for drain insertion. Make a second incision (5 to 8 cm) through abdominal wall lateral to the prepuce over the abscess/cyst cavity. Excise 0.5 to 1 cm of abdominal muscle. Suture capsule or cyst wall to the external rectus fascia. Use continuous or interrupted 3-0 or 4-0 polydioxanone or polyglyconate sutures. Facilitate suturing by having an assistant elevate the prostate toward the abdominal wall. Incise the abscess/cyst wall and suction the contents. Place a second layer of simple continuous or interrupted sutures (e.g., 3-0 or 4-0 nylon, polypropylene) between the skin edge and capsule/cyst edge. Biopsy the prostatic parenchyma. Digitally break down trabeculae and fibrous bands to create a confluent cavity. Lavage the cavity and surgical site, place omentum around the marsupialization, and close the abdomen in three layers.

An alternative technique: incise the ventrolateral aspect of the cyst/abscess wall and suction the cavity before suturing it to the rectus fascia. Then suture the capsule/cyst wall 5 mm from the incised edge of the cavity to the rectus fascia. This variation has a higher risk of abdominal contamination.

V. Postoperative Care and Assessment

A. See Prostatic Abscesses for postoperative care following prostatic or cystic drain placement.

B. Use medical therapy to manage urine retention and constipation.

C. Marsupialization may result in a permanent fistula or may close prematurely.

D. Urine may be voided through the marsupialization for a few days if urethral erosion is present.

VI. Prognosis

A. Inform owners that the prognosis is good to fair after castration and surgical drainage.

B. Some prostatic and periprostatic cysts recur and require repeated drainage; however, this is rare if the dog is castrated.

C. Overzealous resection may cause detrusor atony, incontinence, or bladder ischemia.

Prostatic Neoplasia (*SAS*, pp. 560-562)

I. General Considerations

A. Prostatic neoplasia is the most common prostatic disease in neutered, male dogs, but it is still uncommon in dogs and rare in cats.
   1. Most prostatic tumors are adenocarcinomas. Other tumor types include transitional cell carcinoma, squamous cell carcinoma and undifferentiated carcinoma, leiomyosarcoma, and hemangiosarcoma.
      a. Prostatic carcinomas are locally invasive and metastasize early to regional lymph nodes (iliac, pelvic, and sublumbar), lung, and bone. Other metastatic sites include liver, spleen, kidney, heart, and adrenal glands.

B. Prostatic enlargement causes compression and partial obstruction of the colon, rectum, and sometimes urethra.

C. Pitting edema of the pelvic limbs may occur secondary to lymphatic invasion of the tumor.

D. Most tumors involve the trigone and urethra and have metastasized at the time of diagnosis.

E. Hypertrophic osteopathy has occasionally been associated with prostatic tumors.

F. The behavior of feline prostatic tumors is unknown.

II. Diagnosis

A. Clinical Presentation

1. Signalment.
   a. Eight- to 10-year-old intact and neutered male dogs are most commonly affected.
   b. Medium- to large-breed dogs are overrepresented.
2. History.
   a. A history typically includes weight loss; pelvic limb lameness or weakness; tenesmus; dyschezia; urine retention or incontinence; stranguria; dysuria; polyuria; polydipsia; hematuria; pelvic limb edema; and/or abdominal, pelvic, or lumbar pain.

B. Physical Examination

1. The animal may be debilitated and weak or have pelvic limb edema from lymph node infiltration and lymphatic obstruction.
2. On rectal palpation, the prostate is often asymmetrically enlarged.
   a. Pain, firmness, and nodular irregularity are typical of prostatic neoplasia.
   b. Palpate for sublumbar lymph node enlargement.

C. Radiography/Ultrasonography

1. Evaluate abdominal and pelvic radiographs for prostatic size and

mineralization, lymph node enlargement, colon displacement, and osteolytic or proliferative vertebral or pelvic lesions.
2. Evaluate thoracic radiographs for metastasis.
3. Use retrograde urethrocystography to determine urethral size and mucosal smoothness, prostatic symmetry, and urethroprostatic reflux.
4. Perform ultrasonography to define the prostatic mass as cystic or solid, as well as to evaluate abdominal lymph nodes and guide prostatic biopsy or aspiration.
   a. Most prostatic adenocarcinomas are hyperechoic.
5. Consider nuclear bone scans to locate metastatic sites.

D. Laboratory Findings

1. FNA of prostatic neoplasia may yield a moderately cellular sample with abnormal epithelial cells.
2. Prostatic washes are less reliable in obtaining neoplastic cells.
3. Perform a biopsy for a definitive diagnosis.

III. Medical Management

A. Efficacy of chemotherapy and radiation therapy have not been reported for prostatic tumors. Use of ketoconazole and luteinizing hormone-releasing hormone agonists have been suggested.

IV. Surgical Treatment

A. Treatment is rarely successful.

B. Positioning.
1. Position the animal in dorsal recumbency.

C. Surgical technique.
1. Perform castration to potentially slow tumor growth temporarily.
2. Prostatectomy may be curative if the tumor is diagnosed early; unfortunately, most tumors are advanced when diagnosed.

V. Postoperative Care and Assessment

A. Provide analgesics.

B. Decompress the bladder and divert urine for 4 to 5 days with a urinary catheter or cystostomy tube after prostatectomy.

C. Monitor patients for urine leakage, incontinence, and/or infection.

D. Reevaluate frequently for local recurrence and metastasis.

E. See Prostatectomy for complications and treatment.

VI. Prognosis

A. The prognosis is poor because of metastasis, recurrence, and poor quality of life associated with urinary incontinence.

Testicular and Scrotal Neoplasia (*SAS*, pp. 562-565)

I. Definitions

A. **Sertoli cells** are supporting elongated cells of seminiferous tubules that nourish spermatids.

B. **Leydig cells** are interstitial tissue cells, believed to be responsible for internal secretion of testosterone.

II. General Considerations

A. Scrotal Tumors

1. Mast cell tumors (MCTs).
   a. In dogs, 50% of MCTs are malignant, especially those in the preputial, inguinal, and perineal areas.
   b. They commonly metastasize to regional lymph nodes, spleen, liver, and bone marrow.
   c. MCTs have no distinctive appearance.
   d. Gastroduodenal ulcers occur in up to 80% of dogs with MCTs because of histamine release, potentially causing anorexia, vomiting, diarrhea, and/or melena.
   e. Heparin and proteolytic enzyme release may prolong coagulation and delay wound healing after resection.
2. Melanomas.
   a. Masses may be brown to black or occasionally nonpigmented.
   b. Melanomas are more common in dogs than cats.
   c. Tumors originating in the skin tend to be benign.
   d. Local recurrence and distant metastasis are common with malignant melanomas. Metastasis usually occurs first to the lymph nodes and then to the lungs.

B. Testicular Tumors

1. General considerations.
   a. Sertoli cell tumors, interstitial (Leydig) cell tumors, and seminomas are the most common testicular neoplasms; they occur with equal frequency.
   b. Many old dogs have multiple tumors in one or both testicles.
   c. Tumors involving scrotal testes are usually benign, whereas those in cryptorchid testes may be malignant.
      i. Metastases are slow growing, but are occasionally detected in the lumbar, deep inguinal, and external iliac lymph nodes.
      ii. Visceral metastasis is rare.
2. Sertoli cell tumors.
   a. Normal and neoplastic Sertoli cells produce estrogenic hormones.
      i. Signs of hyperestrogenism (Table 23-6) regress with castration and tumor removal.
      ii. Persistence or recurrence of clinical signs suggests estrogen-producing metastasis.
   b. Sertoli cell tumors have a higher rate of metastasis than other testicular tumors.

Table 23-6
Signs of hyperestrogenism

- Bilateral symmetric alopecia
- Brittle hair
- Poor hair regrowth
- Thin skin
- Hyperpigmentation
- Nipple elongation
- Mammary enlargement
- Penile atrophy
- Preputial swelling and sagging
- Squatting micturition
- Reduced libido
- Male attraction
- Testicular atrophy
- Prostatic atrophy or cystic enlargement
- Myelotoxicosis

3. Interstitial (Leydig) cell tumors.
   a. Most interstitial cell tumors are benign, soft, encapsulated, and rarely exceed 1 to 2 cm in diameter.
      i. They may cause the testicle to enlarge but are difficult to palpate.
   b. These tumors produce androgens or contribute to androgenic hormone imbalance.
   c. Perineal hernia, perianal adenomas and hyperplasia, and prostatic disease have been associated with interstitial cell tumors.
4. Seminomas.
   a. Seminomas can be large, replacing most testicular tissue.
   b. Signs of feminization rarely occur.
   c. They rarely metastasize.

III. Diagnosis

A. Clinical Presentation

1. Signalment.
   a. Dogs older than 10 years are most commonly affected; however, tumors in cryptorchid animals may occur earlier.
   b. Scrotal and testicular tumors are more common in dogs than cats.
2. History.
   a. There is typically a history of a mass that has been seen or felt in the scrotal or inguinal areas.
   b. Animals may also be presented for endocrine abnormalities (e.g., changes in haircoat, infertility, lethargy, feminization [see Table 23-6], perianal tumors, or prostatic disease).

B. Physical Examination

1. Small or deep intraparenchymal testicular tumors are not detectable on palpation, but the testis may be firm and hard.
2. Perform rectal palpation to assess the sublumbar lymph nodes and the prostate.

3. Palpate the abdomen for evidence of metastasis.
4. Observe for signs of feminization (see Table 23-6).

C. Radiography/Ultrasonography

1. Take abdominal radiographs to identify intraabdominal testicles if they are at least twice the diameter of the small intestine. Radiographs also help identify intraabdominal lymph node enlargement and organomegaly.
2. Use ultrasound to delineate scrotal and testicular neoplasia.
   a. Testicular tumors have variable echogenicity.

D. Laboratory Findings

1. Nonregenerative anemia, leukopenia, and thrombocytopenia may be associated with hyperestrogenism and myelotoxicosis.
2. Perform FNA cytology of scrotal and testicular lesions to attempt to identify neoplastic cells, fungal elements, abnormal sperm, bacteria, and inflammation.
   a. FNA cytology is usually diagnostic for MCT.
      i. Evaluate animals with MCTs for disseminated disease.
3. Consider *Brucella canis* infection in animals presented for scrotal dermatitis, orchitis, reproductive failure, epididymitis, or testicular atrophy.

IV. Medical Management

A. MCTs may respond to chemotherapy or radiation therapy.

B. The efficacy of chemotherapy or radiation therapy for other scrotal or testicular tumors is unknown.

V. Surgical Treatment

A. General Considerations

1. Perform castration to treat testicular neoplasia.
2. Perform scrotal ablation in addition to castration to treat scrotal tumors and testicular tumors with scrotal adhesions.
3. Obtain 3-cm margins when removing an MCT.
4. Submit excised tissue for histologic examination.

B. Preoperative Management

1. Administer an antihistamine (e.g., diphenhydramine [Benadryl], 0.5 mg/kg IV, slowly) and an H_2 antagonist (i.e., ranitidine, cimetidine, or famotidine) or a proton pump inhibitor (i.e., omeprazole) to patients with MCTs before surgery.

C. Positioning

1. Position the animal in dorsal recumbency for a prescrotal castration or an exploratory laparotomy.

VI. Postoperative Care and Assessment

A. Provide analgesics.

B. Continue patients with MCT on an H_2 antagonist (see Preoperative

Management), proton pump inhibitor, and/or a protectant if gastrointestinal ulceration occurs.

C. Adjunctive therapy for malignant tumors may prove beneficial.

D. Reevaluate patients with malignant tumors every 3 to 4 months for recurrence or metastasis.

VII. Prognosis

A. Surgery is curative for most testicular tumors.
   1. Inform owners that the prognosis for interstitial cell tumors, Sertoli cell tumors without metastasis or myelotoxicity, and seminomas without signs of hyperestrogenism is excellent.
   2. Myelotoxicity may be fatal despite appropriate therapy, but usually improves within 2 to 3 weeks of tumor removal.

B. Institute chemotherapy if Sertoli cell tumors or seminomas have metastasized.

C. Nonresectable or incompletely resected MCTs may respond to radiation therapy or chemotherapy.

Hypospadias (*SAS*, pp. 565-567)

I. Definition

A. **Hypospadias** is a developmental anomaly in males where the urethra opens ventral and caudal to the normal orifice.

II. General Considerations

A. Hypospadias is rare and many affected animals have other congenital or developmental anomalies.

B. It occurs as a result of failure of the genital folds and genital swellings to fuse normally during fetal development.
   1. The urethra opens anywhere along its length at one or more locations.
   2. The prepuce is similarly affected and ventrally incomplete.
   3. In some cases the penis may be underdeveloped and abnormal (ventral or caudal deviation, blunt) and the scrotum may be divided.
   4. Urine may pool within the prepuce causing irritation and infection of the penis and preputial lining (balanoposthitis).

C. Do not use animals with hypospadias for breeding.

III. Diagnosis

A. Clinical Presentation

1. Signalment.
   a. There is no documented breed predisposition.
   b. The defect is present at birth.
2. History.
   a. There is typically a history of preputial discharge, urinary incontinence, or infection, but small defects may not cause clinical signs.

B. Physical Examination

1. The urethral opening is identified on the ventral aspect of the penis along the normal urethral path.
2. A fibrous band may be noted running from the glans to the urethral opening and deviating the penis.

C. Laboratory Findings

1. Perform a urine culture.

IV. Medical Management

A. Treat urine scalding by frequent bathing and application of water-impermeable ointments near the urethral opening.

B. If urine pooling occurs, flush the prepuce daily with saline solution.

C. Keep the penile mucosa moist with ointments.

V. Surgical Treatment

A. General Considerations

1. Abnormal urethral openings near the penile tip may not require surgery.
2. In other cases, perform reconstruction (with or without penile amputation).
3. Perform excision of the external genitalia for major developmental defects involving the urethra, prepuce, and penis.
4. Delay surgery until approximately 8 weeks of age.

B. Preoperative Management

1. Place a urethral catheter to facilitate urethral identification.

C. Positioning

1. Position the animal in dorsal recumbency unless the urethra opens in the perineal or anal regions and a perineal position is preferred.

D. Surgical Technique

1. Prepuce reconstruction.

Incise the mucocutaneous junction on the caudoventral aspect of the prepuce. Separate mucosa from skin. Reappose the mucosa beginning at a more cranial location with simple interrupted sutures (e.g., 4-0 to 6-0

polydioxanone or polyglyconate). Appose skin with a second layer of simple interrupted sutures (e.g., 3-0 or 4-0 nylon or polypropylene). If this creates an orifice that is too small to allow penile extrusion, incise the dorsocranial aspect of the prepuce and suture the mucosa to the skin on each side with interrupted sutures (e.g., 4-0 nylon or polypropylene).

2. Urethral reconstruction.

Close small urethral defects by incising the margins of the defect and apposing the urethral edges over a urethral catheter. Use 4-0 to 6-0 monofilament absorbable suture (e.g., polydioxanone, polyglyconate) in a simple interrupted or continuous pattern. Close skin over the urethral repair with 3-0 or 4-0 nonabsorbable suture (e.g., nylon or polypropylene) using an appositional pattern.

3. Subtotal penile amputation.

Make an elliptical incision around the prepuce, penis, and scrotum, preserving adequate skin for closure. Dissect the penis from the body wall from cranial to caudal. Ligate or cauterize preputial vessels. Perform a castration as with scrotal ablation. Locate and ligate the dorsal penile vessels just caudal to the desired amputation site. Perform a urethrostomy; scrotal urethrostomy is preferred. Reflect or transect the retractor penis muscle. Make a midline urethral incision over the catheter. Place a circumferential catgut ligature around the penis just caudal to the proposed amputation site and just cranial to the urethrostomy site. Amputate the penis in a wedge fashion. Appose the tunica albuginea to close the end of the penis with 3-0 or 4-0 absorbable suture (e.g., polydioxanone or polyglyconate). Appose urethral mucosa to skin at the urethrostomy site with simple interrupted 4-0 to 6-0 absorbable or nonabsorbable sutures (e.g., polydioxanone, polyglyconate, polypropylene, nylon). Close subcutaneous tissue and skin cranial and caudal to the urethrostomy in two layers.

VI. Postoperative Care and Assessment

A. Provide analgesics.

B. Monitor urination by observing for a nonrestricted urine stream.

C. Hemorrhage may occur from cavernous tissue for days, especially during excitement or urination.

D. Place an Elizabethan collar to prevent self-trauma.

E. Potential incisional complications include hemorrhage, urine leakage, infection, seroma, and dehiscence.

F. Urethral or preputial reconstruction may cause stricture formation.

VII. Prognosis

A. Surgery usually salvages an animal as a pet, improves cosmesis, and reduces urine-induced dermatitis.

Phimosis (*SAS,* pp. 567-569)

I. Definition

A. **Phimosis** is the inability of the penis to protrude from the prepuce or sheath.

II. General Considerations

A. Phimosis is rare.

B. It is usually the result of too small (or absent) a preputial opening, either as a developmental abnormality or because of trauma, neoplasia, or preputial cellulitis.

III. Diagnosis

A. Clinical Presentation

1. Signalment.
   a. There is no known breed predisposition.
   b. Congenital phimosis is recognizable in neonates, but acquired phimosis may occur at any age.
2. History.
   a. There is typically a history of dribbling urine or inability to copulate.

B. Physical Examination

1. Affected animals have a small or nonexistent preputial opening.
2. Manual extrusion or palpation of the penis may reveal a mass preventing advancement of the penis.

IV. Medical Management

A. Relieve phimosis caused by an inflammatory or infectious disease by warm compresses, antibiotic therapy, and urinary diversion with a catheter.

B. Lavage the prepuce daily with physiologic saline solution to reduce urine scalding.

V. Surgical Treatment

A. General Considerations

1. Treat phimosis caused by a developmental anomaly or stricture by reconstruction of the preputial orifice.
2. Neuter animals with small preputial openings.

B. Preoperative Management

1. Lavage the prepuce with a dilute antiseptic solution before surgery.
2. Place a urinary catheter to divert urine.

C. Positioning

1. Position the animal in dorsal recumbency.

D. Surgical Technique

Enlarge the preputial opening by making a full-thickness incision at the craniodorsal aspect of the prepuce. Determine the desired length and width of the preputial incision based on the severity of phimosis. Remove a small wedge (3 to 5 mm) of prepuce with the base at the mucocutaneous junction. Appose mucosa to the ipsilateral skin edge on each side with a simple interrupted suture pattern (e.g., 4-0 to 6-0 polydioxanone or polyglyconate). Extrude the penis completely to examine for other developmental defects, injuries, or masses. Amputate the tip of the prepuce if stenosis is too long to be relieved by incision and adequate preputial length can be maintained. Amputation may cause a shortened prepuce, allowing chronic penile protrusion and exposure. Identify the site of resection and amputate the preputial tip. Circumferentially appose preputial mucosa to skin with a simple interrupted or continuous suture pattern (e.g., 4-0 to 6-0 polydioxanone or polyglyconate). Neuter affected animals.

VI. Postoperative Care and Assessment

A. Provide analgesics.

B. Apply warm compresses and administer antibiotics to treat balanoposthitis.

C. Place an Elizabethan collar to prevent self-trauma.

D. Phimosis may persist if the incision is not long enough.

E. Persistent protrusion of the glans may occur if the ventrocaudal prepuce is incised.

F. Self-trauma may cause dehiscence and stricture formation.

VII. Prognosis

A. Without surgery, balanoposthitis may become severe and cause discomfort.

B. Warn owners that a second surgical procedure may be necessary after the animal matures.

Paraphimosis (*SAS*, pp. 569-572)

I. Definitions

A. **Paraphimosis** is the inability to retract the penis into the sheath/prepuce.

B. **Priapism** is persistent erection of the penis without sexual excitement.

II. General Considerations

A. Paraphimosis may be associated with copulation, trauma, penile hematoma, neoplasia, or foreign bodies.

B. The penis may be unable to retract within the prepuce because the edges of the prepuce roll inward or the preputial orifice is too small to accommodate the swollen or engorged penis.

C. Initially the penis appears normal, but because of trauma and impaired circulation, the penis becomes edematous. A chronically protruded penis becomes dry, fissured, and cornified.

III. Diagnosis

A. Clinical Presentation

1. Signalment.
   a. Dogs are more often affected than cats.
2. History.
   a. There is typically a history of priapism, masturbation, excessive sexual activity, or posterior paralysis.
   b. Long-haired cats may entangle the penis in hair.

B. Physical Examination

1. The exposed, swollen, edematous penis is typically painful.
2. The traumatized penis may be fissured, lacerated, and/or bleeding.

IV. Medical Management

A. Pull the prepuce back until the preputial mucocutaneous junction is identified, allowing restoration of penile circulation and resolution of edema.

B. To reduce edema, gently massage the penis and apply a hypertonic or hygroscopic agent (sugar). Corticosteroids and diuretics may reduce edema after the constriction is relieved.

C. When swelling has decreased, flush the prepuce with a mild antiseptic soap or lubricant.

D. Dilate the preputial edges to allow the penis to retract within the prepuce.

V. Surgical Treatment

A. General Considerations

1. In general, manage patients with acute paraphimosis conservatively.
2. For others, perform preputial reconstruction or penile amputation.
   a. Preputial deficiencies of less than 1 to 2 cm may be corrected by cranial advancement of the prepuce.
   b. Partial amputation of the penis is indicated for severe trauma or abnormalities of the penis or prepuce, neoplasia, recurring urethral prolapse, and recurring paraphimosis.

c. Perform castration to prevent recurrence of paraphimosis caused by sexual activity.

B. Positioning

1. Position the animal in dorsal recumbency.

C. Surgical Technique

1. Preputiotomy.

Make a full-thickness dorsal or ventral linear incision in the prepuce. If the preputial orifice is of normal size, anatomically reappose mucosa (e.g., 4-0 to 6-0 polydioxanone or polyglyconate, approximating sutures) and skin (e.g., 3-0 or 4-0 nylon or polypropylene, approximating sutures) in separate layers.

2. Preputial lengthening.

Lengthen or translocate the prepuce cranially by resecting a crescent-shaped piece of skin from the body wall just cranial to the prepuce. Preserve the preputial vessels. Identify the preputial muscles and shorten them by overlapping and suturing or segmental excision and reapposition. Close subcutaneous tissues and skin in two layers to further advance the skin cranially. Alternatively, the prepuce can be lengthened with a two-stage procedure in which oral mucosa is transplanted cranial to the prepuce and later rolled into a tube to cover the end of the penis.

3. Partial penile amputation.

Place a urethral catheter to facilitate orientation and prevent urethral trauma. Extrude the penis from the prepuce and maintain this position by snugly closing the preputial orifice around the penis with a towel clamp. Place a Penrose drain tourniquet caudal to the proposed amputation site. Make a lateral "V" incision through the tunica albuginea and cavernous tissue on each side of the urethra and os penis. Transect the os penis with bone cutters as far caudally as possible being careful not to traumatize the urethra. Transect the urethra 1 to 2 cm cranial to the penile transection and spatulate the dorsal aspect. Identify and ligate the dorsal artery of the penis after loosening the tourniquet. Fold the spatulated urethra over the transected end of the penis. Appose urethral mucosa to tunic albuginea; include some cavernous tissue with each bite. Use 4-0 to 6-0 polydioxanone or polyglyconate with a swaged-on, taper point needle in a simple interrupted or continuous pattern. Shorten the prepuce if the new penile tip cannot be extruded from the prepuce; the prepuce should extend approximately 1 cm cranial to the retracted penis. Resect an ellipse of prepuce approximately the same length as the amount of penis that was amputated. Make an elliptical, transverse, full-thickness incision in the midportion of the prepuce (beginning approximately 2 cm caudal to the cranial junction of the prepuce and body wall). Remove this ventral skin and mucosal segment, reflect the penis caudally, and resect a similar segment of dorsal preputial mucosa. Close the defect by first apposing the dorsal and then ventral preputial mucosa with 4-0 or 5-0 monofilament absorbable suture (e.g., polydioxanone or polyglyconate) in a simple interrupted or continuous pattern. Then appose skin with approximating 3-0 or 4-0 nonabsorbable sutures (e.g., nylon, polyproylene).

VI. Postoperative Care and Assessment

A. Provide analgesics.

B. Place an Elizabethan collar to prevent self-trauma.

C. Potential complications include dehiscence, stricture, infection, and recurrence.

D. Hemorrhage usually occurs during urination or excitement for several days after penile amputation.

VII. Prognosis

A. Inform owners that the prognosis with manual reduction or reconstruction plus castration is good; however, recurrence is common if the animal is not castrated.

Penile and Preputial Trauma and Neoplasia (*SAS*, pp. 572-574)

I. General Considerations

A. Trauma may cause penile hematomas or os penis fracture. Lacerations or punctures may bleed for days.

B. Neoplasms commonly found on skin occur on the prepuce: hemangiomas, papillomas, histiocytomas, melanomas, mast cell tumors, hemangiosarcomas, squamous cell carcinomas.

C. Neoplasms of the penis and mucosal lining of the prepuce include transmissible venereal tumors (TVTs), squamous cell carcinoma, hemangiosarcoma, and papillomas.

1. TVTs are contagious tumors spread by sexual contact or licking. They are wartlike, friable, and bleed easily.

II. Diagnosis

A. Clinical Presentation

1. Signalment.
   a. Young, intact males are more commonly affected by trauma
   b. Old, intact males are more commonly affected by tumors.
2. History.
   a. There is typically a history of serosanguineous, hemorrhagic, or purulent preputial discharge, inability or unwillingness to copulate, and/or pain.
   b. The urethra may be obstructed or lacerated, causing dysuria, anuria, or urine extravasation.
   c. Many dogs are asymptomatic.

B. Physical Examination

1. Abnormalities involving preputial skin are usually apparent; preputial mucosal lesions may be detected only by palpation.
2. It may be impossible to exteriorize the penis for examination if there is a mass within the prepuce or on the penis. In other cases,

paraphimosis is present because of injury causing inflammation, edema, and engorgement; or a mass prevents penile retraction.

C. Radiography/Ultrasonography

1. Take radiographs to reveal os penis fractures.
2. Perform a urethrogram to assess urethral involvement with penile trauma or tumors.

D. Laboratory Findings

1. Perform cytology of preputial or penile masses to help identify the tumor type.
   a. TVTs have large round cells with numerous mitotic figures.

III. Medical Management

A. Some injuries heal spontaneously.
   1. Allow penile hematomas to resolve spontaneously, unless they cause persistent paraphimosis.

B. Treat TVTs with vincristine, 0.5 mg/m^2 IV, or 0.025 mg/kg up to 1 mg IV, weekly for 3 to 6 weeks.

IV. Surgical Treatment

A. General Considerations

1. Resect tumors other than TVTs.
2. Perform partial or complete penile amputation for severely traumatized, necrotic, or neoplastic lesions.

B. Os Penis Fractures

1. Os penis fractures with minimal displacement require no surgery.
2. Splint displaced fractures with an indwelling polypropylene urethral catheter spanning the os penis and sutured to the tip of the urethra.
3. Stabilize more comminuted fractures with small plates, or amputate the penis.

C. Preoperative Management

1. Lavage the prepuce and penis with dilute antiseptic solutions.

D. Positioning

1. Position the animal in dorsal recumbency.

E. Surgical Technique

1. Preputial lacerations.

Debride, lavage, and appose preputial lacerations. Close full-thickness injuries in two layers, first apposing the preputial mucosa (e.g., 4-0 to 6-0 polydioxanone or polyglyconate) and then skin (e.g., 3-0 or 4-0 nylon or polypropylene) with approximating sutures. Hematomas that cause persistent paraphimosis can be surgically exposed and evacuated. Incise the tunic albuginea over the hematoma. Remove blood clots and fibrin. Lavage the cavity and snugly appose the tunic albuginea. Take care to maintain an adequate preputial orifice and length when reconstructing preputial lacerations.

2. Penile lacerations or punctures.

Suture the tunica albuginea to close penile lacerations or punctures and minimize hemorrhage during excitement or urination. Use 4-0 to 6-0 absorbable (e.g., polyglyconate or polydioxanone), simple interrupted sutures on a swaged-on, taper-point needle. Bleeding from small penile punctures or lacerations during penile engorgement is minimized by suturing the tunica albuginea.

V. Postoperative Care and Assessment

A. Provide analgesics and antibiotics as needed.

B. Monitor for hemorrhage and/or urine leakage.

C. Place an Elizabethan collar to prevent self-trauma.

D. Reevaluate for tumor recurrence or metastasis every 3 to 4 months for 1 year.

E. Potential complications include hemorrhage, seroma, infection, urine leakage, dehiscence, stricture, recurrence, and metastasis. Urethral obstruction may occur because callus formation following os penis fractures.

VI. Prognosis

A. Some injuries heal by second intention without complications; however, nonsutured preputial lacerations may fistulate. In other cases, persistent hemorrhage, urine extravasation, infection, and stricture may cause morbidity.

B. The prognosis is good following appropriate surgical treatment for most injuries.

C. The prognosis following tumor excision depends on the tumor type and stage.

24

Surgery of the Cardiovascular System (*SAS*, pp. 575-608)

General Principles and Techniques (*SAS*, pp. 575-582)

I. Definitions

A. **Closed cardiac procedures** are those that do not require opening major cardiac structures.

B. In **Open cardiac surgery,** a major cardiac structure must be opened to accomplish the repair.

C. **Venous inflow occlusion** provides brief circulatory arrest, allowing short procedures (<5 minutes) to be performed.

D. **Cardiopulmonary bypass** establishes an extracorporeal circulation to maintain organ perfusion during surgery.

II. Preoperative Concerns

A. Correct or control medically any cardiovascular compromise before anesthetic induction, if possible (see Appendix I).
   1. Manage congestive heart failure, particularly pulmonary edema, with diuretics (e.g., furosemide) and ACE inhibitors (e.g., enalapril, lisinopril).
   2. Recognize and treat cardiac arrhythmias (see Postoperative Care, p. 443).
      a. Suppress ventricular tachycardia with class I antiarrhythmic drugs (i.e., lidocaine, procainamide).
      b. For supraventricular tachycardia, use digoxin, β-adrenergic blockers (e.g., esmolol, propranolol, atenolol), or calcium channel blocking drugs (e.g., diltiazem).
      c. Control atrial fibrillation before surgery with digoxin to lower the ventricular response rate below 140 beats per minute. You may need to add a β-adrenergic blocker or calcium channel blocker if digoxin alone does not decrease the ventricular rate sufficiently.
      d. In bradycardic animals, consider an atropine response test. If

bradycardia is not responsive to atropine, consider temporary transvenous pacing or constant intravenous infusion of isoproterenol (see Management of Bradycardia).

e. Perform an echocardiogram before cardiac surgery because an incomplete or inaccurate diagnosis can have devastating consequences. With the advent of Doppler echocardiography, cardiac catheterization is no longer routinely necessary before cardiac surgery.

III. Anesthetic Considerations

A. Preanesthetics (see Appendixes G-24 and G-25)

1. Parenteral opioids (i.e., oxymorphone, butorphanol, buprenorphine, or fentanyl) induce sedation with minimal cardiovascular effects.
   a. Administer atropine or glycopyrrolate as needed to treat bradycardia when using an opioid.
   b. Combine benzodiazepines (i.e., diazepam, 0.2 mg/kg up to 5 mg; or midazolam, 0.2 mg/kg up to 5 mg), which have minimal cardiopulmonary effects with opioids to enhance sedation.

B. Induction of Anesthesia

1. Avoid thiobarbiturates in patients with significant cardiac disease because they cause dose-dependent cardiac depression and are arrhythmogenic.
2. Propofol (Diprivan, Rapinovet) produces rapid induction but causes essentially the same cardiovascular compromise as thiobarbiturates.
3. Consider ketamine combined with diazepam for induction of compromised patients.
   a. Do not use if the animal has mitral insufficiency because it increases the regurgitant fraction.
   b. Diazepam has minimal cardiopulmonary effects and helps offset the negative effects of ketamine (i.e., muscle rigidity and potential for seizures).
4. Consider opioids for induction of very sick and compromised dogs; however, opioids do not truly induce anesthesia, so intubation may be difficult in alert animals.
5. Etomidate is not arrhythmogenic, maintains cardiac output, and offers rapid induction.
6. Do not use mask induction with isoflurane because of the high inspired concentrations and time necessary to achieve intubation.

C. Maintenance

1. For compromised patients, isoflurane is the inhalation agent of choice.
   a. Use adjunct intravenous opioids to decrease the levels of isoflurane necessary to achieve adequate anesthesia.
   b. If further muscle relaxation is needed, use a nondepolarizing muscle relaxant.
      i. Atracurium 0.1 to 0.2 mg/kg IV.
2. Control ventilation.
   a. Manually squeeze the reservoir bag or use a mechanical ventilator.
      i. Ideally, mechanical ventilation should achieve a tidal volume of 10 to 15 ml/kg of body weight at an inspiratory pressure of 20 cm H_2O.
      ii. Ensure adequate ventilation by optimizing tidal volume, inspiratory pressure, and respiratory rate to achieve ventilation with the least risk of causing pulmonary injury or cardiovascular compromise.

iii. Monitor ventilation by measurement of end tidal CO_2 by capnography, or arterial CO_2 by blood gas analysis.

3. Inflow occlusion.
   a. Hyperventilate animals for 5 minutes before inflow occlusion.
   b. Discontinue ventilation during inflow occlusion and resume it immediately upon release of inflow occlusion.
   c. Perform gentle cardiac massage, if necessary, after inflow occlusion to reestablish cardiac function. Digitally occlude the descending aorta during this period to help direct available cardiac output to the heart and brain.
   d. If ventricular fibrillation occurs, perform immediate internal defibrillation as soon as inflow occlusion is discontinued.
   e. Initiate constant intravenous infusion of lidocaine (Table 24-1) before inflow occlusion and continued as needed.
   f. Administer epinephrine as a constant rate infusion as the animal is being weaned off inflow occlusion or a pump (see Table 24-1). If long-term inotropic support is necessary, give dobutamine (see Table 24-1).

IV. Antibiotics

A. Use perioperative antibiotics for cardiac procedures lasting more than 90 minutes.

B. Administer first-generation cephalosporins (e.g., cefazolin sodium, cephapirin sodium) intravenously at induction and repeat once or twice every 4 to 8 hours.

C. For cardiac procedures involving circulatory arrest or cardiopulmonary bypass, administer intravenous cefoxitin sodium before surgery and continue for 24 to 48 hours after surgery (see Appendix I).

V. Surgical Anatomy

A. Except for a portion of the right side of the heart (cardiac notch), most of the heart surface is covered by lung.

B. The phrenic nerves lie in a narrow plica of pleura adjacent to the pericardium at the heart base. Complete pericardiectomy requires that these nerves be elevated to avoid incising them.

C. The vagus nerves lie dorsal to the phrenic nerve.

Table 24-1
Drugs for inflow occlusion

Lidocaine
50-75 µg/kg/min IV infusion (see also Appendix I)
Dobutamine
10 µg/kg/min IV
Epinephrine
0.1-0.4 µg/kg/min IV

D. The left recurrent laryngeal nerve leaves the vagus and loops around the aortic arch distal to the ligamentum arteriosum to run cranially along the ventrolateral tracheal surface.

VI. Surgical Techniques

A. General Considerations

1. Ligature placement using hand ties are useful and the ability to place hand-tied knots (versus instrument tying) is a fundamental skill for cardiac surgeons.
2. Use fine suture with swaged-on atraumatic needles and carefully follow the needle contour when suturing (to minimize the size of needle tracts).
3. "Palming" of needle holders is a good skill for fast suturing, but avoid doing so when suturing inside the thoracic cavity. Finer control is gained by grasping instruments with fingers placed in the instrument rings.

B. Inflow Occlusion (*SAS,* pp. 578-579)

1. Ideally, circulatory arrest in a normothermic patient should be less than 2 minutes, but can be extended to 4 minutes if necessary. Circulatory arrest time can be extended up to 6 minutes with mild, whole-body hypothermia (30° to 34°C).

Depending on the cardiac procedure being done, perform a left or right thoracotomy or median sternotomy. With a right thoracotomy or median sternotomy, occlude the cranial and caudal venae cavae and azygous vein with vascular clamps or Rumel tourniquets. Make a Rumel tourniquet by passing umbilical tape around the vessel, then thread the umbilical tape through a piece of rubber tubing that is 1 to 3 inches long. When the umbilical tape has been adequately tightened to occlude the vessel, place a clamp above the rubber tubing to hold it securely in place. Take care to avoid injuring the right phrenic nerve during placement of the clamps or tourniquets. For left thoracotomies, pass separate tourniquets around the cranial and caudal venae cavae. Then, dissecting dorsal to the esophagus and aorta, occlude the azygous vein by placing a tourniquet around it.

C. Cardiopulmonary Bypass (*SAS,* p. 578)

1. Greatly extends the time available for open cardiac surgery. It can be used to treat dogs with congenital or acquired cardiac defects.
2. Readers are referred to a cardiovascular surgery text for details of performing cardiopulmonary bypass.

VII. Healing of Cardiovascular Structures

A. Vascular structures heal quickly, forming a fibrin seal within minutes.

B. Epithelialization and early endothelial regeneration occur in veins used for grafts.

C. To avoid thrombosis of vascular structures, handle them gently because trauma may lead to the deposition of platelets, fibrin, and red cells on the intimal surface. If the torn intima is lifted upward, a flap may develop that partially or completely occludes the distal lumen. This in turn can lead to accumulation of blood within the vessel wall, vascular sludging, and thrombosis.

VIII. Suture Materials/Special Instruments

A. Suture

1. Polypropylene (3-0, 4-0, and 5-0) is the standard suture used for cardiovascular procedures.
2. Use swaged-on taper-point cardiovascular needles. Some procedures require that suture be double-armed (i.e., with needles at both ends).
3. Use teflon pledgets for buttressing mattress sutures in ventricular myocardium or great vessels.

B. Instruments

1. The standard thoracic retractor is a Finochietto retractor. Have at least two sizes to accommodate different-sized animals.
2. The standard tissue forceps for thoracic surgery is a DeBakey tissue forceps. Have at least two available; it is helpful if one has a carbide inlay for grasping suture needles.
3. Metzenbaum scissors are the standard operating scissors for cardiac surgery. Curved Metzenbaum scissors are more versatile than the straight design.
4. Potts scissors (45-degree angle) are desirable for some cardiac surgery.
5. Needle holders (Mayo-Heger, Crile-Wood, Castroviejo) should be long and available in different sizes to accommodate a variety of suture needle sizes.
6. Have angled thoracic forceps available in a variety of sizes.
7. Vascular clamps are noncrushing clamps used for temporary occlusion of cardiovascular and pulmonary structures. The most versatile shape for most cardiac surgery is a medium-width tangential clamp.

IX. Postoperative Care and Assessment

A. Evaluate ventilation carefully and often.

1. Hypoventilation.
   a. Assessment.
      i. Assess total ventilation directly by measuring the volume of expired gas with a respirometer. Tidal volume should be at least 10 ml per kg of body weight.
      ii. The best measure of alveolar ventilation is arterial CO_2 tension ($Paco_2$). Alveolar hypoventilation is present when $Paco_2$ is increased above 40 mm Hg.
   b. Treatment.
      i. Correct the underlying cause if possible.
      ii. Use drugs that are known to depress ventilation (i.e., opioids and muscle relaxants) with caution in the perioperative period. Weigh the risk of ventilatory depression against the risk of hypoventilation caused by pain.
      iii. Evacuate pleural air or fluid if present.
      iv. Correct injury or dysfunction of the neuromuscular ventilatory apparatus, if possible.

v. If hypoventilation is severe and the cause is not immediately correctable, use positive-pressure ventilation.

vi. Supplement oxygen.

(a) Maintain oxygen saturation (Sao_2) at or above 90%. Measure Sao_2 using pulse oximetry.

(b) On a blood gas keep the Pao_2 above 80 mm of Hg.

(c) Consider positive end-expiratory pressure (PEEP) therapy for patients with severe gas exchange impairment that is not responsive to supplemental oxygen therapy alone.

(d) Maintain the PCV above 30%, especially if cardiopulmonary compromise is present.

2. Hypotension.

a. Measure blood pressure to assess cardiovascular function, especially during and immediately after surgery.

i. Indirect techniques include the oscillometric method, the basis of monitors such as the Dinamap, or Doppler method.

ii. Direct measurement requires placement of an arterial catheter.

b. Maintain a mean blood pressure above 65 mm of Hg and systolic blood pressure above 90 mm Hg. Maintain central venous pressure between 5 and 10 cm H_2O.

i. Elevate blood pressure by increasing either cardiac output or systemic vascular resistance.

(a) Obtain inotropic and pressor support by constant intravenous infusion of epinephrine (see Table 24-1).

(b) Maintain long-term inotropic support by dobutamine (see Table 24-1).

3. Arrhythmias

a. Sinus tachycardia is the most common rhythm disturbance in surgery patients.

i. Direct therapy at correcting its underlying cause and improving cardiac output.

b. Ventricular arrhythmias, including premature ventricular complexes (PVCs) and nonsustained or sustained ventricular tachycardia, are common during and after surgery.

i. Suppress frequent PVCs, particularly when they occur with a short coupling interval (i.e., R on T phenomena), and rapid ventricular tachycardia.

(a) Continuous intravenous infusion of lidocaine is effective in most instances.

c. Have equipment available to defibrillate animals.

X. Complications

A. Hemorrhage

1. Have materials available for blood transfusion. Collect fresh whole blood as close as possible to the time that it is needed. Cooling the blood may reduce platelet content. If possible, identify a compatible donor by crossmatching with the patient before surgery.
2. Consider autotransfusion in animals that are bleeding after surgery by collecting blood from the pleural space directly into CPDA (citrate, phosphate, dextrose, adenine) collection bags and returning the blood to the patient with a standard blood administration filter. In most cases, autotransfusion of bleeding patients is preferred over returning the patient to surgery to control bleeding.

XI. Special Age Considerations

A. Do not withhold food for more than 4 to 6 hours before surgery in young animals. Feed them as soon as they are fully recovered from anesthesia. If they cannot be fed, support glucose concentrations by adding glucose to intravenous fluids and monitor serum glucose concentrations intraoperatively.

B. Hypothermia is common in young patients during thoracotomy and is protective during cardiac procedures. Monitor the temperature closely and actively rewarm them postoperatively.

Specific Diseases

Patent Ductus Arteriosus (*SAS*, pp. 582-585)

I. Definition

A. The **ductus arteriosus** is a fetal vessel that normally closes shortly after birth; continued patency of the ductus arteriosus for more than a few days after birth is termed **patent ductus arteriosus (PDA).**

II. General Considerations and Clinically Relevant Pathophysiology

A. PDA is the most common congenital heart defect of dogs; it also occurs in cats.

B. It causes a left-to-right shunt resulting in volume overload of the left ventricle and produces left ventricular dilation and hypertrophy. Progressive left ventricular dilation distends the mitral valve annulus causing secondary regurgitation and additional ventricular overload. This severe volume overload leads to left-sided congestive heart failure and pulmonary edema, usually within the first year of life. Atrial fibrillation may occur as a late sequela caused by marked left atrial dilation.

C. Rarely, dogs with PDA develop suprasystemic pulmonary hypertension that reverses the direction of flow through the shunt causing severe hypoxemia and cyanosis (Eisenmenger's physiology). Right-to-left PDA can be a late sequela to untreated PDA. In very young animals it may be caused by persistent pulmonary hypertension after birth.

III. Diagnosis

A. Clinical Presentation

1. Signalment.
   a. Most common in purebred, female dogs.

b. Maltese, Pomeranians, Shetland sheepdogs, English springer spaniels, keeshonden, bichons frises, miniature and toy poodles, and Yorkshire terriers are at increased risk for developing PDA.
c. A genetic basis has been established in poodles.

2. History.
   a. Most young animals with PDA are asymptomatic or have only mild exercise intolerance.
   b. The most common complaint in symptomatic animals with left-to-right shunts is cough or shortness of breath (or both) caused by pulmonary edema.
   c. Animals with right-to-left or reverse PDA may be asymptomatic or have exercise intolerance and hind limb collapse on exercise.

B. Physical Examination Findings

1. Auscultation.
   a. The most prominent physical finding associated with PDA is a characteristic continuous (machinery) murmur heard best at the left heart base.
   b. The left apical cardiac impulse is prominent and displaced caudally and a palpable cardiac "thrill" often is present.
2. Femoral pulses are strong or hyperkinetic (water hammer pulse) because of a wide pulse pressure caused by diastolic runoff of blood through the ductus.
3. Tall R waves (greater than 2.5 mV) or wide P waves on a lead II ECG are supportive of the diagnosis, but not always present. Atrial fibrillation or ventricular ectopy may be present in advanced cases.
4. Right-to-left or reverse PDA.
   a. "Differential" cyanosis is typically present (i.e., cyanosis is most apparent in the caudal mucous membranes), but cyanosis may also be noted in the cranial half of the body in some animals.
   b. A systolic cardiac murmur, rather than a machinery murmur, is often present. However, a murmur may not be auscultated if polycythemia is present (see Laboratory Findings later in this section) or if left- and right-sided pressures are nearly equal, and shunting of blood through the ductus is minimal.

C. Radiography/Echocardiography

1. Thoracic radiographs typically show left atrial and ventricular enlargement, enlargement of pulmonary vessels, and a characteristic dilation of the descending aorta on the dorsoventral view.
2. Echocardiographic findings that support a diagnosis of PDA include left atrial enlargement, left ventricular dilation and hypertrophy, pulmonary artery dilation, increased aortic ejection velocity, and a characteristic reverse turbulent Doppler flow pattern in the pulmonary artery.
3. Right-to-left PDA.
   a. Thoracic radiographs show evidence of biventricular enlargement and marked enlargement of the pulmonary artery segment. Pulmonary arteries may also appear tortuous.
   b. Document by performing a saline bubble contrast echocardiogram. Observing bubbles in the descending aorta, but not in any left-sided cardiac chamber, is diagnostic.

D. Laboratory Findings

1. Laboratory abnormalities are uncommon in animals with left-to-right shunting PDA.
2. Animals with right-to-left shunts are commonly polycythemic in response to increased erythropoietin production caused by chronic hypoxemia.

IV. Differential Diagnosis

A. A combination of aortic stenosis/aortic insufficiency or ventricular septal defect/aortic insufficiency results in a to-and-fro murmur that may be difficult to differentiate from continuous PDA murmurs.

B. In some animals in which the diastolic component of the PDA murmur is difficult to detect, other differentials include subaortic stenosis, pulmonic stenosis, atrial septal defect, and ventricular septal defect.

C. Differentials for dogs with right-to-left PDA include tetralogy of Fallot, right-to-left shunting atrial or ventricular septal defects, or other complex forms of cyanotic heart disease (rare).

V. Medical Management

A. Give furosemide for 24 to 48 hours before surgery in animals with pulmonary edema (see Appendix I).

B. If atrial fibrillation is present, control the ventricular response rate using digoxin (with or without β-adrenergic blockers or calcium channel blockers) before surgery (see Appendix I).

C. If hemodynamically significant arrhythmias are present, control them.

VI. Surgical Treatment

A. General Considerations

1. Perform ligation or intravascular occlusion of the PDA as soon as possible after diagnosis.
2. Secondary mitral regurgitation usually regresses after surgery because of reduction in left ventricular dilation.

B. Preoperative Management

1. Control preoperative arrhythmias before surgery.
2. If the animal has signs of congestive heart failure, initiate treatment with positive inotropes (i.e., digoxin), vasodilators (i.e., hydralazine, enalapril), and diuretics (i.e., furosemide) preoperatively (see Appendix I).
3. Avoid excessive diuretics and/or vasodilators that may cause hypotension.

C. Anesthesia

1. Give an anticholinergic (i.e., atropine or glycopyrrolate) if the heart rate drops below 60 beats per minute after ductal occlusion.
2. Have blood available for transfusion if excessive hemorrhage occurs during the surgical procedure.
3. See Appendixes G-24 and G-25 for techniques for anesthetic management of cardiovascular patients.

D. Surgical Anatomy

1. The ductus arteriosus in dogs and cats is located between the aorta

and main pulmonary arteries, caudal to the origin of the brachycephalic and left subclavian arteries.

2. The left vagus nerve always passes over the ductus arteriosus and must be identified and retracted during dissection. The left recurrent laryngeal nerve can often be identified as it loops around the ductus.

E. Positioning

1. Position the animal in right lateral recumbency and prepare the left thorax for aseptic surgery.

F. Surgical Techniques

Perform a left fourth space intercostal thoracotomy. Identify the left vagus nerve as it courses over the ductus arteriosus and isolate it using sharp dissection at the level of the ductus. Place a suture around the nerve and gently retract it. Isolate the ductus arteriosus by bluntly dissecting around it without opening the pericardial sac. Pass a right-angle forceps behind the ductus, parallel to its transverse plane, to isolate the caudal aspect of the ductus. Then dissect the cranial aspect of the ductus by angling the forceps caudally approximately 45 degrees. Complete dissection of the ductus by passing forceps from medial to the ductus in a caudal to cranial direction. Grasp the suture with right-angle forceps. Slowly pull the suture beneath the ductus. If the suture does not slide easily around the ductus, do not force it. Regrasp the suture and repeat the process, being careful not to include surrounding soft tissues in the forceps. Pass a second suture using the same maneuver. Alternatively, the suture may be passed as a double loop and the suture cut so that you have two strands. Slowly tighten the suture closest to the aorta first. Then tighten the remaining suture.

VII. Suture Materials/Special Instruments

A. Use heavy silk (No. 1 or 0) or cotton tape for ductal ligation.

B. For blunt dissection of the PDA and passing ligatures use right-angle forceps.

C. Angled or tangential vascular clamps are required for surgical division of PDA, or for repair of inadvertent ruptures.

D. Use polypropylene mattress sutures (4-0), buttressed with Teflon pledgets to repair ruptured PDAs.

VIII. Postoperative Care and Assessment

A. Treat postoperative pain with systemic opioids and local anesthetic techniques. Consider bupivacaine given intercostally or intrapleurally to supplement analgesia (see Appendix I).

B. Feed young animals as soon as they are fully recovered from surgery.

C. Generally, remove thoracostomy tubes (if used) within 12 to 24 hours after surgery.

IX. Prognosis

A. Seventy percent of dogs with untreated PDA die before 1 year of age.

Pulmonic Stenosis (*SAS*, pp. 585-588)

I. Definition

A. **Pulmonic stenosis (PS)** is a congenital narrowing of the pulmonic valve, pulmonary artery, or right ventricular outflow tract.

II. General Considerations and Clinically Relevant Pathophysiology

A. PS is a common congenital heart defect in dogs and an uncommon defect in cats.

B. In dogs, the condition is usually valvular, although supravalvular and subvalvular defects have been reported.

C. PS causes pressure overload and hypertrophy of the right ventricle. Right ventricular hypertrophy often compounds right ventricular outflow obstruction by narrowing the right ventricular outflow tract. Narrowing of the right ventricular outflow tract is greatest during systole, producing a dynamic obstruction that contributes to the fixed stenosis.

III. Diagnosis

A. Clinical Presentation

1. Signalment.
   a. English bulldogs, beagles, miniature schnauzers, cocker spaniels, Samoyeds, mastiffs, and terrier breeds are at increased risk to develop PS.
   b. English bulldogs and boxers have a high concurrent incidence of aberrant left coronary artery (because of a single right coronary artery), which has important surgical implications.
2. History.
   a. Young animals with PS are often asymptomatic.
   b. Advanced cases may present with exercise intolerance, syncope, or abdominal distention from ascites.

B. Physical Examination Findings

1. The predominate physical finding is a systolic ejection murmur heard best at the left heart base.
2. The ECG may show prominent S waves in leads I, II, III, and a VF indicative of a right axis shift and right ventricular hypertrophy.

C. Radiography/Echocardiography

1. Thoracic radiographs show varying degrees of right ventricular enlargement and main pulmonary artery segment enlargement.
2. Echocardiographic findings include right ventricular hypertrophy, poststenotic dilation of the main pulmonary artery, malformation of the pulmonic valve, and a high pulmonary flow velocity.
3. Cardiac catheterization is usually only necessary if abnormal coronary anatomy is suspected or an intervention procedure (e.g., percutaneous balloon valvuloplasty) is performed.

D. Laboratory Findings

1. Specific laboratory abnormalities are not found in animals with PS.

IV. Differential Diagnosis

A. Differential diagnoses include subvalvular aortic stenosis, ventricular septal defect, atrial septal defect, and tetralogy of Fallot.

V. Medical Management

A. There is no specific medical therapy for PS other than symptomatic treatment for congestive heart failure, if it occurs.

B. Percutaneous balloon valvuloplasty is a nonsurgical alternative for correction of moderate to severe PS, if facilities and expertise for cardiac catheterization are available. Simple valvular PS is more amenable to balloon valvuloplasty than severe pulmonic valve dysplasia or severe PS with dynamic obstruction.

VI. Surgical Treatment

A. Base therapy for PS on its degree of severity and on the type of lesion present. Judge severity by the presence of signs, extent of right ventricular hypertrophy, and magnitude of systolic pressure gradient.

1. Measure systolic pressure gradients in unsedated or unanesthetized animals.
   a. Mild–less than 50 mm Hg.
   b. Moderate–50 to 75 mm Hg.
   c. Severe–greater than 75 mm Hg.
2. Animals with PS that have no signs, mild hypertrophy, and a pressure gradient less than 50 mm Hg generally do not require surgical intervention.
3. If the pressure gradient is greater than 50 mm Hg and right ventricular hypertrophy is significant, surgical correction should be considered.

B. In English bulldogs, the left coronary artery may course across the right ventricular outflow tract and is at risk for injury during valve dilation. Sudden death caused by rupture of the coronary artery has occurred during balloon valvuloplasty. Aberrant left coronary artery also precludes patch-graft valvuloplasty. A valved or nonvalved conduit placed between the right ventricle and pulmonary artery is a possible surgical option for this condition.

C. Preoperative management.
1. Manage right-sided congestive heart failure or cardiac arrhythmias medically before surgery (see previous discussion).

D. Surgical anatomy.
1. The pulmonary valve is approached through a left fourth or fifth intercostal thoracotomy or median sternotomy. The valve consists of right, left, and intermediate semilunar cusps.
2. The area in which sounds associated with lesions of the pulmonary valve may be heard best is located at the fourth intercostal space, slightly below a line drawn through the point of the shoulder.
3. See also previous comments about concurrent aberrant left coronary arteries.

E. Positioning.
1. Position animals in right lateral recumbency and prepare the entire left hemithorax for aseptic surgery.

VII. Surgical Techniques

A. General Considerations

1. Animals with moderate pressure gradients, simple valvular lesions, and moderate infundibular hypertrophy are most likely to benefit from valve dilation techniques.
2. Patch-graft valvuloplasty is indicated for severe PS, particularly if marked infundibular hypertrophy and dynamic stenosis are suspected. Patch-graft valvuloplasty also can be used effectively to relieve concurrent or isolated supravalvular PS.

B. Surgical Techniques

1. Valve dilation.

Perform a left fourth intercostal thoracotomy. Open the pericardium over the right outflow tract and suture it to the thoracotomy incision. Place a buttressed mattress suture in the right ventricular outflow tract and pass it through a tourniquet. Make a stab incision in the ventricle and pass a dilating instrument into the right ventricular outflow tract and across the pulmonic valve (see SAS, Fig. 24-9). Dilate the pulmonic valve several times by opening and closing the dilating instrument. Remove the instrument and close the ventricular incision by tying the mattress suture.

2. Open-patch graft correction.

Perform a left fifth intercostal thoracotomy. Pass tape tourniquets around the vena cavae and azygous vein for inflow occlusion (see p. 441). Make a partial-thickness incision in the right ventricular outflow tract. Suture an autogenous pericardial or synthetic patch to the ventriculotomy incision and the cranial aspect of the pulmonary artery. Initiate venous inflow occlusion and make full-thickness incisions into the pulmonary artery and right ventricle. Incise or excise dysplastic pulmonic valve leaflets, as necessary. Complete suturing of the pulmonary artery to the patch-graft and discontinue inflow occlusion. Resuscitate the heart. It is important to remove air from the heart by discontinuing inflow occlusion just before tying the last suture.

VIII. Suture Materials/Special Instruments

A. Use polypropylene (3-0) suture buttressed with Teflon pledgets for transventricular valve dilation.

B. Accomplish valve dilation with a Cooley or Tubbs valve dilating instrument or with an appropriately sized hemostatic forceps.

C. Synthetic materials such as polytetrafluoroethylene (PTFE) or autogenous pericardium can be used for the patch-graft procedure. Polypropylene (4-0) suture is appropriate for suturing the patch-graft.

IX. Postoperative Care and Assessment

A. Treat postoperative pain with systemic opioids and local anesthetic techniques (see Appendix I).

B. Monitor animals for pulmonary edema after surgery. If pulmonary edema occurs, administer furosemide (see Appendix I).

X. Prognosis

A. Valve dilation is associated with minimal risk of complications and carries a low operative mortality, but is less likely to be effective for severe PS.

B. Operative mortality for patch grafting for this procedure is approximately 15% to 20% in the hands of an experienced surgeon. The most common problem encountered is inability to resuscitate the heart after inflow occlusion.

C. Prognosis for dogs with PS depends on its severity.
   1. Animals with systolic pressure gradients greater than 75 mm Hg are likely to experience heart failure or sudden death early in life.
   2. The prognosis after surgery depends on the degree of gradient reduction achieved.
      a. Valve dilation procedures are effective in relieving moderate to severe stenosis, but may not sufficiently reduce the pressure gradient across severely dysplastic valves.
      b. Patch-graft valvuloplasty is highly effective at relieving the pressure gradient across the pulmonic valve, regardless of severity, but it carries a higher risk of operative mortality.

Aortic Stenosis (*SAS*, pp. 588-591)

I. Definition

A. **Aortic stenosis** is a congenital narrowing of the aortic valve, aorta, or left ventricular outflow tract. The stenosis may be supravalvular, valvular, or subvalvular.

II. General Considerations and Clinically Relevant Pathophysiology

A. Subvalvular aortic stenosis (SAS) is the second most common congenital heart defect of dogs and is the most important defect affecting large-breed dogs. Aortic stenosis (AS) occurs uncommonly in cats.

B. Subvalvular AS accounts for greater than 90% of canine cases. The typical lesion is a discrete subvalvular fibrous ring that courses across the ventricular septum and reflects onto the anterior mitral valve leaflet.

C. Subvalvular AS causes pressure overload of the left ventricle. Varying degrees of left ventricular concentric hypertrophy develop, depending on severity.
   1. Dogs with moderate to severe SAS are at risk for sudden death, presumably the result of myocardial ischemia and malignant ventricular arrhythmias.
   2. Affected dogs may also develop congestive heart failure, particularly if concurrent mitral insufficiency is present.
   3. Affected dogs are at increased risk to develop bacterial endocarditis of the aortic valve because of turbulent blood flow that occurs around the valve.

III. Diagnosis

A. Clinical Presentation

1. Signalment.
   a. Newfoundlands, golden retrievers, rottweilers, German shepherds, boxers, and Samoyeds are at increased risk to develop SAS.
   b. A genetic basis for SAS has been established in Newfoundland dogs.
   c. Subvalvular AS should be considered a progressive lesion until maturity.
2. History.
   a. Dogs with SAS may be asymptomatic or exhibit exercise intolerance, collapse, or syncope.
   b. Lack of clinical signs is not an appropriate reason to delay diagnostic evaluation because the first clinical evidence of SAS may be sudden death.

B. Physical Examination Findings

1. The predominant physical finding in animals with SAS is a systolic ejection murmur heard best at the left heart base. The murmur radiates well to the right base and thoracic inlet.
2. In moderate to severe cases, femoral pulses are noticeably weak or hypokinetic, unless substantial concurrent aortic insufficiency is present.

C. Radiography/Echocardiography

1. Thoracic radiographs may reveal a normal cardiac silhouette or mild left ventricular enlargement. Enlargement of the ascending aorta frequently is evident.
2. Definitive diagnosis of SAS is obtained by echocardiography.
   a. M-mode echocardiography demonstrates variable left ventricular freewall and septal thickening, depending on severity. With

moderate to severe disease, left ventricular diameter is small unless substantial concurrent aortic or mitral insufficiency is present.

b. Systolic anterior motion (SAM) of the mitral valve may cause mitral insufficiency.
c. Early closure of the aortic valve suggests that dynamic obstruction may be present.
d. Doppler-measured aortic velocities are increased (systolic gradients measured in unsedated or unanesthetized animals).
   i. Mild–25 to 50 mm Hg.
   ii. Moderate–50 to 75 mm Hg.
   iii. Severe–greater than 75 mm Hg.

D. Laboratory Findings

1. Specific laboratory abnormalities are not associated with SAS.

IV. Differential Diagnosis

A. Differentiate aortic stenosis from other conditions that may cause systolic murmurs (i.e., pulmonic stenosis, ventricular septal defect, tetralogy of Fallot).

V. Medical Management

A. Consider β-adrenergic blockade therapy with propranolol or atenolol (see Appendix I) because it may reduce the risk for sudden death by decreasing myocardial oxygen requirements and suppressing ventricular arrhythmias during exercise.

B. Treat heart failure symptomatically (i.e., furosemide, enalapril) if it occurs.

VI. Surgical Treatment

A. General Considerations

1. Consider surgical intervention for dogs with substantial left ventricular hypertrophy and systolic gradients above 75 mm Hg. If surgery is undertaken, do it early to minimize degenerative myocardial changes.
2. Surgical options for dogs with SAS include valve dilation and open resection. Open resection during cardiopulmonary bypass is currently the most effective treatment for severe SAS in dogs.

B. Preoperative Management

1. Control arrhythmias with appropriate antiarrhythmic drugs (i.e., atenolol, procainamide, tocainamide, sotolol) before surgery.
2. Discontinue β-adrenergic blockade 24 hours before surgery by gradually tapering the dose over 3 to 5 days.

C. Surgical Anatomy

1. Subvalvular stenosis usually consists of a discrete fibrous ring located 1 to 3 mm below the aortic valve leaflets. The ring generally extends across the septum and reflects onto the anterior mitral valve leaflet.
2. The conduction system (His bundle) courses through the septum at the juncture of the right and noncoronary aortic leaflets.

D. Positioning

1. Position the animal in dorsal recumbency to perform a transventricular aortic valve dilation.
2. Prepare the entire sternum from proximal to the manubrium to distal to the xiphoid cartilage for aseptic surgery.

E. Surgical Techniques

1. Transventricular aortic valve dilation.

Perform a median sternotomy. Open the pericardium and suture it to the incision to elevate the apex of the heart. Place a buttressed mattress suture in the left ventricular apex and pass it through a tourniquet. Pass a Cooley valve dilator through a stab incision in the left ventricle and position it in the left ventricular outflow tract by palpating the ascending aorta. Open the valve dilator several times to widen the outflow tract.

VII. Suture Materials/Special Instruments

A. Accomplish valve dilation by a transventricular approach with a Cooley valve dilator.

B. Use polypropylene (3-0) suture buttressed with Teflon pledgets for the transventricular mattress stitch.

VIII. Postoperative Care and Assessment

A. Monitor ventilation carefully in the early postoperative period. Poor ventilatory efforts may be associated with residual pneumothorax, hemorrhage, anesthetic agents, or pain.

B. Monitor heart rate and rhythm postoperatively for 48 to 72 hours, and treat hemodynamically significant arrhythmias.

C. Measure blood pressure by direct or indirect means until the animal is fully recovered from anesthesia.

D. Give analgesics (local anesthetic techniques and systemic opioids) to decrease postoperative discomfort.

E. Monitor urine output if hypotension occurred during surgery or postoperatively.

IX. Prognosis

A. Retrospective analysis of dogs with SAS suggests that those with systolic gradients above 75 mm Hg have a substantial risk for sudden death in the first several years of life.

B. Valve dilation can be performed at an early age with low operative mortality and without cardiopulmonary bypass.

C. Open resection of SAS under cardiopulmonary bypass may result in a 70% to 90% reduction of the systolic pressure gradient that is sustained for at least several years after. The procedure reduces, but probably does not eliminate, the risk for sudden death.

Ventricular Septal Defect (*SAS*, pp. 591-594)

I. Definition

A. **Ventricular septal defect (VSD)** is a congenital defect that results from failure or incomplete development of the membranous or muscular interventricular septum.

II. General Considerations and Clinically Relevant Pathophysiology

A. VSD is the second most common congenital heart defect in cats and accounts for 5% to 10% of congenital heart defects seen in dogs.

B. The etiology of VSD is incompletely understood, but is suspected to have a genetic component. VSD has been demonstrated to be a polygenic trait in keeshonden.

C. Most ventricular septal defects in small animals occur in the membranous septum.

D. The pathophysiology of VSD depends on the size of the defect and on pulmonary vascular resistance. VSD typically causes a left-to-right shunt.
   1. A typical VSD overloads the left heart and, depending on its size and location, may overload the right heart as well.
   2. A large VSD can progress to left-sided congestive heart failure.
   3. Chronic overcirculation of the lungs can cause progressive pulmonary vascular remodeling leading to severe pulmonary hypertension and right-to-left shunting of blood (Eisenmenger's physiology).

E. Aortic insufficiency is a fairly common secondary abnormality associated with VSD, particularly infundibular VSD.

III. Diagnosis

A. Clinical Presentation

1. Signalment.
   a. No breed predisposition has been clearly determined for VSD; however, English bulldogs may have a higher than expected incidence.
2. History.
   a. Young animals with VSD often are asymptomatic at first presentation.

b. Animals with large VSD may present with signs of left-sided congestive heart failure (i.e., cough and shortness of breath).

B. Physical Examination Findings

1. The most prominent physical finding associated with VSD is a systolic murmur with the point of maximal intensity at the right sternum. The murmur usually also is heard well at the left heart base.
2. Animals with right-to-left VSD may have no murmur because of polycythemia.

C. Radiography/Echocardiography

1. Thoracic radiographs reveal varying degrees of left or biventricular enlargement, depending on the size of the defect. The degree of pulmonary vascular enlargement from overcirculation also depends on the size of the defect and pulmonary vascular resistance.
2. A VSD larger than 5 mm usually can be visualized directly on two-dimensional echocardiography.
3. Color-flow Doppler is particularly useful for detecting small defects. The direction and velocity of shunt flow can be determined by spectral Doppler.
   a. A high-velocity left-to-right shunt suggests that the VSD is "restrictive" or hemodynamically insignificant and warrants a good prognosis.
   b. Large defects are usually associated with lower shunt velocities and suggest the animal is at risk for development of progressive heart failure or pulmonary hypertension.
   c. The pulmonary to systemic flow ratio can be calculated from Doppler analysis of aortic and pulmonary flows. Pulmonary to systemic flow ratios (Q_p:Q_s) greater than 2:1 are indicative of a hemodynamically significant VSD.

D. Laboratory Findings

1. Polycythemia may be present in dogs with right-to-left shunts.

IV. Differential Diagnosis

A. Differential diagnoses include subaortic stenosis, pulmonic stenosis, tetralogy of Fallot, atrial septal defect, and atrioventricular septal defects.

V. Medical Management

A. Medical management for VSD (see Appendix I) consists of symptomatic treatment for congestive heart failure.

B. There is no effective medical management for Eisenmenger's physiology.

C. Use periodic phlebotomy and replacement with crystalloid fluids to keep the hematocrit below 60%.

D. Recommend low-dose aspirin therapy to prevent thromboembolic complications.

VI. Surgical Treatment

A. General Considerations

1. Consider surgical intervention for hemodynamically significant VSD.
2. Concurrent aortic insufficiency usually is progressive and also is an indication for surgical intervention.

B. Preoperative Management

1. If significant heart failure is present, attempt to control it medically.

C. Surgical Anatomy

1. The interventricular septum is composed of a dorsal, thin, membranous part and a large, ventral, muscular part. The membranous part is formed by fusion of the atrioventricular cushions. When the cushions fail to fuse, a ventricular septal defect arises.
2. The AV node and its bundle are usually closely associated with the caudal margin of a perimembranous VSD.

D. Positioning

1. Position the animal in right lateral recumbency for pulmonary artery banding.
2. Prepare the entire left thorax for aseptic surgery.

E. Surgical Techniques

1. Pulmonary artery banding.

Perform a left fourth intercostal thoracotomy. Open the pericardium and suture it to the thoracotomy incision. Separate the pulmonary artery from the aorta using a combination of sharp and blunt dissection. Pass a large cotton or Teflon tape around the pulmonary artery just distal to the pulmonic valve. Tighten the tape to reduce the circumference of the pulmonary artery. Place a purse-string suture in the pulmonary artery wall distal to the ligature and insert a catheter into the pulmonary artery to measure pressures. Constrict the pulmonary artery until the pulmonary artery pressure distal to the band is less than 30 mm Hg. Also, monitor systemic artery pressures, which should increase during the banding. Optimal banding is where the increase in systemic arterial pressures just reaches a plateau.

VII. Suture Materials/Special Instruments

A. Use wide cotton or Teflon tape for pulmonary artery banding.

VIII. Postoperative Care and Assessment

A. Observe the animal closely for worsening of heart failure secondary to anesthesia, surgery, or arrhythmias.

B. If the animal becomes hypoxemic or cyanotic the band may have been placed too tightly.

C. Treat postoperative pain with systemic opioids and local anesthetic techniques.

IX. Prognosis

A. The prognosis for animals with VSD depends on the size of the defect.
   1. Animals with small "restrictive" defects may tolerate the defect without ill effects.
   2. Large defects (i.e., $Q_p:Q_s$ greater than 2:1) will likely result in the development of progressive heart failure or pulmonary hypertension.
   3. Pulmonary artery banding is a reasonably effective procedure for palliation of the consequences of a hemodynamically significant VSD in both dogs and cats. Definitive closure of a VSD under cardiopulmonary bypass is considered curative.
   4. Dogs with uncorrected VSD are potentially at increased risk for development of bacterial endocarditis.
   5. Aortic insufficiency places an added volume load on the left ventricle and is generally indicative of a poor prognosis.

Tetralogy of Fallot (*SAS*, pp. 594-596)

I. Definition

A. **Tetralogy of Fallot** is a complex congenital heart defect that consists of pulmonic stenosis, ventricular septal defect, a dextropositioned overriding aorta, and right ventricular hypertrophy.

II. General Considerations and Clinically Relevant Pathophysiology

A. Tetralogy of Fallot (T of F) is the most common congenital heart defect that causes cyanosis in small animals.

B. It occurs in cats and a variety of canine breeds (see Signalment, directly below).

C. Tetralogy of Fallot can be simplified into two physiologically significant defects: pulmonic stenosis and ventricular septal defect (VSD). The pathophysiologic consequences of T of F depend on the relative magnitude of these two defects.

III. Diagnosis

A. Clinical Presentation

1. Signalment.
   a. Breeds most commonly reported to have T of F include keeshonden, English bulldogs, poodles, schnauzers, terriers, collies, and shelties.
   b. In keeshonden, T of F is genetically transmitted as part of the spectrum of conotruncal defects.
2. History.
   a. Clinical findings at presentation for a typical T of F include

moderate to severe exercise intolerance, exertional tachypnea, collapse, and syncope.

B. Physical Examination Findings

1. Physical findings in animals with T of F include cyanosis unresponsive to supplemental oxygen and systolic murmurs heard well at the left heart base and right sternum.
2. If polycythemia is severe, a murmur may not be heard.

C. Radiography/Echocardiography/Electrocardiography

1. Thoracic radiographs typically show evidence of right ventricular enlargement, with or without main pulmonary artery enlargement. Pulmonary vessels are usually small, suggesting pulmonary undercirculation.
2. Electrocardiograms usually show a right axis shift in the frontal plane suggestive of right ventricular hypertrophy.
3. Two-dimensional echocardiography demonstrates all the elements of T of F, including right ventricular hypertrophy, pulmonic stenosis, ventricular septal defect, and overriding aorta. Doppler interrogation of the pulmonic outflow tract and septal defect is useful in determining the direction and magnitude of the shunt.

D. Laboratory Findings

1. Polycythemia (i.e., PCV >55%) is often present because of the chronic hypoxemia.

IV. Differential Diagnosis

A. Differentials include right-to-left shunting VSD, atrial septal defect, atrioventricular septal defect, complex cyanotic cardiac disease, and patent ductus arteriosus.

V. Medical Management

A. Consider periodic phlebotomy with crystalloid fluid replacement to maintain the hematocrit below 60% in animals with severe cyanosis and progressive polycythemia. Take extreme caution to avoid introducing intravenous air during this procedure to avoid systemic vascular air embolism.

B. Recommend low-dose aspirin therapy to reduce the risk of thromboembolic complications.

C. β-Adrenergic blockade therapy with propranolol or atenolol has been advocated as a palliative treatment for T of F. Possible beneficial effects include reduced dynamic outflow obstruction, decreased heart rate, increased systemic vascular resistance, and decreased myocardial oxygen demand.

VI. Surgical Treatment

A. General Considerations

1. Consider animals with a resting arterial oxygen saturation less than 70% candidates for surgery.

2. Palliative surgeries for T of F include isolated correction of the pulmonic stenosis or creation of a systemic-to-pulmonary shunt (e.g., Blalock-Taussig shunt, explained under Surgical Techniques, directly below). Definitive repair of T of F can be undertaken in medium- to large-breed dogs with cardiopulmonary bypass.

B. Preoperative Management

1. Although arrhythmias are uncommon, perform an ECG and control hemodynamically significant arrhythmias before surgery.
2. Correct severe polycythemia before surgery.

C. Surgical Anatomy

1. With T of F, the parietal portion of the infundibular septum attaches more cranial and leftward than normal, resulting in a narrowing of the right ventricular outflow tract and dextropositioned overriding of the aorta.
2. The VSD is usually located high in the infundibular septum, just below the crista supraventricularis, although supracristal septal defects do occur.

D. Positioning

1. Position the animal in right lateral recumbency for Blalock-Taussig shunt surgery.
2. Prepare the entire left hemithorax for aseptic surgery.

E. Surgical Techniques

1. Modified Blalock-Taussig shunt.

Perform a left fourth intercostal thoracotomy. Harvest an autogenous arterial graft by ligating and dividing the proximal left subclavian artery. Open the pericardium and suture it to the thoracotomy incision. Place tangential vascular clamps on the pulmonary artery and ascending aorta. Make incisions into both vessels by making a longitudinal incision in the vessel wall held within the clamp. Interpose the graft between the aorta and pulmonary artery by end-to-side anastomoses using simple continuous suture patterns. Be sure that the graft is not kinked. Release the clamps and verify hemostasis at the suture sites. Release the pulmonary artery clamp first.

VII. Suture Materials/Special Instruments

A. Use polypropylene (5-0) suture for the vascular anastomoses of the Blalock-Taussig shunt.

B. Have two tangential vascular clamps available to control hemorrhage during the surgery.

VIII. Postoperative Care and Assessment

A. Treat postoperative pain with systemic opioids and local anesthetic techniques.

B. See pp. 442-443 for postoperative care of patients undergoing cardiac surgery.

IX. Prognosis

A. Animals with reasonably balanced acyanotic T of F should be followed for progression, but otherwise generally do not require surgical intervention.

B. The prognosis for animals with cyanotic T of F depends on the shunt fraction, magnitude of hypoxemia, and degree of polycythemia. Some animals may live several years without surgical therapy despite moderate to severe exercise intolerance. Animals with severe hypoxemia and progressive polycythemia will likely succumb to the effects of the disease or will experience sudden death early in life.

C. Modified Blalock-Taussig shunts are reasonably effective at reducing the magnitude of hypoxemia and palliating the consequences of T of F.

Pericardial Effusion and Pericardial Constriction (*SAS*, pp. 596-601)

I. Definitions

A. The **pericardium** is a fibroserous envelope that encompasses the heart and great vessels.

B. **Pericardial effusion** is an abnormal accumulation of fluid within the pericardial sac.

C. **Cardiac tamponade** refers to the decompensated phase of cardiac compression resulting from an unchecked rise in intrapericardiac fluid pressure.

D. **Pericardial constriction** results from a restrictive fibrosis of the parietal and/or visceral pericardium that interferes with diastolic function of the heart.

II. General Considerations and Clinically Relevant Pathophysiology

A. Diseases affecting primarily the pericardium account for approximately 1% of cardiovascular disease.

B. Although primary pericardial disease represents a small percentage of the total number of cardiac diseases in small animals, it is an important cause of right-sided congestive heart failure in dogs.

C. Pericardial diseases of all types are uncommon in cats.

D. Pericardial effusion can be transudative, exudative (inflammatory), or sanguineous.

1. Pericardial transudates.
   a. May be associated with right-sided congestive heart failure, hypoproteinemia, or incarceration of a liver lobe within the pericardial cavity.
2. Infectious pericarditis.
   a. Bacterial pericarditis may arise from bite wounds to the thorax, migrating foreign bodies, or hematogenous seeding.
   b. Coccidioidomycosis is an important cause of pericardial effusion in endemic regions.
3. Inflammatory pericarditis.
   a. In cats, feline infectious peritonitis and toxoplasmosis are potential causes of inflammatory effusions.
4. Neoplastic effusions.
   a. The most common cause of pericardial effusion in dogs.
   b. Neoplasms that produce pericardial effusion in dogs include hemangiosarcoma, chemodectomas, ectopic (heart base) thyroid carcinoma, pericardial mesothelioma, and metastatic carcinoma to the heart.
   c. Neoplastic pericardial effusions usually are sanguineous.
5. Idiopathic (benign) pericardial effusion.
   a. The second most common cause of pericardial effusion in dogs.
   b. Not reported in cats.
   c. The effusion usually appears sanguineous and must be differentiated from neoplastic effusions.
6. Hemorrhagic pericardial effusion.
   a. Coagulopathies or left atrial rupture secondary to chronic mitral insufficiency are rare causes of acute pericardial hemorrhage.
7. Rapid or sudden accumulation of fluid (e.g., pericardial hemorrhage) results in acute cardiac tamponade.
8. Pericardial constriction occurs when visceral or parietal pericardial layers, or both, become fused, thickened, densely fibrotic, or inelastic and form a rigid case around the heart.

E. Diagnosis

1. Clinical presentation.
   a. Signalment.
      i. Idiopathic benign and neoplastic pericardial effusions are more commonly observed in large- and giant-breed dogs.
         (a) Hemangiosarcoma of the right atrium is especially common in German shepherds and golden retrievers.
         (b) Aortic body tumors are most common in aged brachycephalic dogs.
      ii. Idiopathic pericardial effusion has been reported most commonly in golden retrievers, German shepherds, and other large-breed dogs.
      iii. Medium- to large-breed, middle-aged dogs are most commonly affected with constrictive pericardial disease; however, the condition is rare.
2. History.
   a. Presenting complaints associated with pericardial effusion include weakness, lethargy, exercise intolerance, and/or collapse. Often, patients present with right-sided congestion, ascites, and/or pleural effusion.
   b. The most common owner complaint with constrictive pericarditis is abdominal enlargement. Less frequently, dyspnea, tachypnea, weakness, syncope, and/or weight loss may be noted. Occasionally, there will be a previous history of idiopathic pericardial effusion.

F. Physical Examination Findings

1. The classic triad of signs of cardiac tamponade (i.e., rapid and weak arterial pulse, distended systemic veins, and diminished heart sounds) are usually present.
2. Jugular venous distention or a positive hepatojugular reflux will be present, but is commonly overlooked.
   a. Measure central venous pressure to document systemic venous hypertension. It frequently exceeds 10 cm H_2O (normal: 5-6 cm H_2O).
3. Lung sounds may be diminished if pleural effusion is present.
4. Other auscultatory abnormalities (e.g., gallop rhythms, cardiac murmurs, arrhythmias) are uncommon.
5. Ascites, hepatomegaly, and/or peripheral edema may also be noted.
6. Electrocardiographic findings.
   a. Electrical alternans is strongly suggestive of pericardial effusion.
   b. Other findings supportive of pericardial effusion on electrocardiograms are diminished QRS voltages and ST segment depression.
   c. Sinus tachycardia is the predominant rhythm, although nonsustained ventricular tachycardia may be present.

G. Radiography/Echocardiography

1. Radiography.
   a. Thoracic radiography usually demonstrates varying degrees of globoid enlargement (i.e., the cardiac silhouette loses its angles and waists and becomes globe-shaped) of the cardiac silhouette.
   b. Radiographic evidence of pulmonary congestion or edema is not an expected finding, and this helps distinguish pericardial effusion from dilated cardiomyopathy.
   c. If right-sided congestion has developed, distention of the caudal vena cava, hepatomegaly, ascites, and pleural effusion are usually evident.
   d. Heart base tumors may deviate the trachea and produce a mass effect.
   e. Abnormal radiographic findings in animals with constrictive pericarditis are subtle; the cardiac silhouette may be rounded. Dilation of the caudal vena cava may be evident.
   f. Fluoroscopy may demonstrate reduced cardiac motion in animals with pericardial effusion.
   g. Pneumopericardiography is useful for identifying intrapericardial mass lesions.
   h. Angiography will usually show filling defects or tumor vascularity if neoplasia is the cause of the effusion; furthermore, angiography will show increased endocardial-pericardial distance typical of pericardial effusion.
2. Echocardiography.
   a. Definitive diagnosis of pericardial effusion is obtained readily by echocardiography.
   b. The fibrous pericardium is easily identified as a thin echo-dense structure and any degree of separation or echo-free space between the pericardium and underlying cardiac structures on two-dimensional or M-mode echocardiography is diagnostic of pericardial effusion.
   c. Echocardiography is the most reliable procedure for identifying primary cardiac neoplasia, although failure to identify a mass does not rule out neoplasia.
   d. Flattening of the left ventricular endocardium during diastole, abnormal diastolic (early notch) and systolic septal motion are often noted in patients with constrictive pericarditis. Differentia-

tion of constrictive pericardial disease and restrictive myopathy may be difficult with echocardiography.

H. Laboratory Findings

1. With pericardial effusion, the CBC may indicate inflammation or infection.
   a. Increased numbers of circulating nucleated RBCs are suggestive of cardiac or splenic hemangiosarcoma.
2. Cardiac enzymes may be elevated owing to ischemia or myocardial invasion. Other abnormalities may be associated with the primary disease or with CHF.
3. Serum fungal titers (coccidioidomycosis) or ELISA tests for FeLV or FIP (cats) may be positive when pericarditis is related to these infections.
4. Chronic right-sided heart congestion associated with pericardial effusion or constriction can cause splenic dysfunction (functional hyposplenism) and protein-losing enteropathy (intestinal lymphangiectasia). Hyposplenism can result in increased numbers of circulating activated platelets, whereas protein-losing enteropathy may exacerbate the splenic dysfunction and cause reductions in circulating antithrombin III levels. Both conditions promote a hypercoagulable state and may make affected animals prone to pulmonary thromboembolism.
5. Pericardial fluid analysis.
   a. An inflammatory exudate on cytologic examination suggests infectious pericarditis.
   b. Neoplastic effusions are usually sanguineous (i.e., characterized by large numbers of RBCs and variable numbers of neutrophils and mononuclear cells). *Cytology is unreliable in identifying neoplastic effusions because both false positives and false negatives occur.*
   c. Idiopathic pericardial effusion produces a sanguineous effusion that is difficult to distinguish from neoplastic effusions on fluid analysis alone.

III. Differential Diagnosis

A. In addition to pericardial effusion, differentials for a globoid-appearing heart on thoracic radiographs include dilated cardiomyopathy and peritoneopericardial diaphragmatic hernia. The latter may be associated with pericardial effusion, particularly when the liver is herniated.
   1. Ultrasonography is used to detect incongruities in the diaphragmatic silhouette and identify abdominal contents within the pericardial sac.
   2. Echocardiography differentiates diffuse cardiac enlargement from pericardial effusion.
   3. If echocardiography is not available, nonselective angiography can be used.

IV. Medical Management

A. Pericardiocentesis

1. Perform pericardiocentesis in symptomatic animals with suspected pericardial effusion, even if echocardiography is not available to confirm the diagnosis.
2. Procedure.

Shave and surgically prepare a large area of the right hemithorax (sternum to midthorax, third to eighth rib). Perform a local block with lidocaine and, if necessary, sedate the animal with oxymorphone or fentanyl. Be sure to infiltrate the pleura with lidocaine because pleural penetration seems to cause significant discomfort. Place the animal in sternal or lateral recumbency, depending on its demeanor. Pericardiocentesis can be accomplished in the standing animal, but adequate restraint is essential to prevent cardiac puncture or pulmonary laceration. Determine the puncture site based on heart location on thoracic radiographs. Attach a 14- to 18-gauge needle or catheter to a three-way stopcock, extension tubing, and syringe to allow constant negative pressure to be applied during insertion and drainage. Once the catheter has been inserted through the skin, apply negative pressure. If pleural effusion is present, it will be obtained immediately upon entering the thoracic cavity. Pleural effusion associated with heart disease is usually a clear to pale yellow color. Advance the catheter until it contacts the pericardium and a scratching sensation is noticed. Then advance the catheter slightly to penetrate pericardium. Stop advancing the catheter as soon as fluid is obtained. Withdraw the needle immediately if the epicardium is contacted and cardiac motion is felt through the needle. Ultrasound guidance is seldom necessary when performing pericardiocentesis unless the volume of fluid is small or it is compartmentalized.

3. Approximately 50% of dogs with idiopathic effusion are managed successfully by periodic pericardiocentesis and possibly corticosteroids without pericardiectomy. In the remainder, repeat centesis is necessary to control clinical signs.

V. Surgical Treatment

A. General Considerations

1. Although temporary relief of cardiac tamponade is provided by pericardiocentesis, long-term palliation of pericardial effusion often requires pericardiectomy. Removing only a small portion of the pericardium may result in the remaining pericardium adhering to the heart and recurrence of pericardial effusion.
2. Approach.
   a. It is technically easier to perform a pericardiectomy through a median sternotomy than an intercostal thoracotomy because access to both sides of the heart and both phrenic nerves is provided by this approach.
   b. If right atrial hemangiosarcoma is suspected, either a right fifth intercostal thoracotomy or a median sternotomy should be used.
   c. Chemodectomas can arise on either the left or right heart base. Pericardiectomy in these cases should be performed through a thoracotomy on the side where the bulk of the tumor is suspected to be.
   d. If cardiac neoplasia is not identified before surgery and idiopathic pericardial effusion is suspected, then perform pericardiectomy through a right thoracotomy or medial sternotomy so that the right atrium can be examined and resected, if necessary.
3. Although total pericardiectomy can be performed, subphrenic pericardiectomy is usually adequate for animals with pericardial effusion. Total pericardiectomy may be indicated in some animals with neoplasia or infectious processes of the pericardium. Total pericardiectomy is best performed from a median sternotomy approach.

4. Pericardiectomy is the therapy of choice for constrictive pericarditis.

B. Preoperative Management

1. If hemodynamically significant quantities of pericardial effusion are present (i.e., cardiac tamponade as evidenced by jugular vein distention, ascites, and/or pleural effusion), perform pericardiocentesis before surgery.
2. Rule out metabolic causes of pericardial effusion such as hypoproteinemia.
3. Correct electrolyte and acid–base abnormalities, which may be associated with high doses of diuretics, before anesthetic induction.

C. Positioning

1. Position the animal in either lateral recumbency for an intercostal thoracotomy or in dorsal recumbency for median sternotomy.
2. Prep a sufficiently large area to allow intraoperative placement of a thoracostomy tube.

D. Surgical Techniques

1. Subphrenic (subtotal) pericardiectomy via right thoracotomy.

After opening the chest, open the pericardium and submit fluid samples for microbiologic examination, fungal culture, and/or cytology, if indicated. Make a T-shaped incision in the pericardium from cardiac base to apex and across the cardiac base ventral to the phrenic nerve. Extend the circumferential incision at the cardiac base around the venae cavae taking care not to violate the vessel walls. Have an assistant elevate the heart and retract it as the circumferential incision is extended to the opposite side. Take care not to injure the contralateral phrenic nerve. Divide the pericardiophrenic ligament with cautery or between ligatures. Check the remnants of the pericardium to ensure that there is no hemorrhage. Submit pericardium for histologic analyses. Place a thoracostomy tube before thoracic closure.

2. Total pericardiectomy.

Using blunt dissection, carefully elevate the phrenic nerves from the pericardial sac. Make a longitudinal incision in the pericardial sac and resect the pericardium as close to the base of the heart as possible. Place a thoracostomy tube before thoracic closure.

VI. Suture Materials/Special Instruments

A. Electrocautery is useful for pericardiectomy to decrease intraoperative and postoperative hemorrhage.

VII. Postoperative Care and Assessment

A. Aspirate the thoracostomy every hour initially and quantitate the volume of pleural effusion. Once the pleural effusion has decreased to levels consistent with those caused by the thoracostomy tube, remove it.

B. Suspect thromboembolism if the patient develops acute respiratory

distress without evidence of pleural effusion or significant pulmonary infiltrates suggestive of pulmonary edema.
1. Oxygen therapy may be beneficial in such cases.
2. If a definitive diagnosis of pulmonary thromboembolism is made, thrombolytic agents may be used.

C. Treat postoperative pain with systemic opioids and local anesthetic techniques.

VIII. Prognosis

A. Pericardiectomy is palliative for neoplastic pericardial effusion and curative for idiopathic pericardial effusion.

B. Long-term palliation after pericardiectomy is possible for dogs with mesothelioma or chemodectoma.

C. Intracavitary cisplatin has shown promise in achieving long-term remission in dogs with mesothelioma.

D. Chemodectomas are slow-growing tumors and long-term palliation with pericardiectomy and primary mass excision is possible.

E. Median survival for dogs with cardiac hemangiosarcoma is approximately 4 months with pericardiectomy.

Cardiac Neoplasia (*SAS*, pp. 601-603)

I. Definition

A. **Cardiac neoplasia** includes any neoplastic condition involving the heart, great vessels, or pericardium.

II. General Considerations and Clinically Relevant Pathophysiology

A. General Considerations

1. Cardiac neoplasia is relatively uncommon in small animals.
2. The most important cardiac neoplasms in dogs are right atrial hemangiosarcoma and heart base chemodectoma.
3. Lymphosarcoma and metastatic neoplasia are the most frequent causes of cardiac neoplasia in cats.

B. Hemangiosarcoma

1. The right atrium is a common primary site for hemangiosarcoma and accounts for 40% to 50% of canine cases of hemangiosarcoma. Other reported primary cardiac sites for hemangiosarcoma include the right

ventricular free wall, interventricular septum, and main pulmonary artery.

2. Primary cardiac hemangiosarcoma has not been described in cats, but metastasis of hemangiosarcoma to the heart is reported.

C. Chemodectomas

1. May arise from the aortic body at the base of the heart (e.g., between aorta and pulmonary artery, between aorta and right atrium, or between pulmonary artery and left atrium) or from the carotid body in the neck.
2. Aortic body chemodectomas account for approximately 80% of chemodectomas and occur in older dogs.
3. Occur rarely in cats.

D. Ectopic thyroid adenomas and carcinomas account for approximately 5% to 10% of all heart base tumors in dogs.

III. Diagnosis

A. Clinical Presentation

1. Signalment.
   a. German shepherds and golden retrievers have been identified as having increased risk to develop hemangiosarcoma.
   b. Boxers, English bulldogs, and Boston terriers are the most common breeds to develop chemodectomas.
2. History.
   a. Animals with cardiac neoplasia may present for evaluation of dyspnea, cough, syncope, congestive heart failure, or may be asymptomatic.

B. Physical Examination Findings

1. The most common clinical presentation for right atrial hemangiosarcoma is acute or chronic cardiac tamponade resulting from intrapericardial hemorrhage.
2. Animals with chemodectomas may present for evaluation of congestive heart failure, signs of cardiac tamponade, or pleural effusion, or they may be asymptomatic.

C. Radiography/Echocardiography

1. Radiography.
   a. Thoracic radiographs of animals with chemodectomas may show dorsal elevation of the terminal trachea, pleural or pericardial effusion, pulmonary edema, or increased perihilar density.
   b. Selective angiography has been used to identify chemodectomas in dogs.
   c. Suggestive findings on angiography include identifying tortuous, aberrant vessels at the base of the heart, displacement of the aortic arch, and/or filling defects in the left atria.
   d. Angiography is also useful for identifying intracardiac lesions.
2. Echocardiography frequently is useful in identifying masses on the right atrial appendage or at the cardiac base.

D. Laboratory Findings

1. Specific laboratory abnormalities are not found with cardiac neoplasia. Cytologic analysis of the sanguineous effusion obtained by pericardiocentesis is not useful in differentiating neoplastic from idiopathic pericardial effusion.

IV. Differential Diagnosis

A. Differentiate cardiac neoplasia from other causes of pericardial effusion, congestive heart failure, or cardiac arrhythmias.

B. Endomyocardial biopsy may be used to make a definitive diagnosis of intracardiac neoplasia.

C. Differentials for radiographic masses near the heart base include hilar lymphadenopathy, left atrial enlargement, aberrant parathyroid or thyroid tissue, and fibrosing pleuritis or pericarditis.

V. Medical Management

A. Various chemotherapeutic strategies can be employed for cardiac neoplasia, both as a primary therapy or as an adjunct to surgery. Doxorubicin, cyclophosphamide, and vincristine have been reported as the primary treatment of cardiac hemangiosarcoma.

VI. Surgical Treatment

A. General Considerations

1. Pericardiectomy and excision of the right atrial tumor provide palliative relief of signs for atrial hemangiosarcoma.
2. Surgical excision of aortic body chemodectomas is possible depending on size, location, and degree of invasiveness of the tumor. However, many animals with chemodectomas and clinical signs associated with pericardial effusion benefit from pericardiectomy without tumor excision.
3. Surgical excision of intramural or intracavitary primary cardiac tumors has been attempted rarely in small animals. Surgical excision of well-defined primary cardiac tumors utilizing inflow occlusion or cardiopulmonary bypass is possible in selected cases. However, given the high incidence of malignancy of most primary cardiac tumors, consider carefully echocardiographic, angiographic, and endomyocardial biopsy findings in selecting appropriate cases for surgery.

B. Preoperative Management

1. Perform abdominal radiographs or ultrasonography before surgery to detect concurrent intraabdominal neoplasia (e.g., rule out concurrent splenic hemangiosarcoma).
2. If hemodynamically significant quantities of pericardial effusion are present (i.e., cardiac tamponade as evidenced by jugular vein distention, ascites, and/or pleural effusion), perform a pericardial tap before surgery.

C. Positioning

1. Position the animal in dorsal recumbency for median sternotomy or in lateral recumbency for intercostal thoracotomy.
2. Prepare a sufficiently generous area for aseptic surgery to allow a thoracostomy tube to be placed intraoperatively.

D. Surgical Techniques

1. Right atrial hemangiosarcoma.

Perform a median sternotomy or right fourth space intercostal thoracotomy. Clamp the atrial appendage with a tangential vascular clamp and excise the appendage. Close the atriotomy incision with a continuous mattress suture pattern. Remove the vascular clamp and oversew the incision with a simple continuous suture pattern. Perform a pericardiectomy if pericardial effusion is present. Alternatively, the right atrial appendage may be excised with a TA stapling instrument.

2. Chemodectoma.

Determine the surgical approach based on the suspected location of the tumor. Sharply dissect the tumor from the walls of the great vessels and atria. Use care to avoid rupturing these structures during dissection. Use electrocautery to decrease hemorrhage during excision of these highly vascular tumors.

VII. Suture Materials/Special Instruments

A. A tangential vascular clamp is useful for excision of right atrial hemangiosarcoma. Closure of the right atrium can be accomplished with polypropylene (4-0) suture. Electrocautery is useful for excision of chemodectomas.

VIII. Postoperative Care and Assessment

A. Monitor the animal carefully for evidence of hemorrhage (pleural effusion) postoperatively.

B. Monitor for arrhythmias for 36 to 72 hours after surgery.

C. Treat postoperative pain with systemic opioids and local anesthetic techniques.

IX. Prognosis

A. The prognosis for right atrial hemangiosarcoma is poor. Micrometastasis is considered present in virtually all cases at the time of diagnosis. Pericardiectomy and excision of the right atrium is palliative. Median survival after surgery is approximately 4 months.

B. Long-term survival of up to several years is possible after surgical removal of an aortic body chemodectoma. In older animals with incidental asymptomatic chemodectoma, the risks of surgical excision should be weighed against the likelihood that the tumor will be slow growing and can remain asymptomatic for a long period of time.

Bradycardia (*SAS*, pp. 603-608)

I. Definition

A. **Bradycardia** is a slower-than-normal heart rate.

II. General Considerations and Clinically Relevant Pathophysiology

A. Sinus bradycardia results from a predominance of parasympathetic influence and often is accompanied by other parasympathetically mediated rhythms (i.e., sinus arrhythmia, wandering pacemaker, or low-grade, second-degree atrioventricular block). It is generally considered a physiologic rather than pathologic rhythm.

B. Atrial standstill occurs when the atria fail to conduct an electrical impulse.
   1. Transient atrial standstill is caused by hyperkalemia.
   2. Persistent atrial standstill occurs as a result of a heritable muscular dystrophy syndrome that involves the cardiac atria, ventricles, and scapulohumeral skeletal muscles.
   3. Sick sinus syndrome is the clinical result of sinus node malfunction and is characterized by frequent syncopal and near-syncopal episodes. Sick sinus syndrome may also be accompanied by frequent supraventricular tachycardia.

C. Atrioventricular block results when there is a delay or block of cardiac impulse conduction through the AV node.
   1. First-degree AV block is a prolongation of conduction through the AV node and usually results from exaggerated parasympathetic influence on the AV node.
   2. Second-degree (incomplete) AV block is characterized by intermittent failure of impulse conduction through the AV node.
      a. Low-grade (infrequent) second-degree AV block usually results from exaggerated parasympathetic influence on the AV node.
      b. High-grade (frequent) second-degree AV block is more likely the result of intrinsic disease of the AV node.
   3. Third-degree (complete) AV block is a complete failure of conduction through the AV node and strongly implies intrinsic degenerative or infiltrative disease of the AV node. Third-degree AV block causes complete AV dissociation and development of a slow ventricular escape rhythm. The result is low and unresponsive cardiac output.

III. Diagnosis

A. Clinical Presentation

1. Signalment.
   a. English springer spaniels and Siamese cats are predisposed to persistent atrial standstill.
   b. Small-breed dogs, particularly miniature schnauzers, are predisposed to sick sinus syndrome.

c. Third-degree AV block occurs in German shepherds and other large-breed dogs.

2. History.

a. Clinical signs associated with bradycardia include weakness, exercise intolerance, collapse, and syncope. The relatively short duration of syncopal episodes (usually only a few seconds) and lack of tonic-clonic motor activity or postictal signs help distinguish syncope from neurologic seizures, with which it is sometimes confused.

B. Physical Examination Findings/Electrocardiography

1. Electrocardiography.

a. Sinus bradycardia is recognized on the electrocardiogram as a normal but slow rhythm with normal P-QRS-T complexes. It is abolished by exercise or atropine administration.

i. Give atropine–0.02 to 0.04 mg/kg SC or IM.

ii. Wait 15 to 20 min, then recheck rhythm.

b. ECG abnormalities associated with transient atrial standstill are bradycardia, small or absent P waves, and shortening and widening of the QRS complexes.

c. ECG abnormalities associated with persistent atrial standstill are an absence of P waves and a slow supraventricular or ventricular escape rhythm.

d. ECG findings associated with sick sinus syndrome include intermittent severe bradycardia, sinus pauses that last several seconds, supraventricular escape complexes, and occasionally paroxysmal supraventricular tachycardia. Sick sinus syndrome causes frequent syncopal attacks and places the animal at substantial risk for sudden death. Sick sinus syndrome is usually not responsive to acute administration of atropine.

e. First-degree AV block is recognized by a prolongation of the PR interval on an ECG. Second-degree AV block is intermittent failure of impulse conduction through the AV node. It is recognized on an ECG as a P wave that is not followed by a QRS-T complex. Low-grade, second-degree AV block is characterized by occasional "dropped complexes" after several normal complexes and usually is abolished by atropine. High-grade, second-degree AV block is characterized by more dropped complexes than conducted complexes and usually does not respond to atropine. Third-degree AV block is recognized on an ECG by complete dissociation of the P waves and QRS-T complexes and the presence of a slow ventricular escape rhythm. Third-degree AV block is not atropine responsive.

C. Radiography/Echocardiography

1. Thoracic radiographs are usually normal or show mild to moderate cardiomegaly.
2. With transient atrial standstill, echocardiography shows a lack of atrial motion and little or no flow through the mitral valve during the atrial filling phase.
3. Echocardiography is also used to rule out concurrent valvular or congenital abnormalities.

D. Laboratory Findings

1. Hyperkalemia is present with transient atrial standstill; however, with persistent atrial standstill, serum potassium levels are normal.
2. Other specific laboratory abnormalities are not found.

IV. Differential Diagnosis

1. Differentiate other causes of bradycardia (i.e., hyperkalemia, increased intracranial pressures) from intrinsic conduction system dysfunction.

V. Medical Management

A. Direct therapy for atrial standstill secondary to hyperkalemia at immediately lowering serum potassium levels and correcting the underlying cause of hyperkalemia.
1. Administer intravenous fluids (0.9% saline). If the animal has concurrent hyponatremia, avoid 5% dextrose solutions (i.e., D_5W) and half-strength saline.
2. Treat severe hyperkalemia with sodium bicarbonate (see Appendix J) or insulin (0.5-1.0 unit/kg regular insulin IV) and dextrose (2 g per unit of insulin).
3. If the hyperkalemia appears immediately life-threatening, consider giving 10% calcium gluconate slowly intravenously to protect the heart until other therapy lowers the plasma potassium concentration.

B. If the animal presents with severe life-threatening bradycardia, provide emergency therapy to increase the heart rate.
1. Short-term anticholinergic therapy with atropine or glycopyrrolate may be attempted, but most clinically relevant bradycardias are not due to parasympathetic mechanisms and will not be responsive to these drugs.
2. Intravenous adrenergic therapy with isoproterenol (see Appendix I) is sometimes effective as a short-term measure for increasing heart rate associated with persistent atrial standstill or third-degree AV block.
3. Consider temporary intravenous pacing, which is accomplished by percutaneous jugular venous placement of a pacing electrode into the right side of the heart under sedation and local anesthesia (see Anesthesia in the following text). The electrode is then connected to an external pulse generator.
4. Long-term oral anticholinergic therapy with propantheline bromide (see *SAS,* Table 24-16) is sometimes advocated for various bradycardias. However, this drug is seldom effective for clinically relevant bradycardias and often is associated with unpleasant side effects.
5. Animals with sick sinus syndrome may require management of supraventricular tachycardia with digoxin, β-adrenergic blockade, or calcium channel blockade therapy after pacemaker implantation.

VI. Surgical Treatment

A. Cardiac pacemaker therapy is indicated for bradycardias that are the result of intrinsic cardiac disease, are not responsive to atropine, and are associated with clinical signs.

B. Preoperative management.
1. It is necessary to maintain an acceptable cardiac rhythm during permanent pacemaker implantation. Temporary transvenous pacing is the most reliable method of maintaining an adequate heart rate during pacemaker implantation.

2. Administer perioperative antibiotic therapy during pacemaker implantation to reduce the risk of implant-associated infections.

C. Anesthesia.
1. Temporary pacemakers can be implanted in dogs under oxymorphone sedation (0.05-0.1 mg/kg IV) plus diazepam (0.1-0.2 mg/kg IV) and a local anesthetic block with lidocaine. Once the animal is paced, administer etomidate (0.5-1.5 mg/kg IV) for intubation. Maintain anesthesia with isoflurane and oxygen.

D. Positioning.
1. Place the animal in dorsal recumbency for transdiaphragmatic pacemaker implantation.
2. Prep the entire abdomen and caudal thorax for aseptic surgery.

E. Surgical techniques.
1. General considerations.
   a. Epicardial pacemaker implantation in small animals is accomplished through a midline celiotomy diaphragmatic incision. The transdiaphragmatic approach has several advantages, including avoidance of a thoracotomy and abdominal placement of the generator.
2. Surgical technique.

Perform a celiotomy that extends cranially to the level of the xiphoid. Make a vertical midline incision in the diaphragm and expose the cardiac apex. Open the pericardium and retract it gently with tissue forceps to expose the apex of the left ventricle. Implant a screw-in electrode into the left ventricular apex by turning the electrode tip a specified number of rotations (see instruction sheet accompanying pacemaker, usually 2.5 turns). Bring the lead wire into the abdominal cavity through the diaphragmatic incision and connect it to the pulse generator using a small screwdriver. Place the pulse generator in a pocket created between the transverse abdominis and internal abdominal oblique. Avoid using electrocautery once the permanent pacemaker is functioning. Do not suture the pericardium. Close the diaphragm and abdomen in routine fashion.

VII. Suture Materials/Special Instruments

A. The most commonly used pacing mode in small animals is VVI, which stands for ventricular-sensing, ventricular-pacing, inhibited mode. This means that the pacemaker is intended to pace the cardiac ventricles, but will sense naturally occurring ventricular impulses and inhibit its own output when they occur. This demand function prevents competitive rhythms between the heart and pacemaker, should spontaneous intrinsic ventricular activity occur.

B. Most recent-model pulse generators are powered by lithium cells that have a life of 8 to 12 years.

C. Dogs are paced at a rate of 70 to 110 beats per minute, depending on size and nature of the animal. Ideally, the stimulus voltage should be approximately two times the measured stimulus capture threshold.

D. Endocardial leads may be unipolar or bipolar and are intended for placement in the right ventricle via a jugular vein. They may be used for temporary or permanent cardiac pacing.

E. Epicardial leads are unipolar and require open thoracic surgery for implantation on the epicardial surface. The screw-in epicardial electrode has the advantage of not requiring epicardial sutures and allows a minimal thoracic approach for implantation.

VIII. Postoperative Care and Assessment

A. Monitor pacemaker function closely for the first 48 hours postoperatively, and thereafter every 3 to 6 months. Recognition of normal pacemaker function is an important aspect of pacemaker management after surgery.

B. Prognosis.

1. Animals showing clinical signs of severe exercise intolerance or syncope as a result of bradycardia are at risk for sudden death or development of congestive heart failure.
2. Pacemaker therapy is extremely effective in preventing these consequences and restoring reasonably normal activity to animals with clinically relevant bradycardia.

25

Surgery of the Upper Respiratory System (*SAS*, pp. 609-647)

General Principles and Techniques (*SAS*, pp. 609-619)

I. Definitions

A. **Tracheotomy** is an incision through the tracheal wall.

B. **Tracheostomy** (tracheostoma) is the creation of a temporary or permanent opening into the trachea to facilitate airflow.

C. **Tracheal resection and anastomosis** is removal of a segment of trachea and reapposition of the divided tracheal ends.

D. **Ventriculocordectomy** (debarking, devocalization) is resection of the vocal cords.

II. Preoperative Concerns

A. For the initial examination of animals with moderate to severe dyspnea (evidenced by open-mouth breathing, abducted forelimbs, labored breathing, restlessness).
   1. Use minimal restraint and allow the animal to maintain the position in which it feels most comfortable.
   2. Provide supplemental oxygen, if necessary (nasal insufflation, tracheostomy tube or catheter, endotracheal intubation, mask, or cage).
   3. Consider corticosteroids, sedation, or cooling.
      a. Corticosteroids.
         i. Dexamethasone (Azium)–0.5 to 2 mg/kg IV, IM, SC.
      b. Sedation.
         i. Dogs.

(a) Use intravenous oxymorphone or butorphanol plus either acepromazine or diazepam.
(i) Oxymorphone (Numorphan)–0.05 mg/kg, max 4 mg.
(ii) Butorphanol (Torbutrol, Torbugesic)–0.2 to 0.4 mg/kg.
(iii) Acepromazine–0.02 to 0.05 mg/kg, max 1 mg IV.
(iv) Diazepam (Valium)–0.2 mg/kg IV.
(b) Alternatively, fentanyl plus droperidol may be used.
(i) Fentanyl plus droperidol (Innovar-Vet)–1 ml/20 to 40 kg IV or 1 ml/10 to 15 kg IM.

ii. Cats.
(a) Acepromazine or diazepam is recommended. Diazepam may not reliably result in sedation in cats.
(i) Acepromazine–0.05 mg/kg, IV, IM, SC.
(ii) Diazepam (Valium)–0.2 mg/kg IV.

c. Cooling.
i. Direct a fan at the patient.
ii. Apply ice packs to the head, axilla, inguinal area, and extremities.
iii. Administer cooled fluids intravenously.

B. Diagnosis of upper respiratory disease.

1. Clinical signs.
a. Common abnormalities include abnormal respiratory noises (e.g., cough, stridor, wheeze), exercise intolerance, hyperthermia, tachypnea, dyspnea, cyanosis, restlessness, collapse, gagging and regurgitation of secretions, voice change (laryngeal paralysis), dysphagia (supraglottic obstructions), subcutaneous emphysema (penetrating laryngotracheal injuries).
b. Signs may intensify or be precipitated by excitement, stress, eating, drinking, or high ambient temperatures.

2. Laboratory data.
a. Evaluate hematologic and serum biochemical data to determine the presence of underlying metabolic disease and the advisability of general anesthesia.
b. Anemia and bleeding.
i. Animals with nasal neoplasia, fungal infection, or foreign bodies may be anemic due to profuse epistaxis.
ii. Provide blood transfusions preoperatively if the PCV is less than or equal to 20% (Appendix A).
iii. Bleeding during rhinotomy may be severe, requiring intraoperative blood transfusion or carotid artery ligation.
iv. Laboratory tests or findings that may suggested bleeding problems.
(a) Thrombocytopenia.
(b) Bleeding from venipuncture sites.
(c) Presence of ecchymoses, petechiation, melena, hematuria, or retinal hemorrhages.
v. Assess coagulative ability by activated clotting time, prothrombin time, partial thromboplastin time, mucosal bleeding time.

3. Ancillary tests.
a. Tidal-breathing flow volume loops.
b. Pulmonary function tests.
c. Electromyography.
d. Nerve conduction studies.

C. Preoperative drug therapy.

1. Administer antiinflammatory doses of corticosteroids with nasopharyngeal and intraluminal laryngeal procedures to reduce edema.
a. Dexamethasone (Azium)–0.5 to 2 mg/kg IV, IM, SC.

2. Prophylactic antibiotics.
   a. Generally unnecessary in healthy animals (see p. 479).

III. Anesthetic Considerations

A. Laryngeal Examination

1. Avoid drugs that inhibit laryngeal function.
2. Premedicants.
   a. Sedated animals (see pp. 476-477).
      i. Give an anticholinergic.
         (a) Atropine–0.02-0.04 mg/kg IM or SC.
         (b) Glycopyrollate–0.005 to 0.011 mg/kg IM or SC.
   b. Unsedated animals.
      i. Give an opioid.
         (a) Oxymorphone (Numorphan)–0.05 to 0.1 mg/kg IM, max 4 mg.
         (b) Butorphanol (Torbutrol, Torbugesic)–0.2 to 0.4 mg/kg IM or SC.
         (c) Buprenorphine (Buprenex)–5 to 15 μg/kg IM.
3. Induction.
   a. Propofol.
      i. Noncumulative.
      ii. Give in small incremental dosages.
      iii. 4 to 6 mg/kg IV.
   b. Diazepam plus ketamine titrated to effect.
      i. Diazepam (Valium)–0.2 mg/kg IV.
      ii. Ketamine–5.5 mg/kg IV.
   c. Thiobarbiturates.
      i. Induction doses may impair laryngeal function.
         (a) Thiopental–10 to 12 mg/kg IV.
4. Maintenance.
   a. Isoflurane or halothane.
5. Supplement oxygen during the exam and monitor oxygen saturation with pulse oximetry (preferable) or by observation of mucous membrane color.

B. Upper Respiratory Surgery

1. General anesthesia is preferred for most upper respiratory procedures; local anesthesia may allow tracheostomy tube placement when the patient is comatose or cannot tolerate general anesthesia.
2. Preoxygenate dyspneic patients with a face mask, if possible.
3. Affected animals being anesthetized (see above for laryngeal exam) may be premedicated with an opioid, but continuous monitoring is necessary.
4. Anticholinergics are indicated for bradycardia.
5. Induction should be rapid (e.g., propofol, thiobarbiturate, or ketamine plus diazepam; see above) and oxygen should be administered immediately (Appendix G-26). Mask induction is not recommended.
6. Maintain anesthesia with inhalant drugs. Sigh the patient frequently during surgery to renew surfactant.
7. Laryngeal or tracheal procedures may necessitate temporary retraction of the endotracheal tube from the surgical site, placing an endotracheal tube distal to the surgical site through a tracheotomy, or using injectable drugs.
8. Monitor oxygen saturation, blood gases, or both from induction until recovery and correct abnormalities.

IV. Antibiotics

A. Animals with normal immune function undergoing short procedures (e.g., nares resection, laryngeal saccule resection, vocal cordectomy) do not need prophylactic antibiotics.

B. *Streptococcus* spp., *E. coli, Pseudomonas* spp., *Klebsiella* spp., and *Bordetella bronchiseptica* are most commonly isolated from normal dogs.

C. Most canine respiratory tract infections are due to gram-negative organisms, many being resistant to commonly used antibiotics.

D. Base antimicrobial drug selection on cytologic and culture results of tracheobronchial, pulmonary parenchymal, or pleural secretions.

E. Bland aerosol therapy (e.g., sterile 0.9% NaCl) helps loosen secretions and facilitates their clearance in dogs with tracheostomies.

F. Lipid-soluble antibiotics that contain a benzene ring reach highest levels in the normal trachea and bronchus; however, increased permeability associated with inflammation allows numerous antibiotics to achieve high levels during infection.

G. Recommended antibiotics for treatment of respiratory disease include ampicillin, trimethoprim-sulfadiazine, cefazolin (Ancef, Kefzol), amikacin (Amiglyde V), enrofloxacin (Baytril). (see Appendix I)

V. Surgical Anatomy

A. Thyroid Cartilage

1. Forms the ventral and lateral walls of the larynx.
2. Ventrally the cricothyroid ligament joins the caudal border of the thyroid cartilage to the cricoid cartilage.

B. Cricoid Cartilage

1. Forms the dorsal wall of the larynx and cranially lies within the wings of the thyroid cartilage.
2. Articulates at its cranial dorsolateral margin with the arytenoid cartilage, which is paired.

C. Glottis (Laryngeal Inlet)

1. The vocal folds extend dorsally from the vocal processes of the arytenoids to the thyroid cartilage ventrally.
2. Laryngeal ventricles or saccules are rostral and lateral to the vocal folds.
3. The recurrent laryngeal nerve, a branch of the vagus, terminates as the caudal laryngeal nerve, which innervates some intrinsic muscles of the larynx. **Be sure to identify and protect the recurrent laryngeal nerves during cervical surgery to prevent postoperative laryngospasms or paralysis.**

D. Trachea

1. Consists of 35 to 45 C-shaped hyaline cartilages.

2. Joined by annular ligaments ventrally and laterally and trachealis muscle (dorsal tracheal membrane) dorsally.
3. The tracheal vessels and nerves are found in the lateral pedicles and supply the trachea segmentally.

VI. Surgical Techniques

A. Tracheotomy (*SAS*, p. 613).
   1. Indications.
      a. To gain access to the tracheal lumen to remove obstructions.
      b. To facilitate collection of specimens.
      c. To improve airflow.
   2. Surgical technique.

Approach the cervical trachea through a ventral cervical midline incision. Extend the incision from the larynx to the sternum as needed to allow adequate exposure. Separate the sternohyoid muscles along their midline and retract them laterally. Dissect the peritracheal connective tissue from the ventral surface of the trachea at the proposed tracheotomy site. Take care to avoid traumatizing the recurrent laryngeal nerves, carotid artery, jugular vein, thyroid vessels, or esophagus. Immobilize the trachea between the thumb and forefinger. Make a horizontal or vertical incision through the wall of the trachea. Place cartilage-encircling sutures around adjacent cartilages to separate the edges and allow lumen inspection or tube insertion. Suction blood, secretions, and debris from the tracheal lumen. Following completion of the procedure, appose tracheal edges with simple interrupted 3-0 or 4-0 polypropylene sutures. To close the tracheal incision, place sutures through the annular ligaments encircling adjacent cartilages or through the annular ligaments only. Lavage the surgical site with saline. Appose the sternohyoid muscles with a simple continuous pattern of 3-0 or 4-0 absorbable suture (polydioxanone, polyglyconate, polyglactin, or chromic catgut). Appose subcutaneous tissues and skin routinely. Alternatively, allow the tracheotomy to heal by second intention.

B. Tracheostomy (*SAS*, pp. 613-615) allows air to enter the trachea distal to the nose, mouth, nasopharynx, and larynx. May be temporary (tube is inserted) or permanent (a stoma is created).
   1. Temporary tracheostomy.
      a. Indications.
         i. To provide an alternate airflow route during surgery.
         ii. To provide an airway in severely dyspneic patients with upper airway (i.e., above the site of the tracheostomy) obstruction.
         iii. To allow the animal to be placed on a ventilator.
      b. General considerations.
         i. Use a nonreactive tube that is no larger than one half the size of the trachea.
         ii. Select a cuffed or cannulated autoclavable silicone, silver, or nylon tube. Avoid polyvinyl chloride and red rubber tubes.
         iii. Use a cuffed tube if the animal is being placed on a respirator.
      c. Surgical technique.

Make a ventral midline incision from the cricoid cartilage extending 2 to 3 cm caudally. Separate the sternohyoid muscles and make a horizontal (transverse) tracheotomy through the annular ligament between the third and fourth or fourth and fifth tracheal cartilages. Do not extend the incision around more than half the circumference of the trachea. Alternatively, make a vertical tracheotomy across the ventral midline of cartilages 3 through 5. Suction blood and

mucus from the lumen, widen the incision, and insert the tracheostomy tube. Facilitate tube placement by encircling a cartilage distal or lateral to the incision with a long stay suture. Place tension on this suture to open the incision. Alternatively, open a hemostat in the incision or depress the cartilages cranial to the horizontal incision. Resect a small ellipse of cartilage if tube insertion is difficult. Appose the sternohyoid muscles, subcutaneous tissue, and skin cranial and caudal to the tube. Secure the tube by suturing it to the skin or tieing it to gauze that is tied around the neck.

2. Permanent tracheostomy–creation of a stoma in the ventral tracheal wall by suturing tracheal mucosa to skin.
   a. Indications.
      i. Recommended for animals with upper respiratory obstructions causing moderate to severe respiratory distress that cannot be successfully treated by other methods (e.g., laryngeal collapse, nasal neoplasia).
   b. General considerations.
      i. Tracheostomy tubes are not needed to maintain lumen patency following this procedure.
      ii. Warn owners that these animals must be restricted from swimming, and advise them that vocalization is diminished or absent following this procedure.
   c. Surgical technique.

Expose the proximal cervical trachea with a ventral cervical midline incision. Create a tunnel dorsal to the trachea in the area of the third to sixth tracheal cartilages. Using this tunnel, appose the sternohyoid muscles dorsal to the trachea with horizontal mattress sutures to create a muscle sling to reduce tension on the mucosa-to-skin sutures. Beginning with the second or third tracheal cartilages, outline a rectangular segment of tracheal wall 3 to 4 cartilage widths long and one third the circumference of the trachea in width. Incise the cartilage and annular ligaments to the depth of the tracheal mucosa. Elevate a cartilage edge with thumb forceps and dissect the cartilage segment from the mucosa. Place one or two prosthetic tracheal rings cranial and caudal to the stoma if the tracheal cartilages show any weakness or tendency to collapse. Excise a similar segment of skin adjacent to the stoma (excise larger segments of skin if the animal has loose skin folds or abundant subcutaneous fat). Suture the skin directly to the peritracheal fascia laterally and the annular ligaments proximal and distal to the stoma with a series of interrupted intradermal sutures (3-0 or 4-0 polydioxanone or polypropylene). Make an I- or H-shaped incision in the mucosa. Fold the mucosa over the cartilage edges and suture it to the edges of the skin with approximating sutures to complete the tracheostoma. Use simple interrupted sutures at the corners and a simple continuous pattern to further appose skin and mucosa (4-0 polypropylene).

C. Tracheal resection/anastomosis (*SAS*, pp. 615-616).
   1. Indications.
      a. Removal of a tracheal segment may be necessary to treat tracheal tumors, stenosis, or trauma.
      b. Diseased trachea exceeding the limits of resection and anastomosis may be managed with permanent tracheostomy, intraluminal silicone tubes, grafts, or prostheses with variable success.
   2. General considerations.
      a. Depending on the degree of tracheal elasticity and tension, approximately 20% to 60% of the trachea may be resected and direct anastomosis achieved.
      b. The split cartilage technique is preferred because it is easier to

perform and results in more precise anatomic alignment with less luminal stenosis than many other techniques.

3. Surgical technique.

Expose the involved trachea through a ventral cervical, midline, lateral thoracotomy, or median sternotomy approach. Mobilize only enough trachea to allow anastomosis without tension. Preserve as much of the segmental blood and nerve supply to the trachea as possible. Place stay sutures around cartilages cranial and caudal to the resection sites before transecting the trachea. Resect the diseased trachea by splitting a healthy cartilage circumferentially at each end or incising annular ligaments adjacent to the intact cartilages. Use a No. 11 blade to split the tracheal cartilages at their midpoint. Transect the dorsal tracheal membrane with Metzenbaum scissors. Preplace, and then tie, three or four simple interrupted sutures (3-0 or 4-0 polypropylene) in the dorsal tracheal membrane. Retract the endotracheal tube into the proximal trachea during resection and placement of sutures in the dorsal tracheal membrane. Remove blood clots and secretions from the lumen and advance the tube distal to the anastomosis after dorsal tracheal membrane sutures are placed. Complete the anastomosis by apposing the split cartilage halves or adjacent intact cartilages with simple interrupted sutures beginning at the ventral midpoint of the trachea. Space additional sutures 2 to 3 mm apart. Place three or four retention sutures to help relieve tension on the anastomosis. Place and tie these sutures so that they encircle an intact cartilage cranial and caudal to the anastomosis, crossing external to the anastomotic site. Lavage the area and appose the sternohyoid muscles with a simple continuous pattern. Close subcutaneous tissues and skin routinely. If tension-relieving sutures do not adequately relieve tension at the anastomosis, further mobilize the trachea, make partial-thickness incisions through annular ligaments proximal and distal to the anastomosis, or restrict head and neck movement after surgery. Prevent full extension of the neck by placing a suture from the chin to the manubrium or fixing a muzzle to a harness to maintain mild to moderate cervical flexion. Maintain the muzzle for 2 to 3 weeks.

D. Ventriculocordectomy (*SAS,* pp. 616-617).

1. Indications.
   a. To reduce or prevent noise associated with vocalization.
   b. To remove vocal fold masses.
   c. To enlarge the ventral glottis in order to decrease obstruction associated with laryngeal paralysis.
2. General considerations.
   a. Removal of the vocal folds may be performed using an oral or ventral (laryngotomy) approach.
   b. Anesthesia is maintained by using a tube tracheostomy, manipulating the endotracheal tube to the contralateral side of the larynx, or performing the procedure using injectable anesthetic agents.
   c. Ventriculocordectomy performed to widen the ventral glottis requires that more vocal fold be resected than for debarking.
   d. **Webbing is a problem after this procedure. Maintaining 1 to 2 mm of mucosa at the dorsal and ventral aspects of the vocal cord may help prevent this complication.**
   e. Staging the procedure, by waiting 2 to 3 weeks before removing the contralateral vocal fold, helps prevent glottic stenosis.
   f. Be careful to avoid disrupting the blood supply to the larynx and trachea during surgery or necrosis may result.
   g. Reduce inflammation by minimal, gentle tissue manipulation and pretreating with corticosteroids.
3. Surgical technique.

a. Oral approach.

Position the patient in ventral recumbency with the neck extended. Suspend the maxilla and pull the mandible ventrally to maximally open the mouth. Extend the tongue from the mouth to get maximum exposure of the glottis. Retract the cheeks laterally to improve visualization. Avoid placing padding or hands in the region of the larynx because this may distort the nasopharynx. Remove the central margin of the vocal cord for debarking with a laryngeal or uterine cup biopsy forceps. To widen the glottis, use long-handled Metzenbaum scissors and remove as much of the vocal fold extending into the laryngeal lumen as possible. With either technique maintain 1 to 2 mm of mucosa at the dorsal and ventral aspects of the vocal cord. Control hemorrhage with pressure. Remove blood clots and secretions with suction or sponges. Allow the incision to heal by second intention.

b. Laryngotomy approach.

Position the patient in dorsal recumbency with the neck extended over a rolled towel. Expose the larynx using a ventral midline cervical approach beginning rostral to the basihyoid bone and extending caudally to the proximal trachea. Separate and retract the paired sternohyoid muscles. Identify the midline of the thyroid cartilage. Ligate and divide the laryngeal impar vein if necessary. Incise the cricothyroid ligament with a No. 15 or No. 11 blade. Extend the incision along the midline of the thyroid cartilage as needed to expose the vocal folds. Excise the entire vocal fold from the arytenoid cartilage dorsally and the thyroid cartilage ventrally. Close the defect by apposing the mucosa with a simple continuous appositional suture pattern (4-0 polydioxanone). Appose the cricothyroid ligament and thyroid cartilage with simple interrupted sutures. Appose the sternohyoid muscles with a simple continuous pattern (3-0 or 4-0 polydioxanone or polyglyconate). Close subcutaneous tissues and skin routinely.

VII. Healing of the Respiratory Tract

A. Laryngeal Wounds

1. Heal by reepithelialization if mucosal edges are in apposition.
2. Constant motion associated with breathing and head movement inhibits primary healing.
3. Wounds with gaps heal by second intention, first filling with granulation tissue and then reepithelializing.
   a. Second intention healing may result in scarring across the glottis. Scarring may be prevented by restricting surgery to one side of the larynx and leaving intact epithelium at the dorsal and ventral commissures.

B. Trachea

1. Tracheal epithelium responds immediately to irritation or disease by increasing mucus production. If the insult continues, cells desquamate and goblet cell hyperplasia occurs to increase the protective mucous layer.
2. Superficial wounds heal by reepithelialization; full-thickness tracheal mucosal wounds with a gap between mucosal edges fill with granulation tissue before reepithelialization.
3. Full-thickness wounds may heal with scar tissue protruding into the lumen. Scar tissue narrows the lumen and may interfere with mucus transport.

VIII. Suture Material/Special Instruments

A. Long-handled instruments are useful for laryngeal surgery.

B. Skin hooks, laryngeal or uterine cup biopsy forceps, and tracheal prostheses (*SAS,* p. 635) are needed for some procedures.

C. Nonreactive, monofilament suture is recommended for surgery of the upper respiratory tract (e.g., polydioxanone or polypropylene).

IX. Postoperative Care and Assessment

A. General Considerations

1. Closely monitor these patients during anesthetic recovery for hemorrhage, coughing, gagging, or aspiration.
2. Keep patients intubated as long as possible and reintubate or place a tracheostomy tube if respiratory distress occurs following extubation.
3. Provide supplemental oxygen if necessary during recovery. Insert a nasal oxygen catheter at the conclusion of surgery or place the animal in an oxygen cage.
4. Minimize excitement and pain by using postoperative analgesics (Appendix F).
5. Position the patient in sternal recumbency to facilitate respiration.
6. Administer postoperative corticosteroids as necessary to reduce mucosal swelling and edema.
7. Discontinue prophylactic antibiotics immediately after surgery.
8. Offer water 6 to 12 hours after surgery, and if gagging, regurgitation, or vomiting does not occur, offer soft food (e.g., meatballs) 18 to 24 hours postoperatively.
   a. Feeding meatballs one at a time for 5 to 7 days following nasopharyngeal or laryngeal procedures to slow ingestion may be beneficial.
9. Restrict exercise for 4 weeks.
10. Use a harness rather than a collar for 2 to 4 weeks to avoid incisional, tracheal, or laryngeal trauma.
11. Warn clients that surgery may improve, but seldom cures, upper respiratory problems. Continued medical therapy may be required.

B. Tube Tracheostomy

1. Intensive postoperative care is required.
2. Observe the animal closely to prevent asphyxiation secondary to tube obstruction or dislodgement.
3. Tube cleaning.
   a. Mucus clearance is inhibited in these animals, and mucosal irritation leads to increased mucus production.
   b. May be required every 15 minutes if the trachea is irritated.
   c. Use sterile technique (i.e., gloves, instruments) to clean the tubes.
   d. Remove secretions by inserting a sterile suctioning cannula into the tube's lumen and distal trachea.
   e. When using cannulated tubes, remove the inner cannula and clean it while the outer tube is suctioned.
   f. Inject sterile saline (1 ml) into the tube a few minutes before suctioning to help loosen secretions.
   g. Use a new tube if these techniques do not adequately remove secretions.

4. Remove tracheostomy tubes when an adequate airway and spontaneous ventilation are established.
   a. Occasionally, occluding the tube and observing the patient while the animal breathes around the tube are required to determine whether the tube can be removed. Do not do this in animals with cuffed tubes or those that have large tubes that fill the tracheal lumen.
   b. After tube removal, allow the tracheostomy site to heal by second intention.

C. Permanent Tracheostomies

1. Initially, inspect the tracheostoma for mucus accumulation every 1 to 3 hours.
   a. When mucus begins to occlude the tracheostoma or when respiratory effort increases, suction the site as described above for tube tracheostomies.
   b. Mucus at the stoma may be removed by aspiration or by gently wiping with a sponge or applicator stick.
   c. Only a moderate amount of mucus is expected to accumulate during the first 7 to 14 days after surgery unless the animal has severe tracheitis.
   d. By 7 days increase the cleaning interval to every 4 to 6 hours.
   e. After 30 days perform twice-daily stomal cleaning.
   f. Note: Smoke and other noxious stimuli will cause increased mucus production and necessitate more frequent cleaning.
2. Clip hair as needed from around the stoma to prevent hair matting with mucus.
3. Restrict exercise and housing to clean areas.

D. Tracheal Resection and Anastomosis

1. Restrict exercise and neck extension for 2 to 4 weeks.

E. Ventriculocordectomy

1. Keep animals quiet and observe for signs of respiratory distress.
2. Some animals will gag and cough.
3. Vocalization should be discouraged for 6 to 8 weeks.

X. Complications

A. Acute respiratory obstruction may occur because of mucosal swelling, edema, irritation, increased mucus production. Laryngeal or tracheal collapse must be relieved promptly.

B. Use strict aseptic technique and lavage contaminated tissues to prevent infection.

C. Nerve damage.
1. Injury to the recurrent laryngeal nerve may cause laryngeal spasms, paresis, or paralysis leading to aspiration pneumonia.
2. Mucostasis may occur following nerve damage.
3. Nerve damage is prevented by gentle tissue handling, appropriate dissection, and careful tissue retraction.

D. Tube tracheostomy.
1. Complications include gagging, vomiting, coughing, tube obstruction, tube dislodgement, emphysema, tracheal stenosis, tracheal malacia, and tracheocutaneous or tracheoesophageal fistula.

2. Some animals will occlude their tracheostomy tube when their neck is flexed and when they sleep with bedding.
3. Tracheostomy tubes and endotracheal tubes causing pressure necrosis of the tracheal mucosa or cartilages may cause strictures.

E. Permanent tracheostomy.
1. The main complication is stomal occlusion from accumulated mucus, skin folds, or stenosis.
2. Mucus accumulation, coughing, and gagging may occur as a result of tracheal irritation.

F. Tracheal resection and anastomosis.
1. Complications may include hemorrhage, voice change, fistula formation, and cartilage malacia, dehiscence, and stenosis.
    a. Dehiscence occurs following tracheal anastomosis if there is too much tension or neck movement following surgery.
        i. Subcutaneous emphysema, acute respiratory distress, hemoptysis, and subcutaneous swelling are signs of dehiscence.
    b. Excessive anastomotic tension and second-intention healing may lead to tracheal stenosis.
    c. Excessive dissection may cause ischemic necrosis of the remaining trachea.
    d. Traumatizing the recurrent laryngeal nerves may cause laryngospasms, laryngeal paresis, or laryngeal paralysis.

G. Ventriculocordectomy.
1. Scar tissue may form within the larynx and trachea leading to obstruction weeks after surgery.
2. Clinical signs of obstruction are not usually apparent until luminal compromise approaches 50%.
3. Scar tissue forms across the larynx from mucosal damage or when there is second-intention healing near the dorsal and ventral commissures.
4. Other complications include edema, hemorrhage, cough, gag, stenosis, and altered vocalization. Mucosal edema may partially obstruct the glottis and can be reduced by pretreating with corticosteroids.
5. Stenosis may occur at the dorsal or ventral commissures of the glottis following ventriculocordectomy if intact mucosa is not preserved in these areas and healing occurs by second intention.
    a. Approximating mucosa over the ventriculocordectomy sites also minimizes stenosis.
6. Ventriculocordectomy is expected to alter the normal bark, making it lower pitched and harsher.
7. Resumption of a near-normal bark may occur within months after removal of only the vocal fold margin and second-intention healing.

XI. Special Age Considerations

A. Tracheal and laryngeal cartilages of very young animals have a high water content. These cartilages may not hold sutures well.

B. Congenital abnormalities involving the respiratory tract should be treated early in the animal's life (within the first year) to avoid progressive respiratory distress and improve quality of life.

C. Old animals may have ossified, inelastic, brittle cartilages that are difficult to manipulate during surgery.

Stenotic Nares (*SAS*, pp. 620-622)

I. Definitions

A. **Stenotic nares** are nostrils with abnormally narrow openings.

II. General Considerations and Clinically Relevant Pathophysiology

A. Nasal cartilages lack normal rigidity and collapse medially causing partial occlusion of the external nares.
   1. Airflow into the nasal cavity is restricted and greater inspiratory effort is necessary, causing mild to severe dyspnea.
   2. Concurrent soft palate elongation, everted laryngeal saccules, aryepiglottic collapse, or corniculate collapse often contributes to the severity of respiratory distress.

B. Brachycephalic syndrome.
   1. Combination of stenotic nares, soft palate elongation, and laryngeal saccule eversion.
   2. Concurrent tracheal hypoplasia or advanced laryngeal collapse often contributes to the respiratory distress.
   3. Brachycephalic animals typically have a compressed face with poorly developed nares and a distorted nasopharynx. The soft tissues of the head are not proportionally reduced and often appear redundant.

III. Diagnosis

A. Clinical Presentation

1. Signalment.
   a. Brachycephalic breeds (particularly English bulldogs, Boston terriers, pugs, and Pekingese) are predominantly affected.
   b. Feline breeds more commonly affected include Himalayan and Persian.
   c. Either sex may be affected.
   d. Stenotic nares are present at birth; however, many animals present for evaluation between 2 and 4 years of age.
2. Clinical signs.
   a. Noisy (stridulous), difficult breathing.
   b. Frequent retching or gagging up of phlegm.
   c. Trouble swallowing (because the normal occlusion of the airway during deglutition compromises ventilation).
   d. Exercise intolerance.
   e. Cyanosis.
   f. Restless sleeping ("sleep-disordered breathing").
   g. Collapse.
   h. Excitement, stress, and increased heat and humidity frequently exacerbate clinical signs.

B. Physical Examination Findings

1. Nares may be mildly, moderately, or severely deviated medially.
2. Signs of increased inspiratory effort include retraction of lip commissures, open-mouth breathing or constant panting, forelimb abduction, exaggerated use of abdominal muscles, paradoxical movement of the thorax and abdomen, recruitment of accessory respiratory muscles, inward collapse of the intercostal spaces and thoracic inlet, orthopneic posture (extended head and neck and reluctance to lie down).
3. The mucous membranes are normal in color with mild or moderate dyspnea, but pale or cyanotic with severe dyspnea.
4. Affected animals are often restless and anxious, especially when restrained.
5. Hyperthermia is common due to ineffective cooling.
6. Careful thoracic auscultation is difficult because of referred upper airway noise.
7. Gastrointestinal tract distention may occur secondary to aerophagia associated with open-mouth breathing.

C. Radiography

1. Evaluate thoracic radiographs for underlying cardiac (e.g., cardiomegaly, heart failure) or pulmonary (e.g., pulmonary edema, pneumonia) abnormalities.
2. Consider lateral radiographs of the nasopharynx, larynx, and trachea to assess concurrent airway abnormalities.
   a. The soft palate may be thickened and elongated.
   b. Nasopharyngeal, laryngeal, and tracheal masses may be identified.
   c. Determining tracheal-to-thoracic inlet diameter ratios can help assess tracheal size (*SAS,* p. 633).

D. Laboratory Findings

1. Hematology and serum biochemistry values are usually normal.
2. Blood gas evaluation may reveal hypoxemia and respiratory alkalosis.
3. Oxygen saturation acutely falling below 80% may cause signs of syncope and collapse.
4. Polycythemia may occur if hypoxia is chronic.

IV. Medical Treatment

A. Mild Clinical Signs

1. Institute a weight reduction program for obese animals.
2. Restrict exercise.
3. Eliminate precipitating causes.

B. Moderate to Severe Clinical Signs

1. Sedation.
   a. Dogs.
      i. Use intravenous oxymorphone or butorphanol plus either acepromazine or diazepam.
         (a) Oxymorphone (Numorphan)–0.05 mg/kg, max 4 mg.
         (b) Butorphanol (Torbutrol, Torbugesic)–0.2 to 0.4 mg/kg.
         (c) Acepromazine–0.02 to 0.05 mg/kg, max 1 mg IV.
         (d) Diazepam (Valium)–0.2 mg/kg IV.
      ii. Alternatively, use fentanyl plus droperidol.
         (a) Fentanyl plus droperidol (Innovar-Vet)–1 ml/20 to 40 kg IV or 1 ml/10 to 15 kg IM.

b. Cats.
   i. Acepromazine or diazepam is recommended. Diazepam may not reliably result in sedation in cats.
      (a) Acepromazine–0.05 mg/kg, IV, IM, SC.
      (b) Diazepam (Valium)–0.2 mg/kg IV (Appendix G-26).
2. Corticosteroids.
   a. Dexamethasone (Azium)–0.5 to 2 mg/kg IV, IM, SC.
3. Supplement oxygen.
4. Cool the animal.

V. Surgical Treatment

A. Preoperative Management

1. Monitor carefully for decompensation and progressive respiratory distress.
2. Be prepared to provide emergency therapy (e.g., temporary tracheostomy) if dyspnea worsens acutely.
3. Administer antiinflammatory doses of corticosteroids if the animal is undergoing concurrent laryngeal or nasopharyngeal procedures.
   a. Dexamethasone (Azium)–0.5 to 2 mg/kg IV, IM, SC.

B. Anesthesia

1. Sedate or anesthetize these animals carefully (see above).
   a. Virtually all sedatives and anesthetic agents relax the upper airway dilating muscles, while allowing the diaphragm to continue contracting. This allows the upper airway to collapse and reduces respiratory drive. Airway collapse is worsened by negative inspiratory pressure that draws the pharyngeal walls medially.
   b. Anesthesia also relaxes muscles employed by brachycephalics to facilitate breathing (e.g., geniohyoid, genioglossus, sternohyoid).
   c. Oxygen saturation can drop rapidly during anesthesia or sedation; monitor it during induction, oral examination, anesthesia, and anesthetic recovery.
2. Induce anesthesia and intubate the animal as rapidly as possible.
3. See Appendix G-26 for selected anesthetic protocols for animals with upper respiratory disease.

C. Positioning

1. Position the patient in sternal recumbency with the chin resting on a pad.
2. Tape the head to the table to avoid rotation.
3. Scrub the planum nasale with antiseptic soaps and solutions.

D. Surgical Techniques

1. Resect a portion of the dorsal lateral nasal cartilage.

Grasp the margin of the nares with a Brown-Adson thumb forceps. Maintaining this grip, make a V-shaped incision around the forceps with a No. 11 scalpel blade. Make the first incision medially and the second incision laterally. Remove the vertical wedge of tissue. Control hemorrhage with pressure and by reapposing the cut edges. Align the ventral margin of the nares and mucocutaneous junction and place three to four simple interrupted sutures (e.g., polydioxanone, 3-0 or 4-0) to reappose the tissues. Repeat the procedure on the opposite side, being careful to excise the same size tissue wedge.

E. Postoperative Care and Assessment

1. Monitor these animals constantly during recovery from anesthesia (*SAS,* p. 618).
2. Provide nasal insufflation of oxygen.
3. Leave the animal intubated as long as possible–reintubate or place a tracheostomy tube if respiratory obstruction or severe distress occurs.
4. Clean the surgical site (expect slight hemorrhage).
5. Protect the surgical site from the animal by using an Elizabethan collar, if necessary.

F. Prognosis

1. Animals with mild stenosis may do well without surgery; however, those with moderate or severe stenosis and other obstructive problems can develop severe respiratory distress.
2. The prognosis following resection of stenotic nares in animals with brachycephalic syndrome is good if advanced laryngeal collapse is not present and the palate and saccules are concurrently resected.
3. Most animals have reduced inspiratory effort and increased exercise tolerance after surgery.

Elongated Soft Palate (*SAS,* pp. 622-624)

I. Definitions

A. An elongated soft palate is one that extends more than 1 to 3 mm caudal to the tip of the epiglottis.

II. General Considerations and Clinically Relevant Pathophysiology

A. The most commonly diagnosed respiratory problem in brachycephalic dogs.

B. Part of the brachycephalic syndrome in addition to stenotic nares (see pp. 487-490) and laryngeal saccule eversion (see pp. 494-497).

C. Congenital.

D. Effects on respiration.

1. The soft palate is pulled caudally during inspiration, obstructing the dorsal aspect of the glottis.
2. It is sometimes sucked between the corniculate processes of the arytenoid cartilages, which increases inspiratory effort and causes more turbulent airflow.
3. Laryngeal mucosa becomes inflamed and edematous, further narrowing the airway.
4. The tip of the soft palate is blown into the nasopharynx during expiration.

E. Affected dogs may have trouble swallowing because normal occlusion of the airway during deglutition compromises ventilation. Dysfunctional swallowing may result in aspiration pneumonia.

III. Diagnosis

A. Clinical Presentation

1. Signalment.
   a. Uncommon except in brachycephalic breeds (English bulldogs, Boston terriers, pugs, Pekingese).
   b. It affects either sex.
   c. Although the condition is present at birth, many affected animals present for evaluation between 2 and 3 years of age. Older animals often have concurrent, advanced laryngeal collapse.
2. History.
   a. Affected animals typically have a history of noisy (stridulous), difficult breathing (especially inspiratory).
   b. Some animals may retch or gag phlegm because they have trouble swallowing if normal occlusion of the airway during deglutition compromises ventilation.
   c. Exercise intolerance, cyanosis, and collapse are common and may be worsened by excitement, stress, increased heat, and humidity.
   d. Restlessness during sleeping (sleep-disordered breathing) may be noted.

B. Physical Examination Findings

1. Pharyngeal and laryngeal auscultation reveals prominent snoring obscuring other respiratory sounds.
2. Increased inspiratory effort may be noted as retraction of lip commissures, open-mouth breathing or constant panting, forelimb abduction, exaggerated use of abdominal muscles, paradoxical movement of the thorax and abdomen, recruitment of accessory respiratory muscles, inward collapse of the intercostal spaces and thoracic inlet, and orthopneic posture.
3. Animals may be hyperthermic.
4. **Always evaluate these animals for the presence of other upper respiratory abnormalities.**
5. Laryngeal exam.
   a. Sedation or general anesthesia is usually necessary.
      i. It is difficult to visualize the oropharynx and larynx in brachycephalic animals because their tongues are thick and restraint may accentuate respiratory distress.
      ii. Dorsally displace the soft palate to improve visualization of the arytenoid cartilages.
   b. Observations.
      i. An elongated soft palate overlies the epiglottis by more than a few millimeters (i.e., often more than 1 cm).
      ii. The soft palate is often thickened with a roughened and inflamed tip.
      iii. The arytenoids are frequently inflamed and edematous.

C. Radiography

1. Take thoracic radiographs to rule out concurrent diseases such as hypoplastic trachea or cardiomegaly.
2. Pharyngeal radiographs may show an abnormally long, thickened soft palate but are usually unnecessary.

IV. Differential Diagnosis

A. Other causes of upper respiratory obstruction include laryngeal paralysis; masses obstructing the glottis, larynx, or trachea; and traumatic disruption of the airway.

V. Medical Treatment

A. For mildly affected animals.
   1. Institute a weight reduction program for obese animals.
   2. Restrict exercise.
   3. Eliminate precipitating causes.

B. For moderate to severely affected animals.
   1. Consider sedating the animal.
   2. Administer corticosteroids.
   3. Provide supplemental oxygen.
   4. Cool the animal.

C. **Note: Prolonged medical therapy may allow progression of degenerative changes.**

VI. Surgical Treatment

A. Timing of the Surgical Procedure

1. Perform soft palate resection when the animal is young (i.e., 4 to 24 months) to prevent laryngeal cartilage from degenerating and collapsing, if possible.

B. Preoperative Management

1. Pretreat with antiinflammatory doses of corticosteroids to decrease laryngeal swelling and postoperative obstruction.
2. Lavage the oral cavity gently with dilute antiseptic solutions.
   a. Do not scrub the mucosal surfaces to avoid causing irritation and edema.
3. Place sponges around the endotracheal tube at the glottis to prevent fluids from entering the airway.
4. Placement of a tracheostomy tube is usually unnecessary unless other oral procedures are being done concurrently.

C. Surgical Anatomy

1. Soft palate.
   a. Use the tonsillar crypt as a landmark for determining appropriate soft palate length. The soft palate generally extends no further than the mid to caudal aspect of the tonsillar crypt.
   b. The end of the soft palate just covers the tip of the epiglottis in a normal dog.
   c. The distal end of an elongated soft palate is frequently sucked into the larynx, giving it a pointed or pinched appearance.

D. Positioning

1. Position the patient in sternal recumbency with the mouth fully opened.

2. Suspend the maxilla from a bar positioned several feet above the surgery table and secure the mandible ventrally with tape.
3. Do not allow the chin to rest on the table or pads.
4. For maximal visualization, retract the cheeks laterally and pull the tongue rostrally (*SAS,* Fig. 25-8).

E. Surgical Techniques

1. General considerations.
   a. Resect the soft palate with scissors, carbon dioxide laser, or electrosurgery (the latter may increase postoperative swelling).
   b. Control hemorrhage (generally mild to moderate following resection) with gentle pressure.
   c. Shorten the caudal margin of the soft palate so that it contacts the tip of the epiglottis.
      i. Resecting too little soft palate will not optimally relieve respiratory distress.
      ii. Resecting too much soft palate results in nasal regurgitation, rhinitis, and sinusitis.
2. Surgical technique.

Visually mark the site of proposed resection using the tip of the epiglottis and the caudal or midpoint of the tonsils as landmarks. Handle the soft palate gently and as little as possible to avoid excessive mucosal swelling. Grasp the tip of the soft palate with thumb forceps or Allis tissue forceps. Place stay sutures at the proposed site of resection on the right and left borders of the palate. Place hemostats on these sutures and have an assistant apply lateral traction. Transect across one third to one half the width of the soft palate with curved Metzenbaum scissors. Begin a simple continuous suture pattern (4-0 polydioxanone) at the border of the palate, apposing the oropharyngeal and nasopharyngeal mucosa. Continue transecting and suturing until the excess palate has been resected.

VII. Postoperative Care and Assessment

A. Monitor these patients closely for respiratory distress postoperatively.

B. Delay extubation for as long as possible.

C. Keep the animal quiet.

D. Administer oxygen by nasal insufflation.

E. If severe dyspnea occurs, place a tracheostomy tube.
1. Excessive mucosal swelling may cause asphyxiation.
2. Postoperative coughing and gagging are common.

F. Administer corticosteroids postoperatively if swelling is severe and respiratory obstruction persists.

G. Maintain intravenous fluids until oral intake resumes.
1. Offer water when the animal is fully recovered from anesthesia (6 to 12 hours postoperatively).
2. Withhold food for 18 to 24 hours.
   a. Offering food soon after surgery may traumatize swollen tissues, causing swelling, airway obstruction, or aspiration.

H. Observe the animal in the hospital for 24 to 72 hours after surgery.

VIII. Prognosis

A. Without Surgery

1. Poor because laryngeal collapse and respiratory distress will worsen.

B. With Surgery

1. The prognosis is good in young patients having elongated soft palate as the primary problem.
2. Older animals frequently do not respond as well because their laryngeal cartilages have begun to collapse.
3. If advanced laryngeal collapse has developed, the prognosis is poor unless additional surgery is performed.

Everted Laryngeal Saccules (*SAS*, pp. 625-626)

I. Definitions

A. Prolapse of the mucosa lining the laryngeal crypts.

II. Synonyms

A. Laryngeal saccule eversion.

B. Laryngeal ventricle eversion.

C. Stage one laryngeal collapse.

III. General Considerations and Clinically Relevant Pathophysiology

A. Is a component of brachycephalic syndrome.

B. Diagnosed less often than either elongated soft palate or stenotic nares.

C. Is the first stage of laryngeal collapse. Increased airflow resistance and increased negative pressure generated to move air past obstructed areas (stenotic nares, dorsal glottis) pull the saccules from their crypts, causing them to swell.

D. Once everted, the saccules are continuously irritated by turbulent airflow and become increasingly edematous.

1. Everted saccules obstruct the ventral aspect of the glottis and further inhibit airflow.
2. May be difficult to differentiate everted laryngeal saccules from the vocal folds due to their close proximity.
    a. Everted saccules partially or completely obscure the vocal folds.
3. **Because this is usually a "secondary" problem, be sure to identify other concurrent disease.**

IV. Diagnosis

A. Clinical Presentation

1. Breeds.
   a. Most common in brachycephalic dogs.
   b. Chronic barking may cause laryngeal saccule eversion in other breeds.
2. Age of onset.
   a. Most brachycephalic dogs with laryngeal saccule eversion are diagnosed between 2 and 3 years of age, although it may occur at any age.
3. History.
   a. Affected animals have a history of stridulous breathing and respiratory distress as described for animals with stenotic nares and elongated soft palate.
   b. The stridor is most prominent during inspiration.

B. Physical Examination Findings

1. Mild to severe dyspnea.
2. Increased inspiratory effort may be evident as retraction of lip commissures, open-mouth breathing or constant panting, forelimb abduction, exaggerated use of abdominal muscles, paradoxical movement of the thorax and abdomen, recruitment of accessory respiratory muscles, inward collapse of the intercostal spaces and thoracic inlet, or an orthopneic posture.
3. General anesthesia is necessary to evaluate the larynx (see above and *SAS*, p. 610, for general anesthesia during laryngeal exam).
   a. When the saccules are everted they cannot be visualized in their normal position between the vocal folds and the ventricular folds.
   b. Acutely everted saccules are whitish and glistening in appearance.
   c. Chronically everted saccules are pink and fleshy.
   d. Soft palate elongation may make it difficult to visualize and thoroughly evaluate the laryngeal saccules.

C. Radiography

1. Laryngeal saccule eversion is not diagnosed radiographically.
2. Evaluate thoracic radiographs for evidence of cardiac or pulmonary abnormalities or concurrent disease (e.g., hypoplastic trachea, tracheal collapse).

D. Laboratory Findings

1. Laboratory abnormalities are uncommon.

V. Differential Diagnosis

A. Stenotic nares and an elongated soft palate are usually present in animals with laryngeal saccule eversion.

B. Evaluate for advanced laryngeal collapse; laryngeal paralysis; tracheal collapse; and nasopharyngeal, laryngeal, or tracheal masses.

VI. Medical Treatment

A. For mildly affected animals.
   1. Institute a weight reduction program for obese animals.

2. Restrict exercise.
3. Eliminate precipitating causes.

B. For moderate to severely affected animals.
1. Consider sedating the animal.
2. Administer corticosteroids.
3. Provide supplemental oxygen.
4. Cool the animal.

C. **Note: Prolonged medical therapy may allow progression of degenerative changes.**

VII. Surgical Treatment

A. General Considerations

1. Treat everted laryngeal saccules at the same time the stenotic nares and soft palate elongation are corrected.

B. Preoperative Management

1. Monitor continuously before surgery because the severity of respiratory distress may increase.
2. Administer an antiinflammatory dose of corticosteroids before anesthetic induction.
   a. Dexamethasone (Azium)–0.5 to 2 mg/kg IV, IM, SC.

C. Anesthesia

1. If the endotracheal tube obscures visualization of the saccules, use a smaller tube or place the tube via a tracheotomy.
2. Alternatively, maintain these patients on injectable anesthetics (e.g., propofol, thiobarbiturates, diazepam plus ketamine).
3. Anesthesia of animals with brachycephalic syndrome is described in Appendix G-26.
4. General anesthetic recommendations for animals with upper respiratory disease are in *SAS,* p. 610 (see also Appendix G-26).

D. Surgical Anatomy

1. The laryngeal saccule is a slight dorsoventral depression between the vestibular and vocal folds.
2. The everted saccules lie just rostral to the vocal folds and should not be mistaken for the vocal cords.
3. Surgical anatomy of the larynx is provided in *SAS,* p. 611.

E. Positioning

1. Position the patient in sternal recumbency with the mouth fully opened.
2. Suspend the maxilla from a bar positioned several feet above the surgery table and secure the mandible ventrally with tape.
3. Do not allow the chin to rest on the table or pads.
4. For maximal visualization, retract the cheeks laterally and pull the tongue rostrally.

F. Surgical Technique

Retract the endotracheal tube dorsomedially so the saccule on one side can be better visualized. Grasp the everted saccule with long-handled forceps or a tissue hook. Position the tip of a long-handled, curved Metzenbaum scissors at the base of the everted tissue and transect. Biopsy forceps or laryngeal cup forceps may also be used. Control hemorrhage with gentle pressure. Repeat

the procedure on the opposite side. Handle the tissues gently. Excessive manipulation will cause obstructive edema postoperatively.

VIII. Postoperative Care and Assessment

A. Monitor closely for respiratory distress following surgery.

B. Mild hemorrhage from the resection sites may lead to coughing, gagging, and hematemesis.

C. Postoperative swelling and edema may cause severe laryngeal obstruction, requiring temporary tracheostomy.

IX. Prognosis

A. Acute episodes of respiratory distress may be adequately managed with medical therapy alone.

B. Chronic medical management often allows advanced laryngeal collapse to develop because of cartilage degeneration.

C. Partial resection of the laryngeal saccules (in addition to the nares and soft palate when indicated) should relieve moderate to severe signs of respiratory distress in patients who do not have laryngeal collapse.

Laryngeal Collapse (*SAS*, pp. 626-628)

I. Definitions

A. A form of upper airway obstruction caused by loss of cartilage rigidity that allows medial deviation of the laryngeal cartilages.

II. Synonyms

A. Aryepiglottic collapse.

B. Corniculate collapse.

III. General Considerations and Clinically Relevant Pathophysiology

A. Occurs secondary to chronic upper airway obstruction or trauma.
   1. Trauma may fracture or disrupt the laryngeal cartilages and allow medial collapse.

2. It is most commonly due to chronic upper airway obstruction and cartilage fatigue or degeneration.

B. The obstruction causes increased airway resistance, increased negative intraglottic luminal pressure, and increased air velocity.
1. These forces displace laryngeal structures medially with permanent cartilage deformation and fatigue the cartilages.
2. Increased inspiratory effort irritates the mucosa, causing inflammation and edema, which further obstructs the airway, causing more airflow resistance and increasing the effort of breathing.

C. Three stages of laryngeal collapse.
1. Stage 1.
   a. Laryngeal saccule eversion (see pp. 494-497).
2. Stage 2.
   a. Medial deviation of the cuneiform cartilage and aryepiglottic fold or aryepiglottic collapse.
3. Stage 3.
   a. Medial deviation of the corniculate process of the arytenoid cartilages or corniculate collapse.

D. Diagnosis of laryngeal collapse that occurs concurrently with other upper respiratory abnormalities (i.e., elongated soft palate, stenotic nares) is easily overlooked on oral examination. If response to treatment is less than expected following appropriate surgery for these abnormalities, laryngeal collapse may be present.

IV. Diagnosis

A. Clinical Presentation

1. Breeds.
   a. Brachycephalic breeds are most commonly affected.
2. Age of onset of clinical signs.
   a. Usually occurs in animals greater than 2 years of age.
   b. May be diagnosed in younger animals with severe upper airway obstruction.

B. History

1. Stridor and other signs of upper airway obstruction have usually been present in affected animals for years already, but may have gradually or acutely worsened.
2. Laryngeal collapse should be suspected in patients who respond well to surgery for upper airway obstruction but later relapse with moderate to severe respiratory distress.

C. Physical Examination Findings

1. Stridulous labored breathing is the most consistent finding.
2. Animals with advanced laryngeal collapse (stage 2 or 3) usually have moderate to severe respiratory distress.
3. Laryngeal evaluation requires general anesthesia.
4. Patients with laryngeal collapse have a decreased glottic lumen aperture.
   a. Stage 1.
      i. Recognized as prolapsed, edematous mucosa just rostral to the vocal cords at the ventral aspect of the glottis.
   b. Stage 2.

i. One or both aryepiglottic folds are deviated medially and obstruct the ventral aspect of the glottis.

c. Stage 3.

i. Laryngeal collapse occurs when the corniculate processes of the arytenoid cartilages deviate medially from their normal paramedian position and are not adequately abducted during inspiration.

ii. The cartilages often have a flaccid appearance.

5. **Be sure to assess laryngeal function under a light plane of anesthesia before intubation.**

D. Radiography

1. Evaluate the thorax and neck for evidence of concurrent abnormalities.
   a. A lateral radiograph of the pharynx may show cartilage ossification, cartilage fracture, or neoplasia.

E. Laboratory Findings

1. Hematology and serum biochemistry results are usually normal.

V. Differential Diagnosis

A. Laryngeal or Tracheal Masses

B. Laryngeal Paralysis

C. Everted Laryngeal Saccules

D. Elongated Soft Palate

E. Stenotic Nares

VI. Medical Treatment

A. For mildly affected animals.
1. Institute a weight reduction program for obese animals.
2. Restrict exercise.
3. Eliminate precipitating causes.

B. For moderate to severely affected animals.
1. Consider sedating the animal.
2. Administer corticosteroids.
3. Provide supplemental oxygen.
4. Cool the animal.

VII. Surgical Treatment

A. General Considerations

1. In stable patients, treat concurrent abnormalities (e.g., resection of stenotic nares, elongated soft palates, and everted laryngeal saccules).
2. Options.
   a. Resect the aryepiglottic fold in patients with mild to moderate stage 2 laryngeal collapse.
   b. Consider permanent tracheostomy for patients with advanced

laryngeal collapse and moderate to severe respiratory distress who do not or are not expected to respond to resection.

i. Partial laryngectomy or lateralization procedures are seldom beneficial because the weakened cartilages generally continue to collapse medially.

B. Preoperative Management

1. Stabilize the patient before surgery.
2. Observe closely for worsening dyspnea.
3. Pretreat with corticosteroids before aryepiglottic fold resection (see below).

C. Anesthesia

1. See Appendix G-26 for general anesthetic recommendations for animals with upper respiratory disease.
2. See Appendix K for recommended anesthetics for laryngeal examination.

D. Surgical Anatomy

1. See *SAS,* p. 611, for a description of the surgical anatomy of the larynx.

E. Positioning

1. Position the animal in sternal recumbency with the maxilla suspended and the mouth widely opened for resection of the soft palate, laryngeal saccules, and aryepiglottic fold.
2. Perform permanent tracheostomy with the animal in dorsal recumbency.

F. Surgical Techniques

1. Aryepiglottic fold resection is accomplished through an oral approach.
2. It is performed unilaterally in conjunction with resection of the nares, soft palate, and everted laryngeal saccules.

Grasp and stabilize the fold with forceps. Then transect the fold and cuneiform process with Mayo scissors or uterine biopsy forceps. Allow second-intention healing.

G. Postoperative Care and Assessment

1. Monitored continuously during anesthetic recovery for signs of airway obstruction.
   a. Patients with advanced laryngeal collapse may develop acute respiratory obstruction following surgery.
2. Manage tracheostomas as described in *SAS,* p. 618, to prevent occlusion of the stoma with mucus.

VIII. Prognosis

A. Moderate to severe respiratory distress will persist without surgical intervention.

B. Acute inflammation may cause cyanosis, collapse, and respiratory arrest.

C. The prognosis for improvement in advanced laryngeal collapse after surgery is poor if resection of the nares, soft palate, and laryngeal saccules is done.

D. The prognosis is fair to good with concurrent permanent tracheostomy.

Laryngeal Paralysis (*SAS*, pp. 628-632)

I. Definition

A. Complete or partial failure of the arytenoid cartilages and vocal folds to abduct during inspiration.

II. General Considerations and Clinically Relevant Pathophysiology

A. Laryngeal paralysis causes upper respiratory obstruction and mild to severe dyspnea.

B. May be caused by dysfunction of the laryngeal muscles, dysfunction of the recurrent laryngeal or vagus nerves, or cricoarytenoid ankylosis.

C. Acquired or congenital neurologic causes are most common.
1. The intrinsic laryngeal abductor and adductor muscles are innervated by the recurrent laryngeal nerves.
   a. Subsequent atrophy of the cricoarytenoideus dorsalis muscle causes the cartilages to remain in a paramedian position during inspiration, preventing maximal air intake and increasing airflow resistance.
   b. Ineffective laryngeal adduction and closure during swallowing predispose the patient to aspiration of food and secretions causing subsequent aspiration pneumonia.
2. Congenital laryngeal paralysis.
   a. Breeds affected.
      i. Bouvier des Flandres.
         (a) Due to degeneration of the nucleus ambiguus.
      ii. Dalmatians.
         (a) Caused by polyneuropathy associated with dying back of peripheral nerves.
      iii. Bull terriers.
      iv. Siberian huskies.
3. Acquired laryngeal paralysis.
   a. Usually idiopathic.
   b. May occur secondary to trauma, disease (e.g., polyneuropathy, myopathy, Chagas' disease [trypanosomiasis], hypothyroidism, neoplasia), or surgery.
   c. May affect one or both sides of the larynx.
      i. Unilateral paralysis is often asymptomatic.

III. Diagnosis

A. Clinical Presentation

1. Breeds.
   a. Clinical signs are more common in large-breed dogs than small-breed dogs.
   b. Acquired idiopathic laryngeal paralysis is most common in middle-age or older (mean age 9.5 years, range 4 to 13 years). Labrador retrievers, Afghan hounds, and Irish setters.
   c. Congenital laryngeal paralysis should be suspected in young (less than 1 year of age) Bouviers, Siberian huskies, bull terriers, or dalmatians with upper airway obstruction (see above).
2. Sex.
   a. Males are affected two to four times more frequently than females.

B. History

1. Progressive inspiratory stridor, voice change, and exercise intolerance. They may also have increased stridor, dyspnea, cyanosis, coughing, gagging, vomiting, restlessness, and anxiety.
2. Some animals are asymptomatic at rest.
3. Obesity, exercise, excitement, and high ambient temperatures may exacerbate clinical signs.
4. Laryngeal paralysis occurs in approximately one third of dogs with tracheal collapse.
5. All animals with laryngeal paralysis are at risk for inhalation pneumonia from aspirating food and saliva.

C. Physical Examination Findings

1. Physical examination findings are nonspecific. Findings in some animals include labored breathing, continuous panting, hyperthermia, muscle wasting, and weakness.
2. Perform a neurologic exam to detect concurrent abnormalities.
3. To evaluate the larynx use light, general anesthesia (propofol or diazepam plus ketamine; see above).
4. Delay intubation until the larynx has been examined because placement of the endotracheal tube may obscure visualization.
   a. Laryngeal cartilages are located in a paramedian position and do not abduct during inspiration.
   b. Do not mistake fluttering of the vocal folds and arytenoid cartilages during turbulent airflow for purposeful abduction.
      i. Paradoxical vocal fold movement may occur and be confused with normal movement.
      ii. A normal larynx maximally abducts during inspiration, not expiration.

D. Radiography

1. Evaluate lateral cervical and thoracic radiographs to rule out other causes of abnormal respiratory noises and dyspnea.
   a. Evaluate for inhalation pneumonia because affected animals are at increased risk for this.
2. Laryngeal paralysis cannot be diagnosed radiographically.

E. Laboratory Findings

1. Hematology and serum biochemistry values are usually normal (*SAS,* p. 620).
2. Exclude hypothyroidism (*SAS,* p. 428) by evaluating serum thyroid hormone levels.

3. Diagnosis of acquired myasthenia gravis.
   a. Demonstrate circulating antibodies to acetylcholine receptors.
   b. Evaluate clinical signs and response to a cholinesterase inhibitor.
      i. Expect a dramatic, but transient, improvement in voluntary muscle function when you give edrophonium chloride intravenously.
         (a) Dogs–0.1 to 2.0 mg.
         (b) Cats–0.5 to 1.0 mg.
      ii. Use caution when giving edrophonium. Possible complications associated with its use include paralysis.
4. Electromyography.
   a. Use bipolar concentric needle electrodes to diagnose denervation of the laryngeal muscles (dorsal cricoarytenoid, ventricular, and thyroarytenoid).
   b. Consider nerve conduction studies to help rule out generalized neuromuscular disease.
5. Tidal breathing flow volume loops show a reduction in inspiratory flow rate.
6. Histopathology and histochemistry confirm neurogenic laryngeal muscle atrophy.

IV. Differential Diagnosis

A. Brachycephalic Syndrome

B. Laryngeal Collapse

C. Tracheal Collapse

D. Masses or Trauma Involving the Upper Airway

V. Medical Treatment

A. Asymptomatic or mildly affected animals.
1. Maintain a sedentary lifestyle (restrict exercise).
2. Avoid excess weight gain.
3. Reduce weight if animal is obese.
4. Avoid stress.

B. Small dogs are more successfully managed with medical therapy than are large dogs.

C. Acute respiratory distress.
1. Sedate if necessary.
   a. Dogs.
      i. Use intravenous oxymorphone or butorphanol plus either acepromazine or diazepam.
         (a) Oxymorphone (Numorphan)–0.05 mg/kg, max 4 mg.
         (b) Butorphanol (Torbutrol, Torbugesic)–0.2 to 0.4 mg/kg.
         (c) Acepromazine–0.02 to 0.05 mg/kg, max 1 mg IV.
         (d) Diazepam (Valium)–0.2 mg/kg IV.
      ii. Alternatively, use fentanyl plus droperidol.
         (a) Fentanyl plus droperidol (Innovar-Vet)–1 ml/20 to 40 kg IV or 1 ml/10 to 15 kg IM.

b. Cats.
  i. Use acepromazine or diazepam. Diazepam may not reliably result in sedation in cats.
    (a) Acepromazine–0.05 mg/kg, IV, IM, SC.
    (b) Diazepam (Valium)–0.2 mg/kg IV.
2. Cool.
  a. Direct a fan at the patient.
  b. Apply ice packs to the head, axilla, inguinal area, and extremities.
  c. Administer cooled fluids intravenously.
3. Administer corticosteroids.
  a. Dexamethasone (Azium)–0.5 to 2 mg/kg IV, IM, SC.
4. Supplement oxygen.
5. Maintain in a quiet, nonstressful environment.

VI. Surgical Treatment

A. General Considerations

1. Recommend surgery for patients with laryngeal paralysis who have moderate to severe signs of respiratory distress.
2. The goal of treatment is to enlarge the glottis without exaggerating aspiration of food or saliva.
3. Many surgical techniques have been described to treat laryngeal paralysis, including partial laryngectomy, lateralization, castellated laryngofissures, and muscle-nerve pedicle transposition.
  a. Arytenoid lateralization (tie-back).
    i. Technique of choice.
      (a) Consistently good results (greater than 90%).
      (b) Few complications.
  b. Vocal fold excision (ventriculocordectomy).
    i. Enlarges the ventral aspect of the glottis.
    ii. Is effective in mild to moderate cases.
    iii. Relatively easy to perform.
    iv. Glottic stenosis occurs in approximately 20% of the cases and is difficult to treat successfully.
  c. Partial arytenoidectomy (corniculate process).
    i. Enlarges the dorsal aspect of the glottis.
    ii. Success depends on the skill of the surgeon.
    iii. Serious complications and death occur in up to 50% of the cases following this procedure.
  d. Modified castellated laryngofissure technique.
    i. A combination of vocal fold excision, lateralization, and laryngofissure creation to enlarge the glottis.
    ii. Effective but technically difficult.
  e. Muscle-nerve pedicle transposition.
    i. Can successfully reinnervate the larynx and improve function, but the process takes 5 to 11 months before clinical improvement is seen.

B. Preoperative Management

1. Observe closely before surgery for progressive respiratory distress.
2. Keep animals cool, calm, and quiet.
3. Pretreat with an antiinflammatory dose of corticosteroids immediately before surgery.
  a. Dexamethasone (Azium)–0.5 to 2 mg/kg IV, IM, SC.

C. Anesthesia

1. See Appendix G-26 for general anesthetic recommendations for animals with upper respiratory disease.

2. Intubation via a tracheotomy incision may be helpful when performing a partial laryngectomy, but is unnecessary for arytenoid cartilage lateralization.
3. See Appendix K for anesthetic recommendations for laryngeal examination.

D. Surgical Anatomy

1. The cricoarytenoideus dorsalis is the abductor muscle of the larynx.
   a. Extends from the muscular process of the arytenoid cartilage in a dorsomedial direction to the cricoid cartilage.
   b. See *SAS,* p. 611, for surgical anatomy of the larynx.

E. Positioning

1. Arytenoid cartilage lateralization.
   a. Position the animal in lateral or dorsal recumbency with the neck over a rolled towel.
   b. Rotate to elevate the ipsilateral mandible.
   c. Stabilize the head by taping it to the table.
   d. Clip and prepare the entire cervical area for aseptic surgery.
2. Partial laryngectomy via an oral approach.
   a. Position the animal in sternal recumbency with the head suspended by the maxilla.
   b. Have an assistant hold the mandible open or tape it to the table.
3. Partial laryngectomy via a ventral approach.
   a. Position the animal in dorsal recumbency with the head extended and secured to the operating table.

F. Surgical Techniques

1. Unilateral arytenoid lateralization.

Make a skin incision just ventral to the jugular vein beginning at the caudal angle of the mandible and extending over the dorsolateral aspect of the larynx to 1 to 2 cm caudal to the larynx. Incise and retract subcutaneous tissues, platysma, and parotidoauricularis muscles. Retract the sternocephalicus muscle and jugular vein dorsally and the sternohyoid muscle ventrally to expose the laryngeal area. Palpate the dorsal margin of the thyroid cartilage. Incise the thyropharyngeus muscle along the dorsolateral margin of the thyroid cartilage lamina. Place a stay suture through the thyroid cartilage lamina to retract and rotate the larynx laterally. Identify the cricoarytenoideus dorsalis muscle. Disarticulate the cricothyroid articulation with a No. 11 blade or scissors. Palpate, identify, and disarticulate the cricoarytenoid articulation at the muscular process. Using curved Metzenbaum scissors, transect the sesamoid band (interarytenoid ligament) between the two corniculate processes, being careful not to penetrate the laryngeal mucosa. Place a polypropylene suture (2-0 to 2) through the muscular process of the arytenoid cartilage and the caudal one third of the cricoid cartilage near the dorsal midline to mimic the direction of the cricoarytenoid muscle. Alternatively, place the suture through the muscular process and the most caudodorsal aspect of the thyroid cartilage. Muscular process–to–thyroid cartilage sutures tend to pull the arytenoid laterally, and muscular process–to–cricoid cartilage sutures tend to rotate the arytenoid laterally. Tie the suture with enough tension to moderately abduct the arytenoid cartilage. Have an assistant verify abduction by intraoral visualization of the larynx. If abduction is insufficient, the suture can be repositioned to achieve better abduction. Lavage the surgical site. Appose the thyropharyngeus muscle with a cruciate or simple continuous pattern (3-0 polydioxanone). Appose subcutaneous tissues and skin routinely.

2. Partial laryngectomy.
   a. Perform via an oral approach or a ventral laryngotomy approach.
   b. Perform vocal fold resection and unilateral resection of the

corniculate, cuneiform, and vocal processes of the arytenoid cartilage.

c. Note: Partial laryngectomy via an oral approach is extremely difficult in small dogs because of limited exposure.
d. Complications of partial laryngectomy may be severe. Use this technique in large-breed dogs with acquired laryngeal paralysis only.

Via oral approach: ***Grasp the corniculate process and retract it medially with biopsy forceps. Use a long-handled scalpel or scissors to excise the corniculate process and the proximal half and base of the cuneiform process. Do not excise the aryepiglottic fold or the distal half of the cuneiform process. Remove the vocal fold, vocal process, and vocal muscle with biopsy forceps, Metzenbaum scissors, or both. Leave the ventral aspect of the vocal cord intact. Control bleeding by applying pressure with gauze sponges.***

Via laryngotomy approach: ***Make a ventral midline incision over the larynx. Separate the sternohyoid muscles and incise the cricothyroid membrane and thyroid cartilage on the midline. Retract the edges of the thyroid cartilage with small Gelpi forceps. Visualize the arytenoid cartilages and vocal folds. Have an assistant visualize the larynx per os to help determine how much to remove. After incising the mucosa over the corniculate, cuneiform, and vocal processes of one arytenoid cartilage, excise them with scissors or a scalpel. Also excise the vocal fold on that side (if necessary, excise the vocal fold and process on the opposite side). Excise redundant mucosa and suture the defect with 4-0 to 6-0 absorbable suture material in a continuous pattern. Suture the thyroid cartilage with interrupted sutures that do not penetrate the laryngeal lumen. Close subcutaneous tissues and skin routinely.***

VII. Postoperative Care and Assessment

A. Monitor closely for signs of respiratory distress caused by airway obstruction.

B. Provide analgesics as necessary (see Appendix F).

C. Observe for gagging, coughing, swallowing discomfort, and impaired glottic function in the early postoperative period.

D. Maintain intravenous fluids until the animal is drinking.

E. Offer soft food in 18 to 24 hours, but observe the animal for aspiration pneumonia.

F. Restrict exercise for 6 to 8 weeks.

G. Minimize barking for 6 to 8 weeks. The bark is expected to be quiet and hoarse.

VIII. Complications

A. Arytenoid Lateralization

1. Although bilateral arytenoid lateralization enlarges the glottis more than unilateral lateralization, it is not routinely recommended because postoperative coughing, pneumonia, and death are more frequent.

2. Severe mucosal inflammation and swelling are rare following lateralization; therefore acute respiratory distress is unlikely.
3. Mineralization of cartilages.
   a. Cartilages of congenitally affected dogs may be insufficiently mineralized to retain sutures.
   b. Mineralized cartilages of older dogs may fracture or avulse the muscular process, which results in failure of abduction and recurrence of clinical signs.
   c. If these events occur the procedure may be repeated on the opposite side of the larynx.
4. Early complications of suture lateralization (these complications usually resolve within a few days, unless aspiration occurs).
   a. Hematoma formation.
   b. Suture avulsion.
   c. Swallowing discomfort.
   d. Temporary glottic impairment.
   e. Coughing after eating and drinking (may indicate mucosal irritation or aspiration).

B. Partial Laryngectomy

1. Aspiration pneumonia.
   a. Most common complication.
   b. Due to resection of too much tissue, resulting in inadequate closure of the larynx during swallowing.
2. Resection of too little tissue does not allow a functional airway.
3. Intermittent coughing.
4. Production of excessive granulation tissue or a web of scar tissue at the surgery site.

IX. Prognosis

A. Mildly affected animals do well at rest without surgery.

B. Moderate to severely affected animals may develop laryngeal collapse and acute respiratory obstruction. Prognosis after unilateral lateralization is good, with more than 90% having less respiratory distress and improved exercise tolerance.

Tracheal Collapse (*SAS*, pp. 632-637)

I. Definition

A. **Tracheal collapse** is a form of tracheal obstruction caused by cartilage flaccidity and flattening.

B. **Tracheal stenosis** is an abnormal narrowing of the tracheal lumen due to congenital malformation or trauma.

II. Synonyms

A. Tracheal collapse is sometimes erroneously referred to as congenital tracheal stenosis.

III. General Considerations and Clinically Relevant Pathophysiology

A. Etiology

1. Unknown.
2. Probably multifactorial.
3. Proposed etiologies include genetic factors, nutritional factors, allergens, neurologic deficiencies, small airway disease, and cartilage matrix degeneration.
4. Affected tracheal cartilages become hypocellular and their matrix degenerates.
   a. Normal hyaline cartilage is replaced by fibrocartilage and collagen fibers, and there are decreased amounts of glycoprotein and glycosaminoglycans.
   b. The cartilages lose their rigidity and ability to maintain normal tracheal conformation during the respiratory cycle.
5. They usually collapse in a dorsoventral direction.
6. The cervical trachea collapses during inspiration and the thoracic trachea collapses during expiration.
7. Collapse reduces the lumen size and interferes with airflow to the lungs.
8. Abnormal respiratory noises, exercise intolerance, gagging, and varying degrees of dyspnea occur with tracheal collapse.
9. Chronic inflammation of the tracheal mucosa causes coughing, which exacerbates inflammation. Persistent inflammation leads to squamous metaplasia of the respiratory epithelium and interferes with mucociliary clearance. Therefore coughing becomes an important tracheobronchial clearing mechanism.
10. Do not confuse tracheal collapse with tracheal stenosis.
    a. Tracheal stenosis.
       i. Etiology.
          (a) Trauma (e.g., penetrating or blunt wounds, foreign bodies, indwelling tubes).
          (b) Surgery.
          (c) Congenital.
              Tracheal cartilages are abnormally small, abnormally shaped, or malpositioned.
       ii. Treat traumatic stenosis by balloon dilation or resection and anastomosis.
    b. Tracheal hypoplasia.
       i. A form of congenital tracheal stenosis characterized by an abnormally narrow lumen along the entire length of the trachea, rigid tracheal cartilages that are apposed or overlap, and a dorsal tracheal membrane that is narrow or absent.
       ii. Primarily affects brachycephalic breeds, especially English bulldogs.
          (a) Observe for other congenital abnormalities (e.g., stenotic nares, elongated soft palate, aortic stenosis, pulmonic stenosis, megaesophagus).

iii. May be associated with continuous respiratory distress, coughing, and recurrent tracheitis, but may be tolerated in the absence of concurrent respiratory or cardiovascular disease.
iv. Can be identified endoscopically or radiographically.
v. Treatment of symptomatic animals.
(a) Medical therapy (i.e., antibiotics, cough suppressants) and correction of other airway obstructions (e.g., resection of nares, palate, saccules).

IV. Diagnosis

A. Clinical Presentation

1. Signalment.
   a. Occurs typically in toy- and miniature-breed dogs; most commonly toy poodles, Yorkshire terriers, Pomeranians, Maltese, and Chihuahuas.
   b. Males and females are affected equally.
   c. In larger dogs, it is usually associated with trauma, deformity, or intraluminal or extraluminal masses and should not be equated with tracheal collapse in toy-breed dogs.
   d. Classically occurs in middle-age or older toy breeds (average 6 to 8 years of age). However, tracheal collapse is frequently diagnosed in dogs with respiratory problems between 1 and 5 years of age.
2. History.
   a. The onset of clinical signs is often before 1 year of age.
   b. Clinical signs often progress with age.
   c. Clinical signs include the following.
      i. Abnormal respiratory noise.
         (a) Wheezing.
         (b) Hacking.
         (c) Coughing.
            i). May be productive or nonproductive.
            ii). Classically a "goose honk" cough. **Note: Some affected dogs do not have a goose honk.**
            iii). Often becomes cyclic and paroxysmal.
            iv). Gagging after coughing may occur in up to 50% of cases.
         (d) Stridulous breathing.
      ii. Dyspnea.
      iii. Exercise intolerance.
      iv. Cyanosis.
      v. Syncope.
   d. Some dogs do not make abnormal respiratory noises.
   e. Some dogs die of asphyxiation.
   f. Clinical signs are more severe in obese animals.
   g. Signs may be elicited or exacerbated by tracheal infections, tracheal compression, exercise, excitement, eating, drinking, hot, humid weather, and noxious stimuli (e.g., smoke and other respiratory irritants).

B. Physical Examination Findings

1. Palpation of the cervical trachea may reveal flaccid tracheal cartilages with prominent lateral borders.
2. Palpation may elicit paroxysmal coughing.
3. Auscultation may localize abnormal respiratory noises and identify mitral valve disease.

4. A soft end-expiratory snapping together of the tracheal wall may be auscultated in dogs with intrathoracic tracheal collapse.
5. Electrocardiography may reveal sinus arrhythmia or evidence of cor pulmonale or left ventricular enlargement.
6. Hepatomegaly has been associated with this syndrome in some patients and may result from venous congestion caused by cor pulmonale or fatty change.
7. Perform laryngoscopy and tracheoscopy under light anesthesia.
   a. Laryngeal paresis, paralysis, or collapse is present in approximately 30% of dogs with tracheal collapse.
   b. Approximately 50% of affected dogs show evidence of bronchial compression or collapse.
   c. Evaluate tracheal conformation as the scope is withdrawn to determine the location and severity of the collapse.
      i. The entire trachea is usually collapsed; however, one area of the trachea is often more severely affected and is used for classification purposes.
         (a) Grade I tracheal collapse.
            (i) 25% reduction in lumen diameter.
            (ii) Trachealis muscle is slightly pendulous.
            (iii) Cartilages maintain a somewhat circular shape.
         (b) Grade II collapse.
            (i) 50% reduction in lumen diameter.
            (ii) Trachealis muscle is stretched and pendulous.
            (iii) Cartilages beginning to flatten.
         (c) Grade III collapse.
            (i) 75% reduction in lumen diameter.
            (ii) Trachealis muscle stretch and pendulous.
            (iii) Cartilages nearly flattened.
         (d) Grade IV collapse.
            (i) Lumen is essentially obliterated.
            (ii) Tracheal cartilages are completely flattened and may invert to contact the trachealis muscle.
      ii. Obtain tracheal cultures and brushings during tracheoscopy to help select antibiotics.

C. Radiography/Fluoroscopy

1. Perform inspiratory and expiratory lateral radiographs of the neck and thorax.
   a. Diagnostic in approximately 60% of patients with severe (greater than 50%) tracheal collapse.
   b. Cervical trachea is expected to collapse on inspiration and the thoracic trachea is expected to collapse on expiration.
2. Perform fluoroscopy to evaluate dynamic movement of the trachea and mainstem bronchi through all phases of respiration.
3. Thoracic radiographs often reveal cardiomegaly and pulmonary disease.

D. Laboratory Findings

1. Hematology and serum biochemistry values are normal unless concurrent systemic disease is present.
2. Positive tracheobronchial cultures are found in more than 50% of animals with tracheal collapse.

V. Medical Treatment

A. Medical therapy is recommended for all animals with mild clinical signs and those with less than 50% collapse.

B. Medical therapy.
  1. Antitussives.
     a. Butorphanol tartrate (Torbutrol)–0.5 to 1.0 mg/kg PO, BID to TID.
     b. Hydrocodone bitartrate (Hycodan)–0.2 mg/kg PO, TID to QID.
  2. Antibiotics.
     a. Ampicillin–22 mg/kg IV, IM, SC, PO, TID.
     b. Cefazolin (Ancef, Kefzol)–20 mg/kg IV, IM, TID.
     c. Clindamycin (Antirobe, Cleocin)–11 mg/kg PO, IV, IM, BID.
     d. Enrofloxacin (Baytril)–5 to 10 mg/kg PO, IV, BID.
  3. Bronchodilators.
     a. Aminophylline.
        i. Dogs–11 mg/kg PO, IM, IV, TID.
        ii. Cats–5 mg/kg PO, BID.
     b. Oxytriphylline Elixir (Choledyl)–15 mg/kg PO, TID.
  4. Corticosteroids.
     a. Dexamethasone (Azium)–0.2 mg/kg IV, IM, SC, BID up to 6 mg/kg for emergency treatment.
     b. Prednisone–1 to 2 mg/kg PO, SID to BID.

C. Sedate.
  1. Acepromazine–0.05 to 0.2 mg/kg (max 1 mg) IV, IM, SC, TID.
  2. Diazepam–0.2 mg/kg IV BID.

D. Supplement oxygen in severely dyspneic patients.

E. Institute weight reduction for obese patients.

F. Restrict exercise.

G. Maintain affected dogs in an environment free of smoke and other respiratory irritants or allergens.

H. Note: Response to medical therapy is usually transient and the disease typically progresses.

VI. Surgical Treatment

A. General Considerations

1. Recommend surgery in dogs with moderate to severe clinical signs, dogs with a 50% or greater reduction of the tracheal lumen, and dogs that are refractory to medical therapy.
2. Do not delay surgery until the animal is in severe respiratory distress.
   a. Tracheal collapse is often overlooked in young dogs, which allows degenerative changes to progress, clinical signs to worsen, and secondary problems to develop.
3. Note that dogs presenting with laryngeal paralysis or collapse, generalized cardiomegaly, and chronic pulmonary disease are poor surgical candidates.
4. Caution owners that coughing and dyspnea caused by laryngeal, pulmonary, or cardiac disease are not expected to improve without appropriate therapy, and respiratory distress and death may occur in animals with severe laryngeal dysfunction or bronchopulmonary disease.
5. Concurrent mainstem bronchial collapse is present in some dogs.
   a. There is presently no technique to support collapsed mainstem bronchi.

b. Cervical tracheoplasty may not be beneficial if mainstem bronchial collapse is severe.

6. Goal of surgery is to support the tracheal cartilages and trachealis muscle, while preserving as much of the segmental blood and nerve supply to the trachea as possible.
   a. Currently, the only techniques that meet this goal are placement of individual rings or modified spiral ring prostheses.
   b. Generally only the cervical trachea and most proximal portion of the thoracic trachea are supported, even when cervical and thoracic tracheal collapse are both present.
7. Patients with concurrent laryngeal paralysis or laryngeal collapse may also require arytenoid lateralization or permanent tracheostomy, respectively.

B. Preoperative Management

1. Observe closely for signs of progressive dyspnea after hospitalization.
2. Perform surgery immediately after endoscopy to avoid a second complicated anesthetic recovery.
3. Administer prophylactic antibiotics.
   a. Cefazolin 20 mg/kg IV at induction, repeat once or twice at 4- to 6-hour intervals.
4. Administer corticosteroids to dogs with very small tracheas (i.e., less than 2 to 4 kg) to minimize tracheal mucosal swelling.

C. Anesthesia

1. Preoxygenate and induce and intubate quickly.
2. Have an assistant manipulate the endotracheal tube during placement of each ring prosthesis to ensure that sutures have not been placed into the tube.
3. Delay extubation as long as possible after surgery.
4. Supplement oxygen via nasal insufflation (see *SAS,* Table 25-11 on p. 618) if laryngeal paralysis or severe tracheal inflammation occurs.
5. See *SAS,* p. 621, for anesthesia of animals with brachycephalic syndrome.
6. See *SAS,* p. 610, for general anesthetic recommendations for animals with upper respiratory disease.

D. Surgical Anatomy

1. See Appendix G-26 for surgical anatomy of the trachea.
2. The segmental blood and nerve supply to the trachea travels in the lateral pedicles on each side of the trachea.
   a. Use minimal mobilization of the trachea to maintain a good blood supply following surgery.
   b. The left recurrent laryngeal nerve is located in the lateral pedicle; the right is sometimes located within the carotid sheath.

E. Positioning

1. Position in dorsal recumbency with the neck extended and elevated over a pad (to deviate the trachea ventrally).
2. Clip and prepare the caudal mandibular area, ventral neck, and cranial thorax for aseptic surgery.

F. Surgical Techniques

1. Make prosthetic tracheal rings or spirals by cutting 3-ml polypropylene syringe cases.
   a. To create individual rings, use a pipe cutter to divide a syringe case into cylinders 5 to 8 mm wide.
   b. Drill five or more staggered holes through each ring for suture placement.

c. Split the ring ventrally to allow placement.
d. Smooth rough edges of the rings by firing or trimming with a No. 11 blade or file.
e. Autoclave the rings before implantation.
   i. If you gas sterilize the rings, aerate them for at least 72 hours to prevent toxic tissue reactions and tracheal necrosis.

Incise skin and subcutaneous tissues along the ventral cervical midline from the larynx to manubrium. Separate the sternohyoid and sternocephalicus muscles along their midline to expose the cervical trachea. Examine the trachea for evidence of collapse and deformity. Identify and protect the recurrent laryngeal nerves. Place the first tracheal prosthesis one or two cartilages distal to the larynx. Dissect the peritracheal tissues and create a tunnel immediately around the trachea only in the areas of prosthetic ring placement. Guide and position a prosthetic ring through the tunnel and around the trachea with a long curved hemostat. Position the prosthetic ring with the split on the ventral aspect of the trachea. Chondrotomy is occasionally necessary to allow deformed, rigid cartilages to conform to the prosthesis. Secure the prosthesis with sutures ventrally, laterally, and dorsally. Place three to six sutures (3-0 or 4-0 polypropylene) to secure each prosthesis. Direct sutures around rather than through cartilages and engage the trachealis muscle in at least one suture. Place four to six additional ring prostheses 5 to 8 mm apart along the trachea. Cranial traction on the prostheses around the cervical trachea allows one or two rings to be placed at the thoracic inlet or beyond. Preserve the blood vessels and nerves between the rings. Manipulate the endotracheal tube or trachea after the placement of each prosthesis to be sure the tube cuff has not been engaged by a suture. Lavage the surgical site with sterile saline. Appose the sternohyoid and sternocephalicus muscles with simple continuous sutures (3-0 or 4-0 polydioxanone) and appose subcutaneous tissues and skin routinely.

VII. Postoperative Care and Assessment

A. Monitor these animals continuously during recovery.
1. Observe for acute respiratory distress secondary to inflammation, edema, or laryngeal paresis or paralysis.
   a. Administer oxygen via nasal insufflation and give an antiinflammatory dose of corticosteroids in animals with edema and inflammation.
2. Animals with laryngeal paralysis may require surgery to widen the glottis (*SAS,* p. 629), and those with collapse a permanent tracheostomy (*SAS,* p. 614) within the first 24 hours to relieve respiratory distress.

B. Continue antibiotics for 7 to 10 days if bacterial tracheitis is present.

C. Give antitussives, bronchodilators, analgesics, and sedatives as necessary to control coughing and excitement (see above).
1. Expect coughing and lack of improvement in clinical signs for several weeks postoperatively due to tracheitis, peritracheal swelling, and suture irritation.
2. Clinical improvement (e.g., decreased respiratory noise, less respiratory effort, increased exercise tolerance, fewer tracheobronchial infections) should be noted within 2 to 3 weeks of surgery.

D. Restrict exercise (cage rest) for 3 to 7 days, then gradually increase exercise.

E. Use a harness, rather than a collar, for leash walking.

F. Reduce weight in obese patients.

G. Perform tracheoscopy 1 to 2 months after surgery and later if respiratory signs deteriorate.

VIII. Prognosis

A. Clinical signs may be controlled medically in animals with mild clinical signs if patients do not become obese and a sedentary lifestyle is practiced.

B. The prognosis is more dependent on concurrent respiratory problems such as laryngeal paralysis or collapse and bronchial disease than on the location or severity of tracheal collapse.

C. Dogs with laryngeal and bronchial disease do not improve clinically as much as those with tracheal collapse alone.

D. Approximately 80% to 90% of dogs with tracheal collapse improve clinically after tracheoplasty.

Nasal Tumors (*SAS*, pp. 637-644)

I. Definitions

A. **Nasal tumors** arise from the nasal cavity or paranasal sinuses.

B. **Rhinotomy** is an incision into the nasal cavity.

II. Synonyms

A. Sinonasal Tumors

III. General Considerations and Clinically Relevant Pathophysiology

A. Neoplasms of the nasal cavity and paranasal sinuses are rare in most domestic species.
  1. Reported prevalence varies from 0.3% to 2.4% of canine tumors.
  2. They occur more commonly in dogs than cats.

B. May be classified histologically as epithelial, nonepithelial, or miscellaneous.
  1. Epithelial tumors are most common overall.
     a. Dogs–adenocarcinomas are most common.

b. Cats–epithelial tumors and lymphoreticular tumors are most prevalent.
2. Nonepithelial tumors of skeletal origin (e.g., chondrosarcoma and osteosarcoma) account for approximately one fifth of canine nasal tumors.

C. Metastasis.
1. Low.
2. Generally occurs late in the natural course of these tumors.
3. One survey showed metastasis in 49 of 120 dogs with sinonasal tumors that underwent necropsy.
4. Most common sites (decreasing order of frequency).
   a. Brain.
   b. Lymph nodes.
   c. Lungs.
   d. Liver.

IV. Diagnosis

A. Clinical Presentation

1. Signalment.
   a. Male dogs and cats have a higher incidence of sinonasal neoplasms than females, irrespective of histologic diagnosis.
   b. Usually occur in older animals.
      i. Median reported age of approximately 10 years in dogs and cats.
      ii. Mean age varies according to histologic diagnosis.
         (a) Chondrosarcomas often occur in younger dogs (7 years of age or less).
      iii. Soft tissue tumors involving the nasal cavity have even been reported in 1-year-old dogs.
2. History.
   a. Most affected dogs present for evaluation of nasal discharge, often with epistaxis.
   b. Tumors may cause paroxysmal sneezing (which is violent enough to produce epistaxis).
   c. Most cats are evaluated for sneezing and nasal discharge and occasionally epistaxis.
   d. Duration of clinical signs varies, but most animals have them for greater than 1 month and many for greater than 6 months before definitive diagnosis.
   e. Initial clinical signs are often intermittent, gradually becoming persistent as the tumor progresses.
   f. Infections associated with nasal tumors often respond transiently to antibiotics and other drugs, delaying definitive diagnosis.

B. Physical Examination Findings

1. Epistaxis.
2. Swelling of the facial region (including exophthalmos).
3. Nasal discharge.
4. Sneezing or snuffling.
5. Dyspnea.
6. Ocular discharge.
7. Bleeding from the oral cavity.
8. Neurologic signs include seizures, behavior changes, obtundation, paresis, ataxia, circling, visual deficits, and proprioceptive deficits.

C. Radiography

1. Evaluate thoracic radiographs for metastasis.
2. Anesthetize animals for optimal skull radiographs.
3. Perform nasal radiographs before rhinoscopy, nasal flushes, or surgical biopsies.
   a. Take lateral, dorsoventral, open-mouth ventrodorsal, and frontal sinus views.
   b. Oblique views may be necessary occasionally to outline lesions that are masked by, or superimposed over, bony structures.
   c. The open-mouth ventrodorsal view consistently provides the most information.
   d. Evaluate radiographs for increased soft tissue density of the nasal cavity or frontal sinuses, bony lysis, destruction of the normal turbinate pattern, new bone formation, and foreign bodies.
4. Radiographic signs of neoplasia.
   a. Bone destruction.
      i. May also occur with severe bacterial infection or fungal infection.
      ii. Cribriform plate destruction may indicate extension into the brain and a poor prognosis.
   b. Increased soft tissue density.
      i. May occur in both neoplastic and inflammatory diseases.
      ii. Extension into the frontal sinus or the contralateral nasal cavity and destruction of the hard palate indicate an aggressive process.
      iii. Do not interpret increased soft tissue density in the frontal sinus, without bony erosion, as neoplastic extension into the frontal sinus since obstruction of outflow secondary to a nasal tumor often results in fluid accumulation there.
5. Plain and contrast-enhanced x-ray computed tomography (CT) or magnetic resonance imaging.
   a. Helps define the extent of disease in animals with nasal tumors.
   b. Useful in patients with minimal neurologic signs, but with evidence of destruction of the rostral portion of the calvarium.

D. Laboratory Findings

1. Laboratory abnormalities are uncommon.
2. Severe epistaxis may rarely cause anemia.
3. White cell counts are seldom increased, even when a secondary bacterial infection exists.
4. Assess the coagulation system (e.g., platelet numbers, bleeding from venipuncture sites, presence of ecchymoses, petechiation, melena, hematuria, or retinal hemorrhages).
5. Evaluate cats for feline leukemia virus (FeLV) and feline immunodeficiency virus (FIV) infections.

V. Differential Diagnosis

A. Bacterial and fungal infections.

B. Foreign bodies.

C. Bleeding diatheses associated with ehrlichiosis, immune-mediated thrombocytopenia, multiple myeloma, systemic hypertension, polycythemia vera, or hyperviscosity syndrome.

VI. Medical Management

A. Radiation Therapy

1. Appears to be the most effective treatment for nasal tumors.
2. Optimum dosage and method of delivery have not been determined.
3. Radiotherapy of nasal tumors in cats is as effective as, or more effective than, in dogs.
4. Whether radiation therapy should be combined with surgical debulking is controversial.
   a. One reason for doing so is to improve the clinical status of the dog before the radiation therapy.
   b. Prior surgery may reduce dyspnea caused by nasal cavity obstruction, nasal discharge, and epistaxis during radiation therapy.

B. Chemotherapy

C. Immunotherapy

VII. Surgical Treatment

A. Surgery, as the sole treatment of dogs with nasal tumors, has not prolonged survival time.

B. The poor response of dogs with nasal tumors to surgery is due to the following.
   1. The advanced nature of most tumors at the time of diagnosis.
   2. A propensity for these tumors to invade bones that are inaccessible or that cannot be surgically removed.
   3. Lack of appreciable encapsulation.

C. Surgery may palliate clinical signs in some dogs by alleviating obstruction and epistaxis.

D. Permanent tracheostomy may benefit some dogs that have severe respiratory difficulties and in whom other treatment options are not feasible.

E. **Have blood available for transfusion because excessive bleeding may occur.**

F. Preoperative management.
   1. Administer blood if the PCV is less than 20% (see Appendix A).
   2. Preoxygenate.
   3. Administer perioperative antibiotics at anesthetic induction and continue for 12 hours after surgery (optional–may inhibit bacterial growth from tissue obtained at surgery).

G. Anesthesia.
   1. See Appendix G-26 for selected anesthetic protocols for animals undergoing nasal surgery.
   2. Perform biopsy and rhinotomy under general anesthesia.
   3. Use a cuffed endotracheal tube to prevent aspiration of blood or fluids into the airway.
   4. Have blood, hypertonic saline, or both available in the event severe hemorrhage occurs.

5. Place two cephalic catheters to allow simultaneous administration of blood and inotropes, if necessary.
6. Evaluate arterial blood pressure during surgery and avoid acepromazine.
7. Extubate the animal with the cuff slightly inflated to help remove partially aspirated blood and mucus.

H. Surgical anatomy.

1. The nasal cavity extends from the nostrils to the nasopharyngeal meatus and is separated into two halves by the nasal septum.
   a. The septum is mostly cartilaginous, but it also has bony and membranous portions.
2. The nasal conchae develop from the lateral and dorsal walls of the nasal cavity.
   a. The air passages between the conchae are known as meatuses.
3. The paranasal sinuses include a maxillary recess, frontal sinus, and a sphenoidal sinus.
   a. The frontal sinus occupies the supraorbital process of the frontal bone.

I. Positioning.

1. For a dorsal approach.
   a. Position the animal in sternal recumbency with a rolled towel under the neck.
   b. Clip and prepare the entire head and nasal area for aseptic surgery.
2. For a ventral approach.
   a. Position the animal in dorsal recumbency with the mouth tied open maximally.
   b. Flush the oral cavity with sterile saline and swab the palate with dilute betadine or chlorhexidine solution.

J. Surgical techniques.

1. Biopsy.
   a. Anesthetize the animal and intubate with a cuffed endotracheal tube to prevent aspiration of blood or other materials during the procedure.
   b. Visually inspect the palate and posterior nasal area using a flexible fiberoptic endoscope (flexing the scope behind the soft palate) and biopsy if a tumor is seen.
   c. Transnostril core biopsies.
      i. May be obtained using the outer protective shield of a Sovereign catheter with the end cut off at a sharp angle or an alligator forceps.

To prevent inadvertent penetration of the cribriform plate, measure the catheter or forceps with the tip placed at the medial canthus of the eye. Do not advance these instruments past this point. Attach the catheter (with the metal stylet removed) to a 12-ml syringe. Discern the location of the lesion from the radiographs and advance the catheter through the tumor several times while applying negative pressure to the syringe. Upon withdrawal of the catheter from the nare, remove the barrel of the syringe and add a small amount of air to the syringe. Use this air to propel the tissue sample forcefully from the syringe hub onto a microscopic slide or into a formalin-filled container. Repeat sampling at various angles until sufficient tissue is obtained. When biopsying masses in the caudal nasal cavity, be sure to adjust the catheter length so as to prevent perforation of the cribriform plate. When using an Alligator forceps, grasp tissue in the area of the lesion and pull it out through the nostril. This latter technique has been the most successful for the author.

d. Nasal flushes.
   i. Use the same catheter as described for transnostril core biopsies.
   ii. Hemorrhage may occur after this procedure, but it is generally mild and transient.

To prevent inadvertent entry into the calvarium in patients with bony lysis of the cribriform plate, measure the distance from the medial canthus of the eye to the external nare and mark the catheter to correspond to this length. Place gauze sponges above the soft palate and below the external nares to collect fluid and tissues dislodged during flushing. Attach a 35-ml syringe to the catheter and flush 150 to 300 ml of saline into the nasal cavity. Evaluate the gauze sponges for the presence of tissue and debris. Examine the tissues cytologically and save samples for microbiological examination, including fungal and bacterial cultures. If sufficient quantities are obtained, place samples in formalin for histopathology.

2. Rhinotomy.
   a. Generally, diagnostic and therapeutic procedures (rhinotomy and debulking) are combined.
   b. Intraoperative cytology, frozen section examination of tissues, or both, are helpful.
   c. Although rhinotomy may not extend the life of patients with nasal tumors appreciably, it often makes them more comfortable.
   d. Carotid artery ligation may be performed before rhinotomy (see *SAS,* p. 203, for technique).
      i. Note: Temporary carotid artery ligation may not be safe in cats or anemic or hypovolemic dogs.
   e. If bleeding continues after surgery pack the nasal cavity with sterile gauze strips.
      i. Exit the end of the gauze from the nostril or a dorsal stoma and sutured to the side of the face.
      ii. Remove the packing 1 or 2 days after surgery.
   f. Use the dorsal approach for most nasal tumors; however, consider the ventral approach to explore the region caudal to the ethmoid turbinates and the ventral aspect of the turbinates.

Dorsal approach to the nasal cavity and paranasal sinuses: Make a dorsal midline skin incision from the caudal aspect of the nasal planum to the medial canthus of the orbit. Either or both sides of the nasal cavity can be entered through a single midline skin incision. To explore the frontal sinus, extend the incision caudal to a line that connects the zygomatic processes of frontal bone. Incise subcutaneous tissue and periosteum on the midline. Elevate the periosteum and reflect it laterally on either or both sides of the nasal cavity. Use a bone saw to elevate a flap of bone over the proposed site of entry into the nasal cavity. Save the bone flap (if healthy) and replace it after the nasal cavity has been explored. Alternatively, drill a hole to one side of the nasal septum with a Steinmann pin. Use rongeurs to enlarge the hole and discard the bone fragments. Extend the bone removal bilaterally, if necessary. Gently lavage the nasal passages and remove abnormal tissue. Submit tissues for histologic examination and culture. Use cautery, iced saline, or pressure to control hemorrhage. If continued hemorrhage is a problem, pack the nasal cavity with cotton gauze (see below under special instruments). If a bone flap was made, suture it in place with 3-0 or 4-0 wire (do not use wire to replace the bone flap if radiation therapy is planned) placed through predrilled holes in the bone flap and adjacent bone. Close periosteum and subcutaneous tissues with absorbable suture material in a simple continuous pattern. Close the skin routinely. If rongeurs were used, close periosteum and subcutaneous tissues,

leaving a stoma at the caudal aspect of the incision. Close skin similarly, leaving a stoma.

Ventral approach to the nasal cavity: Make a midline incision in the hard palate. Elevate the mucoperiosteum of the hard palate laterally to the alveolar ridge. Be careful to spare the palatine nerves and vessels as they emerge from the major palatine foramen. Incise the mucoperiosteum and soft palate attachments to the caudal edge of the palatine bone and extend the incision as far caudally as necessary into the soft palate (full-thickness). Retract the edges of the incision with stay sutures. Remove the palatine bone with a power-driven burr or rongeurs and discard it. Explore the nasal cavity and remove abnormal tissues. Submit tissues for histologic examination and culture. Close nasal mucosa of the soft palate with absorbable material in a simple continuous or simple interrupted pattern. Then, close submucosa-periosteum of the hard palate with absorbable suture in an interrupted pattern. Last, close oral mucosa of the hard and soft palate with monofilament nonabsorbable sutures in a simple continuous pattern.

VIII. Suture Materials/Special Instruments

A. Use vacuum suction devices and suction tips to increase visualization compromised during rhinotomy.

B. Use an oscillating saw if a bone flap is to be removed; otherwise use a Steinmann pin and rongeurs.

C. Use sterile gauze packing to pack the nose following completion of the procedure.
   1. **Note: Nu-Gauze comes in both plain and Betadine-impregnated variety. Use the plain Nu-Gauze to prevent esophageal irritation from swallowing Betadine.**

IX. Postoperative Care and Assessment

A. Suction the airway to remove blood and fluid before extubation.

B. Recover patients with their heads down to help decrease aspiration of blood.

C. Closely monitor these animals for epistaxis following surgery or biopsy.

D. Evaluate the hematocrit during and after surgery and transfuse if the PCV is less than 20% (see Appendix A).

E. Prevent these animals from banging their heads on the cage during recovery.

F. Administer analgesics if the animal appears excited or in pain during recovery (see Appendix F).

G. Give acepromazine (0.05 mg/kg IV or IM, max of 1 mg total dose) if the patient is normovolemic, not hemorrhaging, does not have a history of seizures, and has been given adequate analgesics.

H. Assess neurologic function postoperatively.

I. After dorsal rhinomoty, observe for subcutaneous air accumulation.

J. After ventral rhinotomy, feed soft food for several days after a ventral approach to the nasal passage and prevent the animal from chewing on hard objects for 3 to 4 weeks.

X. Prognosis

A. The prognosis for dogs with nasal tumors is generally poor.

B. Mean survival time is generally 3 to 5 months.

C. Improvement in this survival period has been accomplished with radiation therapy combined with surgical debulking (see above) with mean reported survival times of 8 to 25 months.

D. The prognosis for carcinomas is better than for sarcomas, and adenocarcinomas appear to have the best overall prognosis.

E. The prognosis for cats with lymphoid neoplasia of the nasal cavity appears good.

F. Note: Many dogs are euthanized because the owners perceive that their quality of life is poor. Surgery can increase patient comfort and prolong life, despite being noncurative.

G. One unusual neoplasm associated with a much better long-term prognosis than those previously mentioned is intranasal transmissible venereal tumor (TVT).

Laryngeal and Tracheal Tumors (*SAS*, pp. 644-647)

I. Definitions

A. Oncocytomas arise from epithelial cells called oncocytes that are found in small quantities in various organs (e.g., larynx, thyroid, pituitary, trachea).

II. General Considerations and Clinically Relevant Pathophysiology

A. Laryngeal tumors.
   1. Rare.
   2. Canine laryngeal tumors.
      a. Malignant.
         i. Squamous cell carcinoma.
         ii. Lymphoma.

iii. Osteosarcoma.
iv. Fibrosarcoma.
v. Rhadbdomyosarcoma.
vi. Melanoma.
vii. Mast cell tumor.
viii. Other sarcomas.
ix. Granual cell myoblastomas.
x. Adenocarcinoma.
(a) Undifferentiated carcinoma.

b. Benign.
i. Lipoma.
ii. Oncocytoma.
iii. Rhabdomyoma.

3. Feline laryngeal tumors.
   a. Lymphosarcoma.
   b. Squamous cell carcinoma.
   c. Adenocarcinomas have also been reported.
4. Rhabdomyomas and oncocytomas are laryngeal tumors that appear histologically similar with light microscopy; electron microscopy and immunocytochemistry are necessary to distinguish them.
5. Oncocytomas have been reported in young dogs and warrant special consideration because long-term survival without evidence of metastasis following surgical resection has been reported.

B. Canine tracheal tumors.

1. Malignant.
   a. Osteosarcoma.
   b. Chondrosarcoma.
   c. Lymphoma.
   d. Mast cell tumor.
   e. Adenocarcinoma.
   f. Squamous cell carcinoma.
2. Benign.
   a. Osteochrondroma.
      i. May occur in dogs less than 1 year of age.
      ii. Probably reflect a malfunction of osteogenesis.
   b. Oncocytoma.
   c. Leiomyoma.
   d. Chondroma.
   e. Polyps.

C. Feline tracheal tumors.

1. Squamous cell carcinomas.
2. Adenocarcinomas.
3. Lymphosarcomas.

D. Metastatic thyroid carcinomas, lymphomas, and pharyngeal rhabdomyosarcomas may also involve the larynx and trachea.

E. Incidence of metastasis of laryngeal and tracheal tumors in dogs and cats is unknown.

F. *Filaroides osleri (Oslerus osleri).*

1. A nematode.
2. Forms nodules in the canine trachea and mainstem bronchi.
3. Must be differentiated from neoplastic lesions.
4. Diagnosis.
   a. Definitive diagnosis is difficult because larvae are intermittently shed in the feces.

   b. Diagnosis is best made by finding larvae or adult worms in bronchoscopically obtained biopsy specimens or by identification of the larvae in feces.
5. Anthelmintic therapy and surgical resection have met with varying success.

G. Laryngeal and tracheal tumors cause luminal obstruction by occupying space or compressing the lumen externally.

III. Diagnosis

A. Clinical Presentation

1. Signalment.
   a. Laryngeal and tracheal tumors occur most commonly in middle-age to older animals (i.e., 5 to 15 years).
   b. Tumors arising in older animals are more likely to be malignant.
   c. Benign tracheal osteocartilaginous tumors (osteochondromas) are most common in animals with active osteochondral ossification.
2. History.
   a. Affected animals may have an acute or a progressive history of upper airway obstruction.
   b. Signs may include stridor, dyspnea, cough, decreased exercise tolerance, voice change, hyperthermia, ptyalism, gagging, dysphagia, cyanosis, and syncope.
   c. Development of a mass in the ventral neck may be reported.

B. Physical Examination Findings

1. Usually normal unless there are concurrent diseases or abnormalities.
2. Occasionally, extraluminal masses may be palpated along the ventral neck and tracheal palpation may elicit coughing or increased dyspnea.
3. A voice change may be noted in animals with laryngeal masses.
4. Visual examination with a laryngoscope or endoscope allows identification and biopsy of the mass.
   a. Most laryngeal and tracheal tumors are inflamed or edematous, pink, fleshy masses protruding into the lumen; however, some laryngeal tumors appear as a diffuse thickening.
   b. Note size, consistency, and nature of attachment of the tumor to the tracheal wall.
5. Definitive diagnosis requires histologic or cytologic evaluation of a biopsy specimen.
   a. Perform biopsy using biopsy forceps or needle biopsy instruments.
   b. Biopsy of tracheal tumors is more difficult than laryngeal tumors but can usually be performed using a bronchoscope.
   c. Aspirate or biopsy enlarged, accessible lymph nodes to help stage the disease.

C. Radiography

1. Evaluate cranium and cervical radiographs to determine the location and extent of the tumor.
   a. Laryngeal and tracheal masses may appear as soft tissue densities within the airway.
   b. Laryngeal distortion and decreased laryngeal space may also be seen.
   c. Extraluminal masses may compress the tracheal lumen.
2. Evaluate thoracic radiographs for metastasis and bronchopneumonia.
3. If necessary, perform contrast esophograms or esophagoscopy to rule out esophageal involvement.

4. Laboratory findings.
   a. Perform a complete blood count, serum biochemistry profile, and urinalysis to evaluate the patient's overall status and evidence of paraneoplastic syndromes.
   b. If lymphoma is suspected, perform a bone marrow aspiration and an FeLV test (in cats).

IV. Medical Management

A. Radiation therapy may help treat squamous cell carcinomas, mast cell tumors, and lymphomas, but little information is available.

B. Some tumors (lymphomas, mast cell tumors, adenocarcinomas) respond to chemotherapy.

C. Permanent tracheostomy can palliate signs of respiratory distress during medical therapy.

V. Surgical Treatment

A. Surgical excision may be curative if the tumor is benign, localized, and small.

B. Complete excision of malignant tumors is rarely possible, but excision may provide palliation by alleviating dyspnea.

C. Laryngeal tumors may be resected via partial or total laryngectomy.

D. For removal of tracheal tumors, a tracheal resection and end-to-end anastomosis are required.
   1. Twenty percent to sixty percent (i.e., usually six to eight rings) of the trachea may be resected depending on the elasticity of the trachea.
   2. Resection of large tumors with a minimum of 1 cm of normal adjacent trachea is not always possible.
   3. Resection of a segment of the tracheal wall without complete transection (i.e., wedge resection) and reapposition of the cut edges is not recommended because it narrows, or kinks, the trachea, which interferes with airflow and mucociliary transport.

E. Preoperative management.
   1. Keep the animal calm to prevent progressive dyspnea; sedation may be necessary in some animals.
   2. Administer an antiinflammatory dose of corticosteroids if dyspnea is severe (see above).
   3. Preoxygenate before surgery if the animal is dyspneic.
   4. Place an emergency tracheostomy in severely dyspneic animals.

F. Anesthesia.
   1. Animals with laryngeal masses may require intubation via a pharyngostomy or tracheotomy incision.
   2. Intubation and ventilation of patients with intraluminal tracheal masses may require insertion of a small-diameter tube or tracheostomy distal to the obstruction.
   3. See Appendix G-26 for specific anesthetic recommendations for animals with respiratory disease.

G. Surgical anatomy.
   1. See *SAS*, page 611.

H. Positioning.
   1. Laryngotomy or cervical tracheal resection.
      a. Position the animal in dorsal recumbency with the neck deviated ventrally with a dorsally placed pad or roll.
      b. Clip and prepare the entire caudal mandibular area, ventral neck, and cranial thorax for aseptic surgery.
   2. Partial laryngectomy.
      a. Position the animal in ventral recumbency with the head suspended and the mouth opened widely, or in dorsal recumbency.
   3. Total laryngectomy.
      a. Position in ventral recumbency for oropharyngeal mucosal incision and then repositioned in dorsal recumbency to allow removal of the larynx and permanent tracheostomy.

I. Surgical techniques.
   1. Partial laryngectomy.
      a. Partial laryngectomy is performed using either an oral or a laryngotomy approach.
      b. Mucosal closure after tumor resection helps prevent scar tissue formation and is more readily achieved when a laryngotomy approach is used.

Remove the mass with a margin of normal tissue by sharp dissection. If possible, preserve the lateral margin of the corniculate process to allow appropriate epiglottic protection of the glottis. Avoid bilateral disruption of the dorsal and ventral laryngeal commissures to reduce the risk of postoperative glottic stenosis.

   2. Complete or total laryngectomy.
      a. Total laryngectomy requires the creation of a permanent tracheostomy.
      b. It is a difficult procedure that has infrequently been performed.

Expose the larynx by a ventral midline cervical incision. Transect the right and left sternohyoideus muscles from their insertion on the basihyoid bone. Disarticulate the hyoid apparatus between the keratohyoid and basihyoid articulations with the thyrohyoid bones. Dissect dorsolaterally and excise the thyropharyngeus and cricopharyngeus muscles bilaterally from their insertion on the thyroid cartilage. Incise the pharyngeal mucosa at the base of the epiglottis preserving as much mucosa as possible while still having tumor-free margins. Free the larynx by transecting between the cricoid and first tracheal cartilage or between the first and second tracheal cartilages. Remove additional tissue as necessary to achieve an en bloc resection. Lavage the surgical field. Begin reconstruction by closing the pharyngeal submucosa with a continuous suture pattern (3-0 polydioxanone). This suture line will be under tension. Attach the sternohyoid muscles to the basihyoid bone dorsal to the trachea. Place a Penrose drain if dead space is not completely eliminated. Alternatively, incise and appose the pharyngeal mucosa through an oral approach.

The technique for permanent tracheostomy must be varied when a complete laryngectomy is performed. This procedure is rarely performed and may be challenging. Either close the end of the proximal trachea with a series of interrupted horizontal sutures and then perform a permanent tracheostomy as described in SAS, p. 614, or divert and incorporate the transected proximal trachea to create the tracheostoma. To close the end of the proximal trachea place a series of interrupted horizontal mattress sutures from the annular ligament or tracheal cartilage through the dorsal tracheal membrane.

Alternatively, preserve a flap of dorsal tracheal membrane during resection, fold it over the end of the trachea, and secure it with interrupted sutures. To incorporate the proximal trachea in the tracheostoma, create the tracheostoma by first apposing the sternohyoid muscles dorsal to the trachea. Remove the ventral third of four to six tracheal cartilages, taking care to preserve the underlying tracheal mucosa. Elevate the dorsal tracheal membrane, apposing and suturing it directly to the skin proximally (4-0 polypropylene). Excise excess skin surrounding the stoma and place intradermal sutures from the skin to peritracheal tissues to create adhesions and prevent skin flaps. Incise mucosa and suture it laterally and distally to the skin using a simple continuous suture pattern.

VI. Suture Materials/Special Instruments

A. Use a laryngoscope, bronchoscope, alligator biopsy instrument, needle biopsy instruments, and endoscopic biopsy forceps for laryngeal and tracheal biopsy.

B. See *SAS*, p. 618, for instruments and suture material for laryngeal and tracheal surgery.

VII. Postoperative Care and Assessment

A. Monitor carefully for signs of airway obstruction.

B. Supplement oxygen.

C. Provide corticosteroids, if needed.

D. Offer water 6 to 12 hours and food 18 to 24 hours postoperatively if gagging, regurgitation, and vomiting do not occur.

E. Keep the animal quiet and restrict exercise for 2 to 4 weeks.

F. Perform endoscopic reevaluation at 4 to 8 weeks to identify areas of tumor recurrence or stenosis.
1. Stenosis of greater than 20% leads to mucostasis and infection.
2. Stenosis of 50% causes respiratory distress.

G. Periodically perform physical and radiographic evaluation to look for metastasis or recurrence.

VIII. Complications

A. Dysphagia, gagging, and pharyngeal dehiscence may occur after complete laryngectomy.

B. Some patients benefit from a gastric feeding tube.

C. Vocalization is absent after laryngectomy.

D. Tracheostomas must be monitored closely to maintain patency and prevent self-trauma.

E. Other complications of laryngectomy include fistula secondary to pharyngeal dehiscence, hypoparathyroidism secondary to ischemia, and tumor recurrence or metastasis.

F. **Note: Monitor these animals carefully after surgery. Airway obstruction may occur.**

G. Dehiscence may occur following tracheal anastomosis if tension is excessive and head and neck motion are not restricted.
   1. To relieve tension, the neck should be kept mildly to moderately ventroflexed by attaching a muzzle to a harness with a lead or placing a suture from the chin to the manubrium for 2 weeks.

H. Subcutaneous emphysema may be evident with dehiscence or anastomotic leakage.

I. Infection and fistula formation are possible.

J. Mild stenosis (less than 10%) is expected with the split cartilage technique where there is minimal anastomotic tension.

IX. Prognosis

A. Although prognosis is undoubtedly related to histologic type, with some tracheal tumors the prognosis is excellent (e.g., oncocytomas, osteochondromas).

B. Little information is available on the biologic behavior of laryngeal tumors; however, the long-term prognosis is generally poor.
   1. Without surgery, complete obstruction of the tracheal or laryngeal lumen and subsequent asphyxiation may occur.
   2. Radiation therapy may be a valuable adjuvant following surgery for patients with malignant tumors.

26

Surgery of the Lower Respiratory System: Lungs and Thoracic Wall (*SAS*, pp. 649-673)

General Principles and Techniques (*SAS*, pp. 649-658)

I. Definitions

A. **Thoracotomy** is a surgical incision of the chest wall.
   1. **Intercostal or lateral thoracotomy:** performed by incising between the ribs (intercostal or lateral).
   2. **Median sternotomy:** a thoracotomy performed by incising the sternum.

B. **Pulmonary lobectomy** is the removal of a lung lobe (complete) or a portion of a lung lobe (partial).

C. **Pneumonectomy** is removal of all lung tissue on one side of the thoracic cavity.

II. Preoperative Concerns

A. Emergency Stabilization

1. Emergency stabilization is often necessary before surgery. Procedures that clinicians should be familiar with include thoracentesis, chest tube placement, and nasal oxygen insufflation.
2. If the animal has a large neoplastic lesion, place it in sternal recumbency, or in lateral recumbency with the affected side down, and provide oxygen.

B. Laboratory Analysis

1. Perform a blood gas analysis or evaluate with pulse oximetry preoperatively to detect and define the severity of respiratory impairment.
2. Correct anemia before surgery, if possible.

III. Anesthetic Considerations

A. General Considerations

1. Identify ventilation abnormalities before anesthetic induction.
   a. Pulmonary neoplasia or other space-occupying lesions may prevent normal lung expansion and produce hypoxemia.
   b. With pneumonia or emphysematous lesions, ventilation/perfusion disturbances are common.
2. Administer oxygen by face mask or nasal insufflation before induction to ensure that hemoglobin is optimally saturated and that hypoxemia does not occur during intubation.
3. Avoid sedation with acetylpromazine in severely affected patients because it may cause hypotension.
4. Consider anticholinergics in animals with bradycardia (i.e., heart rate less than 60 bpm).
5. Avoid nitrous oxide in patients with respiratory compromise.
6. Administer opioids only when oxygen can be provided because they may cause severe respiratory depression.
7. Accomplish endotracheal intubation rapidly in animals with respiratory dysfunction and maintain anesthesia with an inhalation anesthetic (e.g., isoflurane or halothane; see Appendix G-26). Do not use mask or chamber induction.
8. Auscultate both sides of the thorax to ensure that a bronchus was not intubated. In compromised animals, intubation of a bronchus rather than the trachea may be disastrous.
9. Use opioids to supplement anesthesia in animals in which you are having difficulty maintaining an adequate depth of anesthesia with inhalation anesthetics alone.
10. Provide intermittent positive pressure ventilation to animals with open chest cavities (including those with diaphragmatic hernias).
    a. Avoid high ventilatory pressures in patients with chronically collapsed lung lobes, pneumonia, or pulmonary bullae.

B. Analgesia

1. Rationale.
   a. Thoracotomy procedures often produce substantial pain.
   b. Analgesics decrease postoperative pain and promote improved ventilation in the postoperative period.
2. Methods.
   a. Systemic analgesics.
      i. Although opioids are respiratory depressants, their analgesic effects often outweigh their negative respiratory effects. If hypoventilation occurs after administration of these drugs, provide oxygen by nasal insufflation.
      ii. Drugs and dosages.
         (a) Oxymorphone–0.05 to 0.1 mg/kg IV, IM every 4 hours (as needed).
         (b) Butorphanol–0.2 to 0.4 mg/kg IV, IM, or SC every 2 to 4 hours (as needed).
         (c) Buprenorphine–5 to 15 μg/kg IV, IM every 6 hours (as needed).
   b. Local anesthesia for dogs.
      i. Interpleural bupivacaine.
         (a) Place 2 mg/kg in the thoracic cavity after closure.
         (b) Position the patient with the affected side down for 20 minutes.
      ii. Intercostal nerve block.

(a) Inject 2 mg/kg bupivacaine dorsally and ventrally in the incised intercostal space and two intercostal spaces cranial and caudal to the incised space.

iii. Combination intercostal and interpleural blocks.

(a) Give 1 mg/kg bupivacaine interpleurally and 1 mg/kg intercostally.

C. Reexpansion Pulmonary Edema (RPE)

1. Clinical considerations.
   a. RPE may develop in some animals with chronically collapsed lung lobes. It does not appear to be associated with cardiac failure.
   b. Within a few hours of surgery, the patient typically develops progressively worsening dyspnea and tachypnea. Hypoxemia develops and persists despite intense oxygen therapy.
   c. The condition is rapidly fatal in most animals.
2. Pathogenesis.
   a. Reoxygenation of chronically collapsed lungs may release superoxide radicals, which result in increased pulmonary capillary permeability and pulmonary edema.
   b. Chronically collapsed lung tissue may have decreased mitochondrial superoxide dismutase and cytochrome oxidase activity.
3. Prevention.
   a. Prophylaxis and therapy of patients with RPE are difficult and poorly understood.
   b. Reexpand chronically collapsed lung tissue slowly.
      i. Close the thorax with one or two lung lobes collapsed, allowing them to reexpand slowly.
      ii. Avoid high ventilation pressures (i.e., greater than 25 cm H_2O pressure).
4. Treatment.
   a. Positive end-expiratory pressure ventilation.
   b. Drugs that stabilize pulmonary capillary membranes (e.g., methylprednisolone).

IV. Antibiotics

A. Animals with underlying pulmonary disease or trauma (e.g., pulmonary contusions) are at increased risk to develop pulmonary infections.

B. Monitor patients carefully and initiate antibiotics at the earliest sign of infection (i.e., leukocytosis or fever).

C. Young, healthy animals undergoing thoracotomy for relatively short procedures (e.g., ligation of a patent ductus arteriosus) generally do not require prophylactic antibiotics.

D. Use prophylactic antibiotics in debilitated animals undergoing thoracotomy for removal of large neoplastic lesions (which may contain focal areas of necrosis).

V. Surgical Anatomy

A. Sternum

1. Composed of eight unpaired bones and forms the floor of the thorax.
   a. Manubrium: the first sternebrae.
   b. Xiphoid: the last sternebrae.

B. Ribs

1. There are usually 13 pairs of ribs.
2. The 10th, 11th, and 12th ribs do not articulate with the sternum, but instead form the costal arch bilaterally.
3. The cartilaginous portion of the 13th rib terminates free in the musculature.
4. The space between the ribs is known as the intercostal space and is generally 2 to 3 times as wide as the adjacent ribs.
5. The intercostal arteries lie caudal to the adjacent rib, in conjunction with a satellite vein and nerve.
6. A typical intercostal nerve begins where the dorsal branch of the thoracic nerve divides and runs distally among the fibers of the internal intercostal muscle.

C. Muscles of the Thoracic Wall

1. The deepest muscles of the thoracic wall are the intercostal muscles.
   a. External intercostal muscle.
      i. Arises on the caudal border of each rib and run caudoventrally to the cranial border of the next rib.
      ii. Important primarily in inspiration.
   b. Internal intercostal muscles.
      i. Run from the cranial border of one rib to the caudal border of the preceding rib.
      ii. Primarily functioning to aid expiration.
   c. Other inspiratory muscles are the scalenus, serratus dorsalis cranialis, levatores costarum, and diaphragm.
   d. Additional expiratory muscles include the rectus abdominis, external abdominal oblique, internal abdominal oblique, transversus abdominis, serratus dorsalis caudalis, transversus costarum, and iliocostalis.

D. Lungs

1. Have deep fissures that create distinct lobes, which allows the lungs to alter their shape in response to alterations in thoracic cavity shape.
2. Fissures allow individual lobes to be isolated and removed without compromising integrity of the surrounding lobes.
3. Left lungs.
   a. Cranial lobe with a cranial and caudal part.
   b. Caudal lobe.
4. Right lungs.
   a. Cranial, middle, caudal, and accessory lobes.
   b. Larger than the left.
5. Cardiac notch.
   a. A small area overlying the heart where lung tissue is not interposed between the heart and body wall.
   b. Usually located at the ventral aspect of the fourth intercostal space.
   c. Larger on the right side.

E. Vessels

1. Pulmonary arteries.
   a. Function.
      i. Carry nonaerated blood from the right ventricle of the heart to the lungs.
   b. Location.
      i. The left pulmonary artery lies cranial to the left bronchus.
      ii. On the right side, the pulmonary artery lies dorsal and slightly caudal to the right bronchus.
2. Pulmonary veins.
   a. Function.
      i. Return aerated blood from the lungs to the left atrium.

b. Location.
   i. The left pulmonary veins are ventral to the bronchus.
   ii. On the right side, the pulmonary veins lie craniodorsal and ventral to the bronchus.

VI. Surgical Techniques

A. Thoracotomy (*SAS,* pp. 651-655)

1. Determine approach (intercostal or median sternotomy) based on exposure needed and underlying disease process.
   a. A left lateral thoracotomy at the fourth, fifth, or sixth intercostal space will provide adequate exposure for lobectomy (Table 26-1).
      i. A left fourth intercostal space thoracotomy allows exposure of the right ventricular outflow tract, main pulmonary artery, and ductus arteriosus.
      ii. Bilateral removal of the pericardial sac can be difficult from this approach.
   b. A right intercostal thoracotomy provides exposure of the right side of the heart (auricle, atrium, and ventricle), cranial and caudal venae cavae, right lung lobes, and azygous vein.
   c. The ribs cranial to an intercostal incision are more easily retracted than the caudal ribs, so choose the more caudal space if you must choose between two adjacent intercostal spaces.
   d. Median sternotomy affords exposure to both sides of the thoracic cavity.
      i. Bilateral, partial lobectomy is easily performed from a median sternotomy; however, complete lobectomy is often difficult.
      ii. The caudal vena cava, main pulmonary artery, and both sides

Table 26-1
Recommended intercostal spaces for thoracotomy

	Left	Right
Heart	4,5	4,5
PDA	4(5)*	
PRAA	4	
Pulmonic valve	4	
Lungs	4-6	4-6
Cranial lobe	4,5	4,5
Intermediate lobe		5
Caudal lobe	5(6)	5(6)
Esophagus		
Cranial	3,4	
Caudal	7-9	7-9
Cranial vena cava	(4)	4
Caudal vena cava	(6-7)	6-7

Modified from Orton EC: Thoracic wall. In Slatter D, ed: *Textbook of small animal surgery,* ed 2. Philadelphia, 1993, WB Saunders.
*Parentheses indicate alternative surgical site; PDA, patent ductus arteriosus; PRAA, persistent right aortic arch.

of the pericardial sac can be isolated and manipulated via this approach.

iii. Leave two to three sternebrae intact cranially or caudally (depending on where the lesion is located) to decrease postoperative pain and prevent delayed healing caused by sternebral shifting.

(a) To expose the lungs or heart, extend the sternotomy from the xiphoid cartilage cranially to the second or third sternebra.

(b) To expose the cranial mediastinum, extend the sternotomy from the manubrium caudally to the sixth or seventh sternebra.

2. Prepare a large area for aseptic surgery to allow extension of the incision, if needed.
3. Count your sponges at the start of the surgical procedure and before closure of the thoracic cavity: do not leave a sponge in the thoracic cavity.
4. Intercostal thoracotomy.

With the dog in lateral recumbency, select the site for incision (see Table 26-1). Locate the approximate intercostal space and sharply incise the skin, subcutaneous tissues, and cutaneous trunci muscle. The incision should extend from just below the vertebral bodies to near the sternum. Deepen the incision through the latissimus dorsi muscle with scissors, then palpate the first rib by placing a hand cranially under the latissimus dorsi muscle. Count back from the first rib to verify the correct intercostal space. Transect the scalenus and pectoral muscles with scissors perpendicular to their fibers, then separate the muscle fibers of the serratus ventralis muscle at the selected intercostal space. Near the costochondral junction, place one scissor blade under the external intercostal muscle fibers and push the scissors dorsally in the center of the intercostal space to incise the muscle. Incise the internal intercostal muscle similarly. Notify the anesthetist that you are about to enter the thoracic cavity, and, after identifying the lungs and pleura, use closed scissors or a blunt object to penetrate the pleura. This allows air to enter the thorax, causing the lungs to collapse away from the body wall. Extend the incision dorsally and ventrally in order to achieve the desired exposure. Identify and avoid incising the internal thoracic vessels as they course subpleurally near the sternum. Moisten laparotomy sponges and place them on the exposed edges of the chest incision. Use a Finochietto retractor to spread the ribs. If further exposure is needed, a rib adjacent to the incision can be removed; however, this is seldom required. If a chest tube is to be placed, do so before closing the thorax. The tube should not exit from the incised intercostal space. Close the thoracotomy by preplacing four to eight sutures of heavy (3-0 to No. 2, depending on the animal's size) monofilament absorbable or nonabsorbable suture around the ribs adjacent to the incision. Approximate the ribs with a towel clamp or rib approximator, or have an assistant cross two sutures to appose the ribs, then tie the remaining sutures. Tie all the sutures before you remove the rib approximator or towel clamp. Suture serratus ventralis, scalenus, and pectoralis muscles with a continuous suture of absorbable suture material. Appose the edges of the latissimus dorsi muscle similarly. Remove residual air from the thoracic cavity using the preplaced chest tube or an over-the-needle catheter. Close subcutaneous tissues and skin in a routine fashion.

5. Median sternotomy.

With the dog in dorsal recumbency, incise skin on the midline over the sternum. Expose the sternum by a combination of sharp incision and blunt dissection of the overlying musculature. Transect the sternebrae longitudinally on the midline with a bone saw, chisel and osteotome, or bone cutters. In young

animals, heavy scissors may be adequate; however, avoid crushing the bone. Splitting the sternebrae on the midline will facilitate closure. Ensure that the underlying lung and heart are not damaged while completing the sternotomy. Place moistened laparotomy sponges on the incised edges of the sternebrae and retract the edges with a Finochietto rib retractor. If a chest tube is to be placed, do so before closing the sternotomy. Do not exit the tube from between the sternebrae; exit it from between the ribs or through the diaphragm. Close the sternotomy with wires (dogs larger than approximately 15 kg) or heavy suture (cats and dogs smaller than approximately 15 kg) placed around the sternebrae. Suture subcutaneous tissues with a simple continuous suture of absorbable suture material. Remove residual air from the thoracic cavity and close skin routinely.

B. Partial Lobectomy (*SAS*, pp. 655, 656)

1. General considerations.
   a. May be performed to remove a focal lesion involving the peripheral one half to two thirds of the lung lobe, or for biopsy.
   b. Partial lobectomy may be performed via a lateral fourth or fifth space intercostal thoracotomy or median sternotomy.
2. Manual partial lobectomy.

Identify the lung tissue to be removed and place a pair of crushing forceps across the lobe, proximal to the lesion. Place a continuous, overlapping suture pattern of absorbable suture material (2-0 to 4-0) 4 to 6 mm proximal to the forceps. A second row of sutures may be placed in a similar manner to the first. Excise the lung between the suture lines and clamps, leaving a 2- to 3-mm margin of tissue distal to the sutures. Oversew the lung with a simple continuous suture pattern of absorbable suture. Replace the lung in the thoracic cavity and fill the chest cavity with warmed, sterile saline solution. Inflate the lungs and check the bronchus for air leaks. Remove the fluid before closing the thorax.

3. Partial lobectomy using staples.
   a. Partial lobectomy may be performed with stapling devices (e.g., thoracoabdominal [TA] stapler).
   b. The stapling equipment comes in various sizes that produce staple lines 30, 55, or 90 mm long.
   c. The stapling devices compress tissue to a thickness of either 1.5 mm (3.5-mm-long staples) or 2.0 mm (4.8-mm-long staples).
   d. Avoid stapling excessively thick or fibrotic lung because this may result in large air leaks or hemorrhage.

Select the staple size based on the width of the lung so that the staple line extends across the entire width of the lung to be removed, but does not extend beyond the edges. If air leaks or hemorrhage is noted, place a simple continuous suture pattern of absorbable suture material along the lung margin. Check the lung for leaks and close as described above.

C. Complete Lobectomy (*SAS*, pp. 655-656)

1. Best performed through a lateral thoracotomy.
2. If the lung contains large quantities of purulent material, prevent excessive fluid from draining into the proximal bronchi and trachea by clamping the bronchus near the hilus before manipulating the lobe.
3. Torsed lung lobes should be removed without untwisting the pedicle to prevent release of necrotic material trapped in the lung.

4. Dogs can survive acute loss of up to 50% of their lung volume; however, transient respiratory acidosis and exercise intolerance may occur.
5. Stapling devices may be used for complete lobectomy, but ensure that the bronchus and vessels are adequately ligated by the staples.

Identify the affected lobe(s) and isolate them from the remaining lobes with moistened sponges (laparotomy or 4 × 4s depending on the animal's size). Identify the vasculature and bronchus to the lobe. Using blunt dissection, isolate the pulmonary artery supplying the affected lobe and pass a ligature of nonabsorbable or absorbable suture material (2-0 to 3-0) around the proximal end of the vessel. Do not compromise the lumen of the parent vessel from which this vessel arises. Place a second ligature in a similar fashion distal to the site where the vessel is to be transected. A transfixing suture may be placed between these sutures, proximal to the transection site, to prevent the first suture from being inadvertently dislodged. Transect the artery between the distal two ligatures. Ligate the pulmonary vein in a similar fashion. Identify the main bronchus supplying the lobe and clamp it with a pair of Satinsky or crushing forceps proximal and distal to the selected transection site. Sever the bronchus between the clamps and remove the lung. Suture the bronchus proximal to the remaining clamp with a continuous horizontal mattress suture pattern, or in cats and small dogs place a tranfixing ligature around the bronchus. Before removing the clamp, secure a suture in the bronchus distal to the clamp, and after removing the clamp, oversew the end of the bronchus with a simple continuous suture pattern. Fill the chest cavity with warmed, sterile saline solution. Inflate the lungs and check the bronchus for air leaks. Observe lungs that have been "packed-off" to make sure they reinflate and are not twisted before closure. Remove the fluid and close the chest as described above.

VII. Healing of the Lungs and Sternum

A. Following multiple lobectomies or partial lobectomies of several lobes, expansion of the remaining lung may occur in an attempt to restore normal lung volume. Therefore exercise intolerance may decrease in some animals with time after pneumonectomy.

B. Healing of median sternotomies has been of concern; however, if several sternebrae are left intact and the closure is performed properly, these incisions heal readily and without complication, even in animals with pyothorax.

VIII. Suture Materials/Special Instruments

A. Absorbable or nonabsorbable suture material can be used for lobectomy.

B. Avoid braided, multifilament, nonabsorbable suture (e.g., silk) if infection is present.

C. Useful instruments include Finochietto rib retractors, Satinsky clamps (for clamping the bronchus), and right-angled forceps (such as Mixter forceps; also called gallbladder or gall duct forceps or thoracic forceps).

D. A bone saw is recommended for median sternotomy, particularly in medium or large dogs.

E. Vacuum suction devices facilitate removal of the fluid placed in the chest to identify air leaks.

F. Thoracoabdominal (TA) staplers are also useful for lobectomies.

IX. Postoperative Care and Assessment

A. Monitor respiration closely once the animal begins ventilating on its own.
1. If respiratory excursions are inadequate, evaluate the chest to verify that residual air was removed after chest closure. If in doubt, examine thoracic radiographs for evidence of pneumothorax.
2. Evaluate a blood gas to help determine the adequacy of ventilation.
   a. If the animal is hypoxemic, administer oxygen by nasal insufflation or place the animal in an oxygen-enriched environment.
   b. Evaluate animals with severe or progressive hypoxemia for pulmonary edema.
   c. Inadequate ventilation in some animals may be due to pain.
      i. Median sternotomy may result in decreased ventilation as compared to intercostal thoracotomy.
      ii. Administration of analgesics in such patients is needed and should be considered in all patients undergoing thoracotomy procedures (see anesthesia, p. 529).
3. Prevent hypothermia and use warm water bottles and circulating water or air blankets to rewarm these patients.

X. Special Age Considerations

A. Use extra care in anesthetizing young patients.
1. Uptake of inhalation agents in patients younger than 12 weeks of age may be more rapid than in adults, and the level of anesthesia may fluctuate more readily in these patients.
2. Young animals are particularly prone to hypothermia when the chest cavity is opened.
3. Monitor blood glucose and supplement if necessary.
4. Monitor fluid and electrolyte needs.

B. Geriatric patients with compromised pulmonary function or decreased cardiovascular capacity may also have abnormal uptake of inhalation anesthetics.

Thoracic Wall Trauma (*SAS*, pp. 658-661)

I. Definition

A. Flail chest occurs when several ribs on both sides of the point of impact are fractured such that the fractured segment moves paradoxically with respiration.

II. General Considerations and Clinically Relevant Pathophysiology

A. Thoracic wall injury may be due to either blunt (e.g., motor vehicular accidents, being kicked by a horse) or penetrating trauma.

B. The most common causes of penetrating injuries of the thorax in dogs are bite wounds and gunshot injuries.

C. Occasionally, pain associated with muscular tears may lead to altered respiration because the animal is unwilling to breathe deeply.

D. Subcutaneous emphysema.
  1. It may occur with both blunt and penetrating trauma, but is usually of little significance.
  2. The air may reach the subcutaneous tissues through a disruption of the pleura and intercostal muscles, by direct communication with an external wound, or as an extension of mediastinal emphysema.
  3. Treatment of subcutaneous air should be directed at its cause.

E. Rib fractures.
  1. Isolated rib fractures are seldom associated with major morbidity.
  2. Occasionally rib fractures produce sharp fragments that may injure a major vessel or lacerate the lung.
  3. Rib fractures may interfere with ventilation if the animal splints the thorax in an attempt to reduce pain by decreasing motion of the fragments.
  4. Flail chest occurs when several ribs on both sides of the point of impact are fractured such that the intervening rib segments lose their continuity with the remainder of the thorax.
     a. Paradoxical movement of the chest wall occur; the fractured segment moves inward during inspiration and outward during expiration.
     b. Respiratory abnormalities in patients with flail chest may be severe and include decreased vital capacity, reduced functional residual capacity, hypoxemia, decreased compliance, increased airway resistance, and increased work of breathing.

III. Diagnosis

A. Clinical Presentation

  1. Signalment.
     a. Most common in young animals prone to trauma.
  2. History.
     a. A history of trauma may or may not be present.
     b. The animal may be presented for evaluation of respiratory distress, reluctance to move because of pain, depression, lethargy, or anorexia.

B. Physical Examination Findings

  1. Examine for rib fractures or subcutaneous emphysema (see above).
  2. Observe for delayed-onset cardiac arrhythmias.
     a. There may be no external evidence of injury.
     b. May not begin until 12 to 72 hours after the trauma.
     c. May be associated with myocardial contusion, myocardial ischemia secondary to shock, or neurogenic injuries that result in sympathetic overstimulation.
  3. Examine for cardiac contusions.

C. Radiography

1. Evaluate thoracic radiographs of animals with trauma for the presence of pulmonary hemorrhage/contusions or pneumothorax.
2. Check carefully for nondisplaced or minimally displaced rib fractures.
3. Evaluate both radiographic views.
4. Examine the vertebrae, scapula, and proximal forelimb for evidence of bony trauma.

D. Laboratory Findings

1. Nonspecific.
2. Blood gas analysis may show hypoxemia and respiratory acidosis or alkalosis (resulting from hyperventilation).

IV. Differential Diagnosis

A. Neoplasia or infectious processes may cause rib fractures.
   1. Look for lysis or proliferation of the adjacent bone.

V. Medical Management

A. Usually you can stabilize these animals without surgery.

B. Antibiotic therapy is indicated in patients with marked pulmonary contusion/hemorrhage.

C. Identify and treat concurrent pneumothorax.

D. Provide supplemental oxygen if the animal is dyspneic.

E. Flail chest.
   1. Initially stabilize the rib segment by positioning the patient with the affected side down.
   2. Stabilization may prevent further damage to intrathoracic structures, improve pulmonary ventilation, and decrease pain associated with movement of fragments.

VI. Surgical Treatment

A. General Considerations

1. Rib fractures seldom require surgical treatment.
2. Multiple rib fractures may cause a defect in thoracic wall continuity (i.e., concavity) that warrants surgical repair.
3. Open stabilization of rib fractures may be indicated if there is concurrent intrathoracic trauma that requires surgery.
4. Flail chest is generally managed by placing an external splint over the thorax to stabilize the fractured segment (see below).

B. Preoperative Management

1. Stabilize animals with pulmonary contusions before repairing the rib fractures, if possible.

2. Initiate shock treatment (fluids, antibiotics, plus or minus corticosteroids) if necessary.
3. Provide nasal oxygen if the animal is dyspneic.
4. Administer antibiotics if pulmonary contusion or hemorrhage is present.
5. Place the animal with the affected side down if a flail segment is present.

C. Anesthesia

1. A splint may be applied to the flail segment of some animals using an intercostal nerve block rather than general anesthesia.
2. See anesthetic recommendations for animals with respiratory disease, Appendix G-26.
3. If general anesthesia is required, refer to Appendix G-26.

D. Positioning

1. For rib fractures and flail chest, clip and aseptically prepare the lateral thorax encompassing the fractured ribs.

E. Surgical Technique

1. Rib fractures.

Place a small intramuscular pin through the proximal fragment and into the marrow canal. Reduce the fracture and drive the pin into the distal fragment. Exit the pin through the cortex and bend the ends slightly to help prevent migration. Alternatively, use cerclage wires or cross pins.

2. Flail chest.

Secure the affected ribs to a sheet of plastic splinting material (e.g., Orthoplast) that has been molded to conform to the thoracic wall. Using a Steinmann pin, place holes in the splinting material large enough to pass the selected suture (see below) through. Place sutures circumferentially around the affected ribs. Pass the suture ends through the predrilled holes and tie securely. Alternatively, aluminum rods may be substituted for the plastic splinting material.

VII. Suture Materials/Special Instruments

A. Flail chest.

1. Use large (2-0 to No. 2, depending on the animal's size) monofilament suture with an attached large, curved needle to apply the splint.
2. A Steinmann pin and pin chuck are also needed.

B. For rib fracture repair, small IM pins and cerclage wire are needed.

VIII. Postoperative Care and Assessment

A. Monitor closely in the postoperative period for hypoventilation and pneumothorax.

B. Provide analgesics.

IX. Prognosis

A. Prognosis depends on the amount of concurrent pulmonary or cardiac trauma that is present.

B. Most rib fractures heal without surgery.

Pulmonary Neoplasia (*SAS*, pp. 661-664)

I. Definitions

A. **Primary pulmonary neoplasms** originate in pulmonary tissues and may arise as a solitary mass or rarely may be multicentric.

II. General Considerations and Clinically Relevant Pathophysiology

A. Primary pulmonary neoplasia is less common than metastatic neoplasia in dogs and cats.

B. The diaphragmatic lobes are most frequently involved, with the right lung lobes more often affected than the left.

C. Classification of primary lung tumors.
   1. Usually based on the predominant histologic pattern.
   2. Adenocarcinoma is the most common histologic type found in dogs and cats.
   3. Squamous cell carcinoma and anaplastic carcinomas are less common.
   4. Primary pulmonary tumors of connective origin (e.g., osteosarcoma, fibrosarcoma, hemangiosarcoma) are rare.
   5. Although most pulmonary tumors are malignant, benign tumors (e.g., papillary adenoma, bronchial adenoma, fibroma, myxochondroma, and plasmacytoma) have been reported.

D. Pulmonary neoplasms are highly aggressive and tend to metastasize early.
   1. Most anaplastic carcinomas and squamous cell carcinomas have metastasized at the time of diagnosis, whereas approximately one half of adenocarcinomas have done so.
   2. Metastasis is often to the lung itself, regional lymph nodes, or both.

E. Metastatic pulmonary neoplasia is an important differential diagnosis for nodular lung disease.

F. Tumors with a high likelihood of resulting in pulmonary metastasis include mammary carcinoma, thyroid carcinoma, hemangiosarcoma, osteosarcoma, transitional cell carcinoma, squamous cell carcinoma, and oral and digital melanoma.

III. Diagnosis

A. Clinical Presentation

1. Signalment.
   a. Average age of dogs and cats with primary lung tumors is 10 to 11 years and 12 years, respectively.
   b. Anaplastic carcinomas tend to occur at a slightly younger age (8 to 9 years) than adenocarcinomas.
   c. No sex or breed predilection, although boxers may be overrepresented.
2. History.
   a. Nearly 25% of dogs with pulmonary neoplasia are asymptomatic at the time of diagnosis.
   b. Clinical signs may be present for weeks to months before presentation.

B. Physical Examination Findings

1. The most common clinical finding in dogs with primary pulmonary neoplasia is a nonproductive cough.
2. Respiratory signs are present in only one third of affected cats.
3. Other signs include hemoptysis, fever, lethargy, exercise intolerance, weight loss, dysphagia, and anorexia.
4. Lameness may be associated with metastasis to bone or skeletal muscle or with development of hypertrophic osteopathy.

C. Radiography/Ultrasonography

1. Obtain thoracic radiographs in animals with suspected pulmonary neoplasia.
2. The radiographic pattern may be classified as solitary nodular, multiple nodular, or disseminated-infiltrative.
   a. The most common finding with primary pulmonary neoplasia in dogs is a solitary nodular density in the periphery of a dorsocaudal lung lobe.
   b. Multiple, miliary lesions are less common.
   c. Multiple, discrete lesions within a single lobe or multiple lobes usually represent metastatic neoplasia, rather than multicentric primary neoplasia.
3. Take radiographs of ventrodorsal and right and left lateral recumbent views.
   a. Lung lesions may go undetected in recumbent lateral radiographs when the affected lung is dependent due to increased opacity of surrounding lung tissue.
4. Nodules must be at least 1.0 cm in diameter to be reliably recognized.
5. Evaluate radiographs for sternal or hilar lymphadenopathy and pleural effusion.
6. It may be difficult to differentiate metastatic pulmonary neoplasia from pulmonary metastasis of a primary pulmonary tumor.
   a. Metastatic tumors are generally smaller, more well circumscribed, and usually located in the peripheral or middle portions of the lung.
7. Pulmonary perfusion scans.
   a. Sensitive, but relatively nonspecific, for thoracic neoplasia.
   b. May detect lesions at the diaphragmatic border of the lungs that are not readily visualized on thoracic radiographs.

D. Laboratory Findings

1. Laboratory abnormalities are nonspecific but may include nonregenerative anemia, leukocytosis, and hypercalcemia.

IV. Differential Diagnosis

A. Differentials.
   1. Abscess.
   2. Granuloma (fungal, heartworm).

B. Collect samples for cytologic examination by surgical biopsy, percutaneous fine-needle aspiration, transtracheal lavage, or bronchoscopy.

C. Fine-needle aspiration cytology may be the most helpful noninvasive diagnostic tool if the needle can be directed into the nodule.

D. Thoracotomy is often necessary for definitive diagnosis of a pulmonary mass.

V. Medical Management

A. Surgical removal of primary pulmonary neoplasia is the treatment of choice in small animal patients.

B. Chemotherapy is routinely used for some pulmonary neoplasms in human beings; however, there are few reports of its use in similarly affected veterinary patients.

C. Adjunctive chemotherapy may be particularly beneficial in patients with micrometastasis at the time of surgery.

VI. Surgical Treatment

A. Wide Surgical Excision

1. Treatment of choice for solitary nodules and multiple masses involving a single lobe without evidence of distant metastasis or extrapleural involvement.
2. Surgical resection is occasionally indicated for lung metastasis of a distant primary tumor (e.g., limb osteosarcoma).
3. An intercostal thoracotomy is preferred over median sternotomy because it provides adequate exposure for lobectomy and lymph node biopsy.
4. Complete lobectomy should be performed unless the tumor is located at the periphery of the lung lobe.

B. Preoperative Management

1. If the mass is large, position the animal with the affected side down.

C. Positioning

1. Prepare the lateral thorax for aseptic surgery.

D. Surgical Technique

Perform an intercostal thoracotomy and identify the affected lung lobe. Palpate each lung lobe for additional nodules, and biopsy the hilar lymph node for staging purposes. Perform a partial lobectomy if the tumor is located at the peripheral margin of the lobe; otherwise, perform a complete lobectomy. Submit excised tissue for cytologic and histologic examination. If the neoplasm is cavitary, or there is evidence of preexisting pyothorax, submit cultures of the mass. Place a chest tube before thoracic closure if there is evidence of infection, or if pneumothorax or hemorrhage seems likely postoperatively. Remove residual air from the pleural space after closure.

VII. Suture Materials/Special Instruments

A. Avoid nonabsorbable braided suture (e.g., silk) if there is evidence of infection.

VIII. Postoperative Care and Assessment

A. Monitor the animal for dyspnea.

B. Provide oxygen if necessary.

C. Give analgesics.

D. Evaluate ventilation by analysis of blood gas parameters or pulse oximetry.

E. Sudden respiratory distress may be associated with hemorrhage or pneumothorax.

IX. Prognosis

A. Dogs

1. Prognosis is guarded due to the advanced nature of the disease at the time of diagnosis.
2. Over 50% of dogs that have small, solitary lesions (that have not metastasized) and do not have respiratory signs will live for at least a year after surgery.
3. Those with tumors in the lung periphery or near the base of a lung have better survival times than those whose tumors involve an entire lobe.
4. Most important prognostic factor related to survival following surgery is whether or not there is lymph node metastasis.

B. Cats

1. The prognosis is poor due to the advanced nature of disease at the time of diagnosis and the tumors' aggressive metastatic behavior.
2. Most patients will eventually die or be euthanatized with recurrence of the primary tumor or metastatic disease.

Pulmonary Abscesses (*SAS*, pp. 664-665)

I. Definitions

A. An **abscess** is a localized collection of pus that often results in cavitation in the lung.

II. General Considerations and Clinically Relevant Pathophysiology

A. Pulmonary abscesses are rare.

B. May occur as a complication of foreign bodies, neoplasia, bacterial pneumonia, aspiration pneumonia, fungal infections, or parasites.

C. Abscesses secondary to neoplasia may be sterile or infected.

D. The most common organisms cultured from abscesses associated with necrotizing pneumonia in dogs are *Escherichia coli, Pseudomonas* spp., and *Klebsiella* spp.

E. Rupture of pulmonary abscesses may result in pyothorax or pneumothorax.

F. In some parts of the country, pulmonary abscesses are common secondary to inhalation or thoracic penetration of plant material (e.g., foxtails) that migrate through the lung.

III. Diagnosis

A. Clinical Presentation

1. Signalment.
   a. May occur in dogs or cats of any age, breed, or sex.
2. History.
   a. Animal may present with persistent low-grade fever, varying degrees of respiratory distress, weight loss, lethargy, and anemia.
   b. The duration of illness may vary from hours to days or even weeks.
   c. Rupture of a pulmonary abscess that causes pneumothorax may result in acute dyspnea.

B. Physical Examination Findings

1. Vary depending on whether pneumothorax or pleural effusion is present.
2. Most animals are febrile, and moist rales may be heard over the mass.

C. Radiography/Ultrasonography

1. Generally appear as nodular or cavitary radiopaque lesions on thoracic films.
2. Remove pleural effusion before radiographs to better define the lesion.

3. Ultrasound evaluation may help differentiate noncavitary from cavitary lesions.

D. Laboratory Findings

1. White blood cell numbers are variable.
   a. Leukocytosis with a degenerative left shift may be present.
   b. Leukogram may be normal.
2. If the infection is chronic, a nonregenerative anemia may be present.

IV. Differential Diagnosis

1. Differentials.
   a. Granulomas.
   b. *Paragonimus* spp.
   c. Neoplasia.
2. Perform cytology or histologic examination of samples obtained by fine-needle aspiration or surgery.
3. **Use caution in aspirating cavitary lesions to avoid pyothorax or pneumothorax.**
   a. Ultrasound is often useful in locating the appropriate site for aspiration.
4. Some nonneoplastic lesions can be managed without surgery (e.g., *Paragonimus*); however, a definitive diagnosis may require surgical biopsy.

V. Medical Management

A. Stabilize the animal if it is dyspneic.

B. Perform thoracentesis if pleural fluid or air is present.

C. Initiate antibiotic therapy based on results of culture and sensitivity testing. Choose a broad-spectrum antibiotic with a good anaerobic spectrum.

D. Continue antibiotic therapy for 3 to 6 weeks.

E. If pyothorax is present, place chest tubes and lavage the thorax.

VI. Surgical Treatment

A. Perform an intercostal thoracotomy and complete or partial lobectomy for solitary pulmonary abscesses that do not resolve with medical therapy.

B. Perform a median sternotomy approach if multiple opacities are present involving both sides of the thorax.

C. Preoperative management.

1. Perform thoracentesis if the animal is dyspneic.

2. Initiate antibiotic therapy after the mass, pleural space, or both have been cultured.

D. Surgical technique.

Identify and remove the diseased lung. Submit the lung for bacterial or fungal cultures and for histologic examination. Explore the remainder of the chest cavity for the presence of foreign matter. Palpate all the lung lobes that can be reached to identify other pulmonary lesions. Free remaining lung lobes of adhesions so that all lobes are moveable and remove loculated areas of exudate. Remove sheets of fibrin that cover the lung lobes. Place a chest tube before thoracic closure.

VII. Suture Materials/Special Instruments

A. Braided, multifilament, nonabsorbable suture (e.g., silk) should be avoided in the presence of infection.

VIII. Postoperative Care and Assessment

A. Continue appropriate antibiotics for 3 to 6 weeks if infection is present.

B. Consider thoracic lavage if pyothorax is present.

C. Provide postoperative analgesics.

IX. Prognosis

A. Prognosis depends on the underlying cause.

B. With appropriate management, the prognosis of animals with abscesses associated with nonneoplastic disease is good.

Lung Lobe Torsion (*SAS*, pp. 665-667)

I. Definitions

A. **Lung lobe torsion** (LLT) is a rotation of the lung lobe along its long axis, with twisting of the bronchus and pulmonary vessels at the hilus.

II. General Considerations and Clinically Relevant Pathophysiology

A. Potential Causes

1. Any mechanism that increases mobility of a lung lobe seems to favor development of a torsion, including partial collapse of the lung, pleural effusion, pneumothorax (along with subsequent atelectasis of lung lobes), and previous surgery.
2. Although LLT has been reported to cause chylothorax in dogs, it is more likely that the chylothorax caused the LLT.
3. The right middle lung lobe is most commonly affected.

B. Pathophysiology

1. Torsion of a lung lobe results in venous congestion of the affected lobe; however, the arteries remain at least partially patent, allowing blood to enter.
2. As fluid and blood enter the alveoli, lung consolidation occurs and the lobe becomes dark colored and firm, similar in shade to the liver.
3. The shape of the affected lobe is often altered and it may appear displaced from its normal location within the thorax radiographically.
4. Pleural fluid usually accumulates as a result of continued venous congestion.

III. Diagnosis

A. Clinical Presentation

1. Signalment.
   a. Deep-chested, large-breed dogs are more commonly affected.
      i. LLT in Afghan hounds may be associated with chylothorax.
      ii. May occur spontaneously, without previous history of disease or trauma.
   b. Has been reported in small breeds but is usually secondary to primary pleural effusion, thoracic surgery, or trauma.
   c. Rare in cats.
   d. Middle-aged dogs are more commonly affected, but LLT may occur in animals of any age.
2. History.
   a. Respiratory distress.
   b. Coughing (may be chronic).
   c. Hemoptysis (may be chronic).
   d. Anorexia.
   e. Depression.
   f. Often there is a previous history of pleural effusion, pneumothorax, pneumonia, or trauma.

B. Physical Examination Findings

1. Muffled heart and lung sounds.
2. Other findings may include depression, anorexia, coughing, fever, dyspnea, hemoptysis, hematemesis, or vomiting.

C. Radiography/Ultrasonography

1. Thoracic radiographic changes are variable depending on volume of pleural fluid, presence or absence of preexisting disease, and duration of the torsion.

2. The most consistent finding is the presence of pleural effusion accompanied by an opacified lung lobe.
3. Initially, air bronchograms will be present in the torsed lobe and can be seen extending toward the abdomen.
4. Air bronchograms eventually disappear as fluid and blood fill the bronchial lumen.
5. The presence of a noninflated, radiopaque lung lobe that persists after removal of pleural fluid should increase suspicion for LLT.
6. Positional radiographs using horizontal beam x-rays (lateral decubitus or upright VD) are often helpful and may show persistent pleural fluid around the affected lobe (rather than falling to the dependent side) or failure of the lobe to reinflate in the "up" or nondependent hemithorax.

D. Laboratory Findings

1. Fluid analysis may reveal a sterile, inflammatory effusion or chyle, or the fluid may be bloody.
2. The appearance of blood in a previously nonhemorrhagic pleural fluid may indicate occurrence of LLT.
3. An inflammatory leukogram may be present; however, changes in the leukogram may reflect the initial disease process rather than the LLT.

IV. Differential Diagnosis

A. Differentials

1. Pneumonia.
2. Pulmonary thromboembolism.
3. Pulmonary contusion.
4. Pulmonary neoplasia.
5. Atelectasis.
6. Hemothorax.
7. Diaphragmatic hernia.
8. Pyothorax.

B. Bronchoscopy

1. May visualize partial or complete occlusion of the affected bronchus.
2. Bronchial mucosa at the site of obstruction may appear folded and edematous.

C. Surgery

1. Demonstration of LLT at surgery provides the definitive diagnosis.

V. Medical Management

A. Stabilize the animal and alleviate respiratory distress before surgery.

B. Perform thoracentesis to remove pleural fluid.

C. If there is persistent or massive pleural effusion, place a chest tube.

D. Provide oxygen (oxygen cage or nasal insufflation) if the animal is dyspneic.

E. Identify and treat underlying diseases such as pneumonia.

F. Provide intravenous fluid therapy before and during surgery to maintain hydration.

G. **Spontaneous resolution of LLT is extremely uncommon. This is a surgical condition.**

VI. Surgical Treatment

A. The treatment of choice for LLT is lobectomy of the affected lobe.

B. Unless LLT is diagnosed very quickly (i.e., immediately after a surgical procedure), damage to the pulmonary parenchyma is generally severe enough that attempts to salvage the lobe are not warranted.

C. Recurrence has been reported following surgical correction where lobectomy was not performed.

D. Preoperative management.
  1. Administer prophylactic antibiotics.
  2. Remove pleural effusion before anesthetic induction.

E. Positioning.
  1. Prepare the affected lateral thorax for an intercostal thoracotomy.

F. Surgical technique.

Clamp the affected pedicle with a noncrushing forceps to prevent release of toxins into the bloodstream, before attempting to derotate it. Untwisting the lobe before its removal may help facilitate identification of the vascular structures and bronchus for ligation; however, in some cases, the lobe cannot be easily returned to its normal position due to extensive adhesions. Check the remaining lobes for position and normal expansion. Culture pulmonary parenchyma following removal of the lobe. Submit excised tissue for histologic examination to help determine underlying causes (e.g., pneumonia, neoplasia). Place a chest tube before closing the thoracic cavity.

VII. Suture Materials/Special Instruments

A. Avoid braided, multifilament suture because of the risk of infection.

B. Large clamps such as Satinsky clamps are useful for clamping the bronchus.

VIII. Postoperative Care and Assessment

A. Continue antibiotics if there is evidence of infection.

B. Provide postoperative analgesics.

C. Remove the chest tube when the effusion decreases to less than 2.2. ml/kg body weight.

D. Provide oxygen therapy if there is underlying lung disease such as pneumonia.

E. If dyspnea remains after surgery, take thoracic radiographs to rule out LLT in a remaining lobe.

IX. Prognosis

A. The prognosis is good for most animals with LLT if surgery is performed.

B. Pleural effusion usually resolves within a few days of surgery.

Pectus Excavatum (*SAS*, pp. 667-672)

I. Definitions

A. **Pectus excavatum** (PE) is a deformity of the sternum and costocartilages that results in a dorsal to ventral narrowing of the thorax.

B. **Pectus carinatum** is a protrusion of the sternum that occurs much less frequently than PE.

II. General Considerations and Clinically Relevant Pathophysiology

A. The cause or causes of PE in animals are unknown.

B. Theories proposed include shortening of the central tendon of the diaphragm, intrauterine pressure abnormalities, congenital deficiency of the musculature in the cranial portion of the diaphragm, and abnormal respiratory gradients (i.e., brachycephalic dogs are most commonly affected).

C. May be associated with "swimmer's syndrome."

D. Abnormalities of the joints of the limbs and the long bones may occur.

E. Circulatory disorders in animals with PE may occur because of abnormal cardiac positioning resulting in kinking of the large veins and disturbance of venous return, compression of the heart predisposing to arrhythmias (particularly the auricles), restriction of ventricular capacity, or decreased respiratory reserve.

F. Cardiac abnormalities are common (see following text).

G. **Although the etiology of PE is uncertain, multiple animals in some litters have been affected. Breeding should not be undertaken and affected animals should be neutered.**

III. Diagnosis

A. Clinical Presentation

1. Signalment.
   a. In symptomatic animals clinical signs are usually present at birth, or shortly thereafter.
   b. PE may occur in any breed, but brachycephalic dogs appear to be predisposed.
   c. A sex predisposition has not been identified.
2. History.
   a. Many animals with PE are asymptomatic.
   b. Owners may seek veterinary care because they palpate the defect.
   c. Symptomatic animals may present for evaluation of exercise intolerance, weight loss, hyperpnea, recurrent pulmonary infections, cyanosis, vomiting, persistent and productive coughing, inappetence, or mild episodes of upper respiratory disease.
   d. A correlation between severity of clinical signs and severity of anatomic or physiologic abnormalities has not been observed.

B. Physical Examination Findings

1. The sternal deformity is usually palpable.
2. Other physical examination findings may include cardiac murmurs and harsh lung sounds.
3. Dyspnea is variable, but rapid, shallow respirations may be noted.
4. **Do not assume that cardiac murmurs in animals with PE are due to heart disease. They may be due to abnormal positioning of the heart because of the sternal deformity.**

C. Radiography

1. Thoracic radiographs show abnormal elevation of the sternum in the caudal thorax.
2. Objective assessment of the deformity may be determined by measuring the frontosagittal and vertebral indices on thoracic radiographs (Table 26-2).
   a. Frontosagittal index.
      i. Ratio of the width of the chest at the tenth thoracic vertebra, measured on a dorsoventral or ventrodorsal radiograph, and the distance between the center of the ventral surface of the tenth thoracic vertebra and the nearest point on the sternum.
      ii. Vertebral index.
         (a) Ratio of the distance between the center of the dorsal surface of the selected vertebral body to the nearest point on the sternum and the dorsoventral diameter of the center of the same vertebral body.
3. Evaluate thoracic radiographs for evidence of concurrent abnormalities (e.g., tracheal hypoplasia, cardiac abnormalities, pneumonia).
4. Most animals with PE have abnormally positioned hearts, which may cause the heart to appear enlarged radiographically; thus true cardiac enlargement cannot always be distinguished from apparent enlargement caused by abnormal heart position.

D. Laboratory Findings

1. Laboratory abnormalities are uncommon.

Table 26-2
Normal frontosagittal and vertebral indices

Frontosagittal	
Nonbrachycephalic dogs	0.8 to 1.4
Brachycephalic dogs	1.0 to 1.5
Cats	0.7 to 1.3
Vertebral	
Nonbrachycephalic dogs	11.8 to 19.6
Brachycephalic dogs	12.5 to 16.5
Cats	12.6 to 18.8

IV. Differential Diagnosis

A. Cardiac murmurs associated with the cardiac malpositioning often disappear following surgical correction of the defect or a change in the patient's position.

B. Systolic murmurs may be related to kinking of the pulmonary artery or to exaggeration of the artery's normal vibrations resulting from its proximity to the chest wall.

C. Differentiate animals with PE and innocent systolic murmurs from those that have underlying cardiac defects, such as pulmonic stenosis or atrial septal defects.

V. Medical Management

A. Animals with merely a flat chest may contour to a normal or near-normal configuration without surgical intervention.
   1. Encourage owners to regularly perform medial-to-lateral compression of the chest on these young animals.
   2. Animals with severe elevation of the sternum will not benefit from this technique or from splintage that simply provides medial-to-lateral compression and does not correct the malpositioned sternum.
   3. Other medical management includes treatment of respiratory tract infections and, if the animal is severely dyspneic, oxygen therapy.

VI. Surgical Treatment

A. General Considerations

1. Definitive treatment of PE using external splintage is possible because the costal cartilages and sternum are pliable in these young animals and the thorax can be reshaped by applying traction to the sternum using sutures that are placed around the sternum and through a rigid splint.
2. Whether surgical correction of the defect should be performed in asymptomatic patients with moderate or severe PE is unknown. Symptomatic patients that do not have associated cardiac abnormalities will benefit from surgery.

B. Preoperative Management

1. Treat respiratory infections before surgery.
2. Provide oxygen if the animal is severely dyspneic.
3. Administration of prophylactic antibiotics is not necessary. Development of intrathoracic infection associated with surgery is uncommon.

C. Anesthesia (see Appendix G-27)

1. General considerations.
   a. Pay careful attention to airway, ventilation, body temperature, and blood glucose concentration.
   b. Intubate animals and assist ventilation. Provide a high inspired fraction of oxygen.
   c. Administer warm intravenous fluids.
   d. Provide glucose if serum glucose concentrations cannot be monitored.
   e. Insulate the animal from the cool surgical environment.
   f. Fit and form the splint before anesthesia to reduce anesthetic duration.
   g. **Do not use nitrous oxide** in these patients because of the risk of pneumothorax.
   h. Provide postoperative analgesia in puppies with butorphanol, oxymorphone, or buprenorphine and in kittens with butorphanol or buprenorphine (Appendix F).
   i. Do not use chamber or mask induction if the animal is dyspneic.

D. Positioning

1. Place the patient in dorsal recumbency and prepare the ventral thorax for aseptic surgery.

E. Surgical Technique

Fashion a rectangular piece of moldable splinting material into a U shape and mold it to fit the ventral aspect of the thorax. Apply a small amount of adhesive padding to the cranial border and inner surface of the splint, or alternatively, pad the splint with cast padding after it has been positioned. Place two parallel rows of four to six holes in the splint with a small Steinmann pin. Position the holes so that the distance between adjacent holes is slightly greater than the width of the sternum. Pass the selected suture (see under suture materials) around the sternum by maneuvering the needle blindly off the lateral edge of the sternum. Alternatively, pass the needle around the sternebra at a 45-degree angle to incorporate the costocartilage and possibly decrease the chance of the suture pulling through the soft sternebral bone. Sutures must be placed around the sternum and not subcutaneously. Additionally, sutures must be placed in the area of the greatest concavity. If the sutures are placed proximal

to the area with the greatest depression the sternum cannot be pulled into a normal position, resulting in less than optimal correction of the defect. Keep the needle as close as possible to the dorsal aspect of the sternum to avoid piercing the heart or lungs. Leave the suture ends long and tag them. When all sutures have been placed, pass the ends through the predrilled holes in the splint and tie them securely on its ventral aspect. Two sutures may be placed and tied to themselves and then these sutures tied together so that the splint can be adjusted without replacement of sutures or use of anesthesia.

VII. Suture Materials/Special Instruments

A. A taper-point needle is recommended; if suture material with a large, swaged-on needle is not available, a large, eyed, taper-point needle should be selected (to prevent bending and possible breakage as it is passed around the sternum).

B. Large (No. 0-2), monofilament absorbable or nonabsorbable suture material is recommended (polydioxanone, polyglyconate, or nylon suture).

VIII. Postoperative Care and Assessment

A. Evaluate the animal in the early postoperative period for intrathoracic hemorrhage because piercing of the heart, lung, or internal thoracic vessels as the needle is passed around the sternum is possible.

B. Positioning the animal in dorsal recumbency, paying close attention to the phase of respiration, and keeping the needle as close to the sternum as possible will help prevent such complications.

C. Leave the splint in place for 10 to 21 days (although fewer days may suffice).

IX. Complications

A. Suture abscesses, mild superficial dermatitis, and skin abrasions are common, but these are usually minor and heal quickly after splint removal.

B. Adequate padding of the splint may help prevent abrasions.

C. Fatal reexpansion pulmonary edema has been reported in a kitten after correction of PE.

X. Prognosis

A. Excellent for animals without underlying disease in whom surgery is performed at a young age.

B. Older animals with a less pliable sternum may not respond as favorably to external splintage. Partial sternectomy may benefit such animals.

Thoracic Wall Neoplasia (*SAS*, pp. 672-673)

I. Definitions

A. **Chondrosarcomas** are tumors that arise from cartilage.

B. **Osteosarcomas** are tumors that arise from bone.

II. General Considerations and Clinically Relevant Pathophysiology

A. Rib Tumors

1. Primary tumors of the rib have a high metastatic rate and are uncommon in dogs or cats.
2. Osteosarcomas are most common, followed by chondrosarcomas.
   a. Osteosarcomas usually arise at the costochondral junction.

B. Sternal Tumors

1. Both metastatic and primary tumors of the sternum have been reported in dogs.
2. Primary sternal tumors of dogs include chondrosarcoma and osteosarcoma.

III. Diagnosis

A. Clinical Presentation

1. Signalment.
   a. Primary rib tumors generally develop in young and middle-aged dogs.
   b. Rib tumors should be considered as a possible differential for masses involving the thoracic wall, even in young dogs.
2. History.
   a. Animals with rib tumors may present for dyspnea or evaluation of a nonpainful thoracic wall mass.
   b. Animals with sternal neoplasia often present for evaluation of a palpable sternal mass.

B. Physical Examination Findings

1. Rib tumors.
   a. Most rib tumors cause a localized swelling of the thoracic wall.
   b. Pleural effusion without evidence of a thoracic mass occasionally occurs in dogs with small primary rib tumors and metastatic pulmonary lesions.
   c. Other clinical signs are weight loss and dyspnea.

2. Sternal tumors.
   a. Sternal tumors usually cause a localized swelling, but may be associated with dyspnea if they metastasize to the lungs.

C. Radiography

1. Rib tumors are generally expansile masses that cause bone destruction.
2. Sternal tumors may result in lysis of several sternebrae and the adjacent ribs.
3. Evaluate thoracic radiographs for pulmonary metastasis, lymph node involvement, and pleural effusion.

D. Laboratory Findings

1. Laboratory findings are nonspecific.
2. Blood gas analysis may show hypoxemia and respiratory acidosis or alkalosis.

IV. Differential Diagnosis

A. Differentials include osteomyelitis, fungal infections, and abscesses.

B. A tentative diagnosis of the cell type can usually be made by fine-needle aspiration of the mass.

C. Definitive diagnosis usually requires histologic examination of a biopsy specimen.

D. Although pleural effusion is common in dogs with rib tumors, identification of neoplastic cells in the fluid is uncommon.

V. Medical Management

A. Medical management (thoracentesis if pleural effusion exists, oxygen therapy for dyspnea) of animals with rib or sternal tumors is generally palliative only.

B. Pleuroperitoneal shunts may be considered.

VI. Surgical Treatment

A. General Considerations

1. Surgical resection of thoracic wall tumors is the treatment of choice.
2. Full-thickness or "en bloc" resection of three or more ribs for thoracic wall neoplasia requires surgical reconstruction to reestablish thoracic wall continuity.
3. Removal of more than six ribs is not recommended.
4. With tumors of the caudal thorax, advancement of the diaphragm cranial to the resected ribs decreases the need for rigid fixation of the thoracic wall.

5. Partial or complete sternectomy may be curative in dogs with primary sternal neoplasia.
6. Although temporary instability of the thorax may occur following large sternal resections, this does not appear to cause any permanent or significant respiratory dysfunction.

B. Preoperative Management

1. Perform thoracentesis before induction in dogs with pleural effusion associated with thoracic wall neoplasia.

C. Positioning

1. Aseptically prepare a generous area surrounding the tumor to allow for wide resection.
2. Positioning will depend on the site of the lesion.

D. Surgical Technique

1. En bloc resection of thoracic wall neoplasia.

Remove the thoracic wall containing the neoplasm and a margin of normal tissue, leaving a square or rectangular defect. Cut a piece of polypropylene mesh slightly larger than the defect. Fold over the edges of the mesh and suture the double thickness of mesh to the pleural side of the defect. Draw the mesh tightly across the defect when suturing it to prevent it from moving paradoxically with respiration. If more than four or five ribs are removed, support the ribs with plastic spinal plates or rib grafts. Mobilize and advance thoracic wall musculature over the defect, or if there is insufficient muscle, exteriorize an omental pedicle flap through a paracostal abdominal approach and tunnel it subcutaneously to the defect. Alternatively, exteriorize the omental flap through the diaphragm. Place the omental flap over the mesh and suture skin over the defect. For caudal rib tumors, advancement of the diaphragm may be done following "en bloc" resection of the mass and surrounding tissues. Synthetic reconstruction of the rib cage is rarely necessary.

2. Partial sternectomy.

Partial sternectomy should be considered only for relatively small, localized sternal neoplasms that do not appear to have intrathoracic involvement. Sternectomy has been used successfully for extensive sternal osteomyelitis. The entire sternum can be removed in small animals. Incise through the skin overlying the neoplasm (if skin involvement is suspected, resect the skin). Identify rib articulations on the sternum. Use rongeurs to remove the affected sternebrae and ribs. If possible remove one sternebra caudal and one cranial to the lesion. Assess the thoracic cavity for involvement. Avoid lacerating the internal thoracic arteries—ligate them if necessary. Appose the ribs and intercostal muscles with a large (e.g., No. 1) monofilament suture in an interrupted or horizontal mattress suture pattern. Use a simple continuous suture pattern to appose remnants of the rectus abdominis muscle over the junction of the rib ends. Minimize dead space by apposing skin and underlying tissues with walking sutures. Place a thoracostomy tube and evacuate air from the thoracic cavity. Place a light support wrap over the thorax to protect the incision and thoracostomy tube.

VII. Suture Materials/Special Instruments

A. For reconstruction of thoracic wall defects, use monofilament, non-absorbable suture (polypropylene or nylon).

B. Polypropylene (Marlex) mesh may be used for thoracic wall reconstruction.

VIII. Postoperative Care and Assessment

A. Monitor animals with surgically created thoracic wall defects closely in the postoperative period for hypoventilation and development of pneumothorax.

B. Provide analgesics.

IX. Prognosis

A. Because of the high rate of pulmonary metastasis, the prognosis for dogs with rib tumors is poor.

1. In one study of 15 dogs with primary rib tumors, greater than 90% died or were euthanatized within 4 months of the diagnosis.

B. Too few sternal tumors have been reported to define the prognosis in affected animals.

27

Surgery of the Lower Respiratory System: Pleural Cavity and Diaphragm (*SAS*, pp. 675-704)

General Principles and Techniques (*SAS*, pp. 675-682)

I. Definitions

A. **Thoracocentesis** is a surgical puncture of the thoracic wall to remove air (pneumothorax) or fluid (pleural effusion) from the pleural space.

B. **Pleurodesis** is the creation of adhesions between the visceral and parietal pleura caused by instilling irritating agents into the pleural cavity or mechanically damaging the pleura during surgery.

II. Preoperative Concerns

A. Monitor respiratory function carefully, including respiratory rate and pattern and capillary refill time and color, in patients with pleural cavity or diaphragmatic abnormalities.

B. Animals with pleural cavity disease usually exhibit a restrictive respiratory pattern (i.e., rapid, shallow respirations).

C. Arterial blood gas analysis will augment qualitative information concerning the effectiveness of ventilation and gas exchange (Appendix L).

D. Pulse oximetry is a noninvasive tool that provides information regarding the hemoglobin saturation of blood and thus indirectly provides quantitative information regarding oxygenation.

E. Evaluate cardiovascular parameters (i.e., heart rate and rhythm). Perform an ECG in all trauma patients.

F. Provide intravenous fluids to dehydrated animals or those that are not drinking sufficient fluids to maintain hydration.

G. Take care to avoid causing overhydration and pulmonary edema, which will further compromise respiration.

H. Monitoring central venous pressure may be useful in some patients.

I. Animals with pleural effusion or pneumothorax may be extremely dyspneic.
1. In severely dyspneic animals with suspected pleural cavity disease, perform thoracentesis (see p. 562) before radiographs are made.
2. Removal of even small amounts of pleural effusion or air may significantly improve ventilation, allowing safer manipulation of the patient for radiographic procedures.
3. Most dyspneic animals will allow thoracentesis to be performed with minimal restraint. Avoid general anesthetics.
4. Allow the animal to remain in sternal recumbency and provide oxygen by face mask or nasal insufflation if the animal will tolerate it.
5. A negative tap does not rule out pleural effusion; however, if the animal remains dyspneic after thoracentesis, suspect underlying lung disease (e.g., pneumonia, pulmonary edema, pulmonary contusions, pulmonary neoplasia) or loculated fluid.
6. Provide nasal oxygen or place the animal in an oxygen cage while treatment of the pulmonary disease is initiated.

J. Do not attempt chest tube placement in an animal with severe respiratory distress.
1. Remove some pleural air or fluid via needle thoracentesis to improve ventilation.
2. Most animals with pleural cavity disease benefit from intermittent positive pressure ventilation and oxygen supplementation during tube placement.
3. When using general anesthesia, control the airway (via endotracheal intubation and positive pressure ventilation) and administer oxygen.

K. For preoperative concerns of patients with diaphragmatic herniation, see the section on traumatic diaphragmatic hernias later in this chapter.

III. Anesthetic Considerations (see also Chapter 26)

A. Whenever possible, maintain dogs and cats with respiratory insufficiency with inhalation anesthetics (isoflurane or halothane).
1. Manage respiratory patients with extreme care until intubation has been accomplished and ventilation can be assisted.
2. Provide oxygen by face mask until an airway has been secured.
3. Accomplish intubation as rapidly as possible in patients with pleural effusion or pneumothorax; mask induction is not recommended.
4. Maintain an adequate respiratory volume via endotracheal intubation and intermittent positive pressure ventilation in patients whose lungs may not expand normally because of the presence of pleural cavity or diaphragmatic abnormalities.
5. **Do not use nitrous oxide** in patients with pneumothorax or diaphragmatic hernias.

IV. Antibiotics

A. Needle thoracentesis, if performed with proper aseptic technique, is unlikely to induce infection in patients with normal immune function.

Therefore prophylactic antibiotics generally do not need to be provided when performing this procedure.

B. Maintain and handle chest tubes with appropriate precautions (e.g., sterile gloves and syringes, chest bandages) to decrease the potential for iatrogenic contamination.

C. Gram-negative bacteria and anaerobes are common isolates in animals with respiratory disease.

D. Base therapy of pyothorax on culture and sensitivity test results, if possible, because unpredictable antibiotic sensitivity is common with the microorganisms commonly encountered with this condition.

E. For patients with pyothorax, see the discussion of specific antibiotic recommendations in the pyothorax section later in this chapter.

V. Surgical Anatomy

A. Each pleural cavity is only a potential space unless air or fluid collects between the parietal and visceral pleura, preventing normal lung expansion.

B. Thickening of the pleura (i.e., fibrosing pleuritis) may result in decreased reabsorption of pleural effusion.

C. The diaphragm is composed of a central tendinous portion and an outer muscular portion, attached to the last few ribs and extending cranially into the thoracic cavity.

VI. Surgical Techniques

A. General Considerations

1. For traumatic pneumothorax, intermittent needle thoracentesis may be sufficient in some animals to prevent dyspnea while the lung heals, but chest tubes are occasionally required.
2. Chest tube placement and continuous drainage of air in animals with spontaneous pneumothorax that have undergone mechanical pleurodesis are recommended to allow pleurodesis.
3. With some types of pleural effusion (e.g., pyothorax), tube thoracentesis and thoracic lavage are mandatory in the primary treatment of most affected animals.
4. Choose thoracocentesis or chest tube placement site based on radiographs or physical exam.
5. Occasionally, bilateral chest tubes may be necessary; however, in most dogs and cats the mediastinum is permeable to fluid or air, allowing drainage of both hemithoraxes through a single tube.

B. Needle Thoracentesis

1. General considerations.
   a. Perform needle thoracentesis with a small-gauge (No. 19 to No. 23) butterfly needle attached to a three-way stopcock and syringe, or an over-the-needle catheter attached to an extension tubing, three-way stopcock, and syringe.
2. Technique.

Perform thoracentesis at the sixth, seventh, or eighth intercostal space, near the level of the costochondral junction. Clip the selected site and perform a local anesthetic block if needed (rarely). Aseptically prepare the site and introduce the needle into the middle of the selected intercostal space. Be careful to avoid the large vessels associated with the posterior aspect of the rib margins. Advance the needle into the pleural space. Aspirate fluid while the needle is being advanced to allow prompt recognition of the appropriate depth of needle placement. With the bevel of the needle facing inward, orient the needle against the rib cage to prevent damage to the lung surface. Gently aspirate fluid and place 5-ml samples in an EDTA tube and a clot tube for a cell count and biochemical parameters, respectively. Make six to eight direct smears for cytologic evaluation. Submit samples for aerobic and anaerobic cultures.

C. Chest Tube Placement (*SAS,* pp. 678-680)

1. General considerations.
   a. Improperly placed or managed chest tubes are extremely dangerous; be sure to take proper precautions and ensure that the animal cannot remove the tube prematurely or chew on the tube.
   b. Chest tubes simplify the management of some animals with pleural effusion or pneumothorax.
   c. If needle thoracentesis or ultrasonography suggests that the fluid is severely loculated or extensive adhesions are present, surgical placement of the chest tube may be advisable.
   d. Components of a tube thoracostomy include a chest tube, an apparatus to connect the tube to a syringe or to a continuous suction bottle, and a device to collect the drained material (syringe or collecting bottle).
   e. Chest tubes.
      i. Commercial chest tubes come in many sizes, are minimally reactive, and have a metal stylet to aid in placement.
      ii. Red rubber feeding tubes may be less likely to perforate lung tissue during placement, but they cannot be attached to a continuous suction device because they collapse readily and are more difficult to place.
2. Technique.

Clip and prepare the lateral thorax for aseptic surgery. To allow sufficient drainage, place additional holes in the tube by bending it and removing a notch with a pair of sterile scissors. Holes should be no larger than one third the tube's circumference. If using a commercial tube with a radiopaque line, place the last hole through the line to allow identification of its position on a thoracic radiograph. Make a small skin incision in the dorsal one third of the lateral thoracic wall at the level of the tenth or eleventh intercostal space. Advance the tube subcutaneously in a cranioventral direction for three to four intercostal spaces; introduce the tube through the muscle and pleura using the stylet or a large hemostat. When using a trocar tube, firmly grasp the tube 2 to 4 cm from the body wall with one hand while using the other to "pop" the tube through the intercostal musculature and pleura. This prevents the tube from being inadvertently pushed too far into the thorax and thereby damaging the lung or other thoracic structures. Feed the tube in a cranioventral direction to a predetermined point. Before completely removing the trocar, clamp the tube with a hemostat. Place a purse-string suture in the skin around the tube (do not enter the lumen of the tube) and leave both ends of the suture long. Use this suture to perform a "Chinese finger-trap" or "Roman sandal" suture. Connect the chest tube to a three-way stopcock to increase the ease of thoracic drainage. Use a five-in-one (Christmas tree) adapter or a female Luer-Lok (with small tubes) between the tube and the three-way stopcock to ensure an airtight

seal. Use suture to secure the tube to the connecting devices so they will not become inadvertently dislodged, resulting in pneumothorax. For added safety when the chest cavity is not being suctioned, clamp the tube where it exits the body wall with a hemostat or C-clamp. Verify appropriate placement of the chest drain radiographically before covering it with a loose bandage.

Drainage may be either intermittent or continuous. Intermittent pleural drainage is usually adequate, but in some situations (e.g., spontaneous pneumothorax, pleurodesis) continuous suction is preferable. Heimlich valves should be used only in medium to large dogs, because small dogs and cats may not develop sufficient expiratory pressure for effective drainage. Additionally, these valves are prone to malfunction if fluid is aspirated into the apparatus. "Milking" or "stripping" of chest tubes to prevent obstruction of the tube by clots has been recommended in the veterinary literature; however, these techniques generate high intrapleural pressures and may cause pulmonary damage.

D. Chest Tube Removal (*SAS,* p. 680)

With pleural effusion, remove the tube when the drainage decreases to a volume that is consistent with that caused by the presence of the tube itself (i.e., 2.2 ml/kg body weight per day). The tube can be removed in patients with pneumothorax once negative pressure has been achieved for 12 to 24 hours. Culture the end of the tube following removal if the tube has been present for several days or if the animal shows signs of infection. Suture the skin incision with one or two simple interrupted sutures.

E. Continuous Thoracic Suction

1. General considerations.
   a. If fluid accumulation is so rapid that intermittent drainage is not practical, or if adherence of the visceral pleura to the body wall is desired, use continuous suction.
   b. A continuous 10- to 15-cm negative pressure on the thorax effectively aspirates pneumothorax, increasing the likelihood of spontaneous sealing of large pulmonary defects.
   c. Use slightly greater pressures (up to 20 cm H_2O) when draining viscous fluid.
2. Technique.

Connect the chest tube to a bottle that serves as an underwater seal (filled with 2 to 3 cm of sterile water), which in turn is connected to a suction bottle (also partially filled with water) attached to a suction device. Vary the amount of suction by raising or lowering the level of water in the suction bottle. A rigid plastic vent tube opened to room air serves to allow air to be aspirated into the bottle as the vacuum is applied. A third bottle interposed between the chest tube and the underwater seal bottle serves to collect fluid and prevent the level from rising in the underwater seal bottle as fluid is drained from the chest. The bottle is unnecessary in animals with pneumothorax. Alternatively, use a commercial continuous suction device.

VII. Healing of the Pleura

A. Healing or damaged pleura is prone to adhesion formation in some species; however, dogs and cats seem resistant to chemical pleurodesis.

B. Fibrosing pleuritis has been reported in dogs and cats secondary to prolonged exudative or blood-stained effusions.

1. In animals with fibrosis, the pleura is thickened by diffuse fibrous tissue that restricts normal pulmonary expansion (the lungs do not adhere to the body wall in these patients).
2. Exudates are characterized by a high rate of fibrin formation and degradation because chronic inflammation induces changes in mesothelial cell morphologic features that result in increased permeability, mesothelial cell desquamation, and triggering of both pathways of the coagulation cascade.

VIII. Suture Materials/Special Instruments

A. Trocar chest tubes (DekNatel thoracic trocar catheter, Argyle thoracic trocar catheter) and continuous suction devices (DekNatel Pleur-evac chest drainage system, Thora-Seal III three-bottle underwater chest drainage system) are available from several commercial sources.

IX. Postoperative Care and Assessment

A. If dyspnea persists following needle thoracentesis or chest tube placement, administer oxygen therapy (nasal insufflation or oxygen cage).

B. Take thoracic radiographs to assess fluid or air removal or to evaluate chest tube position.

C. Continually monitor animals with chest tubes to prevent iatrogenic dislodgement or damage of the tube or connectors causing pneumothorax.

D. Exercise care when handling tubes to prevent thoracic contamination.

E. Aspirate chest tubes gently so that lung tissue is not suctioned into the tube drainage ports.

X. Special Age Considerations

A. Surgical correction of respiratory abnormalities in young animals requires that special attention be paid to the anesthetic requirements of the young.

B. Diaphragmatic hernia repair is commonly performed in young animals (see discussion of diaphragmatic hernias, below) because they are prone to trauma that may result in such lesions.

C. Peritoneopericardial diaphragmatic hernias are usually diagnosed at a young age (i.e., less than 1 year of age) and concurrent cardiac abnormalities may be present, complicating the anesthetic management of these patients.

D. Geriatric animals may have severe, concurrent underlying pulmonary or cardiac disease that complicates the management of pleural cavity disease in these patients.

Traumatic Diaphragmatic Hernias (*SAS*, pp. 682-685)

I. Definitions

A. **Diaphragmatic hernia** (DH) occurs when continuity of the diaphragm is disrupted such that abdominal organs can migrate into the thoracic cavity.

II. General Considerations and Clinically Relevant Pathophysiology

A. DH is commonly recognized by small animal clinicians and may be congenital or occur following trauma.

B. Most DHs in dogs and cats result from trauma, particularly auto vehicle accidents.
   1. The location and size of the tear(s) depend on the position of the animal at the time of impact and location of the viscera.
   2. Traumatic DH is often associated with significant respiratory embarrassment; however, chronic DH in asymptomatic animals is not uncommon.

III. Diagnosis

A. Clinical Presentation

1. Signalment.
   a. There is no breed predisposition for traumatic DH, but most afflicted dogs are young males between 1 and 2 years of age.
2. History.
   a. The duration of DH may range from a few hours to years.
   b. The animals may be presented in shock following the injury.
   c. The animals often have associated injuries, such as fractures.
   d. With chronic DH, clinical signs are most often referable to either the respiratory or gastrointestinal systems and may include dyspnea, exercise intolerance, anorexia, depression, vomiting, diarrhea, weight loss, or pain following ingestion of food.

B. Physical Examination Findings

1. Animals with traumatic DH are frequently presented in shock; thus clinical signs may include pale or cyanotic mucous membranes, tachypnea, tachycardia, or oliguria.
2. Cardiac arrhythmias are common and are associated with significant morbidity.
3. Other clinical signs depend on which organs herniate and may be attributed to the gastrointestinal, respiratory, or cardiovascular systems.
4. The liver is the most common herniated organ and is often associated with hydrothorax resulting from entrapment and venous occlusion.

C. Radiography/Ultrasonography

1. Make definitive diagnosis of pleuroperitoneal DH via radiography or ultrasonography.
   a. Use ultrasound examination of the diaphragmatic silhouette in animals in which the herniation is not obvious radiographically.

2. Radiographic signs of DH include loss of the diaphragmatic line, loss of the cardiac silhouette, dorsal or lateral displacement of lung fields, presence of gas or a barium-filled stomach or intestines in the thoracic cavity, and pleural effusion.
   a. If significant pleural effusion is present, thoracentesis may be necessary for diagnostic radiographs.
3. Use positive-contrast celiography if needed for the diagnosis.
   a. Inject prewarmed water-soluble contrast agent into the abdominal cavity at a dosage of 1.1 ml/kg (dose is doubled if ascites is present), roll the patient gently from side to side or elevate the pelvis, and take films immediately following the injection and manipulation.
   b. Evaluate these films using the presence of contrast medium in the pleural cavity, absence of a normal liver lobe outline in the abdomen, and incomplete visualization of the abdominal surface of the diaphragm as criteria.
   c. Interpret positive-contrast celiograms cautiously–omental and fibrous adhesions may seal the defect, resulting in false-negative films.

IV. Medical Management

A. If the animal is dyspneic, provide oxygen by face mask, nasal insufflation, or an oxygen cage.

B. Position the animal in sternal recumbency with the forelimbs elevated to help ventilation.

C. If moderate or severe pleural effusion is present, perform thoracentesis.

D. Give fluid therapy and antibiotics if the animal is in shock.

V. Surgical Treatment

A. General Considerations

1. Traumatic DHs have a higher mortality rate when surgery is performed either less than 24 hours or greater than 1 year following the injury.
2. Delay surgical repair of DH until the patient has been stabilized; however, do not unnecessarily delay herniorrhaphy.
3. Evaluate animals with herniation of the stomach carefully for gastric distention and operate as soon as they can safely be anesthetized because acute gastric distention within the thorax may cause rapid, fatal respiratory impairment.

B. Preoperative Management

1. Give prophylactic antibiotics before anesthetic induction in animals with hepatic herniation.
   a. Massive release of toxins into the circulation may occur with hepatic strangulation or vascular compromise.
   b. Premedicating such patients with steroids may be beneficial.
2. Perform an ECG on all trauma patients before surgery.

C. Anesthesia

1. Avoid chamber or mask induction in animals with DH.
2. Before induction, supplement the inspired oxygen to improve myocardial oxygenation.

3. Because of the animal's already compromised ventilation, use drugs with minimal respiratory depressant effects.
4. Use injectable anesthetics, which allow rapid intubation.
5. Use inhalation anesthetics for anesthetic maintenance.
6. Perform intermittent positive pressure ventilation and avoid high inspiratory pressures to help prevent reexpansion pulmonary edema.
7. Allow the lungs to slowly expand after surgery.
8. **Do not use nitrous oxide** in patients with DH.
9. Drugs such as methylprednisolone may be beneficial for preventing reexpansion pulmonary edema in animals with chronic DH.
10. See Appendix G-26 for examples of selected anesthetic protocols that may be used in animals with diaphragmatic hernias.

D. Positioning

1. Place the animal in dorsal recumbency for a midline abdominal incision.
2. Prepare the entire abdomen and caudal one half to two thirds of the thoracic cavity for aseptic surgery.
3. Acute ventilatory compromise may occur during positioning; thus monitor these animals carefully during this period.

E. Surgical Techniques

Make a ventral midline abdominal incision; if increased exposure is needed, extend the incision cranially through the sternum. Replace the abdominal organs in the abdominal cavity (if necessary, enlarge the diaphragmatic defect). If adhesions are present, dissect the tissues gently from thoracic structures to prevent pneumothorax or bleeding. With chronic hernias, debride the edge of the defect before closure. Close the diaphragmatic defect with a simple continuous suture pattern. If the diaphragm is avulsed from the ribs, incorporate a rib in the continuous suture for added strength. Remove air from the pleural cavity following closure of the defect. If continued pneumothorax or effusion is likely, place a chest tube. Explore the entire abdominal cavity for associated injury (e.g., compromise of the vasculature to the intestine, splenic, renal, or bladder trauma) and repair any defects.

VI. Suture Materials/Special Instruments

A. For diaphragmatic closure use either a nonabsorbable suture material such as polypropylene or an absorbable material such as polydioxanone (PDS) or polyglyconate (Maxon) suture.

VII. Postoperative Care and Assessment

A. Monitor postoperatively for hypoventilation; provide oxygen if needed.

B. Reexpansion pulmonary edema (RPE) is a potential complication associated with rapid lung reexpansion following DH repair.

VIII. Prognosis

A. If the animal survives 12 to 24 hours after the operation, the prognosis is excellent, and recurrence is uncommon with proper technique.

Peritoneopericardial Diaphragmatic Hernias (*SAS*, pp. 685-687)

I. Definitions

A. **Peritoneopericardial diaphragmatic hernia** (PPDH) occurs when there is a congenital communication between the abdomen and the pericardial sac.

II. General Considerations and Clinically Relevant Pathophysiology

A. PPDHs are less commonly recognized by small animal clinicians than are traumatic diaphragmatic hernias.

B. They are always congenital in dogs and cats because there is no direct communication between the pericardial and peritoneal cavities after birth.

C. Cardiac abnormalities and sternal deformities often occur concomitantly with PPDH.

D. The combination of congenital cranial abdominal wall, caudal sternal, diaphragmatic, and pericardial defects has been reported in dogs, often associated with ventricular septal defects or other intracardiac defects.

E. It is not known whether this condition is heritable; however, several breed predispositions have been recognized (see following text).

F. Polycystic kidneys have been reported in association with PPDH in cats.

III. Diagnosis

A. Clinical Presentation

1. Signalment.
   a. Although PPDHs are congenital, it is not uncommon for the diagnosis to be made when the animal is middle-aged or older because clinical signs are variable and may be intermittent.
   b. Weimaraners and cocker spaniels may be at increased risk.
2. History.
   a. Clinical signs may be referable to the gastrointestinal, cardiac, or respiratory systems and include anorexia, depression, vomiting, diarrhea, weight loss, wheezing, dyspnea, exercise intolerance, or pain following ingestion of food.
   b. Neurologic signs may occur because of hepatoencephalopathy.

B. Physical Examination Findings

1. Physical examination findings in animals with PPDH may include ascites, muffled heart sounds, murmurs caused by displacement of the heart by visceral organs or caused by intracardiac defects, and concurrent ventral abdominal wall defects.

2. The most commonly herniated organ is the liver, and associated pericardial effusion is common.

C. Radiography/Ultrasonography

1. A tentative diagnosis of PPDH may be made based on history, clinical signs, and physical examination, but radiography, ultrasonography, or both are essential for a definitive diagnosis.
2. Radiographic signs of PPDH include (a) enlarged cardiac silhouette, (b) dorsal elevation of the trachea, (c) overlap of the heart and diaphragmatic borders, (d) discontinuity of the diaphragm, (e) gas-filled structures in the pericardial sac, (f) sternal defects, and (g) dorsal peritoneopericardial mesothelial remnant.
3. Undertake contrast studies (nonselective angiogram, barium contrast study) only if a definitive diagnosis cannot be made on plain films or with ultrasound.
4. A distinct curvilinear radiopacity, termed the *dorsal peritoneopericardial mesothelial remnant,* has been identified between the cardiac silhouette and the diaphragm on a lateral thoracic radiograph in cats with PPDH.
5. Ultrasonography is useful because there is often discontinuity of the diaphragmatic outline. Hepatic herniation is usually evident.

IV. Differential Diagnosis

A. The most common differentials for PPDH are pericardial effusion and cardiomegaly.

B. Ultrasound and echocardiography are useful to distinguish these abnormalities from PPDH.

V. Medical Management

A. If the animal is dyspneic, provide oxygen by face mask, nasal insufflation, or an oxygen cage.

B. Position the animal in sternal recumbency with the forelimbs elevated to help ventilation.

VI. Surgical Treatment

A. General Considerations

1. Perform surgical repair as early as possible (generally when the animal is between 8 and 16 weeks of age), when it is unlikely that adhesions will be present and the pliable nature of the skin, muscles, sternum, and rib cage facilitates closure of large defects.
2. Early correction of PPDH may prevent acute decompensation and the potential development of acute postoperative pulmonary edema.

B. Preoperative Management

1. Give prophylactic antibiotics before anesthetic induction in animals with hepatic herniation.
2. Upon repositioning of the liver into the abdominal cavity of animals with hepatic strangulation or vascular compromise, a massive release of toxins into the bloodstream may occur. Premedicating such patients with steroids may be beneficial.

C. Anesthesia

1. See discussion of anesthesia for traumatic DH, p. 567.
2. See Appendix G-26 for examples of selected anesthetic protocols that may be used in animals with diaphragmatic hernias.

D. Positioning

1. Place the animal in dorsal recumbency for a midline abdominal incision.
2. Prepare the entire abdomen and caudal two thirds of the thoracic cavity for aseptic surgery.

E. Surgical Technique

Make a ventral midline abdominal incision. If increased exposure is needed, extend the incision cranially through the sternum. Enlarge the diaphragmatic defect if necessary, and replace the abdominal organs in the abdominal cavity. If adhesions are present, gently dissect the tissues from thoracic structures, resecting or debriding necrotic tissue as necessary. Debride the edges of the defect and close with a simple continuous suture pattern. Do not close the pericardial sac. Remove air from the pericardial sac or pleural cavity following closure of the defect. If continued pneumothorax or effusion is likely, place a chest tube. Repair concomitant sternal or abdominal wall defects.

VII. Suture Materials/Special Instruments

A. For diaphragmatic closure use either a nonabsorbable suture material such as polypropylene or an absorbable material such as polydioxanone (PDS) or polyglyconate (Maxon) suture.

VIII. Postoperative Care and Assessment

A. See discussion of postoperative care for traumatic DH, p. 568.

B. Pulmonary hypoplasia may be present in patients with PPDH, contributing to the development of high intrapleural pressures and RPE.

IX. Prognosis

A. If the animal survives the early postoperative period (i.e., 12 to 24 hours) the prognosis is excellent, and recurrence is uncommon with proper technique.

B. The prognosis is worse in patients with PPDH who have concurrent cardiac abnormalities.

Pneumothorax (*SAS*, pp. 687-691)

I. Definitions

A. **Pneumothorax** is an accumulation of air or gas within the pleural space.

B. **Traumatic pneumothorax** may be classified as either open or closed.
   1. An **open pneumothorax** is one in which there is free communication between the pleural space and the external environment.
   2. With a **closed pneumothorax,** air accumulates because of leakage from the pulmonary parenchyma, bronchial tree, or esophagus.

C. **Tension pneumothorax** occurs when a flap of tissue acts as a one-way valve so that there is a continuous influx of air into the pleural cavity on inspiration that does not return to the lung on expiration.

D. **Spontaneous pneumothorax** occurs because of air leakage from the lung, but without trauma as a precipitating cause.

E. **Cysts** are closed cavities or sacs lined by epithelium and are usually filled with fluid or semisolid material.

F. **Bullae** are nonepithelialized cavities produced by disruption of intraalveolar septa.

G. A **bleb** is a localized collection of air contained within the visceral pleura.

II. General Considerations and Clinically Relevant Pathophysiology

A. Traumatic pneumothorax is the most frequent type of pneumothorax in dogs.
   1. It most often occurs from blunt trauma, which causes parenchymal pulmonary damage to the lung and a closed pneumothorax.
   2. Alternatively, pulmonary parenchyma may be torn as a result of shearing forces on the lung.
   3. Pulmonary trauma occasionally results in subpleural bleb formation, similar to those seen with spontaneous pneumothorax (see following text).

B. Open pneumothorax is less common, but is also frequently due to trauma (e.g., gunshot, bite or stab wounds, lacerations secondary to rib fractures).
   1. Some penetrating injuries are called "sucking chest wounds" because large defects in the chest wall allow an influx of air into the pleural space when the animal inspires.
   2. These large, open chest wounds may allow enough air to enter the pleural space that lung collapse and marked reduction in ventilation occur.
   3. There is a rapid equilibration of atmospheric and intrapleural pressure through the defect, interfering with normal mechanical function of the thoracic bellows, which normally provides the necessary pressure gradient for air exchange.

C. Pneumomediastinum may be associated with pneumothorax; tracheal, bronchial, or esophageal defects; or subcutaneous air migration along fascial planes at the thoracic inlet.

D. Spontaneous pneumothorax occurs in previously healthy animals without antecedent trauma and may be primary (i.e., an absence of underlying pulmonary disease) or secondary (underlying disease is present).

E. Based on the histologic appearance of the pulmonary lesion, both cysts and bullae have been reported in dogs.

1. Primary spontaneous pneumothorax in dogs may be due to rupture of subpleural blebs–remaining lung tissue may appear normal. These blebs are most commonly located in the apices of the lungs.
2. Secondary spontaneous pneumothorax is more common in dogs than the primary form. In these animals, the subpleural blebs are associated with diffuse emphysema or other pulmonary lesions.

III. Diagnosis

A. Clinical Presentation

1. Signalment.
   a. Traumatic pneumothorax is most common in young dogs because they are more likely to be hit by cars or to receive other trauma resulting in pulmonary damage.
   b. For similar reasons, males may be more commonly affected than females.
   c. Traumatic pneumothorax is less common in cats.
   d. Spontaneous pneumothorax usually occurs in large and "deep-chested" breeds; however, it may occur in small dogs.
   e. Dogs of any age and either sex may develop spontaneous pneumothorax.
2. History.
   a. Pneumothorax secondary to trauma usually results in acute dyspnea.
   b. The history of trauma is often unknown, making the differentiation between traumatic and spontaneous pneumothorax difficult.
   c. Although the history of dogs with spontaneous pneumothorax varies depending on underlying etiology, most animals present with an acute history of dyspnea.
   d. Occasionally a chronic cough or fever may be noted.
   e. Recurrence of dyspnea in an animal previously treated for pneumothorax suggests spontaneous rather than traumatic pneumothorax.

B. Physical Examination Findings

1. Most animals with pneumothorax have bilateral disease and present with an acute onset of severe dyspnea.
2. Other evidence of trauma may be evident in animals with trauma-induced pneumothorax.
3. Most animals with pneumothorax exhibit rapid, shallow respirations.
4. If hypoventilation causes hypoxemia the animal may appear cyanotic, and the heart and lung sounds are often muffled dorsally.
5. Dogs are able to tolerate massive pneumothorax by increasing their chest expansion.
6. Respiration becomes ineffectual in animals with tension pneumothorax as the chest becomes barrel-shaped and fixed in maximal extension. This condition is life threatening.
7. Subcutaneous emphysema will occasionally be noted in animals with pneumomediastinum and pneumothorax.
8. The air may migrate from the mediastinal space to the thoracic inlet and be noticeable under the skin over the neck and trunk.

C. Radiography/Ultrasonography

1. Delay thoracic radiographs until after thoracentesis in dyspneic animals.
2. Pneumothorax usually occurs bilaterally in animals because air diffuses through the thin mediastinum and results in large air-filled spaces within the pleural cavity.

3. The most sensitive view is a horizontal-beam, laterally recumbent thoracic radiograph.
4. On a recumbent lateral thoracic radiograph the lungs collapse and retract from the chest wall and the heart usually appears to be elevated from the sternum.
   a. This apparent elevation of the heart is not noticeable on a standing lateral radiograph.
5. Partially collapsed or atelectatic lung lobes appear radiopaque when compared with the air-filled pleural space.
   a. The vascular pattern will not extend to the chest wall as the lungs collapse.
   b. This may be particularly noticeable in the caudal thorax on a ventrodorsal view.
6. Evaluate radiographs carefully for underlying pulmonary disease or associated trauma.
7. Pulmonary blebs found in some animals with spontaneous pneumothorax are seldom visible radiographically.
   a. This is probably because the large blebs have ruptured, causing the pneumothorax.
   b. In such cases, surgical identification of bullae is necessary.
   c. Air-filled bullae may be incidental findings on thoracic radiographs of some animals.
8. Pneumomediastinum is characterized by the ability to visualize thoracic structures (i.e., aorta, thoracic trachea, vena cava, esophagus) that are not usually apparent on thoracic radiographs.

IV. Medical Management

A. Medical management of an animal with pneumothorax consists of initially relieving dyspnea by thoracentesis.

B. If the pleural air accumulates quickly or cannot be effectively managed with needle thoracentesis, place a chest tube.

C. Tube thoracostomy is typically required in animals with spontaneous pneumothorax.

D. Use intermittent or continuous pleural drainage, depending on the speed with which air accumulates.

E. Continuous drainage may cause quicker resolution of pneumothorax in animals with large, traumatic defects.

F. Providing an enriched oxygen environment may be beneficial, particularly in animals with concurrent pulmonary trauma (e.g., pulmonary contusion or hemorrhage).

G. Providing analgesics to animals with fractured ribs or severe soft tissue damage may improve ventilation.

H. Surgical intervention is seldom required in animals with traumatic pneumothorax.
1. Perform thoracentesis as necessary to prevent dyspnea while the pulmonary lesion heals, usually within 3 to 5 days.
2. Recurrence is uncommon.

I. Conversely, animals with spontaneous pneumothorax commonly have recurrent pneumothorax if they are not operated on.

J. Cover an open chest wound immediately with any available material.
   1. Apply a sterile occlusive dressing as soon as possible and evacuate intrapleural air by thoracentesis or tube thoracostomy.

V. Surgical Treatment

A. General Considerations

1. Animals with traumatic pneumothorax seldom require surgery.
2. However, nonsurgical management of spontaneous pneumothorax usually results in a less than satisfactory outcome.
   a. Mechanical pleurodesis of the lungs (see below) may decrease the recurrence of pneumothorax in animals operated on for spontaneous pneumothorax.
   b. Mechanical pleurodesis damages the pleura such that healing results in adherence to the visceral and parietal pleura.
   c. Prevent postoperative pneumothorax and pleural effusion because they will result in separation of the parietal and visceral pleura, precluding adhesion formation.

B. Preoperative Management

1. Perform an ECG and thoracentesis before anesthetic induction.
2. Preoxygenating these animals is often beneficial.
3. Perioperative antibiotics are seldom warranted and may prevent culturing bacteria from infected pulmonary tissue during surgery.

C. Anesthesia

1. Use care when anesthetizing and ventilating animals with pneumothorax or pulmonary bullae.
2. Intermittent positive pressure ventilation (IPPV) may rupture intact bullae or accelerate air leakage from the damaged lung or bronchial tree.
   a. Do not exceed inspiratory pressures of 10 to 12 cm H_2O pressure in these animals until the chest cavity is opened.
   b. Then reevaluate the adequacy of ventilatory pressures.
3. Because IPPV may induce a tension pneumothorax, anticipate immediate treatment (i.e., needle thoracentesis, chest tube placement).
4. **Do not use nitrous oxide** in patients with pneumothorax.
5. See Appendix G-26 for selected anesthetic protocols for use in animals with respiratory dysfunction.

D. Positioning

1. See intercostal thoracotomy or median sternotomy.

E. Surgical Techniques

1. General considerations.
   a. If an underlying pulmonary lesion is readily identified (i.e., pulmonary abscess or neoplasia) and can be localized to one hemithorax, an intercostal thoracotomy allows lobectomy to be performed more readily than from a median sternotomy approach.
   b. However, diffuse, bilateral pulmonary disease with multiple bullae is usually present in dogs with spontaneous pneumothorax. A median sternotomy allows visualization of all lung lobes, in addition to partial resection of any diseased lobes.
   c. Perform mechanical pleurodesis in dogs with spontaneous pneumothorax to decrease recurrence.
   d. In animals with an open pneumothorax, definitive closure of large thoracic wall defects may require mobilization of adjacent muscles to provide an airtight closure.

2. Technique.

Identify and remove diseased lung. If the source of the pleural air is not evident, fill the chest with warmed, sterile saline or water and look for air bubbles when the anesthetist ventilates the animal. If multiple, partial lobectomies are necessary, use an automatic stapling device to decrease operative time. Perform pleural abrasion using a dry gauze sponge. Gently abrade the entire surface of the lung and parietal pleura. Before closure, fill the chest cavity with warmed fluid and look for air bubbles when the animal is ventilated to ensure that there are no further air leaks. Place a chest tube and remove residual air before recovering the animal. Postoperatively, if continuous air leakage is present, or pleural effusion develops, place the animal on a continuous suction device.

VI. Suture Materials/Special Instruments

A. In animals with spontaneous pneumothorax (where multiple pulmonary bullae may be present), stapling devices allow partial lobectomies to be performed rapidly.

B. Continuous suction devices are available commercially, or three-bottle systems can be made.

VII. Postoperative Care and Assessment

A. Observe the animal postoperatively for pain and hypoventilation.

B. Nasal insufflation is beneficial in most patients, but is especially indicated in those with diffuse underlying pulmonary diseases or those in which significant portions of the lung were resected.

C. Consider analgesic therapy in all animals undergoing thoracotomy.

VIII. Prognosis

A. With appropriate monitoring and care, the prognosis is excellent for animals with traumatic pneumothorax in which therapy is initiated before extreme dyspnea or respiratory arrest.

B. In a recent study of dogs with spontaneous pneumothorax, 100% of those treated with needle thoracentesis alone and 81% of those managed with chest tubes had recurrence of pneumothorax.

Chylothorax (*SAS*, pp. 691-698)

I. Definitions

A. **Chyle** is the term used to denote lymphatic fluid arising from the intestine and therefore containing a high quantity of fat.

B. **Chylothorax** is a collection of chyle in the pleural space.

II. General Considerations and Clinically Relevant Pathophysiology

A. In most animals, abnormal flow or pressures within the thoracic duct (TD) are thought to lead to exudation of chyle from intact, but dilated, thoracic lymphatic vessels (known as thoracic lymphangiectasia).

B. These dilated lymphatic vessels may form in response to increased lymphatic flow (from increased hepatic lymph formation), decreased lymphatic drainage into the venous system caused by high venous pressures, or both factors acting simultaneously to increase lymph flows and decrease drainage.

C. Any disease or process that increases systemic venous pressures may cause chylothorax.

D. Trauma is an uncommonly recognized cause of chylothorax in dogs and cats because the TD heals rapidly following injury and within 1 to 2 weeks the effusion resolves without treatment.

E. Possible causes of chylothorax include anterior mediastinal masses (mediastinal lymphosarcoma, thymoma), heart disease, fungal granulomas, venous thrombi, and congenital abnormalities of the TD.

F. It may occur in association with diffuse lymphatic abnormalities including intestinal lymphangiectasia and generalized lymphangiectasia with subcutaneous chyle leakage.

G. In a majority of animals, despite extensive diagnostic workups, the underlying etiology is undetermined (idiopathic chylothorax).

H. Because the treatment of this disease varies considerably depending on underlying etiology, it is imperative that clinicians identify concurrent disease processes before instituting definitive therapy.

III. Diagnosis

A. Clinical Presentation

1. Signalment.
    a. Any breed of dog or cat may be affected; however, a breed predisposition has been suspected in the Afghan hound for a number of years.
    b. Recently, it has been suggested that the Shiba Inu breed may also be predisposed to this disease.
    c. Although Afghan hounds appear to develop this disease when middle-aged, affected Shiba Inus have been less than 1 year old.
    d. Among cats, Oriental breeds (i.e., Siamese and Himalayan) appear to have an increased prevalence.
    e. Chylothorax may affect animals of any age; however, in one study older cats were more likely to develop chylothorax than were young cats.
    f. A sex predisposition has not been identified.
2. History.

a. Coughing is often the first (and occasionally the only) abnormality noted by owners until the animal becomes dyspneic.
   i. Many owners report that they first noticed coughing months before presenting the animal for veterinary care; therefore evaluate animals that cough and do not respond to standard treatment of nonspecific respiratory problems for chylothorax.
   ii. Coughing may be a result of irritation caused by the effusion, or it may be related to the underlying disease process (e.g., cardiomyopathy, thoracic neoplasia).

B. Physical Examination Findings

1. The most common physical examination finding in animals with pleural effusion is dyspnea.
   a. The dyspnea may be marked by a forceful inspiration with delayed expiration, making the animal appear to be holding its breath. This respiratory pattern is particularly noticeable in cats.
2. Increased bronchovesicular sounds may be heard dorsally.
3. Lung sounds may be absent ventrally (usually bilaterally, but occasionally unilaterally).
4. Most animals with chylothorax present with a normal body temperature, unless extremely excited or severely depressed.
5. Additional findings in patients with chylothorax may include muffled heart sounds, depression, anorexia, weight loss, pale mucous membranes, arrhythmias, murmurs, and pericardial effusion.

C. Radiography/Ultrasonography

1. If the animal is not overtly dyspneic, take thoracic radiographs to confirm the diagnosis of pleural fluid.
2. Taking dorsoventral (rather than ventrodorsal) and "standing lateral" radiographic views, minimizing handling, and supplementing oxygen by face mask during the radiographic procedures may help prevent further compromise of respiration.
3. If the animal is not dyspneic and only small amounts of fluid are suspected, ventrodorsal and expiratory views may help delineate the effusion.
4. Radiographic signs associated with pleural effusion include blurring of the cardiac silhouette, interlobar fissure lines, rounding of lung margins at the costophrenic angles, widening of the mediastinum, separation of the lung borders from the thoracic wall, and scalloping of the lung margins at the sternal border.
5. The scalloping of the lung margins may be the earliest radiographic sign of pleural effusion.
6. Perform ultrasonography before fluid removal because the fluid acts as an "acoustic window" enhancing visualization of thoracic structures.
   a. Ultrasonography is used to evaluate cardiac function, valvular lesions and function, congenital cardiac abnormalities, the presence of pericardial effusion, and mediastinal masses.
7. The presence of pleural fluid will often prevent satisfactory radiographic evaluation of the structures of the thoracic cavity.
   a. Because adequate visualization of the entire thorax is necessary to rule out anterior mediastinal masses such as lymphosarcoma or thymoma, retake radiographs following removal of most of the pleural fluid.
   b. In animals with collapsed lung lobes that do not appear to reexpand after removal of pleural fluid, suspect underlying pulmonary parenchymal or pleural disease, such as fibrosing pleuritis.
      i. Although the etiology of the fibrosis is unknown, it apparently can occur subsequent to any prolonged exudative or blood-stained effusion.

ii. Diagnosis of fibrosing pleuritis is difficult. The atelectatic lobes may be confused with metastatic or primary pulmonary neoplasia, lung lobe torsion, or hilar lymphadenopathy.

8. Consider fibrosing pleuritis in animals with persistent dyspnea in the face of minimal pleural fluid.

D. Laboratory Findings

1. Place fluid recovered by thoracentesis in an EDTA tube, rather than a "clot tube," for cytologic examination to allow the performance of cell counts.
2. Although chylous effusions are routinely classified as exudates, the physical characteristics of the fluid may be consistent with a modified transudate.
3. The color varies depending on dietary fat content and the presence of concurrent hemorrhage.
4. The protein content is variable and often inaccurate because of interference of the refractive index by the high lipid content of the fluid.
5. The total nucleated cell count is usually less than 10,000 and consists primarily of small lymphocytes or neutrophils, with lesser numbers of lipid-laden macrophages.
6. Chronic chylous effusions may contain low numbers of small lymphocytes because of the inability of the body to compensate for continued lymphocyte loss.
7. Nondegenerative neutrophils may predominate with prolonged loss of lymphocytes or if multiple therapeutic thoracenteses have induced inflammation.
8. Degenerative neutrophils and sepsis are uncommon findings because of the bacteriostatic effect of fatty acids but can occur iatrogenically from repeated aspirations.
9. To help determine if a pleural effusion is truly chylous, perform comparison of fluid and serum triglyceride levels, Sudan III stain for lipid droplets, or the ether clearance test.
   a. The most diagnostic test is comparison of serum and fluid triglyceride levels.
   b. If the effusion is truly chylous it will contain a higher concentration of triglycerides than simultaneously collected serum.

IV. Differential Diagnosis

A. *Pseudochylous effusion* is a term that has been misused in the veterinary literature to describe effusions that look like chyle, but in which a ruptured TD is not found.

1. Given the known causes of chylothorax in dogs and cats, reserve this term for effusions in which the pleural fluid cholesterol is greater than the serum cholesterol concentration and the pleural fluid triglyceride is less than or equal to the serum triglyceride.
2. Pseudochylous effusions are extremely rare in veterinary patients, but may be associated with tuberculosis.

V. Medical Management

A. If an underlying disease is diagnosed, treat it and manage the chylous effusion by intermittent thoracentesis.

B. If the underlying disease is effectively treated the effusion often resolves; however, complete resolution may take several months.

C. Consider surgical intervention only in animals with idiopathic chylothorax or those that do not respond to medical management.

D. Place chest tubes only in those animals with suspected chylothorax secondary to trauma (very rare), with rapid fluid accumulation, or following surgery.

E. Monitor electrolytes, because hyponatremia and hyperkalemia have also been documented in dogs with chylothorax undergoing multiple thoracentesis.

F. A low-fat diet may decrease the amount of fat in the effusion, which may improve the animal's ability to resorb fluid from the thoracic cavity.

G. Commercial low-fat diets are preferable to homemade diets; however, if commercial diets are refused, homemade diets are a reasonable alternative (*SAS,* Tables 27-10 and 27-11).

H. Medium-chain triglycerides (once thought to be absorbed directly into the portal system, bypassing the TD) are transported via the TD of dogs. Thus they may be less useful than previously believed.

I. It is unlikely that dietary therapy will cure this disease, but it may help in the management of animals with chronic chylothorax.

J. Inform clients that with the idiopathic form of this disease there is no effective treatment that will stop the effusion in all animals.

K. However, the condition may spontaneously resolve in some animals after several weeks or months.

L. Whether benzopyrone drugs might be effective in decreasing pleural effusion in animals with chylothorax is unknown; however, preliminary findings suggest that greater than 25% of animals treated with Rutin (50-100 mg/kg PO, TID) had complete resolution of their effusion 2 months after initiation of therapy.

M. Whether the effusion resolved spontaneously in these animals or was associated with the drug therapy requires further study.

VI. Surgical Treatment

A. General Considerations

1. Surgical intervention may be warranted in animals that do not have underlying disease and in whom medical management has become impractical or is ineffective.
2. Surgical options in animals that do not have severe fibrosing pleuritis include mesenteric lymphangiography and TD ligation, active pleuroperitoneal or pleurovenous shunting, and pleurodesis (the latter is not recommended by the author).
3. Thoracic duct ligation.
   a. The mechanism by which TD ligation is purported to work is that

following TD ligation abdominal lymphaticovenous anastomoses form for the transport of chyle to the venous system.

b. Unfortunately, TD ligation results in complete resolution of pleural effusion in only about 50% of animals operated on.
c. The advantage of TD ligation is that, if it is successful, it results in complete resolution of pleural fluid (as compared with palliative procedures such as passive or active pleuroperitoneal shunting).
d. Disadvantages include a long operative time (problematic in debilitated animals), a high incidence of continued or recurrent chylous or nonchylous (from pulmonary lymphatics) effusion, and the fact that mesenteric lymphangiography may be difficult to perform (particularly in cats).
e. Without mesenteric lymphangiography, complete ligation of the TD cannot be ensured; however, this technique may not be uniformly successful in verifying complete ligation of the TD.
f. Some small branches of the TD system may be present and yet not fill with dye during lymphangiography.

B. Preoperative Management

1. Withhold food 12 hours before surgery.
2. Feed cream or oil 3 to 4 hours before surgery to help visualize lymphatics, or inject methylene blue into a lymph node at surgery.

C. Anesthesia

1. Refer to Appendix G-26 for selected anesthetic protocols for animals with respiratory disease.

D. Surgical Anatomy

1. The TD is the cranial continuation of the cisterna chyli and is generally said to begin between the crura of the diaphragm.
2. In cats the TD lies between the aorta and azygous vein on the left side of the mediastinum.
3. In dogs, it lies on the right side of the mediastinum until it reaches the fifth or sixth thoracic vertebra, then crosses to the left side.
4. The TD terminates in the venous system of the neck (left external jugular vein or jugulo-subclavian angle).

E. Positioning

1. If a thoracic approach to the TD is used, prepare the left side (cats) or right side (dogs) of the thorax and abdomen for aseptic surgery.
2. If a transdiaphragmatic approach is used, prepare the cranial abdomen and caudal chest.

F. Surgical Techniques

1. Mesenteric lymphangiography.

For a thoracic approach, make a paracostal incision (or for a transdiaphragmatic approach, make a cranial midline abdominal incision), exteriorize the cecum, and locate an adjacent lymph node. If necessary, inject a small volume (0.5 to 1 ml) of methylene blue into the lymph node to increase lymphatic visualization. Avoid repeated doses of methylene blue because of the risk of inducing a Heinz body anemia or renal failure. Find a lymphatic near the node to catheterize by gently dissecting the mesentery. Cannulate the lymphatic with a 20- or 22-gauge over-the-needle catheter and attach a three-way catheter and extension tubing (filled with heparinized saline) to the catheter with a suture (3-0 silk). Place an additional suture around the extension tubing and through a segment of intestine to prevent dislodgement of the catheter. Dilute 1 ml/kg of a water-soluble contrast agent (e.g., Renovist) with 0.5 ml/kg of sterile saline. Inject this mixture into the catheter and take a lateral thoracic radiograph while the last ml is being flushed into the catheter. Use this lymphangiogram to help

identify the number and location of branches of the TD that need to be ligated. Repeat the lymphangiogram following TD ligation (see below) to identify branches that were not occluded. Embolization of the TD with cyanoacrylate injected through a mesenteric lymphatic catheter has been reported in dogs. Advantages of TD embolization are that direct visualization of the TD is not required, which negates the need for a thoracotomy or diaphragmatic incision. Disadvantages of this procedure are the same as those for mesenteric lymphangiography and TD ligation (i.e., not all TD branches may fill with the cyanoacrylate mixture and collateralization may occur past the obstruction).

2. Thoracic duct ligation.

Perform an intercostal thoracotomy (right side for dogs, left side for cats) at the eighth, ninth, or tenth intercostal space or make an incision in the diaphragm (see note above). Locate the TD and use hemostatic clips or silk (2-0 or 3-0) suture to ligate it. Visualization of the TD can be aided by injecting methylene blue into the lymphatic catheter.

G. Active Pleuroperitoneal or Pleurovenous Shunting

1. General considerations.
   a. Commercially made shunt catheters are available and can be used to pump pleural fluid into the abdomen or into a vein (e.g., jugular, azygous, caudal vena cava).
   b. Two types of shunts are available: a pleuroperitoneal shunt and an ascites (peritoneovenous) shunt.
      i. The latter is meant to pump fluid from the abdomen into a vein and does not require manual pumping (i.e., it acts in an active fashion).
      ii. This shunt can be placed from the pleural space into a vein (pleurovenous); when used in this manner, manual pumping is required (the shunt will not act in an active fashion).
      iii. A potential complication of pleurovenous shunt placement is formation of a right atrial or ventricular thrombus. This complication may be life threatening; therefore pleuroperitoneal shunting is preferred if there is no reason to believe that the animal may not reabsorb the fluid from its abdominal cavity (e.g., presence of diffuse lymphatic disease or cardiac disease).
   c. Observe these patients closely for several weeks following pleurovenous shunt placement, and use preoperative heparinization and maintenance on heparin, aspirin, or other anticoagulants if necessary.
   d. Both types of catheters are placed under general anesthesia.
2. Technique.

Place the pump chamber and tubing in a bowl of sterilized, heparinized saline. Prime the pump by compressing the valve repeatedly until the system is filled with fluid and flow is established. Expel any remaining air bubbles from the tubing or valve. Make a vertical incision over the middle of the sixth, seventh, or eighth rib. Bluntly insert the pleural end of the shunt catheter into the thoracic cavity. For a pleuroperitoneal shunt, create a tunnel under the external abdominal oblique muscle using blunt dissection and pull the pump chamber through the tunnel. Place the efferent (peritoneal) end of the catheter into the abdominal cavity just caudal to the costal arch through a small skin incision and a preplaced purse-string suture in the abdominal musculature. For a pleurovenous shunt, tunnel the efferent (venous) end of the catheter over the shoulder to the ventral cervical region. Make a small incision over the jugular vein and insert the venous end of the catheter into the vein. Using fluoroscopy, place the distal end of the catheter at the caudal aspect of the cranial vena cava, just proximal to the right atrium (the venous end of the catheter may be

shortened if necessary). Alternatively, the venous end of the catheter may be placed in the azygous or caudal vena cava through an abdominal incision. Make sure that the pump chamber overlies a rib so that the chamber can be effectively compressed.

VII. Suture Materials/Special Instruments

A. The advantage of using hemoclips is that they can be used as a reference point on subsequent radiographs if further ligation is necessary.

B. However, it is best to also ligate the duct with nonabsorbable suture (i.e., silk) if hemoclips are used.

C. Ordering information for products and supplies (e.g., butterfly catheter; methylene blue, USP 1%; Surflo catheter; Renovist contrast agent; isobutyl 2-cyanocrylate; and hemoclips [medium]) for lymphangiography or TD ligation is provided in the Product Appendix of *Small Animal Surgery*.

D. Shunts for active drainage include Denver double-valve peritoneous and pleuroperitoneal shunts.

VIII. Postoperative Care and Assessment

A. If chylothorax resolves spontaneously or after surgery, periodic reevaluation for several years are warranted to detect recurrence.

B. Fibrosing pleuritis is the most common, serious complication of chronic chylothorax.

C. Immunosuppression may occur in patients undergoing repeated and frequent thoracentesis because of lymphocyte depletion.

IX. Prognosis

A. This condition may resolve spontaneously or following surgery.

B. Untreated or chronic chylothorax may result in severe fibrosing pleuritis and persistent dyspnea.

C. Euthanasia is frequently performed in animals that do not respond to surgery or medical management.

Pyothorax (*SAS*, pp. 698-701)

I. Definitions

A. **Pyothorax** is a suppurative inflammation of the thoracic cavity with resultant accumulation of pus.

II. General Considerations and Clinically Relevant Pathophysiology

A. The route by which the thoracic cavity becomes infected is usually not evident.

B. Exclude immunosuppressive diseases in animals with pyothorax, although there is no evidence that development of pyothorax requires debilitation or an increased susceptibility to infection.

C. Multiple organisms are often cultured from animals with pyothorax; there is, however, a high incidence of obligate anaerobic infections as sole pathogens.

D. Obligate anaerobic infections or gram-positive filamentous organisms (*Nocardia* and *Actinomyces*) are frequently cultured from dogs with pyothorax; obligate anaerobes and *Pasteurella* spp. are the most common isolates in cats.

III. Diagnosis

A. Clinical Presentation

1. Signalment.
   a. There is no breed predisposition, and pyothorax may occur in animals of any age; however, young male cats that fight and receive chest wounds are at increased risk.
   b. Similarly, adult, large-breed dogs (particularly hunting dogs) may be affected because they often inhale plant foreign material and suffer penetrating thoracic wounds.
2. History.
   a. A delay of several weeks between the trauma that induced the pyothorax and the onset of clinical signs is not uncommon.
   b. Most animals are presented for evaluation of respiratory distress, anorexia, or both.

B. Physical Examination Findings

1. Affected animals usually have a restrictive respiratory pattern (i.e., rapid, shallow respirations), and many are febrile.
2. Additional findings in patients with pyothorax may include depression, anorexia, weight loss, dehydration, muffled heart and lung sounds, and pale mucous membranes.
3. The chest wall may seem incompressible in cats with thoracic effusion.

C. Radiography

1. Thoracic radiographs usually diagnose pleural effusion.
2. The cause of the pyothorax is seldom apparent radiographically; however, increased density in the thoracic cavity following thoracentesis may indicate an abscess or foreign body.
3. Consolidated lung lobes that do not reexpand following fluid removal may be indicative of fibrosing pleuritis or lung lobe torsion.

D. Laboratory Findings

1. Neurtrophilia (with or without a degenerative left shift) may be present on a complete blood cell count.

2. Fluid analysis is necessary to differentiate pyothorax from other exudative effusions.
   a. The fluid can range from amber to red or white in color.
   b. Protein content is usually greater than 3.5 g/dl, and the fluid appears turbid or opaque because of the high nucleated cell count.
   c. Nucleated cells consist primarily of degenerative neutrophils, but nondegenerative neutrophils can predominate, depending on the causative agent.
   d. Effusions associated with fungi and higher bacterial agents such as *Actinomyces* and *Nocardia* are often characterized cytologically by nondegenerative neutrophils and macrophages, or they may appear hemorrhagic.
   e. Macrophages and reactive mesothelial cells are present in purulent effusions in variable numbers depending on the cause and the chronicity of the fluid.
   f. Occasionally, fungal elements may be noted in the pleural effusion of animals with fungal disease involving the pulmonary parenchyma.
3. Positive cultures may not be obtained in all animals with pyothorax, particularly if anaerobic organisms are present.

IV. Medical Management

A. Although the cause of the effusion is often not discernible, find and correct, if possible, underlying diseases.

B. Management of these animals must be aggressive.

C. Following diagnosis, place a chest tube.

1. Perform lavage two to three times daily.
   a. Use isotonic fluid, such as saline or lactated Ringer's solution (warmed to room temperature), at a dosage of 20 ml/kg body weight.
   b. Leave the fluid in the thoracic cavity for 1 hour and then remove.
   c. Addition of antibiotics to the lavage fluid offers no advantage over the use of appropriate systemic antibiotics.
   d. The use of proteolytic enzymes is controversial and is no longer recommended by most authors.
   e. The addition of heparin (1500 units/100 ml of lavage) appears beneficial.
   f. Lavage may be required for 5 to 7 days.

D. Base systemic antibiotic therapy on results of microbial culture and sensitivity testing.

1. Prevalence of anaerobic infections is high (see above). Use antibiotics with an anaerobic spectrum (e.g., penicillins or penicillin derivatives, clindamycin, metronidazole) for a minimum of 4 to 6 weeks.
2. Recommended antibiotics for *Actinomyces* and *Nocardia* infections are provided in Table 27-1.

V. Surgical Treatment

A. General Considerations

1. Surgery is indicated in animals that have underlying disease (e.g., lung abscess, lung lobe torsion, foreign body) and in those that do not respond to medical management in 3 to 4 days.

Table 27-1
Selected antibiotics*

Actinomyces:
Ampicillin†
20-40 mg/kg IM, SC, PO or IV, QID
Nocardia:
Trimethoprim-sulfadiazine (Tribrissen)‡
45 mg/kg PO, BID **or**
Amikacin
30 mg/kg IV or SC, SID

*Treat for a minimum of 6 weeks.
†May not be effective against L-phase variants.
‡Observe for side effects (e.g., anemia, thrombocytopenia, keratoconjunctivitis sicca).

2. If the pyothorax is chronic or localized, or if the patient remains dyspneic in the absence of significant volumes of pleural fluid, fibrosing pleuritis may be present.
3. Decortication may be warranted in such patients.

B. Preoperative Management

1. Perform thoracentesis before induction if the animal is dyspneic.
2. Correct hydration and electrolyte and acid–base abnormalities before surgery.

C. Anesthesia

1. Refer to anesthetic management of animals with respiratory impairment in Appendix G-26.

D. Surgical Technique

Approach the thorax via an intercostal thoracotomy if an abnormality can be localized to one hemithorax, or median sternotomy if localization is not possible. Explore the thoracic cavity for abscesses, foreign bodies, or other abnormalities, and remove affected tissues. If possible, remove fibrin covering the lung tissues. Submit appropriate samples for microbiological examination and culture. Place a chest tube for postoperative lavage. Before closure, lavage the thoracic cavity with warmed, sterile saline solution.

VI. Suture Materials/Special Instruments

A. Do not use braided, nonabsorbable, multifilament suture for lobectomy or partial lobectomy in these patients.

B. Absorbable suture (polydioxanone, polyglyconate) is preferred in the presence of infection.

VII. Postoperative Care and Assessment

A. Continue thoracic lavage after surgery until the infection resolves.

B. Monitor serum protein and electrolytes (i.e., potassium) and continue fluid therapy until the animal is eating and drinking normally.

C. Continue antibiotic therapy for 4 to 6 weeks.

D. Refer to the postoperative management of animals undergoing thoracotomy procedures for additional recommendations.

VIII. Prognosis

A. The prognosis for most animals with pyothorax is good if they are managed as described previously.

B. Recurrence is common in animals treated with antibiotics only (i.e., without thoracic lavage).

C. Long-standing empyema may resorb leaving a pleural "peel," which is a thick sheet of fibroblasts and inflammatory cells attached to the visceral pleura.
   1. This pleural peel may inhibit normal expansion of lung tissue (fibrosing pleuritis).
   2. If multiple lung lobes are fibrosed and cannot expand normally, the prognosis may be poor.

D. Decortication is recommended if lung entrapment is suspected.
   1. Decortication is best performed once the empyema is mature, but before it adheres to the pleura and becomes vascularized.

Thymomas and Thymic Branchial Cysts (*SAS*, pp. 701-704)

I. Definitions

A. **Thymomas** are tumors that arise from epithelial tissues of the thymus.

B. **Thymic branchial cysts** develop from vestiges of the fetal branchial arch system.

II. General Considerations and Clinically Relevant Pathophysiology

A. Masses in the mediastinum of dogs and cats are usually neoplastic, although abscesses, granulomas, and cysts are occasionally found.

B. Lymphoma is the most common cranial mediastinal tumor in dogs and cats.

C. Other tumors occasionally found here include thymomas, chemodectomas (aortic and carotid body tumors), and ectopic thyroid and parathyroid tumors.

D. Thymomas are the most common surgically treatable neoplasm of the cranial mediastinum in dogs–most are benign. However, because histological appearance of the tumor correlates poorly with clinical behavior, the terms *invasive* and *noninvasive* are frequently used.
   1. Stage I (noninvasive) thymomas are well circumscribed and do not extend beyond the thymic capsule.
   2. Others may extend beyond the capsule locally or may invade surrounding organs or metastasize to other thoracic or extrathoracic structures.
   3. The clinical signs associated with thymomas may be due to occupation of space, a paraneoplastic syndrome, or both.
   4. As thymomas enlarge they may cause respiratory distress by compressing the lungs or trachea or inducing pleural effusion.
   5. Effusions associated with thymomas may be serosanguineous or chylous.
   6. Nearly 50% of thymomas in dogs are associated with myasthenia gravis (MG).
      a. Myasthenia gravis is an autoimmune neuromuscular disorder that is characterized by muscular weakness.
      b. The weakness is due to a deficiency of functional acetylcholine receptors in the neuromuscular postsynaptic membrane caused by autoantibodies that bind to and block the receptors.
   7. Other paraneoplastic syndromes associated with thymomas are nonthymic cancer and polymyositis.
   8. As thymomas enlarge they may compress the cranial vena cava and other cranial thoracic vessels, causing edema of the head, neck, or forelimbs (cranial vena cava syndrome).

E. Thymic branchial cysts develop from vestiges of the branchial arch system of the fetus.
   1. They may be found in the subcutaneous tissues of the neck or in the thymus.
   2. Rupture of these cysts may result in a chronic inflammatory reaction and abscessation.

III. Diagnosis

A. Clinical Presentation

1. Signalment.
   a. The average age of dogs with thymoma is 8 to 9 years; however, it has been reported in dogs as young as 3 years of age.
   b. Large-breed dogs, particularly German shepherds, golden retrievers, and Labrador retrievers, are more commonly affected than small dogs.
   c. A sex predisposition has not been identified.
   d. Most cats with thymomas have been greater than 8 years of age.
   e. Thymic branchial cysts also occur most commonly in middle-age to older animals.
2. History.
   a. Dogs with thymomas may present for evaluation of dyspnea, coughing, weight loss, lethargy, dysphagia, muscle weakness, vomiting or regurgitation, excessive salivation, or neck edema.
   b. The onset of clinical signs may be acute despite relatively slow tumor enlargement.
   c. Lethargy, anorexia, dyspnea, and pleural effusion are common in cats with thymoma.

d. Occasionally, thymomas are fortuitous findings on thoracic radiographs of asymptomatic animals.
e. Clinical findings in dogs and cats with thymic branchial cysts are similar to those in animals with thymomas.
f. Most are presented for evaluation of progressive dyspnea.
g. Lameness and swelling of the head, neck, and forelimbs are also common.

B. Physical Examination Findings

1. Clinical findings in dogs with thymomas vary among patients.
2. Respiratory abnormalities caused by pleural effusion or aspiration pneumonia may be the predominant finding.
3. Other animals may present for generalized exertional weakness without evidence of respiratory problems.
4. Occasionally, localized forms of myasthenia are found where the weakness is limited to the esophagus, larynx or pharynx, or facial musculature.
5. The most common clinical findings in dogs and cats with thymic branchial cysts are dyspnea and pleural effusion.

C. Radiography/Ultrasonography

1. Dogs with mediastinal masses may have dorsal elevation of the trachea and caudal displacement of the heart on lateral thoracic radiographs.
2. On the ventrodorsal view the mediastinum may appear widened and the heart may be deviated laterally.
3. Pleural effusion is commonly associated with invasive tumors, and pneumothorax is rare.
4. Megaesophagus or secondary aspiration pneumonia may be noted on thoracic radiographs.
5. Ultrasonography is often helpful in ruling out extrathoracic metastasis.

D. Laboratory Findings

1. Specific laboratory abnormalities are not found with thymoma or branchial cysts.
2. Leukocytosis may be present if the animal has aspiration pneumonia.
3. Pleural effusion associated with thymoma or thymic branchial cysts may contain mature lymphocytes; however, the presence of immature lymphocytes indicates lymphoma.
4. Both lymphoma and thymoma may cause chylous effusions.

IV. Medical Management

A. If aspiration pneumonia is present, treat the dog with appropriate antibiotics before surgery.

B. Dogs with megaesophagus sometimes benefit from being fed in an upright position.

C. Perform thoracentesis to remove pleural effusion and provide an oxygen-enriched environment if the animal is dyspneic.

D. Anticholinesterase (pyridostigmine bromide) or corticosteroid therapy may benefit dogs with megaesophagus or weakness secondary to MG.

E. Provide fluid therapy and correct electrolyte abnormalities in animals with severe or frequent regurgitation.

F. Radiation therapy may reduce clinical signs in some animals with thymomas.

V. Surgical Treatment

A. General Considerations

1. Long-term survival without thymectomy (up to 3 years) has been reported in dogs with thymomas.
2. Surgical removal of stage I or stage II thymomas may be indicated.
3. Concurrent MG makes therapy of thymoma more difficult.
4. Surgical removal of thymic branchial cysts is indicated.

B. Preoperative Management

1. Resolve aspiration pneumonia before surgery and treat severe muscle weakness.
2. Before anesthetic induction, remove excess pleural fluid and correct fluid and electrolyte abnormalities.

C. Anesthesia

1. Refer to Appendix G-26 for recommendations for anesthetic management of patients undergoing thoracotomy procedures.
2. Avoid neuromuscular blocking agents (atracurium, pancuronium) in patients with MG.
3. Intubate patients with megaesophagus while positioned sternally, rather than laterally.

D. Surgical Anatomy

1. The thymus is bordered dorsally by the cranial vena cava and trachea.
2. It is closely associated with many smaller blood vessels (e.g., branches of the brachycephalic trunk and internal thoracic arteries), which often require ligation during thymectomy.
3. The phrenic nerve is closely associated with the dorsal border of the thymus.

E. Positioning

1. Depending on surgical approach chosen, prepare either the left thorax or ventral thorax for aseptic surgery.

F. Surgical Techniques

1. General considerations.
   a. Perform thymectomy through a left third or fourth space intercostal thoracotomy if the tumor is small, or a cranial median sternotomy.
      i. If the mass is large, a median sternotomy approach allows improved visualization of surrounding structures such as the cranial vena cava.
   b. Small encapsulated thymomas can usually be removed without difficulty, but cytoreduction is often all that is possible with large, invasive tumors.
   c. Thymomas are often friable and occasionally cystic; handle them with care to avoid seeding the thoracic cavity with tumor cells.
   d. Thymic branchial cysts appear as multilobulated masses containing numerous cysts on transverse section.
2. Technique.

Explore the thoracic cavity for evidence of metastasis. Identify the cranial vena cava and other associated vessels. Locate the phrenic nerve and attempt

to preserve it, if possible. Ligate small vessels and bluntly dissect the mass and its capsule from surrounding tissues. Try to maintain the integrity of the thymic capsule where possible. If complete removal of the mass is not possible, remove as much as can safely be excised. Submit tissues for histologic examination. Place a chest tube before thoracic closure.

VI. Suture Materials/Special Instruments

A. Electrocautery is useful when removing thymomas and other vascular neoplasms.

VII. Postoperative Care and Assessment

A. Animals with thymomas are at great risk to aspirate during the postoperative period; position them with their heads elevated to decrease the risk.

B. Additionally, suction the pharynx before extubation and extubate with the cuff slightly inflated to decrease the risk of aspiration if there has been passive regurgitation during the surgical procedure.

C. Observe the animal for hemorrhage and pneumothorax postoperatively.

D. Adjuvant radiation therapy may be beneficial in animals with invasive tumors that cannot be completely excised.

E. Observe the animal closely for development of paraneoplastic disease following therapy.

F. With thymomas, remove the chest tube within 24 hours if hemorrhage and pneumothorax do not occur.

G. Longer-term tube thoracostomy may be necessary in animals with thymic branchial cysts if rupture of a cyst has caused pleuritis.

VIII. Prognosis

A. The prognosis depends on the invasiveness of the tumor, its size at the time of diagnosis, and the presence or absence of paraneoplastic disease.

B. The prognosis for thymic branchial cysts and noninvasive thymomas is good.

C. If paraneoplastic syndromes are present, the prognosis is guarded.

PART

Orthopedics

28

Fundamentals of Orthopedic Surgery and Fracture Management (*SAS*, pp. 705-765)

Preoperative Concerns (*SAS*, pp. 705-706)

I. Elective Surgery

A. Evaluate younger patients by physical examination and screening laboratory tests, including PCV, serum total solids, and urinalysis.

B. Consider complete blood count and chemistry profile for older patients.

C. Order special diagnostic tests (e.g., coagulation profile) depending on history, signalment, and physical findings.

II. Emergency Surgery

A. An external blow severe enough to disrupt musculoskeletal integrity often injures other organs.
  1. Reevaluate the patient periodically.
  2. Listen to the chest, take thoracic radiographs, and perform an electrocardiogram to detect cardiac and pulmonary injury.
  3. Assess minimum database results before surgery.

B. Abnormalities may necessitate delay of surgical repair or alter the prognosis.

Preoperative Coaptation (*SAS*, pp. 706-708)

I. General Considerations

A. Reduce further injury and increase patient comfort with coaptation of unstable injuries.

B. Use external splints to provide temporary limb support or primary fracture stabilization.

C. Properly apply and carefully monitor external splints to prevent complications.
1. Manage fractures or luxations below the elbow or stifle with a soft padded bandage, with or without a splint.
2. Place a spica splint for fractures above the elbow or stifle joint.

II. Robert Jones Bandages

A. The thick cotton layer provides mild compression of soft tissues and immobilizes fractures without causing vascular compromise.

B. Should extend from the toes to the midfemur or midhumerus.

C. **Use only for injuries below the stifle or elbow joint.**

Prepare the limb by clipping long hair from the midhumerus (midfemur) to the toes, and treat any open wounds. Apply adhesive tape stirrups to cranial and caudal surfaces of the foot from carpus (tarsus) to 6 inches beyond the toes. Wrap 3 to 6 inches of cotton padding (from a 12-inch roll or cast padding) around the limb from toes to midhumerus (midfemur). Ensure that the nails of the third and fourth digits are visible so that limb swelling can be detected. Then wrap elastic gauze firmly over the cotton to compress it. Apply at least two to three layers of gauze to achieve smooth, even tension. Sufficient compression will cause the bandage to sound like a ripe watermelon when tapped with a finger. Invert the tape stirrups and stick them to the outer layer of gauze. Then apply elastic tape (e.g., Elasticon or Vetrap) to the outer surface of the bandage.

III. Metal Spoon Splints

A. Provide support to injuries of the distal radius and ulna, carpus or tarsus, metacarpus or metatarsus, or phalanges.

B. Use to support internal fixation device or as a primary means of fixation when a fracture is expected to heal rapidly with minimal stress.

Clip long hair and treat open wounds before covering them with a sterile dressing. Apply adhesive tape stirrups from the carpus (tarsus) to toes, leaving the ends extending 6 inches beyond the toes. Firmly apply cast padding around the limb in a spiral fashion with a 50% overlap. Begin the padding at the toes and extend it proximally 1 inch beyond the proximal aspect of the splint. Apply just enough cotton to prevent skin abrasions and pressure sores, but do not make the bandage so bulky that it will be awkward for the patient. Cover bony prominences with excess padding. Wrap elastic gauze over the cotton to compress it. Place the padded limb in an appropriate-sized splint and secure it to the limb with Vetrap or elastic adhesive tape. Invert and stick the stirrups to the final wrapping.

IV. Spica Splints

A. Use to temporarily immobilize humeral or femoral fractures or as added stabilization after internal fixation; rarely used as a primary means of stabilization.

Clip long hair, and treat open wounds before covering them with a sterile dressing. Place adhesive tape stirrups on the medial and lateral surface of the limb, and apply cotton cast padding to the limb and torso. Begin the padding at the paw and wrap it proximally in a spiral fashion, overlapping it 50%. When the inguinal or axillary region is reached, wrap the cotton padding around the animal's torso several times alternating cranially and caudally to the affected limb. Next wrap elastic gauze over the cast padding (i.e., 50% overlap). Wrap the gauze firmly around the limb to mildly compress the soft tissues. Reinforce the spica bandage with fiberglass casting material to provide additional stabilization of the fracture ends. Fold the casting tape onto itself to provide a lateral splint that is four to six layers thick, extending from toes to dorsal midline. Use Vetrap or elastic adhesive tape to hold the fiberglass cast to the limb and provide an outer covering for the splint.

V. Postoperative Care of Coaptation Devices

A. Observe toes twice a day for swelling, and limb for swelling or discharge.

B. Keep bandage clean and dry.

Anesthesia (*SAS*, p. 708)

I. Considerations

A. Select from a variety of anesthetic protocols for healthy patients (Appendix G-28).

B. Anesthetize patients with acute traumatic injuries or systemic disease with care.

C. Perform an ECG and thoracic radiographs, and correct hypovolemia before surgery.

D. Give analgesics before surgery based on level of postoperative discomfort expected (Appendix F).

1. Remember, analgesics are most effective when administered before painful stimuli.
2. Administer as part of the preoperative medication and for 12 to 24 hours after surgery.
    a. Use butorphanol or buprenorphine for minimally painful procedures.
    b. Use oxymorphone or morphine for more painful procedures.
    c. Opioid epidurals can supplement systemic opioid analgesia (Appendixes D and E).
        i. For surgery of the rear quarters use oxymorphone, buprenorphine, or morphine epidurally.
        ii. For surgery of the thoracic limb use morphine epidurally.

iii. Adjust the systemic opioid premedication to account for the epidural (calculate total patient dose and divide between systemic and epidural administration).

Antibiotics (*SAS*, pp. 708-709)

I. Prophylactic Antibiotics

A. Administer in contaminated cases, cases with severe trauma, and cases requiring lengthy operative times (2 hours or longer).

B. Consider using them in elective procedures in which postoperative infection would be catastrophic (e.g., hip replacement). See Chapter 10 for general prophylactic antibiotic recommendations.

C. Select the appropriate antibiotics and time the administration.
1. Identify the microorganisms most likely to cause orthopedic wound infections.
   a. Coagulase-positive *Staphylococcus* spp. and *Escherichia coli* are the predominant aerobic bacteria isolated from surgical wounds.
   b. Anaerobic bacteria (e.g., *Bacteroides, Fusobacterium,* and *Clostridium* spp.) are now recognized as important pathogens in orthopedic patients.
   c. Periodically culture surgical tables, instrument stands, and surgical lights to provide insight into potential bacteria in the surgical environment.
2. Know which antibiotics are most likely effective against potential microorganisms.
   a. Cefazolin (20 mg/kg IV) is the antibiotic of choice for prophylaxis in small animal orthopedic surgery.
   b. **The antibiotic must be present within tissues at the time bacteria enter the wound to effectively suppress bacterial growth.**
   c. Administer the antibiotic intravenously at the time of anesthetic induction, repeat every 2 to 4 hours, and discontinue at completion of surgery.

II. Antimicrobial Therapy for Bone Infections

A. The traditional belief that bone infections are difficult to treat because antibiotics exhibit poor bone penetration is invalid.

B. Factors important in treatment of bone infection are fracture stability, presence of surgical implants, and ability of bacteria to colonize inanimate biomaterials.
1. Matrix and serum proteins coat implants. Bacteria possess cell membrane receptors for the matrix protein fibronectin, facilitating adhesion of microorganisms to implant surfaces.
2. Bacteria adhered to biomaterials produce a biofilm composed of polysaccharides, ions, and nutrients, which enhances adherence of bacteria and protects them from host defenses.
3. Beta-lactams (penicillins, cephalosporins) and aminoglycosides readily traverse capillary membranes in bone and are widely distributed in bone interstitial fluid. (See Chapter 23 for treatment of osteomyelitis.)

Bone Healing (*SAS*, pp. 709-716)

I. Blood Supply

A. Repair processes during fracture healing are dependent on an adequate blood supply.

B. Normal circulation of bones.
1. Circulation consists of an afferent supply from the principal nutrient artery, proximal and distal metaphyseal arteries, and periosteal arteries that enter bone at areas of heavy fascial attachment.
2. Blood flows through the diaphysis from medullary canal to periosteum. Under normal conditions, medullary pressure probably restricts periosteal blood flow to the outer third of the cortex.
3. Immature animals have numerous arteries that perforate newly formed appositional bone running longitudinally over the periosteal surface.
4. Separate blood supplies feed the metaphysis and epiphysis.
   a. Interruption of the epiphyseal blood supply results in the death of growing cells and cessation of physeal function.
   b. Interruption of metaphyseal blood flow delays endochondral ossification, resulting in widening of the cartilaginous physis. When circulation is reestablished, endochondral ossification resumes.
5. Flat bones with extensive muscle attachment (i.e., pelvis and scapula) have tremendous extraosseous blood supply in addition to that provided by nutrient arteries.
6. Irregular bones (e.g., carpal and tarsal bones) generally have multiple nutrient arteries.

C. Disruption of blood supply.
1. Most long bone fractures disrupt medullary circulation.
2. A transient extraosseous vascular supply develops to nourish the early periosteal callus.
3. Medullary blood supply is reestablished and extraosseous circulation diminishes as bone healing progresses and stability is restored.

D. Effects of types of fracture reduction and fixation on blood supply.
1. Closed fracture reduction and application of casts or external fixators causes the least disruption to surrounding soft tissues and newly formed extraosseous blood supply.
2. Open reduction disturbs developing extraosseous blood vessels and hinders reestablishment of medullary blood flow.
3. Intramedullary pins disrupt medullary vasculature.
   a. Pins that contact endosteal surfaces block medullary afferent flow.
   b. Stable implants allow new medullary circulation to develop, which supplies the adjacent endosteal surfaces.
4. Cerclage wire applied tightly to cortical surfaces does not significantly impair vasculature.
5. Plate and screw application affords the greatest fracture stability and allows early reformation of medullary circulation.
   a. Plates impair blood supply to outer cortical bone beneath the plates, causing affected cortices to remodel and become more porous.
   b. Newer plate designs (e.g., limited-contact dynamic compression plates) minimize blood supply impairment.
6. Motion of loose implants, especially cerclage wires, disrupts developing vasculature.

E. Blood supply to bone fragments.
   1. Minimally disturbed fracture fragments revascularize and incorporate into callus when major bone segments are stabilized with a plate or external fixator.

II. Types of Bone Healing

A. Indirect Bone Healing

1. This type occurs in fractures with an unstable mechanical environment resulting from the motion of the adjacent bones.
2. Motion at fracture sites affects interfragmentary strain between fragments.
   a. **Strain** is the ratio between the change in gap width to the total gap width.
      i. Excessive strain results in tissue rupture.
      ii. Fragment end resorption increases the width of gaps, decreasing strain.
      iii. Strain decreases with increased fracture rigidity as fractures are bridged by less strain-tolerant tissues.
   b. Decreased motion occurs at fracture sites when external or periosteal callus is produced because increasing the tissue diameter increases the bone's ability to resist bending.
3. Progression of indirect bone healing.
   a. Gaps are initially bridged by tissues that withstand motion (hematoma and granulation tissue). Tissues that increase the bone's rigidity (fibrous connective tissue, fibrocartilage, lamellar bone) replace them. Then fibrocartilage mineralization begins at the fragment surfaces and continues toward the gap center, forming trabecular and woven bone.
   b. Local resorption of initial bone occurs, followed by vascularization of resorption cavities and replacement with lamellar bone, resulting in remodeling of bony callus to cortical bone.

B. Direct Bone Healing

1. Bone forms directly at fracture sites, without an intermediate cartilage stage, when fixation devices maintain absolute fragment stability.
   a. There must be no fracture motion.
   b. Fragments must be in contact or separated by only small (i.e., 150- to 300-μm) gaps.
2. **Gap healing** is direct bone formation in small gaps after rigid fixation.
   a. Gaps initially fill with a network of fibrous bone.
   b. Haversian remodeling begins replacing the mechanically weak fibrous bone within 7 to 8 weeks.
3. Fragments in contact under rigid fixation undergo simultaneous union and reconstruction with haversian remodeling.
4. Haversian remodeling begins with osteoclastic resorption of bone and formation of resorption cavities that penetrate longitudinally through fragment ends and newly formed bone in fracture gaps. The osteoclasts are followed by vascular loops, mesenchymal cells, and osteoblast precursors. Osteoblasts line resorption cavities and secrete osteoid, which is mineralized to bone. This lamellar bone is arranged along the bone's long axis, through the fragment ends and fracture gaps, and results in a strong union of bone fragments.

C. Distraction Osteogenesis

1. Accomplish by application of gradual traction to cortical bone so that sufficient stress is created to stimulate and maintain formation of new bone.

a. Osteoid is laid down in parallel columns that extend from osteotomy surfaces centrally. Lamellar bone develops within the columns.
b. If there is sufficient instability at the fracture site, formation of an intermediate cartilaginous phase may occur.
2. Use with external fixation techniques for limb lengthening, treatment of angular deformities, and transportation of cortical bone.
3. General considerations.
a. Preserve medullary and periosteal blood supply after corticotomy or osteotomy, and stabilize major bone fragments.
b. Ideal distraction rate is 1 mm per day divided into two to four distraction periods.
c. Keep the fixator in place to allow remodeling of new cortical bone after the desired limb length is achieved.

D. Metaphyseal Fractures

1. The fractures heal differently than fractures through cortical bone, because trabecular bone is more stable.
2. They do not heal by periosteal callus formation unless there is tremendous instability.
3. New bone deposits on existing trabeculae, and fracture gaps are filled with woven bone. Bridging between trabeculae occurs before union of the cortical shell.

III. Radiographic Appearance of Bone Healing

A. Assess fracture alignment and implant position with postoperative radiographs.

B. Repeat radiographs every 4 to 6 weeks during healing.
1. Periosteal callus indicates indirect bone formation is occurring.
2. Filling of stable fracture lines with bone indicates direct healing.
3. Trabecular bone healing in metaphyseal fractures appears radiographically as the formation of one or two dense bands at the fracture site. Gradual bridging of these bands occurs until finally the cortical shell is completely spanned by bone.

C. Fixation removal decisions.
1. General considerations.
a. Make decisions after evaluating radiographs of healing fractures.
b. Know the radiographic appearance of bone healing associated with various fixation systems in order to make wise decisions regarding timing of removal.
c. In general, remove fixation systems when there is radiographic evidence of bone bridging the fractures.
d. Casts.
i. Remove casts once the callus has bridged the fracture.
(a) Bridging periosteal and endosteal callus form because of indirect bone formation.
(b) Distal radial and ulnar fractures in toy breeds generally do not produce large amounts of callus.
e. External fixators (EFs).
i. Remove fixators after fracture lines have bridged with bone.
ii. Spectrum of healing ranges from direct to indirect bone healing.
iii. Callus formation.
(a) Rigid stabilization produces little callus; poor fracture

reduction or stabilization produces resorption of bone at fracture lines and callus formation.

(b) In general, EFs produce less periosteal callus formation than casts.

(c) EFs develop more endosteal and uniting callus than periosteal callus.

f. Pins and wires.

i. Remove pins once bone has bridged the fracture.

ii. Do not remove wires unless they cause problems (e.g., migration, interference with fracture healing).

iii. Pins and wires heal by direct bone union if the fracture is rigidly stabilized, or by indirect if unstable.

g. Plates and screws.

i. Wait 6 to 12 months after surgery for implant removal to allow adequate time for bone remodeling.

ii. These fracture heal by direct bone union.

iii. Fracture lines disappear and fractures appear devoid of bridging periosteal and endosteal callus.

iv. Implant acts as buttress to support the fracture during haversian remodeling.

h. Healing of comminuted fractures.

i. Healing depends on how well the biologic environment is preserved and on the rigidity of the fixation.

ii. In severely comminuted fractures, preservation of the biologic environment is often best accomplished with closed reduction or limited exposure and rigid fixation (e.g., external fixators or bridging plates).

iii. Fractures treated by this method heal with endosteal bone formation and bone bridging between fragments, with minimal periosteal callus formation.

Postoperative Care and Assessment (*SAS*, pp. 716-717)

I. Physical Therapy

A. Cold Therapy

1. Use cold therapy in the acute phase of injury or during the first 2 to 3 days after surgery.
2. Controls swelling and provides analgesia.
3. Apply cold packs to the area for 20 minutes three times a day.

B. Heat Therapy

1. Use hot compresses in the chronic phase of healing.
2. Decreases pain and improves circulation.
3. Relaxes muscles before beginning passive physical manipulation.
4. Does not decrease swelling and should not be used in the initial 3 to 4 days after surgery.
5. Heat is most easily applied with moist, hot towels. Avoid scalding the skin.

C. Passive Physiotherapy

1. Involves controlled stretching of muscles, tendons, and ligaments by

2 to 3 minutes of gentle flexion and extension of the joint above or below the area in question.

2. Effective in maintaining joint motion and patient comfort but does not enhance muscle tone and strength; therefore combine with active physical therapy.

D. Active Physical Therapy

1. Allow or help the patient to stand on the operated limb for 1 to 2 minutes during the first postoperative week.
2. Gradually increase the duration of weight bearing until the patient begins to bear weight on the operated limb without coaching.
3. Encourage slow leash walking immediately after surgery.
4. Swimming, beginning with 2 to 3 minutes per session, is excellent active therapy.

II. Bandages

A. Use padded soft bandages, Ehmer slings, Velpeau slings, and 90/90 slings for postoperative comfort and soft tissue compression or immobilization.

1. Ehmer sling.
   a. General considerations.
      i. The sling prevents weight bearing by the pelvic limb.
      ii. Use it to support closed or open reduction of hip luxations.
   b. Application.

Place a thin layer of cast padding around the metatarsal area, and wrap nonadherent gauze (Kling) multiple times over the padding. Maximally flex the stifle and wrap the gauze around the thigh by bringing it medially between the body wall and limb. Pull the gauze firmly and bring it over the front of the knee to maintain flexion. Then wrap the gauze over the lateral surface of the thigh and bring it distally medial to the tarsus and over the padded metatarsal area. Repeat the wrapping three to four times. Finish the bandage by applying elastic adhesive material in the same manner.

2. Velpeau sling.
   a. General considerations.
      i. The sling prevents weight bearing and provides some stability to the proximal forelimb.
      ii. Use to help maintain closed or open reduction of medial shoulder luxations and support scapular fractures.
   b. Application.

With the shoulder and elbow flexed and the limb adducted against the body wall, begin by placing two to three layers of padding around the torso and limb. Wrap layers cranial and caudal to the opposite limb to prevent slippage of the incorporated limb. Place an additional layer in a similar manner with gauze (Kling) to add mild compression. Last, place an outer layer of elastic tape or Vetrap to provide support.

3. 90/90 sling.
   a. General considerations.
      i. The sling provides flexion of the stifle joint and immobilizes the pelvic limb after surgery.
      ii. Use after repair of a distal femoral physeal fracture, to prevent quadriceps contracture.

b. Application.

Place the stifle joint and tarsus in 90-degree flexion. Using cast padding, wrap several layers of padding around the metatarsus area. Wrap elastic adhesive around the flexed tarsus and stifle joints to maintain 90 degrees of flexion.

Complications (*SAS*, pp. 717-718)

I. Nonunions

A. Diagnose by radiographic evidence that bone healing is not occurring.

B. Most nonunions are a result of poor fixation selection or technique.

C. Vascular nonunions.
1. Radiographic appearance is a lucent line through fractures, representing cartilage and fibrous tissue, coupled with callus formation.
2. Vascular nonunions result from inadequate fracture stability. Constant motion at fracture sites prevents cartilage mineralization. Rigid immobilization of fractures with either plates or external fixators usually allows fracture healing to progress.
3. Hypertrophic nonunions (i.e., vascular nonunions with large amounts of callus).
   a. Treat by removal of loose implants, joint alignment, and placement of stable fixation (compression plate).
   b. Cancellous bone grafts may be used; however, the hypertrophic callus usually provides adequate cancellous bone for healing.
   c. Swab for bacterial culture and sensitivity.
   d. If osteomyelitis is present, treat by removing any large pieces of necrotic cortical bone and filling defects with cancellous bone autografts, which may be placed during the plating procedure or after 5 to 7 days of open wound management.
   e. Remove plates after healing occurs in infected nonunions because plates may serve as a nidus for continued infection.

D. Avascular nonunions.
1. Atrophic nonunions are biologically inactive pseudoarthroses.
2. Observe no radiographic evidence of bone reaction, and bone ends appear sclerotic.
3. Histologically, fracture gaps are filled with fibrous tissue and medullary cavities are sealed with cortical bone.
4. Perform surgery to remove fibrous tissues, open medullary canals, and place stable fixation (usually a plate) and cancellous bone grafts.

II. Delayed Unions

A. Delayed unions are fractures that unite more slowly than anticipated.

B. Treat patients with intact implants by confinement of the patient.

Reoperation is not necessary; however, cancellous bone grafts may be added to speed healing.

C. Remove loose or migrating implants, and place stable fixation placed along with cancellous bone autografts.

III. Malunions

A. Malunions are healed fractures in which anatomic bone alignment was not achieved.
   1. Malunions may adversely affect function and precipitate osteoarthritis in adjacent joints.

B. Angular deformities.
   1. Angular deformities are characterized by loss of correct parallel relationships between joints above and below the fractured bone.
   2. Classify as valgus, varus, antecurvatum, or recurvatum.

C. Translational and rotational deformities.
   1. Rotation of femoral fractures may adversely affect hip function.

D. Shortening of affected bones.
   1. Extension of adjacent joints compensates for shortened bone in a single bone system (femur, humerus).
   2. Shortening of a single bone in a paired bone system (radius/ulna, tibia/fibula) causes incongruity in alignment of adjacent joints.

E. Treat malunions with corrective osteotomy if it adversely affects the ability to ambulate.

Special Age Considerations (*SAS*, p. 718)

I. Physeal Fractures

A. Thirty percent of fractures in immature animals occur at the physis.

B. Damage to the hypertrophic zone heals rapidly by continued growth of physeal cartilage and metaphyseal callus formation. Once fracture gaps fill, normal endochondral ossification resumes and physeal function continues.

C. With damage to growing cells (i.e., reserve and proliferating zones), growth of physeal cartilage does not occur; instead, endochondral ossification proceeds bone formation in fracture gaps results in premature physeal closure.

D. Malalignment of the fractured physis allows trabecular bone healing and physeal bridging.

Orthopedic Examination (*SAS*, pp. 719-730)

Problem Identification (*SAS*, pp. 719-722)

I. Signalment and History

A. Use signalment and history to develop a list of differentials, since many orthopedic diseases are predictable within age groups and breeds (Table 28-1).

B. Obtain a complete history to provide clues from which to form a differential list.

II. Physical Examination

A. Evaluate general health before anesthetizing any animal for orthopedic disease.

B. Perform thoracic radiographs and serial electrocardiograms on traumatized animals presenting for fracture evaluation. Evaluation of the abdominal cavity is done initially with palpation and evaluation of serum chemistry tests.

III. General Orthopedic Examination

A. Allow the animal to walk around the examination room and observe for obvious lameness and for more subtle signs, such as reducing the weight placed on the affected limb when standing or sitting.

B. Observe for unilateral or bilateral muscle atrophy and abnormal muscle development.

C. Observe while walking and trotting, preferably outdoors.
   1. Animals quickly shift their weight from the affected limb, making it appear that they are landing heavily on the opposite, or "good," limb.
   2. With forelimb lameness the head will lift after the lame limb strikes the ground.
   3. A short stride occurs with decreased range of motion in a diseased joint.
   4. External swinging occurs when advancing a limb that cannot be adequately flexed.
   5. With bilateral lameness the signs may be subtle (e.g., shifting weight from limb to limb while standing, shortened stride, or bilateral muscle atrophy).

Table 28-1
Differential diagnoses for lameness

Signalment	History	Differential diagnosis
Immature, large dogs Front limb	Acute	Fractured physis* Fractured bone*
	Chronic	OCD shoulder OCD elbow UAP elbow FCP elbow Premature closure of physes Elbow incongruity Retained cartilage cores Panosteitis Hypertrophic osteodystrophy
Immature, large dogs Rear limb	Acute	Fractured physis* Fractured bone*
	Chronic	Hip dysplasia OCD stifle Patellar luxation Avulsion of long digital extensor tendon OCD hock Panosteitis Hypertrophic osteodystrophy
Immature, small dogs Front limb	Acute	Fractured physis Fractured bone
	Chronic	Congenital luxation—shoulder Congenital luxation—elbow Premature closure of physes Atlantoaxial instability
Immature, small dogs Rear limb	Acute	Fractured physis Fractured bone
	Chronic	Avascular necrosis femoral head Patellar luxation*
Adult, large dogs Front limb	Acute	Fractured bone* Luxated shoulder* Luxated elbow*
	Chronic	Degenerative joint disease* Panosteitis Bicipital tenosynovitis Contracture infraspinatus tendon Radius curvus/elbow incongruity Bone/soft tissue neoplasia* Brachial plexus injury* Cervical disk disease Inflammatory joint disease*

*Denotes potential differential diagnoses in cats.

D. Palpation and neurologic exam.
   1. Perform examination without sedation, if possible (Appendix M).
   2. Follow a consistent evaluation pattern.
   3. Begin by examining a sound limb to identify the individual's normal response to manipulation and pressure.
   4. Perform initial examination with the animal standing, to assess muscular symmetry, joint enlargement, and proprioceptive responses.
   5. Note asymmetry (between limbs), response to pain, swelling,

Table 28-1
Differential diagnoses for lameness—cont'd

Signalment	History	Differential diagnosis
Adult, large dogs Rear limb	Acute	Fractured bone* Luxated hip* Luxated stifle* Cruciate/meniscus syndrome* Ruptured Achilles tendon*
	Chronic	Degenerative joint disease* Panosteitis Patellar luxation Cruciate/meniscus syndrome* Bone/soft tissue neoplasia* Lumbosacral syndrome Thoracolumbar disk disease Inflammatory joint disease*
Adult, small dogs Front limb	Acute	Fractured bone Luxated shoulder Luxated elbow
	Chronic	Degenerative joint disease Luxating shoulder Bone/soft tissue neoplasia Inflammatory joint disease Radius curvus/elbow incongruity Cervical disk disease
Adult, small dogs Rear limb	Acute	Fractured bone Luxated hip Luxated stifle Cruciate/meniscus syndrome
	Chronic	Degenerative joint disease Patellar luxation Cruciate/meniscus syndrome Bone/soft tissue neoplasia Lumbosacral syndrome Thoracolumbar disk disease Inflammatory joint disease

abnormalities in range of motion, instability, and crepitation as each bone, joint, and soft tissue area is palpated.

Forelimb (*SAS*, pp. 722-724)

I. Below Carpus

Examine the paw closely for foreign material. Inspect the webbing and pads. Palpate each digit for swelling and to determine if the bones are intact. Extend and flex the phalangeal joints and palpate the corresponding extensor and flexor tendons to see if they relax and tighten appropriately. Test the lateral and medial stability of each joint in extension. Palpate the areas adjacent to the metacarpal pad and over the palmar sesamoids of metacarpophalangeal joints 2 and 5 for sensitivity to pressure. Palpate the metacarpal bones for swelling or instability.

II. Carpus

Palpate the dorsal surface of the carpus gently to determine if there is fluctuant swelling associated with joint effusion. Compare the affected limb with the opposite carpus. May be more easily noted with animal standing. (Note: Bilateral swelling may occur with some diseases, such as rheumatoid arthritis.) Extend and flex the carpus. Maximum extension is about 180 to 190 degrees; maximum flexion about 45 degrees. A decreased range of motion may indicate degenerative joint disease. Note any crepitation. Extend and stress the carpus in the medial to lateral plane to determine if there is joint instability.

III. Radius

Palpate the radius for instability (fracture), swelling (fracture, tumor), and pain response to deep bone palpation (panosteitis).

IV. Elbow

Palpate the elbow for fluctuant swelling in the space between the lateral condyle and over the medial coronoid process. Effusion results from many diseases. May be more easily detected when the animal is standing. Firm swelling indicates degenerative joint disease. Flex and extend the elbow. Normal extension and flexion are about 165 degrees and 40 degrees to 50 degrees, respectively. The carpus should almost touch the shoulder when the elbow is flexed. Decreased range of motion suggests degenerative joint disease, which may occur secondary to a fragmented coronoid process, an ununited anconeal process, or osteochondritis dissecans. While the elbow is in extension, check the integrity of the collateral ligaments by applying medial and lateral force to the radius and ulna.

V. Humerus

Palpate for instability (fracture), swelling (fracture, tumor), and pain response to deep palpation (panosteitis). Palpate in areas not covered by muscles, to differentiate panosteitis from muscular pain.

VI. Shoulder

Move the shoulder through a range of motion, including hyperextension and hyperflexion while stabilizing the scapula. Osteochondritis dissecans of the humeral head elicits a pain response when the shoulder is hyperextended. Hold the acromial process stationary and mobilize the humeral head to detect luxation or subluxation. Many shoulder joints pop or click without significance. Palpate the biceps tendon and apply pressure. A painful response indicates tenosynovitis.

VII. Scapula

Palpate the scapula for instability (fracture) and swelling (fracture, tumor). Palpate the muscle over the scapula and compare it with the opposite side to determine atrophy secondary to disuse or nerve injury. Probe the axillary area for swellings and observe for signs of pain. This can be indicative of a nerve root tumor.

Rear Limb (*SAS*, pp. 724-728)

I. Below Tarsus

A. See the procedure below for carpus in the forelimb section.

II. Hock

Palpate the tarsal joints for fluctuant swelling indicative of joint effusion. May be more easily noted when the animal is standing. Firm swelling suggests degenerative joint disease. Extend and flex the hock. Normal flexion is about 45 degrees. Decreased flexion indicates degenerative joint disease, which may be secondary to osteochondritis dissecans. Pain on manipulation of the joint may indicate a fracture. Extend, adduct, and abduct the hock and metacarpal bones to demonstrate instability of the collateral ligaments. With the stifle in extension and the hock stressed into flexion, palpate the Achilles tendon. Rupture of the entire tendon complex allows hock flexion while the stifle is extended. Rupture of the gastrocnemius tendon and common tendon of the biceps femoris, gracilis, and semitendinous muscles, with preservation of the superficial digital flexor, allows partial flexion of the hock while the stifle is extended and causes simultaneous flexion of the digits.

III. Tibia

Palpate the tibia for instability (fracture), swelling (fracture, tumor), and pain in response to deep bone palpation (panosteitis).

IV. Stifle

With the animal standing, simultaneously palpate both stifles to detect swelling. Swelling usually indicates degenerative joint disease. The patellar ligament becomes less distinct with effusion and the medial aspect of the stifle enlarges.

V. Patella

Extend and flex the stifle while holding one hand over the cranial aspect of the joint to detect crepitation. Extend the stifle, internally rotate the foot, and apply digital pressure in an attempt to displace the patella medially. Slightly flex the stifle, externally rotate the foot, and apply digital pressure to attempt to displace the patella laterally.

VI. Collateral Ligaments

Test their integrity by holding the stifle in full extension and attempting to open the stifle on the medial and lateral aspects. If the stifle is allowed to flex, it may feel as though there is lateral laxity.

VII. Cruciate Ligaments

Test their integrity by trying to elicit a cranial or caudal drawer motion. Immature animals have slight drawer motion, but it stops abruptly as the ligament tightens. To elicit direct drawer motion, place the index finger and thumb of one hand over the patella and lateral fabellar regions, respectively. Place the index finger of the opposite hand on the tibial tuberosity and, with the thumb positioned caudal to the fibular head, slightly flex the stifle. Stabilize the femur, and gently move the tibia cranial and distal to the femur. Do not allow tibial rotation. If the muscles are tense, they may prevent this motion. If this occurs, gently flex and extend the stifle to relax the animal, and repeat the procedure. Test drawer motion with the femur flexed and extended. If the patella is luxated, replace it in the trochlear groove before attempting the drawer motion. Perform the tibial compression test to detect indirect drawer motion. Detect forward motion of the tibia by placing the index finger along the patella and the tibial tuberosity. With the leg in a standing position, flex the hock to tense the gastrocnemius muscle. This compresses the femur and tibia together, causing the tibia to move forward in a cranial cruciate deficient stifle. Sedate large or tense animals to elicit drawer motion, if necessary. Minimal drawer motion may occur with chronic cruciate pathology resulting from fibrosis. Minimal or partial drawer motion also occurs with incomplete tears or stretching. Drawer motion is evident with a torn caudal cruciate ligament. To identify caudal drawer motion, start with the stifle in a neutral position.

VIII. Meniscus

A. Most tears are identified during exploratory arthrotomy. Try to feel a click or pop as the stifle is flexed and extended.

IX. Femur

Palpate the femur for instability (fracture), swelling (fracture, tumor), and pain in response to deep bone palpation (panosteitis).

X. Hip

Extend and flex the hip while a hand is placed over the greater trochanter to detect crepitation. The femur should extend caudally almost parallel to the pelvis, and the stifle should approach the ilium with full flexion. Degenerative joint disease limits the range of motion and may induce pain.

XI. Hip Luxation

In the standing animal, compare the distance from the greater trochanter to the tuber ischium bilaterally. A unilateral increase in that distance indicates hip luxation. Externally rotate the femur while placing the thumb in the space caudal to the greater trochanter; displacement of the thumb should occur. With hip luxation, the trochanter rolls over the thumb.

XII. Hip Laxity

Perform the evaluation under sedation, if possible. With the animal in lateral recumbency, perform the Ortolani maneuver. Grasp the stifle with one hand and hold it parallel with the table surface. Place the other hand over the dorsal pelvis and adduct and push the stifle toward the pelvis. With joint laxity, the hip will subluxate. Maintain the pressure and abduct the stifle. As the femoral head returns to the acetabulum, use the hand stabilizing the pelvis to detect a click. Alternatively, perform the evaluation with the animal in dorsal recumbency, with the stifles held parallel to each other and perpendicular to the table. Apply downward pressure on the stifle to subluxate the hip. Maintain pressure and abduct the stifle. With laxity, a click is noted as the femoral head returns to the acetabulum. The angle of subluxation is the point at which the hip luxates, and the angle of reduction is the point at which the femoral head returns to the acetabulum.

XIII. Pelvis

Examine the pelvic region for evidence of fracture (asymmetry, instability, swelling, crepitation, bruising, or pain). Consider taking radiographs, because they are superior to physical exam for identifying fractures of the pelvis. Perform a rectal examination.

XIV. Neurologic Examination

Perform a complete neurologic examination to differentiate orthopedic from neurologic disease. Evaluate conscious proprioception in all four limbs by gently supporting the animal and individually turning each paw until the dorsal surface of the paw contacts the ground. Normal animals return the paw to the correct position almost immediately. Loss of conscious proprioception usually indicates neurologic disease, but the same lack of response is found with a painful

fractured limb. Differentiate lumbosacral from hip pain. Apply direct pressure on the ventral lumbar musculature to isolate lumbosacral pain. Check for peripheral nerve damage by applying pressure to digits of the affected limb to elicit a response to superficial and deep pain.

Diagnostic Imaging (*SAS*, pp. 728-729)

I. Radiographs

A. Radiographs are essential for a definitive diagnosis and for evaluating fracture healing.

B. Achieve correct patient positioning, and take at least two radiographic views.

C. Use chemical restraint when necessary.

II. Bone Scintigraphy

A. Intravenously administered bone-seeking radiolabeled compound (e.g., technetium-99m linked to methylene diphosphonate) incorporates into actively metabolizing bone over a period of hours and can be visualized with gamma camera scanning.

B. Increased bone turnover may indicate a bone abnormality.

C. Use to pinpoint an obscure lameness in which the origin cannot be identified with physical examination or by radiographs.

III. Computed Tomography

A. Consists of multiple radiographs reconstructed using a computer.

B. Computed tomography (CT) is superior to plain radiographs in identifying neoplastic bone margins, stenosis of the spinal column, small bone fragments within a joint, and bone bridging within a physis.

IV. Magnetic Resonance Imaging

A. Magnetic resonance imaging (MRI) provides superior soft tissue definition, but it does not provide bone detail.

B. Functions by analyzing the energy emitted by hydrogen atoms in tissues subjected to a pulsating magnetic field.

C. MRI is superior in identifying central nervous system changes, including spinal cord compression, and soft tissue components of joints.

Decision Making in Fracture Management (*SAS*, pp. 730-733)

Fracture-Assessment Score (*SAS*, pp. 730-733)

I. General Considerations

A. Consider mechanical, biologic, and clinical parameters, in addition to fracture configuration, when selecting an implant system.

B. Score ranges from 1 to 10. The lower end of the scale represents factors that do not favor rapid bone union and return to function, whereas the upper end of the scale represents those factors that favor rapid bone union and return to function.

II. Mechanical Factors

A. Assessment of these factors estimates stress applied to implant and implant bone interfaces.
   1. Factors include the number of limbs injured, patient size and activity, and ability to achieve load-sharing fixation between the bony column and the implant.
   2. Lower-end score is assigned for injury to multiple limbs, preexisting lameness in another limb, large or active patients, and loads transmitted from bone segment to bone segment through implants rather than through the bony column.

III. Biologic Factors

A. Assessment of these factors estimates length of time implants must be functional.
   1. Factors include age and general health of the patient, degree of soft-tissue injury, degree of comminution, location of injury, whether the injury is closed or open, and whether open reduction is required.
   2. Obtaining desired reduction and stability with minimal soft tissue manipulation and operative time allows greater success than with longer surgeries in which reduction and stability are obtained at the expense of significant soft tissue manipulation.
   3. **Bridging osteosynthesis** is a fracture-management technique in which minimal or no manipulation of the soft tissue envelope is done.

IV. Clinical Factors

A. Assessment of these factors considers the willingness and ability of clients to attend to their pet's postoperative needs, anticipated patient cooperation following surgery, and postoperative limb function.

B. Avoid stabilization systems requiring postoperative maintenance (e.g., external coaptation or external skeletal fixations) with clients unable or unwilling to care for them.

C. Avoid selecting very active, uncontrollable patients as candidates for external stabilization.

D. Weigh patient's ability to cope with discomfort and estimated time to bone union.

Fracture-Assessment Score Interpretation (*SAS*, pp. 732-733)

I. Low Scores (0 to 3)

A. Implants must have sufficient strength to prevent permanent bending or cyclic breakage.

B. Use lengthening bone plates, bone plate/IM rod combinations, bone plate/external skeletal fixator combinations, type II or type III external skeletal fixators, and external skeletal fixator/IM pin combinations.

C. Use implants that purchase bone with raised threads.

II. Midscale Scores (4 to 7)

A. Less implant strength and endurance are required than in patients with low assessment scores because of either immediate load sharing or early callus formation.

B. Use bone plates, type I or type II external skeletal fixators, IM pin/external skeletal fixator combinations, or IM pin/cerclage wire combinations.

C. Use implants with raised threads or combination of thread and friction purchase.

III. High Scores (8 to 10)

A. Strength, stiffness, and length of function of the implant need not be extreme.

B. Use type I external skeletal fixators with smooth transfixation pins, IM pin/cerclage wires, and external coaptation.

C. Use implants that hold bone through friction to provide adequate bone purchase.

Fracture Fixation Systems (*SAS*, pp. 733-756)

External Coaptation—Casts (*SAS*, pp. 733-735)

I. Indications

A. Use casts as a primary means of stabilization or as a supplement to internal fixation devices.

B. Casts are most useful in stable fractures.

C. Use only for fractures of the distal limb.

II. Cast Materials

A. Classic casting material is plaster of paris.

B. Synthetic casts made of fiberglass or polyester fabric impregnated with water-activated polyurethane resin have considerable advantages over plaster casts (i.e., they are lighter, more comfortable, and dry well if they accidentally become wet).

III. Application

A. Apply under general anesthesia to allow fracture reduction.

Suspend the limb using adhesive stirrups applied to the medial and lateral limb surface. If the fractured bone ends cannot be reasonably reduced (i.e., varus-valgus and rotational alignment are maintained with at least 50% contact of major fragment ends), perform surgery. Clip long hair and apply a single layer of cast stockinette onto the limb over the stirrups. Temporarily release the limb to apply the stockinette (alternatively, apply it before reducing the fracture). Extend the stockinette from the toes to 2 inches above the estimated proximal extent of the cast. Fit the stockinette snugly against the limb; do not allow the excess material to fold on itself or wrinkle. Apply cast padding in a spiral fashion to the limb from the toes to the estimated proximal extent of the cast, overlapping the material 50%. Use sufficient cast padding to protect the limb from developing cast sores, but not too much to prevent the cast from resting snugly against and conforming to the limb. Generally, cast padding should be only two layers thick. Place extra padding over bony prominences, if desired. Place a layer of gauze over the cast padding, wrapping from the toes proximally. Immerse the casting tape into cold water, squeeze excess water gently from the roll, and apply it to the limb, beginning at the toes. Wrap the cast material in a similar fashion as the cast padding (i.e., 50% overlap). Encompass the toes, but leave the nails of the third and fourth phalanges exposed, to allow limb swelling to be detected. As the cast tape is applied above the elbow or stifle, use firm pressure to compress the larger muscles and conform the cast to the limb. Use

two layers of cast tape with 50% overlap (i.e., four layers on cross section) in small and medium dogs and three layers (six on cross section) in larger dogs (i.e., more than 30 kg). Apply the cast tape quickly because it will set in 4 to 6 minutes. Before the cast tape sets, roll the edges of the cast outward by pulling the proximal aspect of the stockinette over the end of the cast. Apply elastic adhesive or Vetrap around the cast and stick the stirrups to this layer. Next, fashion a walking bar of aluminum rod into a U shape and tape it to the bottom of the cast so that the animal does not bear weight directly on the cast. Direct weight bearing may cause the cast material to erode, causing abrasions on the dorsal paw.

IV. Cast Removal

A. An oscillating saw is required for cast removal, and sedation facilitates removal.

B. Cut the medial and lateral sides of the cast, and separate the two halves.

C. Avoid frequent removal of a cast used for fracture stabilization, because anatomic fracture reduction may be lost.

D. Bivalve the full cast on initial application if frequent removal is anticipated.
   1. Use the oscillating saw to cut the medial and lateral walls.
   2. Tape the two halves securely with three to four layers of adhesive tape.

V. Postoperative Care

A. Evaluate 24 hours following application and weekly thereafter.

B. Instruct clients to observe the toes daily for evidence of swelling (i.e., spreading of the exposed digits) and to watch for excessive chewing or licking at the cast or a foul odor. Any of these signs require that the animal be evaluated immediately.

C. Keep the cast clean and free of moisture.

D. Change a cast on a growing animal every 2 weeks; with an adult the cast may last 4 to 6 weeks.

External Skeletal Fixators (*SAS*, pp. 735-742)

I. Indications

A. Use external skeletal fixators to stabilize fractures, for joint arthrodesis, and to temporarily immobilize a joint.

II. Equipment/Supplies

A. Transfixation Pins

1. Half pin vs. full pin.
   a. Half pins penetrate both cortices but only one skin surface.
   b. Full pins penetrate both cortices and skin surfaces.
2. Threaded vs. nonthreaded.
   a. Nonthreaded transfixation pins have smooth shafts (e.g., Steinmann IM pins).
   b. Completely threaded pins are weak and tend to break.
   c. Centrally threaded pins are used as full pins with type II or type III external fixator frames.
   d. End-threaded pins are often described according to the number of cortices to be engaged by the threads (i.e., one-cortex or two-cortex end-threaded pins).
      i. One-cortex end-threaded pins engage only the far cortex.
      ii. Two-cortex end-threaded pins have sufficient thread length to engage both cortices.
   e. Thread profile (e.g., negative or positive).
      i. With negative profile pins the core diameter of the threaded section is smaller than the diameter of the smooth section.
      ii. With positive profile pins the core diameter is consistent between smooth and threaded regions.
   f. Thread height and thread pitch are specifically designed to engage dense cortical bone or spongy cancellous bone.

B. External Connectors

1. Materials.
   a. Stainless steel is used for small and medium Kirschner rods.
   b. Aluminum is used for large Kirschner rods.
   c. Acrylic can be used to fashion an external fixator and linkage devices. Use either commercial kits or the polymethylmethacrylate derived from dental acrylic or hoof-repair acrylic.

C. Linkage Devices (Clamps, Pin Grippers)

1. They connect transfixation pins to the external bar.
2. Consist of a single clamp through which the external bar and transfixation pin are placed.

III. Application

A. Apply external fixators to create a stable pin-bone interface.
   1. Stable pin-bone interfaces have fewer fixator-related complications (i.e., pin loosening).
   2. Use stronger fixators when there is a lower patient fracture-assessment score (and vice versa).
   3. Err on the side of increased strength and stiffness rather than on the side of too little, because an overly rigid frame can always be disassembled to a less rigid frame as healing progresses.

B. Fixator configuration.
   1. Apply more or larger external connecting bars to increase strength and stiffness.
   2. Use connecting bars on more than one side for increased strength and stiffness.

a. Classification system of configurations.
   i. Type Ia is unilateral-uniplanar.
   ii. Type Ib is unilateral-biplanar.
   iii. Type II is bilateral-uniplanar.
   iv. Type III is bilateral-biplanar.
   v. Tie-in configuration connects external fixator with an IM pin.

C. Transfixation pin placement.
1. More pins per fragment, up to four, means a more stable fixator. More than four provides negligible additional mechanical advantage.
2. Lower fracture-assessment scores require more pins, whereas higher scores require fewer pins.
3. Place three to four pins in each major fragment when using type I frames, and two to four transfixation pins when applying a type II or type III frame.
4. Use the largest pin diameter that does not exceed 20% of the bone diameter in order to minimize micromotion at the pin-bone interface.
5. Power drill transfixation pins at low revolutions per minute (rpm).
6. Consider predrilling dense bone with a drill bit 0.1 to 1 mm smaller than the transfixation pin's core diameter.
7. Place one pin 2 cm proximal and one pin 2 cm distal to the fracture.
8. Place the most proximal and distal pins in the respective metaphyses, and space the remaining pins evenly in the proximal and distal fragments.
9. Use threaded pins for fixators that will need to remain in place longer (i.e., low patient fracture-assessment score) in order to increase the length of time the bone-pin interface remains stable.

D. Causes of transfixation pin loosening.
1. Micromotion.
2. Thermal or mechanical damage caused by pin insertion.
3. Fatigue failure of the cortex where pin and bone contact.

E. Pin insertion technique.
1. Adhere to the principles of aseptic surgical technique.
2. Optimal technique for pin insertion is controversial; currently preferred technique is direct insertion of pins with a slow-speed drill, or placement of pins with a hand chuck or slow-speed drill after predrilling the bone with a twist drill bit.
3. Drill each transfixation pin into the bone at the point of greatest cross-sectional diameter.
4. Exit the trochar point at the far cortical surface for a distance of 2 to 3 mm.

Suspend the injured limb from hooks in the ceiling or with an intravenous stand. Use a ceiling hook if available, because intravenous stands get in the way during surgery. Scrub the liberally clipped area with an antiseptic soap. If the fixation is being applied to the radius or tibia, leave the limb suspended during application of the external fixator. If the fixation is being applied to the humerus or femur, release the limb from the suspension after it has been draped. Because the external fixator system is only as strong as the connection of the external frame to the bone, insert the pins carefully. Make a small (1-cm) longitudinal skin incision over the proposed pin site. Use a hemostat to bluntly dissect through the soft tissue from the skin surface to bone to create a soft tissue tunnel that allows free gliding motion of surrounding muscles around the transfixation pin. Create the soft tissue tunnel between large muscle bellies rather than through them and avoid neurovascular structures. Protect the soft tissues from trauma by using a drill sleeve, or retract and stabilize the tis-

sue with a hemostat. When the pins are in place, adjust the position of the connecting bar(s) as close to the body as possible without impinging on the skin surface, usually so that one forefinger can be inserted between the clamps and the skin surface (approximately 1 cm).

F. Positive-profile pin placement.
1. Raised threaded section of the pin will not pass through the hole in some pin grippers.
2. Place threaded pins in the most proximal and most distal pin sites because these pins do not require placement through pin grippers.
3. When placing threaded pins in intermediate sites, pins must be placed through pin grippers already positioned on the external bar.
   a. End-threaded pin.
      i. When using an end-threaded pin, first back the nonthreaded end through the hole in the pin gripper, then advance the threaded end into the bone. Position the external bar 4 to 5 cm from the skin surface before placing the pin. Once all pins are in position, slide the external bar down into the recommended position (1 cm from the skin surface). To facilitate this maneuver, place all pins parallel to each other.
   b. Centrally threaded pin.
      i. Must pass from one pin gripper, through the bone, and into the pin gripper on the opposite side of the limb.
      ii. Use visual alignment, or a guide system and pilot hole.

Insert the most proximal and distal pins and connect to the medial and lateral external bars. For each centrally threaded transfixation pin, drill a hole through the bone with a drill bit 0.1 mm smaller than the core diameter of the transfixation pin. Remove one external bar and insert the centrally threaded transfixation pin(s) into the drill hole(s). Replace the external bar.

4. The grooved half clamp is a newly designed pin gripper that simplifies use of raised end-threaded or centrally threaded transfixation pins.
   a. It resembles a standard pin gripper in which the base of the U has been cut, so that a transfixation pin can be inserted before the pin gripper (clamp) is placed on the external bar. After placing the transfixation pin, capture the pin and bar by sliding the half clamp over the end of the pin and onto the external bar. Tighten the nut of the clamp to simultaneously tighten the clamp to the external bar and the clamp to the transfixation pin.

IV. Specific Fixator Configurations

A. Unilateral-Uniplanar (Type Ia) Fixators

1. Apply to the medial surface of the radius and tibia and the lateral surface of the femur or humerus, using half pin transfixation pins.

Begin by placing a half pin in the metaphyses of the proximal and distal bone fragments. Place the pins in the center of the bone, perpendicular to its long axis and through both cortices. Place an appropriate number of pin grippers on the bar to accommodate placement of subsequent pins. Reduce the fracture (open or closed) and connect the two pins to the external bar. Place the additional half pins directly through the pin grippers. Remember the previously discussed insertion technique for a positive-threaded profile pin vs. a smooth or

negative-profile threaded pin. Once all of the intermediate pins have been placed, tighten the pin grippers and make a radiograph examination of the limb to assess fracture reduction and pin placement.

B. Unilateral-Biplanar (Type Ib) Fixators

1. Apply most commonly to the radius and tibia.
   a. With the radius, place one external bar on the craniomedial surface of the bone and a second on the craniolateral surface.
   b. With the tibia, place one external bar on the cranial surface of the bone and a second on the medial surface.

Begin by placing four half pins (two in each plane) in the metaphysis of each major fragment in a similar fashion as described previously. Reduce the fracture (open or closed), place an appropriate number of pin grippers on two external bars, and connect pins in a given plane with external bars. Determine the number of half pins to use, depending on the desired strength and stiffness of the external fixator as determined through the fracture-assessment score. Generally, place four half pins in one plane (craniomedial or medial) and four in the second plane (craniolateral or cranial). Therefore place two empty pin grippers on each connecting bar. Place additional half pins directly through these pin grippers. Once all of the intermediate pins are in place, tighten the pin grippers and make a radiograph examination of the limb.

C. Bilateral-Uniplanar (Type II) Fixators

1. Apply only to the radius or tibia, because the adjacent body trunk means bilateral configurations cannot be placed on the femur or humerus.
2. Place in a medial to lateral plane.

First place full pins in the proximal and distal metaphyses so that they lie in the same plane. Place the pins perpendicular to the bone surface and parallel to the adjacent joint line to facilitate restoring limb alignment. If necessary, use these pins to apply traction to the limb to aid in fracture reduction. Reduce the fracture, place the appropriate number of empty pin grippers on each external bar to accommodate placement of subsequent intermediate pins, and connect the proximal and distal full pins with a medial and lateral connecting bar. Insert intermediate pins as half pins or full pins, using smooth or threaded pins. Determine which pin type to use based on the fracture-assessment score. If intermediate pins are to be positive-profile threaded pins, refer to the special insertion techniques discussed previously under positive-profile pin placement. Once all of the intermediate pins are in place, tighten the pin grippers and take a radiograph of the limb to assess fracture reduction and pin placement.

D. Bilateral-Biplanar (Type III) Fixator

1. Apply to radius or tibia, but not to the femur or humerus because of the position of the body wall.
2. Place a bilateral-uniplanar frame (type II) in a medial-to-lateral plane, and follow it with the application of a unilateral-uniplanar (type I) frame in a cranial-to-caudal plane. Connect the two frames to form the tent configuration of type III external fixator configurations. Remember to slide empty pin grippers onto the external bar to accept placement of intermediate pins, and plan for the application of half pins or full pins if they are to be enhanced threaded pins.

E. External Skeletal Fixators in Combination with IM Pins

1. Use this combination to provide humeral and femoral fractures with additional stabilization, because the most stable frames (type II and type III) cannot be applied to these bones.
2. Limit the number of transfixation pins to one or two pins placed above and below the fracture, in order to decrease the amount of discomfort associated with pins placed through the large muscle groups.
3. Use one of two methods to strengthen an external fixator without increasing the number of pins. Add more external bars; the addition of a single external bar doubles the strength of the system. Alternatively, leave the IM pin protruding above the skin surface at the exit point proximal to the greater trochanter. Then "tie" the IM pin into the external fixator by connecting the two with an additional short segment of external bar.

First, reduce the fracture and insert an IM pin that fills 60% to 75% of the medullary canal. Use cerclage wire to support long oblique fractures, spiral fractures, or comminuted fractures having one or two large fragments. If multiple fragments are present, bridge the comminuted section of bone with the IM pin and external fixator without disturbing soft tissue attachments to small bone fragments. Once the fracture is reduced and the IM pin has been placed, add the external fixator. Use the largest size transfixation pin that does not exceed 20% of the diameter of the bone and will pass adjacent to the IM pin. If unsure of the track of the IM pin inside the bone relative to the chosen site for insertion of a transfixation pin, drill the proposed transfixation pin site with a small Kirschner pin. If the IM pin is encountered, select an alternative location; otherwise insert the transfixation pin at this site. If more than two transfixation pins are being placed, insert the intermediate pins through preplaced pin grippers. Connect the transfixation pins to an external bar placed 1 cm from the skin surface. Increasing the number of transfixation pins strengthens the external fixator, but adding fixator pins increases postoperative discomfort.

F. Acrylic Splints

1. Apply acrylic splints using a single- or two-stage technique.
   a. With the single-stage technique you must remove a small section of the acrylic column if radiographs show unsatisfactory fracture reduction or pin placement.
   b. With the two-stage techniques you can assess pin placement and fracture reduction before the acrylic hardens.

Insert transfixation pins in the bone fragments following the same principles and guidelines used for construction of standard external fixator frames. Place acrylic column molding tubes over the ends of the transfixation pins 2 cm from the skin surface. If using a single-stage technique, reduce the fracture and pour the acrylic into the columns. Allow the acrylic to cure for 5 to 10 minutes. If a two-stage technique is used, place the tubes over the ends of the transfixation pins but do not add acrylic. Instead, reduce the fracture and apply a temporary alignment frame consisting of standard Kirschner clamps and external bars added to the fixation pins outside of the column molding tubes. Take radiographs to assess pin placement and fracture reduction and, if satisfactory, pour acrylic into the columns and allow it to cure. If alignment must be changed after the acrylic has hardened, cut the acrylic column(s) at the fracture line with a saw. Once appropriate adjustments are made, patch the acrylic column by adding new acrylic to fill the gap. Peel the plastic molding back from each end at the gap and drill several holes in the remaining acrylic to provide a site of attachment for the old and new acrylic. Mold a small amount of new acrylic by hand and place it into the gap, then allow the acrylic to cure.

V. Postoperative Care

A. Provide postoperative analgesia.

B. Clean the pin-skin interface with antiseptic solution, using cotton swabs, immediately after surgery.

C. Place sterile gauze sponges around and between transfixation pins and the limb, then wrap with Vetrap or a similar bandage material.

D. Clean the pin-skin interface and change the bandage daily.

E. Discontinue gauze packing after approximately 1 week. Discontinue daily cleaning of the pin-skin interface when little or no serosanguineous transudate is noted at the surface, but continue daily observations.

F. Reevaluate the animal weekly for the first 2 to 3 weeks postoperatively, then once every 2 weeks. Clean areas of skin irritation or drainage, and pack with gauze.

G. Remove the fixator once the bone has healed. Base the time to take radiographs on the estimated time to bone union and the patient fracture assessment.

H. Sedate patients for pin removal. Loosen the pin gripper, and remove transfixation pins with a hand chuck or drill (smooth transfixation pins can also be removed with a pin remover).

Internal Fixation (*SAS*, pp. 742-756)

Intramedullary Pins (*SAS*, pp. 742-744)

I. Indications and Biomechanical Properties

A. Use IM pins for fractures of the humerus, femur, and tibia.

B. Biomechanical advantage.
   1. Pins resist bending loads from all directions equally, in contrast to other implants (e.g., bone plates, external fixators).

C. Biomechanical disadvantages.
   1. Poor resistance to axial (compressive) loads.
   2. Poor resistance to rotational loads.
   3. Lack of fixation (interlocking) with bone.
   4. Friction between pin and bone is the only resistance to rotation or axial loads.

D. Supplement IM pins with other implants (e.g., cerclage wire and external skeletal fixation) to increase rotational and axial support.

E. Using two IM pins together has not been shown to increase rotational support, and there is a high complication rate when double-pin fixation is used. A modest increase in rotational support is seen when more than two pins are stacked into the marrow cavity.

II. Equipment/Supplies

A. Intramedullary pins are smooth, round, 316L stainless steel rods that are inserted into the medullary cavity.

B. Steinmann pins are the most commonly used.
1. Available from 1/16 inch to 1/4 inch in diameter.
2. Number of points.
   a. Single-armed pins have one end with a point and one end blunt.
   b. Double-armed pins have a point at each end.
3. Popular point designs.
   a. Trocar points are most commonly used. They have a triple cutting edge and cut through cancellous bone easily.
   b. Chisel points have a two-sided cutting edge that is slightly more effective in cutting through dense cortical bone.

C. Smooth or end-threaded pin.
1. End-threaded pins were developed to increase the pin's holding power in cancellous bone, but their use is controversial.
   a. The pin must be "screwed out" of the bone on removal, suggesting enhanced bone-holding ability over smooth pins.
   b. There may not be improved holding until bone grows into the threads, which may not occur until after the critical early period of postoperative healing.
   c. When threads are cut into a pin, the pin diameter is greater in the nonthreaded section of the pin than in the threaded section. This concentrates stress at the junction of the two sections, predisposing the pin to premature bending or breakage.

III. Application

A. Use specific techniques for the individual long bone involved described in the next chapter on fracture management.

IV. Postoperative Care

A. Provide postoperative analgesia.

B. See sections on individual long bones for general postoperative care.

C. In general, recheck weekly for 2 to 3 weeks following surgery, then every 2 weeks.

D. Subcutaneous fluid swelling surrounding the pin end is a seroma caused by irritation of the pin moving in soft tissues. It will resolve on its own once the IM pin is removed.

E. Remove the pin once bone union has occurred.

To remove a pin, sedate the patient and clip and aseptically prepare the skin surface overlying the end of the pin. Instill a local anesthetic and make a small skin incision over the palpable end of the pin. Bluntly dissect soft tissues from the pin, grasp it with a pin remover, and extract it from the bone. Place a suture(s) in the skin wound.

Interlocking Intramedullary Pins (*SAS*, pp. 744-745)

I. Indications and Biomechanical Properties

A. Screws are placed through the bone and IM pin. The pin provides bending support, while the interlocking screws provide axial and rotational support.

B. Screw number varies from a single screw proximal and distal to the fracture to three screws proximal and three distal to the fracture.

C. Use primarily for humeral or femoral fractures, but may also be implanted into the tibia.

II. Equipment/Supplies

A. Special instrumentation needed includes a reamer, interlocking nails, interlocking screws, and a guide system for screw placement.

III. Application

Prepare the marrow cavity for pin placement with an instrument that reams the marrow cavity and establishes an avenue for the pin. Once the pin is in place, attach it to a guiding system to place drill holes in the bone for the interlocking screws. The guide system is mandatory to ensure that the drilled hole intersects the bone at a site where a hole exists in the pin. After the hole has been drilled, place a screw through the cortex to interlock with the IM pin. If the screw is self-tapping, place it directly into the drill hole; if the screw is not self-tapping, tap the drill hole before screw placement. See instructions on placement of IM pins in the femur and humerus.

IV. Postoperative Care

A. Provide postoperative analgesia.

B. See the section on individual long bones for postoperative care.

C. In general, recheck weekly for 2 to 3 weeks, then every 2 weeks.

D. Schedule postoperative radiographs depending on the estimated time to bone union, based on the patient fracture assessment.

E. Remove interlocking IM pins when the bone has healed. Use general anesthesia.

Clip and aseptically prepare the skin surface and make small skin incisions over the interlocking screws. Remove the screws and make an incision over the end of the pin. Apply the distraction device and remove the pin.

Orthopedic Wire (*SAS*, pp. 745-747)

I. Definitions

A. **Cerclage wire** is orthopedic wire placed around the circumference of the bone.

B. **Hemicerclage** is orthopedic wire placed through predrilled holes in the bone.

II. Indications

A. Provide stability to long oblique fractures, spiral fractures, and comminuted fractures.

B. Use together with other implants to supplement axial, rotational, and bending support of fractures.

C. Alternatively, use to hold fracture fragments in alignment (adaptation) while the other implants provide stability.

D. Three criteria must be followed in order to achieve the necessary compression to stabilize a fracture with cerclage wire.
   1. The fracture line should be three times the diameter of the marrow cavity.
   2. Use with a maximum of three (preferably only two) fracture fragments. Use with multifragmented fractures is the number one reason for cerclage wire failure.
   3. The fracture must be anatomically reduced.

E. Cruciate hemicerclage wire pattern is most effective in resisting rotation and bending.
   1. Use only with transverse fractures, because if the fracture is oblique and collapses even a small amount, the wire will loosen.

III. Equipment/Supplies

A. Orthopedic wire is made from 316L stainless steel.

B. The wire is available in sizes ranging from 22 gauge (0.64 mm) to 18 gauge (1.0 mm).
   1. Use 22- or 20-gauge wire for cats and small dogs, and 18-gauge wire for larger dogs.
   2. Use 18- or 20-gauge wire for hemicerclage wire.

C. Many instruments are available to secure wire around the bone.
   1. Some instruments simultaneously tension and secure with a twist or loop knot (single-phase tighteners).
   2. Others instruments tension first and then secure with a twist or loop knot (two-phase tighteners).

IV. Application

A. Cerclage Wire

Use a wire passer to place the wire around the bone without extensively reflecting soft tissue. Do not entrap tissue between the wire and periosteum. Use a minimum of two wires placed 3 to 4 mm from each end of the fracture line. Place additional wires 1 cm apart and within the boundaries of the most proximal and distal wires. To prevent slippage and loosening of the wire, place the wires perpendicular to the bone surface. If the bone changes diameter at the placement site, the wire will tend to slip toward the area of smaller diameter. To prevent slipping, place a Kirschner wire across the fracture and leave the ends of the Kirschner wire protruding 1 mm beyond the bone surface at both the near and far cortex. Place the cerclage wire around the bone such that the loop rests above the Kirschner pin at the far cortex and below the Kirschner pin at the near cortex. Alternatively, make a small notch in the bone surface with the point of a pin or small file. Place the wire loop within the notch to prevent slippage. The instrument used for tightening the wire is not critical; however, the wire must be tight after securing the knot. Ascertain the degree of tightness by feel and check it by attempting to move the wire with a pair of needle holders. Replace the wire if it is loose. If a twist knot is used, do not bend the twist over because significant tension is lost in the wire loop by this maneuver. Instead, leave the twist in the extended position and cut it near the third twist. A fibrous cap will rapidly form over the protruding end of the wire, providing protection from soft tissue irritation. When all of the wires have been placed, recheck the tightness of each wire because loosening of the initial wires may occur with subsequent wire placement.

B. Hemicerclage Wire

Drill small holes through the bone 1 cm above and 1 cm below the fracture. Drill the holes so that the wire rests on the tension surface of the bone (e.g., in the femur, drill the holes near the lateral cortex in a cranial-to-caudal direction). Pass one end of a piece of wire through the hole proximal to the fracture and the other end through the distal hole. Twist the free ends of the wire such that a cruciate pattern is formed on the tension surface of the bone. Cut the ends of the twist knot but do not bend them.

V. Postoperative Care

A. Provide postoperative analgesia.

B. Special postoperative care is not required for cerclage/hemicerclage wire.

C. Wire is generally not removed once the fracture has healed, unless it causes problems.

Tension Bands (*SAS*, p. 747)

I. Indications

A. Use a tension band to counteract the tension of a muscle group pulling on its point of insertion or origin. It converts distractive tensile forces into compressive forces.

II. Equipment/Supplies

A. Tension band placement requires Steinmann pins or Kirschner wire and orthopedic wire.

III. Application

When using pins and wire to apply a tension band, first reduce the fracture and place two small pins or Kirschner wires across the fracture to maintain reduction. Place the pins perpendicular to the fracture line and parallel to each other. Drill a small hole through the bone 1 to 2 cm below the fracture line such that the wire will rest on the bone's tension surface when tightened (i.e., in the femur, drill the hole from cranial to caudal so that the wire will rest on the lateral or tension surface of the femur). Pass the wire through the drill hole and around the two small pins used to stabilize the fracture. Twist the ends to form a figure-eight from the pins to the drill hole. The twist portion of the wire should be on top of the flat portion of the wire. Wind the twist knot to tighten the arms of the tension band. As the wire is tightened, tension is created that opposes that generated by muscle contraction.

IV. Postoperative Care

A. Provide postoperative analgesia.

B. Special postoperative care is not required for tension bands.

C. Tension bands are not removed once the fracture has healed, unless pins irritate soft tissues.

Bone Plates and Screws (*SAS*, pp. 747-754)

I. The AO/ASIF System

A. Although several companies market varied designs of equipment, the AO/ASIF system will be used to describe the principles of application in this text. The Swiss group Arbeitsgemeinschaft fur Osteosynthesefragen (AO) is referred to as the Association for the Study of Internal Fixation (ASIF) in the United States.

II. Indications

A. Use bone plates and screws to stabilize fractures of the long bone or axial skeleton.

B. They are particularly useful when postoperative comfort and early limb use are critical.

III. Equipment/Supplies

A. Screws.
   1. Screws are made of 316L stainless steel or titanium.
   2. Self-tapping vs. non–self-tapping.
      a. Which is best is controversial, but the most commonly used ASIF screws are non–self-tapping.
   3. Cortical vs. cancellous screws.
      a. Cortical screws are fully threaded and designed for use in compact cortical bone. The pitch of the screw (number of threads per inch) is greater than that of a cancellous screw.
      b. Cancellous screws are either completely or partially threaded and are used primarily in the epiphysis or metaphysis. The thread height (difference between the core diameter and outer screw diameter) of cancellous screws is greater than the thread height of cortical screws, allowing deep purchase into the soft spongy epiphyseal or metaphyseal bone.
   4. Screws are named for their outside diameter, and are available in sizes from 1.5 to 6.5 mm.
   5. Plate screws are bone screws used to anchor bone plates to bone.
   6. Position screws are bone screws used to hold bone fragments in place. They can be inserted through a plate hole or placed in bone independent of the plate.
   7. Lag screws (also called compression screws) apply compression between fragments.

B. Drill bits corresponding to the inner core diameter (shaft) of the screw and to the outer diameter are available, as are taps corresponding to the threads of the screw.

C. A depth gauge is used to measure the length of screw desired.

D. Countersink cuts a groove in the cortex to accept the head of the screw used when the screw is inserted independent of a bone plate.

E. Bone plates.

1. Bone plates are made of 316L stainless steel or titanium (more expensive).
2. Plates are designated by plate length, cortical screw size that the plate hole will accept, plate and screw hole configuration, and function.
3. Plate holes can be round (e.g., veterinary cuttable plate) or oblong (e.g., dynamic compression plate). Plates with oblong holes are dynamic compression plates (DCPs) because compression can be applied to the bone by tightening the screws.
4. Drill guides are used to center the drill hole in either a loading or neutral position. Loading position applies approximately 1 mm of compression for each screw tightened, whereas neutral position applies approximately 0.1 mm of compression.
5. Broad plates are wider than standard plates, giving them increased strength and stiffness.
6. Titanium plates are designed as limited-contact plates (LCPs). They are made to limit contact between the plate and bone to minimize interruption of blood flow. The screw holes are oblong and inclined from both ends, allowing compression to be applied in either direction.
7. Specialized bone plates (e.g., reconstruction plates, angled plates, and condylar screw plates) are available.

F. Plates specifically for small animals.

1. Veterinary cuttable plates (VCPs) are available in varying lengths up to 50 screw holes (300 mm) and may be cut to desired length. They are available in two sizes, 2.0/2.7 and 1.5/2.0, designated by the size screw that the plate hole will accept. The plates can be stacked to increases strength and stiffness.
2. Canine acetabular plates are made to conform to the dorsolateral surface of the canine acetabulum and are available in two sizes.
3. Canine distal radial plates are made for distal radial and ulnar fractures in small breeds. The T configuration allows an adequate number of screws to be placed in the short metaphyseal segment.

G. Plates can function as compression plates, neutralization plates, or buttress plates regardless of plate configuration (DCP, broad plate).

1. Place a DCP to function as a compression plate only if the fracture line is transverse or short oblique (no greater than 45 degrees).
2. Place a neutralization plate to neutralize physiologic forces acting on a section of bone that has been repaired with screws, wire, or both.
   a. Use a neutralization plate for comminuted fractures in the diaphysis that can be reconstructed with bone screws or cerclage wire, and for oblique fractures in which the fracture line exceeds 45 degrees.
3. Place a buttress plate to bridge a fragmented section of bone or hold a collapsed epiphysis in position.
4. A neutralization plate-bone construct is mechanically more stable and prone to fewer complications than is a buttress plate-bone construct. Use a neutralization plate whenever possible, but use a buttress plate if reduction and stabilization of fragments is not feasible.

H. Select a plate size (2.0 mm, 2.7 mm, 3.5 mm, 4.5 mm) depending on patient weight and bone dimensions. ASIF/AO has charts to use to select a suitable plate.

1. Minimum plate length allows purchase of six cortices (three screws if

both cortices are purchased by each screw) above and six below the fracture. This number is often exceeded to ensure that the plate spans the diaphyseal length.

I. Place plates on tension surfaces of long bones. All long bones are subject to bending forces because physiologic loads are applied eccentrically to the bone center. This causes compression of one cortex and tension on the other. Plating the tension side counters the force pulling the fracture apart.

IV. Application

A. Compression Plates

To apply a plate as a compression plate, contour it so that the plate remains slightly offset (1 to 2 mm) from the surface of the bone at the fracture line. If contoured to the bone, compression will occur on the near cortex and distraction on the far cortex. Offsetting the plate from the bone pulls each bone fragment up to the plate and compresses the far cortex. Insert the two plate screws nearest the fracture first. Place both screws in a loaded position and tighten them to achieve compression of the fracture line. Insert subsequent plate screws in holes in an alternating fashion on either side of the fracture, working toward the plate ends. Adequate compression of the fracture is generally achieved with loading of the first two screws. If you desire greater compression, place an additional screw on each side of the fracture in the loaded position (insert the remaining screws in a neutral position).

B. Neutralization Plates

First reduce and stabilize the fracture with a series of lag screws, multiple cerclage wires, or a combination of both. Because the screws and wire are not sufficiently strong to resist physiologic forces generated by weight bearing, use a bone plate to bridge the area and neutralize those forces that would act to collapse the fracture. As with a compression plate, apply a neutralization plate to the tension surface of the bone but contour it to the anatomic surface of the bone. The recommended number of cortices (six) engaged on each side of the fracture is the same as for a compression plate. However, with a neutralization plate, insert all screws in the neutral position, beginning from the end of the plate and working toward the center. If a plate screw cannot be inserted because it lies over a fracture line, leave the hole empty. If the plate hole lies over a lag screw placed through the bone, leave the hole empty or insert a screw that purchases only the near cortex.

C. Buttress Plates

Apply a buttress plate to the tension surface of the bone and contour it to the anatomic shape of the bone. Use a radiograph of the intact bone of the opposite leg as a template to help contour the plate if the affected bone is severely comminuted. All applied loads will be carried by the plate and screws during the early postoperative period, causing greater stress on the bone screws than occurs with compression or neutralization plates, which share loads with the bone. Therefore purchase a minimum of eight cortices, rather than six, and use a stronger and stiffer plate. For optimal strength and stiffness use a broad plate, lengthening plate, or stacked VCP, rather than a standard plate. Alternatively, support the plate with ancillary implants (IM pins or external

skeletal fixators) that share the applied loads during the early healing period. With a plate/IM pin combination, insert an IM pin approximately 50% of the diameter of the marrow cavity, being careful to maintain the rotational alignment and axial length of the bone. Contour a plate of appropriate length and apply it to the tension surface of the bone. Insert the most proximal and distal plate screws so that they avoid the IM pin and engage both near and far cortices. Insert the plate screws near the center of the plate so that they engage only the near cortex (monocortical screws). With a plate/external skeletal fixator combination, contour the plate and apply it to the tension surface of the bone. Insert the transfixation pins proximal and distal to the plate and connect them with an external bar. With either system, methods to enhance the formation of callus are as important as the mechanical properties of the plate-bone construct. Use autogenous cancellous bone and avoid manipulating the fragmented section of bone.

D. Screws

1. Follow a precise order when inserting a screw.
2. Plate screw placement in the diaphysis.

When inserting a plate screw in the diaphysis, drill a thread hole through the near (cis) and far (trans) cortices, using the appropriate drill guide. To create a thread hole where the screw purchases bone when tapped, use a drill bit corresponding to the inner core diameter of the screw. To insert a 3.5-mm plate screw, use a drill bit that corresponds to the inner core diameter (shaft) of the screw (2.5 mm) and a tap that corresponds to the outer thread diameter of the screw (3.5 mm). Determine the length of screw needed with the depth gauge and cut threads into the near and far cortices with a tap. Use a tap sleeve when cutting threads, to maintain axial alignment relative to the thread hole and to prevent soft tissue from winding around the tap threads. Remove the tap and flush the hole with sterile saline to eliminate bone debris and lubricate the hole. Insert a cortical screw and use fingers only on the screw-driver to tighten it. In spongy metaphyseal or epiphyseal bone, use a cancellous bone screw as a plate screw and place in a similar fashion.

3. Lag screw placement.
   a. Insert a lag screw so that it bisects the angle formed between a line perpendicular to the fracture surface and a line perpendicular to the long axis of the bone. The drill hole in the near cortex must be a glide hole (a hole equal in diameter to the outside diameter of the screw), whereas the drill hole in the far cortex must be a thread hole (a hole equal in diameter to the inner core diameter or shaft of the screw).

To insert a lag screw, use a drill bit that corresponds to the outer diameter of the screw to create a glide hole through which the screw will pass without purchasing bone. Drill using a drill guide to maintain alignment and protect soft tissues. Insert a drill sleeve into the glide hole in preparation for creating the thread hole in the far cortex (the drill sleeve insert centers the thread hole in the far cortex relative to the glide hole, which prevents stripping the thread hole on screw insertion). Then use a countersink to prepare a site for the screw head in the cortex and use a depth gauge to determine the appropriate length screw to use. Tap the thread hole through a tap sleeve to maintain alignment and protect soft tissues. Insert the appropriate length screw and tighten it with your fingers only on the screwdriver. The threads of the screw will glide through the hole in the near cortex (glide hole) and purchase the bone in the far cortex (thread hole). As the threads purchase the far cortex, the fracture line is compressed.

4. Lag screw placement through a plate hole.
   a. A lag screw can be placed through a plate hole by following the same procedure, except no countersink in the near cortex is made. Fully threaded cancellous screws can also be inserted as lag screws, either through the plate or independent of the plate, by following the same procedures. The only difference is the instrumentation needed to match the screw size.
5. Threaded cancellous screw placement as a lag screw.

To place partially threaded cancellous screws as lag screws, drill the near and far cortices as thread holes. Use a depth gauge to determine the appropriate length screw and tap both cortices before inserting the screw. Because the screw is only partially threaded, there are no threads to engage the bone on the near side of the fracture and bone is purchased only in the far cortex. As the screw head contacts bone and the screw is tightened, compression is achieved. It is critical that the smooth shaft of the screw crosses the fracture line; if threads are present at the fracture line, compression cannot be achieved.

6. Position screw placement.
   a. Either a cortical screw or fully threaded cancellous screw can function as a position screw, which holds two bone fragments in anatomic alignment.

Hold the fragments in position with bone-holding forceps, and drill a thread hole through the cortex of each fragment with a drill bit corresponding to the inner core diameter (shaft) of the screw. Use a depth gauge to determine the appropriate length screw, and cut threads in both cortices with the appropriate tap. Insert the screw, using bone-holding forceps to hold the fragments in position and prevent distraction at the fracture line. Gently tighten the screws ("finger-tight") until the screw head rests adjacent to the near cortex (or bone plate).

V. Postoperative Care

A. Provide postoperative analgesia.

B. See sections on individual long bones for general postoperative care.

C. In general, recheck weekly for 2 to 3 weeks following surgery; then every 2 weeks.

D. Schedule postoperative radiographs depending on the estimated time to bone union, based on the patient fracture assessment.

E. Remove plates 3 to 4 months following radiographic bone union, if plates are to be removed.

F. Remove plates applied to long bone fractures in younger patients, and plates applied in areas with limited soft tissue covering (e.g., radius, tibia), where cold conduction may cause discomfort. Use aseptic technique with the patient under general anesthesia.

Incise the skin overlying the plate screws and bluntly dissect through soft tissues to the head of the screw. Once all plate screws are removed, lift the plate from the bone surface at one end and extract it.

Fracture Reduction (*SAS*, pp. 756-760)

I. Definition

A. Reduction is the process of reconstructing fractured bones to their normal anatomic configuration or restoring normal limb alignment (length, spatial orientation, and alignment of joints).

II. Closed Versus Open Reduction

A. Closed reduction refers to reducing fractures without surgically exposing fractured bones.
   1. Advantages.
      a. Preservation of soft tissues and blood supply, which accelerates healing.
      b. Decreased possibility of inducing infection.
      c. Reduced operating time.
   2. Disadvantage.
      a. It is difficult to gain accurate fracture reduction.

B. Open reduction refers to using a surgical approach to expose fractured bone segments and fragments so they can be anatomically reconstructed and held in position with implants.
   1. Advantages.
      a. Visualization and direct contact with bone facilitates fracture reconstruction.
      b. Direct placement of implants is possible.
      c. Bone reconstruction allows bone and implants to share loads, which results in stronger fracture fixation.
      d. Cancellous bone grafts can be used to enhance bone healing.
   2. Disadvantages.
      a. Increased surgical trauma to soft tissues and blood supply.
      b. Greater opportunity to introduce bacterial contamination.

Closed Reduction (*SAS*, p. 756)

I. Indications

A. Perform closed reduction with greenstick and nondisplaced fractures of bones distal to the elbow and stifle.
   1. Realign limb and immobilize fracture with a cast or external fixator.

B. Simple, easily palpable, femoral or humeral fractures in young animals can be repaired with an IM pin placed normograde through the proximal segment and seated into the distal segment.

C. Use closed reduction with severely comminuted fractures (particularly tibial and radial fractures) that are difficult or impossible to anatomically reconstruct.

1. Align the limb, and rigidly stabilize with an external fixator.

II. Goals of Closed Reduction

A. Restore bone length and limb alignment.

B. Eliminate rotation and angular deformity of distal segments.

C. Align joints above and below the fracture parallel to each other and in correct rotational alignment. Check the alignment with radiographs.

Open Reduction (*SAS*, pp. 756-757)

I. Indications

A. Perform open reduction with fractures that can be anatomically reconstructed or those that are displaced and involve joint surfaces.

II. Surgical Approaches

A. See subsequent chapters for surgical approaches for exposing individual bones for repair.

1. Follow normal separations between muscles.
2. Obtain adequate exposure of fractured bones.
3. Handle soft tissues gently and preserve soft tissue attachments to bone fragments.
4. Avoid trauma to major nerves and vessels.

III. Techniques for Biological Fracture Treatment of *Comminuted Fractures*

A. Avoid surgical techniques and implants that compromise surrounding soft tissues and interfere with vasculature, because it delays bone union.

B. Consider the concepts developed by Perron and co-workers: "It is better to trade some stability to achieve optimal biologic response" and "single fractures concentrate tissue strain but multiple fractures distribute and thus reduce tissue strain."

C. Radial and tibial comminuted fractures can be treated with closed reduction, but comminuted femoral or humeral fractures are harder to reduce; closed and external fixators are less suitable for these bones.

D. When using internal implants with a comminuted fracture adopt an "open but do not touch" philosophy. After exposing the major bone segments, and distracting them to length, apply a precontoured, buttress plate. Do not disturb the fracture fragments.

E. Use the same criteria used to evaluate the reduction as with closed reduction.

Anesthesia (*SAS*, pp. 757-758)

I. General Considerations

A. Maintain on inhalant anesthesia for adequate muscle relaxation for fracture reduction.

B. Epidural anesthesia (Appendix E) with general anesthesia provides profound relaxation of rear limb muscles.

Surgical Fracture Reduction (*SAS*, pp. 758-761)

I. Techniques

A. Use slow manipulation to counteract muscle contraction and allow reduction of overriding bone segments.
   1. Transverse fractures.
      a. Lift the bone ends out of the incision, bring them into contact, and replace the bones into normal position.
      b. Alternatively, use a lever placed between overriding bone segments to help distract and reduce the fracture.
   2. Long oblique fractures.
      a. Move the bone segments into close approximation with bone-holding forceps, then use two self-retaining reduction forceps applied perpendicular to the fracture line to slowly force distraction of segments until reduction is achieved.

B. Inspect bone for fissure fracture lines, and support with cerclage wires before attempting reduction.

C. Reconstruct fractures with more than two pieces that can be completely reconstructed by first securing loose fragments to one segment with lag screws or cerclage wire. Then carefully distract and align the resulting two-piece fracture.

D. Use fracture distractors attached by fixation pins to the proximal and distal metaphyses of fractured bones (or to intact bones adjacent to the fracture) to facilitate fragment distraction of open or closed fractures.

E. Another method of fracture distraction is to drive an IM pin normograde through the proximal bone segment, then drive it into the distal segment until it engages metaphyseal bone and distracts the fracture. Steady the proximal segment with bone-holding forceps while the pin is advanced.

F. Suspend the limb from the ceiling to use the animal's own weight to distract the fracture.

Bone Grafting (*SAS*, pp. 761-765)

I. Considerations

A. Bone grafts are named to indicate their structure and source.
   1. **Autografts** are transplanted from one site to another in the same animal.
   2. **Allografts** are transplanted from one animal to another of the same species.
      a. Cellular antigens of these grafts may be recognized as foreign by host immune systems, resulting in graft rejection.
      b. **Alloimplants** are bone treated by freezing, freeze-drying, autoclaving, chemical preservation, or irradiation so that they are devoid of cellular activity.
      c. Allografts reinforced with cancellous autografts are **composite grafts.**
   3. **Xenografts** are transplanted from one animal to another of a different species.
   4. Bone substitutes of β-tricalcium phosphate ceramics are available as extenders for cancellous bone grafts.

B. Bone grafts can be sources of osteoprogenitor cells (osteogenesis), either providing cells directly or inducing formation of osteoprogenitor cells from surrounding tissues (osteoinduction).

C. Bone grafts provide varying degrees of mechanical support, ranging from forming space-occupying trellises for host bone invasion (osteoconduction) to supplying weight-bearing struts within fractures.

D. Select a bone graft to augment fracture repair based on the function required to optimize healing.
   1. Cancellous autografts are highly cellular (superior osteoinduction), but mechanically weak.
   2. In contrast, cortical alloimplants provide excellent mechanical support but in most cases are acellular and stimulate little osteogenic response.

Cancellous Bone Grafts (*SAS*, pp. 761-762)

I. Harvesting

A. Harvest cancellous bone from the proximal humerus, the proximal tibia, and the ilial wing, because they are accessible and contain large amounts of cancellous bone.

B. In general, harvest after fracture stabilization, but harvest first if concerned with tumor or bacterial contamination of the donor site.

II. Proximal Humerus

Prepare the graft site for aseptic surgery. Perform a craniolateral approach to the proximal humerus by incising through skin and subcutaneous tissues. Retract the acromial head of the deltoid muscle caudally and expose the flat aspect of the craniolateral metaphysis, just distal to the greater tubercle. Make a round hole in the bone cortex, using an intramedullary pin or drill bit. A round hole is made through the cortex to minimize formation of a stress riser that could contribute to fracture through the cortical defect. After penetrating bone cortex, insert a bone curette and harvest cancellous bone. Place the cancellous bone directly into the recipient bed or store it in a blood-soaked sponge or stainless steel cup. Add blood to the graft if it is placed in a cup, to keep it moist. The blood will clot and form a moldable composite with the graft, which facilitates handling. Do not store cancellous bone grafts in saline or treat them with antibiotics because this may kill cells. Secure stored grafts on the instrument table to avoid inadvertent disposal. Flush the fracture site and loosely pack all defects and fracture lines with graft material. Close subcutaneous tissues around the graft to hold them in position. Close subcutaneous tissues and skin of the graft site routinely.

III. Proximal Tibia

Make a craniomedial skin incision over the medial surface of the proximal tibia. After incising subcutaneous tissues, harvest cancellous bone as described above.

IV. Ilial Wing

Make a skin incision over the craniodorsal iliac spine. Incise subcutaneous tissues and expose the dorsal surface of the ilial wing. Elevate gluteal musculature from the lateral surface and harvest cancellous bone as described above. Alternatively, obtain a corticocancellous graft by using rongeurs to remove a cortical wedge from the ilial wing. Macerate the wedge with rongeurs and place it into the recipient site.

V. Other Considerations

A. Incorporation of the cancellous bone graft progresses from vascularization of the graft, to osteoinduction, to osteoconduction, to remodeling.

B. The process of healing the defect at the donor site takes approximately 12 weeks to complete.

C. Complications associated with autogenous cancellous bone grafting are uncommon, and include donor site pain, seroma formation, wound dehiscence, infection or seeding of tumor to donor sites, and fractures through the donor site.

Cortical Bone Autografts (*SAS*, p. 762)

I. Considerations

A. Harvest from areas where cortical bone can be removed without adversely affecting function (i.e., ribs, ilial wing, distal ulna, and fibula).

B. Incorporate the graft into the fracture site as a segmental graft (i.e., it is placed between fracture segments) or as a sliding onlay graft (i.e., it is placed over the fracture site).

C. Hold in place with the same implant used to stabilize the fracture.

Cortical Bone Allografts (*SAS*, pp. 763-765)

I. Graft Harvest

A. Transplant immediately or bank for future use.

B. Use radiographs of the contralateral matching bone to determine graft size and length and to serve as a model for precontouring plates.

Euthanize the donor animal and prepare the femur, tibia, or humerus for aseptic surgery. Make surgical approaches to the bone diaphyses, elevate soft tissues, and isolate the bones. Use an oscillating bone saw to resect the diaphyses, then clean the marrow canals and flush them with saline. Immediately transplant the bones into the fracture site or store them for future use. To bank bones, double-package them in presterilized containers and store at 0° C for up to 6 to 12 months. Radiograph them so you will have a record of bone sizes available in the bank. Before use, culture one of the harvested bones to check sterility of the harvesting technique. Alternatively, cleanly harvest cortical bones and double-wrap them in semipermeable packaging material. Sterilize them with ethylene oxide. Following sterilization, aerate the bones to eliminate toxic residues and store at 0° C for up to 6 to 12 months.

II. Graft Placement

A. Adhere to aseptic technique.

Prepare the affected limb and cancellous bone autograft site for aseptic surgery. Approach the fracture, remove fragments, and resect bone segments proximally and distally to uninjured bone. Use an oscillating bone saw to cut the bones perpendicular to their long axes. Cut the graft to an appropriate length in a similar manner (i.e., perpendicular to its long axis) in order to allow 360-degree

contact of graft and host bone. Determine the appropriate number and length of cortical bone screws for the graft length and secure the graft to the center of the precontoured plate. Place the graft-plate composite in the fracture gap and reduce bone segments to the plate. Secure the plate to host bone segments using cortical bone screws. To achieve compression of host-graft interfaces, insert those screws that are immediately proximal and distal to the graft into the host bone in a loaded fashion. Insert the remaining screws in a neutral position. Flush the fracture with sterile saline. Then harvest a cancellous bone autograft and place it at host-graft interfaces. Obtain samples for microbiologic culture and close the skin and subcutaneous tissues routinely. Document allograft and metal implant positioning with postoperative radiographs.

III. Graft Healing

A. Fracture healing with cortical allografts or alloimplants consists of filling host-graft interfaces with bone, followed by graft vascularization, graft resorption, and graft replacement with host bone.

B. Host-graft interfaces heal within 1 to 3 months; however, graft remodeling takes months to years.

C. Monitor the process of remodeling radiographically.
   1. Host-graft interfaces initially fill with the cancellous bone. As resorption and remodeling proceed from host-graft interfaces toward the graft center, grafts change from cortical structures to porous, cancellous bone. Eventually the cancellous bone remodels into cortical bone.
   2. Because the amount of graft that has been remodeled may be difficult to ascertain, leave the plate in place unless complications occur.

IV. Complications

A. Complications associated with cortical allografts include infection, graft rejection, failure of fracture repair, and graft fracture. Infection usually results from graft or fracture site contamination, coupled with instability.

29

Management of Specific Fractures (*SAS*, pp. 767-882)

Maxillary and Mandibular Fractures (*SAS*, pp. 767-778)

I. General Considerations

A. These fractures occur secondary to trauma, severe periodontitis, or neoplasia.
   1. Check for concurrent injuries when fracture is secondary to trauma. Delay fracture repair until animal is stable.
   2. Avoid fractures from bone loss associated with severe periodontitis by performing teeth extraction with care in older patients with oral disease.
      a. Extract diseased teeth before fracture stabilization.
      b. Bone healing may be impaired.
   3. Perform histopathology to identify pathologic fractures secondary to neoplasia.

B. Preserve normal teeth involved in fractures unless loose, and assess need for endodontic therapy.

C. Treat teeth fractured above gumline with endodontic therapy. Extract teeth fractured below the gumline.

D. Avoid tooth roots when placing implants, because damage to them may necessitate extraction after fracture healing.

II. Diagnosis

A. Clinical Presentation

1. Signalment.
   a. Young dogs are at a greater risk of trauma.
   b. Geriatric small and toy breed dogs that have not had regular dental prophylaxis and are fed soft food are at greater risk of pathologic fractures.

2. History.
   a. There is typically a history of trauma or tooth extraction.

B. Physical Examination

1. Observe for excessive drool, reluctance to open the mouth, reluctance to eat, and blood-tinged saliva. Profuse bleeding is uncommon.
2. Use anesthesia to enable complete oral examination.
3. Biopsy fractures that are associated with marked bony lysis or proliferation.

C. Radiography/Computed Tomography

1. Use anesthesia or heavily sedate patients for radiographs of the mandible and maxilla.
2. Take five radiographic views (i.e., dorsoventral, lateral, right and left oblique, and intraoral).
3. Use computed tomography to identify fractures in the caudal mandible that may be difficult to detect radiographically.

III. Medical or Conservative Management

A. Tape Muzzle

1. Use a tape muzzle to support a minimally displaced mandibular fracture with adequate dental occlusion and favorable fracture-assessment score (see Chapter 28).
2. Dogs with mandibular plus maxillary fractures may not tolerate tape muzzles because the muzzle may put pressure on the maxillary fracture.
3. Tape muzzles are difficult to apply on cats and brachycephalic dogs.

Make a circle to fit around the dog's nose from two pieces of tape placed with the sticky sides together. Similarly, make a piece of tape extending from the circle around the head and behind the ears. Fit the muzzle to allow the dog to open its mouth enough to lap water and eat gruel. Keep the muzzle on for 6 weeks.

IV. Surgical Treatment

A. General Considerations

1. Mandibular fractures.
   a. Fracture-assessment score (FAS) 8-10.
      i. For example, simple fractures in young animals.
      ii. Treat with tape muzzles, interdental wiring, or interfragmentary wiring techniques.
   b. FAS 4-7 or bilateral fractures that can be anatomically reconstructed.
      i. Use interfragmentary wires, external fixation, or bone plates and screws.
      ii. Consider placing a cancellous bone autograft to promote rapid bone union.
   c. FAS 0-3 and/or comminution, bone loss, or severe soft tissue damage.
      i. Use closed reduction and EF application.
      ii. Treat severely comminuted fractures of the vertical ramus with a tape muzzle.

2. Maxillary fractures.
   a. If nondisplaced use conservative therapy. Treat segmental maxillary fractures or depressed fracture lines with repositioning and surgical stabilization.
   b. Reduce and stabilize mandibular or maxillary fractures that alter normal occlusion. Malocclusion can lead to temporomandibular arthritis, impaired mastication, abnormal tooth wear, plaque and tartar accumulation, and periodontitis. Treat mild malocclusion with interference of teeth by remodeling the teeth to allow clearance.
   c. Reduce and stabilize maxillary fractures that result in nasal malpositioning or instability. Interfragmentary wires are most often used to stabilize maxillary fractures.
3. Interarcade wiring (mandibular-maxillary wires) can be used in some cases to maintain mandibular and maxillary alignment. Most cats tolerate it, but dogs are more difficult to manage.

B. Application of Interdental Wires

Place around teeth adjacent to fracture lines. Position securely in the bone around the tooth's neck to prevent sliding off the crown. Drill guide holes between the teeth and through the superficial cortical bone surface. Pass wire through the guide holes, circle the teeth, and tighten. Bend wire ends into the mucosa.

C. Application of Interfragmentary Wires

1. Use large-gauge wire (18 to 22 gauge) to stabilize simple, reconstructible mandibular and maxillary fractures. Use a long segment of wire to facilitate passage.
2. Locate wires near the oral margin to neutralize forces that disrupt fractures. Avoid tooth roots. When using multiple wires, place all wires before any wires being tightened, then tighten beginning at the caudal fracture line and working forward.
3. Use Kirschner wires with figure-eight-patterned orthopedic wire if bending or slippage occurs with oblique fractures.

Use Kirschner wire to place drill holes in the bone, 5 to 10 mm from the fracture line, positioned so the wire will be perpendicular to the fracture line when tightened. Slope the drill holes toward the fracture line to facilitate wire tightening. Tighten using either a twist knot or a tension loop, applying even tension to both strands. Apply leverage under the twist to eliminate slack. Bend the wire away from the gingival margin and cut. Twist the cut ends and bend into the bone.

D. Application of Bone Plates and Screws

1. Apply bone plates to the ventrolateral mandibular surface after contouring the plate.
2. Avoid tooth roots when placing screws.

E. Application of External Skeletal Fixators (EFs)

1. Kirschner fixators.
   a. Use Kirschner fixators to stabilize mandibular body fractures. Place positive profile end-threaded pins percutaneously through the mandibular body, avoiding tooth roots.
   b. Apply type I fixators to the ventrolateral mandibular surface with at least two pins on either side of the fracture.
   c. Apply type II fixator for bilateral mandibular body fractures, using

bilateral and unilateral pins and a connecting bar on either side of the jaw.

2. Acrylic fixators (dental acrylic).
   a. Use acrylic as a versatile connecting bar for mandibular fractures, especially severely comminuted ones.

After placing pins, bend the pin ends parallel to the skin. Evaluate dental occlusion and reduce fractures with the animal's mouth closed. Place temporary Kirschner clamps and a connecting bar if necessary to hold the fracture in reduction while molding the acrylic. Protect soft tissues by laying wet sponges beneath the pins. Mix the acrylic and mold it over the bent pins to form a connecting bar; or, alternatively, impale plastic tubing over the pins (do not bend them) and used as a mold for the liquid phase acrylic. The acrylic splint can be curved around the rostral portion of the mandible.

F. Preoperative Management

1. Reduce and hold mandibular fractures in position with a tape muzzle until surgery. Cats and brachycephalic dogs may have to be left untreated until surgery.
2. Administer antibiotics.

G. Anesthesia

1. If using dental occlusion to guide mandibular realignment with complex fractures or cortical bone loss, place the endotracheal tube through a pharyngotomy incision in order to allow the mouth to close completely during surgery. Remove the tube after surgery and allow the incision to granulate closed.

H. Surgical Anatomy

1. To approach the ramus and temporomandibular joint, dissect and elevate the masseter muscle. Avoid the parotid duct and gland and facial nerve, which are dorsal and superficial to the masseter muscle.
2. The shape of the mandibular canal and the presence of major vessels and nerves preclude intramedullary (IM) pin fixation of mandibular fractures.

I. Positioning

1. Place the animal in ventral recumbency for maxillary fractures.
2. Place the animal in dorsal recumbency for mandibular fractures.
3. If planning a cancellous bone graft, position in dorsal recumbency with forelimbs tied caudally to allow access to the proximal humeral metaphysis and oral cavity.

J. Surgical Techniques

1. Open reduction of mandibular fractures.

With bilateral mandibular fractures, make a ventral midline incision in the skin between the mandibles. Move this incision in either direction to expose both mandibles. If only one mandible is involved, make a ventral skin incision directly over that mandible. Elevate soft tissues from the mandibles to expose the fracture(s). Maintain the digastricus muscle attachment. Reduce and stabilize the fracture. If there is a segmental fracture of the mandibular body, stabilize the caudal fracture first. Because there is little musculature around the mandibular body, reduction is usually easily accomplished. Open reduction of the mandibular cortex will realign the teeth. Evaluate the oral cavity for open wounds. If large wounds are present, close the mucosa partially to decrease their size. Do not completely close contaminated wounds so that postoperative drainage may be allowed. Place a Penrose drain if infection is present or likely.

2. Open reduction of fractures of the vertical ramus and temporomandibular joint.

Make a skin incision over the ventrolateral border of the caudal mandibular body and separate the platysma muscle to expose the digastricus muscle. Elevate the masseter muscle from the ramus to expose its lateral mandibular surface and angular and coronoid processes. Reduce the fracture and stabilize it. Repair large, open wounds of the oral cavity as described above.

3. Open reduction of maxillary fractures.

Make a skin incision over the fracture(s) and gently elevate the soft tissues from the bone. Reduce the fracture and stabilize it. Repair large, open wounds to the oral cavity as described previously.

4. Stabilization of mandibular symphyseal fractures.
   a. Treat symphyseal fractures with a single cerclage wire encircling the mandible caudal to the canine teeth.
   b. Remove the wire once the fracture has healed, generally 6 to 8 weeks.

Make a small nick in the skin overlying the ventral aspect of the symphysis. Insert a 16- or 18-gauge hypodermic needle through this nick and along one lateral mandibular surface (under the subcutaneous tissues). Exit the needle in the oral cavity caudal to the canine tooth and thread an 18- or 20-gauge wire through the needle. Reposition the needle on the opposite side of the mandible, and curve the wire across and behind the canine teeth and reinsert it through the hypodermic needle. Exit the wire from the skin incision at the original insertion point. Once the fracture is reduced, tighten the wire. Leave the ends of the wire exposed through the skin incision and bend them to decrease the possibility of injury to the owner.

5. Stabilization of mandibular transverse fractures.
   a. Realign and compress transverse fractures with one or two interfragmentary wires applied perpendicular to the fracture line. For more rigid fixation use an external fixator or compression bone plate.
6. Stabilization of oblique fracture lines.
   a. Prevent oblique fractures from overriding.
      i. Stabilize caudal-to-rostral oblique fractures with two wires placed at right angles to each other. Two wires may be placed through a single drill hole.
      ii. Stabilize medial-to-lateral oblique fracture with two wires placed perpendicular to each other in two perpendicular planes.
   b. Incorporate butterfly fragments into the fixation if they are large and relatively stable.
7. Stabilization of comminuted fractures.
   a. Stabilize these fractures with interfragmentary wires if they have long fracture lines and can be anatomically reconstructed. Bridge with a plate or external fixator if fractures cannot be reconstructed. Pay attention to proper dental occlusion.

V. Postoperative Care and Assessment

A. Take postoperative radiographs to evaluate implant position. However, dental occlusion is more important than accurate fragment reduction and is more readily determined by physical examination than with radiographs.

B. Consider using a tape muzzle to support the fixation postoperatively.

C. Evaluate external fixators to ensure that the clamps or acrylic is not too close to the skin.

D. Feed soft food until the fracture heals. Avoid chew toys and tug-of-war games.

E. Clean the skin beneath a tape muzzle and the area around external fixation pins daily.

F. Reevaluate 10 days postoperatively and radiograph every 6 weeks until healed.

G. Remove intraoral wires, external fixators, and plates when fractures are healed. Do not remove interfragmentary wires unless they cause problems.

VI. Prognosis

A. Inform owners that the prognosis is generally excellent.

B. Mandibular and maxillary fractures generally heal without a large callus.

Scapular Fractures (*SAS*, pp. 778-784)

I. General Considerations

A. Scapular fractures are uncommon in dogs and cats.

B. Assess animals for concurrent injuries such as pulmonary contusions, pneumothorax, rib fractures, traumatic cardiomyopathy, and nerve injury (i.e., suprascapular nerve).

C. Typically, scapular body and spine fractures are minimally displaced and require only conservative therapy. However, transverse fractures of the scapular body and spine may allow the scapula to fold on itself, resulting in a poor cosmetic appearance if not reduced and stabilized.

D. Avulsions of the supraglenoid tuberosity occur in immature dogs and are physeal separations. Reduce and internally stabilize fractures of the scapular neck and glenoid cavity because they may affect scapulohumeral joint function.

II. Diagnosis

A. Clinical Presentation

1. Signalment.
   a. Traumatic fractures occur at any age, but young animals are at increased risk.

2. History.
   a. There is usually a history of trauma.

B. Physical Examination

1. Most animals present with a non–weight-bearing lameness.
2. Assess for swelling and crepitation.

C. Radiographs

1. Obtain lateral and caudal-cranial views. Extend the contralateral forelimb during the lateral projection to avoid superimposing scapulae. A distal-proximal or axial projection provides a skyline view of the scapular spine and cranial and caudal scapular borders.
2. Use sedation as necessary.

III. Medical or Conservative Management

A. Treat most closed, minimally displaced fractures of the scapular body and spine with conservative treatment with a Velpeau sling. Leave the sling on for 2 to 3 weeks or until there is radiographic evidence of the fracture bridged with bone.

B. Treat fractures of the articular surface with open reduction, alignment, and rigid fixation.

IV. Surgical Treatment

A. Application of Orthopedic Wire

1. Use orthopedic wire as interfragmentary wire for fractures of the scapular spine and body, and in conjunction with Kirschner wires as a tension band for avulsions of the supraglenoid tuberosity.
2. Select large-gauge wire (18 to 22 gauge) for interfragmentary fixation, and smaller-gauge wire (20 to 24 gauge) for a figure-eight pattern. Portions of the scapula are thin, and large-gauge wire may pull through when tightened.

B. Application of Kirschner Wires

1. Use as crossed pins to stabilize transverse fractures of the scapular neck.
2. To stabilize moderately comminuted neck and glenoid fractures, place multiple Kirschner wires at diverging angles while holding the fracture lines in reduction with reduction forceps.
3. Use Kirschner wires with figure-eight orthopedic wire for tension band fixation of avulsion fractures or repair of acromial osteotomies.

C. Application of Bone Plates and Screws

1. Use inverted small, semitubular plates to stabilize fractures of the scapular spine and body.
2. Use small (2.7 and 2.0 mm) angle and T plates to stabilize neck fractures. With neck fractures, place plates under the suprascapular nerve and protect the nerve from trauma while positioning the plate.
3. Use cancellous and cortical bone screws as lag screws to stabilize avulsion fractures of the supraglenoid tuberosity and T fractures of the neck.
4. Articular fractures are best treated with anatomic reconstruction and lag screw compression.

D. Surgical Anatomy

1. The suprascapular nerve and artery course over the scapular notch and under the acromial process.

E. Positioning

1. Place the animal in lateral recumbency with the affected side up.
2. Prepare the ipsilateral proximal humerus if planning on performing a cancellous bone graft.

F. Surgical Techniques

1. Approaches to the scapulohumeral joint, excision arthroplasty, and shoulder arthrodesis are described in Chapter 30.
2. Approach to the scapular spine and body.

Make a lateral skin incision extending the length of the spine distally to the shoulder joint. Transect the omotransversarius muscle from the spine and reflect it cranially. Incise trapezius and scapular parts of the deltoideus muscles from the spine and reflect them caudally. Incise the supraspinatus and infraspinatus muscular attachments to the spine and elevate these muscles from the scapular body.

3. Approach to the scapular neck and glenoid cavity.

Make a lateral skin incision from the middle portion of the scapular spine and extend it distally to the shoulder joint. Expose the acromion process by incising attachments of the omotransversarius, trapezius, and scapular head of the deltoideus muscles to the scapula. Osteotomize the acromial process and reflect it distally with the acromial head of the deltoideus muscle. Reflect the supraspinatus and infraspinatus muscles away from the scapular spine and neck. Take care to identify and protect the suprascapular nerve. If needed for complete joint exposure, tenotomize the infraspinatus muscle. Incise the joint capsule to observe the articular surface during reduction of fractures involving the glenoid cavity. For additional exposure, osteotomize the greater tubercle of the humerus and reflect the supraspinatus muscle. Close the joint capsule with interrupted sutures of 3-0 absorbable suture material. Reappose the infraspinatus tendon with a tendon suture (three-loop pulley suture, Bunnell, or locking loop), and support it with interrupted 0 or 2-0 nonabsorbable sutures. Repair the osteotomies with tension band wire. Suture deep fascia, subcutaneous tissues, and skin separately.

4. Stabilization of scapular body and spine fractures.
   a. FAS 0-3.
      i. Treat severely comminuted fractures of the scapular body and spine that cannot be reconstructed conservatively if severe angulation of the joint is not present.
      ii. Use a bone plate if the animal must bear weight on the limb in the immediate postoperative period.
      iii. Reduce and stabilize articular fractures with plate or screw fixation.
   b. FAS 4-7.
      i. Select open reduction and plate and screw fixation.
      ii. Reduce and stabilize articular fractures with plate or screw fixation.
   c. FAS 8-10.
      i. Select conservative therapy.
      ii. If grossly displaced or there is folding of the body, perform open reduction and stabilize with interfragmentary wiring instead.
      iii. Reduce and stabilize articular fractures with Kirschner wires or a tension band wire.

5. Stabilization of avulsion fractures of the supraglenoid tuberosity and fractures of the scapular neck and articular surface.
   a. General considerations.
      i. Treat avulsion fractures of the supraglenoid tuberosity with open reduction and placement of a lag screw or tension band wire.
      ii. Treat simple fractures of the scapular neck and articular surface with open reduction and stabilization with crossed Kirschner wires, lag screws, or a small plate.
      iii. Reconstruct and buttress severely comminuted fractures involving the neck and glenoid with a small plate.
      iv. Use cancellous bone autografts in conjunction with open reduction.

V. Postoperative Care and Assessment

A. Take radiographs to evaluate fracture reduction and implant position. Repeat every 4 to 6 weeks until fractures are healed.

B. Apply a Velpeau sling if you are concerned about implant stability during full weight bearing; however, with joint fractures strive for early return to function. Observe the animal daily for bandage slippage or irritation.

C. Limit the animal's activity until radiographic signs of fracture bridging with bone. Instruct owners to confine the animal to a small area (preferably a cage).

D. Implant removal is usually unnecessary.

VI. Prognosis

A. Most fractures heal without complications.

B. Prognosis for normal limb function is excellent unless malunion leads to scapulohumeral joint incongruity and secondary degenerative joint disease.

Humeral Fractures

Humeral Diaphyseal and Supracondylar Fractures (*SAS*, pp. 784-795)

I. General Considerations

A. Assess the patient for concurrent injuries when high-velocity trauma has occurred.
   1. Take chest radiographs before anesthesia.

2. Assess neurologic function of the radial nerve, which courses from medial to lateral in the musculospiral groove of the distal humerus.
   a. Reflexes and proprioception may be difficult to assess, but superficial pain sensation should be easily elicited on the dorsum of the paw if the radial nerve is functional.

II. Diagnosis

A. Clinical Presentation

1. Signalment.
   a. Any age or breed dog or cat may be affected.
2. History.
   a. Usually there is a history of a motor vehicle accident, but gunshot or fall should be considered.

B. Physical Examination

1. Swelling, pain, and crepitation are typical.
2. Abnormal proprioception is generally due to reluctance to move the limb.
3. Assess for concurrent injuries caused by trauma.

C. Radiography

1. Sedate or take radiographs under anesthesia for proper positioning and quality radiographs.
2. Obtain craniocaudal and lateral radiographs.
3. Take radiographs of the contralateral limb as a template for bone length and shape.

III. Medical or Conservative Management

A. Conservative management is not indicated, because the scapulohumeral joint cannot be effectively immobilized with casts or splints.

IV. Surgical Treatment

A. Application of Intramedullary (IM) Pins in the Canine Humerus

1. General Considerations.
   a. Use one of two methods: either wedge the pin into the most narrow part of the marrow cavity (isthmus), or guide the pin through the epicondyloid ridge to seat into the medial epicondyle.
   b. Estimate pin size from the preoperative radiograph.
   c. Place an IM pin either retrograde or normograde in the humerus. In general, if performing open reduction place the pin retrograde; if performing closed reduction place the pin normograde.
2. Technique.

To retrograde an IM pin in the humerus, drive the pin in a proximal direction from the fracture surface toward the shoulder joint. To ensure that the pin exits at the proper site proximally, press the shaft of the pin against the caudomedial surface of the marrow cavity. This forces the point of the pin to glide along the craniolateral cortex and exit craniolateral to the shoulder joint.

i. To wedge the pin above the supratrochlear foramen, drive a pin close to the diameter of the isthmus to the level of the lateral epicondyloid ridge.
ii. To seat the pin into the medial epicondylar ridge, drive a pin equal in diameter to the width of the epicondylar ridge to the level of the medial epicondyle.

To normograde an IM pin in the humerus, drive it from proximal to distal beginning at the craniolateral aspect of the greater tubercle. Make a small skin incision at the point of pin entry over the greater tubercle and drive the pin in line with the marrow cavity to exit 3 to 5 mm beyond the fracture surface. Toggle the distal fragment over the end of the pin point, align for proper reduction, and then drive the pin distally. Apply one of the same two methods for distal seatage and choice of pin size as discussed previously for normograde placement.

B. Application of Intramedullary (IM) Pins in the Feline Humerus

1. General considerations.
   a. Follow the same placement guidelines as for dogs. Normograde placement is easier in cats because the marrow cavity has a uniform diameter, there is less bone curvature, and there is less soft tissue covering.
   b. Do not enter the supratrochlear foramen because the median nerve is in this area.

C. Application of IM Pins with External Skeletal Fixation

1. General considerations.
   a. First, insert an IM pin that occupies 50% to 60% of the medullary cavity in a normograde or retrograde manner. Then apply an appropriate number of transfixation pins and the external frame.
   b. Use a single external bar with one transfixation pin placed proximal to the fracture and one placed distal to the fracture for moderately stable fractures that are expected to heal in a relatively short time period (i.e., less than 6 weeks).
   c. Be careful to avoid the radial nerve in the distal third of the humerus.
2. Techniques.

Place the proximal transfixation pin craniolaterally, approximately 3 cm distal to the greater tubercle. Use a small Kirschner wire as a "feeler" pin to identify the proper angle of insertion for the transfixation pin to avoid intersecting the IM pin. Predrill the condyles because of the dense cancellous bone. Insert the distal transfixation pin laterally across the humeral condyles and center within the condyles. Palpate the lateral epicondyle and insert the pin 1 to 2 mm cranial and distal to the epicondylar prominence. Exit the transfixation pin medially from the bone near the medial epicondylar prominence.

   a. For unstable fractures add additional transfixation pins, or place an additional external bar or connect the IM pin to the EF frame to make a "tie-in" configuration. To construct a type Ib EF, place an additional transfixation pin proximally at a 60- to 90-degree angle to the transfixation pin already in place. Then construct the external bars to form a triangular shape.

D. Application of External Skeletal Fixation

1. General considerations.
   a. Adhere to the principles of EF application to avoid fixator-related

complications. There is extra stress on transfixation pins, because of the long distance between connecting bar and bone.

b. Consider using open reduction and a temporary IM placed retrograde to achieve adequate spatial alignment. Do not reduce or manipulate bone fragments in the area of comminution. Place the most proximal and distal transfixation pins as half-pins into their respective metaphyseal-epiphyseal junctions. If difficulty bypassing the IM pin is encountered, use a Kirschner wire to feel for an appropriate site for the transfixation pin. Connect the external bar to the proximal and distal transfixation pin to maintain alignment of the humerus once the temporary IM pin is removed. Place remaining transfixation pins and connect to the external bar, taking care in the distal third of the humerus not to damage the radial nerve.

c. Select the number and type of transfixation pins depending on the rigidity and duration of function needed. It is better to err on the side of being too rigid, because it can be destabilized if necessary as the fracture heals.

E. Application of Bone Plates and Screws

1. General considerations.
   a. Use bone plates when the time to bone union will be lengthy or early return to function is critical. Base selection of plate size on intended function (i.e., compression, neutralization, or buttress plate) and patient size.
   b. Place the plate on the craniolateral, caudolateral, caudomedial, or medial surfaces of the humerus. Craniolateral plate placement is easiest with proximal and midshaft fractures; medial and caudomedial placement is easiest with distal fractures.
   c. Use a minimum of three plate screws (six cortices) proximal and three distal to the fracture for compression or neutralization plates, and a minimum of four plate screws (eight cortices) proximal and distal to the fracture for buttress plates.

F. Preoperative Management

1. Apply a spica splint before surgery for patient comfort and to protect soft tissues.
2. Examine the animal for concurrent traumatic injuries.
3. Provide analgesics.

G. Surgical Anatomy

1. During a craniolateral approach the humeral diaphysis, identify the radial nerve and protect it during fracture reduction and stabilization. It lies superficial to the brachialis muscle and deep to the lateral head of the triceps.
2. In cats, take care to avoid entering the supratrochlear foramen because of the presence of the median nerve.

H. Positioning

1. Position the animal in lateral recumbency with affected leg up.
2. Perform a hanging-leg preparation.

I. Surgical Technique

1. Surgical approach to the humeral diaphysis.
   a. Craniolateral approach to the proximal and central humeral diaphysis.

Make a skin incision from the cranial border of the tubercle of the humerus to the lateral epicondyle distally. The incision should follow the normal

curvature of the humerus. Incise the subcutaneous fat and brachial fascia along the same line, being careful to isolate and protect the cephalic vein. The cephalic vein may be ligated if necessary to achieve the desired exposure. Incise the brachial fascia along the border of the brachiocephalicus muscle and the lateral head of the triceps. Use caution when incising the fascia along the cranial border of the triceps overlying the brachialis muscle until the radial nerve is visualized. Once the nerve is isolated, make an incision through the periosteal insertion of the superficial pectoral and brachiocephalicus muscles at their insertion on the humeral shaft. Reflect these two muscles cranially and the brachialis muscle caudally to expose the proximal and central humeral shaft. To gain further exposure of the distal humeral shaft reflect the brachialis muscle cranially and the lateral triceps muscle caudally. Release the origin of the extensor carpi radialis muscle from the ridge of the lateral epicondyle for maximum exposure. To close, suture the brachiocephalicus muscle and superficial pectoral muscles to the fascia of the brachialis muscle. Suture the subcutaneous tissue and skin using standard methods.

b. Medial exposure of the distal one third of the humerus.

Make an incision from the greater tubercle proximally to the medial epicondyle distally. Incise the deep brachial fascia along the caudal border of the brachiocephalicus muscle. Take care distally to preserve and isolate the neurovascular structures (i.e., median, musculocutaneous, and ulnar nerves and brachial artery and vein). Reflect the brachiocephalicus muscle cranially and incise through the insertion of the superficial pectoral muscle. For exposure of the midportion of the humerus, reflect the superficial pectoral muscle cranially and the biceps brachii and neurovascular structures caudally. For exposure of the distal humerus, reflect the biceps brachii, neurovascular structures, and superficial pectoral muscle cranially. To close, suture the superficial pectoral to the brachiocephalicus fascia. Suture the remaining deep fascia, subcutaneous tissue, and skin in a routine fashion.

2. Stabilization of midshaft transverse or short oblique fractures.
   a. FAS 0-3.
      i. Use a bone plate and screws inserted to function as a compression plate.
      ii. Or use a six-pin type Ib EF with raised threaded transfixation pins "tied in" with an IM pin.
   b. FAS 4-7.
      i. Use a compression plate.
      ii. Or use an IM pin "tied in" with a three-pin, type Ib EF.
      iii. Or use an IM pin and cruciate hemicerclage wire combined with an EF.
   c. FAS 8-10.
      i. Use an IM pin/cruciate hemicerclage wire.
      ii. Or use an IM pin, two-pin type Ia EF.
      iii. Consider using a single IM pin placed closed in a normograde fashion in small patients who are less than 4 to 5 months of age, because rapid callus formation will provide support.
3. Stabilization of midshaft long oblique fractures or comminuted fractures with a large butterfly fragment.
   a. FAS 0-3.
      i. Use neutralization plates. First achieve interfragmentary compression with wire or compression screws to reconstruct the cylinder of bone, and then bridge the area with a bone plate.
      ii. Or use an IM pin initially and apply interfragmentary compression with cerclage wire. Then supply additional support with an EF, with or without a tie-in to the IM pin.

b. FAS 4-7.
   i. Use a neutralization plate or an IM pin plus cerclage wire for interfragmentary compression combined with a two-pin, type Ia EF. Use threaded transfixation pins.
c. FAS 8-10.
   i. Use an IM pin combined with cerclage wire for interfragmentary compression.

4. Stabilization of midshaft comminuted fractures with multiple fragments.
   a. General considerations.
      i. These fractures cannot be reduced without significant soft tissue manipulation, so there is no load sharing between the implant and bone until biologic callus forms. Expect high stresses on the implant.
      ii. In keeping with the concept of bridging osteosynthesis, do not attempt to reduce the fragments.
      iii. Insert an autogenous cancellous bone graft when appropriate.
   b. FAS 0-3.
      i. Use a bone plate/pin combination.
      ii. Or use a rigid type Ib EF tied in to an IM pin.
      iii. Or use a type Ib EF.
      iv. The transfixation pins should have a raised thread and at least three pins proximal and two pins distal to the area of comminution. Err on the side of too much rigidity, because the fixator can be destabilized postoperatively.
   c. FAS 4-7.
      i. Use a bone plate functioning as a buttress plate (lengthening plate or broad plate). Apply the plate to the cranial, medial, or lateral surface dependent on the location of the fracture and surgeon preference.
      ii. Or use an EF, with or without a tie-in to the IM pin. The choice of frame, number of pins, and pin design for the EF depend on the fracture assessment.
      iii. Or use an interlocking nail.
   d. FAS 8-10.
      i. Use an IM pin with or without a tie-in to a type Ia or type Ib EF. Use smooth or threaded transfixation pins.

5. Stabilization of supracondylar fractures.
   a. General considerations.
      i. These fractures are commonly transverse or short oblique, but are occasionally comminuted. When comminuted, the length of bone involved is usually limited to a small area. Either bridge the fracture with an implant to serve as a buttress or collapse the fracture to resemble a load-sharing transverse or short oblique fracture.
      ii. Transverse or short oblique fractures require rotational and bending support, whereas comminuted fractures require axial, rotational, and bending support.
   b. FAS 0-3.
      i. Use a caudolateral plate combined with a caudomedial plate.
      ii. Or use a caudolateral plate combined with a medial IM pin.
      iii. Use a neutralization plate combined with lag screws for intrafragmentary compression with long oblique fractures or comminuted fractures where reconstruction of the bony column is feasible.
   c. FAS 4-7.
      i. Use a medial plate or caudolateral plate.
      ii. Or use an IM pin supported with an EF. Select the fixator frame, number of pins, and pin design based on the fracture

assessment. Use a biplanar frame with threaded pins when the fixator will remain in place for an extended period. Tie in the IM pin to increase rigidity.

d. FAS 8-10.
   i. Use a medial and lateral IM pin.

V. Postoperative Care and Assessment

A. Allow leash walking only until there is radiographic evidence of fracture healing.

B. Perform passive flexion and extension of the elbow to maintain range of motion.

C. Remove IM pins and EF when healing occurs; do not remove bone plates unless they cause a problem.

VI. Prognosis

A. Poor implant choice relative to the fracture assessment is the most common reason for fixation failure.

B. If the initial implant system fails, apply a bone plate as a compression plate or neutralization plate, or a plate/rod construct if a zone of comminution must be bridged.

Humeral Epiphyseal and Metaphyseal Fractures (*SAS*, pp. 795-803)

I. General Considerations

A. Proximal humeral growth plate fractures are uncommon, but they occasionally occur in young animals.
   1. They result from minimal external force and may exhibit only slight displacement.
   2. To diagnose, examine the lateral radiograph and compare to contralateral limb.

B. Distal epiphysis (elbow) fractures are common. Lateral condylar fractures predominate over medial and frequently occur in young, toy breed dogs that jump from the furniture or owner's arms with the elbow extended.

C. Isolated medial condylar fractures are not common. More common is a T or Y fracture where separation between the medial and lateral condyles occurs in conjunction with a transverse (T) or oblique (Y) fracture through both medial and lateral epicondyloid ridges.

II. Diagnosis

A. Clinical Presentation

1. Signalment.
   a. Frequently young, toy breed dogs are affected; however, Salter fractures may occur in any animal that has open growth plates.
   b. Any adult animal may sustain an epiphyseal (elbow) fracture.
2. History.
   a. Salter fractures usually occur following a fall, but they may also be caused by automobile accidents.
   b. Elbow fractures or proximal humeral fractures in adult animals are usually associated with vehicular trauma.

B. Physical Examination

1. Typically there is a non–weight-bearing lameness, pain and crepitus on manipulation, and a swollen limb if the fracture is secondary to an automobile accident.

C. Radiography

1. Take craniocaudal and medial to lateral radiographs.
2. In spaniels, if a fracture of the intercondylar articular surface is suspected but not evident, take oblique views.

III. Medical or Conservative Management

A. Do not manage fractures involving or close to a joint with conservative treatment.

IV. Surgical Treatment

A. General Considerations

1. Use the fracture-assessment score to determine the rigidity of stabilization needed.

B. Preoperative Management

1. Stabilize the patient and provide analgesia.

C. Surgical Anatomy

1. Start surgical dissection proximal or distal to the area of soft tissue bruising and swelling to make identification of landmarks easier.
2. Avoid the radial nerve, which lies beneath the lateral head of the triceps. Carefully dissect the tissue plane between the brachiocephalicus and triceps muscles to avoid radial nerve injury.

D. Positioning

1. Place in lateral recumbency for all lateral approaches and for olecranon osteotomy.
2. Perform a hanging-leg preparation.

E. Surgical Techniques

1. Surgical approach to the proximal epiphysis.

Make an incision over the craniolateral region of the proximal humerus. Begin the incision 2 to 3 cm proximal to the greater tubercle and extend it distally to a point near the midshaft of the humerus. Incise through the subcutaneous tissue along the same line to expose deep fascia along the lateral border of the brachiocephalicus muscle and insertion of the deltoid muscle. Elevate and reflect the brachiocephalicus muscle from the cranial surface of the bone. Elevate the deltoid muscle and retract it caudally to expose the insertions of the teres minor and infraspinatus muscles. Make an incision through the insertions of these two muscles to expose the lateral surface of the proximal humerus. If increased exposure of the craniomedial surface of the proximal humerus is needed, release the insertion of the superficial pectoral muscle deep to brachiocephalicus muscle. To close, suture the fascia of the superficial pectoral muscle to the fascia of the deltoid muscle. Appose the fascia of the brachiocephalicus muscle, then suture subcutaneous tissue and skin.

2. Surgical approach to the lateral condyle and epicondyle.

Make a lateral incision beginning over the distal third of the humerus and extending to a point 4 to 5 cm distal to the joint line overlying the ulna. Incise the subcutaneous tissue to expose the deep brachial fascia. Incise the deep fascia along the cranial border of the lateral triceps muscle and continue this incision across the joint line over the extensors. Incise the intermuscular septum between the extensor carpi radialis and the common digital extensor muscle and continue the incision proximally through the periosteal origin of the extensor carpi radialis muscle. Retract the muscle cranially to expose the joint capsule and underlying lateral condyle. For further exposure of the epicondyle, incise through the anconeus muscle at its origin on the epicondylar ridge. Incise the joint capsule with an L-shaped incision to visualize the lateral humeral condyle. To close the incision, suture the joint capsule with interrupted sutures and close the intermuscular septum with a continuous suture pattern. Suture the origins of the external carpi radialis and anconeus muscles together with interrupted sutures, and then suture subcutaneous tissue and skin.

3. Surgical approach to the elbow via olecranon osteotomy.

Make an incision from the distal third of the humerus to the proximal third of the ulna. Center the incision at the level of the olecranon process over the caudolateral region of the leg. Undermine the subcutaneous tissue such that the caudal skin margin can be reflected over the olecranon process to expose the medial epicondyle. Laterally, free the cranial border of the lateral head of the triceps near its tendinous insertion at the olecranon. Next, flex the elbow and palpate the ulnar nerve as it courses in the deep fascia along the cranial edge of the medial head of the triceps. The nerve should be isolated and protected during the osteotomy procedure. Incise the fascia along the cranial border of the medial head of the triceps near its insertion at the olecranon. Pass a Gigli wire through the lateral fascial incision so that it exits through the medial fascial incision. Pull the wire caudally next to the olecranon beneath the tendon of the triceps. Make sure the ulnar nerve is free from the wire and then osteotomize the olecranon process with the Gigli wire. Incise and retract the anconeus muscle from the lateral and medial epicondylar ridges, then reflect the olecranon process and triceps muscle proximally to visualize the caudal surface of the elbow joint. For closure, reduce and stabilize the olecranon process with a tension band wire. Suture the border of the triceps to the deep fascia on the medial and lateral sides of the leg and close the subcutaneous tissue and skin.

4. Surgical approach to the elbow joint through osteotomy of the proximal ulnar diaphysis.

Begin the incision 6 to 7 cm above the olecranon in the space between the lateral epicondyle and the olecranon process. Extend the incision distally along the caudolateral border of the proximal olecranon. Incise the subcutaneous tissue along the same line to expose the deep fascia. Make two incisions in the deep fascia to expose the shaft of the ulna. Make the first incision distally between the ulna and ulnaris lateralis; extend this incision proximally through the insertion of the anconeus muscle on the lateral surface of the olecranon process. On the medial surface of the ulna, incise between the flexor carpi ulnaris and bone. Reflect and retract the medial and lateral muscles and place Hohmann retractors in the interosseous space between the radius and ulna to protect soft tissues. Perform an oblique osteotomy of the ulna with a power saw. The cranial cortex of the ulna can be cut with an osteotome. On the lateral surface at the joint line, incise the ulnar collateral ligament and annular ligament to allow medial rotation of the proximal ulnar segment. This will allow visualization of the elbow joint. To close, reduce and stabilize the osteotomy with an IM pin and figure-eight wire. Do not suture the annular or collateral ligaments. Suture the fascia of the lateral and medial musculature with an interrupted pattern. Suture subcutaneous tissue and skin routinely.

5. Stabilization of proximal epiphyseal and metaphyseal fractures.
   a. FAS 0-3.
      i. Use a buttress plate, a buttress plate/rod construct, or a buttress plate/external skeletal fixator construct.
      ii. Or use a type Ib EF, with or without an IM pin tie-in.
      iii. If lacking intact bone for screws, transfixation pins, or an IM pin proximally, use a combination of implants (plate/rod, EF/rod, EF/plate).
   b. FAS 4-7.
      i. With a comminuted fracture use a buttress plate or a type Ia or type Ib EF, with or without an IM pin tie-in.
      ii. With a simple fracture pattern use a compression plate or neutralization plate. Or use an IM pin combined with cerclage wire supported with a type Ia EF.
   c. FAS 8-10.
      i. With physeal fractures of the proximal humerus in juvenile patients, perform closed reduction and stabilize with diverging Kirschner wires or small Steinmann pins.
      ii. If closed reduction is not possible, perform open reduction and pinning. Enter the bone proximally at the greater tubercle and drive the pins distocaudally to cross the fracture line and into the caudal metaphysis.
6. Lateral or medial condyle fractures.
   a. General considerations.
      i. In adults, stabilize condylar with an intercondylar compression screw combined with a pin bridging the fracture of the epicondyloid crest.
      ii. In older patients, or those with injury or disease of another limb, stabilize with a compression plate placed across the epicondyloid crest.
      iii. Achieve intercondylar compression in one of three ways:
         (a) A partially threaded cancellous bone screw placed so the threads purchase bone on only one side of the fracture plane.
         (b) A cortical screw placed using a glide hole drilled in the lateral condyle and a thread hole drilled in the medial condyle.
         (c) A position screw placed after the fracture is reduced and compressed with bone holding forceps.

iv. Immature toy breeds of dogs with lateral condylar fractures have fracture assessments favorable for rapid bone union.
   (a) Stabilize with a bone screw for intercondylar compression and a small pin crossing the epicondyloid crest for rotational support.
   (b) Alternatively, stabilize with small pins placed at diverging angles. Choose patients for this method carefully. If patients are hyperactive and difficult to confine, premature pin migration and fracture displacement may occur.
   (c) Attempt either method by closed reduction with implant positioning identical to that described previously for adult patients. If postoperative radiographs show unsatisfactory alignment, perform open reduction. Alternatively, perform open reduction and stabilization as the primary method of treatment.

b. Fixation using a partially threaded cancellous screw or a position screw.

Reduce the fracture and hold in position with bone-holding forceps while placing Kirschner pins perpendicular to the fracture surface. Take care not to place the Kirschner pins where they will interfere with the bone screw. Drill the thread hole for the screw and measure and tap it. Start the thread hole at a point 1 to 2 mm cranial and distal to the lateral epicondyle and exit it near the medial epicondyle. Place the screw and remove the Kirschner pins or leave them in place if they are not interfering with normal function of the elbow joint.

c. Fixation using a cortical screw as a compression screw.

Drill the glide hole before reducing the fracture. The glide hole may be drilled from the fracture surface to exit at the lateral epicondyle or, alternatively, from the lateral epicondyle to exit at the fracture surface. Reduce the fracture and hold it in position with bone-holding forceps and Kirschner pins placed perpendicular to the fracture surface. Take care not to place the Kirschner pins where they will interfere with the bone screw. Place an appropriately sized drill sleeve in the glide hole and drill, measure, and then tap the thread hole to accept the appropriate screw. Place a cortical screw. As before, the Kirschner pins can be left in place or removed. Additional rotational support can be achieved by placement of a small pin or caudal bone plate across the lateral epicondyloid crest.

7. T or Y fractures of the elbow.
   a. General considerations.
      i. These fractures commonly occur in a motor vehicle accident or a fall from a height.
      ii. The intercondylar fracture is accompanied by a transverse, oblique, or comminuted fracture through the medial and lateral epicondyloid crests. Open reduction is necessary for accurate alignment of the intercondylar fracture.
   b. FAS 0-3.
      i. Use a compression screw for the intercondylar fracture.
      ii. Affix the condyles to the humerus with a plate/rod combination or medial or lateral plates. When using a plate/rod system, place the IM pin in the medial position and the bone plate caudolaterally.
   c. FAS 4-7.
      i. Use an intercondylar compression screw.
      ii. Affix the condyles to the humeral diaphysis with a medially applied bone plate or two IM pins. Pass one pin through the medial epicondyloid crest, across the fracture plane, and into the proximal segment of the humerus. The pin will exit the

bone near the greater tubercle. Place a second pin in the lateral epicondyloid crest and across the fracture to exit the metaphysis of the proximal segment of the humerus.

d. FAS 8-10.
   i. Use an intercondylar compression screw and two pins placed as described previously.
   ii. Substitute small diverging pins for the compression screw if the patient is young and not too active.

V. Postoperative Care and Assessment

A. Restrict activity to leash walking until the fracture has healed.

B. Take radiographs to assess healing.

C. Perform physical therapy (i.e., gentle flexion and extension of the joints above and below the fracture and muscle massage) once or twice daily.

VI. Prognosis

A. Epiphyseal fractures of the humerus generally heal without complication, especially in young patients.

B. If the initial implant system fails, apply a compression bone plate or a plate/rod construct.

Radial and Ulnar Fractures

Radial and Ulnar Diaphyseal Fractures (*SAS*, pp. 803-811)

I. General Considerations

A. They are common and usually involve the middle to distal diaphysis of both bones.

B. They are often secondary to trauma, so evaluate the patient for concurrent injuries.

II. Diagnosis

A. Clinical Presentation

1. Signalment.
   a. Any age or breed dog or cat may be affected.
   b. Young animals sustain vehicular trauma more often.
2. History.
   a. Expect the animal to be non-weight bearing after trauma.

B. Physical Examination

1. Palpate the limb for swelling, pain, and crepitation.
2. These fractures may be open because of minimal soft tissue coverage of the bone.
3. Abnormal proprioception generally is due to a reluctance to move the limb.

C. Radiography

1. Take craniocaudal and lateral views, including the proximal and distal joints.
2. Provide sedation as long as there are no contraindications.

III. Medical or Conservative Management

A. Provide analgesics, and administer antibiotics for open fractures.

B. Reserve conservative management of radial and ulnar diaphyseal fractures with splints and casts for closed nondisplaced or greenstick fractures in immature animals.

IV. Surgical Treatment

A. General Considerations

1. Consider open reduction and stabilization with internal fixation, EF, or a combination of techniques, for simple or moderately comminuted fractures with large fragments that can be anatomically reconstructed to establish the bone column.
2. Consider closed reduction and external skeletal fixation or open reduction and application of a buttress plate and cancellous bone autograft for severely comminuted fractures that cannot be completely reconstructed.
3. Because the ulna is supported indirectly by radial stabilization, stabilize the ulna only to add support to a comminuted radial fracture, to provide additional support for a large dog, and to achieve anatomic reduction of radius and ulna of an athlete.
4. Use casts, intramedullary pins (ulna), external skeletal fixation, and plates and screws for fractures of the radial and ulnar diaphysis.

B. Application of Casts

1. Cast stable fractures in young dogs or cats when the fracture will maintain reduction and heal quickly.
2. Be sure to immobilize the carpus and elbow.
3. Apply the cast with slight carpal flexion and varus angulation.
4. To "bivalve" a cast, apply over extra cast padding, cut longitudinally along the medial and lateral surfaces, and then tape in position. Not as rigid as a cylinder cast, but useful as additional support with pin or plate fixation and easily changed to allow wound treatment.

C. Application of Intramedullary (IM) Pins

1. General considerations.
   a. IM pins are poorly suited to use in the radius because of the narrow radial medullary canal and necessity of invading the carpal joint to position the pin.
   b. Expect a high rate of complications, including angulation, distraction, rotation, osteomyelitis, delayed union, nonunion, and degenerative joint disease.

2. Technique.

Use IM pins to align the ulna, stabilize a simple ulnar fracture, and add support to the primary fixation of a comminuted radial fracture. Introduce it into the medullary canal from the proximal surface of the olecranon and drive it in an antegrade manner to the fracture surface. Parallel the lateral cortex of the ulna to maintain the pin within the medullary canal. Drive the pin distally as far as possible without penetrating the cortex. Cut the pin below the level of the skin.

D. Application of External Skeletal Fixators

1. Type Ia or Ib frames.
   a. An EF is useful for radial diaphyseal fractures, particularly with open fractures because an EF avoids metal implants at the fracture site.
   b. Construct the fixator to suit the patient and the fracture. A lower fracture-assessment score requires a stiffer fixator.
   c. Apply a type Ia (unilateral external fixation splint) to the cranial medial surface of the radius to avoid penetration of the major muscle masses with the fixation pins.
   d. Apply a type Ib fixation splint placing the fixation pins in areas of bone that have minimal muscle coverage.
2. Type II frames.
   a. General considerations.
      i. Penetration of major muscle masses is unavoidable with type II (bilateral) fixation splint, but they are used because of their increased stiffness.
      ii. Use an open reduction with a limited approach to facilitate reconstruction of the bone column in simple fractures, and use a closed reduction with severely comminuted fractures.
   b. Technique.

Span the length of the bone with the fixator, with the most proximal and distal pins placed in the metaphyses and the central pins placed about 1 to 2 cm from the fracture line. Place additional pins when there is adequate bone. Use smaller fixation pins to the medial or lateral surface of the radius to avoid splitting the bone. Place the initial pins in the proximal and distal metaphyses of the radius, centered in the bone on the medial to lateral plane and parallel to the respective joint surfaces. Reduce the fracture by distracting the transfixation pins manually, using the weight of the animal in the hanging limb position, or with a fracture distractor placed on the concave side of the fracture. Apply medial and lateral connecting bars containing the predetermined number of clamps to the transfixation pins. Secure a third connecting bar with three clamps to the transfixation pins on one side of the limb. Place the remaining pins using the guide bar to ensure proper alignment of the pins with the clamps. Place at least two pins, preferably three, proximal and distal to the fracture. If the anterior curve of the radius precludes the placement of bilateral transfixation pins, apply unilateral pins to the diaphysis of the radius. If additional rigidity is needed, construct a type III EF.

3. Methylmethacrylate fixators.
   a. These fixators allows pins of any size to be directed at angles.
   b. Useful to rigidly stabilize distal diaphyseal fractures in toy breed dogs.

E. Application of Bone Plates and Screws

1. Use wide, flat plates on the cranial surface of the radius, or apply plates to the medial surface of the distal radius to stabilize transverse distal diaphyseal fractures.
2. Apply as compression plates to transverse fractures. Reconstruct long

oblique or spiral fractures, compress with lag screws, and protect with a neutralization plate. Bridge comminuted diaphyseal fractures that cannot be reconstructed with a buttress plate after distracting the fracture and realigning the limb.
3. Consider using an autogenous cancellous bone graft if performing open reduction.

F. Preoperative Management

1. Manage open wounds, swab for bacterial culture, and temporarily stabilize with a Robert Jones bandage.

G. Positioning

1. Prepare any cancellous bone graft donor sites.
2. Suspend the leg to facilitate visualization of correct joint alignment if performing closed reduction or limited open reduction.

H. Surgical Technique

1. Craniomedial approach to the radius.

Make an incision through skin and subcutaneous tissue of the craniomedial radius to expose the diaphysis. Extend the incision distally and elevate the extensor tendons to expose the cranial surface of the distal metaphysis of the radius.

2. Stabilization of midshaft transverse or short oblique radial fractures.
   a. FAS 0-3.
      i. Use a bone plate as a compression plate and screws.
      ii. Or use a type II or III EF with raised threaded transfixation pins.
      iii. Even young, toy-breed dogs have a high complication rate with this type of fractures, and so often have an FAS of 0-3.
   b. FAS 4-7.
      i. Use a compression plate.
      ii. Or use a type II EF or type Ia or Ib EF.
   c. FAS 8-10.
      i. Use a four- to six-pin type Ia EF.
      ii. Or use a cast.
3. Stabilization of midshaft long oblique radial fractures or comminuted fractures with a large butterfly fragment.
   a. FAS 0-3.
      i. Use wire or compression screws to achieve interfragmentary compression area then bridge the area with a neutralization plate.
      ii. Or use cerclage wire for interfragmentary compression and an EF for additional support.
   b. FAS 4-7.
      i. Use lag screws or cerclage wire for interfragmentary compression combined with a neutralization plate or type Ia, Ib, or II EF. Transfixation pins should have a raised thread or have a negative thread profile.
   c. FAS 8-10.
      i. Use cerclage wire for interfragmentary compression combined with a type Ia EF.
4. Stabilization of midshaft comminuted radial fractures with multiple fragments.
   a. These fractures cannot be reduced without significant soft tissue manipulation, so there is no load sharing between the implant and bone until biologic callus forms. Expect high stresses on the implant.
   b. In keeping with the concept of bridging osteosynthesis, do not attempt to reduce the fragments.

c. FAS 0-3.
   i. Use a bone plate used in a buttress fashion.
   ii. Or use a type II or III EF. Apply threaded transfixation pins, at least three pins and two pins below the area of comminution (or vice versa). Err on the side of too much rigidity, as the fixator can be destabilized postoperatively.
d. FAS 4-7.
   i. Use a bone plate functioning as a buttress plate.
   ii. Or use a type II or Ib EF.
e. FAS 8-10.
   i. Use a type II or type Ib EF.

V. Postoperative Care and Assessment

A. Take postoperative radiographs to assess reduction, alignment, and implant position.

B. Frequently evaluate casts. Clean wounds caused by pressure from the cast and remove the cast or replace it with a bivalve cast. Early destabilization of the fracture to treat wounds can cause delayed unions and nonunions.

C. After external skeletal fixation cover the incision. Treat open wounds daily with wet-to-dry dressings until a granulation bed has formed, then cover with a nonadhesive pad and change as needed. Daily hydrotherapy aids in cleaning open wounds, reduces postoperative swelling, and cleans pin sites. Instruct the owner to limit exercise, and administer daily hydrotherapy with a handheld shower massage.

D. Recheck the EF at 2 weeks, and then every 4 or 6 weeks for radiographic evaluation. Destabilization is usually done at 6 to 8 weeks. Identify some radiographic evidence of bone formation and bridging of the fracture site before destabilizing. Remove one half of a type Ib EF or selected transfixation pins from a type I or type II EF to decrease rigidity. Remove the EF when there is radiographic evidence of bone bridging of the fracture lines. After removal a support bandage or a splint may be used to protect the healing bone for a few weeks.

E. Apply a padded bandage for a few days after plate application to control swelling. Expect full weight bearing within 2 to 3 weeks. Confine until there are radiographic signs of bone union. Remove plates after bone union to avoid tissue irritation and cold sensitivity.

Radial and Ulnar Metaphyseal and Epiphyseal Fractures (*SAS*, pp. 811-814)

I. General Considerations

A. Fracture of the proximal ulna may occur singularly or in combination with luxation of the radial head (i.e., Monteggia fracture).

B. Fractures of the proximal radius are rare.

C. Fractures of the distal radius may be extraarticular or intraarticular. Intraarticular fractures usually disrupt the medial epicondyle and result in loss of ligamentous support for the carpus. The ligamentous attachment on the epicondyle causes displacement of the fragment that must be neutralized with internal fixation.

D. Fractures of the styloid process of the ulna cause similar disruptions to the lateral aspect of the carpus.

II. Diagnosis

A. Clinical Presentation

1. Signalment.
   a. Any age or breed dog or cat may be affected.
2. History.
   a. Typically the animal presents with a non–weight-bearing lameness after trauma.

B. Physical Examination

1. Assess for swelling, pain, crepitation, and apparent instability of the adjacent joint.
2. Abnormal proprioception generally is due to reluctance to move the limb.
3. Assess for concurrent injuries caused by trauma. Degloving injuries may be present.

C. Radiography

1. Take craniocaudal and lateral radiographs.
2. Provide sedation as long as there are no contraindications.
3. Take thoracic radiographs to identify pulmonary changes.

III. Surgical Treatment

A. Application of Bone Plates and Screws

1. Apply the plate to the caudal surface of the ulna to function as a tension band plate. With comminuted fractures, apply the plate to the lateral surface of the proximal ulna to function as a buttress plate.

B. Preoperative Management

1. Temporarily stabilize the fracture with a Robert Jones bandage.

IV. Positioning

A. Position the animal in lateral recumbency for proximal fractures and dorsal recumbency for distal.

B. Prepare donor site if planning a cancellous bone graft.

V. Surgical Technique

A. Caudal approach to the ulna.

Palpate the caudal border of the ulna directly under the skin and subcutaneous tissue on the caudal surface of the limb. Make an incision through skin and subcutaneous tissues along the ulnar diaphysis. Elevate the flexor carpi ulnaris and deep digital flexor muscles medially and the ulnaris lateralis muscle laterally to expose the bone surface. Reflect the origin of the flexor carpi ulnaris muscle to expose the trochlear notch.

B. Stabilization of proximal radial and ulna fractures.

1. FAS 0-3.
   a. Use plates and screws for proximal ulnar fractures.
2. FAS 4-7.
   a. Use crossed Kirschner wires or small intramedullary pins for extra-articular fractures of the proximal and distal radius.
3. FAS 8-10.
   a. Use pins and wires.
4. Anatomically reduce and stabilize articular fractures with tension band wires or lag screws to restore joint continuity and function and limit development of degenerative joint disease.
5. Technique.

To place a tension band wire, reduce the fracture (i.e., proximal ulna, styloid process of the ulna, or medial epicondyle of the radius) and start two Kirschner wires in the fragment. Drive the wires across the fracture line to lodge in the major bone segment. Place a transverse drill hole in the major bone segment, pass a figure-eight wire through the hole and around the Kirschner wires, and tighten.

C. Stabilization of distal radial and ulnar fractures.

1. Stabilize distal radial and ulnar fractures with a lag screw or tension band wire.

To place a lag screw, reduce the fracture and hold it in place with a Kirschner wire. Drill a gliding hole (equal to the diameter of the threads on the screw) in the epicondylar fragment. Insert a drill sleeve into the gliding hole and drill a smaller hole (equal to the core diameter of the screw) across the radius. Measure and tap the hole and select and place the appropriate length screw in it. Compression of the fracture should occur. The Kirschner wire may be left to provide rotational stability.

VI. Postoperative Care and Assessment

A. Take postoperative radiographs to assess fracture reduction, alignment, and implant position.

B. Perform physical therapy (range-of-motion exercises for 10 to 15 minutes, two to three times a day) to help restore joint function.

C. Treat open wounds daily with wet-to-dry dressings until a granulation bed has formed, then cover with a nonadhesive pad and change as needed. Perform daily hydrotherapy to aid in cleaning open wounds and reducing postoperative swelling.

D. Limit exercise until radiographic evidence of bone healing is apparent.

E. Recheck at 2 weeks, then every 4 or 6 weeks for radiographic evaluation.

F. Remove implants after bone healing if the implants interfere with or irritate soft tissues.

VII. Prognosis

A. Expect trabecular bone to heal quickly with minimal callus formation, but comminuted proximal ulnar fractures may require long healing periods.

B. Degenerative joint disease (DJD) may occur after articular fractures, especially if anatomic reduction and rigid fixation are not achieved.

Radial and Ulnar Physeal Fractures (*SAS*, pp. 814-818)

I. General Considerations

A. Separation should occur at the weakest portion of the physis, which is the zone of hypertrophying cells. However, with severe trauma the fracture can damage growing cells in the zone of proliferating cells, resulting in premature physeal closure.

B. Fractures of the proximal and distal radial physis are usually radiographically classified as Salter-Harris type I or II (Table 29-1).

C. Be aware that occult type V fractures of the radial physes and distal ulnar physis can occur and are diagnosed after closure of the physis and alteration of forelimb growth.

II. Diagnosis

A. Clinical Presentation

1. Signalment.
   a. These fractures occur in immature dogs or cats with open physes.

Table 29-1
Salter-Harris classification

Type I fractures involve only the cartilaginous physis.
Type II fractures involve the physis and metaphyseal bone.
Type III fractures involve the physis and epiphyseal bone.
Type IV fractures involve metaphyseal and epiphyseal bone and cross the physis.
Type V fractures crush the physis.

2. History.
   a. These animals present with a non–weight-bearing lameness after trauma.

B. Physical Examination

1. Assess for swelling, pain, crepitation, and apparent instability of the adjacent joint.
2. Abnormal proprioception generally is due to reluctance to move the limb.
3. Assess for concurrent injuries caused by trauma.

C. Radiography

1. Take craniocaudal and lateral radiographs of the affected radius and ulna, including the proximal and distal joints.
2. Compare radiographs of the contralateral bone to detect subtle changes in the physis.
3. Radiographs made at the time of injury do not give information about Salter V fractures or damage to the physeal blood supply, making accurate prognosis for growth at the time of injury difficult.

III. Surgical Treatment

A. General Considerations

1. Most physeal fractures have fracture-assessment scores between 8 and 10; therefore the implant system does not need to function for a long time.

B. Application of Casts

1. Apply casts, which immobilize the carpus and elbow, as the sole method of fixation for nondisplaced physeal fractures.
2. Position the limb with slight carpal flexion and varus (inward) angulation.

C. Application of Crossed Kirschner Wires or IM Pins

1. Perform reduction carefully to avoid injuring the physeal cartilage.
2. Use smooth pins when crossing the physis.
3. Proximal radial physeal fractures.
   a. Technique.

Drive a Kirschner wire from the lateral surface of the proximal radial epiphysis across the physis, into the radial metaphyses, and through the medial cortex. Drive a second wire from the lateral proximal radial metaphysis across the fracture into the epiphysis. Avoid penetrating the articular surface.

4. Distal physeal fractures.
   a. Technique.

Drive a Kirschner wire from the medial styloid process across the physis, into the radial metaphyses, and through the lateral cortex. Drive the second wire from the lateral aspect of the distal radial epiphysis, across the fracture into the metaphysis, and through the medial cortex, avoiding the articular surface.

D. Preoperative Management

1. Stabilize the limb temporarily with a Robert Jones bandage to immobilize the fragments, decrease soft tissue swelling, and protect open wounds.

E. Surgical Anatomy

1. Avoid the radial nerve because it lies deep to the extensor carpi radialis muscle.

F. Positioning

1. Position the animal in lateral recumbency for proximal radial physeal fractures.
2. Position the animal in dorsal recumbency for distal radial and ulnar physeal fractures.

G. Surgical Techniques

1. Approach to the proximal radial physis.

Make a skin incision over the lateral humeral condyle, extending over the proximal third of the radius. Continue the incision through subcutaneous tissues and brachial and antebrachial fascia. Identify and separate the lateral digital extensor and ulnaris lateralis muscles to expose the proximal radius. Close the wound by suturing fascia, subcutaneous tissues, and skin in separate layers.

2. Approach to the distal radial physis.
   a. See the craniomedial approach to the radius.
3. Approach to the distal ulnar physis.
   a. See the approach for ulnar ostectomy.
4. Stabilization of nondisplaced physeal fractures.
   a. Treat fractures of the radial physes and distal ulnar physis that are nondisplaced with a cast.
5. Stabilization of displaced physeal fractures.
   a. Use Kirschner wires or small Steinmann pins as crossed pins to stabilize physeal fractures that require open reduction.

IV. Postoperative Care and Assessment

A. Take postoperative radiographs to assess fracture reduction and implant position.

B. After internal fixation, apply a padded bandage for a few days to control swelling.

C. Perform physical therapy (range of motion exercises for 10 to 15 minutes, two to three times a day) to help restore joint function.

D. Limit exercise for 4 to 6 weeks.

E. Recheck at 2 weeks, then at 4 to 6 weeks for radiographic evaluation of fracture healing.

F. Compare radiographs of injured and contralateral limb as early as 2 to 3 weeks after injury to assess physeal function.

G. Remove implants after physeal healing to allow bone growth.

V. Prognosis

A. Inform owners that most traumatically induced physeal fractures sustain damage to the growing cells and have a guarded prognosis for growth.

B. Damage to one physis of a paired bone system such as the radius and ulna can cause shortened limbs, angular deformities, rotational deformities, and disruption of normal joint anatomy resulting in degenerative joint disease.

C. Expect younger animals with greater growth potential to have more severe sequelae.

Radial and Ulnar Growth Deformities (*SAS*, pp. 818-826)

I. General Considerations

A. Recognize that asynchronous growth of the ulna and radius results in growth deformities.

B. The radius receives 40% of its length from the proximal physis and 60% from the distal, whereas 85% of the ulna arises from its distal physis.

C. With premature closure of the distal ulnar physis expect a shortened ulna, with cranial bowing and shortening of the radius, valgus angulation, external rotation, and carpal and elbow incongruity.

D. With symmetric closure of either radial physis expect elbow incongruity and varus angulation of the carpus.

E. Asymmetrical physeal closure of the radius results in various deformities depending on location of the closure.

F. Retained cartilage core, which occurs in the distal ulnar physis of fast-growing dogs, results in a deformity clinically identical to premature closure of the distal ulnar physis. The etiology is unknown.

II. Diagnosis

A. Clinical Presentation

1. Signalment.
   a. Occurs in young dogs, rarely in cats.
2. History.
   a. There is typically a history of a fracture of the radius and ulna, or in some animals there is an obscure history of trauma.

B. Physical Examination

1. Palpate joints for pain resulting from joint incongruity.
2. Observe for growth deformity; direction depends on location of initial physeal closure physis and symmetry of closure.

C. Radiology

1. Take craniocaudal and lateral radiographs of affected limb, including elbow and carpus.

2. Always compare with contralateral limb. Take measurements from the lateral radiographic view of the contralateral limb.
3. Remember that a physis that has recently been halted in its growth will be radiolucent until endochondral ossification is complete.
4. Examine for radiolucent retained cartilage core in the center of the distal ulnar physis extending into the metaphysis.

III. Medical Management

A. No medical therapy is available for deformities from premature physeal closure.

B. With mild deformities from retained cartilage cores, try diet limitations. Monitor the animal weekly, and if the deformities do not correct themselves, perform an ulnar ostectomy.

IV. Surgical Treatment

A. General Considerations

1. Perform surgery on growth deformities of the radius and ulna.
2. Allow as much natural growth of the limb as possible by using ostectomy techniques in growing animals. Animals must have growth potential for ostectomy to be effective. Treat partial premature closure of distal radial physis by resecting the bone bridge area of the physis.
3. Treat growth deformities in mature animals with a corrective osteotomy if the deformity has an adverse effect on limb function.
4. Inform the owner that prognosis for normal appearance and function is guarded.
5. Treat deformities of the tibia with the same principles as the radius. Treat deformities of the femur and humerus with plate fixation.

B. Positioning

1. For ulnar ostectomy, position animal in lateral recumbency and prepare both the limb and ipsilateral flank.
2. For oblique osteotomy and possible cancellous bone graft, position the animal in dorsal recumbency with limb suspended.

C. Surgical Technique

1. Ulnar ostectomy and free autogenous fat graft.

Make a lateral skin incision extending over the mid to distal ulna. Incise subcutaneous tissues and identify and separate the lateral digital extensor muscle from the extensor carpi ulnaris muscle to expose the ulna distal metaphysis. Isolate 1 to 2 cm of the ulna metaphysis immediately proximal to the physis by elevating surrounding musculature and fascia. Make sure the ostectomy is below the interosseous ligament to maintain elbow stability. Ensure that all of the periosteum, with its osteogenic potential, remains with the segment of bone to be resected. Failure to remove all periosteum causes premature bone bridging of the ostectomy. Resect a 1- to 2-cm segment of ulna with bone cutters or an oscillating bone saw cooled with a saline flush. If the

interosseous artery is cut, achieve hemostasis by clamping the vessel, if possible, or applying pressure for 5 minutes. To harvest the fat graft, make a 2- to 3-cm skin incision in the ipsilateral flank to expose the subcutaneous fat. Using sharp dissection, free a large, single piece of fat and place it in the ostectomy gap. Close the flank wound by suturing subcutaneous tissues and skin. Close the limb wound over the fat graft by suturing adjacent soft tissues. Close subcutaneous tissue and skin separately.

2. Partial physeal resection.

Surgically expose the closed and bridged portion of the distal radial physis. Determine the limitations of the bone bridge by exploring the area with a hypodermic needle, recognizing that a needle easily penetrates cartilage of the normal physis and resistance will be felt against bone bridge. Remove the bone bridge with a curette or a high-speed burr. Curettage is complete when normal physeal cartilage is observed or probed with the needle. Harvest free autogenous fat from the flank as described above and place it within the physeal defect. Close soft tissue and skin over the transplanted fat.

3. Radial ostectomy and free autogenous fat graft.

Expose the middiaphysis of the radius using a craniomedial approach. Isolate 1 to 2 cm of the radial diaphysis by elevating surrounding musculature and fascia. Ensure that all periosteum, with its osteogenic potential, remains with the segment of bone to be resected. Resect a 1- to 2-cm segment of the radius with bone cutters or an oscillating bone saw cooled with a saline flush. If the interosseous artery is cut, achieve hemostasis by clamping the vessel, if possible, or applying pressure for 5 minutes. Harvest a free autogenous fat graft from the flank and place it in the defect to prevent bone union. Close the wound over the fat graft.

4. Transverse radial osteotomy with continuous distraction.
   a. Inform the owner that continuous distraction requires commitment to intensive aftercare and frequent reevaluations.

Place a centrally threaded positive profile fixation pin through the proximal radius from the lateral aspect so that the pin parallels the proximal radial articular surface and is within the lateral transverse plane of the proximal radius. Place an identical pin through the distal radius from the lateral aspect. The pin should parallel the distal radial articular surface and be within the lateral transverse plane of the distal radius. Make a lateral approach to the distal ulna and resect a 1- to 2-cm segment of bone with bone cutters or an oscillating saw cooled with a saline flush. Then make a craniomedial approach to expose the middiaphysis of the radius. Perform a middiaphyseal radial osteotomy with an osteotome or an oscillating saw. If there is an angular deformity of the radius, make an oblique osteotomy at the point of greatest curvature of the radius that parallels the distal articular surface. Realign the radius and ulna using the proximal and distal transfixation pins as guides to eliminate any angular or rotational deformity. Place threaded or turnbuckle distraction bars with single fixation clamps on the lateral and medial aspect of the limb. Drive additional fixation pins through single clamps placed on the medial and lateral bars. At least one additional pin should be placed in each radial segment. Harvest an autogenous fat graft from the flank and place it in the ulnar ostectomy gap. Close the wound to hold the fat in place. Close the radial incision by suturing the subcutaneous tissue and skin separately. Tighten the clamps and cut the fixation pins to the correct length.

5. Oblique osteotomy.

Place a centrally threaded positive profile fixation pin through the proximal radius from the lateral aspect. The pin should parallel the proximal radial articular surface and be within the lateral transverse plane of the proximal radius. Place an identical pin through the distal radius from the lateral aspect. The pin should parallel the distal radial articular surface and be within the lateral transverse plane of the distal radius. The transfixation pins serve as landmarks: pay special attention to correct placement. Make a lateral approach to the distal ulna and cut the bone with an osteotome or oscillating saw. Make a craniomedial approach to the distal radius at its point of greatest curvature. Perform an oblique osteotomy of the radius with an osteotome or an oscillating bone saw, directing the osteotomy line parallel to the distal radial articular surface in both the craniocaudal and mediolateral planes. Lower the operating table so that the weight of the animal distracts the distal radius and helps to align the proximal and distal joint surfaces parallel to each other. Realign the radius and ulna using the proximal and distal transfixation pins to eliminate any angular or rotational deformity. Place a connecting bar with single fixation clamps on the lateral and medial aspect of the limb. Drive additional fixation pins through single clamps placed on the medial and lateral bars. At least one additional pin should be placed in each radial segment. Harvest an autogenous cancellous bone graft from the proximal humerus and place it at the radial osteotomy site. Close the wounds by suturing the subcutaneous tissue and skin separately. Tighten the clamps and cut the fixation pins to the desired length.

6. Transverse lengthening osteotomy.

Place a centrally threaded positive profile fixation pin through the proximal radius from the lateral aspect. The pin should parallel the proximal radial articular surface and be within the lateral transverse plane of the proximal radius. Place an identical pin through the distal radius from the lateral aspect. The pin should parallel the distal radial articular surface and be within the lateral transverse plane of the distal radius. Use a craniomedial approach to expose the middiaphysis of the radius. Cut the radius with an osteotome or an oscillating saw. Distract the proximal and distal segments of the radius until the head of the radius has contacted the capitulum of the humerus. Place a connecting bar with single fixation clamps on the lateral and medial aspect of the limb. Drive additional fixation pins through single clamps placed on the medial and lateral bars. At least one additional pin should be placed in each radial segment. Harvest an autogenous cancellous bone graft from the proximal humerus and place it at the radial osteotomy site. Close the wounds by suturing the subcutaneous tissue and skin separately. Tighten the clamps and cut fixation pins to the desired length.

Obtain postoperative radiographs to document the position of the radial head and location of fixation pins. Some correction of the radial segment location can be made at this time by adjusting the external fixator. If the radial head does not appear to contact the humeral capitulum, place a transverse bilateral fixation pin through the olecranon proximal to the most proximal transverse pin in the radius. Loosen the external fixator clamps proximal to the radial osteotomy. Connect the ulnar pin and proximal radial pin bilaterally with elastic bands, placing tension on the proximal radius and pulling it toward the humerus.

When using a plate to stabilize the osteotomy, approach the lateral aspect of the elbow to visualize joint congruity before the plate is secured.

b. Proximal ulnar ostectomy.
    i. For the procedure see the section on treatment of elbow subluxations in Chapter 30.
    ii. Use this procedure if shortening the leg will not affect limb function.

V. Postoperative Care and Assessment

A. After ulnar ostectomy, take radiographs to assess location and length of the ostectomy. Apply a padded bandage or splint to protect the limb for 2 weeks if the procedure was bilateral. Limit activity. Recheck monthly, taking radiographs to evaluate correction of angular deformity. If an ostectomy prematurely bridges with bone, perform a second ostectomy.

B. After partial physeal resection, take radiographs to document complete resection of the bone bridge. Apply a padded bandage postoperatively. Limit exercise. Recheck monthly, including radiographs to assess correction of angular deformity and patency of the resected area.

C. After radial ostectomy, take radiographs to document location and length of the ostectomy and to verify that the joints have reestablished normal position. Place a padded bandage or splint. Inform the owner that a second surgery may be necessary to bridge the ostectomy gap with autogenous cancellous bone graft.

D. After transverse radial osteotomy with continuous distraction, take radiographs to assess the correction and the position of the fixation pins. Confirm that the radial joint surfaces are parallel and the segment surfaces are in the same transverse plane. Readjust fixator if not.
   1. On the fifth day after surgery start distraction at the rate of 1 mm per day, ideally divided into 0.5 mm BID or 0.25 mm QID. Reevaluate weekly.
   2. After distraction is complete, leave the fixator in place to allow the osteotomy to heal. Postoperatively, manage the same as a fracture of the radius.

E. After oblique osteotomy, take radiographs to assess the correction and the position of the fixation pins. Confirm that the radial joint surfaces are parallel and the segment surfaces are in the same transverse plane. Readjust fixator if not. Postoperatively, manage the same as a fracture of the radius.

F. After transverse lengthening radial osteotomy and placement of the external fixation pins in the ulna, radiograph the limb within 24 to 48 hours, and remove the pin and elastic bands once the articulation is correct. Postoperatively, manage the same as a fracture of the radius.

VI. Prognosis

A. Inform the owner that prognosis for normal appearance and function is guarded in immature animals after ulnar ostectomy. Normal length and some correction of angulation is possible, but not rotational deformities. Additional surgeries may be indicated, such as corrective radial and ulnar osteotomies.

B. Inform the owner that prognosis is guarded after partial physeal resection until there is radiographic evidence of physeal function, and that additional surgeries may be necessary.

C. Inform the owner that prognosis for normal appearance and function is guarded after radial ostectomy. Additional surgeries may be necessary, such as repeating the ostectomy if it heals prematurely.

D. Inform the owner that prognosis after transverse osteotomy with continuous distraction is guarded because of the complexity of the technique and potential complications (pin track drainage, pin loosening, and premature loss of stability of the fixator).

E. Inform the owners that after oblique osteotomy and transverse lengthening osteotomy the prognosis is good for bone union, but function depends on the amount of correction achieved and presence of degenerative joint disease. Complications are the same as with external fixation of radial fractures.

F. Inform the owner that prognosis after ulnar ostectomy to treat radial head subluxation is good for bone union at the ostectomy site, but function depends on the amount of correction achieved and presence of degenerative joint disease. Remove pin if it irritates soft tissues.

Carpal and Tarsal Fractures (*SAS*, pp. 826-829)

I. Definitions

A. **Plantigrade** stance occurs when the plantar surface of the calcaneus contacts the ground.

B. **Valgus** is an outward deviation of the limb; **varus** is inward deviation.

II. General Considerations

A. Carpal and tarsal fractures are rare in companion animals.
   1. Treat these fractures to avoid joint incongruity and subsequent osteoarthritis that lead to severe lameness.
   2. Radial carpal bone fractures are the most common carpal fracture in companion animals. Accessory carpal bone fractures occur in racing greyhounds and sled dogs.
   3. Transverse fracture of the calcaneus is the most common tarsal fracture in companion animals.
   4. Racing greyhounds often fracture the central tarsal bone.

III. Diagnosis

A. Clinical Presentation

1. Signalment.
   a. Any age or breed dog or cat may be affected.
   b. Racing greyhounds may have central tarsal or accessory carpal bone fractures.
2. History.
   a. Typically there is a history of an acute onset of non–weight-bearing lameness.
   b. If the calcaneus is fractured the animal is partially weight bearing with a plantigrade stance.

B. Physical Examination

1. Attempts to place weight cause the carpus/tarsus to collapse in a plantigrade stance. With calcaneus fracture, the animal may walk plantigrade or be non–weight bearing.
2. Pain, swelling, and crepitus are typically present in the affected limb.
3. Varus or valgus deviation of the foot is usually present.

C. Radiography

1. Take craniocaudal and mediolateral radiographs.
2. To delineate fractures of articular surfaces of the tibial tarsal bone take oblique radiographs.

IV. Surgical Treatment

A. General Considerations

1. Rigidly stabilize radial carpal bone fractures with compression screws or a combination of compression screws and Kirschner wire. Remove chips that are too small to stabilize.
2. Place a tension band to resist the pull of the gastrocnemius muscle with calcaneal fractures.
3. Reduce and rigidly stabilize fractures of the talus, or perform joint arthrodesis.

B. Positioning

1. For carpal fractures place in dorsal recumbency and perform a hanging-leg preparation.
2. For tarsal fractures place in lateral recumbency with the affected limb up for calcaneal fractures and the affected leg down for fractures of the talus.

C. Surgical Techniques

1. Stabilization of radial carpal bone fracture.

Make a craniomedial incision beginning 3 to 4 cm proximal to the radiocarpal joint. Extend the incision distally to the midmetacarpus and incise subcutaneous tissues along the same line. Continue deep dissection medial to the extensor carpi radialis tendon to expose the joint capsule. Incise joint capsule and identify the fracture plane through the radial carpal bone. Reduce the fracture and stabilize fragments with one or more compression screws. Close the joint capsule and subcutaneous tissue with absorbable suture and close skin with nonabsorbable suture.

2. Stabilization of calcaneal fractures.

Make an incision along the lateral surface of the calcaneus. Begin the incision along the common calcanean tendon, just proximal to the tuber calcanei. Continue the incision distally to the level of the tarsometatarsal joint. Incise superficial and deep fascia overlying the caudal border of the calcaneus. Identify the lateral aspect of the superficial digital flexor tendon and make an incision parallel to this border. Retract the tendon medially to expose the caudal surface of the calcaneus. Reduce the fracture fragments and place two small pins or Kirschner wires to maintain reduction. Drill a hole from lateral to medial in the distal fragment to accept orthopedic wire. Proximally, pass the wire around the ends of the pins or through a second predrilled hole positioned through the body of the calcaneus proximal to the fracture. Tighten the wire to

complete the tension band procedure. Replace the superficial digital flexor tendon and suture surrounding deep fascia with absorbable suture to maintain the position of the tendon. Next, suture superficial fascia and skin using standard techniques.

3. Stabilization of talus bone fractures.

Expose the trochlea for visualization of the fracture by an osteotomy of the medial malleolus. Center the skin incision over the medial malleolus. Begin 5 cm proximal to the malleolus and carry the incision distally to the tarsometatarsal joint. Incise through superficial and deep fascia to identify the long component of the medial collateral ligament. Make a transverse, caudal to cranial incision through joint capsule overlying the distal tibia to allow visualization of landmarks for completion of an osteotomy of the medial malleolus. Retract the malleolus and attached ligaments to expose the talus. Reduce fracture fragments and stabilize each with a lag screw or Kirschner wire. Once fracture reduction and stabilization are satisfactory, reduce and stabilize the medial malleolus with a tension band. Suture superficial and deep fascia with absorbable suture and close skin with nonabsorbable sutures.

V. Postoperative Care and Assessment

A. Allow leash walking only until healing is complete. Gradually increase distance walked.

B. Perform passive flexion and extension to maintain joint motion.

C. Remove pins used in tension bands following healing, and screws only if causing a problem.

VI. Prognosis

A. Prognosis for return to function with calcaneal fractures is excellent, and with carpus/tarsus fractures is fair to good.

Metacarpal, Metatarsal, Phalangeal, and Sesamoid Bone Fractures and Luxations (*SAS*, pp. 829-834)

I. General Considerations

A. Metacarpal and metatarsal bone fractures, usually of the second and fifth bones, are common in dogs and cats.

B. Phalangeal fractures occur as frequently, but are often smaller and difficult to secure.

C. The two palmar/plantar sesamoid bones per metacarpal/metatarsal phalangeal joint are numbered 1 through 8 from the medial side. Fractures occur most commonly to 2 and 7.

D. Luxations of the metacarpophalangeal joints or interphalangeal joints occur in working dogs or racing greyhounds. Perform surgical repair rather than closed reduction and splintage because chronic instability leads to degenerative joint disease.

II. Diagnosis

A. Clinical Presentation

1. Signalment.
   a. Any age or breed dog or cat may be affected.
   b. Racing greyhounds typically fracture the second metacarpal or third metatarsal of the right foot, or both, and luxate the distal interphalangeal joints.
   c. Fractured sesamoids are most common in large-breed dogs.
2. History.
   a. Typically there is a history of trauma.
   b. With sesamoid fractures the animal may have had acute lameness that subsided, but recurs with exercise.

B. Physical Examination

1. With fractures expect a non–weight-bearing lameness, except with fractures of sesamoid bones, which cause a less obvious, weight-bearing lameness.
2. Examine for soft tissue swelling, crepitation, and pain on palpation.
3. Dogs with joint luxations present with lameness, swelling over the affected joint, medial or lateral deviation of the digit, joint instability, and pain on palpation.

C. Radiographs

1. Take lateral and caudal-cranial views.
2. Take oblique views to isolate individual bones and stress radiographs to show joint instability.

III. Medical or Conservative Management

A. Treat closed nondisplaced metacarpal and metatarsal diaphyseal fractures affecting one or two bones with bivalve cast or metasplint. Also use a bivalve cast or metasplint for phalangeal and acute sesamoid bone fractures.

1. Do not use casts and splints when three to four metacarpal or metatarsal bones are fractured.
2. Remove the cast or splint when radiographs show bone bridging the fracture, usually in 4 to 8 weeks.

B. Chronic sesamoid fractures do not usually respond to conservative therapy.

C. Treat acute luxations surgically in working or racing dogs. Treat chronic luxations with arthrodesis or amputation.

IV. Surgical Treatment

A. General Considerations

1. Reduce and rigidly stabilize (plates and screws) metacarpal or metatarsal fractures in athletic dogs. Treat avulsed fragments from the base of the second and fifth metacarpals/metatarsals with lag screws.
2. Treat fracture of the shaft of one or two metacarpal or metatarsal bones with external coaptation, and more than two with internal fixation.
3. Treat fractures of phalanges similarly to metacarpal and metatarsal fractures.
4. Treat sesamoid bone fractures by removing fragments.
5. Treat acute luxations by open reduction and suturing of the joint capsule and collateral ligaments. Treat failed surgical stabilization or chronic luxations with amputation (second or fifth toe) or arthrodesis (middle weight-bearing third and fourth digits).

B. FAS 0-3

1. For example, severely comminuted fractures of the diaphysis of three or four metacarpal or metatarsal bones, or multiple limb fractures.
2. Use bridging bone plates, or use external fixation with small pins and acrylic.
3. Use cancellous bone autografts with open reduction.

C. FAS 4-7

1. For example, older or larger dogs, displaced comminuted fractures of the diaphysis of three or four metacarpal or metatarsal bones, or multiple limb fractures.
2. Use open reduction and plate and screw fixations.

D. FAS 8-10

1. Use conservative therapy, unless three or four bones are affected, then consider open reduction and stabilization with IM pins.
2. For athletic dogs, accurate reduction and plate and screw fixation offer the best chance for return to normal function.

E. Preoperative Management

1. Protect the fracture by applying a padded bandage or splint.
2. Manage open wounds after performing culture and sensitivity.

F. Surgical Anatomy

1. The third and fourth digits bear most of the weight.
2. In general, make skin incisions on the dorsal surface of the paw, and retract extensor tendons and ligaments to expose the bones or joints. Only make ventral approaches to the digits to expose the proximal sesamoid bones.

G. Positioning

1. Place the animal in dorsal recumbency with the entire distal leg prepared.
2. Prepare a site for harvesting a bone graft, if necessary.

H. Surgical Techniques

1. Stabilization of transverse metacarpal or metatarsal fractures.
   a. Repair multiple, simple transverse (or very short oblique) metacarpal bone fractures with IM pins.

Incise skin over the dorsal surface of the third and fourth bones. Incise subcutaneous tissues and elevate and retract extensor tendons to expose the fractures. Introduce the pin into the distal, dorsal surface of the bone to avoid the joint (use a high-speed burr to develop a slot in the bone). Blunt the tip of the pin to prevent it from penetrating the intact opposite cortex. Drive the pin through the slot and proximally across the fracture line and seat it in the proximal bone segment. Bend the distal end of the pin to prevent migration and simplify removal. Repeat the procedure for at least the third and fourth metacarpal or metatarsal bone, preferably all four bones. Protect the fixation with a splint or cast for 4 to 6 weeks. If more rigid fixation is required, apply bone plates as compression plates.

2. Stabilization of avulsion fractures and oblique diaphyseal fractures.
   a. For avulsion fractures use lag screws or orthopedic wire with Kirschner wires as tension band wire with patient fracture assessment of 8 to 10. Use lag screw for simple, oblique fractures of the diaphyses. Support with a splint or bivalve cast. Use a bone plate if diaphyseal fractures require additional support.
   b. Use lag screws for best results in athletic dogs.
3. Stabilization of comminuted diaphyseal fractures.
   a. Repair these fractures with small, dynamic compression plates (2.7 mm or 2.0 mm) or veterinary cuttable plates. Do not disturb fragments. Splint or cast after surgery.
   b. Alternatively, use multiple Kirschner wires or IM pins connected with acrylic to form an external fixator. This method is useful for treating open fractures.
4. Sesamoid bone excision.

Incise the skin adjacent to the large central pad directly over the ventral aspect of the affected joint. Continue the incision through subcutaneous tissues and identify the fractured sesamoid. Sharply dissect the sesamoid fragments from their ligamentous attachments. If the fragment is less than one third of the sesamoid bone, remove only the fragment. If the fragment is larger, remove the entire sesamoid bone. Suture subcutaneous tissues and skin separately.

5. Suture repair of luxations.

Incise skin and subcutaneous tissue dorsally over the affected joint to expose the torn joint capsule and collateral ligaments. Use multiple absorbable horizontal mattress sutures to repair the joint capsule and ligament. Continue to imbricate the capsular tissues until the joint is stable. Repair the capsule bilaterally if necessary. Also inspect the extensor tendon retinaculum for tears and stabilize it with interrupted sutures. Suture subcutaneous tissues and skin.

6. Digit amputation.

Make an elliptical skin incision paralleling the long axis of and around the digit, starting proximodorsally and ending distally on the palmar or plantar surface. Preserve the pad if amputating at the interphalangeal joints. Disarticulate the joint with sharp dissection. Remove the sesamoid bones (metacarpophalangeal or metatarsophalangeal joint amputation). Resect the distal end of the proximal remaining bone. Make a transverse osteotomy line for

the interphalangeal joints and third and fourth metacarpal or metatarsal bones, but bevel the osteotomy distally toward the midline for the second and fifth metacarpal or metatarsal bones. Suture soft tissues and skin, taking care to obtain a cosmetic closure.

7. Arthrodesis.

Expose the joint using the approach described for suturing joint luxations. Open the joint capsule and remove the articular cartilage with rongeurs. Conform the surfaces to get good contact at a functional angle (determined by observing adjacent toes). Temporarily hold the bones in position by driving small K-wires from the dorsal surface of each bone across the joint surface. Contour a small plate (2.0 mm) to the dorsal surface of the bones. Attach the plate using at least one lag screw across the joint surface. Alternatively, stabilize the arthrodesis with the small K-wires and a tension band wire in small dogs or cats in which rapid healing is anticipated.

V. Suture Materials/Special Instruments

A. Use a tourniquet to control hemorrhage during surgery, but maintain it only for 1 hour.

VI. Postoperative Care and Assessment

A. Take radiographs to assess fracture and luxation reduction and implant position and alignment of arthrodeses. Repeat every 4 to 6 weeks until the fracture(s) or the arthrodesis is healed. Until healing occurs support the repair in a splint or bivalve cast.

B. Instruct owner to limit activity and confine the animal until fracture bridges with bone.

C. After digit amputation, support the paw in a soft bandage for 1 to 2 weeks.

D. After healing, remove IM pins, plates, and external fixators, but unless complications arise leave wire and screws in place.

VII. Prognosis

A. Prognosis for normal function after healing or removal of sesamoid bones is good.

B. Base prognosis after surgical repair of joint luxations on the stability of the repair. Unstable joints develop progressive degenerative joint disease.

C. Function after amputation of the second and fifth digit is usually good, as is function after arthrodesis.

Pelvic Fractures

Acetabular Fractures (*SAS*, pp. 834-838)

I. General Considerations

A. Displaced acetabular fractures that heal without surgical reduction and stabilization result in degenerative joint disease.

B. Classify acetabular fractures as cranial transacetabular, central transacetabular, caudal transacetabular, or comminuted transacetabular. Central transacetabular fractures are the most common.

II. Diagnosis

A. Clinical Presentation

1. Signalment.
   a. Any age or breed dog or cat may be affected; acetabular fractures are rare in cats.
2. History.
   a. These fractures typically occur as a result of motor vehicle accidents or other blunt trauma.

B. Physical Examination

1. Expect these animals to have a non–weight-bearing lameness, although they may bear weight if the displacement is minimal.
2. Pain can generally be elicited, but crepitation may not be present.

C. Radiography

1. Take ventrodorsal and lateral radiographs. Take medial to lateral or oblique views if further delineation is needed.
2. A single fracture through the articular surface may appear comminuted because of bone fragments from a non–weight-bearing surface.

III. Medical or Conservative Management

A. Perform surgical reduction and stabilization of all acetabular fractures.

B. Consider conservative management only if surgery is not an option (e.g., because of financial constraints). Conservative treatment is similar to that described for ilial fractures.

IV. Surgical Treatment

A. Preoperative Management

1. Monitor urination and defecation.

2. Take chest radiographs and perform an ECG.
3. Provide analgesics.

B. Surgical Anatomy

1. Recognize that the sciatic nerve runs dorsomedial to the acetabulum.
2. Fractures cause the caudal acetabular segment to displace medial and cranial to the cranial segment, and may place the sciatic nerve dorsal or dorsolateral to the caudal segment.

C. Positioning

1. Position the animal in lateral recumbency with the dorsum raised 30 degrees from the table.
2. Perform a hanging-leg preparation.

D. Surgical Technique

Make a skin incision centered over the cranial border of the greater trochanter. Begin the incision 3 to 4 cm proximal to the dorsal ridge of the greater trochanter and curve it distally 3 to 4 cm following the cranial border of the femur. Incise the superficial leaf of the fascia lata at the cranial border of the biceps femoris muscle and retract the muscle caudally. Incise the deep leaf of the fascia lata and carry the incision proximally through the insertion of the tensor fasciae latae muscle at the greater trochanter and along the cranial border of the superficial gluteal muscle. Incise through the insertion of the superficial gluteal muscle at the third trochanter. Reflect the superficial gluteal muscle proximally and the biceps femoris caudally to find and visualize the course of the sciatic nerve. Perform an osteotomy of the greater trochanter with an osteotome and mallet. Position the osteotome just proximal to the insertion of the superficial gluteal muscle at the third trochanter. Angle the osteotome 45 degrees to the long axis of the femur to remove the trochanter with the insertions of the deep gluteal and middle gluteal muscles. Reflect the gluteal muscles and greater trochanter from the joint capsule with a periosteal elevator. Visualize the insertions of the gemellus muscle and tendon of the internal obturator and preplace a suture through the two near the trochanteric fossa. Incise both structures together at the trochanteric fossa and elevate the gemellus muscle from the caudolateral surface of the acetabulum with a periosteal elevator. Use the suture to retract the muscle proximally and caudally. When reducing the fracture, pay particular attention to the alignment of the articular surface (which is facilitated by incising the joint capsule). Place a specially designed canine acetabular plate (a metacarpal plate or mandibular reconstruction plate can work as well) on the dorsolateral surface of the acetabulum. Attempt to place two plate screws in the caudal fragment and three plate screws in the cranial fragment. After reduction and stabilization, suture the gemelli and internal obturator tendon to their point of insertion. Reduce and stabilize the greater trochanter with two Kirschner wires and a tension band wire. Place interrupted sutures in the insertion of the superficial gluteal muscle and a continuous suture in the insertion of the tensor fasciae latae muscle and deep leaf of the fascia lata. Use a continuous suture in the superficial leaf of the fasciae latae and the subcutaneous tissue. Suture skin with an interrupted suture pattern.

V. Postoperative Care and Assessment

A. Leash walk only until radiographic evidence that the fracture has healed, usually in 4 to 8 weeks.

B. Implants are not routinely removed unless they cause irritation.

VI. Prognosis

A. Prognosis is good to excellent if the fracture is anatomically reduced and appropriately stabilized.

Ilial, Ischial, and Pubic Fractures (*SAS*, pp. 839-844)

I. General Considerations

A. The pelvis is a boxlike structure, and for displacement of bone fragments to occur the hemipelvis must be fractured at three different sites.

B. Be sure to perform a complete physical exam to identify concurrent abnormalities such as bladder or urethral rupture.

C. Isolated ischial or pubic fractures are rare, and surgery is commonly performed if there is an associated soft tissue herniation.

II. Diagnosis

A. Clinical Presentation

1. Signalment.
   a. Any age or breed dog or cat may be affected.
2. History.
   a. There is typically a history of a vehicular accident, but gunshots and blunt trauma may also be the cause.

B. Physical Examination

1. Expect the animal to have a non–weight-bearing lameness; however, with little displacement there might be partial weight bearing.
2. Bruising is common, but if ventral abdominal bruising is severe or progresses, suspect urethral trauma.

C. Radiography

1. Take ventrodorsal and lateral radiographs.
2. Consider a urethrocystogram.

D. Laboratory Findings

1. Evaluate for azotemia and hyperkalemia if you suspect a bladder or urethral rupture.

III. Medical or Conservative Management

A. Treat minimally displaced, relatively stable ilial fractures (or cases in which owners are unable to afford surgery) conservatively. Use conservative treatment for isolated ischial or pubic fractures also.

B. Conservative therapy consists of strict rest for 3 weeks, then leash walks with gradual increase in activity for 4 weeks. Provide nonsteroidal anti-inflammatory drugs; maintain animal on clean, well-padded bedding; and monitor urination and defecation. Perform physical therapy to prevent joint and muscle contracture. Warn owners that limb manipulation may be painful for the animal.

IV. Surgical Treatment

A. General Considerations

1. Perform surgery with ilial fractures when suspecting nerve entrapment or with moderate to severe displacement and instability.
2. Inform owners that although many fractures heal adequately with conservative therapy, surgery will shorten the rehabilitation time.
3. Perform surgery with ischial or pubic fractures associated soft tissue herniation, or to reestablish integrity of the pelvic girdle in females that are to be bred.

B. Preoperative Management

1. Monitor urination, defecation, and respiration.
2. Perform chest radiographs and ECG.
3. Provide analgesics.

C. Surgical Anatomy

1. With ilial fractures the caudal fragment is often displaced medially and cranially to the wing of the ilium. Use caution when dissecting near the dorsal ilial border to prevent injury to the sciatic nerve.
2. Be cautious of the sciatic nerve when dissecting in the area of the ischial notch.
3. If dissecting near the obturator foramen, use caution with lateral surgical dissection because the obturator nerve passes through the foramen in this region.

D. Positioning

1. Position the animal in lateral recumbency for ilial and ischial fractures.
2. Use dorsal recumbency for pubic fractures.

E. Surgical Techniques

1. Approach to the ilial body.

Make an incision from the cranial extent of the iliac crest to 1 to 2 cm beyond the greater trochanter caudally. Center the incision over the ventral third of the ilial wing. Incise subcutaneous tissues and gluteal fat along the same line to visualize the intermuscular septum lying between the middle gluteal muscle and long head of the tensor fasciae latae muscle. Visualize the intermuscular septum between the superficial gluteal and short part of the tensor fasciae latae caudally. Continue the incision to separate the tensor fasciae latae muscle and middle gluteal muscle cranially and the tensor fasciae latae and superficial gluteal muscle caudally. Sharply dissect cranially to separate the middle gluteal muscle and long head of the tensor fasciae latae muscle. Palpate the ventral border of the ilium and make an incision at the border through the middle gluteal muscle. Isolate and ligate the iliolumbar vessel and reflect the deep and middle gluteal muscles from the lateral surface of the ilium. If additional exposure is needed, incise the branch of the cranial gluteal nerve that innervates the tensor fasciae latae muscle. For increased exposure so that

compression screws may be inserted, incise through the origin of the iliacus muscle along the ventral border of the body of the ilium.

2. Stabilization of the ilium with a bone plate.

Reduce the fracture by placing bone-holding forceps over the dorsal edge of the caudal ilial fragment and retracting it caudally. Be careful not to injure the sciatic nerve when manipulating the fracture fragments. Contour a plate to fit the normal curvature of the lateral surface of the bone. Use a ventrodorsal radiograph of the opposite ilium as a guide for plate contouring preoperatively. Reduce the fragment with bone-holding forceps and attach the plate to the caudal fragment first to allow the contour of the plate to assist in reduction of the cranial fragment. Then place screws in the cranial fragment. Caudal distraction of the ilial fragment is readily achieved, but lateral distraction of the caudal fragment can be difficult. Use the contour of the plate to aid in mediolateral reduction of the fracture. As the screws in the cranial fragment are tightened, the shape of the precontoured plate helps bring the caudal fragment into position. Place at least three plate screws in the cranial fragment and two in the caudal fragment. To close the incision, place sutures between the fascia of the middle gluteal muscle and tensor fasciae latae muscle cranially and the superficial gluteal muscle and tensor fasciae latae caudally. Approximate deep gluteal fat, subcutaneous tissue, and skin routinely.

3. Stabilization of the ilium with compression screws.

Reduce the fracture as described above and temporarily stabilize it with bone-holding forceps. Rotate the hemipelvis to visualize the ventral surface of the body of the ilium and insert two small Kirschner pins from ventral to proximal. To achieve additional stability place two compression screws in a ventral to proximal direction.

4. Approach to and stabilization of ischial fractures.

Make a skin incision adjacent to the caudal border of the greater trochanter. Reflect the biceps femoris muscle caudally to expose the sciatic nerve and external rotators as they insert into the trochanteric fossa. Incise and reflect the insertions of the external rotators caudally to expose the ischial body. Reduce and stabilize the fragments with a small bone plate and screws or a tension band.

5. Approach to and stabilization of pubic fractures.

Make a skin incision along the ventral midline (in the male dog adjacent to the penile sheath). Visualize the midline cranial to the pubic brim and incise through the tissues overlying the pubic symphysis. If herniated tissues are present, be careful to avoid inadvertently incising vital structures. Replace the herniated tissues into the abdominal cavity. Use a periosteal elevator to reflect adductor muscles from the pubis. Reduce the fragments and drill holes in adjacent fragments for placement of orthopedic wire. Place and tighten the wire to stabilize the fragments.

V. Suture Materials/Special Instruments

A. Use 20-gauge orthopedic wire for pubic fractures in small and medium-sized dogs and 18-gauge wire in larger dogs.

VI. Postoperative Care and Assessment

A. Radiograph at 6 to 8 weeks. Leash walks only until there is radiographic evidence of healing.

B. Do not remove implants unless they cause irritation.

VII. Prognosis

A. Prognosis is excellent for return to normal function after surgery with most ilial fractures, as is the prognosis for isolated pubic and ischial fractures.

Sacroiliac Luxations/Fractures (*SAS*, pp. 844-846)

I. General Considerations

A. The sacroiliac joint is commonly injured when the pelvis is fractured.

B. Recognize that the femoral and sciatic nerves are in close proximity to the sacroiliac joint and concurrent nerve damage may occur. Assess neurologic function before surgery.

II. Diagnosis

A. Clinical presentation

1. Signalment.
   a. Any age or breed dog or cat may be affected.
2. History.
   a. There is typically a history of a motor vehicle accident.

B. Physical Examination

1. Unless there is a contralateral limb injury, expect the animal to be non–weight bearing or minimally weight bearing on the affected limb.
2. When the patient is sedated, dorsoventral movement of the ilium can be detected.

C. Radiography

1. Take ventrodorsal and lateral radiographs.
2. Measure the width of the pelvic canal.

III. Medical or Conservative Management

A. Treat conservatively when there is little patient discomfort and minimal displacement of the hemipelvis, or when financial limitations preclude surgery. See conservative management of ilial fractures.

B. Expect lameness to persist for up to 12 weeks, but the majority of animals regain normal function.

C. Perform surgery if narrowing of pelvic outlet is expected to lead to constipation.

IV. Surgical Treatment

A. General Considerations

1. Stabilize sacroiliac luxations/fractures with bone screws or small intramedullary pins.

B. Preoperative Management

1. Assess lower urinary tract and neurologic status before surgery.

C. Positioning

1. Position the animal in lateral recumbency with the dorsal midline raised 45 degrees from the table.

D. Surgical Technique

1. Surgical approach.

Make a skin incision beginning over the dorsal iliac crest and continue it caudally parallel to the spine to a point even with the hip joint. Incise subcutaneous tissues and pelvic fat along the same line to expose the iliac crest. Incise through the periosteal origin of the middle gluteal muscle on the lateral ridge of the iliac crest. Make a second incision through the deep gluteal fascia and periosteal origin of the sacrospinalis muscle on the medial ridge of the iliac crest. The incisions merge caudally, where it may be necessary to incise through fibers of the superficial gluteal muscle. The supporting ligamentous tissues between the sacrum and ilium are usually separated with the impact of the original trauma. Therefore incision of the lumbar fascia allows lateral reflection of the ilium and exposure of the sacroiliac joint. Elevate the middle gluteal muscle from the lateral surface of the ilium to further expose the ilium for placement of implants. To close the incision, suture fascia of the middle gluteal and sacrospinalis muscles with an absorbable suture in an interrupted pattern. Next, suture subcutaneous tissues and skin using standard methods.

2. Stabilization using a screw.

Once the joint is exposed, position a blunt Hohmann retractor between the ilium and ventral bony shelf of the sacrum. Reflect the ilium ventrally with the retractor. This maneuver exposes the crescent-shaped articular cartilage and fibrocartilaginous joint surfaces of the sacrum. To position a screw properly in the sacrum, direct visualization of the lateral surface of the sacral wing is preferred. Use the appropriately sized drill bit to drill a thread hole 2 mm cranial and 2 mm proximal to the center of the crescent-shaped articular cartilage. The depth of the thread hole in the sacral body should be such that the screw tip

will extend to the midline of the sacral body. Determine the proper location of the glide hole in the ilium by palpating the articular prominence on the medial surface of the ilial wing. Drill the glide hole at the predetermined position with the appropriately sized drill bit. A glide hole is not needed if a partially threaded cancellous screw is used. Advance the proper length screw through the glide hole until the tip appears on the medial surface of the ilium. Bring the ilium caudally in alignment with the articular surface of the sacroiliac joint. Visually guide the screw tip into the prepared thread hole in the sacrum and tighten the screw.

V. Postoperative Care and Assessment

A. Allow leash walking only for 3 weeks; then gradually increase activity over the next 3 weeks.

B. Do not remove implants unless they cause a problem.

VI. Prognosis

A. Prognosis for return to normal activity is excellent after surgical stabilization.

Femoral Fractures

Femoral Capital Physeal Fractures (*SAS*, pp. 846-851)

I. General Considerations

A. These fractures can occur without significant trauma.

B. The femoral neck is usually displaced and lies adjacent to the ilial wing. If the physis of the greater trochanter is also fractured, the femoral shaft will be more dorsal.

II. Diagnosis

A. Clinical Presentation

1. Signalment.
    a. These fractures typically occur in animals less than 10 months of age.
    b. Young, male dogs are more likely to sustain trauma resulting in this type of fracture.

2. History.
   a. There is typically an acute non–weight-bearing lameness.

B. Physical Examination

1. There is usually a non–weight-bearing lameness with pain and crepitation on manipulation of the hip joint. If the fracture is minimally displaced these signs may be absent.

C. Radiography

1. Take ventrodorsal and medial to lateral radiographs. If displacement is difficult to detect, take a ventrodorsal view with the limbs in a "frog" position.
2. Provide sedation for proper positioning.
3. With a concurrent greater trochanter physeal fracture the cap of the greater trochanter will be superimposed over the shaft of the femur and appear as a half-moon radiodense object on a ventrodorsal radiograph. On a lateral projection, the cap of the trochanter will appear as a radiodense fragment caudal to the femur.

III. Medical or Conservative Management

A. Perform surgery to prevent severe degenerative joint disease and lameness.

IV. Surgical Treatment

A. General Considerations

1. Anatomic reduction is critical for optimal outcome.
2. Stabilize with either a compression screw or three triangulated Kirschner pins.
3. If the physis of the greater trochanter is separated, reduce and stabilize with Kirschner wires or a tension band (depending on the weight of the patient).

B. Surgical Anatomy

1. The blood supply to the femoral epiphysis is through a series of cervical ascending vessels lying outside the femoral neck that cross the physis and then penetrate the epiphysis.
2. The physis functions until approximately 8 months of age.

C. Positioning

1. Position the animal in lateral recumbency with the affected limb up.
2. Perform a hanging-leg preparation.

D. Surgical Techniques

1. Surgical approach.

Incise the skin 5 cm proximal to the greater trochanter. Curve the incision distally adjacent to the cranial ridge of the trochanter, and extend it distally for 5 cm over the proximal femur. Incise subcutaneous tissues and the juncture at the superficial leaf of the fasciae latae and cranial border of the biceps femoris muscle. Incise the deep leaf of the tensor fasciae latae between the tensor fasciae latae muscle and deep border of the biceps femoris muscle and superficial gluteal muscle. Reflect the tensor fasciae latae muscle cranially and the superficial gluteal and biceps femoris muscles caudally. Visualize the

tendinous insertion of the deep gluteal muscle by retracting the middle gluteal muscle proximally. Place a periosteal elevator beneath the deep gluteal muscle near its insertion and separate the deep gluteal muscle from the joint capsule using a sweeping motion with the elevator. Incise the deep gluteal tendon for one third to one half of its width at its point of insertion onto the greater trochanter. Leave 1 to 2 mm of tendon on the trochanter for closure, but make the incision through the tendon close to the bone. The joint capsule is commonly lacerated exposing the fracture surface of the femoral neck. If this is the case, enlarge the opening in the joint capsule with an incision from the rim of the acetabulum laterally through the point of origin of the vastus lateralis. If the joint capsule is intact, incise it parallel to the long axis of the femoral neck near its proximal ridge. Continue the joint capsule incision laterally through the point of origin of the vastus lateralis muscle on the cranial face of the proximal femur. It is important to keep this cut at the proximal point of origin just under the cut edge of the deep gluteal tendon. Reflect the vastus lateralis distally to expose the hip joint.

2. Fracture reduction.

Proceed in a stepwise manner. Recognize that the femoral epiphysis remains in the acetabulum because of its attachment to the round ligament, and the femoral neck is displaced cranial and dorsal to the acetabulum. To reduce the fracture, first bring the femoral neck distally so it lies cranial to and level with the acetabulum. Next, derotate the femur to correct for the abnormal anteversion, and third, slide the fracture surface of the femoral neck caudally into the matching surface of the femoral epiphysis.

E. Application of a Compression Screw

Initially, place two Kirschner pins in the femoral neck in a lateral to medial direction so that they lie parallel to one another. Position them so that one pin lies in the superior section of the femoral neck and one pin lies in the inferior section of the femoral neck. Drill a glide hole between the two pins to emerge at the center of the fracture surface. Angle the Kirschner pins and glide hole to correct for normal anteversion of the femoral neck. Reduce the fracture and drive the Kirschner pins into the femoral epiphysis. Place a drill insert into the glide hole for accurate drilling of the thread hole. The thread hole can penetrate the femoral epiphysis. Countersink the glide hole and determine the appropriate screw length by measuring the distance from the lateral surface of the greater trochanter to the femoral epiphyseal articular surface. Choose a screw that is 2 mm shorter than that measured with the depth gauge. Tap the thread hole and insert the screw. Remove one or both Kirschner pins and close the wound routinely.

1. Application of triangulated Kirschner pins.

With this technique, place three Kirschner pins through the femoral neck parallel to one another and positioned in the femoral neck so that they lie in a triangle. Avoid penetrating articular cartilage where it cannot be visualized at surgery. To determine the proper length of pins, place the first pin in the periphery of the femoral epiphysis so that it penetrates the articular cartilage where it is visible. Estimate the length of this pin that would not penetrate the articular cartilage and use it as a gauge for the remaining pins. Drive the remaining pins into the femoral epiphysis and place the joint through a normal range of motion to ensure that a pin has not penetrated the articular surface. Close the wound routinely.

V. Postoperative Care and Assessment

A. Allow leash walking only until healing has occurred, generally in 5 to 6 weeks.

B. Take ventrodorsal and medial to lateral radiographs to assess healing.

C. Do not remove implants unless clinical problems arise.

VI. Prognosis

A. Prognosis for pain-free function is good if the fracture is adequately reduced and stabilized.

B. Animals less than 5 months old may have a shortened femoral neck from closure of the capital physis. This may lead to hip subluxation and development of degenerative joint disease.

Femoral Neck Fractures (*SAS*, pp. 851-853)

I. General Considerations

A. Typically these fractures are a single basilar fracture, but comminution can occur.

B. They are mechanically unstable fractures because of the long moment arm and high shear stress.

II. Diagnosis

A. Clinical Presentation

1. Signalment.
   a. Any age or breed dog or cat may be affected, but it is more often mature animals.
2. History.
   a. Typically there is a history of a motor vehicle accident or a fall.

B. Physical Examination

1. Expect the animal to have a non–weight-bearing lameness and pain and crepitation on manipulation of the hip joint.

C. Radiography

1. Take ventrodorsal and lateral radiographs. The diagnosis can be missed on lateral alone.

III. Medical or Conservative Management

A. Surgical intervention is required. Conservative management is not an option.

IV. Surgical Treatment

A. General Considerations

1. Treat single fracture plane with a compression screw or triangulation of Kirschner wires.
2. With irreparable comminution perform a total hip replacement or femoral head ostectomy.

B. Surgical Anatomy

1. Approximate the normal angle of inclination, the femoral neck/ femoral shaft junction in the frontal plane (135 degrees), when performing surgical reduction.
2. Consider the normal angle of anteversion, 15 to 20 degrees, when inserting screws or pins into the femoral neck.

C. Positioning

1. Position the animal in lateral recumbency with the affected leg up.
2. Perform a hanging-leg preparation.

D. Surgical Techniques

1. General considerations.
   a. Perform a craniolateral approach to the hip joint as described for capital physeal fractures.
   b. Stabilize the fracture with a compression screw, unless biological assessment is extremely favorable, in which case Kirschner wires should be used.
2. Application of a partially threaded cancellous compression screw.

Place two Kirschner pins so they lie at the most proximal and distal level of the fracture surface. Drive the pins from medial to lateral, beginning at the fracture surface or from the lateral surface medially to exit at the fracture surface. Reduce the fracture and drive the Kirschner pins into the femoral epiphysis. Take care to avoid penetrating the articular surface. Drill a thread hole through the femoral epiphysis with the appropriate size drill bit parallel to and centered between the Kirschner pins. Measure the length of screw needed and tap the thread hole. Insert a partially threaded cancellous screw 2 mm shorter than the length measured so that all the threads cross the fracture plane and are seated into the femoral head. Leave one or both pins in place to serve as antirotational devices.

3. Application of triangulated Kirschner fins.

Insert three Kirschner pins from the fracture surface parallel to one another to form a triangle. Retrograde the pins to exit the bone near the third trochanter. Alternatively, normograde the pins so that they enter the bone at the third trochanter and exit at the fracture site. Reduce the fracture and drive the pins into the femoral epiphysis. Take care not to penetrate the articular surface.

V. Postoperative Care and Assessment

A. Allow leash walking only until healing has occurred, generally in 5 to 10 weeks.

B. Do not remove implants unless they cause a problem.

VI. Prognosis

A. The most common problems are inappropriate reduction and poor implant choice.

B. Avoid early loosening by using a compression screw and antirotational pin or two compression screws except where the biologic assessment indicates rapid healing.

Femoral Diaphysial Fractures (*SAS*, pp. 853-863)

I. General Considerations

A. If a patient presents with an acute femur fracture without discernible trauma, suspect preexisting bone pathology, such as a bone tumor. Check radiographs for cortical lysis or new bone formation.

B. Check for concurrent injuries because most femur fractures are from high-velocity injuries.

C. Assess for concurrent coxofemoral luxations and pelvic girdle injuries.

II. Diagnosis

A. Clinical Presentation

1. Signalment.
   a. Any age or breed dog or cat may be affected; however, young, male dogs are more likely to sustain trauma resulting in femoral fractures.
2. History.
   a. There is usually a history of trauma, or the animal may be found with a non–weight-bearing lameness.

B. Physical Examination

1. Expect the animal to have a non–weight bearing lameness with limb swelling. Pain and crepitus may be present on limb manipulation.
2. Abnormal proprioception generally is due to reluctance to move the limb.

C. Radiography

1. Take craniocaudal and lateral radiographs. Radiograph the contralateral limb to assess bone length and shape if anticipating bone plate fixation.
2. Provide sedation or general anesthesia for proper positioning.

III. Medical or Conservative Management

A. Perform stabilization to allow adequate healing. Casts and splints are not recommended.

B. Provide analgesics before definitive treatment.

IV. Surgical Treatment

A. Application of Intramedullary (IM) Pins

1. Use an IM pin equal to 70% to 80% of the diameter of the marrow cavity placed normograded or retrograded.
2. Normograde placement of an IM pin.
   a. There is less soft tissue to pass through, and the pin can be placed more laterally to avoid the sciatic nerve. However, the entry point into the bone is difficult to identify because insertion is generally done blindly.

Make a small skin incision at the point of pin entry over the bony prominence of the greater trochanter. If limb swelling makes the greater trochanter difficult to palpate, make a limited surgical exposure to locate the greater trochanter prominence. Push the point of the pin through soft tissues until it contacts the most proximal trochanteric ridge. Walk the point off the medial edge of the greater trochanter until it falls into the trochanteric fossa. Drive the pin in a slightly caudomedial direction. As the pin point emerges at the fracture site, overreduce the fracture and drive the pin into the distal fragment.

3. Retrograde placement of an IM pin.
   a. Allows visualization of the site of pin insertion; however, the point of pin exit is difficult to control.

So that the pin will exit more laterally in the trochanteric fossa, use a pin that is approximately 70% of the diameter of the isthmus, and as the pin is being retrograded force the shaft of the pin against the caudomedial cortex of the proximal fragment. Once the pin has exited through the trochanteric fossa, overreduce the fracture and seat the pin in the distal fragment.

4. Overreduce the fracture by bringing the distal fragment forward using the cranial cortex as a fulcrum point to compensate for the normal craniocaudal femoral curvature and allow the pin to be seated better in the distal extremity.
5. Always estimate proper pin length using a second pin of equal length as a reference outside the limb. Locate the distal pin tip near the level of the proximal pole of the patella. Perform routine closure, and verify proper placement with radiographs.
6. In cats, use normograde or retrograde placement. Overreduction of the distal fragment is not necessary.

B. Application of IM Pin Plus External Skeletal Fixation

1. Insert an IM pin that occupies 50% to 60% of the medullary cavity in

a normograde or retrograde manner. Place a selected number and type of transfixation pins dependent on the rigidity of fixation desired and the length of time the fixator must remain in place.

2. For stable fractures use a single external bar on the lateral side with one transfixation pin placed proximal to the fracture at the level of the third trochanter and one placed distal to the fracture 2 to 3 cm proximal to the femoral condyles.
3. For unstable fractures add additional transfixation pins. Distal pins cause more discomfort than proximal. Place the third pin craniolateral at the level of the third trochanter at a 60-degree angle to the first transfixation pin. Connect the two proximal and one distal pins, forming a triangular external frame that enhances the strength of the fixation system.

C. Application of External Skeletal Fixation

1. Expect high stress on transfixation pins because of the long distance from the external bar to the point where the transfixation pin enters the bone and the inability to use the stronger bilateral frames. Plan accordingly.
2. Achieve adequate spatial alignment by open reduction and placement of a temporary IM pin. Do not manipulate fragments in the area of comminution.
3. Place the most proximal and distal transfixation pins as half-pins, connect to the external bar, and then remove the temporary IM pin. Place the remaining transfixation pins depending on rigidity and duration needed of the fixator. Err on the side of being too rigid, because the fixator can be destabilized as the fracture heals. However, keep in mind that multiple transfixation pins increase morbidity and may reduce postoperative limb function.

D. Application of Bone Plates and Screws

1. Use bone plates for complex fractures or when prolonged healing is expect.
2. Place plates on the craniolateral tension surface of the femur with a minimum of three plate screws (six cortices) proximal and distal to the fracture with compression or neutralization plates, and a minimum of four plate screws (eight cortices) proximal and distal to the fracture for buttress plates.
3. Use a compression plate with transverse or short oblique fractures. Use a neutralization plate with long oblique fractures or comminuted fractures where the bone fragments can be reduced and stabilized with compression screws or cerclage wire. Use a buttress plate with comminuted fractures that cannot be reduced and stabilized.
4. Contour the plate using a craniocaudal radiograph of the contralateral limb.
5. Assist spatial alignment of the bone by inserting an IM pin.
6. Do not disturb bone fragments in the comminuted area.
7. Attach the bone plate with bicortical plate screws at the most proximal and distal plate holes. If removing the IM pin, use bicortical plate screws. If leaving the alignment pin in place, use monocortical screws centrally. The plate/pin combination increases the strength and fatigue life of the fixation, protecting the plate from premature breakage. It can be destabilized at 6 to 8 weeks by removing the IM pin.
8. Consider placing a cancellous bone graft in the fracture zone.

E. Preoperative Management

1. Immobilization of the fracture is difficult because of the location and generally is not performed. Contracture of thigh muscles helps immobilize bone fragments.

2. Stabilize and confine the animal before surgery.
3. Provide analgesics.

F. Surgical Anatomy

1. Consider the narrowest area of the marrow cavity, the isthmus, when choosing an IM pin. In the femur the isthmus is located within the proximal third of bone, just distal to the third trochanter, and can be estimated from radiographs.
2. The canine femur is normally curved in a cranial to caudal direction. Curvature varies by breed, but the curve is greatest in the distal third of the femur. The greater the curvature or the more distal the fracture, the smaller the IM pin.
3. The feline femur is uniform from proximal to distal and has little or no cranial to caudal bend.

G. Positioning

1. Position the animal in lateral recumbency.
2. Perform a hanging-leg preparation.

H. Surgical techniques

1. Surgical approach to the femoral diaphysis.

Make an incision along the craniolateral border of the thigh. Be careful to ensure that the incision is made slightly more cranial than lateral because the exposure plane will be at the cranial border of the biceps. Select the incision length based on the implant to be used, with bone plates or comminuted fractures requiring a longer incision. Incise the superficial leaf of the fascia lata along the cranial border of the biceps femoris muscle for the length of the incision. Retract the biceps femoris caudally to expose the vastus lateralis muscle. Incise the fascial septum of the vastus lateralis as it inserts at the caudal lateral border of the femur. Reflect the vastus lateralis from the surface of the femur to expose the femoral diaphysis. Carefully manipulate soft tissues and fracture hematoma to allow fracture reduction and application of a fixation system.

2. Stabilization of midshaft transverse or short oblique fractures.
   a. General considerations.
      i. These fractures require rotational and bending support.
      ii. Load will be shared between bone and implant following surgery. Use patient fracture assessment to determine length of time implant will need to function. With prolonged healing, 8 weeks or more, use implants that purchase the bone with threads.
   b. FAS 0-3.
      i. Use a bone plate and screws applied as a compression plate.
      ii. Or use a six-pin type Ia or type Ib EF with raised threaded transfixation pins.
      iii. Or use an IM pin tied in with an EF having raised thread transfixation pins.
   c. FAS 4-7.
      i. Use bone plate and screws.
      ii. Or use an IM pin combined or tied in with an EF with smooth or threaded pins.
   d. FAS 8-10.
      i. Use an IM pin with a cruciate hemicerclage wire.
      ii. Or use an IM pin with two-pin EF with smooth or threaded pins.

iii. In small patients less than 4 to 5 months of age, use a single IM pin placed closed in a normograde fashion.

3. Stabilization of midshaft long oblique fractures or comminuted fractures with one or two large butterfly fragments.
   a. FAS 0-3.
      i. Use interfragmentary compression with lag screws combined with neutralization plates to protect the reconstruction.
   b. FAS 4-7.
      i. Use an IM pin combined with cerclage wire for interfragmentary compression, with or without an EF with threaded transfixation pins.
   c. FAS 8-10.
      i. Use an IM pin combined with cerclage wire to compress the fracture lines.
4. Stabilization of midshaft comminuted fractures with multiple fragments.
   a. FAS 0-3.
      i. Use bone plate/pin combinations.
      ii. Or use rigid type Ib EF tied in to an IM pin with at least two threaded transfixation pins above and one below the area of comminution. Err on the side of too much rigidity, because the fixator can be destabilized postoperatively.
   b. FAS 4-7.
      i. Use bone plates functioning as a buttress plate. Use lengthening plates, broad plates, or in small patients stacked veterinary cuttable plates.
      ii. Or use type Ia or Ib EF (with or without a tie-in to an IM pin). Select threaded pins.
      iii. Or use an interlocking nail.
   c. FAS 8-10.
      i. Use an IM pin tied in to a two-pin, type Ia EF with smooth or threaded pins to bridge the area of comminution.
5. Stabilization of intertrochanteric fractures, which include fractures of the femoral neck, greater trochanter, and proximal metaphysis.
   a. In the immature patient with a favorable biological assessment, use multiple small pins in the femoral neck and femoral metaphysis.
   b. In adult patients, do not use IM pins because the screw securing the femoral head traverses the proximal metaphysis and does not allow placement of an IM pin; instead use a bone plate.
   c. If the metaphyseal fracture is a transverse or short oblique fracture, apply as a compression plate. If the area of comminution is reconstructed with cerclage wire or compression screws, apply as a neutralization plate. Otherwise, bridge the area of comminution with a buttress plate or a plate/rod combination.
   d. Place the compression screw used for stabilization of the femoral neck fracture through a plate hole or offset caudally to the plate.

V. Postoperative Care and Assessment

A. Allow leash walking only until the fracture has healed.

B. Take radiographs to assess healing.

C. Perform physical therapy to maintain joint motion.

D. Communicate with the client weekly about patient progress and activity restriction.

VI. Prognosis

A. These fractures generally heal without complication unless the implant loosens prematurely, which is usually a result of poor implant choice relative to the fracture-assessment score.

B. Fatigue breakage can occur. It is most often noted with bone plates when reduction and stabilization of a zone of comminution with cerclage wire or lag screws are unsuccessful.

Distal Femoral Physeal Fractures (*SAS,* pp. 863-867)

I. General Considerations

A. Classify these fractures according to the Salter-Harris scheme for physeal fractures (see Table 29-1). Most of them are Salter II.

B. A combination of a Salter II fracture and Salter IV fracture also occurs.

II. Diagnosis

A. Clinical Presentation

1. Signalment.
   a. These fractures typically occur with dogs or cats less than 9 months of age.
2. History.
   a. They most often occur from motor vehicle accidents but can also result from minor trauma.

B. Physical Examination

1. Expect these animals to have a non–weight-bearing lameness, with swelling, pain, and crepitus elicited on stifle manipulation.

C. Radiography

1. Take craniocaudal and lateral to medial radiographs. Always take two views because superimposition can cause fractures to be missed with a single radiograph.
2. Take additional oblique and skyline projections to evaluate the articular surfaces if fissures or fractures are suspected.

III. Medical or Conservative Management

A. Externally splint the leg in flexion or at a normal standing angle when financial restraint precludes surgery and there is minimal fracture separation.

IV. Surgical Treatment

A. Surgical Anatomy

1. Recognize that the distal femoral growth plate is shaped like a W and lies at the joint capsule reflection. The shape provides a degree of fracture stability, but the location requires arthrotomy for exposure.

B. Positioning

1. Position the animal in lateral recumbency with the affected leg up, or position the animal in dorsal recumbency.

C. Surgical Techniques

1. Surgical approach.

Palpate the distal end of the femoral shaft, and use this point as the center of the incision. Make the incision on the craniolateral surface of the stifle. Begin the incision 4 to 5 cm proximal to the center point and extend it 4 to 5 cm distally. Incise the subcutaneous tissue along the line and identify the fasciae latae and patellar tendon. Make a parapatellar arthrotomy through the distal fasciae latae and joint capsule. Make the incision along the caudal border of the vastus lateralis muscle through the intermuscular septum of the fasciae latae. Most often the distal femoral metaphysis lies cranial and lateral to the femoral condyles and will be exposed as the incision is made through the joint capsule and fasciae latae. Reflect the quadriceps muscles, patella, and patella tendon medially to expose the articular surface of the femoral condyles. To reduce the fracture, lever the condyles cranially and distally with a "spoon" Hohmann retractor placed between the fracture fragments.

2. Stabilization of Salter I or Salter II fractures with Steinmann pins.

With Salter I or Salter II fractures, use Steinmann pins alone or in combination with small Kirschner pins placed either as IM pins or cross pins. When Steinmann pins are used as IM pins they should be retrograded such that they enter the bone at the distal end of the femoral shaft. Insert one pin in the lateral metaphysis in line with the caudolateral cortex and the other in the medial metaphysis in line with the caudomedial cortex. Use small-diameter pins so they can bend with the curvature of the femoral canal as they pass proximally. Exit the pins through the bone and skin at the hip joint. Overreduce the fracture and drive the lateral pin into the lateral condyle and the medial pin into the medial condyle. When a single pin is used, retrograde the pin from the center of the fracture surface. Overreduce the fracture and insert the pin into the condyle. When placing Steinmann pins as cross pins, position them so that they enter the epiphysis and drive them proximally to a point where they are just visible at the fracture surface. Overreduce the fracture and drive the pins into the metaphysis. Suture joint capsule using an interrupted suture pattern. Close subcutaneous tissues and skin routinely.

3. Stabilization of Salter III or Salter IV fractures with Steinmann pins or bone plates and screws.

Reduce the femoral condyles and apply compression with a partially threaded cancellous bone screw placed across the fracture. In patients less than 4 months of age, diverging Kirschner pins may be used instead of a compression screw. After condylar reduction and stabilization, insert two small Steinmann pins as described for stabilization of Salter I and II fractures.

4. Stabilization of comminuted distal femoral physeal fractures.

Expect fractures to involve the trochlea and articular surface of the femoral condyles. Gain surgical exposure through a combination of the standard approach described with osteotomy of the tibial crest (see Chapter 30) and a medial arthrotomy. Reflect the patellar tendon, patella, and quadriceps muscle group proximally. Reconstruct the articular surface using a combination of partially threaded cancellous screws serving as compression screws and Kirschner pins. Once the articular fractures have been reconstructed, reduce the femoral condyles and stabilize them with Steinmann pins or a reconstruction plate. Steinmann pins are more commonly used, but in large and medium-sized dogs nearing maturity use a reconstruction plate. Contour the reconstruction plate to the lateral surface of the distal femur and femoral condyles.

V. Postoperative Care and Assessment

A. Place a 90/90 bandage for 7 days to reduce the incidence of quadriceps contracture.

B. Perform gentle flexion and extension of the joint to maintain range of motion.

C. Allow leash walking only until healing has occurs, usually 4 to 5 weeks.

D. Remove pins and plates that lie within the joint once healing has occurred.

VI. Prognosis

A. Prognosis for normal limb use is excellent with Salter I or Salter II fractures, despite likely premature closure of the distal femoral growth plate. The exception is in the large- or giant-breed dogs when the injury occurs at 3 to 5 months of age, when considerable growth potential is still present.

B. Prognosis for Salter III, Salter IV, and comminuted Salter fractures is good if anatomic reduction is achieved. However, inform owner of the potential development of secondary degenerative joint disease.

Patellar Fractures (*SAS*, pp. 867-868)

I. General Considerations

A. Patellar fractures are uncommon, but they can occur from direct trauma or from indirect trauma from forceful contraction of the quadriceps muscle group.

B. With these fractures quadriceps function and the ability to bear weight on the limb are lost.

C. Without treatment, forces separate the fragments of the patella resulting in continued loss of function. Loss of articular surface congruity results in degenerative arthritis.

D. Small fragments of the patella may not disable the animal if the quadriceps muscle group insertion remains functional.

II. Diagnosis

A. Clinical Presentation

1. Signalment.
   a. Any breed or age dog may be affected.
   b. Breeds afflicted with congenital myotonia and sporting breeds are most prone to fractures from forceful contraction of the quadriceps.
2. History.
   a. There is usually a history of trauma or an acute onset of lameness during strenuous exercise.

B. Physical Examination

1. Expect the animal to have a non–weight-bearing lameness with pain and swelling of the stifle.
2. Usually there is no crepitation, but there may be a palpable void in the quadriceps-patella-tendon mechanism.

C. Radiography

1. Take craniocaudal and medial to lateral radiographs.

III. Surgical Treatment

A. Preoperative Management

1. Confine to a cage until surgery.

B. Positioning

1. Position the animal in ventral recumbency.
2. Perform a hanging-leg preparation.

C. Surgical Technique

Make a craniolateral skin incision 1 cm lateral to the patella. Begin the incision 5 cm proximal to the patella and extend it distally to the tibial crest. Incise subcutaneous tissues overlying the patella and patellar tendon to expose the fragment ends. Place the limb in extension to reduce the fracture and then stabilize the fragments with a tension band placed over the cranial surface of the patella. If possible, drill small holes through the bone at the superior and inferior poles for wire placement; if this is not feasible because of patient size or comminution, place the wire deep within the fibrous tissue adjacent to the superior and inferior poles of the patella. Visualize the articular surface of the patella to ensure anatomic reduction after tightening the wire.

IV. Postoperative Care and Assessment

A. Allow leash walk only until radiographic union, usually 6 to 12 weeks.

V. Prognosis

A. Prognosis for return to athletic function is good to excellent if integrity of the patella-femoral joint is maintained.

Tibial and Fibular Fractures

Tibial and Fibular Diaphyseal Fractures (*SAS*, pp. 868-876)

I. General Considerations

A. Fractures of the tibia are usually the result of trauma, so evaluate for concurrent injuries. The fibula is usually fractured too, but rarely needs to be stabilized.

B. Minimal soft tissue covering makes open fractures common.

II. Diagnosis

A. Clinical Presentation

1. Signalment.
   a. Any age or breed dog or cat may be affected.
2. History.
   a. There is usually a history of non–weight-bearing lameness after trauma.

B. Physical Examination

1. There is usually a non–weight-bearing lameness with palpable swelling and crepitation.

C. Radiography

1. Take craniocaudal and lateral radiographs, including the proximal and distal joints.
2. Provide sedation if necessary, after ruling out contraindications for administration.
3. Take thoracic radiographs to evaluate pulmonary changes from trauma.

III. Medical Management

A. Use analgesics and provide antibiotics for open fractures.

B. Use splints and casts only for closed, nondisplaced, or greenstick fractures in immature animals. Immobilize the joint above and below the fracture. Be sure the animal will be able to bear weight on the opposite limb when applying a cast.

IV. Surgical Treatment

A. General Considerations

1. Use open reduction for simple or moderately comminuted fractures with large fragments that can be anatomically reconstructed to establish the bone column.
2. With severely comminuted fractures that cannot be completely reconstructed, use closed reduction and external fixation or open reduction and application of a buttress plate.
3. Select reduction method and fixation technique depending on fracture type and location, signalment, fracture-assessment score, and presence of additional skeletal injuries.

B. Application of Casts

1. Apply for fixation for stable fractures in young dogs or cats when the fracture will maintain adequate reduction and heal quickly.
   a. Immobilize the stifle and hock. Apply with the limb positioned in slight extension with varus angulation.
   b. Bivalve casts are occasionally used to support internal fixation, but they are not as rigid a fixation as cylinder casts.

C. Application of IM Pins

1. General considerations.
   a. With transverse or short oblique fractures, use unilateral external fixation with an IM pin to control rotation. With spiral or oblique fractures, where the fracture length is 2 to 3 times the diaphyseal diameter, use an IM pin and multiple cerclage wires.
   b. Always manipulate the hock to ensure the pin does not interfere with the joint.
2. Technique.

Place pins in a normograde manner starting at the proximal tibia. Insert through the skin on the medial aspect of the proximal end of the tibia so that they penetrate the bone at a point midway between the tibial tubercle and the medial tibial condyle on the medial ridge of the tibial plateau. Select a pin diameter that allows the pin to traverse the curve of the medullary canal without disrupting fracture reduction and, if used with an external skeletal fixator, allows fixation pins to be placed through the tibial metaphysis.

D. Application of External Skeletal Fixation

1. General considerations.
   a. Use external fixation to avoid invading the fracture site with metal implants with open fractures.
   b. Apply type Ia or unilateral external fixators to the cranial medial surface of the tibia where major muscle masses are avoided.
   c. Apply a type Ib EF in areas with minimal muscle coverage.
   d. With type II or bilateral fixation splints, penetration of major muscle masses is unavoidable, but use for increased stiffness.
   e. Place the most proximal and distal pins in the metaphyses and the central pins 1 to 2 cm from the fracture line. Place additional pins when there is adequate bone.

2. Type Ia and Ib frames.
   a. General considerations.
      i. Types Ia and Ib EFs are use with closed reduction or limited open reduction.
      ii. Use positive-profile thread pins to increase the stability of the fixator.
   b. Technique.

For a type Ia, place a unilateral fixation pin from the medial aspect of the proximal tibial metaphysis through the lateral cortex. Predrill for threaded pins. Repeat at distal metaphysis. Connect external connecting bar with pin gripping clamps in place, then place the rest of the fixation pins. Place type Ib frames cranially and medially on the tibia.

3. Type II frames.
   a. General considerations.
      i. After placing the fixator, take radiographs to ensure that proximal and distal joint surfaces are parallel to each other and there is no rotational malposition.
   b. Technique.

Place the initial transfixation pins in the proximal and distal metaphyses medial to lateral and parallel to their respective joint surface. Then reduce the fracture by distracting the transfixation pins manually, using the weight of the animal in the hanging-limb position, or using a fracture distractor. Perform a closed reduction or a limited open approach. Attach the medial and lateral connecting bars containing the predetermined number of clamps. Add a third connecting bar with three clamps to the transfixation pins on one side of the limb. Place the remaining pins using the guide bar to ensure proper alignment of the pins with the clamps. Place at least two pins proximal and distal to the fracture. For additional stiffness, construct a type III EF.

E. Application of Bone Plates and Screws

1. Apply bone plates to the wide, flat, medial surface of the tibia via a wide exposure.
2. Make the skin incision cranial to the position of the plate to avoid the implant irritating healing tissues.
3. Apply as a compression plate to transverse fractures. With long oblique or spiral fractures, reconstruct and compress the fracture with lag screws, then protect with a neutralization plate. With comminuted fractures that cannot be reconstructed, leave the fragments undisturbed and apply a buttress plate or a plate/rod combination.
4. With comminuted fractures, carefully contour the plate to match the craniocaudal radiographic view of the contralateral tibia. Failure to reproduce the normal curve of the tibia will result in valgus angulation of the limb.
5. Place autogenous cancellous bone during open reductions.

F. Preoperative Management

1. Manage open wounds and provide antibiotics after bacterial culture and sensitivity. Place a Robert Jones bandage to immobilize the fragments until surgery.

G. Positioning

1. Prepare a donor site if harvesting a cancellous bone graft.
2. For limited open or closed reduction and external skeletal fixation, position with the leg suspended from the ceiling.

3. For open reduction position the animal in dorsal recumbency with access to the medial surface of the leg.

H. Surgical Techniques

1. Craniomedial approach to the tibia.

Make a craniomedial skin incision parallel to the tibial crest, which extends the entire length of the tibia. Continue dissection through the fascia, avoiding the medial saphenous vein and nerve crossing the middle to distal third of the tibial diaphysis.

2. Stabilization of midshaft transverse or short oblique fractures.
   a. FAS 0-3
      i. Use a bone plate and screws inserted to function as a compression plate.
      ii. Or use a type II EF with raised threaded transfixation pins.
   b. FAS 4-7.
      i. Use a compression plate.
      ii. Or use a type II EF.
      iii. Or use an IM pin and two-pin, type Ia EF, with the transfixation pins either smooth or threaded.
   c. FAS 8-10.
      i. Use a cast.
      ii. Or use a type Ia four- to six-pin EF.
      iii. Or use an IM pin, two-pin type Ia EF.
3. Stabilization of midshaft long oblique fractures or comminuted fractures with a large butterfly fragment.
   a. FAS 0-3.
      i. Use a neutralization plate. Achieve interfragmentary compression first with wire or compression screws.
      ii. Or insert an IM pin initially and apply interfragmentary compression with cerclage wire. Then attach an external skeletal fixator with threaded pins.
   b. FAS 4-7.
      i. Use a neutralization plate.
      ii. Or use an IM pin plus cerclage wire for interfragmentary compression combined with a two-pin, type Ia EF with threaded pins.
   c. FAS 8-10.
      i. Use an IM pin combined with cerclage wire for interfragmentary compression.
4. Stabilization of midshaft comminuted fractures with multiple fragments.
   a. General considerations.
      i. If the biologic assessment is not favorable, consider that extended stresses on the implant may lead to implant failure. Use closed reduction, or insert an autogenous cancellous bone graft if open reduction is used.
   b. FAS 0-3.
      i. Use a bone plate/pin combination.
      ii. Or use a rigid type II or III EF with raised threaded pins. Err on the side of too much rigidity because the fixator can be destabilized postoperatively.
   c. FAS 4-7.
      i. Use a bone plate as a buttress plate.
      ii. Or use a type II EF applied with closed reduction.
   d. FAS 8-10.
      i. Use a type II EF with smooth or threaded pins.

V. Postoperative Care and Assessment

A. Follow care instructions as described for radial diaphyseal fractures.

B. Remove EF devices when there is radiographic evidence of bridging callus.

C. Remove IM pins after the fracture has healed, and plates as well, because minimal soft tissue coverage over the plate tissue can cause irritation and cold sensitivity.

Tibial and Fibular Metaphyseal and Epiphyseal Fractures (*SAS*, pp. 876-879)

I. General Considerations

A. Fractures of the distal tibia in mature animals usually involve the malleoli. Perform accurate alignment and rigid fixation to achieve joint stability and decrease subsequent development of degenerative joint disease.

II. Diagnosis

A. Clinical Presentation

1. Signalment.
   a. Any age or breed dog or cat may be affected.
2. History.
   a. Typically there is a history of a non–weight-bearing lameness after trauma.

B. Physical Examination

1. Expect there to be swelling, pain, crepitation, and apparent instability of the adjacent joint.
2. Abnormal proprioception is generally due to reluctance to move the limb.

C. Radiography

1. Take craniocaudal and lateral radiographs, including the proximal and distal joints.
2. Use sedation for proper positioning, provided no contraindications to sedation exist.
3. Take thoracic radiographs to evaluate pulmonary changes.

III. Surgical treatment

A. Application of an IM Pin and Figure-Eight Kirschner Wire for Transverse or Short Oblique Proximal Tibial Fractures

Reduce and stabilize with IM pins as described for diaphyseal fractures of the tibia. If the fracture is not rotationally stable, angle a Kirschner wire across the fracture line. Place a figure-eight orthopedic wire around both ends of the Kirschner wire to provide compression to the fracture line.

B. Application of Crossed Kirschner Wires or IM Pins for Transverse or Short Oblique Proximal or Distal Tibial Fractures

Reduce the fracture and drive a Kirschner wire from the lateral surface of the tibial epiphysis, across the fracture into the tibial metaphysis, and exit the medial cortex. Drive a second wire from the medial tibial epiphysis, across the fracture into the metaphysis, and exit the lateral cortex. Take care to avoid penetrating the articular surface. Alternatively, drive the Kirschner wires from the metaphysis to the epiphysis. This technique can also be used for transverse fractures of the distal tibial metaphysis.

C. Preoperative Management

1. Manage open wounds after taking a culture for microbial sensitivity testing.
2. Temporarily stabilize the fracture with a Robert Jones bandage.

D. Surgical Anatomy

1. Avoid the saphenous nerve that lies caudal to the medial surface of the proximal tibia.

E. Positioning

1. Prepare donor site if harvesting a cancellous bone graft.
2. Position the animal in lateral or dorsal recumbency for proximal tibial and fibular fractures.
3. Position the animal in dorsal recumbency for distal tibial and fibular fractures.

F. Surgical Techniques

1. Surgical approach to the proximal tibia.
   a. Follow the craniomedial approach to the tibia and extend proximally to include the metaphysis. For fibular head stabilization use the lateral approach to the stifle.
2. Surgical approach to the distal tibia.
   a. Follow the craniomedial approach to the tibia and extend distally to expose the medial malleolus. Approach the lateral malleolus via a lateral skin incision over the malleolus and blunt and sharp dissection of surrounding tissues to expose the bone.
3. Stabilization of proximal tibial and fibular metaphyseal fractures.
   a. Stabilize the tibia with a cast if the fracture can be reduced closed, is stable, and will heal rapidly.
   b. If open reduction is necessary, stabilize tibia with an IM pin and adjunct wire fixation. If you elect to use crossed Kirschner wires or cancellous lag screws, additional external support may be required.
   c. Stabilize the fibula if stability of the stifle is impaired because of

disruption of the lateral collateral ligament. Secure the fibular head to the tibia with a screw and Teflon washer.

4. Stabilization of malleolar fractures.
   a. Treat malleolar fractures with open reduction and internal fixation with a tension band, or consider placing a cancellous screw in lag fashion if the fracture-assessment score is low.
   b. Support the repair with additional external fixation or coaptation as necessary.
5. Application of a tension band.

Reduce the fracture (i.e., medial malleolus of the tibia or lateral malleolus of the fibula) and start two Kirschner wires in the fragment. Drive the wires across the fracture line to lodge in the major bone segment. Place a transverse drill hole in the major bone segment and pass a figure-eight wire through the hole, around the Kirschner wire, and tighten it.

6. Application of lag screws.

For the medial malleolus, reduce the fracture and drill a gliding hole (equal to the diameter of the threads on the screw) in the malleolar fragment. Place an insert drill sleeve into the gliding hole and drill a smaller hole (equal to the core diameter of the screw) across the tibia. Measure, tap, and select and place the appropriate length screw. Compression of the fracture should occur. When stabilizing the proximal or distal fibula to the tibia, treat the fibula as the fragment by drilling the gliding hole through the fibula and the tapped hole in the tibia.

IV. Postoperative Care and Assessment

A. Take radiographs to assess fracture reduction, bone alignment, and implant position.

B. After internal fixation apply a padded bandage for a few days.

C. Perform physical therapy (range-of-motion exercises for 10 to 15 minutes, two to three times a day).

D. Treat open wounds daily with wet-to-dry dressings until a granulation bed has formed.

E. Perform daily hydrotherapy to aid in cleaning open wounds and reduce swelling.

F. Limit exercise until bone heals.

G. Recheck at 2 weeks, then every 4 to 6 weeks for radiographic evaluation.

H. Remove implants after bone healing if they irritate soft tissues.

V. Prognosis

A. Tibial and fibular metaphyseal and epiphyseal fractures usually heal quickly.

B. Complications include malunion or degenerative joint disease if articular cartilage is involved in the fracture.

Tibial and Fibular Physeal Fractures (*SAS*, pp. 879–882)

I. General Considerations

A. Use Salter-Harris classification to categorize physeal fractures (see Table 29-1).

B. Tibial physeal fractures may not always be displaced.

C. Proximal fractures are usually Salter type I or II, rarely Salter III or IV.

D. With Salter I or II fractures, look for the epiphysis to be displaced caudolateral to the tibial diaphysis with possible injury to collateral ligaments. Perform open reduction and internal fixation.

E. Distal tibial physeal fractures are also usually Salter type I or II.

II. Diagnosis

A. Clinical Presentation

1. Signalment.
   a. Immature dogs or cats with open physes may be affected.
2. History.
   a. There is typically a history of a non–weight-bearing lameness after trauma.

B. Physical Examination

1. There is usually swelling, pain, crepitation, and apparent instability of the adjacent joint.
2. Abnormal proprioception generally is due to reluctance to move the limb.

C. Radiography

1. Take craniocaudal and lateral radiographs, including proximal and distal joints. With minimally displaced fractures, it may be difficult to determine if the normally radiolucent physis is fractured. Compare with radiographs of the opposite limb.
2. Use sedation for proper positioning, provided no contraindications to sedation exist.
3. Take thoracic radiographs to evaluate pulmonary changes from trauma.
4. Remember that radiographs at the time of injury do not provide information about crushing injuries to the physis or damage to the physeal blood supply.

III. Surgical Treatment

A. General Considerations

1. Treat physeal fractures with external coaptation or internal fixation, recognizing that internal fixation may affect physeal function.
2. Threads of a pin or screw placed across the physis will not allow continued growth; therefore place a smooth IM pin or Kirschner wire perpendicular to and across the physis to allow proliferating cartilage to slide along the pin.

B. Application of Casts

1. Apply from the toes to above the stifle. To avoid angular limb deformities place the animal in lateral recumbency with the affected limb down, holding the limb in slight extension with the hock in slight varus while the cast hardens.

C. Application of Crossed Kirschner Wires or IM Pins

1. General considerations.
   a. Avoid traumatizing the physis when reducing the fragments.
   b. Use smooth implants when crossing the physis.
   c. Use this technique for physeal fractures of the distal tibia even though the Kirschner wire or pin driven from the lateral aspect of the tibia penetrates the fibular malleolus.
2. Technique.

Drive one Kirschner wire from the lateral surface of the tibial epiphysis across the physis, into the tibial metaphysis, and through the medial cortex. Drive the second wire from the medial tibial epiphysis across the physis, into the metaphysis, and through the lateral cortex. Avoid penetrating the articular surface.

D. Application of a Tension Band Wire

1. General considerations.
   a. Use a tension band wire to stabilize tibial tubercle physeal fractures.
2. Technique.

Reduce and start two Kirschner wires in the fragment. Drive the wires across the physis to lodge in the proximal tibia and check if stabilization is sufficient to prevent avulsion of the fracture. If not, use a tension band wire even though it may prevent physeal growth. Drill a transverse hole in the major bone segment and pass a figure-eight wire through the hole and around the Kirschner wire. Tighten the wire.

E. Preoperative Management

1. Temporarily place a Robert Jones bandage.

F. Positioning

1. Position the animal in dorsal recumbency.

G. Surgical Technique

1. Surgical approach to the craniomedial tibia.
   a. Use the craniomedial approach to the tibia described in the section on tibial and fibular diaphyseal fractures extended proximally to include the metaphysis.

2. Surgical approach to the distal physis.
   a. Approach distal physeal fractures with a distal extension of the craniomedial approach to the tibia or by a cranial skin incision and retracting the extensor tendons.
3. Stabilization of nondisplaced fractures.
   a. Treat with closed reduction and a cast that immobilizes the stifle and the hock.
4. Stabilization of displaced fractures.
   a. Perform internal fixation for proximal physeal fracture in immature dogs with Kirschner wires or small IM pins.
   b. Perform closed reduction and stabilize minimally displaced distal tibial fractures with a cast.
5. Stabilization of avulsion fractures of the tibial tubercle.
   a. Reduce and stabilize to restore quadriceps muscle function and stifle extension.
   b. Perform open reduction, then place two Kirschner wires or a tension band wire.
   c. Occasionally, closed reduction can be performed by sufficiently extending the stifle. Then cast the limb in extension for 2 to 3 weeks.

IV. Postoperative Care and Assessment

A. Take radiographs to assess fracture reduction and implant position.

B. After internal fixation, place a padded bandage for a few days.

C. Perform physical therapy (range-of-motion exercises for 10 to 15 minutes, two to three times a day).

D. Limit exercise for 4 to 6 weeks.

E. Recheck in 2 weeks, and at 4 to 6 weeks for radiographic evaluation.

F. Compare radiographs to contralateral bone for length as early as 2 to 3 weeks after the injury to determine physeal function. If the physeal line appears as a bone density, endochondral ossification has occurred and continued physeal function is unlikely.

G. Remove implants after healing to allow bone growth if the physis is functional. Perform early removal of tension band wires used to stabilize the tibial tubercle to encourage physeal function (i.e., 3 to 4 weeks postoperatively).

V. Prognosis

A. Prognosis for healing is excellent, but continued growth of the physis depends on the amount of damage sustained by the zone of proliferating cells.

B. Premature closure of the proximal or distal tibial physis usually results in a short (but straight) limb for which the animal compensates by extending the stifle. Premature closure of the tibial tuberosity physis can alter the conformation of the proximal tibia and result in impaired function and degenerative joint disease of the stifle.

30

Management of Joint Disease (*SAS*, pp. 883-998)

General Principles, Techniques, and Nonsurgical Joint Disease (*SAS*, pp. 883-898)

I. Definitions

A. **Osteoarthritis** is noninflammatory degenerative joint disease (DJD) characterized by degeneration of articular cartilage, hypertrophy of marginal bone, and synovial membrane changes.

B. **Synovial joints** are lined with synovial membrane and allow relatively free movement.

C. **Fibrous joints** (i.e., skull, tooth sockets) and **cartilaginous joints** (i.e., mandibular symphysis, growth plates) allow for little or no movement.

II. General Considerations

A. Most dogs with joint disease are managed medically rather than surgically.

B. Joint disease can be categorized as inflammatory (infectious or noninfectious) or noninflammatory. Noninfectious arthropathies may be erosive or nonerosive (Table 30-1).

III. Medical Management of Joint Disease

A. Be aware that some nonsteroidal antiinflammatory drugs (NSAIDs) (e.g., salicylates, fenoprofen, ibuprofen) affect articular cartilage by inhibiting net proteoglycan synthesis. However, they also reduce pain, encourage joint motion, and decrease synovitis.

B. Other NSAIDs do not appear to have negative effects on proteoglycan synthesis (e.g., piroxicam, naproxen, and diclofenac).

Table 30-1
Classification of arthropathies in dogs and cats

INFLAMMATORY
Infectious
Bacteria
Rickettsia
Spirochetes
Fungi
Mycoplasma
Protozoa
Noninfectious
Erosive
Rheumatoid arthritis
Feline chronic progressive polyarthritis
Erosive polyarthritis of greyhounds
Periosteal proliferative arthropathy
Nonerosive
Idiopathic immune-mediated polyarthritis
Chronic inflammatory-induced polyarthritis
Plasmacytic-lymphocytic synovitis
Systemic lupus erythematosus
NONINFLAMMATORY
Degenerative joint disease
Trauma
Neoplasia

C. Corticosteroids depress chondrocyte metabolism and alter the matrix composition by decreasing proteoglycan and collagen synthesis; therefore avoid using corticosteroids to treat cartilage injury or DJD.

D. Polysulfated glycosaminoglycans induce articular cartilage matrix synthesis and decrease matrix degradation; however, these effects appear to be more beneficial in prophylaxis than in treatment of ongoing osteoarthritis.

IV. Antibiotics

A. For infectious arthritis administer antibiotics based on culture and sensitivity for 4 to 6 weeks, and at least 2 weeks after cessation of clinical signs.

V. Surgical Techniques

A. Synovial Fluid Collection

1. General considerations.
   a. Synovial fluid collection is essential to differentiate arthropathies.

b. Provide sedation.
c. Use sterile gloves, 25-gauge needles, 22-gauge 1½-inch needles (for shoulder, elbow, and stifle joints in larger dogs), 3-inch needles (for the hip joint), and 3-ml syringes.
d. To improve reliability, incubate sample for 24 hours in blood culture medium before culturing on blood agar plates.

2. Procedure.

Select the joint(s) that are swollen for initial taps. Clip the appropriate area over the joint and prepare the site for an aseptic procedure. Use a gloved hand to palpate landmarks. Insert a needle attached to a syringe into the joint. Apply gentle suction to the syringe. After the fluid has been collected, release the negative pressure on the syringe and withdraw the needle. If blood appears in the syringe, withdraw the syringe immediately; contamination with blood can alter cell counts. If only a few drops of fluid are obtained (common in small dogs and cats), spray the material directly onto a slide and examine it cytologically. Estimate viscosity as the fluid drops from the needle to the slide. Normal joint fluid is viscous and forms a long string. Place a drop of fluid on a slide and make a smear for an estimated complete cell count and a differential cell count. Culture fluid for bacterial and mycoplasmal growth.

VI. Healing of Cartilage Defects and Response of Cartilage to Treatment

A. With reversible damage, as with some inflammation, chondrocytes may replace the lost matrix components, once the insult is removed.

B. With superficial lacerations (not down to subchondral bone) a standard inflammatory response does not occur because inflammatory cells cannot gain access to the joint. Nearby chondrocytes respond, but not enough to heal; however, superficial lacerations seldom progress.

C. With a full-thickness cartilage defect, a fibrin clot forms and is replaced within 5 days by fibroblast-like cells and collagen fibers. After 2 weeks, metaplasia of the fibroblast-like cells into chondrocytes occurs. These chondrocytes do not function normally, and the tissue is thinner than articular cartilage and prone to fibrillation and erosive changes.

D. Joint stabilization.

1. Perform joint stabilization in animals with acute joint instability with the goal of recreating normal anatomic relationships and permitting normal joint function. Cartilage will be repaired if irreversible damage is not present and if cartilage was normal before injury.
2. Cranial cruciate ligament injuries are often repaired after changes have already occurred, and most techniques do not restore normal anatomic relationships. Degenerative joint disease is then progressive despite surgical treatment.

E. Joint immobilization.

1. Avoid prolonged immobilization of synovial joints because it causes progressive proteoglycan loss and decreased synthesis, which leads to cartilage softening.
2. Allow limited activity; forced activity after immobility may further damage softened cartilage.

F. Continuous passive motion.

1. Experimentally, early motion and weight bearing are beneficial for

repair of full-thickness cartilage defects. Continuous passive motion also appears to accelerate repair of full-thickness cartilage defects with tissue more similar to hyaline cartilage.

Selected Nonsurgical Diseases of Joints (*SAS*, pp. 888-898)

I. Degenerative Joint Disease

A. DJD is a noninflammatory, noninfectious degeneration of articular cartilage accompanied by subchondral bone sclerosis, osteophyte formation, periarticular soft tissue fibrosis, and synovial membrane inflammation.

B. Primary DJD is a disorder of aging in which cartilage degeneration occurs for unknown reasons.

C. Secondary DJD occurs in response to recognizable joint disease.
   1. The signalment depends on the underlying etiology.
   2. The presenting clinical sign is usually lameness, which may be acute or chronic and persistent or intermittent. Joint swelling may be due to effusion, but is more likely due to periarticular fibrosis from chronic disease. Decreased range of motion, crepitus, and joint instability are common.
   3. Findings that support a diagnosis.
      a. Radiographs reveal subchondral bone sclerosis, articular and periarticular osteophyte formation, joint-space narrowing, joint effusion, and increased prominence of periarticular soft tissues.
      b. Rheumatoid factor, systemic lupus erythematosus (SLE) preparations, and antinuclear antibody (ANA) test results are usually normal.
      c. Synovial fluid analysis may reveal decreased synovial fluid viscosity, increased synovial fluid volumes, and increased numbers of mononuclear phagocytic cells (6000 to 9000 WBC/ml).

D. Correct the underlying problem.

E. Perform surgical therapy and medical treatment to reduce or eliminate clinical signs. However, expect degenerative changes to progress.

F. Keep in mind that asymptomatic dogs may not ever develop lameness. Such animals do not need treatment just because they have radiographic signs of DJD.

G. Medical management includes weight loss/control, physical therapy, antiinflammatory drugs (see Appendix I), and rest during acute clinical signs.
   1. Inform owner of potential side effects of NSAIDs. They vary with the drug, but many can cause gastrointestinal irritation, anorexia, vomiting, diarrhea, or melena. Try Ascriptin instead of plain aspirin, discontinue use, or use misoprostol concurrently to help prevent gastric erosion/ulceration.
   2. Do not give NSAIDS concurrently with steroids.

3. Use steroids for DJD only as a last resort. Administer infrequently and restrict exercise for several weeks after treatment to protect the cartilage.

H. When medical management is unsuccessful, consider surgical treatment to salvage limb function, such as arthrodesis. Reserve amputation for a non–weight-bearing limb with unrelenting pain that has been unresponsive to other therapies.

II. Septic (Bacterial) Arthritis

A. Septic arthritis is joint infection from hematogenous spread or direct inoculation of bacteria.

B. Diagnose septic arthritis based on synovial fluid analysis, radiographic changes, and positive bacterial cultures.
1. With acute disease expect severe lameness with a swollen, painful, or warm joint, potentially with a reduced range of motion. With chronic disease expect single or multilimb weight-bearing lameness with joint swelling and subclinical endocarditis.
2. Systemic signs (pyrexia, lethargy, and anorexia) occur in only a small percentage of animals. Chronic disease is essentially walled off within the joint.
3. Dogs with infection from bacterial endocarditis often have multiple joint involvement, lameness, pyrexia, lethargy, anorexia, and/or cardiac murmurs.
4. Findings that support a diagnosis.
   a. Early radiographic signs of septic arthritis are joint effusion and soft tissue swelling. Later changes include bone lysis, periosteal new bone formation, joint surface irregularities, subchondral bone sclerosis, and joint subluxation.
   b. Echocardiography may demonstrate valvular lesions confirming bacterial endocarditis.
   c. Arthrocentesis may reveal increased numbers (40,000 cells/ml to more than 100,000 cells/ml) of polymorphonuclear leukocytes and bacteria.
   d. Fifty percent of cultures of septic joints are negative; use blood culture media.

C. Differentiate bacterial causes from other infectious agents causing arthropathies (e.g., spirochetes, rickettsiae, fungi, bacterial L-forms, mycoplasmas, and protozoa).

D. Treat with appropriate antibiotic for 4 to 6 weeks, and at least 2 weeks after cessation of clinical signs. Use tetracycline when bacterial L-forms are suspected.

E. Debride and lavage joints with postoperative joint infections, penetrating joint wounds, or septic joints in which treatment was delayed longer than 72 hours, or that have not responded to 72 hours of appropriate medical therapy.
1. Acute septic arthritis is a surgical emergency.
2. Do not perform surgery if the disease is secondary to bacterial endocarditis.
3. Explore the joint and place ingress-egress drains, or leave incision open for lavage.

4. Perform saline lavage two to three times daily, with or without 0.1% povidone-iodine.
5. Use oral antibiotics, daily wound management, and passive range of motion.
6. Keep the limb in a bandage or splint for 4 weeks to allow cartilage healing before full weight bearing.

F. Prognosis for normal joint function depends on the amount of cartilage destruction.

III. Rickettsial Polyarthritis

A. Riskettsial polyarthritis is caused by rickettsiae transmitted by arthropods.

B. Rocky Mountain spotted fever (RMSF), caused by *Rickettsia rickettsii,* typically presents with an acute onset of multilimb lameness, joint pain, fever, petechial hemorrhages, lymphadenopathy, neurologic signs, facial edema, and edema of the extremities.

C. Ehrlichiosis, caused by *Ehrlichia canis,* can be acute or chronic and typically presents with fever, anorexia, lymphadenopathy, weight loss, lameness, joint pain, petechiation, and neurologic signs.

D. Findings that support a diagnosis.

1. Paired serologic testing is recommended.
2. On radiographs there is typically joint effusion and periarticular soft tissue swelling. Bones and cartilage should appear normal. There may be a thrombocytopenia and increased nondegenerate polymorphonuclear leukocytes in the joint fluid.

E. Treat with doxycycline (10 mg/kg PO, SID), tetracycline (22 mg/kg PO, BID), or chloramphenicol (50 mg/kg PO, TID). Surgery is not indicated.

F. Prognosis with RMSF depends on clinical signs. If not treated until late, generalized CNS signs; uveitis; necrosis of affected tissues; and chronic, progressive polyarthritis may develop. Ehrlichia infections generally respond well to medical therapy.

IV. Lyme Disease

A. Lyme disease is caused by the tick-borne spirochete *Borrelia burgdorferi.* Recognize that it takes several hours of feeding to transmit the spirochete.

B. There is little evidence that cats exhibit clinical disease.

C. Intermittent episodes that may include multilimb lameness, fever, lymphadenopathy, and anorexia are common with the animal appearing normal between acute exacerbations. Glomerulonephritis, renal tubular damage, or cardiac abnormalities may occur with chronic infection.

D. Findings that support a diagnosis:

1. Radiographs are generally normal during the acute phase. Synovial fluid from affected joints is less viscous and has increased numbers of

nondegenerate neutrophils. The organism can be visualized using phase-contrast or dark-field microscopy. Attempts to culture are usually unsuccessful.
2. Positive serologic findings reflect exposure to the organism, not necessarily active infection. An extremely high titer or dramatic increase in a convalescent titer, coupled with clinical signs and a response to antibiotic therapy is diagnostic.

E. Treat with doxycycline (10 mg/kg PO, SID).

F. Surgery is generally not indicated; however, with chronic severe synovitis a subtotal synovectomy may be beneficial.

G. Inform owners the prognosis is excellent for acute infections if treated promptly, but uncertain for dogs with chronic infections.

V. Nonerosive Idiopathic Immune-Mediated Polyarthritis

A. Diagnose nonerosive idiopathic immune-mediated polyarthritis by ruling out all other causes of polyarthritis: septic arthritis, rickettsial arthritis, rheumatoid arthritis, other inflammatory nonerosive polyarthropathies and DJD. The etiology is presumed to be associated with immune complex formation.

B. There is typically a history of acute or chronic single or multilimb lameness, stiffness, difficulty rising, pyrexia, anorexia, and/or lethargy. Other systemic abnormalities (dermatitis, glomerulonephritis, uveitis) may occur.

C. Diagnose this polyarthritis by synovial fluid analysis, by joint radiographs that do not show erosive or proliferative bone lesions, and by eliminating other known causes.

D. Findings that support a diagnosis.
1. Joint radiographs do not show erosive or proliferative bone lesions.
2. Synovial fluid is thin and turbid, with a normal mucin clot test. Nucleated cell counts are markedly elevated with predominately nondegenerate neutrophils.
3. Most dogs test negative for antinuclear antibody (ANA) and rheumatoid factor.

E. Treat with glucocorticoids starting at 2 to 4 mg/kg/day for 2 weeks, then gradually decrease the dosage to the lowest amount that will prevent clinical signs. Many animals require lifelong therapy. Try cyclophosphamide or azathioprine if clinical signs persist despite corticosteroids.

F. Prognosis for remission is good, but expect side effects from long-term corticosteroids.

VI. Chronic Inflammatory-Induced Polyarthritis

A. Nonerosive inflammatory polyarthritis may occur secondary to any chronic inflammatory disorder or persistent antigenic stimulus. The synovium becomes thickened, but typically the cartilage and bone are unaffected.

B. There is typically a history of either acute or chronic lameness, stiffness, difficulty rising, pyrexia, anorexia, and/or lethargy, along with clinical signs of the inciting disease.

C. Findings that support a diagnosis.
1. Radiographs typically reveal no abnormalities, or show joint effusion and periarticular soft tissue swelling.
2. Synovial fluid is thin and turbid, with a normal mucin clot test. Nucleated cell counts are markedly elevated, with predominately nondegenerate neutrophils.
3. Most dogs test negative for ANA and rheumatoid factor.
4. Joint fluid is sterile.

D. Treat chronic inflammatory-induced polyarthritis by eliminating the underlying disease. Consider oral glucocorticoids for short-term control of severe synovitis.

VII. Plasmacytic-Lymphocytic Synovitis

A. Plasmacytic-lymphocytic synovitis is an immune-mediated arthropathy associated with plasmacytic and lymphocytic infiltration of the synovium, often affecting stifle joints, that leads to cruciate ligament degeneration and rupture and DJD.

B. There is typically a history of unilateral or bilateral rear limb lameness of either acute onset or chronic duration, similar to that of cranial cruciate ligament rupture. Cranial drawer sign is usually present once cruciate ligament rupture has occurred. Joint effusion and periarticular soft tissue fibrosis are usually present.

C. Biopsy during surgery for cranial cruciate rupture to differentiate from ruptures associated with trauma.

D. Findings that support the diagnosis.
1. Radiographs of the stifles reveal joint effusion and varying signs of DJD.
2. Synovial fluid is usually thin and turbid with an increased nucleated cell count comprised primarily of lymphocytes and plasma cells.
3. Synovial biopsy typically reveals villus hyperplasia and infiltration of the synovium and cruciate ligament with lymphocytes and plasmacytes.

E. Perform surgical stabilization of the stifle, and consider a subtotal synovectomy. Treat medically as for idiopathic immune-mediated polyarthritis.

F. Inform owners that the prognosis is generally good for achieving remission of clinical signs.

VIII. Systemic Lupus Erythematosus-Induced Polyarthritis

A. Recognize that systemic lupus erythematosus (SLE) is a multisystemic disease caused by autoantibodies against tissue protein and DNA. Circulating immune complexes cause inflammation and eventual organ dysfunction. The synovium is thickened and discolored, but cartilage and bone are less affected.

B. There is generally a history of generalized stiffness, shifting leg lameness, swollen joints, pyrexia, anorexia, or lethargy. Other organ systems can be affected, resulting in glomerulonephritis, myositis, scaly crusting cutaneous lesions, hemolytic anemia, or thrombocytopenia.

C. Findings that support a diagnosis.

1. Radiographs either reveal no abnormalities or show joint effusion and soft tissue swelling.
2. Synovial fluid is usually thin and turbid. Nucleated cell counts are markedly elevated with predominately nondegenerate neutrophils. Lupus erythematosus (LE) cells are rarely in joint fluid.
3. ANA test results should be positive at high dilutions, and rheumatoid factor is usually normal. The ANA test is sensitive but nonspecific for SLE. Anemia, a positive Coombs' test, leukopenia, thrombocytopenia, and proteinuria may be present.
   a. Diagnose SLE with involvement of more than one body system and a positive ANA.
   b. Suspect SLE if serologic tests are normal, but two or more body systems are involved.
4. Joint fluid is sterile.

D. Treat with glucocorticoids starting at 2 to 4 mg/kg/day, then gradually decrease the dosage to the lowest amount that will prevent clinical signs. Many animals require lifelong therapy. Try cyclophosphamide or azathioprine if clinical signs persist despite prednisone.

E. Inform owners that the prognosis is good for control of the polyarthritis; however, other organ abnormalities may progress.

IX. Rheumatoid Arthritis

A. Rheumatoid arthritis is an erosive, noninfectious inflammatory joint disease characterized by chronic bilaterally symmetrical, erosive destruction of the joints. Immune complexes, with altered host immunoglobulins as antigens, deposit in the synovium and initiate an inflammatory response. This leads to cartilage and subchondral bone destruction, rupture of the collateral ligaments, and eventually to a nonfunctional joint.

B. There is typically a history of stiffness after rest, limping, difficulty walking, and joints enlarged with periarticular soft tissue swelling and joint effusion.

C. Findings that support a diagnosis.

1. Radiographs generally show a loss of mineralization, radiolucent foci, and irregular joint margins. Bone proliferation, soft tissue swelling, and joint effusion may occur.
2. Synovial fluid is yellow, turbid, and increased in volume. The mucin clot may be poor and friable. Nucleated cell counts are markedly elevated with predominately degenerate neutrophils.
3. Between 20% and 70% of affected dogs test positive for rheumatoid factor; most show normal ANA levels.
4. Joint fluid is sterile.

D. Classic rheumatoid arthritis requires the presence of destructive lesions seen radiographically, a positive rheumatoid factor, characteristic histopathologic changes in the synovial membrane, plus four additional criteria listed in Table 30-2.

E. Treatment.

1. Start with prednisone at 2 to 4 mg/kg/day for 2 weeks.
2. At 2 weeks, add drugs (i.e., azathioprine [2 mg/kg/day PO for 2-3 weeks; then 2 mg/kg EOD] and/or cyclophosphamide [50 mg/m^2 up to 4 consecutive days each week for up to 4 months]) and give prednisone at 2 mg/kg/day for 2 weeks. Reevaluate monthly.
3. After the first month, decrease the prednisone to 1 to 2 mg/kg every 48 hours and continue the azathioprine or cyclophosphamide.
4. If inflammation persists, add gold salts (1 mg/kg IM once a week for 10 weeks or until remission). Gold salts can be toxic, so monitor hematology at least every 2 weeks.
5. Use aspirin to alleviate joint pain.

F. Perform arthrodesis on joints that have lost all collateral ligament support.

G. Inform owners that rheumatoid arthritis is progressive, and dogs rarely if ever make a full recovery.

X. Feline Chronic Progressive Polyarthritis

A. Feline chronic progressive polyarthritis is an immune-mediated disease of male cats associated with progressive periosteal-proliferative and erosive polyarthritis. The etiology may involve feline syncytium-forming virus (FeSFV) and feline leukemia virus (FeLV).

B. There are two forms of the disease.

1. The **periosteal-proliferative** form results in osteoporosis and periosteal new bone formation around the joint. Periarticular erosions and collapse of the joint space with fibrous ankylosis occur with time.
2. The **erosive** form causes joint changes similar to canine rheumatoid arthritis.

Table 30-2
Characteristics of rheumatoid arthritis

Stiffness after rest
Pain in at least one joint
Swelling in at least one joint
Swelling of at least one other joint within 3 months
Symmetrical joint swelling
Subcutaneous nodules over bony prominence, extensor surfaces, or in juxtaarticular regions
Destructive radiographic lesions
Positive rheumatoid factor
Poor mucin precipitate from synovial fluid
Characteristic histopathologic changes in the synovial membrane
Characteristic histopathologic changes in subcutaneous nodules

C. Typical clinical signs include lameness, reluctance to move, depression, anorexia, weight loss, pyrexia, depression, lymphadenopathy, and multiple joint involvement. Joints can be painful, swollen, and deformed.

D. Consider the differential diagnoses of septic arthritis, DJD, and hypervitaminosis A.

E. Findings that support a diagnosis.
   1. Changes on radiographs of affected joints include proliferative new bone formation on the periphery of the joints, generalized loss of density of the subchondral bone, and the loss of the joint space. Radiolucent foci in the subchondral bone and irregular joint margins may also occur. Periarticular soft tissue swelling and joint effusion may be noted.
   2. Results of tests for FeSFV and feline leukemia virus (FeLV) may be positive.
   3. Although only small amounts of synovial fluid can be obtained, typically the fluid is thin with an increased nucleated cell count of predominately nondegenerate neutrophils.
   4. Joint fluid is sterile.

F. Treatment.
   1. Start with prednisone at 4 to 6 mg/kg/day PO.
   2. Decrease to 2 mg/kg/day in 2 weeks if cat improves.
   3. Expect maintenance therapy of 1 to 2 mg/kg EOD to be needed for the lifetime of the cat.
   4. Try cyclophosphamide (6.25-12.5 mg/cat PO up to 4 consecutive days each week for up to 4 months) or azathioprine (0.3 mg/kg PO, EOD) to aid in long-term control. Assess hematologic values frequently because cats are very sensitive to the myelosuppressive effects of these drugs.

G. Inform owners that the prognosis is good for remission of signs, but guarded for complete control of the disease.

Temporomandibular Joint Luxations (*SAS*, pp. 898-900)

I. General Considerations

A. Temporomandibular joint (TMJ) luxations typically result from head trauma.

B. Luxations occur unilaterally or bilaterally and may be associated with mandibular fractures.

C. Mandibular condyles can displace cranially or caudally, but craniodorsal displacement is most common.

II. Diagnosis

A. Clinical Presentation

1. Signalment.
   a. Any breed or age dog or cat may be affected.
2. History.
   a. Typically there is a history of recent trauma.

B. Physical Examination

1. Generally the animal will be presented with its mouth open.
2. Determine the direction of the luxation by jaw position.
   a. With unilateral craniodorsal luxations the mandible shifts toward the opposite side of the mouth.
   b. With bilateral craniodorsal luxations the mandible protrudes forward.
   c. With caudal condylar luxations the mandible shifts caudally and toward the side of the luxation.
3. Inspect the mandible and maxilla for wounds and fractures.

C. Radiography

1. Take skull radiographs under anesthesia or heavy sedation
2. Assess for increased joint space and concurrent fractures.

III. Differential Diagnosis

A. Differentiate TMJ luxations from mandibular or maxillary fractures and TMJ dysplasia.

IV. Medical or Conservative Management

A. Reduce most luxations without surgical intervention. Use general anesthesia.

Place a wooden dowel rod transversely between the mandibular and maxillary molars while squeezing the rostral mandible and maxilla together. Manipulate the mandible to move the condyle into place.

B. Once the luxation is reduced, palpate to determine stability. Support unstable joints with tape muzzles or interarcade wiring for 7 to 14 days until fibrosis occurs.

C. If unable to reduce or maintain reduction, perform open reduction and stabilization.

V. Surgical Treatment

A. Perform open reduction if concurrent fractures are present or luxations are unstable after closed reduction.

B. Anesthesia.
   1. Temporarily remove the endotracheal tube or place it through a pharyngotomy incision if it interferes with reduction.

C. Surgical anatomy.
   1. Elevate the masseter muscle off the zygomatic arch to expose the joint. Avoid the parotid duct and gland and facial nerve located dorsally and superficially to the masseter muscle.

D. Positioning.
   1. Position the animal in lateral recumbency for a unilateral approach and in ventral recumbency for a bilateral approach.

E. Surgical techniques.

Make a skin incision following the ventral border of the caudal zygomatic arch and centered over the TMJ. Avoid the parotid duct and gland and facial nerve. Elevate the caudal periosteal insertion of the masseter muscle from the zygomatic arch to expose the joint capsule. Incise the joint capsule and mandibular ligament to expose the articular surfaces. Irrigate the joint and remove any bone fragments or debris that may have interfered with reduction. Reposition the mandibular condyle in the fossa. To hold the condyle in position, suture the joint capsule (use absorbable suture material) and mandibular ligament. Suture the masseter muscle to the fascia on the dorsal edge of the zygomatic arch. Close platysma muscle and skin in separate layers.

VI. Postoperative Care and Assessment

A. Take radiographs to evaluate position of the mandibular condyles.

B. If the joints are stable, feed only soft food for 2 to 3 weeks. If unstable, support with a tape muzzle for 1 to 2 weeks. For cats, consider interarcade wiring. Feed liquid diet until muzzles or interarcade wires are removed; then, soft food for 1 to 2 weeks.

VII. Prognosis

A. Inform owners the prognosis is good for normal function if luxations are reduced and joints stabilized.

B. Complications include failure to reduce the joint, repeated luxation, and joint ankylosis.

C. Perform a mandibular condylectomy if joints remain or become unstable, painful, fibrotic, or stiff after surgery.

Temporomandibular Joint Dysplasia (*SAS*, pp. 900-902)

I. General Considerations

A. Recognize TMJ dysplasia as a disease of unknown etiology affecting young, adult dogs. Deformation of the mandibular condyloid processes and mandibular fossa allow subluxation and recurrent locking of the mandible in an open-mouthed position. Joint instability leads to osteoarthrosis.

B. Observe for mandibular symphyseal laxity, which allows independent movement of the mandibles and results in malpositioning of coronoid processes lateral to the zygomatic arch, further promoting open-mouth locking.

II. Diagnosis

A. Clinical Presentation

1. Signalment.
   a. Coronoid process malpositioning has been reported in basset hounds, Irish setters, and a Saint Bernard.
   b. Pain and occasional open-mouth locking without malposition of the coronoid process has been reported in retriever and boxer breeds.
   c. Typically the first clinical signs are noted when the dogs are young adults.
2. History.
   a. Typically there is a history of open-mouth locking after yawning.
   b. Sometimes there is pain on jaw manipulation.
   c. Generally there is no history of trauma.

B. Physical Examination

1. The animal is generally presented with jaws locked in an open-mouth position. There may be pain on palpation of the TMJ.
2. If the coronoid process is locked outside of the zygomatic arch, note a bulge in the subcutaneous tissues overlying the zygomatic arch.

C. Radiography

1. Take a standard skull series.
2. Evaluate lateral views for increased or irregular joint spaces, shallow mandibular fossae, and secondary osteoarthritis.
3. Evaluate ventral dorsal projections for condyles more oblique than normal and coronoid processes positioned lateral to the zygomatic arch when the mouth is opened.

III. Medical or Conservative Management

A. Attempt manual reduction. Use general anesthesia if the dog resists manipulation.

IV. Surgical Treatment

A. Perform a partial resection of the zygomatic arch if the coronoid process locks outside it, or mandibular condylectomy if the coronoid process does not.

B. Surgical anatomy.
1. See Temporomandibular Joint Luxations for surgical anatomy of the TMJ.

C. Positioning.
1. Position the animal in lateral recumbency with the affected side up.

D. Surgical techniques.

1. Partial resection of the zygomatic arch.

Make an incision in the skin and subcutaneous tissues overlying the ventral border of the rostral portion of the zygomatic arch. Elevate the fascial attachments to the arch while preserving the dorsal buccal branch of the facial nerve. Open the mouth widely to induce coronoid process displacement in order to identify the portion of the arch that obstructs replacement of the process. Resect the obstructing portion of the arch with a rongeur or high-speed burr. Before closure, ensure that the coronoid process is normally positioned. Close the subcutaneous tissues and skin separately.

2. Mandibular condylectomy.

Make a skin incision along the ventral border of the caudal zygomatic arch, centered over the TMJ. Elevate the caudal periosteal insertion of the masseter muscle from the zygomatic arch to expose the joint capsule. Identify the joint by palpating it while an assistant moves the mandible. Incise the joint capsule between the meniscus and condyle and elevate the capsule. Identify the condylectomy site at the base of the condylar neck (at the level of the mandibular notch). First, resect the lateral portion of the condyle with a rongeur, then make a cut along the osteotomy line with a high-speed burr. Fracture the remaining portion of the condyle with an osteotome, but leave the meniscus intact. Close the masseter fascia, subcutaneous tissues, and skin separately.

V. Postoperative Care and Assessment

A. No exercise or dietary restrictions are necessary.

VI. Prognosis

A. Expect normal jaw function after surgery; however, recurrence can occur if the opposite TMJ is affected.

B. Inform the owner that potential complications include seroma formation and infection.

Scapulohumeral Joint

Osteochondritis Dissecans of the Proximal Humerus (*SAS*, pp. 903-909)

I. Definition

A. **Osteochondritis dissecans (OCD)** is a manifestation of a general syndrome called **osteochondrosis** in which a flap of cartilage forms because of a disturbance in endochondral ossification.

II. General Considerations

A. OCD occurs bilaterally in the shoulders, elbows, stifles, and hocks of immature, large- and giant-breed dogs.

B. With OCD of the shoulder, look for the cartilage flap to be on the midline or lateral aspect of the dorsocaudal humeral head. A detached flap may be in the caudoventral joint pouch.

C. Once a flap forms, cartilage degradation products induce joint inflammation. Degenerative joint disease results.

D. Council owners against breeding dogs with OCD because it has a hereditary component.

III. Diagnosis

A. Clinical Presentation

1. Signalment.
   a. Typically OCD occurs in large- and giant-breed dogs between 4 and 8 months of age.
   b. Males are more commonly affected than females.
2. History.
   a. Typically there is a history of unilateral forelimb lameness that had a gradual onset and improves with rest and worsens after exercise.

B. Physical Examination

1. Examine for pain when the shoulder is moved into extreme extension.

C. Radiography

1. Diagnose OCD on lateral projections of the shoulder joint. Position the animal in lateral recumbency with the shoulder of interest down and the head elevated. Retract the upper forelimb caudally. Slight external rotation of the humerus may silhouette the affected portion of the humeral head.
2. Radiograph both shoulders because OCD is often bilateral.
3. Provide sedation.
4. Look for flattening of the subchondral bone of the caudal humeral head, the earliest sign of OCD. As the disease progresses, look for a saucer-shaped radiolucent area in the caudal humeral head. Calcification of the flap may allow visualization.
5. To locate cartilage flaps try contrast arthrography using 1.5 to 4 ml of a 25% solution of meglumine-sodium diatrizoate with an admixture of 0.2 mg of epinephrine.

D. Laboratory Findings

1. Analysis of synovial fluid reflects underlying inflammation.

IV. Medical or Conservative Management

A. Attempt a therapeutic trial of exercise restriction (brief leash walks only) for a minimum of 6 weeks, and administer buffered aspirin. If lameness resolves, surgery may not be indicated.

V. Surgical Treatment

A. Perform arthrotomy to remove the cartilage flap in dogs with persistent lameness that is unresponsive to conservative treatment. Remove the cartilage flap and curette the edges of the bony defect and subchondral bone that appears pale and sclerotic. Alternatively, perform arthroscopy.

B. Approaches.
   1. Infraspinatus tenotomy.
      a. Exposes the humeral head.
      b. Provides access to both the cranial and caudal joint compartments.
   2. Caudal approach.
      a. Affords good exposure of the humeral head.
      b. Allows excellent access to the caudal ventral joint compartment.
      c. Does not allow the cranial aspect of the joint to be explored.

C. Surgical anatomy.
   1. Avoid the omobrachial vein located over the acromial head of the deltoid muscle. Protect the caudal circumflex humeral artery and vein and axillary nerve during the caudal approach to the shoulder.

D. Positioning.
   1. Position the animal in lateral recumbency with the affected limb up.

E. Surgical techniques.
   1. Infraspinatus tenotomy.

Make an incision in skin and subcutaneous tissues from just proximal to the acromial process to the proximal humerus. Curve the incision over the joint along the palpable cranial margin of the deltoid muscle's acromial head. Incise the deep fascia along the cranial margin of the acromial portion of the deltoid muscle and retract the muscle caudally. Isolate the infraspinatus tendon and place a stay suture in its proximal portion. Incise the tendon 5 mm from its insertion on the humerus and retract it caudally. Incise the joint capsule midway between the glenoid rim and humeral head. Internally rotate the humerus until the head subluxates, exposing the caudal surface of the humeral head. Remove the cartilage flap from the humeral head and curette the edges of the bony defect to ensure removal of all affected cartilage. Flush all parts of the joint thoroughly to remove any cartilage debris or joint mice. Close the joint capsule with 3-0 absorbable sutures in a simple interrupted pattern. Reappose the infraspinatus tendon with an absorbable suture in a Bunnell or locking-loop pattern. Close muscular fascia, subcutaneous tissues, and skin separately.

   2. Caudal approach.

Make an incision in skin, subcutaneous tissues, and deep fascia that extends from the midscapular spine to midhumeral diaphysis. Incise the intermuscular septum between the caudal border of the scapular portion of the deltoid muscle and the long head of the triceps muscle, and separate the muscles. Use blunt dissection to free the deltoid muscle and expose the caudal circumflex artery and vein, muscular branch of the axillary nerve, and teres minor muscle. Elevate and retract the teres minor muscle cranially, exposing the axillary nerve and joint capsule. Place a Penrose drain around the nerve and gently retract it caudally. Incise the joint capsule 5 mm from and parallel to the glenoid rim to expose the humeral head. To expose OCD lesions of the humeral head, internally rotate the humerus and flex the shoulder. Explore the joint and remove the cartilage as described above. Close joint capsule with interrupted

sutures of 3-0 absorbable suture material. Then suture the intermuscular septum, deep fascia, subcutaneous tissues, and skin as separate layers.

VI. Postoperative Care and Assessment

A. Limit activity for 1 month then gradually return to full activity.

B. Observe the incision site for seroma formation, which usually resolves without therapy.

VII. Prognosis

A. Inform owners that the prognosis for normal limb function is good, but despite the absence of lameness degenerative joint disease may develop.

Scapulohumeral Joint Luxations (*SAS*, pp. 909-915)

I. General Considerations

A. Differentiate traumatic from congenital luxations because treatment and prognosis are different.

B. Luxations occur when supporting structures (ligaments, joint capsule, and tendons) are torn or deficient.

C. Medial or lateral deviations are the most common.

D. The glenoid cavity may be sufficiently deformed or hypoplastic to prevent reduction of the humeral head.

E. This condition often occurs bilaterally in affected animals.

II. Diagnosis

A. Clinical Presentation

1. Signalment.
   a. Traumatic luxations may occur in any dog; they are rare in cats.
   b. Congenital, medial luxations usually occur in small and miniature dog breeds; lameness appears when young.
2. History.
   a. Trauma or chronic forelimb lameness is generally first evident at a young age.

B. Physical Examination

1. With traumatic luxations, there is typically a non–weight-bearing lameness and the limb is carried in a flexed position. Pain and crepitation are evidenced with shoulder manipulation.
2. With chronic, congenital medial luxations, there is generally lameness. The joint is easily luxated and reduced, but manipulation does not usually cause pain. If the glenoid cavity is deformed, reduction of the humeral head may be impossible.

C. Radiography

1. Take lateral and craniocaudal radiographs of the scapula to confirm the diagnosis.

III. Medical or Conservative Management

A. Manage chronic medial luxations with mild intermittent lameness and minimal degenerative joint disease with exercise restriction and aspirin during acute exacerbations.

B. Attempt closed reduction under general anesthesia for traumatic luxations soon after injury.

C. Verify that the humeral head will remain in place during gentle normal range of motion. If the joint appears stable:
1. Apply a lateral spica splint for 10 to 14 days for lateral luxations.
2. Use a Velpeau sling for medial luxations.

IV. Surgical Treatment

A. General Considerations

1. Perform open reduction and stabilization with capsulorrhaphy or tendon transposition if a traumatic luxation is unstable after closed reduction, or if the luxation is chronic.
2. Perform surgery with congenital luxations that cause severe or persistent lameness.
3. If severe joint dysplasia or degenerative joint disease is present, consider salvage procedures (glenoid excision or arthrodesis).

B. Positioning

1. Position the animal in dorsal recumbency.

C. Surgical Techniques

1. Stabilization of medial luxations.

Reduce the joint before the approach to reestablish normal anatomic relationships. Beginning at the medial aspect of the acromion, incise skin and subcutaneous tissue over the greater tubercle and continue the incision medially to the midhumeral diaphysis. Incise the fascia along the lateral border of the brachiocephalicus muscle and retract the muscle medially. Incise the insertions of the superficial and deep pectoral muscles from the humerus and retract them medially. Carefully incise the fascial attachment between the deep pectoral muscle and supraspinatus muscle to avoid causing trauma to the suprascapular nerve. Retract the supraspinatus muscle laterally. Transect the tendon of the coracobrachialis muscle to expose the subscapularis muscular tendon. If the joint capsule is not torn, incise it to inspect the joint and assess

the condition of the humeral head and medial labrum of the glenoid. If the labrum is worn, the prognosis for successful stabilization of the shoulder is poor. The tendon of the coracobrachialis muscle may be torn and retracted with traumatic luxations. Reduce the joint and imbricate the capsule and subscapularis tendon with nonabsorbable mattress sutures. If this does not sufficiently stabilize the joint, incise the transverse humeral ligament over the biceps tendon. Make a small incision in the joint capsule under the biceps tendon to free it and move the tendon medially. Secure it to the humerus with a bone screw and spiked washer. To prevent external rotation of the humeral head during healing, place a rotational suture of heavy nonabsorbable material from the medial labrum of the glenoid through a bone tunnel in the greater tubercle. For closure, suture the joint capsule, and then suture pectoral muscles to deltoid fascia. Suture subcutaneous tissues and skin separately.

2. Stabilization of lateral luxations.

Reduce the joint before the approach to reestablish normal anatomic relationships. Incise skin and subcutaneous tissues and deepen the incision through the pectoral muscles as described above for medial luxations. Perform an osteotomy of the greater tubercle that includes the supraspinatus muscular insertion. If the joint capsule is not torn, incise it to inspect the joint and assess the condition of the humeral head and lateral labrum of the glenoid. If the labrum is worn, the prognosis for successful stabilization of the shoulder is poor. Reduce the joint and imbricate the capsule with nonabsorbable mattress sutures. If sufficient stabilization is not achieved, incise the transverse humeral ligament over the biceps tendon. Make a small incision in the joint capsule under the biceps tendon to free it and move the tendon laterally across the osteotomy site. While the tendon is held in place, reduce and stabilize the osteotomy with Kirschner wires and a tension-band wire or lag screw. Suture the biceps tendon to the deltoid fascia. Close as previously described.

3. Shoulder arthrodesis.

Perform a combined craniolateral and cranial approach to the shoulder with osteotomy of the acromial process (see Chapter 29) and greater tubercle (see previous discussion). Detach the biceps tendon from the supraglenoid tubercle. Using an oscillating saw or osteotome, perform ostectomies of the glenoid process and humeral head; they are parallel to each other when the humerus is held at an angle of 105 degrees to the scapula. Take care to preserve the suprascapular nerve and caudal circumflex humeral artery. Oppose the flat surfaces and temporarily stabilize the bones with a Kirschner wire driven through the cranial aspect of the humerus and into the glenoid. Contour an 8- or 10-hole plate to fit from the dorsocranial junction of the spine and scapula, over the cranial aspect of the humerus. Be sure that the plate does not impinge on the suprascapular nerve. If necessary, contour the cranial humerus with rongeurs to obtain a better fit for the plate. Insert one of the screws across the opposed ostectomy lines as a lag screw. Remove the Kirschner wire and attach the biceps tendon to the surrounding fascia, or attach it to the humerus with a bone screw and spiked washer. Secure the greater tubercle to the humerus lateral to the plate with Kirschner wires or bone screws. Suture the soft tissues and close skin routinely.

4. Excision arthroplasty.

Perform a craniolateral approach to the shoulder with osteotomy of the acromial process. Detach the biceps tendon from the supraglenoid tubercle and incise the joint capsule. Using an oscillating saw or osteotome, perform an ostectomy of the glenoid. Be careful to preserve the suprascapular nerve and

caudal circumflex humeral artery when performing the excision. Bevel the glenoid so that the lateral edge is longer than the medial edge. Part of the humeral head can be ostectomized to create a vascular surface to promote pseudoarthrosis. Pull the teres minor muscle over the glenoid ostectomy site and suture it to the medial joint capsule and biceps tendon to provide soft-tissue interposition between bone surfaces. Pull the acromial process proximally until the deltoid muscle is taut. Wire the process to the scapular spine, then close soft tissues.

V. Postoperative Care and Assessment

A. Take radiographs to assess joint alignment and position of any implants.

B. After lateral luxations, place a spica splint for 10 to 14 days. After medial luxations place a Velpeau sling. Limit activity until 3 to 4 weeks after bandage removal.

C. After shoulder arthrodesis, place a spica splint until radiographic bone union, in 6 to 12 weeks.

D. After excision arthroplasty, encourage early postoperative limb use. Expect lameness for 4 to 8 weeks.

VI. Prognosis

A. Inform the owner that after closed reduction the prognosis is good for return of limb function if joints are stable, but guarded if joints are unstable. Reluxation is the major complication.

B. With traumatic luxations some degenerative joint disease may occur.

C. Recognize that the prognosis is guarded with congenital or developmental medial luxations.

Scapular Luxations (*SAS*, pp. 915-916)

I. General Considerations

A. Scapular luxations are rare.

B. Luxations allow upward displacement of the scapula.

C. Concurrent injuries to ribs and lungs are common.

II. Diagnosis

A. Clinical Presentation

1. Signalment.
   a. Cats are more commonly affected than dogs.
2. History.
   a. There is typically a history of recent trauma.

B. Physical Examination

1. Examine the animal when weight bearing for dorsal displacement of the scapula.

C. Radiography

1. Observe thoracic radiographs for signs of thoracic trauma.

III. Medical or Conservative Management

A. Perform surgical stabilization for a good cosmetic and functional result.

B. Consider closed reduction and a Velpeau bandage in cats with acute luxations.

IV. Surgical Treatment

A. General Considerations

1. Reattaching torn muscles is usually insufficient to allow weight bearing.
2. Repair by affixing the scapula to an adjacent rib using wire.

B. Preoperative Management

1. Assess thoracic radiographs and electrocardiogram before anesthesia.

C. Anesthesia

1. Have equipment available for ventilating the animal if the chest is opened inadvertently.

D. Surgical Anatomy

1. Refer to Chapter 29 for a detailed discussion of the anatomy of the scapula.

E. Positioning

1. Position the animal in lateral recumbency with the affected side up.

F. Surgical Technique

After repositioning the scapula to its normal position, incise through skin and subcutaneous tissues along the dorsal caudal scapular margin to expose the caudal scapular border. Identify the torn edges of the muscles, if possible. Elevate a small portion of the teres major muscle from the caudal scapular border and identify the underlying rib. Elevate periosteum from the rib surface, using care to avoid penetrating the parietal pleura. Use a wire passer to position

a piece of wire around the rib. Use 18- to 20-gauge wire to secure the scapula to the rib. Drill two holes in the caudal scapular border adjacent to the exposed rib and pass the free ends of the wire through these holes in a medial-to-lateral direction. Tighten the wire by twisting the ends to secure the scapula to the rib. If you have identified the torn muscle edges, reattach them before closing subcutaneous tissues and skin.

V. Postoperative Care and Assessment

A. Observe for normal ventilation postoperatively.
   1. If ventilatory difficulties are observed, suspect a pneumothorax from inadvertent penetration of the pleura. Take thoracic radiographs and perform thoracentesis.

B. Place a spica splint to immobilize the limb for 3 weeks after surgery. Change the bandage every 5 to 7 days.

C. Confine the animal until bandage removal. Resume normal exercise at 6 weeks.

VI. Prognosis

A. Inform the owner that chronic luxations will not resolve without surgical intervention.

B. Be aware of potential rare complications of surgery that include fixation failure, iatrogenic infection, and eventual wire fatigue and breakage with migration.

Bicipital Tenosynovitis (*SAS*, pp. 916-917)

I. Definition

A. **Bicipital tenosynovitis** is an inflammation of the biceps brachii tendon and its surrounding synovial sheath.

II. General Considerations

A. The etiology is direct or indirect trauma to the bicipital tendon.

B. Chronic inflammation may cause synovial hyperplasia and dystrophic mineralization of the tendon.

C. The tendon may be partially or completely ruptured.

D. Proliferative fibrous connective tissue and adhesions between the tendon and sheath limit motion and cause pain.

E. Osteophytes may form in the intertubercular groove.

III. Diagnosis

A. Clinical Presentation

1. Signalment.
   a. Typically medium- to large-sized, and middle-aged or older dogs are affected.
2. History.
   a. There is generally a history of intermittent or progressive forelimb lameness, which worsens after exercise.

B. Physical Examination

1. Typically there is a lameness of one forelimb during gaiting, but it can be bilateral.
2. Assess for pain on palpation of the bicipital tendon, especially with concurrent flexion and extension of the shoulder.
3. Attempt to palpate atrophy of the supraspinatus and infraspinatus muscles.

C. Radiography

1. Take radiographs of both shoulders, a lateral and a cranial-caudal projection of the humerus with the shoulder flexed. Assess for calcification of the biceps tendon and osteophytes in the intertubercular groove.
2. Perform arthrography to outline the tendon and reveal irregularities and filling defects suggestive of synovial hyperplasia, tendon rupture, and joint mice.
3. Do not perform arthrography if sepsis is present.

D. Laboratory Findings

1. Results of arthrocentesis are normal or suggest mild inflammation and degenerative joint disease, with higher concentrations of monocytes and macrophages in the joint fluid.

IV. Medical Management

A. Inject methylprednisolone acetate (10 to 40 mg) into the bicipital tendon sheath or, alternatively, into the scapulohumeral joint. Do not perform corticosteroid therapy if sepsis is present. Oral administration of corticosteroids is not effective.

B. Follow the steroid injection by 6 weeks of confinement, then gradually increase the amount of exercise.

V. Surgical Treatment

A. General Considerations

1. Move the bicipital tendon from the intertubercular groove (bicipital tendon tenodesis) to eliminate movement of the biceps tendon in the inflamed tendon sheath.

2. Use surgical treatment with ruptured bicipital tendons and chronic bicipital tenosynovitis if they have not responded to medical therapy.

B. Positioning

1. Position the animal in dorsal recumbency.

C. Surgical Techniques

Use an approach to the cranial region of the shoulder joint to expose the bicipital tendon and bicipital groove (see Scapulohumeral Joint Luxations). Incise the transverse humeral ligament and joint capsule to expose the tendon and intertubercular groove. Transect the tendon near the supraglenoid tubercle. Reattach the tendon to the humerus distal to the groove with a bone screw and spiked Teflon washer. Alternatively, redirect the tendon through a bone tunnel created in the humerus and suture it to the supraspinatus muscle.

VI. Postoperative Care and Assessment

A. Support the limb in a Velpeau sling for 2 to 3 weeks after surgery.

B. Confine the animal for 6 weeks, then gradually resume normal activity.

VII. Prognosis

A. Inform owners that results of medical treatment range from excellent to poor, and results of surgical treatment are generally good to excellent.

B. Expect dog to regain optimal function in 2 to 9 months.

Elbow Joint

Osteochondritis Dissecans of the Distal Humerus (*SAS*, pp. 918-922)

I. Definition

A. **OCD** is a manifestation of a general syndrome called **osteochondrosis** in which a flap of cartilage forms because of a disturbance in endochondral ossification.

II. General Considerations

A. Osteochondrosis has been implicated in the pathophysiology of OCD, fragmented coronoid process (FCP), and ununited anconeal process of the elbow (UAP).

1. Identify loss of range of motion in an immature dog as evidence of DJD, suggesting the presence of OCD, FCP, or UAP.
2. Radiograph both elbows and use careful positioning to identify subtle lesions.
3. Surgically remove bone and cartilage pieces before secondary DJD develops in order to improve limb function; however, the progression of DJD will not change.

B. With OCD of the distal humerus, look for a flap of cartilage covering a defect in the surface of the trochlear ridge of the medial humeral condyle. Opposing joint cartilage of the coronoid process may be eroded.

III. Diagnosis

A. Clinical Presentation

1. Signalment.
   a. Typically large dogs (Labrador retrievers, golden retrievers) are affected.
   b. The age of onset of lameness is generally 5 to 7 months.
2. History.
   a. Generally, there is an acute or chronic forelimb lameness, which worsens after exercise. There may be stiffness in the morning or after rest.

B. Physical Examination

1. Observe for lameness of one forelimb, or a stiff or stilted gait if the lameness is bilateral.
2. Elicit pain on elbow extension and on lateral rotation of the forearm.
3. Flex and extend the elbow. Less than normal flexion indicates secondary DJD. Crepitation, joint effusion, and periarticular swelling may be noted with DJD.
4. Avoid motion in the shoulder joint when manipulating the elbow.

C. Radiography

1. Take a standard lateral of the elbow, a flexed lateral to expose the anconeal process, and a cranial-caudal view made while the elbow is flexed 30 degrees and slightly rotated medially. Radiograph both elbows because OCD is often bilateral.
2. Try oblique views to demonstrate the lesion on the humeral condyle.
3. Identify a radiolucent concavity on the distal trochlear ridge of the medial humeral condyle for a definitive radiographic diagnosis of OCD.

D. Laboratory Findings

1. Arthrocentesis may reveal decreased synovial fluid viscosity, increased fluid volume, and increased numbers (up to 5000 WBC/ml) of mononuclear phagocytic cells.

IV. Medical Management

A. Do not treat dogs with radiographic abnormalities that are asymptomatic.

B. Provide medical therapy (confinement and aspirin administration) for occasional lameness.

C. Implement weight control.

V. Surgical Treatment

A. General Considerations

1. Surgically remove the cartilage flap in young animals when the disease is diagnosed before the onset of DJD.
2. Consider treating animals with chronic, moderate to severe lameness.

B. Surgical Anatomy

1. Avoid the median nerve and brachial artery and vein because they course cranially to the medial epicondyle. Identify and protect them in the surgical field. The ulnar nerve courses caudally to the medial epicondyle, over the anconeus muscle.

C. Positioning

1. Position the animal in dorsal recumbency.
2. Perform a hanging-leg preparation.

D. Surgical Techniques

1. General considerations.
   a. To expose the medial portion of the elbow joint.
      i. Tenotomize the pronator teres muscle and incise the medial collateral ligament for good exposure at the expense of the supporting structures.
      ii. To preserve the supporting structures, try a muscle-splitting technique that provides limited exposure.
      iii. Perform an osteotomy of the medial epicondyle for the most extensive exposure, but recognize that it requires implantation of a lag screw or wire to replace the epicondyle.
   b. Examine the medial condyle of the humerus and remove the cartilage flap. Curette only to remove fragments of cartilage from the edges of the lesion. Inspect and remove the coronoid process if fragmented. Finally, flush the joint.
2. Transection of the pronator teres muscle.

Make an incision on the medial surface of the joint, starting at the medial epicondylar crest and extending distally over the medial epicondyle to the proximal radius. Incise subcutaneous tissues along the same line. Identify the pronator teres muscle, median nerve, and brachial artery and vein. Gently retract the nerve and vessels cranially. Transect the pronator teres tendon and retract the muscle distally, exposing the joint capsule and collateral ligament. Make an incision parallel to the humeral condyle through the joint capsule and collateral ligament to expose the joint. Curette the edges of the lesion and flush the joint. Close the joint capsule with interrupted absorbable sutures. Place several nonabsorbable sutures in the collateral ligament. Reattach the pronator teres tendon with a Bunnell or locking-loop nonabsorbable suture. Suture fascia, subcutaneous tissue, and skin in separate layers.

3. Muscle splitting.

Incise skin and subcutaneous tissues as described above. Identify the demarcation between the flexor carpi radialis and superficial digital muscles and separate and retract them. Expose the joint capsule and incise it parallel to

the muscle-splitting incision to expose the medial humeral condyle and coronoid process. Curette the lesion and flush the joint. Suture the joint capsule with interrupted absorbable sutures. Suture fascia, subcutaneous tissue, and skin in separate layers.

4. Epicondyle osteotomy.

Incise skin and subcutaneous tissues as previously described. Expose the epicondyle and plan the osteotomy to include the origin of the pronator teres and flexor carpi radialis muscles. If the proposed method of epicondylar reattachment is a lag screw, drill the hole before cutting the epicondyle. Make three cuts with an osteotome. First, make proximal and caudal cuts perpendicular to the epicondyle to a depth of 5 mm. Then, make a cranial cut parallel to the surface of the condyle and connect it with the previous cuts to produce a segment of bone. Take care to avoid damaging the articular surface when making your cuts. Retract the bone piece distally to expose the joint. Curette the lesion and flush the joint. Reattach the bone piece with a large screw or tension-band wire. Close the wound as described above.

VI. Postoperative Care and Assessment

A. Take radiographs immediately postoperatively if implants are used, and repeat in 6 weeks.

B. Bandage the limb for up to 2 weeks after surgery and confine the animal for 4 weeks. Gradually return to normal activity.

C. Remove implants if necessary.

VII. Prognosis

A. Expect dogs treated conservatively to have intermittent lameness and progressive DJD.

B. Expect dogs treated surgically to have improved limb function; however, lameness may be evident after exercise. DJD still requires medical treatment. Inform owners of potential surgical complications that include iatrogenic infection and implant irritation of the soft tissues.

Fragmented Coronoid Process (*SAS*, pp. 923-925)

I. Definition

A. **Fragmented coronoid process (FCP)** is the separation of the medial coronoid process from the ulna that results in lameness and degenerative joint disease.

II. General Considerations

A. Although the etiology of FCP is unknown, two theories have been proposed.
   1. It may result from an OCD lesion in which disruption of endochondral ossification of the coronoid process leaves it vulnerable to cartilage degeneration, necrosis, and fissure formation.
   2. It may result from developmental elbow incongruity in which the ulna grows longer than the radius, resulting in an increase of weight-bearing forces on the medial coronoid process that precipitates fragmentation.

B. FCP results in joint instability and degenerative joint disease (DJD). The coronoid fragment may erode the opposing medial humeral condyle.

III. Diagnosis

A. Clinical Presentation

1. Signalment.
   a. Large dogs are usually affected.
   b. Clinical signs generally arise at 5 to 7 months of age.
2. History.
   a. Typically there is a history of an acute or chronic forelimb lameness that worsens after exercise. There may be stiffness in the morning or after rest.

B. Physical Examination

1. The signs of FCP are typically identical to OCD of the elbow with the addition of pain on palpation of the medial coronoid process.

C. Radiography/Computed Tomography

1. Take a standard lateral of the elbow, a flexed lateral to expose the anconeal process, and a cranial-caudal view made with the elbow flexed 30 degrees and slightly rotated medially. Radiograph both elbows because bilateral disease is common.
2. Assess the radiographs for blunting, visible fragments, and osteophytes associated with the coronoid process. If the FCP is not observed, infer the diagnosis from the presence of DJD.
3. The earliest radiographic signs are osteophytes on the anconeal process. Later signs are subchondral bone sclerosis, articular and periarticular osteophyte formation, joint space narrowing, joint effusion, and an increase in periarticular soft tissues.
4. Consider computed tomography (CT scan) to identify FCP.

D. Laboratory Findings

1. Arthrocentesis may reveal decreased synovial fluid viscosity, increased fluid volume, and an increase (up to 5000 WBC/ml) in mononuclear phagocytic cells.

IV. Medical Management

A. Treat dogs with mild clinical signs and radiographic evidence of advanced

DJD with cage confinement for 2 to 3 weeks and antiinflammatory drug therapy. After inflammation is controlled, gradually increase exercise.

B. Do not treat asymptomatic dogs, regardless of radiographic signs of DJD.

V. Surgical Treatment

A. General Considerations

1. Consider surgery when dogs are persistently lame and have mild degenerative changes, or occasionally when animals with advanced DJD and persistent lameness are not amenable to medical therapy. Despite bilateral DJD, perform surgery only on the lame leg.
2. Inform the client that surgical treatment does not halt the progression of DJD, and continued medical therapy may be required in these patients.

B. Positioning

1. Position the animal in dorsal recumbency.
2. Perform a hanging-leg preparation.

C. Surgical Techniques

1. Expose the medial coronoid process with the same basic approaches as for surgery for OCD of the elbow.
2. Transection of the pronator teres muscle.

Make an incision on the medial surface of the joint, starting at the medial epicondylar crest and extending distally over the medial epicondyle to the proximal radius. Protect the median nerve and brachial artery. Make an incision to the humeral condyle through the joint capsule and collateral ligament to expose the joint. Identify the coronoid process and any lesions on the medial humeral condyle. Remove the coronoid fragment. In chronic cases, if osteophytes obscure the line of cleavage, remove them with rongeurs. Use rongeurs to remove the base of the medial coronoid process so that it matches the level of the radial head. This eliminates excessive forces on the medial coronoid process that are present when incongruities in radial and ulnar length exist. Close the wound by suturing the joint capsule with simple interrupted absorbable sutures. Place several nonabsorbable sutures in the collateral ligament. Reattach the pronator teres tendon with a Bunnell or locking-loop nonabsorbable suture. Suture fascia, subcutaneous tissue, and skin in separate layers.

3. Muscle splitting.

Incise skin and subcutaneous tissues as previously described. Identify the demarcation between the flexor carpi radialis and superficial digital muscles and separate and retract them. Expose the joint capsule and incise it parallel to the muscle-splitting incision to expose the coronoid process. Remove the fragmented coronoid as previously described. Suture the joint capsule with interrupted absorbable sutures. Suture fascia, subcutaneous tissue, and skin in separate layers.

4. Epicondyle osteotomy.

Incise skin and subcutaneous tissues as previously described. Expose the epicondyle and perform an osteotomy. Predrill the hole for the lag screw before

making the osteotomy. Remove the fragmented coronoid as previously described. Reattach the bone piece with a lag screw or tension-band wire. Close the wound as described above.

VI. Postoperative Care and Assessment

A. Take radiographs immediately postoperatively if implants are used, and repeat in 6 weeks.

B. Bandage the limb for up to 2 weeks after surgery and confine the animal for 4 weeks. Gradually return to normal activity.

C. Remove implants if necessary.

VII. Prognosis

A. Inform owners that the prognosis for return to full function is guarded because progressive DJD develops regardless of treatment method.

B. Also inform owners of potential surgical complications, including iatrogenic infection and soft-tissue irritation by implants.

Ununited Anconeal Process (*SAS*, pp. 925-928)

I. Definition

A. **Ununited anconeal process (UAP)** is a disease of large, growing dogs in which the anconeal process does not form a bony union with the proximal ulnar metaphysis.

II. General Considerations

A. Because the anconeal process arises as a secondary center of ossification in the elbow at 11 to 12 weeks of age and does not fuse to the ulna until 4 to 5 months of age, do not diagnose ununited anconeal process (UAP) before 6 months of age.

B. The UAP is usually attached to the ulna with fibrous tissue, but it may be free within the joint. The instability causes secondary degenerative joint disease (DJD) with joint effusion, chondromalacia, periarticular fibrosis, and osteophyte formation.

III. Diagnosis

A. Clinical Presentation

1. Signalment.
   a. Large- to giant-breed male dogs are most commonly affected.
   b. The age of presentation is usually 6 to 12 months.
2. History.
   a. Typically there is a history of intermittent lameness of one or both forelimbs that worsens after exercise. There may be stiffness in the morning or after rest.

B. Physical Examination

1. There is typically lameness of one forelimb. Observe the elbow to circumduct laterally during the swing phase of the gait, and the paw to be externally rotated when the animal sits or stands.
2. Pain is evident during joint manipulation, particularly during palpation over the anconeal process.
3. Avoid motion in the shoulder joint when manipulating the elbow.

C. Radiography

1. Take a standard lateral of the elbow, a flexed lateral to expose the anconeal process, and a cranial-caudal view of the elbow made while the elbow is flexed 30 degrees and slightly rotated medially. Take radiographs of both elbows, because UAP is often bilateral.
2. Identify UAP on a flexed lateral view as a lucent, indistinct line separating the anconeal process from the ulna. Be sure the animal is old enough for physeal closure before diagnosing UAP. Look for concurrent FCP.
3. Signs of secondary DJD include subchondral bone sclerosis, articular and periarticular osteophyte formation, joint space narrowing, joint effusion, and an increase in periarticular soft tissues.

D. Laboratory Findings

1. Arthrocentesis may reveal decreased synovial fluid viscosity, increased fluid volume, and increased numbers (up to 5000 WBC/ml) of mononuclear phagocytic cells.

IV. Medical Management

A. Limit exercise for dogs less than 5 or 6 months old with suspected UAP. Take monthly radiographs to document fusion or UAP.

B. Provide medical therapy for older dogs with established DJD, since surgery does not stop the progression of osteoarthritis after extensive development of DJD. Use aspirin or other antiinflammatory drugs. Confine during lameness, then gradually increase exercise. Implement weight control.

V. Surgical Treatment

A. General Considerations

1. Surgically remove the anconeal process if UAP is diagnosed before extensive DJD.

2. Alternatively, consider an ulnar osteotomy to relieve pressure on the anconeal process, which may allow spontaneous healing of the fragment to the ulna in chondrodystrophic dogs, and potentially in other dogs.

B. Surgical Anatomy

1. During a lateral approach avoid the deep branch of the radial nerve that runs under the proximal-cranial border of the extensor carpi radialis muscle. Visualize the superficial branch of the radial nerve between the lateral head of the triceps and the brachialis muscle at the proximal portion of the incision.
2. During a medial approach identify and protect the median nerve and brachial artery and vein, which course cranial to the medial epicondyle and run under the pronator teres muscle. Visualize the ulnar nerve as it courses caudal to the medial epicondyle over the anconeus muscle.

C. Positioning

1. Position the animal in lateral recumbency for a lateral approach, and dorsal recumbency for a medial approach and for ulnar osteotomy.
2. Perform a hanging leg preparation.

D. Surgical Techniques

1. Removal of the anconeal process: lateral approach.

Make an incision in the skin, starting proximal to the lateral humeral epicondyle. Curve the incision to follow the epicondylar crest and end it over the proximal portion of the radius. Incise subcutaneous tissues to expose the cranial border of the lateral head of the triceps muscle. Retract the cranial border of the triceps muscle caudally to expose the anconeus muscle. Fibrous tissue attachments to the ulna may have to be incised before the anconeal process can be mobilized. Incise the anconeus muscle and joint capsule along the epicondylar crest and retract them caudally to expose the anconeal process. Grasp the process with towel forceps or an Oschner forceps and remove it. If necessary, smooth the remaining bone surface with a file. Flush the joint. Suture the joint capsule and anconeus muscle to the extensor carpi radialis muscle. Suture subcutaneous tissues and skin in separate layers.

2. Removal of the anconeal process and medial coronoid process: combined medial approach.

Expose the medial coronoid process using one of the techniques described under OCD of the Distal Humerus. After closing the craniomedial compartment of the elbow, approach the caudomedial compartment by retracting the ulnar nerve cranially and exposing the cranial border of the medial head of the triceps muscle. Retract the triceps muscle caudally to expose the caudal border of the medial epicondylar crest and origin of the anconeus muscle. Incise the anconeus muscle and joint capsule parallel to the medial epicondylar crest, leaving 2 to 4 mm of tissue attached to the crest for closure. Remove the anconeal process. Suture the anconeus muscle and joint capsule in one layer to close the joint.

3. Ulnar osteotomy.

Make a skin incision along the caudal border of the ulna, beginning medial to the tuber olecranon and ending at the middiaphysis of the ulna. Incise subcutaneous tissues and fascia along the same line. Incise attachments of the flexor carpi ulnaris and ulnaris lateralis along the medial and lateral borders of the ulna and elevate the muscles to expose the joint capsule. Incise the joint

capsule on both sides of the ulna to expose the distal trochlear notch area. Make an oblique osteotomy of the ulna distal to the trochlear notch, running from cranial-distal to caudal-proximal with an oscillating saw or Gigli wire. A gap should occur at the osteotomy site. If necessary, elevate the interosseous ligament to free the proximal ulna so it can move into position. Drive a small, smooth pin or Kirschner wire from the tuber olecranon down the medullary canal, across the fracture gap, and into the medullary canal of the distal ulna. The smooth pin and direction of the oblique osteotomy allow the proximal ulna to slide into position with the humerus, without the muscles causing angular distraction of the proximal ulna. Suture the joint capsule. Suture flexor carpi ulnaris fascia to the ulnaris lateralis fascia over the caudal border of the ulna. Suture subcutaneous tissue and skin separately.

VI. Postoperative Care and Assessment

A. If implants are used, take postoperative radiographs immediately and at 6 weeks.

B. Bandage the limb for 2 weeks after surgery and confine the animal for 4 weeks.

C. Remove implants if necessary.

VII. Prognosis

A. Inform owners that the prognosis is guarded for normal limb function because secondary DJD will occur. When treated with surgical removal of the anconeal process, dogs less than 1 year old have good prognosis for limb function; however, progressive DJD will occur.

B. Also inform owners of potential surgical complications, including iatrogenic infection and irritation of the soft tissues by implants.

Traumatic Elbow Luxations (*SAS*, pp. 928-933)

I. General Considerations

A. Recognize that rupture or avulsion of one or both collateral ligaments allows luxation of the radius and ulna. The trauma may also cause the origins of the extensor or flexor muscles to be ruptured or avulsed.

B. The radius and ulna typically luxate laterally.

C. Attempt closed reduction as soon as possible, and evaluate stability after reduction because chronic luxation results in chondromalacia, articular cartilage destruction, and secondary DJD. If the joint is stable despite collateral ligament damage, immobilization will allow periarticular fibrosis and some degree of stability; however this may not provide sufficient stability for large, active dogs.

II. Diagnosis

A. Clinical Presentation

1. Signalment.
   a. Any breed or age dog or cat may be affected, but it is rare in cats.
2. History.
   a. Typically there is a history of trauma with lameness of the affected limb.

B. Physical Examination

1. There is generally a non–weight-bearing lameness and the elbow is carried in a flexed position.
2. Palpate a prominent radial head and laterally displaced olecranon.

C. Radiography

1. Identify displacement of the radius and ulna with a cranial-caudal view. The lateral view shows an uneven joint space. Check for avulsion fractures of the medial or lateral condyle of the humerus.
2. Take thoracic radiographs to check for concurrent lung injury.

III. Medical Management

A. Perform closed reduction within the first few days of injury. With avulsion fractures, consider open reduction and stabilization of the fracture for greater immediate stability.

B. Closed reduction.

For closed reduction, suspend the limb from an intravenous-drip stand for 5 to 10 minutes to allow muscle relaxation, then place the animal in lateral recumbency with the affected limb up. To reduce the elbow, determine the position of the anconeal process in relation to the humeral condyles. Flex the elbow to about 100 degrees and inwardly rotate the antebrachium. After the anconeal process hooks over the lateral condyle, extend the elbow slightly. Abduct and inwardly rotate the antebrachium while placing medial pressure over the head of the radius to force it under the humeral capitulum and into the reduced position.

C. Evaluate stability provided by the collateral ligaments after reduction.

1. Flex the elbow and paw to 90 degrees and rotate the paw medially and laterally.
   a. If the lateral collateral ligament is intact, the paw can be rotated medially to about 70 degrees (versus 140 degrees if it is ruptured).
   b. If the medial collateral ligament is intact, the paw can be rotated laterally to 45 degrees; rupture allows the paw to be rotated laterally to about 90 degrees.

D. Take radiographs after reduction.

1. Typically, mild subluxation or widening of the joint space responds to immobilization.
2. With marked subluxation, perform open reduction and internal stabilization.

E. Immobilize with the elbow in extension and support with a padded bandage and spica splint for 2 weeks. After bandage removal limit exercise for 3 to 4 weeks and perform range of motion exercises.

F. Inform owners that complications may include reluxation and DJD.

IV. Surgical Treatment

A. General Considerations

1. Perform open reduction when closed reduction is impossible to achieve, when the elbow is unstable after closed reduction, or when stabilization of an avulsion fracture will improve joint stability.
2. Consider elbow arthrodesis as a salvage procedure when there is severe damage to the cartilage.

B. Anesthesia

1. Use general anesthesia to provide the muscle relaxation needed for closed reduction. Consider neuromuscular blockage if necessary (see Chapter 12).

C. Positioning

1. Position the animal in lateral recumbency.

D. Surgical Techniques

1. Open reduction of elbow luxations.

Make a lateral approach to the caudal compartment of the elbow (see Ununited Anconeal Process). Reduce the elbow as described for closed reduction. Protect the articular cartilage during reduction. If muscle contraction and subsequent overriding are severe, use a blunt instrument to gently lever the radial head into position. If reduction is not achieved, perform an olecranon osteotomy to eliminate the pull of the triceps muscle, or use a fracture distractor with pins placed in the humeral diaphysis and proximal ulna. After reduction, flush the joint and assess stability. Stability may be enhanced by primary repair of the lateral collateral ligament. Identify the ends of the ligaments and appose them with nonabsorbable sutures in a locking-loop or Bunnell pattern. If the ligament has torn from its attachment to the bone, secure it to the bone with a screw and spiked Teflon washer. If the collateral ligament is beyond repair, replace it with two screws and a figure-8 wire or heavy (No. 1 or No. 2) nonabsorbable suture. Reduce avulsion fractures of the humeral condyle and secure them with a lag screw or tension-band wire technique. Suture torn muscles. Suture fascia, subcutaneous tissue, and skin in separate layers. If additional stability is necessary, expose the medial surface of the elbow (see Ununited Anconeal Process) and repair or replace the medial collateral ligament.

2. Elbow arthrodesis.

Predetermine the angle of arthrodesis by measuring the standing angle of the opposite elbow. Make a caudolateral approach to the joint (see Ununited Anconeal Process) and osteotomize the olecranon. Expose the joint by incising the lateral collateral ligament and elevating the origins of the extensor muscles. Remove the cartilage from the distal humerus, radial head, and coronoid process with a high-speed burr. Follow the contours of the joint. Temporarily stabilize the elbow in the correct position with a pin placed through the humerus and into the ulna. Contour a plate to fit onto the caudal surface of the humerus, over the joint, and onto the caudal surface of the ulna. Place at least three screws in the humerus and three in the ulna. Use additional screws as lag screws to gain compression where they cross the arthrodesis site. Check limb

alignment, rotation, and angulation before securing fixation. Harvest and place a cancellous bone graft at the arthrodesis site. The most accessible site for cancellous bone harvest is the ipsilateral proximal humerus. Reattach the olecranon to the ulna on either side of the plate with a tension-band wire.

V. Postoperative Care and Assessment

A. Take radiographs after open reduction or arthrodesis.

B. After open reduction, position the elbow in extension and support with padded bandage for several days. If stability is questionable apply a spica splint for 2 weeks. After bandage removal, limit exercise for 3 to 4 weeks and perform daily range of motion exercises. Inform owners of potential complications, including recurrent luxation, infection, decreased range of motion, irritation or migration of implants, and secondary DJD.

C. After arthrodesis, apply a padded bandage for a few days. If stability of the implants is questionable, apply a spica splint for 6 weeks or until radiographic evidence of bone healing. Limit activity until the arthrodesis has healed. Inform owners of complications, including iatrogenic infection, delayed union or nonunion, implant migration, implant irritation to soft tissues, fracture of the bone at either end of the plate, and increased degenerative changes in the limb's distal joints.

VI. Prognosis

A. Inform owners that the prognosis after a stable closed reduction is good for normal limb function; however, there will be variable development of DJD and limited range of motion. Prognosis is better for smaller dogs.

B. Inform owners that the prognosis after surgical reduction depends on chronicity of the luxation and severity of joint damage. Most dogs have good limb function; smaller, less active dogs do better. Expect varying degrees of DJD to develop.

Elbow Luxation/Subluxation Caused by Premature Closure of the Distal Ulnar or Radial Physes (*SAS*, pp. 933-936)

I. General Considerations

A. Two syndromes are grouped under elbow subluxation or incongruity.
   1. Premature closure of the distal ulnar or radial physes after trauma in immature dogs.

2. Asynchronous growth of the radius and ulna in chondrodystrophic breeds with no apparent injury to the growth plate.

B. When the ulna is too short, the trochlear notch is pulled distally and the anconeal process impinges on the humeral trochlea. In some dogs this may be associated with an UAP.

C. When the radius is too short, the radial head is pulled distally and does not articulate with the humeral capitulum. The trochlea of the humerus then rests directly on the coronoid process of the ulna, which transmits all of the force of weight bearing.

II. Diagnosis

A. Clinical Presentation

1. Signalment.
   a. Immature dogs of any breed with past trauma to an open physis may be affected.
   b. Alternately, chondrodystrophic dogs may have asynchronous growth of the radius and ulna.
2. History.
   a. Typically there is a history of intermittent lameness.

B. Physical Examination

1. There are generally varying degrees of lameness and potential gross deformity of the limb.

C. Radiography

1. Take radiographs of the radius and ulna that include the carpus and elbow.
2. Radiograph the contralateral forelimb as a normal for comparison or to assess bilateral disease.

III. Medical Management

A. Use medical management to treat the resultant DJD, but it will not affect the primary problem.

IV. Surgical Treatment

A. General Considerations

1. Perform a corrective osteotomy of either the radius or ulna to restore elbow congruity.
   a. Use an ulnar lengthening osteotomy when the ulna is too short.
   b. Use an ulna-shortening ostectomy when subluxation (widening) of the humeroradial joint is caused by radial shortening. Alternatively, use a lengthening osteotomy of the radius if limb shortening would be detrimental.

B. Positioning

1. Position the animal in dorsal recumbency.
2. Perform a hanging leg preparation.

C. Surgical Techniques

1. Ulnar-lengthening osteotomy.

Make a skin incision along the caudal border of the ulna, beginning medial to the tuber olecranon and ending at the ulnar middiaphysis. Incise subcutaneous tissue and fascia along the same line. Incise the attachments of the flexor carpi ulnaris and ulnaris lateralis along the medial and lateral borders of the ulna and elevate the muscles to expose the joint capsule. Incise the joint capsule on both sides of the ulna to expose the distal trochlear notch area. Make an oblique osteotomy of the ulna distal to the trochlear notch, running from cranial-distal to caudal-proximal, with an oscillating saw or Gigli wire. A gap should form at the osteotomy site. If necessary, elevate the interosseous ligament to free the proximal ulna so that it can move into position. Drive a small, smooth pin or Kirschner wire from the tuber olecranon down the medullary canal, across the fracture gap, and into the medullary canal of the distal ulna. The smooth pin and direction of the oblique osteotomy allow the proximal ulna to slide into position with the humerus, without the muscles causing angular distraction of the proximal ulna. Suture the joint capsule. Suture the flexor carpi ulnaris fascia to the ulnaris lateralis fascia over the caudal border of the ulna. Suture the subcutaneous tissue and skin separately.

2. Ulnar-shortening ostectomy.

Shortening the ulna allows the radial head to come into contact with the humeral capitulum. Approach the ulna as described earlier for the ulnar-lengthening osteotomy. Using an oscillating saw or Gigli's wire, resect a segment of ulna that is greater in length than the measured distance from the radial head to the humeral capitulum. Drive a small, smooth pin or Kirschner wire from the tuber olecranon down the medullary canal, across the fracture gap, and into the medullary canal of the distal ulna. The smooth pin allows the forces of the surrounding musculature to exert a dynamic effect on the proximal ulna, causing it to collapse into the ostectomy site.

V. Postoperative Care and Assessment

A. Take postoperative radiographs. Obvious changes in position of the ulna may not be evident until several days after surgery. Take serial radiographs until the ostectomy has healed. Remove implants after healing if necessary.

B. Apply a padded bandage postoperatively. Encourage leash activity because early joint motion is important.

VI. Prognosis

A. Expect DJD and lameness if surgery is not performed. Inform owners the prognosis is good for relatively normal function if surgery is performed before DJD is established, although some DJD will usually occur.

B. Inform owners of potential surgical complications, including iatrogenic infection, implant migration, delayed union or nonunion of the osteotomy, and implant irritation of soft tissues.

Congenital Elbow Luxation (*SAS*, pp. 936-938)

I. General Considerations

A. Although the etiology is unknown, recognize that the bone malpositioning occurs at a young age, and because the bones do not articulate normally, congruent joint surfaces do not form. Degenerative changes begin at approximately 3 months of age.

B. In addition to the olecranon rotated lateral to the distal humerus, and the trochlear notch not in contact with the humeral condyles, look for the following possible pathology.
   1. Hypoplasia and remodeling of the trochlea and trochlear notch.
   2. Hypoplasia of the medial humeral condyle, with stretching of the medial collateral ligament and joint capsule.
   3. Hyperplasia of the lateral humeral condyle, with contracture of the lateral joint capsule and lateral collateral ligament.
   4. Contracture and displacement of the triceps muscle.
   5. Degenerative changes of the articular cartilage.

II. Diagnosis

A. Clinical Presentation

1. Signalment.
   a. Small breeds of dogs (pugs, Yorkshire terriers, Boston terriers, miniature poodles, Pomeranians, Chihuahuas, cocker spaniels, and English bulldogs) are typically affected.
2. History.
   a. Generally there is a history of an inability to extend the front leg(s) and difficulty with walking because of the crouching position. It is noticed from when the puppy begins to walk at 3 to 6 weeks old.

B. Physical Examination

1. Generally the puppies do not experience pain, but they carry the affected forelimb in flexion. The elbows cannot be extended.

C. Radiography

1. Take lateral and craniocaudal radiographs to show lateral displacement and rotation of the olecranon. Identify secondary degenerative joint disease (DJD) in chronic cases.

III. Medical Management

A. Do not attempt conservative therapy because it does not alter the course of disease.

B. Perform joint reduction and stabilization before secondary DJD and joint remodeling occur (usually before the animal is 4 months of age).
   1. Attempt closed reduction in dogs with only mild changes in bone and soft tissue.

2. Rotate the olecranon medially into position and secure by placing a transarticular pin from the caudal aspect of the olecranon, through the olecranon, and into the humerus. Leave the pin in place for 10 to 14 days.

IV. Surgical Treatment

A. General Considerations

1. Perform open reduction and corrective osteotomy when the joint cannot be manually replaced. Provide immediate treatment for best results, but decreased range of motion and DJD will still occur.
2. Select techniques based on the degree of pathology. Consider lateral release of soft tissues, including joint capsule and anconeus muscle; medial support of the olecranon using capsular imbrication and stay sutures; olecranon or ulnar osteotomy, and transposition to reconstruct the joint; or redirection of the pull of the triceps muscle to allow joint extension. Stabilize the osteotomy with Kirschner wires and, if necessary, a tension-band.

B. Surgical Anatomy

1. Identify and protect the ulnar nerve on the medial aspect of the surgical site.

C. Positioning

1. Position the animal in dorsal recumbency.

D. Surgical Technique

Make an incision on the lateral surface of the joint, starting on the lateral epicondylar crest and extending distally over the lateral epicondyle to the proximal. Incise subcutaneous tissues and retract the skin medially and laterally to expose both medial and lateral surfaces of the elbow. Incise soft tissues on the lateral aspect of the humeroulnar joint (including the anconeus muscle and joint capsule) to expose the joint and reposition the ulna. If repositioning is possible, stabilize the ulna by imbricating the medial joint capsule, and placing a large (No. 0 to No. 2) nonabsorbable suture from the proximal ulna to the humeral condyle through tunnels drilled in the bone with the needle or a small Kirschner wire. Perform an olecranon osteotomy and transpose the osteotomized bone to a position on the ulna that best redirects the pull of the triceps muscle to extend the joint. Stabilize the osteotomy with Kirschner wires and possibly a tension-band wire. Reposition the skin to the lateral aspect of the elbow and close subcutaneous tissues and skin with interrupted sutures.

V. Postoperative Care and Assessment

A. Take radiographs to evaluate the position of the ulna and any implants.

B. Bandage and splint the elbow in a functional position for 2 to 3 weeks.

C. Allow leash walking only for 4 to 6 weeks.

D. Remove the pins and Kirschner wire when the osteotomy has healed.

VI. Prognosis

A. Inform owners that without surgery, the dog may compensate by relying on the rear limbs for support and locomotion, but ambulation will always be abnormal.

B. Expect a good prognosis for return of satisfactory function after surgery, but poor for development of a normal joint. Inform owners of potential surgical complications, including loss of joint reduction, iatrogenic infection, implant migration, and irritation of soft tissues.

Carpal Luxation/Subluxation (*SAS*, pp. 938-942)

I. Definition

A. **Carpal luxation/subluxation** results from a loss of collateral and/or palmar ligamentous support of the antebrachial, middle carpal, and/or metacarpal joints.

II. General Considerations

A. Carpal hyperextension injuries are divided into three categories.
   1. **Type I injuries** are subluxations or luxations of the radiocarpal joint.
   2. **Type II injuries** are subluxations of the middle carpal and carpometacarpal joints with dorsal displacement of the free end of the accessory carpal and ulnar carpal bones.
   3. **Type III injuries** are subluxations of the carpometacarpal joint without disruption and displacement of the accessory carpal and ulnar carpal bones.

III. Diagnosis

A. Clinical Presentation

1. Signalment.
   a. Any breed or age dog or cat may be affected.
2. History.
   a. There is typically a history of a non–weight-bearing lameness.

B. Physical Examination

1. With acute injuries, there is generally swelling, pain, and instability. The extent of hyperextension may not be apparent initially when the animal is not using the limb.
2. With Type I injuries, the animal is usually unable to bear weight until definitive treatment is performed. With Type II or III injuries, the animal may bear minimal weight after the injury.

C. Radiography

1. Take craniocaudal and medial-to-lateral radiographs to identify fractures or joint malalignment. To assess carpal integrity, take a standing lateral radiograph while the animal is bearing weight on the limb as a stress radiograph. If the animal refuses to bear weight, position in lateral recumbency and stress the foot.

IV. Medical Management

A. Medical management is not recommended. Consider external coaptation in younger patients, but be aware that gradual hyperextension often occurs as weight bearing returns.

V. Surgical Treatment

A. General Considerations

1. Treat Type I injuries with a pancarpal arthrodesis. Treat Type II injuries with pancarpal arthrodesis or a partial carpal arthrodesis. Make sure the partial arthrodesis reestablishes the accessory carpal moment arm by fusion of the accessory carpal–ulnar carpal articulation or the arthrodesis may eventually fail because of breakdown of the radiocarpal joint.
2. Stabilize Type I injuries with a bone plate on the cranial surface, and Type II injuries with a bone plate, cross pins, or placement of longitudinal metacarpal pins. Remove the articular cartilage, place cancellous bone in the fusion site, and stabilize with cross pins. Combine multiple cross pins and external coaptation for the simplest method.
3. Treat Type III injuries with fusion of the carpometacarpal joint and middle carpal joint. Remove the articular cartilage, place cancellous bone in the fusion site, and stabilize with cross pins.

B. Preoperative Management

1. Protect the limb with a splint or bandage until surgery.

C. Positioning

1. Position the animal in dorsal recumbency.
2. Perform a hanging leg preparation.

D. Surgical Techniques

1. Expect collagenous and bony tissue proliferation and increased vascularity with carpal luxation/subluxation. Consider using a tourniquet.
2. Approach to the carpal bones.

Make a skin incision over the midline of the dorsal surface of the carpus, extending from 4 cm proximal to the radiocarpal joint line to 4 cm distal to the carpometacarpal joint line. Incise subcutaneous tissues; proliferative fibrous tissue; and joint capsule overlying the radiocarpal, middle carpal, and carpometacarpal joints. The proliferative fibrous tissue will be confluent with the joint capsule proximally and distally. Reflect the synovial joint capsule incision from the cranial face of the carpal bones both medially and laterally using sharp dissection. Place Gelpi retractors to maintain exposure of the joint

surfaces and position a small Hohmann retractor between joint surfaces to help visualize the articular cartilage of each joint. Use a low-speed power burr to remove articular cartilage from the surface of the carpal bones in each joint. Be sure to preserve the tendon of the extensor carpi radialis muscle because it crosses the craniolateral aspect of the joint. Harvest a cancellous bone graft and insert the graft within the denuded surfaces of each joint. Stabilize the arthrodesis with an implant as explained later in this chapter.

3. Pancarpal arthrodesis.

Expose the joint surfaces of the radiocarpal, middle carpal, and carpometacarpal articulations and remove articular cartilage. Use a small Kirschner wire to drill multiple holes through the distal radial epiphysis into the marrow cavity to aid vascularization of the fusion. Stabilize the fusion with a bone plate applied as a compression plate to the dorsal surface of the radius. Contour the plate 5 to 10 degrees. Apply the plate so that the proximal three plate screws enter the distal radius and the distal three plate screws enter the third metacarpal bone. Place one intermediate plate screw in the radial carpal bone and the others where bone stock is available. Because the plate is not positioned on the tension surface of the joint, it should be supported with small Steinmann pins and/or external coaptation. If pins are selected, place one pin from medial to lateral, entering the bone near the head of the second metacarpal and exiting through the distal ulna. Place a second pin from lateral to medial, entering the bone near the head of the fifth metacarpal and exiting through the distal radius.

4. Partial carpal arthrodesis used for Type II injuries.

Expose the joint surfaces of the carpal and metacarpal joints and remove articular cartilage as previously described. Harvest and insert a cancellous bone graft. Stabilize the fusion by placing a pin from medial to lateral, entering the bone near the head of the second metacarpal and penetrating the radial carpal bone. Place a second pin from lateral to medial, entering the bone near the head of the fifth metacarpal and penetrating the ulnar carpal bone. Fuse the accessory carpal–ulnar carpal articulation by removing articular cartilage between joint surfaces of the accessory carpal bone and ulnar carpal bone, placing a cancellous bone graft, and stabilizing it with a compression screw. Make an incision lateral to the base of the accessory carpal bone. Incise subcutaneous tissues and deep fascia adjacent to the lateral accessory carpal ligament. (The medial and lateral accessory carpal ligaments will be torn.) Continue the incision lateral to the abductor digiti quinti muscle to the joint capsule. Incise the joint capsule to expose and remove articular cartilage from the ulnar carpal and accessory carpal bones. Insert a cancellous bone graft and stabilize the fusion with a compression screw and wire. Insert the compression screw from the cranial face of the ulnar carpal bone into the accessory carpal bone. Place a wire from the base of the accessory carpal bone through the head of the fifth metacarpal bone.

5. Partial carpal arthrodesis used for Type III injuries.

Expose the joint surfaces of the carpal and metacarpal joints and remove articular cartilage as previously described. Harvest and insert a cancellous bone graft. Stabilize the fusion by placing a pin from medial to lateral, entering the bone near the head of the second metacarpal and penetrating the radial carpal bone. Place a second pin from lateral to medial, entering the bone near the head of the fifth metacarpal and penetrating the ulnar carpal bone.

VI. Postoperative Care and Assessment

A. Apply a coaptation splint for 6 to 8 weeks then remove the splint and allow the internal fixation to support the arthrodesis until radiographic evidence of fusion, usually 12 to 16 weeks. Strictly control activity until bone union is achieved.

VII. Prognosis

A. Expect pancarpal and partial carpal arthrodeses to result in excellent limb function in the majority of patients treated with Type I, Type II, or Type III hyperextension injuries.

Coxofemoral Joint

Hip Dysplasia (*SAS*, pp. 942-949)

I. Definitions

A. **Hip dysplasia** is an abnormal development of the coxofemoral joint characterized by subluxation or complete luxation of the femoral head in younger patients and degenerative joint disease (DJD) in older patients.

B. The **angle of inclination** is the angle formed between the long axis of the femoral neck and the femoral diaphysis in the frontal plane.

C. The **angle of anteversion** is the angle formed between the long axis of the femoral neck and the transcondylar axis.

II. General Considerations

A. The etiology of hip dysplasia is multifactorial and includes both hereditary and environmental factors.
   1. One potential factor is rapid weight gain and growth through excessive nutrition.
   2. Another potential factor is synovial inflammation caused by mild, repeated trauma and/or viral or bacterial synovitis.

B. Subluxation causes pain from stretching of the joint capsule, deforms acetabular cancellous bone, and potentially fractures acetabular trabecular cancellous bone also causing pain.

C. The physiologic responses to joint laxity, proliferative fibroplasia of the joint capsule, and increased trabecular bone thickness, relieves the pain associated with capsular sprain and trabecular fractures. However, premature wear of articular cartilage still occurs, and exposure of subchondral pain fibers results in lameness.

III. Diagnosis

A. Clinical Presentation

1. Signalment.
   a. The dogs most commonly affected are Saint Bernards and German shepherds, but most sporting breeds may be affected as well. The animals are presented between 5 to 10 months of age or later in life when chronic DJD has developed.
   b. Hip dysplasia is rare in cats.
2. History.
   a. Typically there is a history of difficulty rising after rest, exercise intolerance, intermittent or continual lameness, muscle atrophy, and/or waddling gait.

B. Physical Examination

1. Generally the first episode of lameness occurs between 5 and 10 months of age. In young dogs there is typically poorly developed pelvic musculature and pain on external rotation and abduction of the hip joint.
2. When presented with an acute, unilateral non–weight-bearing lameness, suspect a torn round ligament and sprained joint capsule.
3. Under general anesthesia, obtain abnormal angles of reduction and subluxation indicating joint laxity.
   a. The **angle of reduction** is the point where the femoral head slips back into the acetabulum on abduction of the limb.
   b. The **angle of subluxation** is the point where the femoral head slips out of the acetabulum on adduction of the limb.
4. Anticipate that many dogs spontaneously improve with age and conservative management.
5. Older animals have pain during extension of the hip joint, reduced range of motion, atrophy of the pelvic musculature, and exercise intolerance. Do not expect joint laxity because of the proliferative fibrous response.

C. Radiography

1. Evaluate the hips with one or more of the established radiographic methods.
   a. The Orthopedic Foundation for Animals (OFA) grades radiographic congruity between the femoral head and acetabulum.
      i. "Normal" hips are classified as excellent, good, fair, or near normal.
      ii. "Dysplastic" hips are categorized as mild, moderate, or severe.
   b. Stress radiographs comparing neutral stance position to distracted (obtained by levering a custom-designed distractor between the legs) are used to calculate a distraction index. The index predicts the likelihood of developing DJD secondary to hip laxity. Certification must be obtained in order to perform the evaluation.

IV. Medical or Conservative Management

A. When considering conservative and surgical options, keep in mind that many young patients treated conservatively return to acceptable clinical function with maturity. Select surgery when conservative treatment is not effective, when athletic performance is desired, or to slow the progression of DJD in a young patient.

B. Treat initially with complete rest for 10 to 14 days. Stress to owners that they must enforce rest even if the animal feels like exercising. Apply moist heat over the joint, and then once the joint is warm perform passive movement.

C. Prescribe NSAIDs (see Appendix I).

1. Caution owners about potential side effects, including gastrointestinal ulceration. Use the lowest effective dose, and consider using carprofen, which causes less gastrointestinal injury, or concurrent use of sucralfate or the cytoprotective agent misoprostol.
2. Most NSAIDs interfere with chondrocyte glycosaminoglycan synthesis; therefore use continuously only for a short time.
3. For long-term treatment advise weight control, moderate exercise, and administration of NSAIDs only as needed.

V. Surgical Treatment

A. Pelvic osteotomy.

1. Consider for younger patients with minimal radiographic evidence of DJD, an angle of reduction less than 45 degrees, and an angle of subluxation less than 10 degrees.
2. The procedure axially rotates and lateralizes the acetabulum in an effort to increase dorsal coverage of the femoral head.

B. Consider a proximal femoral varus osteotomy, derotational osteotomy, or a combination of the two to increase joint stability.

1. Varus osteotomy involves intertrochanteric osteotomy with removal of a wedge-shaped piece of bone to decreases the angle of inclination to result in a more stable hip.
2. A derotational femoral osteotomy also increases stability by decreasing the amount of anteversion, which is reported to be large in dogs with hip dysplasia.

C. Consider a total hip replacement (THR) for mature patients for which conservative treatment is not effective.

1. The hip joint is replaced with a prosthetic acetabular cup and femoral component.
2. The success rate is excellent, but the surgery should only be performed by surgeons trained in the procedure.

D. Consider a femoral head and neck excision (FHO) for young patients or older patients for which a THR is not financially possible.

1. Excision limits bony contact between the femoral head and acetabulum and allows formation of a fibrous false joint.
2. Clinical function is unpredictable because an unstable joint is created; however, most patients have improved limb function and quality of life.

E. Preoperative management.

1. Perform complete orthopedic and neurologic examinations to confirm the diagnosis.
2. Provide intraoperative antibiotics for a pelvic osteotomy or total hip replacement.

F. Positioning.
   1. Position the animal in lateral recumbency for pelvic osteotomy and for FHO.
   2. Perform a hanging-leg preparation.

G. Surgical techniques.
   1. Pelvic osteotomy.

Pelvic osteotomy requires that an incision be made through the pubic brim, ischial floor, and ilial body. Recent studies show the optimal position for pubic osteotomy is adjacent to the medial walls of the acetabulum. With the patient in lateral recumbency, abduct the leg while maintaining the femur perpendicular to the acetabulum. Locate the origin of the pectineus muscle and center a 6-cm skin incision over this point. Incise subcutaneous tissues to further isolate the origin of the pectineus muscle at the ilieopectineal eminence. Release the origin of the pectineus muscle to expose the cranial brim of the pubis. Reflect the periosteum from the cranial, lateral, and caudal pubic surfaces. To protect soft tissues during the osteotomy, place spoon Hohmann retractors cranial to the pubis and within the obturator foramen caudally. Perform a pubic osteotomy adjacent to the medial wall of the acetabulum. Suture soft tissues and skin using standard methods. Next perform an osteotomy of the ischial floor. Make a skin incision midway between the medial prominence of the ischium and lateral tuberosity. Make the incision in the vertical plane, beginning 4 cm proximal to the ischial floor and extending 3 cm distally. Incise subcutaneous tissues and deep fascia. Make a 3-cm incision through the periosteal insertion of the internal obturator muscle at the dorsal crest of the ischial floor. Elevate the internal obturator muscle cranially to the obturator foramen. Then, incise the periosteal origin of the external obturator muscle at the ventral crest of the ischial floor and reflect the muscle from the ventral surface of the ischium cranially to the obturator foramen. Place two spoon Hohmann retractors to protect the soft tissue; insert one into the obturator foramen dorsally and one into the foramen ventrally. Direct an osteotome caudal to cranial in line with the center of the Hohmann retractors; this will center the osteotomy line into the obturator foramen. Close the incision after the osteotomy of the ilium is completed. At that time, drill two small holes on either side of the osteotomy adjacent to each other. Place orthopedic wire through the holes and twist them in a figure-8 fashion to stabilize the osteotomy. Suture the fascia of the internal obturator muscle to that of the external obturator muscle, then close subcutaneous tissue and skin using standard methods. Next perform an osteotomy of the ilium to allow axial rotation of the acetabulum. Make an incision from the cranial extent of the iliac crest caudally 1 to 2 cm beyond the greater trochanter. Center the incision over the ventral third of the ilial wing. Incise subcutaneous tissues and gluteal fat along the same line to visualize the intermuscular septum between the superficial gluteal muscle and the short part of the tensor fascia lata muscle. Incise the muscular septum to separate the tensor fascia lata muscle and middle gluteal muscle cranially and tensor fasciae latae and superficial gluteal muscles caudally. Cranially, use sharp dissection to separate the middle gluteal muscle and long head of the tensor fascia lata muscle. Palpate the ventral border of the ilium and make an incision to the bone near the ventral insertion of the middle and deep gluteal muscles. Isolate and ligate iliolumbar vessels and reflect the deep gluteal muscle from the lateral surface of the ilium. Incise the origin of iliacus muscle at the ventral border of the ilium and reflect the muscle from the ventral surface. Elevate periosteum from the medial surface of the ilium with a periosteal elevator. Place two spoon Hohmann retractors to protect soft tissue during the osteotomy: place one medial to the ilium to reflect the iliacus muscle and one over the dorsal crest of the ilium to retract the gluteal muscle mass. Judge the cranial position of the osteotomy by placing the osteotomy plate such that the most caudal plate hole is 1 to 2 cm cranial to the acetabulum. Perform the ilial osteotomy with a power saw on a line perpendicular to the long axis of the hemipelvis. Lateralize the

caudal segment with bone-holding forceps and secure an appropriate osteotomy plate to this segment. Next reduce the osteotomy and apply plate screws in the cranial segment. To close the incision, place sutures between the fascia of the middle gluteal muscle and that of the tensor fascia lata muscle cranially and between the superficial gluteal muscle and tensor fascia lata caudally. Approximate deep gluteal fat, subcutaneous tissue, and skin, using standard methods.

2. Femoral head and neck ostectomy.

Make a craniolateral approach to the hip joint and luxate the hip (see Chapter 29, Femoral Capital Physeal Fractures). If the round ligament is intact, incise it. Incising the round ligament is facilitated by placing lateral traction on the greater trochanter with bone-holding forceps and subluxating the femoral head. This allows curved scissors to be placed into the joint to cut the ligament. Perform the osteotomy by externally rotating the limb to the point at which the joint line of the stifle is parallel to the operating table. Identify the line of osteotomy perpendicular to the operating table at the junction of the femoral neck and femoral metaphysis. To ensure accuracy of the bony cut, the surgeon can predrill a series of three or more holes along the line of the osteotomy. Use an osteotome and mallet to complete the cut. Ventral reflection of the vastus lateralis muscle facilitates proper placement of an osteotome during this procedure. Once the femoral neck and head are removed, palpate the cut surface of the femoral neck for irregularities. The most common finding is a shelf of femoral neck left on the caudal surface of the femur. Remove edges with rongeurs. Suture the joint capsule over the acetabulum, if possible. Alternatively, fashion a proximally based biceps femoris muscle pedicle and pass it from caudal to cranial across the excision site. To close, reposition the vastus lateralis and deep gluteal muscles with absorbable suture using a simple interrupted pattern. Suture fascia lata with absorbable suture using a simple continuous pattern. Suture skin with nonabsorbable suture using a simple interrupted pattern.

VI. Postoperative Care and Assessment

A. After pelvic osteotomy allow leash walking only until radiographic evidence of complete healing, generally in 6 weeks. During healing, gradually increase length of exercise and perform passive flexion and extension of the hip. Perform surgery on the other side when discomfort associated with the first surgery is tolerated by the dog. Inform owners of potential complications, including implant failure, loss of limb abduction, and pelvic outlet narrowing.

B. After FHO, stress early active use of the limb with passive flexion and extension of the hip two to three times daily and frequent leash walks beginning immediately after surgery. Encourage running and swimming after suture removal. Good return of active limb function is dependent on the length of time the hip joint pathology was present and on severity of the degenerative changes. Patients with chronic lameness are slower to return to function than patients with acute lameness.

VII. Prognosis

A. The prognosis after pelvic osteotomy is determined by case selection, with best results in patients with few or no degenerative changes. Long-term function is good to excellent, and degenerative changes are less than would be expected without surgery.

B. Expect long-term function after varus osteotomy to be good, and degenerative changes to progress radiographically less than what would be expected without surgery.

C. Expect excellent return to normal function with a THR.

D. Expect results after FHO to depend a great deal on patient size and postoperative physical therapy. More small and medium patients have good or excellent limb function.

Coxofemoral Luxations (*SAS*, pp. 949-955)

I. General Considerations

A. Expect dorsal displacement of the femoral head relative to the acetabulum. Ventrocaudal displacements occur less frequently.

B. Recognize that the round ligament of the femoral head always fails and the joint capsule tears completely. The ligament either ruptures or is avulsed from the fovea capitis.

C. Treat hip luxation as quickly as possible. Reduction prevents further soft tissue damage and allows synovial fluid to provide nutrients to the cartilage again.

D. Assess the patient for concurrent trauma.

II. Diagnosis

A. Clinical Presentation

1. Signalment.
   a. Any breed or age dog or cat may be affected.
2. History.
   a. Typically there is a history of a unilateral non–weight-bearing lameness, following a traumatic episode.

B. Physical Examination

1. There is generally a non–weight-bearing lameness associated with trauma.
   a. Observe the limb carried adducted with the stifle externally rotated when the femur is displaced craniodorsally.
   b. Observe the limb carried abducted with the stifle internally rotated when the femur is displaced caudoventrally.
2. Identify crepitus or pain on manipulation of the limb.
3. Palpate the greater trochanter relative to the tuber ischii and the crest of the ilium.
   a. With craniodorsal displacement, the greater trochanter is dorsal to

an imaginary line drawn from the crest of the ilium to the tuber ischii and the distance between the tuber ischii and greater trochanter is larger than that in the normal limb.

b. With a ventrocaudal luxation palpate the opposite of above.

C. Radiography

1. Confirm the diagnosis with ventrodorsal and lateral radiographs.
2. Evaluate for avulsion of the fovea capitis, associated hip joint fractures, and the presence of degenerative changes secondary to poor joint conformation.

III. Medical or Conservative Management

A. Attempt closed reduction before performing open reduction in most animals, unless there is radiographic evidence of severe hip dysplasia or a fracture.

B. Closed reduction of craniodorsal luxations.

Place the patient in lateral recumbency under general anesthesia. Grasp the affected limb with one hand near the tarsal joint and place the other hand under the limb against the body wall to provide resistance. Externally rotate the limb and pull it caudally to position the femoral head over the acetabulum. When the femoral head lies lateral to the acetabulum, internally rotate the limb to seat the femoral head within the acetabulum. Apply medial pressure to the greater trochanter while flexing and extending the joint to help expel debris from the acetabular cup. Place the limb in an Ehmer bandage. Limit the animal to controlled activity on a leash until the bandage is removed in 4 to 7 days. After bandage removal, limit activity to controlled leash activity for an additional 2 weeks.

C. Closed reduction of caudoventral luxations.

Place the patient in lateral recumbency with the limb held perpendicular to the spine. Grasp the limb at the tarsal joint with one hand and place the other hand under the limb medial to the hip joint. Place traction on the limb while simultaneously abducting the leg to pull the femoral head beyond the medial rim of the acetabulum. Once the femoral head has cleared the acetabular rim, exert lateral pressure medial to the hip joint to position the femoral head lateral to the acetabulum. Push proximally and allow the femoral head to fall into the acetabulum. After reduction, place the patient in hobbles to prevent abduction of the limb. Limit activity to controlled activity on a leash until the bandage is removed in 4 to 7 days. Limit activity to leash walking for an additional 2 weeks after the hobbles have been removed.

IV. Surgical Treatment

A. General Considerations

1. Perform open reduction when avulsion of the fovea capitis is present or when closed reduction has failed.
2. Explore the joint to assess the soft-tissue injury. If a reconstructive procedure is unlikely to maintain reduction, consider an alternate procedure such as a femoral head ostectomy or total hip replacement.

B. Positioning

1. Position the animal in lateral recumbency.
2. Perform a hanging-leg preparation.

C. Surgical Techniques

1. Stabilize the hip with capsular reconstruction if the joint capsule is intact, or with joint reconstruction and/or translocation of the greater trochanter if capsular reconstruction is not feasible or stable.
2. Exploration of the hip joint.

Perform a craniolateral exposure to the hip joint (see Chapter 29, Femoral Capital Physeal Fractures); if additional exposure is necessary, perform a trochanteric osteotomy (see Chapter 29, Acetabular Fractures). Reflect the deep gluteal muscle and visualize the femoral head craniodorsal to the hip joint. Externally rotate the limb to visualize and remove remnants of round ligament and debris from the femoral head and acetabulum; this allows the femoral head to completely seat within the acetabulum. Once the hip is reduced, assess stability by viewing the acetabular coverage of the femoral head and placing the hip joint through a complete range of motion. Perform the chosen stabilization technique.

3. Capsule reconstruction.
   a. If the joint capsule is intact except for a small rent, the acetabular coverage is adequate, and the joint is stable through a range of motion, suture the capsule as the sole reconstructive procedure.

Use nonabsorbable monofilament suture material in an interrupted pattern. If the capsule has torn from its insertion site, drill small holes in the femoral neck through which to pass suture, or reattach with screws and spiked washers.

4. Translocation of the greater trochanter.
   a. Consider a trochanteric osteotomy to translocate the greater trochanter distally and slightly caudally if the joint capsule is injured beyond repair but the gluteal musculature is not compromised. Relocation enables the gluteal muscles to abduct and internally rotate the femoral head.

Perform a trochanteric osteotomy (see Chapter 29, Acetabular Fractures) and reflect the gluteal musculature proximally. Once the hip has been cleaned of debris and reduced, place the limb in abduction. Use an osteotome and mallet to create a new surface caudal and distal to the point where the greater trochanter normally seats. Reposition the greater trochanter at its new attachment site and secure it in place with a tension band.

5. Joint reconstruction.
   a. If the joint capsule is shredded and the gluteal muscle mass is compromised, use a prosthetic capsule or transacetabular pin to maintain reduction during the healing of the fibrous joint capsule.

Place two screws with flat metal washers in the dorsal rim of the acetabulum. Insert one screw at the 10 o'clock position and one at the 1 o'clock position. Place a third screw and washer in the trochanteric fossa (alternatively, drill a hole through the femoral neck in the trochanteric fossa to accept suture). Pass heavy nonabsorbable suture in a figure-8 pattern between the acetabular screws and trochanteric fossa.

Alternatively, place a transacetabular pin through the femoral neck into the medial wall of the acetabulum. Predrill a hole, slightly smaller than the diameter of the pin to be used, from the third trochanter and through the femoral head to

exit from the femoral head where the round ligament inserts. Insert the smooth pin through the drill hole until the pin point is visible just beneath the articular surface of the femoral head. Reduce the luxation and place the limb in abduction and slight internal rotation. While exerting medial pressure on the greater trochanter, drill the pin into the nonarticular wall or the acetabular fossa. Bend the pin at the third trochanter to prevent medial migration. Place the patient in an Ehmer bandage until the transacetabular pin is removed.

6. Placement of an elastic external fixator.
   a. If immediate weight bearing is necessary consider placing an elastic external fixator instead of an Ehmer sling.

Reduce the hip through either closed reduction or open reduction. Make a small incision overlying the greater trochanter and prepare a tunnel through the soft tissue to the trochanteric fossa. Protect the soft tissue while inserting an end-threaded pin into the marrow cavity of the femur. The pin need not extend beyond the proximal one third of the femur. Insert a second end-threaded pin from proximal to distal across the body of the ilium 2 cm cranial to the acetabulum. Connect the pins outside the skin margins with a heavy elastic band. You may wish to place a Kirschner clamp on the pin as it exits the skin surface to help prevent the elastic band from placing pressure on the skin and potentially causing necrosis. Postoperatively, maintain the skin-to-pin interface with daily cleansing and application of an antiseptic. Remove the pins in 10 to 14 days.

V. Suture Material/Special Instruments

A. For capsule reconstruction, select either No. 1 or No. 2 nonabsorbable suture.

B. For prosthetic capsule reconstruction, use screws and stainless steel washers, and for transacetabular pin reconstruction use a small Steinmann pin.

C. For an elastic external fixator use end-threaded pins, Kirschner clamps, and an elastic band (bicycle tubing or a heavy rubber band).

VI. Postoperative Care and Assessment

A. Apply an Ehmer bandage for 4 to 7 days. Leash walk only for an additional 3 weeks, and follow by gradual return to full activity over 2 more weeks.

B. Reexamine 3 days after bandage removal and before unsupervised activity is resumed.

VII. Prognosis

A. There is generally a 50% success rate for maintaining reduction and regaining good to excellent limb function with closed reduction, and an 85% to 90% success rate with open reduction. Failure of closed reduction does not affect the success rate of subsequent open reduction, so attempt closed reduction first if the option is available.

B. A lower success rate is common with poor conformation of the hip joint.

Legg-Perthes (*SAS*, pp. 956-957)

I. Definition

A. **Legg-Perthes** is a noninflammatory aseptic necrosis of the femoral head, occurring in young patients before closure of the capital femoral physis.

II. General Considerations

A. The cause of Legg-Perthes is an interruption in blood flow that results in collapse of the femoral epiphysis. The reason for the loss of blood flow is unknown, but theories center on increased intraarticular pressure (from synovitis or abnormal limb position) collapsing the epiphyseal vessels that are extraosseous and the sole blood supply.

B. During repair, normal physiologic weight-bearing forces may cause collapse and fragmentation of the femoral epiphysis, resulting in DJD.

C. Advise owners to neuter affected animals, because the disease has been linked to an autosomal recessive gene.

III. Diagnosis

A. Clinical Presentation

1. Signalment.
   a. Small-breed dogs (i.e., under 10 kg) between 6 to 10 months old are typically affected. The disease is occasionally bilateral.
   b. Cats are not affected.
2. History.
   a. There is typically a history of a slow-onset of a weight-bearing lameness that worsens over 6 to 8 weeks; however, it may progress to non–weight-bearing status and some clients report acute onset of lameness.
   b. Irritability, reduced appetite, and chewing at the skin over the affected hip may also occur.

B. Physical Examination

1. There is generally pain on manipulation of the hip joint. There may be limited range of motion, muscle atrophy, and crepitus with advanced disease.

C. Radiography

1. Assess radiographs for deformity of the femoral head, shortening of the femoral neck, and foci of decreased bone density within the femoral epiphysis.

IV. Medical or Conservative Management

A. Use antiinflammatory medication for pain relief, but definitive treatment requires surgery.

V. Surgical Treatment

A. Preoperative management

1. Limit activity and provide antiinflammatory medications until surgery is performed.

B. Positioning

1. Position the animal in lateral recumbency.
2. Perform a hanging-leg preparation.

VI. Surgical Techniques

A. Perform excision of the femoral head and neck (FHO) (see Hip Dysplasia).

VII. Postoperative Care and Assessment

A. Encourage limb use immediately after surgery. Perform passive flexion and extension of the hip joint twice daily as soon as the animal will tolerate it.

VIII. Prognosis

A. Inform owners the prognosis for normal limb use is good to excellent with an FHO.

Stifle

Cranial Cruciate Ligament Rupture (*SAS*, pp. 957-966)

I. Definition

A. **Cranial drawer** describes the excessive craniocaudal movement of the tibia relative to the femur as a result of cruciate ligament injury.

II. General Considerations

A. Recognize that the cranial cruciate ligament (CCL) is divided into craniomedial and caudolateral bands. The craniomedial band is taut during all phases of flexion and extension; the caudolateral band is taut in extension but becomes lax in flexion.

B. Remember that the CCL is a check against craniocaudal motion, but it also functions to limit internal rotation of the tibia and provide a limited degree of varus-valgus support to the flexed stifle joint.

C. Injury is the result of violent internal rotation of the leg or hyperextension of the stifle.

D. Histologic and conformational abnormalities may predispose to CCL rupture. For example, the larger stifle angle in some breeds (i.e. rottweiler and chow chows) may play a role.

III. Diagnosis

A. Clinical Presentation

1. Signalment.
   a. Any breed or age dog may be affected.
   b. Cruciate ligament rupture is rare in cats.
2. History.
   a. With acute tears there is typically a sudden onset of a non–weight-bearing or partial–weight-bearing lameness that usually resolves within 3 to 6 weeks, particularly in patients less than 10 kg.
   b. With chronic lameness, DJD is typical.
   c. With partial cranial cruciate ligament, there is generally a mild weight-bearing lameness associated with exercise.

B. Physical Examination

1. With acute tears, there is generally little pain reaction on flexion and extension of the joint. Cranial drawer motion may be difficult to elicit if the patient resists because of nervousness.
2. With chronic tears, assess for thigh muscle atrophy and crepitus when the stifle is flexed and extended. If a clicking or popping is heard and felt, suspect a meniscal injury. Palpate an enlargement along the medial joint surface that is caused by osteophyte formation along the trochlear ridges. Expect craniocaudal instability to be difficult to elicit because of the proliferation of the fibrous joint capsule.
3. With partial tears of the craniomedial band, assess for stability in extension, but instability during flexion.
4. Compare the affected leg with the opposite limb if instability is questionable.
5. See Chapter 28, Orthopedic Examination, for the procedure for eliciting cranial drawer motion. If necessary use sedation. Craniocaudal movement greater than the 0 to 2 mm found in normal stifle joints indicates ligament rupture. Be aware that in younger patients, craniocaudal translation may be as great as 4 to 5 mm, but ligament rupture is confirmed by the absence of an abrupt stop at the cranial extent of movement.

C. Radiography

1. Take radiographs to help rule out other causes of stifle joint lameness.
2. With chronic ligament tears, look for osteophyte formation along the trochlear ridge, caudal surface of the tibial plateau, and inferior pole of the patella. Also assess thickening of the medial fibrous joint capsule and subchondral sclerosis.

D. Laboratory Findings

1. Arthrocentesis may reveal increased amounts of joint fluid and a twofold to threefold increase in cell numbers (6000 to 9000/µl), indicating secondary DJD.

IV. Medical or Conservative Management

A. Although surgical stabilization is recommended for all patients, with conservative treatment (i.e., rest and antiinflammatory drugs) the lameness often resolves within 6 weeks in small patients. Patients weighing less than 10 kg tolerate conservative treatment best. However, instability persists and secondary degenerative joint disease develops.

B. Be aware that abnormal stress, coupled with the increasing mechanical weakness of the cruciate ligament associated with aging, may lead to rupture of the cruciate ligament in the opposite stifle joint within 12 to 18 months. Therefore surgery is recommended in all patients.

V. Surgical Treatment

A. General Considerations

1. Treat with a reconstruction technique or a primary repair with augmentation supplemented with a reconstructive technique. Success rate is the same regardless of method performed.
2. Select among intracapsular and extracapsular techniques for reconstruction of the cranial cruciate ligament.
   a. With intracapsular reconstructions pass autogenous tissue through the joint.
   b. With extracapsular reconstructions place sutures outside the joint or redirect the lateral collateral ligament.
   c. Consider combining intracapsular and extracapsular techniques in large breed dogs.
3. Regardless of technique selected, inspect the meniscus for tears and excise the torn portion.

B. Preoperative Management

1. Limit activity to prevent further damage to the articular cartilage.

C. Surgical Anatomy

1. Have a working knowledge of the origin and insertion of normal ligamentous structures in the stifle joint before surgery.
   a. The CCL originates from the medial surface of the lateral femoral condyle. The ligament fibers course distal and medial, spiral 90 degrees, and insert onto the craniomedial surface of the tibial plateau beneath the intermeniscal ligament.
   b. The medial and lateral menisci are fibrocartilaginous disks that have a semilunar shape. The medial meniscus is often injured with cruciate ligament damage.

D. Positioning

1. Position the animal in dorsal or lateral recumbency.
2. Perform a hanging-leg preparation.

E. Surgical Techniques

1. Lateral approach to the stifle joint.

Make a craniolateral skin incision centered over the patella. Begin the incision 5 cm proximal to the patella and continue it distally 5 cm below the tibial crest. Incise subcutaneous tissues along the same line to visualize the septum between the superficial leaf of the fascia lata and the biceps femoris muscle proximally and the lateral retinaculum distally. Make an incision through the fascia lata proximally and carry the incision through the fascia lata and lateral retinaculum distally. Make an incision through the joint capsule, beginning 1 cm distal to the patella. Continue the incision proximally, along a line adjacent to the patella tendon, to the inferior pole of the patella. Then incise along the border of the vastus lateralis muscle toward the fabella. Displace the patella medially to expose the cranial surface of the joint.

2. Medial approach to the stifle joint.

Make a craniomedial incision centered over the patella. Begin the incision 5 cm proximal to the patella and continue distally 5 cm below the tibial crest. Incise subcutaneous tissues along the same line to expose the parapatellar medial retinaculum. Make an incision through the medial retinaculum and joint capsule adjacent to the medial ridge of the patella tendon. Continue the incision proximally and distally to equal the extent of the subcutaneous tissue incision.

3. Intracapsular repair.
   a. Consider the placement of an autogenous tissue graft through the joint to mimic the course of the cranial cruciate ligament. The technique described here uses the lateral one third of the patella tendon and distal fascia lata.

Place the tissue through a tibial tunnel, through the joint, and over the top of the lateral condyle. Alternately, place the graft through a tibial and femoral tunnel. Perform a lateral approach to the stifle joint as described previously. Free the superficial surface of the patella tendon from all loose connective tissue and flex the limb to tighten the patella tendon and lateral retinacular tissue. Make an incision beginning at the lateral edge of the distal pole of the patella and extend it through the lateral one third of the patella tendon and retinaculum to the tibial crest distally. Use the palpable tuberosity cranial to the groove of the long digital extensor muscle as the landmark for the most distal extent of the incision. Place a periosteal elevator in the incision and separate the patella tendon and fascia lata from the joint capsule. As the graft is freed from the joint capsule near the patella, use the lateral edge of the elevator to reflect the graft from the lateral patella surface. Use scissors to incise the fascia lata along the medial edge of the cranial sartorius muscle. Carry the incision through the fascia lata proximally the full length of the skin incision. When the proximal extent of the incision is reached, incise the fascia lata caudally to the cranial border of the biceps femoris muscle. Continue the incision distally along the cranial edge of the biceps muscle to the tibial plateau. When bringing the fascial incision distally, it is extremely important to maintain equal width of the fascial graft along its entire length. Incise the joint capsule from the distal pole of the patella to the tibial crest. At the level of the patella, direct the capsule incision proximally and caudally along the border of the vastus lateralis muscle to the region of the lateral fabella. Luxate the patella medially to expose the cranial view of the stifle. Remove remnants of the torn cruciate ligament with a

scalpel and examine the internal structures of the joint. To visualize the caudomedial compartment of the joint, place the tip of a Hohmann retractor on the caudal tibial spine and force the body of the retractor against the distal femoral trochlea. Place caudal pressure on the retractor handle to force the tibia forward and down, exposing the medial meniscus. Inspect the meniscus for damage. If it is torn, grasp the torn section of meniscus with a forceps and excise the medial and lateral attachments. Widen the roof and lateral wall of the intercondylar notch to ensure adequate space for the graft (notchoplasty). Next, free the insertion of the fascial graft from the tibial plateau with a small osteotome and mallet. Place an osteotome behind the tibial tuberosity just cranial to the muscular groove of the long digital extensor muscle. Free the graft from this site by removing a small section of bone. Cranially, use the osteotome to free the patella tendon part of the graft from the craniolateral tibial crest. Remove a thin layer of bone with the tendon to free this section of the graft. Use a periosteal elevator to reflect the cranial tibialis muscle from the craniolateral face of the proximal tibia. Drill a tunnel, large enough to accept the graft, from the cranial surface of the tibia to the insertion of the cranial cruciate ligament inside the joint. Place a wire loop through the tunnel from inside the joint to exit laterally. Pull the graft through the tunnel into the joint with the aid of the wire loop. Be sure that the bone is seated well inside the tunnel. Then pass the graft through the joint by passing it "over the top" of the lateral condyle or by passing it through a drill hole in the femur. To perform the over-the-top maneuver, pass a curved forceps over the top of the fabella from caudal to cranial. Glide the forceps next to the lateral condyle and penetrate the caudal joint capsule. Grasp the free end of the graft and pull it through the joint. Make an incision through the femoral fabellar ligament and pass the graft through the ligament. Secure the fascial graft to the lateral femoral condyle with a spiked polyacetyl washer and bone screw, or suture it to the femoral fabellar ligament, fibrous joint capsule, and patella tendon. When the graft is being secured to the femoral condyle, do not attempt to eliminate all the cranial drawer; this would place excessive tension within the graft. Eliminate all but 2 to 3 mm of cranial drawer while the leg is positioned in normal standing angle. Suture the fibrous joint capsule, cut edge of fascia lata, and subcutaneous tissues with absorbable suture using a simple interrupted pattern. Suture skin with nonabsorbable suture in a simple interrupted pattern.

4. Lateral retinacular stabilization.

Perform a lateral approach to the stifle joint, open the joint, and inspect the meniscus for tears or damage. Remove the damaged meniscus, if present, and close the arthrotomy with absorbable suture using a simple interrupted pattern. Alternatively, perform a medial approach to the stifle joint and displace the patella laterally, remove remnants of the cranial cruciate ligament, and inspect the internal structures of the stifle. Treat meniscal tears. Replace the patella in the trochlear groove and suture the arthrotomy with absorbable suture using an interrupted pattern. Reflect the skin laterally and make an incision through the distal fascia lata. Elevate the biceps femoris muscle from the lateral surface of the joint capsule to expose the gastrocnemius muscle. Pass polyester suture or monofilament wire through the femoral-fabellar ligament and around the fabella. Next, pass the suture or wire through a predrilled hole through the tibial crest. Flex the stifle to 90 degrees or to a normal standing angle and hold the tibia caudally to remove drawer motion and tie the suture (or twist the wire) until it engages the joint capsule. The extracapsular sutures can be augmented with tissue advancements. Commonly, advancement of the biceps femoris muscle by suturing the cranial edge of the biceps fascia incision to the patella tendon will aid in restricting cranial drawer. In addition to the stabilizing suture,

place a series of imbricating sutures through the fibrous joint capsule with nonabsorbable suture. Place each suture through the fibrous capsule caudal to the arthrotomy line, cross superficial to the arthrotomy, and penetrate the fibrous capsule cranial to the arthrotomy. Preplace individual sutures and do not tie until the sutures in the series are in place. Consider augmenting the extracapsular sutures with tissue advancement, such as advancement of the biceps femoris muscles by suturing the cranial edge of the biceps fascia incision to the patella tendon. Close as previously described.

5. Fibular head advancement.
   a. General considerations.
      i. Use extreme care to identify and protect the peroneal nerve throughout the procedure.

Perform a lateral approach to the stifle joint and arthrotomy as described above and inspect the meniscus for tears or damage. Remove the damaged meniscus, if present, and close the arthrotomy with absorbable suture using a simple interrupted pattern. Reflect the fascia lata caudally. To facilitate reflection of the fascia lata, make a craniocaudal transverse incision of the fascia lata 2 to 3 cm distal to the joint line. Free the fibular head cranially and caudally from the tibial epiphysis with sharp dissection and elevation. Make an incision along the cranial and caudal edges of the lateral collateral ligament to allow cranial transposition of the ligament-bone complex. While being careful not to injure the popliteal tendon or lateral meniscus, free the deep surface of the ligament from its origin at the femoral epicondyle to its insertion at the fibular head. This is most easily accomplished with a small periosteal elevator. Incise the fibularis longus muscle and lateral digital extensor muscle at the joint line and reflect them craniodistally to allow cranial redirection of the fibular head. Externally rotate the tibia and advance the fibular head and collateral ligament cranially using bone-holding forceps. Stabilize the fibular head with a small Steinmann pin and tension-band wire. Suture extensor muscles and fascia lata with absorbable suture using a simple interrupted pattern. Repair subcutaneous tissues and skin incisions as previously described.

6. Primary repair with augmentation.
   a. General considerations.
      i. Reserve primary repair for the small percentage of patients with failure of the cruciate ligament at the point of insertion on the tibial plateau or failure from the origin of the ligament on the femur.
      ii. Use the same surgical exposure as described for intracapsular or extracapsular reconstruction, and always use a reconstructive procedure in addition to primary repair.

Perform either a medial or lateral approach to the stifle joint as described above. Once the arthrotomy is made, identify the cranial cruciate ligament. A small piece of cancellous bone often remains attached at the site of failure. Pass nonabsorbable suture through the ligament using a locking-loop pattern. Make two small parallel drill holes from the medial tibial metaphysis to exit within the joint at the insertion point of the cranial cruciate ligament. Place wire loops through the holes and pass the free ends of the suture through the wire. Pull the wire through the predrilled holes to exit laterally. Perform a reconstructive procedure to augment the primary repair. Once the reconstruction is completed, tie the sutures from the ligament outside the joint. Close the surgical wound using the technique previously described.

VI. Suture Materials/Special Instruments

A. For extracapsular repairs, select nonabsorbable suture (usually No. 2 to No. 5 polyester or nylon, depending on the weight of the patient) or orthopedic wire (18- to 20-gauge).

VII. Postoperative Care and Assessment

A. Limit exercise to leash walking only for 6 weeks.

B. If wire is used, expect it to break after periarticular fibrous tissue has formed to stabilize the joint. If lameness results when the wire breaks, which happens occasionally, expect it to resolve in 2 weeks with antiinflammatory drugs and rest.

C. Following fibular head advancement, place the limb in a padded bandage for 10 to 14 days. Limit exercise to leash walking only for an additional 3 weeks.

D. For intracapsular repairs maintain a soft bandage for 2 weeks. Restrict activity to leash walking for a minimum of 12 weeks, but gradually increase distance of walks. Perform passive flexion and extension of the joint. Remove the screw and washer 2 to 3 months postoperatively if used.

VIII. Prognosis

A. Inform owners that long-term function is generally good regardless of which surgical procedure performed. Outcome is influenced by the dog's size, activity, and intended use. Larger, active patients have a poorer prognosis for acceptable long-term function.

B. Warn the owner that a significant percentage injure the ligament in the opposite knee within 3 years.

Caudal Cruciate Ligament Injury (*SAS*, pp. 966-969)

I. General Considerations

A. Isolated caudal cruciate ligament tears are rare in small animals. Caudal cruciate ligament injuries are more common with severe derangement of the stifle joint with multiple structures ruptured following a severe traumatic episode.

B. Nonathletic dogs often function normally with caudal cruciate tears.

II. Diagnosis

A. Clinical Presentation

1. Signalment.
   a. Any breed or age dog or cat may be affected. Isolated tears are more frequent in large breeds of dogs.
   b. In cats, caudal cruciate and medial collateral ligaments commonly occur concurrently.
2. History.
   a. Typically there is a history of a non–weight-bearing lameness that progressively improves, but returns during strenuous activity.

B. Physical Examination

1. There is generally cranial-caudal instability with isolated tears. Differentiate caudal cruciate rupture from cranial cruciate rupture in several ways.
   a. When the joint is held in extension, expect the degree of instability to be less with caudal cruciate ligament tears.
   b. With the patient in dorsal recumbency and the limb positioned such that the stifle is flexed and the tibia is parallel to the ground, the tibial tuberosity forms a distinct prominence cranial to the patella. If a caudal cruciate ligament injury is present, observe the weight of the limb to cause a caudal "sag" of the tibia, resulting in loss of the tuberosity prominence.
   c. When the tibia is moved forward, experience a distinct endpoint to the cranial movement when the caudal cruciate ligament is ruptured.
   d. With the tibia in an extended position, observe a distinct caudal subluxation of the tibia when the stifle joint is flexed and internally rotated if the caudal cruciate ligament is torn.
2. There is typically severe instability with caudal cruciate ligament tears that are part of a multiple ligament injury.

C. Radiography

1. Observe radiographs for caudal displacement of the tibial plateau and for small bone densities, which may be apparent on the lateral projection just behind and distal to the femoral condyles.

III. Medical or Conservative Management

A. Consider conservative management (only leash walking for 8 weeks) of isolated caudal cruciate tears as an option for smaller dogs or cats and for dogs leading inactive lives.

IV. Surgical Treatment

A. General Considerations

1. Repair the tear by one of several extracapsular reconstruction techniques: suture stabilization, redirection of the medial collateral ligament, or popliteal tendon tenodesis.
   a. For suture stabilization imbricate the caudomedial joint capsule and place a medial or lateral stabilizing suture.
   b. For redirection repair use existing autogenous tissue such as the medial collateral ligament.

B. Positioning

1. Position the animal in lateral recumbency with the affected limb up or in dorsal recumbency.

C. Surgical Techniques

1. Suture stabilization.

Make a standard craniomedial approach to the stifle joint (see Cranial Cruciate Ligament Rupture). Drill a hole in the caudomedial corner of the tibial epiphysis. Place a stabilizing suture, of heavy (No. 2) nonabsorbable suture material, from the proximal patella tendon through the predrilled hole. On the lateral side, imbricate the caudal joint capsule and place a stabilizing suture from the proximal patella tendon through a predrilled hole in the fibular head.

2. Use of autogenous tissue.

Make a standard craniomedial approach to the stifle joint (see Cranial Cruciate Ligament Rupture). Incise through the insertion of the caudal sartorius muscle and medial fascia along the tibial metaphysis. Reflect the muscle and fascia caudally to expose the medial collateral ligament. Free the body of the ligament with a periosteal elevator and direct the ligament caudally to course in the same sagittal plane as the caudal cruciate ligament. Secure the ligament in this position with a bone screw and spiked washer.

3. Entrapment (tenodesis) of the popliteal tendon.

Make a lateral approach to the stifle joint (see Cranial Cruciate Ligament Rupture) and reflect the fascia lata to isolate the popliteal tendon as it passes beneath the lateral collateral ligament. Entrap the popliteal tendon with a screw and Teflon or polyacetyl washer as it passes caudal and proximal to the fibular head.

V. Postoperative Care and Assessment

A. Allow leash walking only for 8 weeks, then gradually return the animal to unsupervised activity over a 4-week period. Perform passive flexion and extension of the stifle joint.

VI. Prognosis

A. Inform owners that the prognosis is good to excellent for return to normal limb function in most animals after surgery or conservative treatment as appropriate.

Collateral Ligament Injury (*SAS*, pp. 969-972)

I. General Considerations

A. The medial collateral ligament forms a strong attachment to the joint capsule and medial meniscus as it crosses the medial joint surface. This stabilizes the medial meniscus, but also predisposes the caudal body of the meniscus to injury from the medial femoral condyle when the cranial cruciate ligament ruptures.

B. Both the medial and lateral collateral ligaments function to limit varus-valgus motion of the stifle joint. They are both taut when the stifle joint is extended. As the stifle joint flexes, the medial collateral ligament remains tight but the lateral collateral ligament relaxes to allow internal tibial rotation.

C. Isolated collateral ligament tears are rare in small animals. Instead, expect multiple-ligament injuries resulting from severe trauma.

II. Diagnosis

A. Clinical Presentation

1. Signalment.
   a. Any breed or age dog or cat may be affected.
2. History.
   a. Typically there is a history of an acute onset of a non–weight-bearing lameness after exercising or after a vehicular accident.

B. Physical Examination

1. Apply valgus and varus stress to the stifle joint while the joint is held in extension.
   a. If the lateral joint restraints are torn, expect opening of the lateral joint to be apparent. Isolated tears show minimal opening, whereas obvious opening occurs with more extensive injuries (lateral collateral ligament, joint capsule, and peripheral meniscal ligaments).

C. Radiography

1. Assess radiographs for bone chips associated with ligament damage and bony avulsions.
2. Perform stress radiographs to demonstrate increased medial or lateral joint space.

III. Medical or Conservative Treatment

A. Base the decision to use conservative or surgical treatment on the degree of injury to the ligament and secondary joint restraints. Consider conservative treatment with minimal swelling and only slight opening of the joint space when the joint is placed under stress.

B. Apply a fiberglass cast for 2 weeks, followed by controlled activity for 6 additional weeks.

IV. Surgical Treatment

A. General Considerations

1. Perform surgery if there is moderate to severe swelling and significant opening of the joint space when the joint is placed under stress.
2. Reconstruct the collateral ligament, meniscocapsular ligaments, and joint capsule. Repair all injured restraints.

B. Preoperative Management

1. Allow leash walking only to avoid additional damage to the articular cartilage or menisci.
2. Provide NSAIDs to control acute discomfort.

C. Surgical Anatomy

1. When dissecting near the lateral collateral ligament avoid the peroneal (fibular) nerve because it obliquely crosses the distal aspect to the stifle joint. It lies superficial to the gastrocnemius muscle and sends an articular branch to the lateral collateral ligament.

D. Positioning

1. Position the animal in lateral recumbency with the affected leg up to repair a lateral ligament and the affected leg down for a medial ligament.
2. Perform a hanging-leg preparation.
3. If multiple ligament tears are present, consider positioning in dorsal recumbency.

E. Surgical Techniques

1. Medial collateral ligament.

Make a medial parapatellar incision. Use a medial approach to expose the medial collateral ligament (see Cranial Cruciate Ligament Rupture). Incise the insertion of the caudal head of the sartorius muscle and deep fascia along the craniomedial border of the proximal tibia. Retract the muscle and fascia caudally to expose the collateral ligament and medial joint capsule. Reposition the ligament to its anatomic site and secure it with a screw and polyacetyl spiked washer. If the ligament injury is an intrasubstance tear, perform primary repair by suturing the ligament ends; use a locking-loop suture pattern with small nonabsorbable suture. Supplement the primary repair with screws and figure-8 support. Following repair of the collateral ligament, carefully reconstruct the meniscocapsular ligaments and joint capsule using interrupted sutures of small nonabsorbable suture material (polypropylene or nylon).

2. Lateral collateral ligament.

Use a craniocaudal approach to expose the lateral collateral ligament (see Cranial Cruciate Ligament Rupture). Make a proximal-to-distal parapatellar incision through the fascia lata. Continue the incision distally 4 cm below the tibial crest, parallel to the joint line. Use caution in isolating the peroneal nerve and protect it carefully during surgery. Reflect the fascia lata caudally to expose the collateral ligament and lateral joint capsule. Repair the ligament as previously described.

V. Postoperative Care and Assessment

A. Apply a bandage for 10 days. Restrict the animal to leash walking only for 8 weeks. Perform passive flexion and extension for 10 minutes, twice a day.

VI. Prognosis

A. Inform owner that the prognosis for isolated collateral ligament tears is good to excellent. If multiple ligaments are torn, prognosis is fair.

Multiple Ligament Injuries (*SAS*, pp. 972-974)

I. Definitions

A. **Varus angulation** is an inward rotation of the leg (toward the midline of the body).

B. **Valgus angulation** is an outward rotation (away from the midline of the body).

II. General Consideration

A. Expect these types of injury to result from car accidents, but they may result from catching a foot jumping a fence.

B. A common triad of injuries includes cranial and caudal cruciate ligament tears, failure of the primary and secondary medial restraints, and peripheral medial meniscal tears.

III. Diagnosis

A. Clinical Presentation

1. Signalment.
   a. Any breed or age dog or cat may be affected.
2. History.
   a. There is typically a history of an acute, non–weight-bearing lameness following trauma.

B. Physical Examination

1. There is generally marked craniocaudal movement of the tibia relative to the femur when both cranial and caudal cruciate ligaments are torn.
2. Varus and valgus stress applied to the joint in full extension reveals collateral ligament damage.

C. Radiography

1. Assess radiographs for small bone chips at the origin or insertion of ligaments.

IV. Medical or Conservative Management

A. Do not attempt external coaptation with splint or casts. Surgery is required.

V. Surgical Treatment

A. Repair the cranial and caudal cruciate ligaments, collateral restraints, and menisci. Start with the collateral ligaments, then reconstruct the cruciate ligaments.

B. Preoperative management.
   1. Apply a padded bandage and limit activity to prevent further damage to the articular surfaces of the joint.

C. Positioning.
   1. Position in dorsal recumbency with the affected limb up.
   2. Perform a hanging-leg preparation.

D. Surgical techniques.
   1. See the sections for cruciate ligament repair, collateral ligament repair, and meniscal injuries.

E. Postoperative care and assessment.
   1. Place in a support bandage for 3 to 4 weeks. Have the bandage in place before the patient recovers from anesthesia. Change the bandage under sedation weekly, or as necessary.
   2. After bandage removal, perform passive flexion and extension of the stifle.
   3. Allow leash walking only for 8 weeks.

VI. Prognosis

A. Inform owners the prognosis is good for return to nonathletic performance. However, loss of flexion tighter than 110 degrees and mild to moderate instability are common after surgery, limiting athletic performance.

Meniscal Injury (*SAS*, pp. 974-976)

I. General Considerations

A. Recognize that menisci function in load transmission and energy absorption, help provide rotational and varus-valgus stability, lubricate the joint, and render joint surfaces congruent.

B. Isolated meniscal injuries are uncommon in dogs. Most tears occur in conjunction with cranial cruciate ligament ruptures.
   1. Tears most often involve the caudal body of the medial meniscus with a "bucket-handle" tear, a transverse tear in the caudal body of the medial meniscus that extends from medial to lateral.
   2. Peripheral meniscal tears are the second most frequent type of meniscal injury.

II. Diagnosis

A. Clinical Presentation

1. Signalment.
   a. Any breed or age dog may be affected.
   b. Meniscal injury is rare in cats.

2. History.
   a. Instability of the stifle is typical because of cranial cruciate ligament rupture.

B. Physical Examination

1. Examine for a popping sound when checking for cranial drawer motion. The sound is caused by movement of the "free" section of the bucket-handle tear.
2. Do not expect all patients with meniscal tears to have an audible or palpable click.

C. Radiography

1. Take standard craniocaudal and medial-to-lateral radiographs to evaluate the stifle; however, radiographic findings do not correlate with meniscal injury.

D. Laboratory Findings

1. Arthrocentesis may show cell counts that are slightly higher than those in patients with ligament tears alone.

III. Medical or Conservative Management

A. Do not perform conservative treatment because a torn meniscus accelerates degenerative joint disease.

IV. Surgical Treatment

A. Partial meniscectomy involves removal of the torn section of the meniscus, and experimentally carries less morbidity than does a total meniscectomy.

B. Primary repair is advocated by some human orthopedic surgeons, but is reserved for peripheral tears of the meniscocapsular ligaments in dogs. Meticulous repair with absorbable sutures will allow meniscocapsular tissue to heal.

C. Consider a total meniscectomy only when the peripheral rim of the meniscus is damaged to where primary suturing of the meniscocapsular tissue is not possible.

D. Preoperative management.
   1. Limit activity to prevent further damage to the meniscus and articular surfaces.

E. Positioning.
   1. Position the animal in lateral recumbency.
   2. Perform a hanging-leg preparation.

F. Surgical techniques.
   1. Partial meniscectomy.

Facilitate exposure with suction and by levering the tibial plateau down and forward. Lever the tibia forward by placing the tip of a small Hohmann retractor behind the caudal edge of the tibial plateau and forcing the body of the retractor against the nonarticular portion of the trochlear groove. Once the

damaged section of meniscus is visualized, remove it with a No. 11 scalpel blade. Incise the most medial attachment of the bucket handle first, then incise the most lateral attachment. After removal of the torn section of meniscus, inspect the remaining meniscus for additional tears.

V. Postoperative Care and Assessment

A. Follow recommendations for reconstruction of the cranial cruciate ligament.

VI. Prognosis

A. Partial meniscectomy or primary repair lessens the degree of degenerative joint disease and makes the prognosis for return to normal function more favorable.

Medial Patellar Luxation (*SAS*, pp. 976-983)

I. General Considerations

A. The majority of patients with patellar luxation have associated musculoskeletal abnormalities: medial displacement of the quadriceps muscle group, lateral torsion of the distal femur, a lateral bowing of the distal one third of the femur, femoral epiphyseal dysplasia, rotational instability of the stifle joint, or tibial deformity.

B. Recognize that torsional and angular deformities associated with patella luxations are secondary to abnormal pressures exerted on the growth plates by displacement of the quadriceps muscle group.
1. The torsional force with medial luxation is in a lateral direction, resulting in a lateral torsion of the distal femur.
2. The medial malalignment of the quadriceps muscles in dogs with medial patella luxation produces increased pressure on the medial aspect of the growth plate retarding growth, and decreased pressure on the lateral aspect of the growth plate, allowing accelerated growth. This results in bowing of the distal femur.
3. Abnormal growth continues as long as the quadriceps is displaced medially and the growth plates are active. Therefore the degree of lateral bowing depends on the severity of patellar luxation and the patient's age at the onset of luxation.
4. There are generally tibial deformities from abnormal forces acting on the proximal and distal growth plates, including medial displacement of the tibial tuberosity, medial bowing (varus deformity) of the proximal tibia, and lateral torsion of the distal tibia.
5. The trochlear groove may develop abnormally because it is the continued pressure of the patella that is responsible for the normal depth of the groove. The amount of abnormality varies from near

normal to an absent trochlear groove. Immature patients with severe luxations may have an absent trochlear groove.

6. Because the degree of skeletal pathology associated with patella luxation varies considerably, refer to the established grading system (Table 30-3).

II. Diagnosis

A. Clinical Presentation

1. Signalment.
   a. Any breed or age dog may be affected, but small- and toy-breed dogs are more frequently affected.
2. History.
   a. There is typically a history of intermittent weight-bearing lameness. The dog may occasionally hold the leg in a flexed position for one or two steps.

B. Physical Examination

1. Patients with grade I luxations generally exhibit no lameness.
2. Patients with grade II luxations exhibit occasional "skipping" when walking or running.
3. Patients with a grade III patella luxation exhibit varying signs from an occasional skip to a weight-bearing lameness.
4. Patients with grade IV luxations walk with the rear quarters in a crouched position because of inability to extend the stifle joints fully.

C. Radiography

1. With grade III or grade IV luxations locate the patella displaced medially on standard craniocaudal and medial-to-lateral. With grade I

Table 30-3
Grades of patella luxation

Grade I

The patella can be luxated, but spontaneous luxation of the patella during normal joint motion rarely occurs. Manual luxation of the patella may be accomplished during physical examination, but the patella reduces when pressure is released. Flexion and extension of the joint are normal.

Grade II

Angular and torsional deformities of the femur may be present to a mild degree. The patella may be manually displaced with lateral pressure or may luxate with flexion of the stifle joint. The patella remains luxated until it is reduced by the examiner or is spontaneously reduced when the animal extends and derotates its tibia.

Grade III

The patella remains luxated medially most of the time, but may be manually reduced with the stifle in extension. However, after manual reduction, flexion and extension of the stifle result in reluxation of the patella. There is a medial displacement of the quadriceps muscle group. Abnormalities of the supporting soft tissues of the stifle joint and deformities of the femur and tibia may be present.

Grade IV

There may be an 80- to 90-degree medial rotation of the proximal tibial plateau. The patella is permanently luxated and cannot be manually repositioned. The femoral trochlear groove is shallow or absent, and there is medial displacement of the quadriceps muscle group. Abnormalities of the supporting soft tissues of the stifle joint and deformities of the femur and tibia are marked.

or II luxations the patella may be within the trochlear sulcus or may be displaced medially.

III. Medical or Conservative Management

A. Select between conservative and surgical treatment based on clinical history, physical findings, and patient's age. Surgery is seldom warranted in asymptomatic older patients.

IV. Surgical Treatment

A. Recommend surgery in symptomatic and asymptomatic immature or young adult patients because intermittent patellar luxation may prematurely wear the articular cartilage of the patella. Surgery is indicated at any age in patients exhibiting lameness, and is strongly advised in those with active growth plates because skeletal deformity may worsen rapidly.

B. In growing animals, use surgical techniques that will not adversely affect skeletal growth.

C. In general, use a combination of surgical techniques to restrain the patella within the trochlear groove. Techniques include, tibial tuberosity transposition, medial restraint release, lateral restraint reinforcement, trochlear groove deepening, femoral osteotomy, and tibial osteotomy. First identify the abnormalities associated with a given stifle then select which technique(s) to use.

1. Tibial crest transposition is an effective method of treatment for grades II, III, and IV patella luxations.
2. Reinforce the lateral retinaculum with suture placement and imbrication of the fibrous joint capsule, placement of a fascia lata graft from the fabella to the parapatellar fibrocartilage, or excision of redundant retinaculum. Do not use reinforcement techniques alone because they will not permanently prevent reluxation.
3. Deepen the trochlear groove if the medial and lateral trochlear ridges do not constrain the patella. Perform a trochlear wedge recession or a trochlear resection. A trochlear wedge recession is technically more demanding but preserves the articular cartilage.
4. Only perform an osteotomy of the femur in patients with severe skeletal deformity that make it impossible to maintain patellar reduction with other techniques. Deformities are usually varus bowing of the distal femur and medial torsional deformity of the proximal tibia. The goal of surgery is to realign the stifle joint in the frontal plane where the transverse axis of the femoral condyles is perpendicular to the longitudinal axis of the femoral diaphysis. This procedure should be performed by a specialist and should be combined with other procedures.

D. Positioning.

1. Position the animal in lateral or dorsal recumbency.
2. Perform a hanging-leg preparation.

E. Surgical techniques.

1. Tibial tuberosity transposition.

Make a craniolateral skin incision 4 cm proximal to the patella and extend the incision 2 cm below the tibial tuberosity. Incise subcutaneous tissues along the same line. Make a lateral parapatellar incision through the fascia lata and carry the incision distally onto the tibial tuberosity below the joint line. Reflect the cranialis tibialis muscle from the lateral tibial tuberosity and tibial plateau to the level of the long digital extensor tendon. Use sharp dissection to gain access to the deep surface of the patellar tendon for placement of an osteotome. Beginning at the level of the patella, make a medial parapatellar incision through the fascia and distally through the periosteum of the tibial tuberosity. Position an osteotome beneath the patellar tendon 3 to 5 cm caudal to the cranial point of the tibial tuberosity. Use a mallet to complete the osteotomy in a proximal to distal direction. Do not transect the distal periosteal attachment. Base the degree of lateral movement of the tibial tuberosity on the longitudinal realignment of the tuberosity relative to the trochlear groove. Once the site of relocation is chosen, remove a thin layer of cortical bone with a rasp or osteotome. Lever the tibial tuberosity into position and stabilize it with one or two small Kirschner wires directed caudally and slightly proximally. Engage the caudal cortex, but do not exit the pin from the tibia caudally; if the pin protrudes too far from the caudal cortex of the tibia, persistent lameness will result. Suture the arthrotomy with absorbable suture material using a simple interrupted pattern. Appose subcutaneous tissues with a continuous pattern using absorbable suture and then suture the skin with nonabsorbable suture material.

2. Lateral reinforcement.

For suture reinforcement, place a polyester suture through the femoral-fabellar ligament and lateral parapatellar fibrocartilage. Next, place a series of imbrication sutures through the fibrous joint capsule and lateral edge of the patella tendon. With the leg in slight flexion, tie the femoral-fabellar suture and imbrication sutures. To transpose the fascia lata, isolate a section of fascial lata equal in width to the patella and twice the length of the distance from the patella to the fabella. Free the graft proximally and leave it attached to the proximal pole of the patella distally. Pass the free end of the graft deep to the femoral-fabellar ligament and back to the lateral parapatellar fibrocartilage. Suture the graft to itself and the femoral-fabellar ligament with the leg in slight flexion. If the patella is out of position most of the time, the retinaculum opposite the side of the luxation will be stretched; with medial luxations, there is redundant lateral retinaculum. Once the patella is reduced, excise the excess retinaculum and joint capsule allowing tight closure of the arthrotomy.

3. Release of the medial joint capsule.

Expect patients with grade III or grade IV patella luxations to have a thicker than normal and contracted joint capsule. Release the medial joint capsule and retinaculum to allow lateral placement of the patella. Using a scalpel, make a medial parapatellar incision through the medial fascia and joint capsule. Begin the incision at the level of the proximal pole of the patella and extend it distally to the tibial crest. Allow the incision to separate and do not suture the cut edges when surgery is completed. Rather, suture medial subcutaneous tissue to the cranial cut edge of the incision. If dynamic contraction of the cranial sartorius muscle and vastus medialis muscle directs the patella medially, release the insertions of these muscles at the proximal patella. Redirect the insertions and suture them to the vastus intermedius muscle.

4. Deepening of the trochlear groove.
   a. With medial luxations, take more bone from the lateral side of the

groove in order to preserve as much of the medial ridge as possible.

b. Trochlear wedge recession.
   i. In larger patients, use an oscillating saw if available, but in smaller breeds and toy breeds a fine-toothed hand-held saw (No. 12 X-acto saw, available at most hobby shops), or a No. 20 scalpel blade and mallet work just as well to make the cuts in the trochlea.

Cut into the articular cartilage of the trochlea, making a diamond-shaped outline. Be sure that the width of the cut is sufficient at its midpoint to accommodate the width of the patella. Remove an osteochondral wedge of bone and cartilage by following the outline previously made. Make the osteotomy so that the two oblique planes that form the free wedge intersect distally at the intercondylar notch and proximally at the dorsal edge of the trochlear articular cartilage. Remove the osteochondral wedge and deepen the recession in the trochlea by removing additional bone from one or both sides of the newly created femoral groove. The wedge remains in place because of friction and compressive force of the patella. If necessary, remodel the free osteochondral wedge with rongeurs to allow the wedge to seat deeply into the new femoral groove. Rotate the wedge 180 degrees if doing so will aid in heightening the medial ridge when it is returned to the femoral groove. Replace the free osteochondral wedge when the depth is sufficient to house 50% of the height of the patella. Close the arthrotomy as described for lateral approach to the stifle joint under Cranial Cruciate Ligament Rupture.

c. Trochlear resection.
   i. The advantage of this technique is its simplicity.
   ii. The disadvantage is that it removes the articular cartilage of the trochlea and allows articulation of the patella on the rough cancellous surface, which results in wearing of patellar articular cartilage. Nevertheless, the trochlear groove eventually fills with a combination of fibrous tissue and fibrocartilage and the patients appear to have acceptable limb function.

Measure the width of the articular surface of the patella and use this measurement to determine the proper width of the trochlear resection. Remove articular cartilage and bone with a bone rasp, power burr, or rongeurs. Make the length of the trochlear resection extend to the proximal margin of articular cartilage and distally to the cartilage margin just above the intercondylar notch. The depth of the groove should be such to accommodate 50% of the height of the patella and allow the parapatellar fibrocartilage to articulate with the newly formed medial and lateral trochlear ridges. Make the medial and lateral trochlear ridges parallel to each other and the base of the groove perpendicular to each trochlear ridge.

V. Postoperative Care and Assessment

A. Apply a padded bandage for 3 days.

B. Allow leash walking only for 6 weeks.

VI. Prognosis

A. Expect the overall prognosis for patients undergoing surgical correction of a patella luxation to be excellent for return to normal limb function, despite mild or occasional reluxation in about half of the cases.

Lateral Patellar Luxation (*SAS*, pp. 983-985)

I. Definitions

A. **Anteversion** is excessive external rotation of the proximal femur relative to the distal femur.

B. **Coxa valga** is an abnormal increase in the angle formed by the femoral neck and shaft in the frontal plane.

II. General Considerations

A. Lateral patellar luxation generally occurs in large-breed dogs, less often in small and toy breed dogs.

B. Medial patella luxations are more common than lateral luxations in dogs of all sizes.

C. The cause is unknown, but it is thought to be related to anteversion or coxa valga of the coxofemoral joint.

D. Abnormal force placed on the growth plates of immature patients causes skeletal abnormalities that are mirror images of those seen with medial patella luxation.

III. Diagnosis

A. Clinical Presentation

1. Signalment.
   a. Any breed or age dog may be affected, but large-breed dogs are more frequently affected.
2. History.
   a. There is typically a history of intermittent, weight-bearing lameness.
   b. The dog may occasionally hold the leg in a flexed position for one or two steps.

B. Physical Examination

1. Patients with grade I luxations generally exhibit no lameness.
2. Patients with grade II luxations exhibit occasional "skipping" when walking or running.
3. Patients with a grade III patella luxation exhibit varying signs from an occasional skip to a weight-bearing lameness.
4. Patients with grade IV luxations walk with the rear quarters in a crouched position because of inability to extend the stifle joints fully.

C. Radiography

1. With grade III or grade IV luxations locate the patella displaced laterally on standard craniocaudal and medial-to-lateral radiographs.
2. With grade I or II luxations the patella may be within the trochlear sulcus or may be displaced laterally.

IV. Medical or Conservative Management

A. Select between conservative and surgical treatment based on clinical history, physical findings, and patient's age. Surgery is seldom warranted in asymptomatic older patients.

V. Surgical Treatment

A. Refer to Medial Patella Luxation for goals and treatment methods.

1. Perform the osteotomy of the tibial tuberosity in the same manner as with medial patellar luxation, except reposition and stabilize the tuberosity medially.
2. Reinforce the medial retinaculum, instead of the lateral, with suture reconstruction, fascia lata transposition, and/or excision of redundant joint capsule.
3. Release lateral restraints to help neutralize lateral forces acting on the patella.
4. Deepen the trochlear groove by the same methods described for medial patella luxation.
5. For severe angular and/or torsional deformities, have a specialist with the proper training and equipment perform osteotomies of the femur and tibia.

B. Positioning.

1. Position the animal in lateral or dorsal recumbency.
2. Perform a hanging-leg preparation.

C. Surgical Techniques

1. Use the techniques described in Medial Patella Luxation.

VI. Postoperative Care and Assessment

A. Apply a padded bandage for 3 days.

B. Allow leash walking only for 6 weeks.

VII. Prognosis

A. The prognosis is less optimal in large dogs with lateral patellar luxations than in smaller dogs with medial patella luxations; however, the prognosis is good for a return to functional activity.

Osteochondritis Dissecans of the Stifle (*SAS*, pp. 985-986)

I. Definition

A. Osteochondritis Dissecans (OCD) is a manifestation of a general syndrome called **osteochondrosis** in which a flap of cartilage forms because of a disturbance in endochondral ossification.

II. General Considerations

A. OCD occurs more commonly in the shoulder, elbow, and hock.

B. The medial surface of the lateral femoral condyle is most frequently affected.

III. Diagnosis

A. Clinical Presentation

1. Signalment.
   a. Large dogs (Labrador retrievers, golden retrievers) are typically affected.
   b. The onset of lameness is generally at 5 to 7 months.
2. History.
   a. There is typically a history of an acute or chronic rear limb lameness, which worsens after exercise.
   b. There may be stiffness in the morning or after rest.

B. Physical Examination

1. There is generally lameness in one rear limb, and potentially joint effusion and crepitation, especially if degenerative joint disease (DJD) is progressing.

C. Radiography

1. Take radiographs of both stifles including the standard lateral view.
2. Diagnose OCD based on a radiolucent concavity on the medial or lateral femoral condyle. More subtle radiographic signs include flattening of the articular surface and subchondral sclerosis.
3. Expect to visualize signs of secondary DJD.

D. Laboratory Findings

1. Arthrocentesis may reveal decreased synovial fluid viscosity, increased fluid volume, and increased numbers (up to 5000 WBC/ml) of mononuclear phagocytic cells.

IV. Medical Management

A. Use medical management for older dogs with established DJD.

B. Confine the animal until after the lameness has subsided, then gradually increase the amount of exercise. Prescribe NSAIDs (see Appendix I) and recommend weight control.

V. Surgical Treatment

A. General Considerations

1. Consider surgery in young animals before the onset of DJD and in lame animals that are unresponsive to medical therapy. Surgery usually does not alter the progression of DJD.
2. Remove the cartilage flap to allow the defect to heal by outgrowth of fibrocartilage from underlying subchondral bone.

B. Positioning

1. Position the animal in dorsal recumbency.
2. Perform hanging-leg preparation.

C. Surgical Techniques

1. Select the surgical approach depending on the preference of the surgeon as discussed in Cranial Cruciate Ligament Rupture (either lateral parapatellar approach or medial parapatellar approach).
2. Examine the appropriate femoral condyle and remove the flap of cartilage. Curette only to remove fragments of cartilage from the edges of the lesion. Flush the joint before closure.

VI. Postoperative Care and Assessment

A. Apply a bandage for 3 to 5 days.

B. Allow leash walking only for 4 to 6 weeks, then gradually return to normal activity.

VII. Prognosis

A. Expect dogs treated conservatively to have continued intermittent lameness and progressive DJD. Those treated surgically may have improved limb function, but DJD still progresses. Lameness may be evident after exercise and require occasional medical treatment.

Tarsus

Ligamentous Injury of the Tarsus (*SAS*, pp. 986-993)

I. General Considerations

A. Ligamentous injuries generally result from severe trauma such as vehicular accidents.

B. Shearing injuries usually involve the tarsocrural joint and are associated with severe abrasion of the soft tissues and malleoli.

C. With subluxation, examine for injury of the medial or lateral collateral ligament complex or fracture of the medial or lateral malleolus.

D. With luxation, examine for injury of both the medial and the lateral collateral ligament complexes, fracture of both malleoli, or fracture of one malleolus with injury to the contralateral collateral ligament complex.

E. Recognize that a number of intertarsal injuries can result from disruption of various ligament complexes between tarsal bones. Proximal intertarsal subluxation, proximal intertarsal luxation, and tarsometatarsal luxation are the most common.

F. Always place the joint in extension to evaluate medial or lateral restraint injury.

II. Diagnosis

A. Clinical Presentation

1. Signalment.
   a. Any breed or age dog or cat may be affected.
2. History.
   a. There is typically a non–weight-bearing lameness.
   b. There may be an open wound over the tarsus.

B. Physical Examination

1. With complete tarsocrural joint luxation, there is generally a non–weight-bearing lameness, and the paw deviates at an unnatural angle. Pain, swelling, and crepitus is typically present.
2. With complete subluxations, the animal is generally unable to bear weight and the paw deviates to the direction opposite the ligamentous damage.
3. When partial tears of the collateral complex are suspected, apply varus and valgus forces to the joint while it is extended and flexed. Laxity in extension denotes injury to the long components of the collateral ligament complex, whereas laxity in flexion only denotes injury to the short component.
4. With shearing injuries, there is generally soft-tissue abrasion and bone loss.
5. With intertarsal luxations and tarsometatarsal subluxation, the animal is usually in pain and unable to bear weight on the affected limb. There will generally be an abnormal rotation and deviation of the foot.

C. Radiography

1. Take standard craniocaudal and medial-to-lateral radiographs.
2. Take standing lateral and varus-valgus stress films if instability is suspected but not confirmed.

III. Medical Management

A. Perform surgery to restore functional integrity of the joint.

IV. Surgical Treatment

A. General Considerations

1. Perform a thorough neurologic and vascular evaluation on each patient to determine the feasibility of treatment.
2. With tarsocrural luxation or subluxation, treat to reestablish joint stability to achieve pain-free weight bearing. Reconstruct the short and long collateral ligament components for optimal results. With severe ligamentous injuries or severe bone and cartilage damage consider partial or complete fusion of the tarsus or limb.

B. Proximal Intertarsal Subluxation with Plantar Instability

1. Occurs when excessive dorsal flexion and causes disruption of the plantar ligament complex between the calcaneus and fourth tarsal bones. Treat by selective fusion of the joint surfaces between the calcaneus and fourth tarsal bones.

C. Proximal Intertarsal Subluxation

1. Results from hyperextension-caused damage to the dorsal ligaments and dorsal joint capsule between the talus and central tarsal bone. Treat with rigid coaptation. If not successful, perform selective fusion of the talocentral joint.

D. Proximal Intertarsal Luxation

1. Occurs when excessive dorsal flexion causes disruption of the plantar ligament complex, both between the calcaneus and fourth tarsal bones and between the talus and the central tarsal bone. Treat by selective fusion of the proximal intertarsal joint.

E. Tarsometatarsal Luxation

1. Occurs when excessive dorsal flexion causes disruption of the plantar ligaments and fibrocartilage. The luxation occurs between the distal row of tarsal bones and metatarsal bones. Treat with selective fusion of the distal intertarsal joint (tarsometatarsal joint).
2. Occasionally, the luxation occurs laterally between the fourth tarsal bone and adjacent metatarsal bones, with the medial separation occurring between the second and third tarsal bones and the central tarsal bone. Treat with selective fusion of the joint space between the fourth tarsal and adjacent metatarsal bones using a bone plate secured to the fourth tarsal bone and fifth metatarsal bone. Medially, secure a small bone plate to the central tarsal bone proximally and the second tarsal and second metatarsal bones distally.

F. Preoperative Management

1. Bandage to support the limb and confine the animal to prevent further joint damage.

G. Positioning

1. Clip the hair from the coxofemoral joint to the digits so that the paw can be included in the sterile field.
2. Perform a hanging-leg preparation.

H. Surgical Techniques

1. Tarsocrural luxation or subluxation.

Depending on which side is injured, make a curved incision centered over the medial or lateral malleolus. Begin the incision 4 cm above the joint line and continue distally to a point 4 cm below the tarsometatarsal joint line. Incise

subcutaneous tissues and deep fascia along the same line to expose remnants of the collateral ligament complex, joint capsule, and the articular surface. Reduce and align the joint surfaces. Suture the joint capsule and injured ligaments with small-sized, nonabsorbable suture. Protect the repair with nonabsorbable, heavy (No. 2 to No. 5, depending on the animal's size) figure-8 sutures strategically placed to mimic the short and long components of the collateral ligament complex. Drill bone tunnels in the malleolus where the ligament complex originates. Next, drill tunnels where the short and long components of the collateral ligament complex insert. Place two strands of nonabsorbable polyester suture through the predrilled holes in the malleolus. Pass one end of the suture strand through the tunnel drilled to mimic the insertion of the short component and pass the end of the other strand through the tunnel drilled to mimic the insertion of the long component of the collateral ligament complex. Place the sutures in a figure-8 pattern and tie them such that the suture placed as the short component is tied with the joint in 90 degrees of flexion. Tie the suture placed to simulate the long component with the joint in a normal standing angle.

2. Shearing injuries.

When the animal is first seen, cover the wound with a sterile dressing and temporarily immobilize the limb with an external splint. Once the animal is stable enough to be anesthetized, debride the wound. Liberally flush the wound with 0.05% chlorhexidene. Fill the wound with sterile KY jelly and clip the surrounding area. Transfer the patient to the operating room and debride obvious necrotic tissue and remove foreign material. If the medial surface is abraded, perform ligament reconstruction by inserting bone screws in the malleolus and talus to mimic the origin and insertion of the medial collateral ligament complex. If the lateral surface is abraded, place bone screws in the malleolus and calcaneus to mimic the origin and insertion of the lateral collateral ligament complex. Place figure-8, heavy, nonabsorbable sutures between the screws. Tie the suture used to mimic the short component of the ligament complex with the joint at 90 degrees, and tie the suture used to mimic the long component of the ligament complex with the tarsus in a normal standing angle. If malleolar fracture is present, rather than ligament injury, reduce and stabilize the fracture with a tension-band technique. Immobilize the reconstruction for 2 to 4 weeks with a transarticular external skeletal fixator. Place one full pin 6 to 7 cm proximal to the malleolus and one full pin through the metatarsal bones, just below the tarsometatarsal joint line. Contour medial and lateral external bars to an angle simulating the standing angle of the tarsal joint. Place a half pin 2 to 3 cm above the malleolus and a second half pin through the central and fourth tarsal bones. Tighten the pin clamps. After placement of the medial and lateral bars, place an additional external bar if further resistance to craniocaudal bending is desired.

3. Proximal intertarsal subluxation with plantar instability.

Expose the joint through a caudolateral incision. Remove articular cartilage from the articular surface of the calcaneus and fourth tarsal bones with a curette or pneumatic burr. Place a Steinmann pin from the proximal calcaneus down the calcaneal shaft to the point where the tip of the pin can be seen exiting where the cartilage was removed. Harvest a cancellous bone graft and pack it into the space between the calcaneus and fourth tarsal bone. Reduce the joint and drive the pin across it to seat in the body of the fourth tarsal bone. Drill a transverse hole across the distal quadrant of the fourth tarsal bone and drill a second transverse hole in the proximal quadrant of the calcaneus. Place orthopedic wire through the drill holes in a figure-8 pattern to complete a tension-band wire. Use 20-gauge orthopedic wire for small and medium-sized dogs and cats and 18-gauge for large dogs.

4. Proximal intertarsal luxation.

Make a lateral incision beginning at the proximal end of the calcaneus and extending distally 3 to 4 cm below the tarsometatarsal joint line. Remove articular cartilage from the joint surfaces and insert a cancellous bone graft. Apply a compression plate to the lateral surface of the calcaneus, fourth tarsal bone, and fifth metatarsal bone.

5. Tarsometatarsal luxation.

Expose the articular surfaces of the joint through a cranial incision. Reflect extensor tendons laterally to gain adequate exposure. Remove articular cartilage and insert a cancellous bone graft. Reduce the joint and stabilize with cross pins. Place one pin so that it enters the base of the fifth metatarsal bone, crosses the joint, and is seated in the central tarsal bone. Place the second pin so that it enters the base of the second metatarsal bone, crosses the joint, and is seated in the fourth tarsal bone. If the luxation occurs laterally, between the fourth tarsal bone and adjacent metatarsal bones, with the medial separation occurring between the second and third tarsal bones and central tarsal bone, expose the tarsometatarsal joint with two incisions. Make a lateral incision extending 5 cm proximal and distal to the tarsometatarsal joint line. Make a similar incision medially. Remove articular cartilage from all exposed joint surfaces and insert a cancellous bone graft. Stabilize the fusion with small bone plates. Laterally secure a plate to the fourth tarsal and fifth metatarsal bones. Medially, secure a small bone plate to the central tarsal bone proximally and to the second tarsal and second metatarsal bone distally.

6. Tarsocrural joint arthrodesis.
   a. Perform when there is severe injury of the tibial cochlea and condyles of the talus. Use in conjunction with tarsocrural, proximal intertarsal, and distal tarsometatarsal joint fusion.

Determine the normal standing angle of the opposite limb before surgery and use it to approximate the fusion angle during arthrodesis of the injured limb. Make an incision over the cranial surface of the joint. Begin the incision over the distal one third of the tibia and extend it distally midway down the metatarsal bones. Enter the tarsocrural joint to expose the articular surfaces. With a power saw remove the articular surface of the distal tibia by cutting perpendicular to the long axis of the bone. Cut the trochlea of the talus to achieve the appropriate fusion angle when the cut surfaces rest flush with each other. Use the normal standing angle of the opposite limb to approximate the fusion angle. Maintain reduction of the cut surfaces with small Kirschner pins and pack a cancellous bone graft around the joint. Open the joint capsule of the proximal intertarsal and tarsometatarsal joints to expose the articular surfaces. Remove the cartilage with a pneumatic burr and insert a cancellous bone graft. Stabilize the joints with a bone plate applied to the cranial surface. Bend the plate to conform to the established fusion angle and secure it proximally by placing three screws in the distal tibia, two to four screws in the tarsal bones, and three screws in the third metatarsal bone. Alternatively, if a lengthening plate is used to bridge the tarsus, attach the plate to the distal tibia and metatarsus with three or four screws in each bone.

V. Postoperative Care and Assessment

A. After repair of tarsocrural luxations or subluxations, immobilize the tarsus in a normal standing angle with rigid external coaptation or a transarticular external skeletal fixator for 3 weeks. Allow leash walking only and check coaptation frequently. After splint removal, perform passive flexion and extension of the joint and slowly increase activity over 6 weeks.

B. Treat shearing injury as an open wound with daily changes of a sterile adherent dressing and liberal flushing with 0.05% chlorhexidene. Apply a nonadherent sterile dressing once healthy granulation tissue is formed.

C. After arthrodesis, protect the repair with external coaptation or an external skeletal fixator for 4 to 6 weeks, and restrict activity until there is radiographic evidence of bone union.

VI. Prognosis

A. Inform owners that adequate limb function can be expected in most patients with tarsal injuries after appropriate surgical intervention; however, the prognosis depends on the severity of ligamentous injury, cartilage damage, and the joint involved.

Osteochondritis Dissecans of the Tarsus (*SAS,* pp. 993-998)

I. General Considerations

A. OCD also occurs in the shoulder, elbow, and stifle.

B. For pathogenesis of OCD see OCD of the Distal Humerus.

C. Usually involves the medial trochlear ridge.

II. Diagnosis

A. Clinical Presentation

1. Signalment.
   a. Large dogs (Labrador retrievers, golden retrievers) are typically affected.
   b. The onset of lameness is generally at 5 to 7 months.
2. History.
   a. There is typically a history of an acute or chronic rear limb lameness, which worsens after exercise. There may be stiffness in the morning or after rest.

B. Physical Examination

1. There is generally lameness of one rear limb.
2. Observe for hyperextension of the hocks and a stiff or stilted gait because of bilateral lameness. Palpate and flex the hock to detect decreased range of motion secondary to DJD, and to assess for pain and crepitation on flexion.

C. Radiography

1. Take multiple radiographic views including a standard lateral of the hock, flexed lateral to expose the proximal portion of the talus, a cranial-caudal view of the hock (made while the hock is extended, to visualize the proximal portion of the trochlear ridges), and a cranial-caudal view (made with the hock flexed, to visualize the cranial portion of the trochlear ridges and to visualize the lateral condylar ridge without superimposition of the calcaneus). Radiograph both hocks because bilateral disease is common.
2. Diagnose OCD based on a radiolucent concavity on the medial or lateral trochlear ridge.
3. Expect to visualize signs of secondary DJD.

D. Laboratory Findings

1. Arthrocentesis may reveal decreased synovial fluid viscosity, increased fluid volume, and increased numbers (up to 5000 WBC/ml) of mononuclear phagocytic cells.

III. Medical Management

A. Medically manage older dogs with established DJD.

B. Confine the animal until after the lameness has subsided, then gradually increase the amount of exercise. Prescribe NSAIDs (see Appendix I) and recommend weight control.

IV. Surgical Treatment

A. General Considerations

1. Consider surgery in young animals before the onset of DJD, and in lame animals that are unresponsive to medical therapy. Surgery usually does not alter the progression of DJD.
2. Remove the cartilage flap to allow the defect to heal by outgrowth of fibrocartilage from underlying subchondral bone.
3. Use approaches to the lateral and medial trochlear ridge that do not involve osteotomy of the epicondyle or collateral ligament transection for less postoperative morbidity and faster return to function.

B. Positioning

1. Position the animal in dorsal recumbency.
2. Perform a hanging-leg preparation.

C. Surgical Techniques

1. General considerations.
   a. For lesions of the medial trochlear ridge use a dorsomedial and/or plantaromedial surgical approach.
   b. For lesions of the lateral trochlear ridge use a dorsolateral and/or plantarolateral surgical approach.
   c. Examine the appropriate trochlear ridge and remove the flap of cartilage. Curette only to remove fragments of cartilage from the edges of the lesion. Flush the joint before closure.
2. Dorsomedial approach to the tarsus.

Extend the hock and palpate the dorsal portion of the medial trochlear ridge. Make a skin incision starting proximal to the trochlear ridge and extending

distally over the trochlear ridge. Incise subcutaneous tissues along the same line. Identify the tendon of the tibialis cranialis muscle, saphenous nerve, cranial tibial artery and vein, and dorsal branches of the saphenous artery and vein and retract them laterally. Incise the deep fascia and joint capsule along the midline of the palpable portion of the medial trochlear ridge. Extend the incision proximally into the periosteum of the distal tibia. Visualize the cranial and distal part of the medial trochlear ridge. Extend the hock to increase the amount of visible trochlear ridge. Identify and remove the cartilage flap. Curette the edges of the lesion and flush the joint. Close the wound by suturing fascia and joint capsule with simple interrupted absorbable sutures. Suture subcutaneous tissues and skin in separate layers.

3. Plantaromedial approach to the tarsus.

Flex the hock and palpate the proximal or plantar aspect of the medial trochlear ridge. Incise skin and subcutaneous tissues caudal to the medial malleolus over the trochlear ridge. Identify the tendon of the long digital flexor muscle and the distal attachment of the caudal tibial tendon and retract them cranially. Identify the tendon of the flexor hallucis longus muscle, tibial nerve, plantar branches of the medial saphenous vein and saphenous artery, and superficial plantar metatarsal vein and retract them laterally. Incise the deep fascia and joint capsule longitudinally along the midline of the palpable portion of the medial trochlear ridge. Identify and remove the cartilage flap. Flex the hock to increase the amount of medial trochlear ridge visible. Curette the edges of the lesion and flush the joint. Close the wound by suturing fascia and joint capsule with simple interrupted absorbable sutures. Suture subcutaneous tissues and skin in separate layers.

4. Dorsolateral approach to the tarsus.

Extend the hock and palpate the cranial portion of the lateral trochlear ridge. Make a skin incision starting proximal to the trochlear ridge and extending distally over the trochlear ridge. Incise subcutaneous tissues along the same line. Identify the tendons of the long digital extensor muscle, cranial tibial muscle, and extensor hallucis longus muscle, the dorsal branch of the lateral saphenous vein, and the superficial peroneal nerve and retract them medially. Identify the tendons of the peroneus longus, lateral digital extensor, and peroneus brevis muscles and retract them in a plantar direction. Incise the deep fascia and joint capsule longitudinally along the midline of the palpable portion of the lateral trochlear ridge. Visualize the cranial and distal part of the lateral trochlear ridge. Extend the hock to increase the amount of visible trochlear ridge. Identify and remove the cartilage flap. Curette the edges of the lesion and flush the joint. Close the wound by suturing fascia and joint capsule with simple interrupted absorbable sutures. Suture subcutaneous tissues and skin in separate layers.

5. Plantarolateral approach to the tarsus.

Flex the hock and palpate the proximal or plantar aspect of the lateral trochlear ridge. Incise skin and subcutaneous tissues plantar to the lateral malleolus over the trochlear ridge. Retract the tendons of the peroneus brevis muscle, lateral digital extensor muscle, and peroneus longus muscle dorsally. Expect difficulty retracting the tendons of the peroneus brevis, lateral digital extensor, and peroneus longus muscles very far because they are firmly embedded in deep fascia over the lateral malleolus. Retract the plantar branch of the lateral saphenous vein and a branch of the caudal cutaneous sural nerve in a plantar direction, and the tendon of the flexor hallucis longus in a medial direction. Incise the deep fascia and joint capsule longitudinally along the

midline of the palpable portion of the lateral trochlear ridge. Identify and remove the cartilage flap. Flex the hock to increase the amount of lateral trochlear ridge visible. Curette the edges of the lesion and flush the joint. Close the wound by suturing fascia and joint capsule with simple interrupted absorbable sutures. Suture subcutaneous tissues and skin in separate layers.

V. Postoperative Care and Assessment

A. Apply a bandage for 3 to 5 days.

B. Allow only leash walking for 4 to 6 weeks, then gradually return to normal activity.

VI. Prognosis

A. Expect dogs treated conservatively to have continued intermittent lameness and progressive DJD. Those treated surgically may have improved limb function, but DJD still progresses and lameness may be evident after exercise and require occasional medical treatment.

31

Management of Muscle and Tendon Injury or Disease (*SAS*, pp. 999-1008)

Muscle Contusions and Strains (*SAS*, pp. 999–1001)

I. Definitions

A. A **contusion** is a bruise of the muscle with hemorrhage and fiber disruption caused by external trauma.

B. A **strain** is a longitudinal stretching or tearing of muscle fibers caused by overstretching.

II. General Considerations

A. With mild damage, muscle will regenerate and heal completely.

B. With severe damage, expect healing with fibrous interposition between the muscle ends.

III. Diagnosis

A. Clinical Presentation

1. Signalment.
   a. Any dog or cat may be affected, but it usually occurs in athletic dogs.
   b. Rare in cats.
2. History.
   a. Typically there is a history of strenuous activity.

B. Physical Examination

1. Signs depend on the severity and chronicity of injury, and range from mild contusions to severe pain and swelling.

C. Radiography

1. Take craniocaudal and medial-to-lateral radiographs to rule out bone injury.

IV. Differential Diagnosis

A. Differentiate from joint sprains, fractures, polymyopathies, and polyarthropathies.

V. Medical Management

A. Enforce rest for a minimum of 3 weeks. *Warn owners that animals may feel like exercising before they should be allowed to, especially if antiinflammatories are given.*

B. Within the first 24 hours of injury apply cold compresses for 15 minutes, three to four times a day.

C. After 24 hours apply topical heat.

D. Provide NSAIDs for the initial 3 to 4 days.

VI. Surgical Treatment

A. General Considerations

1. Perform surgery if pressure from interstitial fluid accumulation compromises blood flow.

B. Preoperative Management

1. Confine the animal before surgery.
2. Perform surgery as soon as possible.

C. Surgical Anatomy

1. Skeletal muscle is made of long cylindrical fibers encased within connective tissue sheaths.
2. Each individual muscle fiber is enclosed within a sheath called the endomysium. Each fiber bundle is also enclosed within a sheath (perimysium), as is the entire muscle (epimysium).

D. Surgical Technique

Make an incision through the skin and subcutaneous tissues overlying the muscle to be exposed. Once the muscle group is identified, make an incision through the fascia to decompress the muscle compartment. Suture subcutaneous tissues and skin using standard methods.

E. Prognosis

1. Expect the animal to return to normal function in most cases.
2. Repeat injury is likely if adequate rest is not provided.

Muscle-Tendon Unit Laceration (*SAS*, pp. 1001–1003)

I. Definition

A. **Lacerations** are tears within the muscle-tendon unit.

II. General Considerations

A. Lacerations most commonly involve the tendons near the carpometacarpal and tarsometatarsal joints.

III. Diagnosis

A. Clinical Presentation

1. Signalment.
   a. Any dog or cat may be affected.
2. History.
   a. There is usually an open wound and a non–weight-bearing lameness.

B. Physical Examination

1. Explore extent of internal damage after acute penetration of a muscle-tendon in order to diagnose a laceration requiring surgical repair.

C. Radiography

1. Take craniocaudal and medial-to-lateral radiographs to identify foreign bodies or concurrent fractures.

IV. Medical Management

A. Perform surgery on lacerations that involve a tendon. Medical management is not indicated.

V. Surgical Treatment

A. General Considerations

1. In muscle, use appositional sutures supported with deeper stent sutures.
2. In tendon, use delicate manipulation and apposition with small-diameter suture.

B. Preoperative Management

1. Clean wounds and bandage before surgery.

C. Surgical Anatomy

1. Tendons are longitudinally oriented bundles of collagen fibers that are surrounded by loose connective tissue sheaths. The entire tendon is surrounded by the epitenon, which is enveloped by an outer connective tissue sheath called the paratenon.
2. Tendons crossing joint surfaces are often encased in a tendon sheath.
3. Tendon ends may retract within a tendon sheath and require longitudinal incision to identify the severed ends.

VI. Surgical Technique

A. Muscle Laceration

Thoroughly debride the wound edges to fresh, bleeding muscle tissue. Debride carefully to avoid excess removal of tissue, which will make apposition of the severed ends difficult. Place interrupted sutures in the outer muscle sheath around the circumference of the muscle. Support the appositional sutures with heavy stent sutures placed in a cruciate pattern.

B. Tendon Laceration

Delicately manipulate and debride the tendon ends. With small, flat tendons, use small-diameter, nonabsorbable material placed in a series as interrupted vertical mattress or cruciate sutures. For larger tendons, select the largest suture diameter that will readily pass through the tendon atraumatically. A locking-loop suture pattern is recommended. Place each loop of the pattern in a slightly different plane (i.e., a near-far, middle-middle, and far-near pattern). Alternatively, use a three-loop pulley, Bunnell-Mayer, or far-near, near-far suture pattern. Use adjoining fascia to support the tendon appositional sutures.

VII. Suture Materials/Special Instruments

A. Select nonabsorbable or absorbable suture material that maintains its mechanical strength for at least 3 to 4 weeks for muscle repair. Use nonabsorbable suture for tendon repair.

B. Self-retaining retractors are helpful.

VIII. Healing of Tendons and Muscles

A. As healing occurs, undifferentiated mesenchymal cells migrate into the wound and produce collagen and matrix that lend strength to the entire wound. The resultant scar unites the tendon ends. Function is regained through use of the limb postoperatively.

IX. Postoperative Care and Assessment

A. Immobilize the limb for 3 weeks after tendon repair using rigid external coaptation, then place a heavy padded bandage for an additional 3 weeks. Limit activity to leash walks.

B. Perform physical therapy for 4 weeks once the bandage has been removed. Gradually return to normal activity.

X. Prognosis

A. Expect return to normal function.

B. Failure occurs with premature return to exercise.

Muscle-Tendon Unit Rupture (*SAS,* pp. 1003–1005)

I. Definition

A. **Rupture** of the muscle-tendon units is a complete or partial loss of integrity of the muscle-tendon unit caused by extreme overstretching.

II. General Considerations

A. Ruptures result from a powerful contraction occurring during forced hyperextension. Achilles tendon injury is most common.

B. Acute tendon trauma usually occurs from a fall or penetrating injury.

C. Chronic stretching injury occurs in sporting breeds of dogs. The injuries are often bilateral.

III. Diagnosis

A. Clinical Presentation

1. Signalment.
   a. Any dog or cat may be affected.
   b. Athletic dogs are most commonly affected.
2. History.
   a. There is usually a weight-bearing lameness after strenuous activity.

B. Physical Examination

1. Observe for tarsal hyperflexion.
   a. With acute trauma, the animal will be unable to bear weight and the Achilles tendon will be flaccid upon passive dorsal flexion of the tarsus when the stifle is extended.
   b. With chronic stretching of the Achilles tendon, the animal will be weight bearing, but will walk plantigrade.

C. Radiography/Ultrasonography

1. Use ultrasonography to assess extent of tendon fiber disruption.
2. Take craniocaudal and medial-to-lateral radiographs to determine presence or absence of bone avulsion.

IV. Differential Diagnosis

A. Differentiate from sciatic nerve injury and congenital tarsal hyperflexion by palpating loss of tendon continuity and performing a neurologic examination.

V. Medical Management

A. Perform surgical repair of completely ruptured tendons.

B. With partial ruptures, external coaptation may be tried, but the results are usually unsatisfactory.

VI. Surgical Treatment

A. Preoperative Management

1. Clean wounds and bandage.
2. Limit activity until definitive treatment.

B. Surgical Anatomy

1. The Achilles tendon unit is composed of tendons arising from the gastrocnemius, superficial digital flexor, semitendinosus, gracilis, and biceps femoris muscles.
2. With chronic injuries in which fibrous tissue makes identification of individual tendons impossible, treat the complex of fibrous scar and Achilles tendon as a single structure.

C. Positioning

1. Position the animal in lateral recumbency and perform a hanging-leg preparation.

D. Surgical Technique

1. Achilles tendon rupture.

Make an incision over the site of injury on the caudolateral surface of the limb. If the injury is acute, identify the three tendons composing the Achilles complex and suture each tendon separately with an interrupted far-near, near-far pattern using nonabsorbable, small-diameter (3-0 to 4-0, depending the animal's size) monofilament suture. If the injury is chronic, identification of individual tendon units is not possible; continue surgical dissection to expose the circumference of the thickened fibrous band. Then, sequentially remove sections of scar tissue from the center of the mass. Remove enough tissue so that tension is present in the Achilles complex when the stifle joint is in a normal standing position and the tarsus is slightly extended. Be careful not to remove too much of the proliferative fibrous tissue. If excess fibrous tissue is excised, apposition of the cut ends will be difficult. Suture the cut ends with a three-loop pulley pattern or maintain apposition with tendon plating. For tendon plating, appose the cut ends of the tendon with nonabsorbable monofilament suture. Use 3-0 suture for small dogs and cats, 2-0 for medium-sized dogs, and 0 for large dogs. Support the anastomosis by placing a small bone plate adjacent to the tendon. Place interrupted sutures through the plate holes into the body of the tendon. Use large-diameter, nonabsorbable monofilament suture. Support of the tendon anastomosis is critical for a favorable outcome.

Immobilize the tarsal joint in slight extension. Place a raised, threaded transfixation pin threaded through the free end of the calcaneus into the distal tibia. Cut through the pin shaft to leave the pin just below the skin surface. Provide additional support with a fiberglass cast.

VII. Suture Materials/Special Instruments

A. Use nonabsorbable suture.

B. Have an air-driven or battery-operated drill for screw or transfixation pin insertion.

VIII. Postoperative Care and Assessment

A. Leave the cast and transfixation pin in place for 3 weeks. Remove them both, then support the limb in a padded bandage preventing full dorsal flexion of the tarsus.

B. Limit activity to leash walking for 10 weeks.

C. If a plate is used, remove it 8 to 10 weeks after surgery.

IX. Prognosis

A. The animal is unlikely to be able to return to strenuous athletic activity.

Muscle Contracture and Fibrosis (*SAS*, pp. 1005-1008)

I. Definition

A. **Muscle contracture** occurs when normal muscle-tendon unit architecture is replaced with fibrous tissue, shortening the muscle or tendon.

II. General Considerations

A. This condition most commonly affects the infraspinatus and quadriceps muscle-tendon units.
   1. Look for occurrences following distal femoral fractures in young dogs; however, congenital contracture has been reported.
   2. Avoid inadequate fracture stabilization, excessive tissue trauma during surgery, and prolonged limb immobilization; each may contribute to quadriceps contracture, although the etiology is unknown.

3. Infraspinatus muscle contracture occurs most frequently in hunting dogs after irreversible muscle fiber injury. The cause is unknown, but it appears to be a primary muscle disorder.

III. Diagnosis

A. Clinical Presentation

1. Signalment.
   a. Any dog may develop quadriceps muscle contracture, but most commonly affected are immature patients following distal femoral fracture. The condition is rare in cats.
   b. Young, adult, sporting breeds of dogs are more likely to develop contracture of the infraspinatus muscle. It has not been reported in cats.
2. History.
   a. Typically there is femoral trauma 3 to 5 weeks before quadriceps muscle contracture, and likely a previous attempt at stabilization.
   b. An acute lameness following strenuous activity in the 3 weeks before evaluation for infraspinatus muscle contracture is common.

B. Physical Examination

1. Quadriceps muscle contracture
   a. There is a limited range of motion in the stifle or even hyperextension.
   b. Cranial thigh muscles may be atrophied.
2. Infraspinatus muscle contracture
   a. There is initially a weight-bearing forelimb lameness and soft tissue swelling at the shoulder joint.
   b. The lameness resolves for 3 to 4 weeks, but then expect mild lameness and gait abnormality to develop secondary to fibrosis and contracture of the infraspinatus muscle.
   c. Look for external rotation of the shoulder.

C. Radiography

1. Radiographs will not show abnormalities of the muscle-tendon unit.

IV. Surgical Treatment

A. Treat quadriceps contracture by releasing the fibrous thickening and adhesions between the joint capsule and femur and between the quadriceps muscle and femur. If a functional range of motion is not achieved following adhesion release, lengthen the quadriceps muscle-tendon unit by a Z-plasty, or release of the origin of each muscle.

B. Expect recurrence if preventive rehabilitation measures are not taken after surgery, such as application of a transarticular fixator or a 90/90 bandage.

C. Treat infraspinatus contracture by releasing the fibrotic, myotendinous infraspinatus muscle as it crosses the shoulder joint.

V. Surgical Anatomy

A. With quadriceps muscle contracture there is atrophy of the quadriceps muscle-tendon unit, which is composed of the vastus medialis, vastus intermedius, rectus femoris, and vastus lateralis muscles.

B. Normal range of motion in the stifle joint is from 180 degrees to 30 degrees.

C. With infraspinatus muscle contracture there is atrophy of the muscle and the tendon is off-white color. The infraspinatus muscle is a cuff muscle of the shoulder joint that lies just caudal to the spine of the scapula. Its tendon crosses the joint craniolaterally to insert onto the lateral tuberosity of the proximal humerus.

D. Positioning.

1. For quadriceps contracture, position the animal in lateral recumbency and perform a hanging-leg preparation.
2. For infraspinatus muscle contracture, position the animal in lateral recumbency.

E. Surgical Technique.

1. Quadriceps release.

Expose the stifle joint and distal femur through a liberal craniolateral incision. Elevate and release adhesions between the quadriceps muscle group and femur with sharp dissection. Release adhesions between the fibrous joint capsule and femoral condyles. Luxate the patella medially and flex the joint to its full extent. If a functional range of motion (greater than 40 degrees) is not achieved after releasing the adhesions, perform a quadriceps muscle-tendon-unit lengthening procedure.

2. Quadriceps muscle-tendon-unit lengthening.
   a. Z-plasty.

Make a longitudinal incision through the center of the muscle-tendon unit beginning 8 to 10 cm proximal to the patella. Extend the incision distally to a point 3 cm proximal to the patella. At the proximal extent of the longitudinal incision, make a transverse incision laterally through the muscle and fibrous tissue. At the distal extent of the longitudinal incision, make a transverse incision medially through the muscle and fibrous tissue. Flex the stifle and allow the cut edges of the longitudinal incision to slide on each other. When a functional range of flexion is achieved, place interrupted sutures across the longitudinal incision to maintain the desired length of the quadriceps muscle-tendon unit.

   b. Muscle release.

Extend the lateral incision to expose the proximal femur. At the level of the third trochanter, elevate the quadriceps from the medial, lateral, and caudal surfaces of the femur. Incise through the origins of each muscle group to release the quadriceps and allow distal sliding of the muscle group. Release the vastus intermedius near its point of origin on the ilium. Close the surgical wound using standard methods.

3. Transarticular fixator.

Insert a half pin just below the third trochanter of the femur using an end-threaded transfixation pin and insert a full pin through the tibia 4 cm above the tarsus using a centrally threaded transfixation pin. Maximally flex the stifle joint and maintain this position with a heavy rubber band connecting the proximal and distal transfixation pins. Fashion a bandage and connect it to the distal transfixation pin to maintain a functional angle of the tarsus.

4. Infraspinatus release.

Perform a craniolateral approach to the shoulder joint. Isolate the circumference of the infraspinatus muscle with sharp dissection. Transect the fibrotic muscle and any fibrous bands restricting movement of the joint. Once the fibrous contracture is incised, the limb will assume a normal position and a normal range of motion of the shoulder will be possible.

VI. Suture Materials/Special Instruments

A. Self-retaining retractors and a periosteal elevator assist tissue retraction and reflection.

B. Have instruments for pin placement if placing a transarticular fixator.

VII. Postoperative Care and Assessment

A. Perform passive flexion and extension of the stifle joint and tarsus as soon as the patient will allow. Repeat 20 to 30 times, at least three times daily.

B. Maintain the external fixator for 3 to 5 weeks, cleaning the pin-to-skin interfaces daily. After removal, continue physical therapy for an additional 5 weeks.

C. If a 90/90 bandage is applied, maintain it for 3 weeks, then perform passive flexion and extension of the joint as described previously.

D. No special postoperative care is required after surgery for infraspinatus muscle contracture. Expect use of the limb within a few days after surgery.

VIII. Prognosis

A. Prognosis for limb use after surgery for quadriceps muscle contracture is fair, but contracture may recur, and stifle flexion of more than 45 to 90 degrees is seldom achieved.

B. Expect return to preinjury function after surgery for infraspinatus muscle contracture.

32

Other Diseases of Bones and Joints (*SAS*, pp. 1009-1030)

Hypertrophic Osteopathy (*SAS*, pp. 1009–1011)

I. Definition

A. **Hypertrophic osteopathy** is a diffuse periosteal reaction resulting in new bone formation around the metacarpal, metatarsal, and long bones.

II. General Considerations

A. It generally affects all four limbs.

B. It is a paraneoplastic syndrome associated with other primary disease processes (e.g., neoplasia, including lung tumors; granulomatous lesions; bacterial endocarditis; and heartworm disease).

C. Although the pathophysiology is unknown, alterations in pulmonary function may lead to increased peripheral blood flow, with the periosteum responding by forming new bone.

III. Diagnosis

A. Clinical Presentation

1. Signalment.
   a. Any breed of dog may be affected, but because it is often associated with neoplasia, expect to see it mainly in older dogs.
   b. It has been reported in a cat.
2. History.
   a. There is usually an acute or gradual onset of lethargy, reluctance to move and swelling of the distal extremities.

B. Physical Examination

1. Examine the animal for warm swollen limbs.
2. Attempt to identify the primary (underlying) disease process.

C. Radiography/Ultrasonography

1. Take radiographs to reveal irregular periosteal new bone formation. The periosteal reaction involves the phalanges, metacarpal, and metatarsal bones initially and later the more proximal long bones.
2. Articular surfaces appear normal.
3. Take thoracic and abdominal radiographs and perform abdominal ultrasonography to help identify the primary disease.

IV. Medical Management

1. Treat the underlying disease process.
2. Analgesics may be beneficial if the animal appears to be in pain.

V. Prognosis

A. If the primary disease can be effectively treated the bony lesions often resolve.

Panosteitis

I. Definition

A. **Panosteitis** is a disease of young dogs causing lameness, bone pain, endosteal bone production, and occasionally subperiosteal bone production.

II. General Considerations

A. It is a disease of unknown etiology.

B. Endosteal and periosteal new bone formation occur (mostly endosteal because the marrow is invaded by bone trabeculae).

III. Diagnosis

A. Clinical Presentation

1. Signalment.
   a. Usually affects male large-breed dogs.
   b. Most affected animals are less than 2 years of age.
2. History.
   a. A shifting leg lameness is typical.
   b. Owners often believe these dogs have hip dysplasia or OCD.

B. Physical examination

1. A pain response is usually elicited on firm palpation of affected long bones.

C. Radiography

1. Recognize that clinical signs may precede radiographic abnormalities by as many as 10 days.
2. Look for the early findings of widening of the nutrient foramen and blurring and accentuation of trabecular patterns.
3. Later, identify radiodense, patchy, or mottled bone within medullary canals.

IV. Medical Treatment

A. Prescribe NSAIDs (i.e., aspirin or Ascriptin) (see Appendix I).

B. Warn owners about potential gastrointestinal side effects.

V. Surgical Treatment

A. Surgical treatment is not indicated.

VI. Prognosis

A. Advise owners that panosteitis will probably recur but usually resolves by the time the dog is 2 years of age.

Craniomandibular Osteopathy (*SAS,* pp. 1011–1012)

I. Definition

A. **Craniomandibular osteopathy** is a proliferative bone disease of immature dogs involving the occipital bones, tympanic bullae, and mandibular rami.

II. General Considerations

A. The etiology is unknown, but because West Highland white terriers, cairn terriers, and Scottish terriers are most frequently affected, suspect a genetic predisposition.

B. There is proliferation of new, coarse, trabecular bone adjacent to the mandibular rami, occipital bones, and tympanic bullae.

C. The bony proliferation occurs typically at 5 to 7 months of age and is accompanied by intermittent fever, discomfort when eating, and pain when the mouth is forced open.

D. Warn owners that multiple relapses may occur, but bone proliferation will decrease as dogs reach maturity.

III. Diagnosis

A. Clinical Presentation

1. Signalment.
   a. West Highland white terriers, cairn terriers, or Scottish terriers are typically affected.
   b. Affected animals are usually 5 to 7 months of age.
2. History.
   a. Affected animals are usually reluctant to eat.
   b. Occasionally, swelling of the mandibular rami is noted.

B. Physical Examination

1. Bilaterally enlarged mandibles and tympanic bullae may be palpated.
2. Observe for pain on opening of the mouth and for fever.

C. Radiography

1. Skull radiographs reveal increased irregular bone density of the caudal mandibles and tympanic bullae.

IV. Medical Management

A. Provide analgesics to control pain until the animal reaches maturity.

B. Provide nutrition for animals that cannot open their mouths enough to eat solid foods.

C. Administering antibiotics and/or corticosteroids will not alter disease progression.

V. Surgical Treatment

A. Surgery is not indicated.

VI. Prognosis

A. Inform owners that prognosis is guarded until maturity when the extent of bone production is known.

B. Warn owners that multiple relapses may occur until maturity.

C. Do not breed affected dogs.

Hypertrophic Osteodystrophy (*SAS*, pp. 1012–1013)

I. Definition

A. **Hypertrophic osteodystrophy** is a disease that causes disruption of metaphyseal trabeculae in long bones of young, rapidly growing dogs.

II. General Considerations

A. Proposed etiologies include vitamin C deficiency, oversupplementation of dietary calcium, and infectious organisms.

B. Delayed ossification of the physeal hypertrophic zone results.

C. This condition is identified grossly as widened metaphyseal regions of long bones and perimetaphyseal soft tissue swelling, with a line of separation of metaphyseal trabeculae parallel to the growth plate.

D. Typically, the acute phase lasts 7 to 10 days. Animals may exhibit signs ranging from mild lameness to anorexia, pyrexia, lethargy, severe lameness, refusal to rise, and weight loss.

E. Clinical signs may wax and wane.

F. Provide severely affected animals with intense supportive care.

III. Diagnosis

A. Clinical Presentation

1. Signalment.
   a. Young, rapidly growing, large-breed dogs as young as 2 months of age are affected.
   b. Relapse may occur as late as 8 months.
2. History.
   a. There is usually a history of acute onset of lameness, with inappetence and lethargy.
   b. Diarrhea may precede lameness.

B. Physical Examination

1. Mild to severe lameness affecting all four limbs may be noted.
2. The long bone metaphyses are swollen, warm, and painful on palpation.
3. Provide intense supportive care to severely affected dogs that are depressed, anorexic, and pyrexic (up to 106° F).

C. Radiography

1. Take radiographs to reveal an irregular radiolucent zone in the metaphysis, parallel and proximal to the physis, that gives the appearance of a double physeal line.
2. Observe also for flaring of the metaphysis with increased bone density caused by periosteal proliferation.

D. Laboratory Findings

1. The animal may be hypocalcemic; the significance of this is unknown.

IV. Medical Management

A. Provide analgesics.

B. Administer fluids to severely debilitated animals.

C. Corticosteroids, antibiotics, and vitamin C have no proven effect.

V. Prognosis

A. Expect full recovery of most animals within 7 to 10 days.

B. Warn owners that multiple relapses may occur and that interference with normal physeal development may result in permanent deformity of long bones.

Bone Neoplasia (*SAS*, pp. 1014-1025)

I. Definitions

A. **Primary bone neoplasia** arises from cells located within the bone structure.

B. Soft tissue tumors that spread to bone **(metastatic bone tumors)** may occur in either the **appendicular** skeleton (i.e., long bones) or **axial** skeleton (skull, vertebrae, ribs, and pelvis).

II. General Considerations

A. Primary tumors of the appendicular skeleton often arise at the distal radial metaphysis, proximal humerus, proximal or distal femur, and proximal or distal tibia.

B. Refer to Tables 32-1 and 32-2 for malignant bone tumor types and recommended treatment.

C. Benign bone tumors (i.e., osteoma, ossifying fibroma, multilobular osteomas and chondromas, osteochondromas, enchondromas, and chondromas) are generally slow growing, and complete surgical excision is usually curative.

D. Obtain an accurate diagnosis in order to provide appropriate treatment.

E. Osteosarcoma is the most common primary bone neoplasm.

1. Seventy-five percent originate in the appendicular skeleton, most

commonly in the metaphyses of the proximal humerus, distal radius, and distal femur.

2. Metastasis is common and occurs early.
3. Ninety percent of affected animals die or are euthanized within 1 year of diagnosis.
   a. Survival may be improved with amputation or limb-sparing combined with chemotherapy.
4. Osteosarcoma is also the most common tumor of the axial skeleton.
5. Use osteosarcoma as a model for evaluation and diagnosis. Remember that treatment and prognosis vary depending on tumor type (see Tables 32-1 and 32-2).

III. Diagnosis

A. Clinical Presentation

1. Signalment.
   a. Primary bone tumors of the axial skeleton generally occur in medium-sized and large-breed dogs.
   b. Median age is 8.7 years in dogs.
   c. They occur more often in females than males.
   d. Older cats are also affected.
2. History.
   a. Most dogs with primary bone neoplasia affecting the appendicular skeleton present for lameness and/or localized limb swelling.
   b. Most dogs with primary bone tumors of the axial skeleton present for pain, reluctance to eat or walk, visible swelling, and/or bleeding from tumor surfaces.

B. Physical Examination

1. Appendicular bone tumors.
   a. Lameness is often the first sign.
   b. The limb may be enlarged and firm.
   c. Rarely are cutaneous fistulae present.
2. Axial skeleton tumors.
   a. Often noted as palpable firm swellings.
   b. Lameness or paralysis can result from tumors affecting the vertebral column.

C. Radiography

1. Take radiographs to assess cortical lysis, periosteal bone proliferation, and soft-tissue swelling.
2. Evaluate a dorsoventral or ventrodorsal view and both lateral views of thoracic radiographs for tumor metastasis.

IV. Differential Diagnosis

A. Differentiate from bacterial osteomyelitis, fungal osteomyelitis, metastatic bone tumor, direct extension of soft tissue tumors, hypertrophic pulmonary osteopathy, bone infarcts, hypervitaminosis A, periosteal response to trauma, and aneurysmal bone cysts.

B. Biopsy.

1. Obtain a definitive diagnosis by submitting a biopsy or excision for histologic evaluation to a pathologist experienced in evaluating bone samples.

Table 32-1
Malignant bone neoplasia in dogs

Tumor	Incidence	Metastasis	Treatment	Prognosis
Osteosarcoma of the appendicular skeleton	75% of all bone tumors	High rate of early metastasis to lungs and soft tissues. Bone metastasis is a late complication.	Amputation and chemotherapy with cisplatin and/or doxorubicin Limb sparing in select cases Palliative radiation therapy for painful bone lesions	Mean survival time with amputation alone is 12-16 weeks, median survival time with limb sparing or amputation plus cisplatin and doxorubicin is about 300 to 400 days
Osteosarcoma of the axial skeleton	Less common than appendicular tumors	Highly metastatic, local recurrence except for mandible, which is slower to metastasize	Local resection of tumor (i.e., mandible, rib) Cisplatin, local radiation as adjunct to surgery to reduce local recurrence	Median survival time is 22 weeks, 1 year survival is 26.3%, rate of tumor recurrence is 66.7%
Fibrosarcoma	<5% of bone tumors	Slower to metastasize than osteosarcoma	Amputation (chemotherapy not of proven benefit) Limb sparing in select cases	Poor prognosis (but complete excision of low-grade tumors without metastases may be curative)
Chondrosarcoma	5%-10% of bone tumors	Slow to metastasize	Amputation (chemotherapy not of proven benefit)	May be good after amputation or resection of lesion

Hemangiosarcoma	<5% of bone tumors	May be multicentric, often involve spleen and right atrium, highly metastatic	Amputation (chemotherapy not of proven benefit) Limb sparing in select cases	Poor prognosis because of multiple organ involvement, mean survival time less than 5 months
Giant cell tumor	Rare	Metastasis to lymph nodes, lung, and bones	Amputation	Poor prognosis
Liposarcoma	Rare	Metastasis to lung, liver, and lymph nodes	Amputation or local resection	Poor prognosis
Fracture-associated sarcoma	Uncommon, associated with fractures in which healing has been complicated; represents 5% of osteosarcomas	Metastasis has occurred in 14% of reported cases	Amputation Limb-sparing techniques Chemotherapy	Same as osteosarcoma

Table 32-2
Malignant bone neoplasia in cats

Tumor	Incidence	Metastasis	Treatment	Prognosis
Osteosarcoma	Most common primary bone tumor in cats (70%-80%)	Metastasis is uncommon	Amputation, radiation therapy, or excision of skull tumors	Median survival time is 24-50 months; greater than 50% of cats are alive at 64 months
Fibrosarcoma	Rare, more often due to secondary invasion of bone from soft tissue	Incidence is unknown	Amputation	Long disease-free intervals reported (e.g., 10-18 months)
Chondrosarcoma	4% of bone tumors, reported in the scapula	Incidence is unknown	Amputation	Prognosis guarded
Squamous cell carcinoma	Local bone invasion, occurs in oral cavity and digits	See section on oral tumors (see *SAS,* p. 222)	Amputation, mandibulectomy, maxillectomy, +/– radiation therapy, see section on oral tumors (see *SAS,* p. 222)	See section on oral tumors (see *SAS,* p. 222)
Multiple cartilaginous exostosis	Uncommon, usually FeLV positive	Multiple sites common, scapula, vertebra, mandible	Palliative removal of painful lesions	Guarded

a. Take multiple samples from the center rather than the periphery of the lesion because biopsies from the periphery are more frequently interpreted as reactive bone.
b. Radiograph after biopsy to confirm biopsy site.

V. Medical or Conservative Management

A. Use multiple modality treatment (e.g., amputation and chemotherapy) to improve survival time. Refer to medical text for specific treatment recommendations.

VI. Surgical Treatment

A. General Considerations

1. Treat appendicular bone tumors with limb amputation or tumor resection combined with limb salvage techniques and chemotherapy. Be aware that after amputation, dogs with severe concurrent orthopedic disease may have difficulty ambulating.
2. Treat maxillary and mandibular tumors by mandibulectomy or maxillectomy, plus appropriate chemotherapy or radiation therapy.
3. Treat spinal tumors and rib tumors with en bloc resection.

B. Preoperative Management

1. Hydrate animals well before amputations.
2. Provide broad-spectrum antibiotics perioperatively during mandibulectomy, maxillectomy, and limb-sparing techniques.

C. Positioning

1. For bone biopsy, place the animal in lateral recumbency with the affected leg up.
2. For scapulectomy, limb-sparing of the forelimb, or forelimb or rear limb amputation place in lateral recumbency with the affected leg up.

VII. Surgical Techniques

A. Bone Biopsy

1. General considerations.
   a. Use either a Michele trephine or Jamshidi needle to obtain a biopsy. With Michele trephines a larger sample of bone is obtained; however, there may be an increased risk of fracture through the biopsy site. Jamshidi needles secure a smaller sample that may decrease the risk of pathologic fracture after biopsy.
2. Technique.

Make a small skin incision over the center of the lesion. Locate the skin incision so that biopsy tracts that may be seeded with tumor during the biopsy can be removed during the definitive treatment procedure (position the biopsy tract so that it does not interfere with skin flaps developed to cover the amputated bone end, should amputation be necessary). Push the trephine or needle through soft tissues to the bone cortex. Remove the stylet and advance the trephine or cannula through the bone. Remove the cannula and push the specimen out by inserting the probe into it. Repeat the procedure to obtain multiple specimens.

B. Amputation

1. General considerations.
   a. Consider a total or partial scapulectomy for tumors involving only the scapula.
   b. Perform a forelimb amputation by removing the scapula or, alternatively, by resecting the distal humerus. Forequarter amputation eliminates the need to cut through bone and avoids unsightly muscular atrophy around the scapular spine.
   c. Perform rear limb amputation at the midfemoral diaphysis, or by disarticulating the coxofemoral joint. Perform coxofemoral joint disarticulation when tumors affect the femur.
   d. Submit the entire tumor for histologic evaluation to confirm diagnosis after amputation.
2. Scapulectomy.

Make a skin incision from several centimeters dorsal to the dorsal border of the scapula, over the scapular spine, to the middle third of the humerus. Transect superficial muscles (i.e., omotransversarius muscle, trapezius muscle) as close to their origin on the lateral surface of the scapula as the tumor will allow. Expose the medial scapular surface by transecting the rhomboideus muscle and elevating the serratus muscle from the scapula. Protect the brachial plexus and axillary artery and vein during dissection. Transect the suprascapular and subscapular nerves. Transect the teres major and long head of the triceps muscles from their origins on the caudal border of the scapula. Transect the coracobrachialis tendon, teres minor, infraspinatus, supraspinatus, and subscapularis muscles close to their humeral origin. Incise the joint capsule. Osteotomize the supraglenoid tubercle and remove the scapula. To close the wound, suture the tendon origin of the biceps brachii muscle to the joint capsule. Attach the free muscle flaps to adjacent musculature. Suture subcutaneous tissue and skin. Perform partial scapulectomy similarly, but osteotomize the scapula proximal to the scapular notch.

3. Forequarter amputation.

Make a skin incision from the dorsal border of the scapula, over the scapular spine, to the proximal third of the humerus. Continue the skin incision around the forelimb at this level. Transect the trapezius and omotransversarius muscles at their insertions on the scapular spine. Transect the rhomboideus muscle from its attachment on the dorsal border of the scapula and retract the scapula laterally to expose its medial surface. Next, elevate the serratus ventralis muscle from the medial surface of the scapula. Continue to retract the scapula to expose the brachial plexus and axillary artery and vein. Ligate the axillary artery and vein with a three-clamp and transfixation suture technique. Transect the brachial plexus. Transect the brachiocephalicus muscle, deep and superficial pectoral muscles, and latissimus dorsi muscle near their humeral insertions. Remove the forelimb. To close the wound, approximate the muscle bellies to cover the brachial plexus and vessels and suture subcutaneous tissues and skin.

4. Midhumeral amputation.

Make a skin incision around the forelimb at the level of the distal third of the humerus. The lateral portion of the skin incision should extend further distally than the medial portion. Dissect subcutaneous tissues in the same plane. Abduct the limb and separate the biceps brachii muscle and medial head of the triceps muscle to expose the brachial artery and vein and median, ulnar, and musculocutaneous nerves. Ligate the artery and vein with a three-clamp and transfixation suture technique. Transect the nerves, then transect the triceps

tendon and reflect the muscles proximally to expose the humerus. Transect the biceps brachii and brachialis muscles at their insertions on the radius and ulna. Ligate the cephalic vein and transect the radial nerve. Elevate the brachiocephalicus muscle from the humerus. Osteotomize the humerus with an oscillating saw, Gigli wire, or osteotome and remove the distal forelimb. Close the wound by suturing the triceps tendon around the humeral stump to the biceps and brachialis muscles. Suture subcutaneous tissues and skin.

5. Coxofemoral disarticulation.

Make a skin incision around the rear limb at the level of the middle third of the femur. The lateral aspect of the skin incision should extend further distally than the medial aspect. On the medial side, open the femoral triangle by incising between the pectineus muscle and caudal belly of the sartorius muscle to expose and ligate the femoral artery and vein using a three-clamp technique. Transect sartorius, pectineus, gracilis, and adductor muscles approximately 2 cm from the inguinal crease. Isolate the medial circumflex femoral vessels over the iliopsoas muscle and ligate them. Transect the iliopsoas muscle at its insertion on the lesser trochanter and reflect it cranially to expose the joint capsule. Incise the joint capsule and cut the ligament of the head of the femur. On the lateral side, transect biceps femoris muscle and tensor fasciae latae at midfemoral level and reflect them proximally to expose the greater trochanter and sciatic nerve. Sever the nerve distal to its muscular branches to the semimembranosus, semitendinosus, and biceps femoris muscles. Transect the gluteal muscles insertions close to the greater trochanter. Transect semimembranosus and semitendinosus muscles at the level of the proximal third of the femur. Sever the external rotator muscles and quadratus femoris muscle at their attachments around the trochanteric fossa. Elevate the rectus femoris muscle from its origin on the pelvis. Incise the joint capsule circumferentially and remove the limb. Close the wound by flapping the biceps femoris muscle medially and suturing it to the gracilis and semitendinosus muscles. Flap the tensor fascia lata caudally and suture it to the sartorius muscle. Suture subcutaneous tissues and skin.

6. Midfemoral amputation.

Make a skin incision around the rear limb at the level of the distal third of the femur. The lateral aspect of the skin incision should extend further distally than the medial aspect. On the medial side, transect the gracilis muscle and the caudal belly of the sartorius at the midfemoral level. Isolate and ligate the femoral vessels. Transect the pectineus muscle through its musculotendinous junction. Transect the cranial belly of the sartorius muscle. Transect the quadriceps muscle proximally to the patella. Transect the biceps femoris muscle at the same level as the quadriceps muscle. Isolate and cut the sciatic nerve at the level of the third trochanter. Transect the caudal muscles, including the semimembranosus, semitendinosus, and adductor muscles at midfemoral level. Elevate the insertion of the adductor muscle from the linea aspera of the femur. Cut the femur at the junction of the proximal and middle thirds of the diaphysis and remove the limb. Close the wound by flapping the quadriceps muscle caudally to cover the femoral stump and suturing it to the adductor muscle. Flap the biceps muscle medially and suture it to the gracilis and semitendinosus muscles. Appose muscles to completely protect the distal end of the femur. Suture subcutaneous tissues and skin.

7. Limb-sparing techniques.
   a. In cases in which owners will not permit or when preexisting orthopedic or neurologic disease contraindicates amputation, consider limb-sparing techniques that involve en bloc resection of

the tumor and replacement with a bone. Dogs with osteosarcoma affecting less than 50% of the distal radius may be candidates.

Position the dog in lateral recumbency. Dissect around the pseudocapsule of the tumor. Osteotomize the bone 2 to 3 cm proximal to the radiographic margin of the tumor. Transect the extensor carpi radialis muscle and remove it with the tumor (along with any other muscles or tendons that are involved). The distal margin of resection is the joint surface. Incise the joint capsule and dissect the tumor free. Remove the articular cartilage of the carpal bones in preparation for carpal arthrodesis. Replace the resected bone with a cortical allograft stabilized with a long, dynamic compression plate. Make sure that the plate is of sufficient length that at least four screws can be positioned in the proximal radius and three positioned distal to the graft. Harvest autogenous cancellous bone and place it at the host-graft interface and at the arthrodesis site. If desired, insert a closed suction drain adjacent to the graft before closing the wound. Close subcutaneous tissues and skin routinely.

VIII. Suture Materials/Special Instruments

A. Use a Michele trephine or Jamshidi needle for bone biopsy.

B. Use an osteotome and mallet, oscillating saw, or Gigli wire to sever the bone for midhumeral or midfemoral amputation, and use plating equipment for limb sparing.

IX. Postoperative Care and Assessment

A. After biopsy, apply pressure bandages if there is excessive bleeding.

B. After amputation, if hemorrhage or seroma formation is noted, apply pressure to the surgical site by applying a circumferential bandage around the thorax or pelvis. Take sequential thoracic radiographs to detect metastasis. Warn owners of potential complications, including seroma formation, bleeding, infection, and suture line dehiscence.

C. After limb-sparing, maintain closed suction drainage system (if used) and remove drain when drainage subsides (usually 1 day after surgery). Support and protect the leg in a padded bandage to control postoperative swelling. Decrease exercise for 3 to 4 weeks, but instruct owner to perform physical therapy to prevent flexure contracture of digits.

X. Prognosis

A. Survival time for osteosarcoma can be nearly doubled by combining amputation with chemotherapy, but 1-year survival is still less than 50%.

B. Inform the owner that there does not appear to be a difference in survival rates between dogs treated with amputation in conjunction with chemotherapy and those treated with limb-sparing procedures in conjunction with chemotherapy.
   1. Complications associated with limb-sparing include local tumor recurrence, implant failure, and allograft infection.
   2. Warn that infection can require allograft removal or amputation.

Joint Neoplasia (*SAS*, pp. 1025-1026)

I. Definition

A. **Primary joint neoplasms** are tumors that arise from synovial linings of diarthrodial joints, tendon sheaths, and/or bursae.

II. General Considerations

A. Synovial cell sarcomas are rare tumors arising from synovioblastic mesenchyme in deep connective tissues around joints.

B. They are more common at joints above the carpus and tarsus than at distal joints.

C. Consider the biologic behavior to range from slow growth to aggressive invasion of adjacent tissues.

D. Look for metastasis to regional lymph nodes, lungs, and other locations, including bone.

III. Diagnosis

A. Clinical Presentation

1. Signalment.
   a. Large, middle-aged dogs are usually affected.
   b. Females are more commonly affected than males.
2. History.
   a. Affected animals are often lame.
   b. A mass may be noted near a joint.

B. Physical Examination

1. Expect masses to be nonpainful and firm with some fluctuant areas.

C. Radiography

1. Take radiographs to evaluate the extent of bone and soft-tissue involvement.
2. Theres is typically evidence of lobulated soft-tissue masses in the joint region and bone changes often on either side of the joint. This contrasts with the appearance of primary bone tumors, which seldom appear to "cross a joint."
3. Take thoracic radiographs to evaluate for pulmonary metastasis.

IV. Differential Diagnosis

A. Differentiate from synovial cysts, which are well-circumscribed masses attached to joint capsule, tendon sheath, or bursa. Also differentiate from fungal and infectious joint diseases and other tumors. Perform a biopsy for definitive diagnosis.

V. Surgical Treatment

A. Perform amputation. Concurrent chemotherapy may be beneficial.

B. Do not perform local excision because of the high recurrence rate.

VI. Postoperative Care and Assessment

A. See Bone Neoplasia for recommendations for the postoperative care of animals following amputation.

B. Reexamine periodically for early detection of local recurrence or metastasis.

VII. Prognosis

A. Inform the owner that prognosis is guarded after limb amputation. Although historically considered slowgrowing tumors that metastasize late in the course of disease, a recent study suggests that metastasis is common following amputation.

Synovial Cyst (*SAS*, pp. 1026-1027)

I. Definitions

A. **Synovial cysts** are benign, well-circumscribed masses attached to joint capsule, tendon sheath, or bursa.

II. General Considerations

A. Clinical signs are often limited to localized enlargement of the joint or surrounding tissues.

B. Diagnose on histologic findings of a synovial cell lining supported by a zone of collagen, typically without inflammatory cells present.

III. Diagnosis

A. Clinical Presentation

1. Signalment.
   a. Affected animals are typically over 5 years of age.
2. History.
   a. The typical history is a mass near a joint (typically carpus, elbow, or tarsus).
   b. The mass is seldom associated with lameness.

B. Physical Examination

1. Palpate a small, well-circumscribed mass firmly attached to deeper tissues.

C. Radiography

1. Take radiographs to document soft-tissue swelling around the joint without associated bone lysis or proliferation.

IV. Surgical Treatment

A. Excise the cyst by carefully dissecting it from surrounding soft tissues. The cyst will recur if it is drained without removal.

V. Prognosis

A. Cysts seldom recur after complete surgical excision.

Osteomyelitis (*SAS*, pp. 1027–1030)

I. Definitions

A. **Osteomyelitis** is inflammation of bone.
   1. **Acute osteomyelitis** is characterized by systemic illness, pain, and soft-tissue swelling without visible radiographic alterations in bone.
   2. **Chronic osteomyelitis** exists when acute and systemic clinical signs have subsided, but infection manifested by draining sinuses; recurrent cellulitis; abscess formation; and progressive, destructive, and proliferative osseous changes is present.

B. **Sequestra** are fragments of necrosed bone that have become separated from surrounding tissue.

II. General Considerations

A. Bacterial Origin

1. Monomicrobial infections, usually β-lactamase–producing *S. intermedius* or *S. aureus* may occur. Polymicrobial infections may be mixtures of *Streptococcus* spp., *Proteus* spp., *E. coli, Klebsiella* spp., and *Pseudomonas* spp.
2. Anaerobic bacteria, including *Actinomyces* spp., *Clostridium* spp., *Peptostreptococcus* spp., *Bacteroides* spp., and *Fusobacterium* spp. are an important cause of osteomyelitis.
3. When treatment fails, investigate lack of identification and inappropriate treatment of anaerobic bacteria.

4. Recognize that bacteria alone will not necessarily cause osteomyelitis. Other important factors in the pathogenesis of posttraumatic osteomyelitis.
   a. Extent of soft-tissue damage and alteration of blood supply.
   b. Formation of a biofilm (glycocalyx).
   c. Stability of fracture repair.

B. Mycotic

1. May be acquired through hematogenous dissemination of inhaled spores.
2. Organisms include *Coccidiodes immitis, Blastomyces dematiditis, Histoplasma capsulatum,* and *Cryptococcus neoformans.*

C. Other

1. Other causes include viruses, parasites, foreign bodies, and corrosion of metallic implants.

III. Diagnosis

A. Clinical Presentation

1. Signalment.
   a. Any dog or cat may be affected.
2. History.
   a. There may be a history of recent open reduction and stabilization of a fracture, bite wounds, or open traumatic wound.

B. Physical Examination

1. Expect clinical features to vary, depending on the stage of the disease.
   a. For initial response look for signs of inflammation–redness, heat, swelling, and pain. The animal is often pyrexic, depressed, and anorexic.
   b. Consider persistence of an elevated temperature for longer than 48 hours postoperatively or a neutrophilic left shift a sign that infection is present rather than only manifestations of surgically induced trauma. However, lack of either of these findings does not rule out infection.
   c. With chronic osteomyelitis, do not expect draining tracts and/or lameness, pyrexia, anorexia, and other clinical signs associated with systemic disease because they are frequently lacking.

C. Radiography

1. Expect specific radiographic findings to vary depending on the stage of disease, site of infection, and pathogenicity of infective organism.
   a. Anticipate radiographic changes in bone not being present before 2 weeks postinfection.
   b. Identify early radiographic bone changes, including a periosteal shadow with deposition of new bone in a lamellar pattern oriented perpendicular to the long axis of the bone.
   c. Identify lysis of the medullary cavity, sequestra and as involucra (new bone formation around a sequestrum), and bone sclerosis and lysis as the infection progresses. Radiographically, sequestered bone appears more dense than surrounding bone.
2. If draining and skeletal lesions are not confluent, perform fistulography to confirm that the draining tracts lead to the bone lesion. Use a diluted water-soluble contrast agent in order to not obscure identification of associated foreign bodies.

D. Laboratory Findings

1. An elevated WBC count with a neutrophilic left shift may be noted with acute osteomyelitis.
2. With chronic osteomyelitis, the white cell count is usually normal.

IV. Differential Diagnosis

A. Obtain definitive diagnosis by aerobic and anaerobic cultures from bone at the time of surgical intervention, or via deep fine-needle aspiration of material directly surrounding the involved bones.

B. Do not culture draining tracts.

C. If fungal osteomyelitis is suspected, perform fungal cultures, titers, and histologic evaluation of biopsies.

V. Medical or Conservative Management

A. Provide antibiotic therapy as determined by culture and sensitivity, and continue for at least 4 weeks.

B. Apply warm packs in patients with hematogenous osteomyelitis or those having postoperative osteomyelitis.

C. Do not use medical therapy when sequestra, necrotic tissue, pockets of exudate, or unstable surgical implants are present.

VI. Surgical Treatment

A. General Considerations

1. Provide drainage and perform debridement if sequestra or pockets of exudate are present.
2. Stabilize fractures and provide appropriate antibiotic therapy.
3. For chronic osteomyelitis, maintain or provide fracture stability, remove loose implants and sequestered bone, use cancellous bone grafting of bony deficits, and administer appropriate antimicrobial therapy.

B. Preoperative Management

1. With acute osteomyelitis initiate broad-spectrum antibiotic therapy, then change to definitive therapy as necessary based on culture and sensitivity testing.
2. With chronic osteomyelitis wait until intraoperative cultures have been obtained before administering antibiotics.

VII. Surgical Technique

A. Acute Osteomyelitis

Open infected wounds and debride necrotic tissues. If a fracture is present, stabilize bone fragments with an appropriate implant system (bone plates and

screws or external skeletal fixators are usually preferred). Stabilization of fractures is the key to successful treatment of osteomyelitis. Bone union will occur in the presence of infection if fragments are stable. If previous surgery was performed and the fracture remains stable, leave the original implants in place. If the implants have loosened, choose another fixation system to provide rigid fixation. Establish drainage by treating the surgical site as an open wound. Irrigate the wound with 0.05% chlorhexidine and then pack it with sterile gauze soaked with 0.05% chlorhexidine. Cover wounds with a sterile outer dressing that will absorb drainage products accumulated between bandage changes. Once the infection is eliminated, suture the wound.

B. Chronic Osteomyelitis

Determine the degree of fracture stability by palpation and radiographic assessment. If fractures and original implants are stable, leave them in place. However, if implants are loose and fractures have not healed, remove the loose implants and rigidly stabilize the fracture. Identify and remove sequestered bone through radiographic imaging and surgery. At surgery, sequestered bone is recognized by a yellowish discoloration and has no soft tissue attachments. Do not try to stabilize sequestered bone fragments; instead, remove them and place an autogenous cancellous bone graft in areas devoid of bone. Establish drainage as previously described.

VIII. Postoperative Care and Assessment

A. With acute osteomyelitis continue antibiotic therapy for 3 to 4 weeks. With chronic osteomyelitis continue for 4 to 6 weeks.

B. If managing an open wound, irrigate the area with 0.05% dilute chlorhexidine twice daily and pack with a chlorhexidine-soaked sponge. If desired, use umbilical tape secured to the skin on either side of the incision that can be tied over the gauze packing to facilitate frequent changing of the packing materials. Continue bandaging until the wound is closed.

C. If a fracture is present, perform postoperative care depending on the fracture configuration and stabilization procedure used.

D. Observe daily for signs of recurring fever, pain, swelling, and/or draining tracts.

IX. Prognosis

A. Inform the owner the prognosis for resolving the infection is good if all bone sequestra are removed and fractures are adequately stabilized.

B. Be aware that removal of all implants following bone union may be necessary to completely resolve the infection.

PART

IV

Neurosurgery

33

Fundamentals of Neurosurgery (*SAS*, pp. 1031-1048)

I. Definitions

A. **Plegia** and **paralysis** are a complete loss of motor function to the affected extremity, whereas **paresis** is partial loss of motor function.
   1. With **tetraparesis/tetraplegia** all four limbs are affected.
   2. With **paraparesis/paraplegia** both pelvic limbs are affected.
   3. With **hemiparesis/hemiplegia** the front and hind limbs on one side are affected.
   4. With **monoparesis/monoplegia** one limb is affected.

B. **Proprioception** is the ability to recognize the location of limbs in relation to the rest of the body.

C. **Ataxia** is lack of coordination without paretic, spastic, or involuntary movements (although these may be seen in association with ataxia).

D. **Dysmetria** is characterized by movements that are too long **(hypermetria)** or too short **(hypometria).**

Problem Identification (*SAS*, pp. 1031-1039)

I. Signalment

A. Use the signalment (i.e., age, sex, breed, use of animal) together with anatomic location of the lesion to refine differential diagnoses.

II. History

A. Use the history to characterize the disorder as acute or chronic, progressive or static, and persistent or intermittent (Table 33-1).

Table 33-1
Etiology of spinal lesions based on history of pain and/or paresis

Acute/Static	Acute/Progressive	Chronic/Progressive
Vascular	Degenerative	Degenerative
Fibrocartilaginous emboli	IVD—type I	IVD—type I and II
Infarction	Inflammatory	Cauda equina
Trauma	Diskospondylitis	Wobbler syndrome
Fracture/luxation	Vertebral osteomyelitis	Degenerative myelopathy
Degenerative	Trauma	Inflammatory
IVD—type I	Fracture/luxation	Diskospondylitis
	Anomalous	Vertebral osteomyelitis
	Atlantoaxial instability	Neoplastic
	Neoplastic	Meningeal tumors
	Spinal cord tumors	Spinal cord tumors
	Vertebral tumors	

B. Historical data may suggest the lesion's location within the spinal canal.
1. Patients with extradural spinal lesions have an acute onset of persistent and sometimes progressive pain and paresis.
2. Patients with intradural-extramedullary spinal lesions generally have histories of chronic, dull pain with slowly progressive paresis.
3. Patients with intramedullary spinal lesions generally have an acute onset of sudden pain and paresis; the pain is short lived and the paresis is persistent, but not progressive.

III. Physical Examination

A. As part of a general physical examination observe the animal as it moves around the examination room while obtaining the history from the owner.

IV. Neurologic Examination

A. General Considerations

1. Establish the presence of neurologic disease and determine its neuroanatomic location.
2. Perform serial neurologic examinations to assess patient status (i.e., improving, static, deteriorating).

B. Observation

1. Mental status.
   a. Alert (normal).
   b. Depressed (conscious, but inactive).
   c. Unresponsive to environment.
      i. These animals usually have diffuse cerebral cortical disease.
   d. Stuporous (sleeps when undisturbed; will not respond to harmless stimuli such as noise but will awaken with a painful stimulus).
      i. These animals generally have diffuse cerebral disorders or brainstem compression.
   e. Comatose (cannot be aroused, even with painful stimulus).

2. Posture.
   a. Evaluate posture while the animal is free to move about the examination area.
   b. Further assess by moving the animal into different positions and observing its ability to regain normal posture.
   c. Abnormalities include head tilt, abnormal truncal posture, improper positioning of limbs (proprioceptive deficits), decreased muscle tone in a limb (flaccidity), or increased muscle tone (spasticity).
3. Gait.
   a. Evaluate the animal's gait in an area with good footing.
   b. Proprioception (position sense).
      i. Deficits cause knuckling, misplacement of the foot, and/or scuffing of the toenails.
      ii. Deficits may be associated with lesions at any level of the spinal cord.
   c. Paresis.
      i. Is caused by disruption of the voluntary motor pathways, which extend from the cerebral cortex through the brainstem and out to the peripheral nerves.
   d. Circling in tight circles.
      i. Usually caused by caudal brainstem lesions; an associated head tilt usually indicates involvement of the vestibular system.
   e. Ataxia.
      i. Can be caused by lesions at any level, but usually involves cerebellar, vestibular, or spinal cord lesions.
   f. Dysmetria.
      i. Usually caused by cerebellar lesions.
4. Palpation.
   a. Examine for worn toenails, deep and cutaneous masses, deviation of normal contour, abnormal motion, or crepitation, and evaluate for muscular size, tone, and strength.
   b. Compare one side to the other to check for symmetry.

C. Postural Reactions

1. Postural reactions are complex responses that maintain an animal's normal upright position.
2. Proprioceptive positioning.
   a. Flex the paw so that the dorsal surface is on the floor.
   b. Delayed or absent correction of the knuckled paw indicates neurologic disease.
   c. Check for worn dorsal toenails, skin abrasions, or calluses on the dorsum of the foot that may signify long-standing proprioceptive deficits.
3. Purposeful movement.
   a. This is an animal's conscious attempt to move the legs.
   b. Assess in nonambulatory paraparetic animals by grasping the base of the tail with one hand, lifting the animal, and walking it around.
4. Wheelbarrowing.
   a. Perform by having the animal bear weight on the thoracic limbs while supporting it under the abdomen.
   b. Normal animals walk forward with coordinated movements of both thoracic limbs.
5. Hopping.
   a. Test hopping with the animal supported as for wheelbarrowing, except lift one thoracic or pelvic limb from the ground. The entire weight of the animal is supported on one limb as you move the patient medially and laterally.

   b. Poor initiation of hopping suggests proprioceptive deficits, whereas poor movement suggests motor deficits.
   c. Generally, testing thoracic limbs yields more reliable information than pelvic limbs.
6. Extensor postural thrust.
   a. Perform by supporting the animal under the thorax while lowering it to the floor.
   b. When the pelvic limbs touch the floor they should move caudally in symmetric walking movements to achieve a position of support.
7. Hemistanding/hemiwalking.
   a. Perform by elevating the front and rear limbs of one side so that all the animal's weight is supported by the opposite limbs.
8. Placing.
   a. Tactile placing (perform before visual placing).
      i. Perform by supporting the animal under the thorax and covering its eyes with one hand. Bring the distal thoracic limbs (at or below the carpi) in contact with the edge of a table.
      ii. The normal response is immediate placement of the feet on the table surface in a position that will support weight.
   b. Visual placing.
      i. Test by allowing the animal to see the table surface.
      ii. Normal animals reach for the surface before the carpus touches the table.

D. Spinal Reflexes

1. General considerations.
   a. Spinal reflexes (myotactic reflexes) test the integrity of sensory and motor components of the reflex arc and the influence of descending motor pathways on the reflex.
   b. Three kinds of responses may be seen (Table 33-2).

Table 33-2
Comparison of common neurologic findings in UMN and LMN disease

Spinal reflexes	LMN	UMN
Patellar	Absent or depressed	Normal or exaggerated
Triceps	Absent or depressed	Normal or exaggerated
Biceps	Absent or depressed	Normal or exaggerated
Pelvic limb withdrawal	Absent or depressed	Normal or exaggerated
Thoracic limb withdrawal	Absent or depressed	Normal or exaggerated
Crossed extensor	Absent or depressed	Normal or exaggerated
Anal sphincter	Absent or depressed	Normal or exaggerated
Tail wagging	Absent or depressed	Normal or exaggerated
Strength	Poor	Variable but stronger than with LMN
Muscle tone	Flaccid	Spastic
Muscle fasciculation	Present	Absent
Muscle atrophy	Early, neurogenic	Late, disuse
Clonus	Absent	Present
Bladder expression	Easy	Difficult
Root signature	Present	Absent

i. Absent or depressed reflex indicates complete or partial loss of either the sensory or motor nerves responsible for the reflex (lower motor neuron or LMN).
ii. Normal reflex indicates sensory and motor nerves are intact.
iii. Exaggerated reflex indicates an abnormality in the descending pathways from the brain and spinal cord that normally inhibit the reflex (upper motor neuron or UMN).

2. Pelvic limb.
 a. Patellar reflex.
  i. The most reliable pelvic limb reflex.
  ii. Perform with the animal in lateral recumbency. Support the uppermost leg by the hock, with the stifle slightly flexed. Strike the patellar ligament briskly with a reflex hammer.
  iii. Normal.
   (a) The normal response is a single, quick extension of the stifle.
  iv. Abnormal.
   (a) Absence or depression of the patellar reflex (hypopatellar reflex) and decreased muscle tone (flaccidity) indicate a lesion of the sensory or motor component of the reflex arc (LMN).
    (i) Unilateral loss of the reflex suggests a femoral nerve lesion.
    (ii) Bilateral loss suggests a segmental spinal cord lesion involving spinal cord segments L4-L6.
   (b) Exaggerated reflexes (hyperpatellar reflex) and increased muscle tone (spasticity) suggest a lesion cranial to the L4 spinal cord segment (UMN).
 b. Withdrawal reflex.
  i. Perform with the animal in lateral recumbency. Apply the least harmful stimulus possible to the foot.
  ii. Reflex primarily involves spinal cord segments L6-S1 and the sciatic nerve.
  iii. Normal.
   (a) Flexion of the entire limb.
  iv. Abnormal.
   (a) Absence or depression of the reflex indicates lesion of these spinal cord segments or nerves (LMN).
    (i) Unilateral absence of the reflex is most likely the result of a peripheral nerve lesion.
    (ii) Bilateral absence or depression is more likely the result of a spinal cord lesion.
   (b) An exaggerated withdrawal reflex indicates a lesion cranial to spinal cord segment L6 (UMN).
3. Thoracic limb.
 a. Triceps reflex.
  i. Perform the triceps reflex with the animal in lateral recumbency. Support the limb under the elbow; maintain flexion of the elbow and carpus. Strike the triceps tendon with a reflex hammer just proximal to the olecranon.
  ii. The triceps muscle is innervated by the radial nerve, which originates from spinal cord segments C7-T1.
  iii. Normal.
   (a) The normal response is slight extension of the elbow.
  iv. Abnormal.
   (a) The triceps reflex is difficult to elicit in normal animals; thus absent or depressed reflexes may not indicate an abnormality.
   (b) An exaggerated reflex indicates a lesion cranial to C7 (UMN).

b. Biceps reflex.
   i. Perform the biceps reflex by holding the animal's elbow and placing the index finger of the same hand on the biceps tendon cranial and proximal to the elbow. Extend the elbow slightly and strike the finger with the reflex hammer.
   ii. Normal.
      (a) Slight flexion of the elbow.
   iii. Abnormal.
      (a) This reflex is difficult to elicit in the normal animal.
      (b) Absent or decreased reflexes suggest a lesion involving spinal cord segments C6-T8 (LMN), but may be normal in some animals.
      (c) An exaggerated reflex indicates a lesion cranial to spinal cord segment C6 (UMN).
c. Withdrawal reflex.
   i. Perform the thoracic limb withdrawal reflex in a manner similar to the pelvic limb withdrawal reflex.
   ii. This reflex primarily involves spinal cord segments C6-T1.
   iii. Abnormal.
      (a) Absent or depressed reflexes indicate a lesion of these spinal cord segments or of the peripheral nerves (LMN).
      (b) Exaggerated reflexes indicate a lesion cranial to spinal cord segment C6 (UMN).

4. Other reflexes.
   a. Anal sphincter reflex.
      i. Elicit the perineal or anal sphincter reflex by gentle perineal stimulation with a needle or forceps.
      ii. Sensory and motor innervation occurs through the pudendal nerve and spinal cord segments S1 to S3.
      iii. The anal sphincter reflex is the best indication of functional integrity of sacral spinal cord segments and sacral nerve roots.
      iv. Normal.
         (a) Contraction of the anal sphincter muscle is normal.
   b. Bladder expression.
      i. The two general components of urinary bladder innervation are autonomic (hypogastric and pelvic) and somatic (pudendal) nerves.
      ii. Clinical observations of bladder dysfunction can be attributed to spinal cord injury based on the pudendal nerve (S2-3). The pudendal nerve innervates urethral striated muscle and helps maintain urinary continence.
         (a) A lesion above the S2-3 spinal cord segments causes spasm of bladder outflow, making the bladder difficult to express (UMN).
         (b) A lesion involving S2-3 spinal cord segments causes lack of sphincter tone and an easily expressible bladder (LMN).
   c. Crossed extensor reflex.
      i. The crossed extensor reflex may be observed when withdrawal reflexes are elicited. With the animal in lateral recumbency and legs relaxed, gently pinch the toes of the down limb (thoracic or pelvic), eliciting a withdrawal reflex.
      ii. Abnormal.
         (a) Extension of the upper limb.
      iii. The crossed extensor reflex results from a lesion that affects descending inhibitory pathways of the spinal cord (UMN).
      iv. This reflex is frequently associated with severity or chronicity, but does not constitute a poor prognosis.
   d. Tail wag reflex.
      i. Animals with a completely transected spinal cord above the

sacral and caudal spinal cord segments can wag their tails. This reflex wag is often observed when expressing the bladder or eliciting the anal sphincter reflex.

ii. Tail wagging as a conscious response to pleasurable stimuli such as petting the head, calling the animal's name, or seeing the owner, implies that some spinal cord pathways are intact.

e. Panniculus reflex.

i. Elicit the panniculus reflex (cutaneous trunci reflex) by applying a pinprick stimulus to the skin over the back, beginning in the region of the fifth lumbar vertebra and continuing cranially.

ii. Normal.

(a) The normal response is twitching of the cutaneous trunci muscle on both sides of the dorsal midline, at the point of stimulation and cranial.

iii. Abnormal.

(a) Absence of a response occurs one or two segments caudal to the spinal cord lesion.

f. Clonus.

i. Refers to a sustained after-contraction or quivering that may be seen or felt when performing spinal reflexes, especially patellar and crossed extensor reflexes.

ii. The hand supporting the extremity being tested may feel this reaction; this reflex is often not visual.

iii. Presence of clonus implies a chronic condition.

E. Sensory Evaluation

1. As a general rule, perform sensory evaluation last.
2. Deep pain perception.

a. Testing for deep pain is the most important prognostic test of the neurologic examination, and is a reliable indicator of spinal cord integrity.

b. Perform by applying painful stimuli to each limb and the tail using progressively stronger painful stimuli (e.g., hemostatic forceps).

i. A significant behavioral response (e.g., animal attempts to vocalize, turns to look or bite, or attempts to get away from the examiner) indicates the presence of sensation.

ii. Withdrawal of a limb is not a behavioral response.

c. Loss of deep pain indicates a severely damaged spinal cord and a poor prognosis.

d. As a general rule, loss of function after spinal cord injury develops as follows.

i. Loss of proprioception.

ii. Loss of voluntary motor function.

iii. Loss of superficial pain sensation.

iv. Loss of deep pain sensation.

e. As an animal recovers from spinal cord injury, sensation returns first, followed by motor function and lastly proprioception.

3. Hyperpathia.

a. Hyperpathia is noted when pressure applied to spinous processes and paraspinal muscles of the thoracic and lumbar region and transverse processes and paraspinal muscles of the cervical region results in pain and a behavioral response (see previous discussion).

F. Cranial Nerve (CN) Examination

1. Olfactory nerve (CN I).

a. CN I is sensory for conscious perception of smell.

b. Rhinitis, tumors of the nasal passages, and diseases of the cribriform plate are the most common causes for loss of olfaction.

2. Optic nerve (CN II).
    a. CN II is the sensory pathway for vision and pupillary light reflexes.
    b. Examine CN II by means of three major tests.
        i. Menace response.
            (a) Perform by making a threatening gesture with the hand at each eye; the animal should blink and retract the globe.
        ii. Visual placing reaction (see Postural Reactions).
        iii. Ophthalmoscopic examination.
    c. Abnormalities include loss of vision, dilated pupils, and loss of pupillary light response (direct and consensual) when light is shined in the affected eye.
3. Oculomotor nerve (CN III).
    a. CN III contains parasympathetic motor fibers for pupillary constriction.
    b. It is motor to the extraocular eye muscles and levator muscle of the upper eyelid.
    c. Evaluate by shining a light into each eye (pupillary light reflex), and observing pupils for size and symmetry. Both pupils should constrict symmetrically when a light is shined into either eye (consensual response).
    d. Abnormalities include loss of pupillary light reflex on the affected side (even if light is shined in the opposite eye), fixed lateral deviation (strabismus) of the eye, and dilated pupil.
4. Trochlear nerve (CN IV).
    a. CN IV innervates the dorsal oblique muscle of the eye.
    b. Lesions of the trochlear nerve cause lateral strabismus of the eye.
5. Trigeminal nerve (CN V).
    a. CN V innervates muscles of mastication and is sensory to the face.
    b. Test motor function by assessing muscle mass and jaw tone of the masticatory muscles.
    c. Assess sensory function by checking pain perception of the face, eyelids, cornea, and nasal mucosa.
6. Abducent nerve (CN VI).
    a. CN VI innervates the lateral rectus and retractor bulbi muscles.
    b. Lesions of the abducent nerve cause medial strabismus, loss of gaze, and inability to retract the globe.
7. Facial nerve (CN VII).
    a. CN VII is motor to the muscles of facial expression and sensory to the palate, the rostral two thirds of the tongue, and the inside of the pinnae of the ears.
    b. Facial paralysis generally causes facial asymmetry (e.g., lips, eyelids, and ears may droop) and loss of ability to blink or retract the lips.
8. Vestibulocochlear nerve (CN VIII).
    a. CN VIII has two divisions.
        i. The vestibular portion provides information about the orientation of the head with respect to gravity.
        ii. The cochlear portion functions in hearing.
    b. Abnormalities associated with nerve dysfunction include ataxia, head tilt, circling, nystagmus, and loss of hearing.
9. Glossopharyngeal (CN IX) and vagus nerves (CN X).
    a. CN IX and CN X control swallowing.
    b. Elicit the swallowing reflex by gentle external pressure on the hyoid region.
    c. Elicit the gag reflex by inserting a finger into the caudal pharynx.

d. The glossopharyngeal nerve is motor to pharyngeal muscles.
e. The vagus nerve is motor to pharyngeal and laryngeal muscles, and sensory to the caudal pharynx and larynx.
f. Abnormalities caused by glossopharyngeal and vagus nerve dysfunction include loss of the gag reflex, dysphagia, and laryngeal paralysis.

10. Hypoglossal nerve (CN XII).
    a. The hypoglossal nerve is motor to muscles of the tongue.
    b. Observe for abnormalities by wetting the animal's nose and watching its ability to extend the tongue.
    c. Evaluate strength of tongue retraction, tongue deviation, and presence or absence of atrophy.

Lesion Localization (*SAS*, pp. 1039-1040)

I. General Considerations

A. Localize lesions suspected of being above the foramen magnum to one of five locations in the brain (Table 33-3).
1. Cerebral Cortex
2. Diencephalon (thalamus, hypothalamus)
3. Brainstem (pons, medulla oblongata)
4. Vestibular
5. Cerebellum

B. Localize lesions suspected of being below the foramen magnum to one of five locations in the spinal cord on the basis of spinal reflexes.
1. Cranial cervical (C1-C5)
2. Caudal cervical (C6-T2)
3. Thoracolumbar (T3-L3)
4. Lumbosacral (L4-S3)
5. Sacral (S1-S3)

C. If an animal has both an UMN and an LMN lesion to a specific site, LMN reflex changes predominate.

Differential Diagnosis of Spinal Disorders and Diagnostic Methods (*SAS*, pp. 1040-1048)

I. Differential Diagnosis

A. Establish a list of differential diagnoses by incorporating historical as well as physical and neurologic examination findings.

Table 33-3
Abnormal neurologic findings that help localize brain lesions

Cerebral Cortex

Altered mental status

Ipsilateral circling, pacing, head pressing

Contralateral postural and proprioceptive deficits

Contralateral cortical blindness (normal pupils and pupillary light reflexes)

Contralateral UMN hemiparesis

Seizures

Diencephalon (Thalamus and Hypothalamus)

Altered mental status: aggression, disorientation, hyperexcitability, coma

Contralateral postural and proprioceptive deficits

Bilateral visual deficits

Abnormalities of eating, drinking, sleeping, and temperature (hypothalamus)

Muscle tone, segmental reflexes, and sensation are unaltered

Brainstem (Pontomedullary)

Mental status may be unaltered, to severe depression and coma

Ipsilateral UMN hemiparesis or tetraparesis; may circle if ambulatory

Cranial nerve deficits involving cranial nerves V through XII

- Trigeminal—motor and sensory
- Abducent—medial strabismus
- Facial—facial paralysis
- Vestibulocochlear—central vestibular signs; hearing loss
- Glossopharyngeal/vagus—dysphagia, reduced gag reflex, laryngeal dysfunction
- Hypoglossal—abnormal tongue movement

Vestibular

Disoriented or unaltered mental status

Ipsilateral head tilt, circling, rolling, falling, asymmetric ataxia, incoordination

Nystagmus (spontaneous or positional) with fast phase away from the side of the lesion

Ipsilateral ventrolateral strabismus

Must differentiate central from peripheral vestibular disease

Cerebellum

Unaltered mental status

Ataxic gait, wide-based stance, dysmetria, head tremor, intention tremor, truncal ataxia

Visual but may have ipsilateral loss of menace response

Hypermetric postural reactions, goose-stepping gait

Muscle tone, segmental reflexes, and sensation are unaltered

Table 33-4
Etiology of spinal lesions based on lesion location

Extradural	Intradural-Extramedullary	Intramedullary
Intervertebral disk extrusion	Meningeal neoplasia	Vascular insult
Vertebral fracture/luxation	Meningioma	Fibrocartilaginous embolus
Extradural neoplasia	Neurofibroma	Parenchymal neoplasia
Wobbler syndrome		
Atlantoaxial instability		
Diskospondylitis		
Vertebral osteomyelitis		

II. Diagnostic Plan

A. Obtain the minimum data required: hematology, serum chemistry, and urinalysis.

B. Consider obtaining additional data: electrocardiogram, echocardiogram, and chest and abdominal radiographs.

C. For patients suspected of having an intracranial lesion consider: additional serum chemistry tests, cerebrospinal fluid analysis (CSF), electroencephalography, skull radiographs, computed tomography (CT scan), and/or magnetic resonance imaging (MRI).

D. For patients suspected of having a spinal lesion consider: spinal series of survey radiographs, myelography, electromyography, CT scan, and/or MRI.

III. Diagnostic Tests

Diagnostic tests should localize an intracranial or spinal lesion (extradural, intradural-extramedullary, or intramedullary), help determine the most effective treatment (medical or surgical), and may suggest an etiology (Tables 33-4 and 33-5).

IV. Imaging the Spine

A. General Considerations

1. Use spinal radiographs and myelography for accurate localization of most spinal disorders.
   a. Use general anesthesia.
   b. Use symmetric positioning (carefully supporting the spine during repositioning).
   c. Obtain lateral and ventrodorsal projections of each section of the spine.
   d. Use high-quality radiographic film, and high-contrast radiographic technique (less than 60 kVp) with narrow collimation.
   e. Radiograph each section of the spine separately.

Table 33-5
Differential diagnosis of spinal cord disorders based on DAMNIT-V scheme

D—Degenerative
Intervertebral disk disease
Wobbler syndrome
Cauda equina syndrome
Degenerative myelopathy
A—Anomalous
Atlantoaxial instability
M—Metabolic
N—Neoplastic
Spine
Spinal cord
Meninges
I—Inflammatory/Infections
Diskospondylitis
Vertebral osteomyelitis
T—Traumatic
Vertebral fracture/luxation
V—Vascular
Fibrocartilaginous embolism
Spinal cord infarction

B. Survey Radiographs

1. Survey radiographs allow accurate lesion localization if vertebrae or their ligamentous attachments are directly involved (i.e., congenital anomalies, vertebral fracture/luxation, vertebral body neoplasia, diskospondylitis, vertebral body osteomyelitis, extruded calcified intervertebral disk).
2. Lesion localization in patients with spinal disorders that do not cause visible changes in the vertebrae (i.e., fibrocartilaginous emboli, neoplasia of the spinal cord or meninges, intervertebral disk extrusion, cauda equina syndrome, wobbler syndrome) requires myelography, CT scan, or MRI.

C. Stress Radiography

1. Perform stress radiography (to exacerbate or relieve compressive lesions) by placing various sections of the vertebral column in gentle dorsal hyperextension, ventral flexion, and/or linear traction.
2. May be important in establishing lesion location (i.e., atlantoaxial instability, cervical vertebral instability, lumbosacral instability) and planning therapy.
3. Perform carefully, so as not to exacerbate the patient's neurologic deficits.

D. Myelography

1. Indications.
   a. A visible lesion is not identified on survey radiographs.
   b. Multiple lesions compatible with the neurologic examination are observed.

   c. A lesion is visualized that is not compatible with the neurologic examination.
2. Myelography requires subarachnoid injection of contrast media (lumbar or cisternal) to outline the spinal cord.
   a. Use contrast agents that are radiopaque, water soluble, miscible with CSF, nontoxic, and rapidly absorbed from the subarachnoid space:
      i. Iopamidol (Isovue)–0.33 mg/kg.
      ii. Iohexol (Omnipaque)–0.33 mg/kg.
3. Lumbar puncture (L4-5 or L5-6)
   a. Advantages.
      i. Contrast flows forward under pressure to outline lesions.
      ii. Typically results in the most diagnostic myelogram.
   b. Disadvantages.
      i. More difficult to perform.
      ii. Needle often penetrates spinal cord.
      iii. More likely to deposit contrast epidurally.
      iv. A successful lumbar puncture requires practice and a lumbar spine skeleton for constant referral to anatomic structures.
   c. Fluoroscopy simplifies accurate needle placement.
   d. Technique.

Position the patient in lateral recumbency. Flex the spine, palpate the caudal dorsal spinous process of L5 or L6 (L5 in a L4-5 puncture and L6 in a L5-6 puncture), and place a 20- to 22-gauge, 2.5- to 3.5-inch spinal needle with stylet at its caudal aspect. Place the needle at a 45-degree angle caudally, and slowly advance cranioventrally and toward the midline in the direction of the L4-5 or L5-6 interspace. A characteristic "pop" will be felt as the needle penetrates ligamentum flavum and dura. At this point withdraw the stylet to examine for flow of CSF. If CSF is visible remove some for analysis, then slowly inject the calculated dose of contrast. If CSF is not visible, advance the needle through the spinal cord until it contacts the floor of the spinal canal; occasionally, a tail twitch or leg jerk will result. Withdraw the needle slightly until the flow of CSF is visible. Place the bevel of the spinal needle in the direction of desired flow of contrast and slowly inject the calculated dose.

4. Cisternal puncture.
   a. Advantages.
      i. Easier to perform.
      ii. Excellent view of cervical spine.
   b. Disadvantages.
      i. Distribution of contrast depends on gravity and CSF flow.
      ii. Contrast may not pass by compressive lesions.
      iii. Contrast may migrate into the brain.
   c. Technique.

Position the patient in lateral recumbency. Palpate the wings of the atlas with the thumb and middle finger, and palpate the occiput with the index finger, making a triangle. Gently flex the head and place a 20- to 22-gauge, 11.5- to 2.5-inch spinal needle with stylet in the center of the triangle. Place the bevel of the spinal needle in the direction of desired flow of contrast medium. As the needle is advanced a "pop" is felt as it penetrates the dura and enters the subarachnoid space. Return of CSF confirms proper location of the spinal needle. Slowly withdraw a volume of CSF for analysis, followed by injection of contrast. Elevate the head for 2 to 4 minutes to enhance flow of contrast caudally through all sections of the spine.

5. Complications associated with myelography using iohexol or iopamidol are infrequent (less than 10%) and include exacerbation of

neurologic abnormalities, seizures, cardiopulmonary alterations, and death.

6. Lesion classification.
   a. Extradural.
      i. Extradural lesions cause the "contrast column" (subarachnoid space) to be elevated away from the spinal canal on at least one projection (ventrodorsal or lateral).
      ii. On the opposite view, the contrast column may appear narrower because of spinal cord swelling.
   b. Intradural-extramedullary.
      i. Intradural-extramedullary lesions cause the contrast column to become wider on one projection; this widening may resemble a "golf tee" in appearance.
      ii. From the opposite view the contrast column may appear narrower because of spinal cord swelling.
   c. Intramedullary.
      i. Intramedullary lesions cause the contrast column to become narrower on ventrodorsal and lateral projections because of generalized spinal cord swelling.
7. Stress myelography.
   a. Perform stress myelography by placing segments of the vertebral column in dorsal hyperextension, ventral flexion, and linear traction, thus exacerbating or relieving compressive lesions.
   b. It is most commonly used in the diagnosis of Wobbler syndrome.
   c. Perform carefully so as not to exacerbate the patient's neurologic deficits.

E. Other Spinal Imaging Techniques

1. Diskography.
   a. General considerations.
      i. Is the intradiskal injection of a nonionic contrast medium into the nucleus pulposus and recording the image with radiography.
      ii. Most commonly used in the diagnosis of cauda equina syndrome.
      iii. Significant complications have not been reported.
      iv. Do not perform in patients with diskospondylitis.
   b. Technique.
      i. Place a spinal needle into the nucleus pulposus of the affected disk and inject 0.1 to 0.3 ml of contrast medium (normal disks cause back pressure after 0.1 ml).
   c. Radiographic abnormalities.
      i. Extravasation of contrast medium indicates disk protrusion.
      ii. An irregular contrast pattern within the nucleus pulposus and injection of greater than 0.1 ml volume of contrast medium indicates disk degeneration.
2. Epidurography.
   a. General considerations.
      i. Inject a nonionic contrast medium into the caudal epidural space and record the image with radiography.
      ii. Most commonly used in the diagnosis of cauda equina syndrome.
      iii. Significant complications have not been reported.
   b. Technique.
      i. Insert a 20- to 22-gauge spinal needle between the dorsal lamina of the caudal (coccygeal) vertebra 3-4 or 4-5 and inject 0.15 mg/kg of contrast medium. Take lateral and ventrodorsal views; inject additional contrast at the rate of 0.1 mg/kg if necessary. A lateral view of the lumbosacral spine in hyperextension may accentuate a subtle lesion.

c. Radiographic abnormalities.
    i. Abnormalities include elevation or compression of the contrast column by the spinal lesion.

3. Computed tomography (CT).
    a. Use CT to detect subtle changes conventional radiography cannot reveal, such as the cause of spinal stenosis (soft tissue or osseous), and intervertebral foraminal masses (neoplasia, intervertebral disk [IVD], bony proliferation), and to help define the extent and invasiveness of a lesion (i.e., infection, neoplasia, trauma).
4. Magnetic resonance imaging.
    a. MRI of the spine results in enhanced soft-tissue contrast that enables direct visualization of the spinal cord, epidural space, intervertebral disks, and ligaments of the spine.
    b. Most useful in the diagnosis of lumbosacral stenosis and intramedullary tumors.

V. Imaging the Skull and Brain

A. Survey Radiographs

1. Use survey radiographs to help assess patients with trauma to the calvarium, middle ear infection, neoplasms invading or causing mineralization of the calvarium, or any lesion causing direct involvement of the osseous structures of the skull.
2. Guidelines.
    a. Use general anesthesia.
    b. Position the patient carefully to display bilateral symmetry.
    c. Take lateral and ventrodorsal projections.
    d. Use high-quality radiographic film.
3. Survey radiographs may be normal in patients with significant neurologic deficits secondary to intracranial disorders.

B. Computed Tomography

1. CT provides excellent detail of bone and soft tissue, and allows identification and precise localization of most intracranial lesions.
2. Contrast medium can be used to enhance identification of intracranial neoplasia.

C. Magnetic Resonance Imaging

1. MRI has advantages over CT, including improved anatomic detail of soft tissue structures and absence of image degradation caused by the thick canine calvarium.

34

Surgery of the Cervical Spine (*SAS*, pp. 1049-1099)

General Principles and Techniques (*SAS*, pp. 1049-1063)

I. Definitions

A. **Dorsal laminectomy** is removal of dorsal spinous processes, lamina, and portions of the pedicles to expose the dorsal aspect of the spinal cord and nerve roots.

B. **Hemilaminectomy** and **dorsolateral hemilaminectomy** refer to unilateral removal of the lateral and dorsolateral lamina, respectively, in addition to removal of the pedicles and articular facets.

C. **Foramenotomy** refers to the removal of the roof of the intervertebral foramen.

D. **Facetectomy** is the complete excision of the cranial and caudal articular facets. Unilateral facetectomy and foramenotomy are commonly performed with dorsolateral hemilaminectomy to expose nerve roots.

E. **Ventral slot** refers to the creation of a bony defect in the ventral aspect of a cervical intervertebral space to gain entrance to and visualization of the ventral spinal canal.

F. **Fenestration** is the creation of a window or fenestra in the lateral or ventral annulus fibrosus to remove nucleus pulposus from the intervertebral space.

G. **Tetraparesis** is the loss of conscious proprioception and variable motor weakness of all four limbs.

H. **Tetraplegia** is the loss of conscious proprioception, motor function, and the ability to perceive superficial and deep pain in all four limbs.

II. Preoperative Concerns

A. Assess neurologic function and ambulation carefully in patients that require cervical spinal cord surgery.

B. Weakly ambulatory or nonambulatory tetraparetic patients often have subclinical respiratory compromise and require ventilatory support during surgery.

C. Preoperative care of patients with unstable cervical fractures, luxations, or subluxations (i.e., palpable crepitus, instability) includes cage rest and serial neurologic examinations. Use a neck brace to prevent movement of the cervical spine.

D. Preoperative administration of corticosteroids may provide some protection to these structures during surgery; however, use them cautiously because they may predispose to gastrointestinal ulceration/perforation.

E. During cervical fracture reduction, hemorrhage as a result of laceration of one or both vertebral venous sinuses may be fatal. Have blood available for transfusion, and employ techniques to control venous sinus hemorrhage promptly.

III. Anesthetic Considerations

A. Place two cephalic catheters in animals undergoing cervical spinal surgery to allow rapid fluid administration if venous sinus hemorrhage occurs.

B. Have blood for transfusion and mechanical ventilatory support available.

C. Administer a balanced electrolyte solution intravenously during surgery.

D. Intraoperative measurement of direct arterial blood pressure is recommended.

E. Administer hypertonic saline (4 to 5 ml/kg IV) or positive inotropes (dobutamine or dopamine; Appendix I) if bleeding is severe or hypotension profound.

F. A syndrome characterized by paradoxical bradycardia associated with hypotension (acute sympathetic blockade) can occur intraoperatively in dogs with acute cervical spinal cord trauma. No effective treatment has yet been described.

G. Premedicate animals undergoing surgery of the cervical spinal cord with corticosteroids (methylprednisolone sodium succinate or dexamethasone phosphate).

H. Premedicate dogs with an anticholinergic plus oxymorphone, butorphanol, or buprenorphine and induce with a thiobarbiturate or propofol. Isoflurane or halothane is preferred for anesthetic maintenance.

I. Avoid acepromazine because of the risk of hypotension. Acepromazine is also contraindicated in animals undergoing myelography because it may promote seizures.

J. Manipulate the neck carefully in these patients during anesthetic induction and positioning for surgery or radiographs, especially if instability is present.

IV. Antibiotics

A. Use prophylactic antibiotics in cervical surgery if there are one or more of the following factors: geriatric patient (greater than 7 years old); debilitated patient; patient with clean, open wounds associated with surgery site; estimated surgical time longer than 90 minutes; or a "break" in aseptic surgical technique.

1. Select prophylactic antibiotics that are effective against common causes of postoperative infection (e.g., coagulase-positive *Staphylococcus, E. coli*).
2. Cefazolin (20 mg/kg IV at induction, repeat at 4- to 6-hour intervals for 24 hours) is the antibiotic of choice because of its low toxicity and excellent in vitro activity against these bacteria.

B. Use therapeutic antibiotics if there are one or more of the following factors: nonspinal infection that cannot be treated before surgery; spinal infection requiring surgical intervention (e.g., diskospondylitis, vertebral osteomyelitis); or contaminated open wounds associated with the surgical site (e.g., open vertebral fracture/luxation).

1. Base selection of an appropriate antibiotic for therapeutic use (i.e., treatment extending for 7 to 10 days after surgery) on the most probable pathogen.
2. The most common causes of postoperative wound infection in neurologic surgery are *Staphylococcus* spp.; therefore antibiotics of choice include cefazolin, amoxicillin-clavulanate, enrofloxacin, or cephalothin.

V. Surgical Anatomy

A. There are seven cervical vertebrae.

B. Dorsal landmarks.

1. The dorsal spine of C2 is a distinguishing landmark. It is the most prominent of the dorsal cervical spinous processes.
2. C6 and C7 have fairly prominent dorsal spinous processes that slope cranially.
3. The dorsal spinous process of T1 is prominent, is easy to palpate, and allows identification of the adjacent (but much shorter) cranially facing dorsal spinous process of C7.

C. Ventral landmarks.

1. The transverse processes (wings) of C6 and the ventral spinous process of C1 are prominent.
2. The prominent ventral annulus of the C5-C6 intervertebral space lies on the midline at the most cranial aspect of the transverse process of C6.
3. The prominent ventral spinous process of C1 is palpable just cranial to the C1-C2 intervertebral space.

D. Refer to *Small Animal Surgery* or to an anatomy text for more detailed information.

VI. Surgical Techniques

A. Position patients with cervical disk extrusion or cervical vertebral instability with the neck in linear traction to enhance visualization of herniated disk material by widening the intervertebral space or to decompress the spinal cord during surgery in animals with cervical vertebral instability.

B. Position patients with atlantoaxial instability or cervical fracture/luxation so as to reduce the subluxation or fracture (e.g., linear traction, gentle flexion, or extension) and encourage decompression of spinal cord and nerve roots.

C. Position patients requiring dorsal or dorsolateral decompression with the neck gently flexed to open the articular facets and interarcuate spaces facilitating laminectomy, foramenotomy, and facetectomy.

VII. Ventral Slot

A. General Considerations

1. Ventral slot procedures require minimal dissection through normal tissue planes and minimal disruption of normal anatomical structures.
2. They provide adequate visualization of the spinal canal and access to the intervertebral foramina.
3. Minimal manipulation of the spinal cord is necessary and recovery is generally rapid with few complications.
4. Operative time is less than that required for dorsal exposure of the cervical spine.
5. Ventral slots are often combined with stabilization procedures in animals with cervical vertebral instability.
6. Surgical exposure of the ventral aspect of the cervical spine without creating a slot is used for cervical disk fenestration and some cervical stabilization techniques (e.g., atlantoaxial instability, fracture/luxation).
7. Ventral slots may be combined with fenestration.

B. Technique

Clip and prepare the neck from midmandible to caudal to the manubrium sterni for aseptic surgery. Position the animal in dorsal recumbency with the chest in a "V" trough. Tape the front legs caudally and tie the head cranially. Apply mild linear neck traction to help stabilize the cervical spine and slightly distract the intervertebral spaces. Make a midline ventral incision from the caudal aspect of the thyroid cartilage to the manubrium sterni (determine the exact length of the incision by the location of the involved intervertebral space or spaces). Separate the paired sternohyoid and sternomastoid muscles on their midline. Identify the esophagus and trachea and digitally retract them to the left. Locate the carotid sheaths bilaterally and digitally retract them. Determine the location of the affected intervertebral space by palpating the prominent transverse processes (wings) of C6. Locate the prominent ventral annulus of the C5-C6 intervertebral space just midline of the most cranial aspect of the transverse process of C6. Alternatively, identify the affected intervertebral space by palpating the prominent ventral spinous process of C1 (thus identifying the C1-C2 intervertebral space) and counting caudally. Once the involved intervertebral space has been located, bluntly separate the longus colli muscles along their median raphe when the spinal canal is reached. To prevent inadvertent laceration of vertebral venous sinuses, extend the slot no more than one quarter of the length of the vertebra cranially or caudally. Gauge the depth of the slot by visualizing three distinct layers of bone while drilling. First, penetrate the hard outer cortical layer of the vertebral body (the white cortical bone exposed when the longus colli muscle is elevated from the vertebral body). Next, visualize the softer, more hem-

orrhagic, marrow layer just below the outer cortical layer. This layer is more easily drilled than the outer cortical layer. Drill the outer cortical and marrow layers with 4- to 5-mm-diameter carbide burrs. Finally, visualize the 1- to 2-mm-thick inner cortical layer of the vertebral body. Once this layer has been reached, drill carefully, using gentle "paintbrush" strokes with a 2- to 3-mm-diameter diamond burr. Take care not to break into the spinal canal abruptly. After penetrating the inner cortical layer, use a 3-0 or 4-0 bone curette to enlarge the defect. Carefully curette the dorsal annulus fibrosus and periosteum to expose the dorsal longitudinal ligament. Curette the inner cortical layer of bone to a diameter sufficient to allow removal of the herniated disk, but avoid excessive lateral curettage lest laceration of a vertebral venous sinus occur. Once exposure is adequate, carefully remove the dorsal longitudinal ligament with fine ophthalmic forceps and a No. 11 scalpel blade, allowing access to the spinal canal. Determine adequate decompression of the spinal cord by visualizing the characteristic bluish hue of dura mater (spinal cord) through the slot. Ensure adequate visualization during manipulation of neural structures. Before closure, irrigate the wound with physiologic saline solution to dislodge any remaining bone fragments from soft tissues. Do not fill the slot with bone graft, fat, or Gelfoam. Appose paired longus colli muscles with simple interrupted sutures. Close subcutaneous tissues and skin routinely.

VIII. Cervical Disk Fenestration

A. General Considerations

1. Cervical disk fenestration is performed from intervertebral spaces C2-C3 through C6-C7.
2. There is some suggestion that fenestration of alternate disk spaces after ventral slot may decrease recurrence of disk herniation; however, this is controversial.

B. Technique

Position and prepare the patient for surgery as described above. Make an incision from the thyroid cartilage cranially to the manubrium sterni caudally. Expose each intervertebral space in a similar fashion as the ventral slot; however, separate longus coli muscle only at each intervertebral space. Expose ventral annulus fibrosus with a periosteal elevator. Use a No. 11 scalpel blade to excise a large wedge-shaped piece of ventral annulus fibrosus. Hold the scalpel at the proper cranial-to-caudal angle to facilitate excision of ventral annulus and removal of nucleus pulposus. Remove nuclear material with an ear loop, tartar scraper, or small bone curette (4-0 or 5-0). Take care to prevent dorsal extrusion of disk fragments into the spinal canal. Close as described above for ventral slot.

IX. Dorsal Cervical Laminectomy and Hemilaminectomy

A. General Considerations

1. Dorsal cervical laminectomy is the removal of dorsal lamina from cervical vertebrae to expose the spinal cord.
2. Use laminectomy when lesions are located in the dorsal or lateral spinal canal; use ventral slot (described above) when the compressive lesion is located in the ventral spinal canal.

3. The specific laminectomy procedure used (i.e., cranial cervical, midcervical, caudal cervical) depends on location and etiology of the compressive lesion.
4. Dorsolateral hemilaminectomy and facetectomy is removal of right or left dorsal lamina, a portion of the right or left pedicle, and portions of the articular facet from affected vertebrae.
   a. It is indicated in patients with compressive lesions of the lateral aspect of the spinal canal and intervertebral foramen.
   b. Performing a dorsolateral hemilaminectomy and facetectomy with rongeurs requires careful dissection and visualization of the lateral aspect of the facet joint.

B. Dorsal Approach to the Cranial Cervical Spine (C1-C2)

Perform cranial cervical laminectomy with the patient in sternal recumbency, head gently flexed in a neutral position, and head and neck supported by a rolled fleece or rigid vacuum type of apparatus. Make a dorsal midline incision from the occipital protuberance to the dorsal spinous process of C4. Expose the median fibrous raphe between paired splenius muscles and dorsal cutaneous branches of the cervical nerves. Use these structures as a guide to perform midline dissection. Divide the splenius muscles over the spinous process of C2 and retract them laterally. Incise paraspinal epaxial muscles on each side of the spinous process of C2 and reflect them from the spine and dorsal laminae with a periosteal elevator. Elevate muscle to the level of C2-C3 articular facets caudally and the ventral aspect of the C1-C2 intervertebral foramina cranially. If a hemilaminectomy is performed, elevate muscle only on the side to be exposed. Use self-retaining retractors to facilitate exposure. At the cranial end of the dissection, elevate muscles from the dorsal atlantoaxial ligament; wide elevation of muscles from the dorsal arch of C1 may be performed, depending on needed exposure. Caudally, elevate muscle until the multifidus muscle and nuchal ligament are exposed. From this point, perform a hemilaminectomy, dorsal laminectomy, or axial laminotomy, as needed. Specific laminectomy techniques are described below. Close the surgical wound by suturing muscles to the tendinous raphe in their respective layers. Close subcutaneous tissues and skin routinely.

C. Dorsal Approach to the Midcervical Spine (C2-C5)

Position the patient in sternal recumbency. Place rolled padding under the neck at the midcervical region. Flex the neck over the padding to elevate the cervical vertebrae and open interarcuate spaces. Position the patient carefully to improve palpation of important anatomical landmarks and enhance visualization of interarcuate ligaments. Make a dorsal midline incision from the occiput to the spinous process of the first thoracic vertebra. Identify the median fibrous raphe and use it as a landmark for midline dissection to the nuchal ligament. Incise along one side of the nuchal ligament and between paired bellies of epaxial muscles. Identify appropriate anatomical landmarks, and use a periosteal elevator to remove epaxial muscles from dorsal spinous processes and lamina of affected vertebrae. Dissect to the level of the articular processes; this depth is sufficient to perform deep dorsal laminectomy and avoid the vertebral arteries. Specific laminectomy techniques are described below. Close epaxial muscles to the tendinous raphe or nuchal ligament in their respective layers. Close subcutaneous tissue and skin routinely.

D. Dorsal Approach to the Caudal Cervical Spine (C5-T3)

Position the patient in sternal recumbency. Because the scapulae are closely associated with the caudal cervical spine and the vertebral laminae are located

deep in epaxial muscles, position to enhance exposure. To encourage elevation of the C6 and C7 dorsal spinous processes and laminae, cradle the neck by gently flexing and elevating it over rolled fleece, sandbags, or a rigid vacuum type of apparatus. Position the front legs against the body to encourage abduction of the scapulae from the midline. Do this either by positioning the legs close to the body with sandbags or by tieing the front legs across the table. Make a dorsal midline skin incision from the midcervical region to the dorsal spinous process of T3. Locate the fibrous median raphe and continue midline dissection through epaxial muscles. Retract epaxial muscles with self-retaining retractors to enhance exposure of dorsal spinous processes. Palpate the prominent dorsal spinous process of T1 and cranially slanted smaller dorsal spine of C7 (about half of the height of T1) to determine specific anatomical location. Use a periosteal elevator to expose dorsal spinous processes and laminae of affected vertebrae. Remove dorsal spines of T1 through T3 (as needed) for dorsal laminectomy. This will have minimal effect on spinal stability as the nuchal ligament is continuous with the supraspinous ligament. Excise interarcuate ligaments between C6 and T1 (as needed) with a No. 11 scalpel blade to expose the spinal cord. Specific laminectomy techniques are described below. Close the surgical wound by suturing epaxial muscles to the tendinous raphe or nuchal ligament in their respective layers. Close subcutaneous tissues and skin routinely.

E. Dorsolateral Approach to the Cervical Spine

Position the patient in sternal recumbency with the head and neck slightly flexed and elevated. Make a dorsal midline skin incision centered over the affected vertebrae. Identify the median fibrous raphe and expose the dorsal spinous processes via midline dissection. Elevate epaxial muscles from the dorsal spinous processes, lamina, and dorsal articular facets of affected vertebrae. Continue dissection and periosteal elevation on the lateral aspect of the articular facet and intervertebral foramen to provide full visualization of the lateral aspect of the vertebral body. Carefully dissect and identify the vertebral artery before examination of the intervertebral foramen. Specific laminectomy techniques are described below. Close epaxial muscles to the tendinous raphe in their respective layers. Close subcutaneous tissues and skin routinely.

F. Laminectomy and Laminotomy Techniques

1. General considerations.
   a. Laminar thickness varies with patient size; larger patients generally have thicker lamina. Vertebral and laminar density varies with age; older animals tend to have denser, more compact bone.
   b. Disadvantages of dorsal laminectomy and dorsolateral hemilaminectomy include severe disruption of hard and soft tissues, prolonged operating times, poor visualization of ventral and ventrolateral lesions, and excessive spinal cord manipulation to approach the floor of the spinal canal.
2. Technique.

Remove dorsal spinous processes of affected vertebrae with rongeurs. When using a high-speed drill, identify laminectomy depth by visualizing the white outer cortical layer; the softer, red medullary layer; and the white inner cortical layer. Drill the first two layers using 4- to 5-mm carbide burrs. Once the inner cortical layer is reached, use a gentle paintbrush technique with a 2- to 3-mm diamond tip burr to expose inner periosteum. Gently elevate periosteum and remaining interarcuate ligament with a dental spatula to expose spinal canal and spinal cord. When performing C2 laminotomy, use a high-speed drill with a 2-mm carbide burr to make fine laminar cuts as necessary to elevate the dorsal

spinous process and allow its replacement after exposure of the spinal canal and spinal cord. When performing dorsolateral hemilaminectomy, use a high-speed drill with 4- to 5-mm carbide and 2- to 3-mm diamond burrs to remove lamina and articular facets. Carefully identify outer cortical, marrow, and inner cortical layers of lamina and articular facets while drilling. Once the inner periosteal layer is reached, use a dental spatula and fine ophthalmic forceps to explore the spinal canal and intervertebral foramen. Identify the vertebral artery located ventral to the intervertebral foramen before manipulating the nerve roots and spinal cord. When using rongeurs to perform laminectomy procedures, carefully dissect the interarcuate ligament with a No. 15 blade and ophthalmic forceps to expose the intervertebral space and laminar edge. Accentuate the exposed laminar edge by grasping its dorsal spinous process with towel clamps and gently elevating the lamina. Carefully place rongeurs on this edge and remove lamina to expose the spinal canal and spinal cord. Dissect interarcuate ligaments from C6 to T1 to expose the spinal canal and spinal cord. Use of a high-speed drill is recommended.

X. Cervical Spinal Stabilization

A. Is used to repair a cervical fracture/luxation, malformation, malarticulation, or congenital subluxation resulting in spinal instability.

B. Accomplish stabilization by various techniques, including pins and methylmethacrylate bone cement, screws and Lubra plate, cross pins, and orthopedic wire. The specific technique used generally depends on location of the instability (see subsequent sections).

C. Perform surgical exposure by either a dorsal or ventral approach as described above.

XI. Healing of the Spinal Cord

A. Three basic categories of change occur following acute injury to the spinal cord: direct morphologic distortion of neuronal tissue, vascular changes, and biochemical and metabolic changes.

B. In the case of reversible spinal cord injury, a characteristic series of events occurs during the repair process.
   1. Approximately 2 days after injury, a heterogenous population of small cells (most likely of hematogenous origin), including polymorphonuclear, lymphocyte, macrophage, and plasma cells, invade the traumatized tissue.
   2. In 7 to 20 days, fibroblasts appear and begin laying down scar tissue. A concurrent glial reaction consisting of astrocyte proliferation and expansion of processes occurs.
   3. Depending on the extent of spinal cord injury, moderate to extensive fibrosis, nerve fiber degeneration, and multifocal malacia may be seen. Axons that have been severed, compressed, or stretched start to regrow, but will reach the edges of the scar mass and stop.
   4. Regeneration of spinal cord axons sufficient to restore function has not been achieved; however, if enough axons remain intact, return to clinically acceptable motor function can be expected.

XII. Suture Materials/Special Instruments

A. See Table 34-1.

XIII. Postoperative Care and Assessment

A. For the first 24 hours postoperatively, monitor respiration, administer analgesics, and observe for gastric dilatation-volvulus and seizure activity (particularly if the patient had preoperative myelography).

B. Use blood gas analysis in animals with ventilatory compromise. Respiratory depression or arrest secondary to cervical spinal cord manipulation has been reported; monitor patients carefully for this event.

C. Use low doses of opioids to provide postoperative analgesia.

D. Because postoperative pain can result in vocalizing and swallowing air, perform periodic abdominal girth measurements to assess presence of gastric dilatation.

E. Administer fluids at maintenance rates and turn the patient every 2 hours until sternal.

F. Discontinue corticosteroid administration postoperatively. If neurologic status deteriorates after surgery, give corticosteroids until the cause is determined and corrected.

G. Discharge ambulatory patients 24 to 48 hours after surgery. Confine for 2 to 3 weeks, and walk them on a harness for 4 to 8 weeks.

H. Treat nonambulatory patients with frequent hydrotherapy, physiotherapy, elevated padded cage rack, frequent turning, and bladder expression

Table 34-1
Special instruments necessary to perform cervical spinal surgery

Procedure	Instruments
Special instruments needed for most procedures	High-speed pneumatic or electric drill burrs: carbide and diamond tip, cautery unit (monopolar, bipolar), periosteal elevator/osteotome, suction, hemostatic sponge (Gelfoam), bone wax, dental spatula, dural hook
Ventral slot	Micro suction tip, 3-0 or 4-0 bone curette, vertebral spreaders
Dorsal laminectomy, axial laminotomy, dorsolateral hemilaminectomy, facetectomy	Duck-bill, double-action rongeurs, Lempert rongeurs
Fenestration	Tartar scraper, ear curette, No. 7 Bard-Parker scalpel handle
Spinal stabilization	Steinmann pins, methylmethacrylate bone cement, small fragment reduction forceps, vertebral spreaders

three to four times a day. Keep them clean and dry to prevent decubital ulcers.

I. Avoid indwelling urinary catheters because they are a frequent cause of urinary tract infection.

J. Use a supporting cart or sling to help nurse patients to an ambulatory status. Advantages of a cart include unhindered eating, drinking, micturition, and defecation. Additionally, animals with motor function are encouraged to ambulate, and an erect position facilitates physiotherapy.

K. Discharge nonambulatory patients when owners are able to care for them.

XIV. Special Age Considerations

A. Softer cortical bone of lamina, pedicles, and vertebral bodies of young animals requires less aggressive drilling and rongeuring than the denser, more compact bone of older dogs.

Specific Diseases (*SAS*, pp. 1063-1099)

Cervical Disk Disease (*SAS*, pp. 1063-1071)

I. Definitions

A. **Cervical disk disease** is associated with disk degeneration and extrusion causing spinal cord compression, nerve root entrapment, or both.

B. **Hansen type I disk degeneration** is characterized by chondroid degeneration of the nucleus pulposus, whereas **Hansen type II disk degeneration** is characterized by fibrinoid degeneration of the nucleus pulposus.

C. **Radiculopathy** is pain associated with nerve root compression.

D. **Myelopathy** is a general term denoting functional disturbances or pathological changes in the spinal cord.

E. **Diskogenic pain** is caused by derangement of an intervertebral disk.

II. General Considerations and Clinically Relevant Pathophysiology

A. Intervertebral disk disease is the most common neurological disorder diagnosed in veterinary patients.

B. Cervical disk disease accounts for approximately 15% of all canine intervertebral disk extrusions.

C. The most common site of disk extrusion is the C2-C3 intervertebral space; frequency of involvement decreases from C3-C4 to C7-T1.

D. Hansen type I disk extrusions are most common in the cervical region. With cervical disk protrusion, the nucleus pulposus undergoes degenerative changes and loses its ability to absorb shock. Continued degeneration and subsequent protrusion (Hansen type II) or extrusion (Hansen type I) of disk fragments occur spontaneously or secondary to trauma.

E. Location and force of the extrusion or protrusion dictate the degree of neurologic deficits.

III. Diagnosis

A. Clinical Presentation

1. Signalment.
   a. Middle-aged (i.e., 4 to 9 years), chondrodystrophoid breeds are most commonly affected.
   b. Eighty percent of cervical disk protrusions occur in dachshunds, beagles, and poodles.
   c. There is no sex predilection.
2. History.
   a. Most animals with cervical disk disease have acute neck pain.
   b. A stiff, stilted gait, reluctance to move the head and neck, lowered head stance, and muscle spasm of the neck and shoulder muscles are common.
   c. Approximately 10% of affected patients are tetraparetic (ambulatory or nonambulatory).

B. Physical Examination Findings

1. The location of extruded disk fragments within the spinal canal is the most important factor in determining whether affected animals have pain or tetraparesis.
2. If disk material extrudes in a dorsolateral direction (i.e., between the dorsal longitudinal ligament and vertebral venous sinus), nerve root compression and pain occur. This is the most common location of cervical disk extrusion in dogs.
3. If disk material extrudes directly on the midline (i.e., between fibers of dorsal longitudinal ligament), it causes spinal cord compression and subsequent tetraparesis. These patients may also exhibit neck pain as a result of tethering of nerve roots in the intervertebral foramina.
4. If disk material protrudes against (but not through) the dorsal longitudinal ligament, pain may result from pressure on pain-sensitive fibers of the dorsal annulus fibrosus and dorsal longitudinal ligament (diskogenic pain). Diskogenic pain rarely occurs in dogs.
5. Occasionally, patients suffer neck pain and front leg lameness (monoparesis) as a result of a dorsolateral disk extrusion in the lower cervical spine (C4-C7) that entraps a nerve root supplying the brachial plexus.
6. Pressure from disk material on the nerve root causes nerve root ischemia and severe pain and muscle spasm. Pain is often intermittent and generally manifests as a foreleg lameness.

7. Carefully evaluate patients with forelimb lameness to exclude cervical disk disease. Dogs with nerve root signatures (forelimb lameness) are often misdiagnosed as having orthopedic rather than neurologic disease. Perform a complete neurologic examination to distinguish between the two.

C. Radiography/Myelography

1. Well-positioned lateral and ventrodorsal survey radiographs of the cervical spine may be diagnostic for cervical disk disease.
2. Classical findings on plain radiographs include a narrowed intervertebral space, collapse of the articular facets, "fogging" of the intervertebral foramen, and "trailing" of calcified disk material into the spinal canal.
3. Use general anesthesia to obtain diagnostic radiographs in animals with disk protrusion.
4. Myelography.
   a. Use if there are no visible narrowed interspaces, if no disk material is visible within the spinal canal or intervertebral foramen, if a lesion is identified that is not compatible with the neurologic examination, or for precise localization of the disk, which is necessary to determine the appropriate surgical approach (e.g., ventral slot vs. fenestration, dorsolateral hemilaminectomy vs. ventral slot).
   b. Myelography is indicated in 90% to 95% of cervical disk patients.
5. Oblique radiographs.
   a. An intraforaminal or lateral disk extrusion is present in some animals with severe neck pain. Intraforaminal disk fragments cannot be seen on plain or contrast ventrodorsal or lateral projections; an oblique cervical radiograph is necessary.
   b. To obtain oblique cervical radiographs, place the patient in dorsal recumbency, with the entire cervical spine positioned at a 45- to 60-degree angle to the table. The left intervertebral foramina are viewed when the spine is obliqued to the right and vice versa. Fogging of the foramen is diagnostic for intraforaminal disk extrusion.

D. Laboratory Findings

1. Patients presenting with cervical disk disease rarely have abnormalities on CBC or biochemical profile.
2. Because most affected patients have severe neck pain, a stress leukogram may be seen.
3. Patients recently treated with corticosteroids may have elevated hepatic enzymes.

IV. Medical Management

A. Conservative vs. surgical treatment of patients with cervical disk disease is dictated by the patient's history and presenting neurologic signs.

B. Conservative management.

1. Patients treated conservatively that fail to respond may still benefit from surgery. Therefore treat most patients with mild to moderate neck pain from cervical disk extrusion conservatively before surgical intervention.
2. The most important aspect of conservative management in patients with cervical disk disease is strict cage confinement for 3 to 4 weeks. After this period, return to normal activity gradually over 3 to 4

weeks. Restrict walks to a leash and harness; avoid collars that encircle the neck.

3. This duration of forced rest allows resolution of inflammation and facilitates stabilization of the ruptured disk by fibrosis.
4. Strict confinement and exercise control may or may not be accompanied by administration of antiinflammatories or muscle relaxants.
   a. Commonly used antiinflammatories and muscle relaxants and their dosages are provided in Table 34-2. Use antiinflammatory drugs and muscle relaxants independently or in combination. Choosing the proper drug regimen is dictated by the patient's clinical signs and knowing the outcome of therapeutic trials.
   b. Recommended corticosteroid dosages vary dramatically among clinicians. Taper dosages over a 6-day period, and follow with serial neurologic examinations. If there is no response, consider repeat corticosteroid therapy, combination therapy, or surgery.
   c. Nonsteroidal antiinflammatory drugs may cause severe gastric irritation and ulceration, particularly if the dosage is above

Table 34-2
Dosages and regimens of drugs used in patients with cervical or thoracolumbar disk disease

Corticosteroids
Dexamethasone (Azium)
0.2 mg/kg PO or IM BID for 3 days, then SID for 3 days; reevaluate; may repeat treatment once or twice and consider combining with a muscle relaxant; if no response, consider surgery
Prednisolone
0.5 to 1.0 mg/kg PO BID for 3 days, then SID for 3 days; reevaluate; may repeat treatment once or twice; consider combining with a muscle relaxant; if no response, consider surgery
Methylprednisolone (Solu-Medrol)
30 mg/kg IV given once at anesthetic induction; discontinue after 1 dose
Nonsteroidal Antiinflammatories
Aspirin
10 mg/kg PO BID for 7 days; reevaluate; if no response, consider alternative medical therapy or surgery
Phenylbutazone (Butazolidin)
22 mg/kg PO TID (not to exceed 800 mg/day) for 7 days; reevaluate; if no response, consider alternative medical therapy or surgery (not recommended in cats)
Flunixin meglumine (Banamine)
0.5 mg/kg IV, IM, or SC BID for 2 days maximum; reevaluate; if no response, consider alternative medical therapy or surgery
Muscle Relaxants
Methyocarbamol (Robaxin-V)
22 mg/kg PO once as a loading dose, then 11 mg/kg PO TID for 10 days; reevaluate; may repeat treatment once or twice and consider combining with steroids; if no response, consider surgery
Diazepam (Valium)
1.1 mg/kg PO BID (not to exceed 20 mg/day) for 10 days; reevaluate; may repeat once or twice; consider combining with steroids; if no response, consider surgery

recommended levels, given for extended periods, or given in combination with corticosteroids.

d. Do not use nonsteroidal antiinflammatory drugs (NSAIDs) in combination with corticosteroids. Monitor these patients carefully for depression, anorexia, abdominal pain, melena, and vomiting undigested or digested blood (coffee grounds).
e. Muscle relaxants are generally unsuccessful when used alone to treat patients with severe neck or back pain; combine them with corticosteroids initially. Give muscle relaxants in combination with prednisolone, dexamethasone, aspirin, or phenylbutazone. Use a muscle relaxant alone in patients with mild or moderate neck or back pain, or in those with moderate to severe neck or back pain that are improving but require further treatment.
f. Knowledge of the potential side effects of commonly used antiinflammatory drugs (or combinations of drugs) is important.
g. If gastrointestinal lesions are suspected, discontinue corticosteroids and NSAIDs immediately because gastrointestinal ulceration associated with antiinflammatory medication, spinal cord injury, and stress of hospitalization may be fatal.

5. Educate the client about potential euphoric effects of antiinflammatory drugs. If strict confinement is not maintained during drug therapy, the patient could potentially worsen because of increased activity leading to further disk extrusion.
6. Antiinflammatory management of patients presenting with pain alone may be instituted multiple times without fear of inducing tetraparesis.

V. Surgical Treatment

A. General Considerations

1. The objective of surgery in patients with cervical disk disease is to remove extruded disk fragments from attenuated nerve roots or spinal cord. This may result in immediate pain relief and eventual restoration of normal motor function.
2. Ventral slot.
   a. Perform a ventral slot for removal of disk material in the cervical region.
   b. During ventral slot procedures adequate decompression of the spinal cord is achieved when the characteristic bluish hue of the dural tube is identified through the slot.
3. Use midcervical or caudal cervical hemilaminectomy and facetectomy for removal of disk fragments from the intervertebral foramen.
4. Fenestration.
   a. Recurrence of cervical disk extrusion at an alternate intervertebral space is rare; routine fenestration of unaffected disks after ventral slot is unnecessary.
   b. Use cervical disk fenestration to treat patients with neck pain secondary to cervical disk disease.
   c. Fenestration relieves pain in some patients, but does not adequately remove compressive disk material from the spinal canal or intervertebral foramen. Patients that undergo fenestration for cervical disk disease exhibit longer morbidity than those treated with ventral decompression (ventral slot).
   d. Tetraparesis may occur from overaggressive fenestration.

B. Preoperative Management

1. Give intravenous fluids and steroids before surgery. In addition to their therapeutic effect, intravenous steroids may protect the spinal

cord from the effects of surgical manipulation. Use methylprednisolone sodium succinate (30 mg/kg IV).

C. Anesthesia

1. Selected anesthetic protocols for animals undergoing cervical spinal cord surgery are provided in Appendix G-29.
2. Consider the animal's neurologic status and positioning required for surgery. If the patient is exhibiting motor weakness (e.g., weakly ambulatory or nonambulatory tetraparesis), or will require positioning that may cause respiratory compromise, consider mechanical ventilatory support.

D. Surgical Anatomy

1. Unique anatomical features of the cervical spine include the following.
   a. C1-C2 does not have an intervertebral disk.
   b. C6 has a prominent transverse process.
   c. C1 has a prominent ventral spinous process.
   d. Each vertebral body has a characteristic midline ventral ridge.
   e. Presence of transverse foramen (for vertebral artery and vein) in each cervical vertebra except C7.
   f. Characteristic cranial-to-caudal slant of each intervertebral space.
   g. Location of the vertebral venous sinuses and dorsal longitudinal ligament on the floor of the spinal canal.

E. Positioning

1. Place patients undergoing a ventral slot or fenestration procedure in dorsal recumbency with their chest in a V-trough. Carefully secure them with sandbags or a rigid vacuum type of apparatus to prevent lateral motion.
2. Tape the front legs caudally and tie a loop of rope around the muzzle, caudal to the maxillary canine teeth. Secure the rope to the table and pull the front legs caudally to apply linear traction to the cervical spine.
3. Linear traction stabilizes the spine and opens intervertebral spaces and foramina, improving exposure during the ventral slot procedure.
4. Prepare an area from cranial to the laryngeal cartilages to caudal to the manubrium sterni for surgery (i.e., ventral midline cervical incision).
5. Position patients diagnosed with intraforaminal disk extrusion in sternal recumbency with the neck elevated, cradled, and gently flexed.

F. Surgical Technique

Perform a ventral slot as described earlier in the chapter. Once the spinal canal has been reached, remove disk material located on the ventral midline first because removal of laterally located disk material increases the risk of lacerating a venous sinus. A dull, flat dental spatula is best suited for removal of foramenal disk material. Bend the dental spatula at a 60-degree angle to facilitate removal of laterally extruded disk material and reduce venous sinus laceration. Gently sweep the spatula along the lateral aspect of the spinal canal. Gently tease to loosen disk material from the foramen and encourage fragments to move toward the slot margin where they can either be suctioned using a small suction tip or removed with fine ophthalmic forceps. Take special care when old, calcified disks are encountered because they may be adhered to venous sinus or dura. Carefully tease and manipulate these disks away from the dura with a dental spatula. If severe hemorrhage from a lacerated venous sinus occurs, discontinue manipulation in the spinal canal and consider closing the incision. If hemorrhage can be lateralized to one side of the slot, it may be possible to manipulate and remove the disk from the opposite side of the slot, but take care to ensure adequate visualization before manipulation in the spinal canal.

VI. Postoperative Care and Assessment

A. Monitor respiration and observe animals for seizures for 24 hours after surgery.

B. Provide analgesics as necessary and discontinue corticosteroids immediately postoperatively.

C. Perform neurologic examinations twice daily.

D. Discharge ambulatory patients 24 to 48 hours postoperatively.

E. Base discharge of nonambulatory patients on the owners' ability to care for the animal.

F. Fit all patients with harnesses; avoid neck collars.

G. Restrict exercise of ambulatory patients for 3 to 4 weeks, then gradually increase exercise over the subsequent 3 to 4 weeks.

H. Stable interbody fusion after ventral slot requires 6 to 8 weeks; after this time gradually return the animal to normal activity.

I. Return of neurologic function is difficult to predict postoperatively; it may take 6 to 8 weeks (or longer) for the animal to regain the ability to ambulate.

J. Significant complications in patients treated surgically for cervical disk disease are uncommon. Possible complications include continued neck pain and deteriorating motor status. Treatment of the complication is determined by the cause and surgical treatment used.

VII. Prognosis

A. Prognosis for patients treated medically or surgically for cervical disk disease depends on neurologic signs, anatomical location of the disk extrusion, and medical or surgical treatment used, but is generally favorable.

B. Expect ambulatory patients with mild, moderate, or severe neck pain to be pain free or significantly improved by 24 to 48 hours postoperatively.

C. Expect ambulatory, tetraparetic patients (with or without neck pain) to be pain free 24 to 48 hours postoperatively and motor dysfunction to resolve by 7 to 10 days.

D. Expect weakly ambulatory tetraparetic patients (with or without neck pain) to be pain free 24 to 48 hours postoperatively and motor dysfunction to resolve by 3 to 4 weeks.

E. Expect nonambulatory tetraparetic patients (with or without neck pain) to be pain free 24 to 48 hours postoperatively and motor dysfunction to resolve by 4 to 6 weeks. Nonambulatory tetraparetic patients have a better prognosis if they do not have foreleg sensory deficits preoperatively, have a C2-C3 or C3-C4 lesion, and regain ambulation within 96 hours postoperatively.

Wobbler Syndrome (*SAS*, pp. 1071-1084)

I. Definitions

A. **Wobbler syndrome** is a disorder of the caudal cervical vertebrae and intervertebral disks (i.e., spondylopathy) that causes spinal cord compression (i.e., myelopathy).

II. General Considerations and Clinically Relevant Pathophysiology

A. The etiology is unknown but may be nutritional, traumatic, hereditary, or acquired.

B. Wobbler syndrome has been subdivided into five classifications distinguished by the location of the compressive lesion with respect to the spinal canal. The classifications are chronic degenerative disk disease, congenital osseous malformations, vertebral tipping, hypertrophied ligamentum flavum/vertebral arch malformations, and "hourglass" compression.

C. Chronic degenerative disk disease may originate from either vertebral instability (i.e., stress) or primary degeneration of the intervertebral disk (i.e., Hansen type II disk protrusion).
1. The degenerating annulus fibrosus undergoes hypertrophy, hyperplasia, or both.
2. Spinal cord compression occurs when the disk space collapses and buckles the redundant annulus fibrosus dorsally.
3. The dorsal longitudinal ligament (located dorsal to the annulus fibrosus on the floor of the spinal canal) compresses the dura.
4. Spinal cord compression in chronic degenerative disk disease is dynamic in that flexion and extension of the neck may vary the degree of spinal cord compression.
5. Generally, dorsal extension of the neck increases spinal cord compression; ventral flexion and linear traction decrease compression.

D. Congenital osseous malformations may occur anywhere along the cervical spine in one or multiple (most common) vertebrae.
1. Malformed vertebrae cause narrowing of the spinal canal as a result of stenosis of the cranial vertebral canal orifice, articular facet deformities, malformation of vertebral pedicles, or deformation of vertebral arches.
2. Congenital osseous malformations may be related to disorders of endochondral ossification.

E. Vertebral tipping is characterized by displacement (tipping) of the craniodorsal surface of the vertebral body (generally C6 or C7) into the spinal canal, causing spinal cord compression.

1. Instability secondary to chronic degenerative disk disease (or vice versa) may be the predisposing factor that allows the vertebral body to become malpositioned.

F. The compressive lesion in hypertrophied ligamentum flavum/vertebral arch malformations occurs on the dorsal aspect of the spinal cord. Patients with isolated ligamentum flavum abnormalities will probably develop hypertrophy or hyperplasia secondary to instability.
1. Vertebral arch malformations may be genetic or nutritional in origin. Whatever the cause, the vertebral arch, articular processes, and facets become plump, deformed, and asymmetric.
2. Spinal cord compression is not the result solely of deformation, but of a combination of static deformation and dynamic compression.
3. In dorsal extension, the cranial tip of the deformed vertebral arch of one vertebra is brought closer to the caudodorsal rim of the body of the adjacent cranial vertebra, increasing spinal cord compression.
4. When the neck is flexed ventrally, the cranial tip of the elongated vertebral arch is retracted, decreasing spinal cord compression.

G. Hourglass compression occurs because the spinal cord compression occurs dorsally, ventrally, and laterally.
1. Annulus fibrosus hypertrophy or hyperplasia causes ventral spinal cord compression, whereas hypertrophy or hyperplasia of the ligamentum flavum produces dorsal spinal cord compression. Degenerative joint disease or malformation/malarticulation of the articular facets causes lateral spinal cord compression.
2. Dynamic hourglass lesions may occur at any level of the cervical spine.

III. Diagnosis

A. Clinical Presentation

1. Signalment.
   a. Doberman pinschers and Great Danes account for 80% of the cases.
   b. The incidence of chronic degenerative disk disease is twice as great in males than females.
2. History.
   a. Affected animals generally become less coordinated over months to years.
   b. All four limbs are affected, but signs are generally initiated and more pronounced in the rear legs.
   c. Occasionally, an acute exacerbation precipitated by minor trauma may be noted.
   d. Approximately 40% of cases have a history of neck pain.

B. Physical Examination Findings

1. General physical examination findings are normal in the majority of patients with Wobbler syndrome.
2. Upper motor neuron signs (including a crossed extensor reflex) generally occur in the rear limbs of dogs with chronic disease. A broad-based stance is often noted in the rear legs.
3. Thoracic limb reflex changes are generally mild.
4. A stiff, straight-legged gait and atrophy of the supraspinatus and infraspinatus muscles are common with chronicity.

5. The neck is often carried in ventral flexion because this position produces the least amount of spinal cord compression.
6. Dorsal extension of the neck may cause pain or accentuate spinal cord compression, with resultant increased motor signs. Therefore take care when manipulating the head and neck.
7. Abnormalities noted on neurologic examination vary and may include pain alone, paraparesis, ambulatory tetraparesis, weakly ambulatory tetraparesis, or nonambulatory tetraparesis.

C. Radiography/Myelography

1. Plain radiographs of the neck are not diagnostic for the affected vertebra, intervertebral space (IVS), or location of the compressive mass within the spinal canal (i.e., dorsal, ventral, or lateral).
2. Although plain radiography may help diagnose Wobbler syndrome, myelography is essential to determine location and number of affected vertebrae or intervertebral spaces; location of lesion(s) within the spinal canal (i.e., dorsal, ventral, lateral); degree of spinal cord compression; and occurrence of dynamic compression.
3. Stress myelography is radiographic imaging of the cervical spine in various stressed positions (i.e., ventral flexion, dorsal extension, and linear traction) during myelography. It is essential to diagnose dynamic compressive lesions.
4. Classically, spinal cord compression with chronic degenerative disk disease is worsened with the neck in dorsal extension and improved in ventral flexion and linear traction.
5. *Do not* use dorsal extension in radiographic evaluation of patients with Wobbler syndrome because it may exacerbate spinal cord compression.
6. A complete myelographic examination, including linear traction, allows formulation of a rational therapeutic approach.

IV. Differential Diagnosis

A. Degenerative

1. Cervical disk disease.
2. Bilateral hip dysplasia.
3. Bilateral ruptured cruciate.

B. Anomalous

1. Atlantoaxial subluxation.

C. Metabolic

1. Any disorder causing generalized weakness (e.g., Addison's disease).

D. Nutritional

1. Nutritional secondary hyperparathyroidism.

E. Neoplastic

1. Tumors of the cervical spine, spinal cord, or nerve roots.

F. Immunologic

1. Polyarthritis.
2. Polymyositis.

G. Infectious

1. Cervical diskospondylitis.
2. Meningitis.

H. Traumatic

1. Cervical spinal fracture/luxation.

I. Vascular

1. Fibrocartilaginous embolism.

V. Medical Management

A. Wobbler syndrome is a chronic, progressive disorder characterized by subtle hindlimb weakness that often progresses to nonambulatory tetraparesis.

B. Medical therapy may cause temporary improvement; however, progression to an unacceptable neurologic status is common.

C. Conservative treatment.
1. Whether or not a patient is treated conservatively depends on classification of the disorder, degree of neurologic dysfunction, and number of affected vertebrae or intervertebral spaces.
2. The most important aspect of conservative management is strict confinement for 3 to 4 weeks, followed by a gradual return to normal activity over the next 3 to 4 weeks. Restict walks to a leash and harness; avoid neck collars.
3. Although this duration of forced rest allows resolution of spinal cord inflammation, the long-term beneficial effect on cervical spinal stabilization, malformations, disk degeneration, and tissue hypertrophy and hyperplasia is unknown.
4. Strict confinement, use of a neck brace, and exercise control may or may not be accompanied by antiinflammatory therapy.
   a. Educate clients about the potential euphoric effects of antiinflammatory drugs. If strict confinement is not maintained during drug therapy, the patient may become too active and have increased paresis as a result of acute spinal cord contusion.
   b. Commonly used antiinflammatory drugs and their dosages are listed in Table 34-2.
   c. Nonsteroidal antiinflammatory drugs may cause severe gastric irritation and ulceration, particularly if given above recommended doses or for excessive durations or when given in combination with corticosteroids.
   d. *Do not* use nonsteroidal antiinflammatory drugs in combination with corticosteroids.
5. If conservative treatment is successful, spinal cord edema resolves, remyelination occurs, and the animal recovers function.

D. If no improvement is noted by 3 to 4 weeks, or if neurologic deterioration occurs, consider surgical intervention.

VI. Surgical Treatment

A. General Considerations

1. The objectives of surgery in patients with Wobbler syndrome are relief of spinal cord compression, cervical spinal stabilization (where necessary), and reversal of neurologic deficits.
2. Although numerous surgical techniques (e.g., ventral slot, ventral stabilization, ventral traction-stabilization, and dorsal laminectomy)

have been described for treatment of Wobbler syndrome, only a few have long-term prognostic merit.

3. Base the surgical technique used on classification, clinical presentation, vertebral body or interspace affected, number of lesions present, location of the lesion within the spinal canal, and the presence or absence of a dynamic lesion.
4. The major disadvantages of ventral slot decompression are difficulty in adequately removing the entire compressive lesion and possible instability caused by the slot.
5. Techniques that employ decompression and stabilization have improved the outcome of patients with dynamic lesions.
6. Based on pathophysiology of the compressive lesion, techniques using linear traction stretch the annulus fibrosus, thus relieving spinal cord compression. Once the spine is stabilized in traction, the spinal cord remains decompressed and eventually atrophy of the annulus fibrosus occurs, further improving decompression.
7. Several ventral traction-stabilization techniques have been successfully used to treat patients with Wobbler syndrome, particularly those with chronic degenerative disk disease. These include Steinmann pins and methylmethacrylate bone cement, polyvinylidine spinal plates, and Harrington rods.
8. The initial approach for decompression and stabilization is as described for ventral slot; however, once the affected IVS is located, expose the IVS and vertebral bodies cranial and caudal to the affected interspace. This increased exposure is necessary for placement of the chosen stabilizing device.

B. Preoperative Management

1. Premedicate the dog with methylprednisolone sodium succinate (30 mg/kg IV).
2. Administer intravenous fluids throughout the procedure.

C. Anesthesia

1. Anesthesia considerations are described in Appendix G-29.
2. Consider neurologic status and positioning required for surgery.
3. If the patient has motor weakness (e.g., weakly ambulatory tetraparetic or nonambulatory tetraparetic) or will require positioning that may cause respiratory compromise (e.g., flexion of the neck, lateral compression of the chest), consider mechanical ventilatory support.

D. Surgical Anatomy

1. Refer to *Small Animal Surgery* or an anatomy text.

E. Positioning

1. For a ventral approach, position the animal in dorsal recumbency in a V-trough and carefully secure it to the table to prevent lateral motion.
2. Secure patients with a dynamic lesion (e.g., chronic degenerative disk disease, hourglass compression, vertebral arch malformation, redundant ligamentum flavum) to the table with the neck in linear traction. This positioning results in spinal cord decompression.
3. Place patients requiring a dorsal approach in sternal recumbency. Position patients requiring dorsal decompression with the neck elevated and flexed over a rolled fleece or rigid vacuum type of apparatus.

F. Surgical Techniques

1. Decompression via a ventral slot.

Perform a ventral slot as described earlier in the chapter. Once the spinal canal is reached, carefully remove redundant dorsal annulus fibrosus (i.e., dynamic lesion) or disk material (i.e., static lesion). Remove the ventral midline annulus or disk material first so as not to lacerate the vertebral venous sinus. Use ophthalmic forceps and a dental spatula to remove laterally located annular or disk fragments. Continue to remove tissue until the bluish hue of the spinal cord is visible, ensuring adequate decompression of the spinal cord. Lavage the surgical wound and close as described for ventral slot.

2. Stabilization with pins and methylmethacrylate.
   a. Use this technique to distract and stabilize up to two affected intervertebral spaces.
   b. Advantages of this technique include complete spinal cord decompression without entering the spinal canal and reduced risk of iatrogenic cord trauma.

Perform a ventral slot at the affected IVS(s), to the level of the inner cortical layer (i.e., 75% transdiskal slot). Drill the slot no more than half the width of the vertebral body; slot length is determined by the thickness of the vertebral endplates. Discontinue burring once the cortical endplate of each vertebral body is removed. Place a modified Gelpi retractor (see below under the discussion of special instruments) in defects burred in the vertebral bodies, cranial and caudal to the affected vertebral bodies. Create the defects just large enough to accept the blunted tips of the modified Gelpi retractor. Engage the retractor and distract the affected IVS 2 to 3 mm. Harvest autogenous cancellous bone from the heads of the humeri and place it into the distracted slot. Insert two 7/64- or 1/8-inch Steinmann pins into the ventral surface of the vertebral body cranial to the affected IVS. Insert the pins on the ventral midline of the vertebral body and direct them 30 to 35 degrees dorsolateral, to avoid entering the spinal canal. It is important to engage two cortices with each pin. Cut the pins, leaving approximately 1.5 to 2 cm exposed. Notch the exposed portion of each pin with pin cutters to allow the bone cement to grip the pin and prevent migration. Mix sterile methylmethacrylate bone cement powder with liquid monomer until it reaches a doughy consistency and can be handled without sticking to surgical gloves. Meticulously mold the cement around each pin; make sure each pin is completely surrounded and covered with bone cement. Irrigate the bone cement with sterile saline solution for 5 to 10 minutes to dissipate the heat of polymerization. Remove the vertebral spreaders after the cement has hardened. Close the paired longus colli muscles cranial and caudal to the cement mass. Close the remainder of the incision routinely.

3. Stabilization with polyvinylidine spinal plates.
   a. Advantages of this technique over ventral slot decompression alone include adequate spinal cord decompression without entering the spinal canal, reduced risk of iatrogenic spinal cord trauma, and improved recovery.
   b. Disadvantages include high incidence of implant failure in patients that do not tolerate a neck brace, need for a donor or bone bank, time necessary for allograft incorporation into an interbody fusion, and inability to provide adequate stabilization in patients with multiple lesions.

Identify the affected IVS and perform a ventral slot as described earlier in the chapter; however, carry the slot only to the level of the inner cortical layer (i.e., 75% transdiskal slot). Place the affected IVS in approximately 2- to 3-mm linear traction using modified Gelpi retractors as described for pins and bone cement stabilization. Create the slot configuration to precisely accommodate a full cortical allograft harvested from the distal third of the tibia of a 15- to 20-lb

donor. The graft maintains the IVS in linear traction, resulting in spinal cord decompression. Pack the cortical allograft with autogenous cancellous bone harvested from the heads of the humeri before placement in the slot. Once the graft is in place, remove the vertebral spreader. Place the polyvinylidine spinal plate on the ventral surface of the adjacent vertebral bodies to secure the bone graft in the slot. Secure the plate with two screws placed in each vertebral body. Drill and tap holes at a 20- to 25-degree angle from the midline to prevent spinal canal penetration. Determine screw length by assessing vertebral body width and depth from cervical spinal radiographs. Place autogenous cancellous bone on the ventral surface of the plate. Suture the paired longus colli muscles over the autogenous cancellous bone to hold it in place. Close the remainder of the incision routinely.

4. Stabilization with Harrington spinal distraction rods.
   a. Harrington spinal distraction rods provide distraction and stabilization in Wobbler patients without the use of a vertebral spreader.
   b. Advantages of this technique include adequate spinal cord decompression of two adjacent intervertebral disk spaces without entering the spinal canal, reduced risk of iatrogenic spinal cord trauma, and improved recovery of patients with two lesions.
   c. Disadvantages include inability to distract and stabilize only one IVS, implant cost, and possibility of implant failure in patients that do not tolerate a neck brace.
   d. This technique is most useful in patients with two adjacent lesions (generally C5-C6 and C6-C7).

Approach the ventral aspect of the affected vertebrae as described for ventral slot. Fenestrate the intervertebral disk spaces of affected vertebrae. Create slots in the vertebral endplates of affected vertebrae with a high-speed burr to precisely accept the tips of the distraction hooks. Turn the centrally placed nuts such that one nut moves toward each end to contact the hooks. Tighten the nuts to distract both hooks and intervertebral disk spaces. Place the IVS in 2 to 3 mm of distraction, and crimp the nuts or secure cerclage wire to the bolt adjacent to each nut to prevent loosening. Place cancellous bone in the slotted defects to promote interbody fusion. Approximate longus colli muscles over the cancellous graft and close the remainder of the incision routinely.

5. Decompression via dorsal laminectomy.

Identify and expose the dorsal aspect of affected vertebrae as described for dorsal laminectomy. After exposure of the cervical vertebrae, identify affected vertebrae (see the discussion of unique anatomical landmarks of the cervical spine). Remove dorsal spinous processes and laminae with rongeurs and a high-speed surgical burr, respectively. The laminectomy defect may be from three quarters the length of each vertebra to a continuous laminectomy extending from C4 to C7, depending on the extent of the compressive lesion. Limit the width of the laminectomy to the medial aspect of the articular facets of the cranial vertebra. First burr the lamina to the level of the periosteum of the inner cortical layer. Use a dental or iris spatula to carefully penetrate the periosteal layer and enter the spinal canal. Use an ophthalmic forceps and No. 11 scalpel blade to gently excise and remove the ligamentum flavum en bloc. If lateral compression exists, use rongeurs to resect the lateral aspects of the vertebral arches to the level of the vertebral artery and vein. Resect hypertrophied joint capsule and ligamentum flavum to achieve lateral decompression of the spinal cord. Place transarticular lag screws for vertebral stabilization if necessary. Drill an appropriate size hole through the cranial and caudal articular facets, bilaterally. Remove articular cartilage using a high-

speed surgical burr, tap the hole, and place a lag screw. Place cancellous bone around the joints to promote arthrodesis. Place an autogenous fat graft over the laminectomy site to help prevent formation of a fibrous laminectomy membrane that could result in spinal cord compression. Approximate paraspinal muscles and fascia; close remaining tissues routinely.

VII. Suture Materials/Special Instruments

A. Modified Gelpi retractors with blunted ends are useful for distracting affected vertebrae during stabilization procedures and are made by removing the hooked tips of a Gelpi retractor.

VIII. Postoperative Care and Assessment

A. Administer intravenous fluids and analgesics, monitor respiration, measure abdominal girth every 4 hours for 24 hours (for gastric dilatation-volvulus), and monitor for seizures (particularly if the patient had immediate preoperative myelography).

B. Discontinue steroids immediately after surgery and replace the neck collar with a body harness.

C. Postoperative use of a neck brace is generally dictated by the technique chosen and patient cooperation.
   1. Use a neck brace for the first 4 to 6 weeks postoperatively with patients that have ventral traction-stabilization using plastic spinal plates or Harrington rods.
   2. Do not use neck braces in patients that do not tolerate them because they may damage the implant while fighting the presence of the neck brace. Strictly confine these patients to cages.

D. For ambulatory patients, use strict confinement with harness walks two to three times daily for the first 2 to 3 weeks, then increase to normal exercise over the next 6 to 8 weeks. Avoid slippery surfaces.

E. For nonambulatory patients, use physiotherapy (passive range-of-motion exercises), hydrotherapy (swimming), and a supporting cart or sling until the dog has regained the ability to walk.

F. Pay special attention to good nursing care of recumbent patients to avoid decubital ulcers, urinary tract infections, and pneumonia. Use heavily padded, dry bedding or waterbeds to prevent decubital ulcers.

G. Assess patients initially by immediate postoperative radiographs to evaluate implants and by neurologic examination 48 hours after surgery.

IX. Complications

A. The most common long-term complication in patients treated with ventral slot or ventral traction-stabilization for chronic degenerative disk disease, vertebral tipping, or hourglass compression is development of a second compressive lesion at the interspace adjacent to the previously affected interspace.

B. It is presumed that once an IVS is fused, stress at the adjacent interspaces is increased. It is possible that this increased stress encourages development of spinal instability and subsequent spinal cord compression in some patients or that some patients have a predisposition to disk degeneration in the lower cervical spine that encourages a second lesion.

C. Whatever the cause, this phenomenon is referred to as the *domino effect* and has been reported to occur in 25% of patients at 5 to 60 months postoperatively.

X. Prognosis

A. Prognosis for patients treated conservatively is guarded, but also depends on classification, severity of neurologic signs, and number of lesions.

B. The prognosis for surgically treated patients depends on disease classification, severity of neurologic deficit, number of lesions, method of therapy available, and quality of aftercare.

Atlantoaxial Instability (*SAS*, pp. 1084-1088)

I. Definitions

A. **Atlantoaxial instability** is an alteration of the dens, ligaments, or both that span the multifaceted, diarthrodial atlantoaxial articulation and cause instability, vertebral subluxation, and subsequent spinal cord and nerve root compression.

II. General Considerations and Clinically Relevant Pathophysiology

A. Atlantoaxial instability is probably a congenital or developmental problem resulting in an unstable articulation between the first two cervical vertebrae.

B. Laxity may result from fracture, absence, hypoplasia, or malformation of the dens, resulting in a nonfunctional attachment of alar, apical, or transverse ligaments or improper formation, laxity, or rupture of the alar, apical, transverse, or dorsal atlantoaxial ligaments, resulting in lack of ligamentous support between the atlas and axis.

C. Trauma may elicit clinical signs in animals with laxity as a result of these causes.

D. Instability predisposes the patient to spinal cord and nerve root compression, often resulting in neck pain and ambulatory to nonambulatory tetraparesis.

III. Diagnosis

A. Clinical Presentation

1. Signalment.
   a. Atlantoaxial instability primarily occurs in toy-breed dogs. It has occasionally been reported in large-breed dogs and rarely in cats.
   b. It generally occurs in dogs younger than 1 year of age.
   c. Dogs that present with clinical signs at an older age generally have had instability since birth, but recent trauma has caused significant spinal cord and nerve root compression.
2. History.
   a. Progressive tetraparesis and incoordination, often associated with neck pain, are expected.
   b. Acute presentations can occur after seemingly minor trauma. Owners may report that the dog dislikes having its head touched.

B. Physical Examination Findings

1. General physical examination findings are usually normal.
2. Neurologic examination reveals a dog with motor weakness and UMN signs to the front and hindlegs.
3. Patients have varying degrees of neck pain.
4. Ventral flexion of the head will often exacerbate neck pain and may worsen the neurologic condition.
5. Exercise care during cervical flexion because the dens (if present) can cause spinal cord compression. Avoid forceful flexion at all times.
6. Do not forcefully flex the head of these patients, because it may exacerbate neurologic deficits.

C. Radiography

1. A preliminary lateral radiograph without anesthesia allows diagnosis of atlantoaxial instability with significant subluxation.
2. Use a flexed lateral view of the anesthetized animal to reveal increased laxity and subluxation of C1-C2. The instability is most pronounced dorsally.
3. A gap of 4 to 5 mm between the lamina of C1 and dorsal spine of C2 is diagnostic.
4. Ventrodorsal and open-mouth views may show absence or fractionation of the dens. Because the open-mouth view requires flexion of the neck, it is not routinely recommended.

IV. Medical Management

A. Medical treatment consisting of strict confinement for 3 to 4 weeks, a neck brace that maintains the neck and head in extension, and short-term corticosteroids may alleviate symptoms.

B. The neck brace, constructed of padded splint material, such as x-ray film or fiberglass casting material, must be worn during the 3 to 4 weeks of confinement, ensuring maximum scar tissue formation. Use corticosteroids (dexamethasone, prednisolone, or methyl-prednisolone) for 24 to 48 hours.

C. Recurrence is common.

V. Surgical Treatment

A. General Considerations

1. Use surgical correction of atlantoaxial instability when neurologic dysfunction is mild to severe (i.e., severe neck pain or weakly ambulatory to nonambulatory tetraparesis [with or without neck pain]) or a course of medical therapy has failed.
2. Objectives of surgery include reduction of atlantoaxial subluxation, decompression of spinal cord and nerve roots, and atlantoaxial joint stabilization.
3. Surgical techniques for decompression and stabilization fall into two major categories (i.e., dorsal and ventral).

B. Preoperative Management

1. Give the animal intravenous fluids and administer steroids before surgery (methylprednisolone sodium succinate, 30 mg/kg IV) to protect the spinal cord from the possible effects of surgical manipulation.
2. Assess serum glucose concentrations before, during (every 30 to 60 minutes), and after surgery in toy breeds. Supplement with dextrose-containing fluids during surgery, if necessary.

C. Anesthesia

1. Consider the patient's neurologic status and positioning required for surgery.
2. If the patient has motor weakness or will require positioning that may cause respiratory compromise, consider mechanical ventilatory support.
3. Trauma to the cranial cervical spinal cord during reduction of the atlantoaxial instability may cause transient respiratory arrest; therefore support ventilation during surgical manipulation of atlantoaxial subluxation.
4. Take care to avoid hypothermia and actively rewarm animals after surgery.
5. Use extreme care during intubation to avoid excessive neck manipulation in these patients.

D. Surgical Anatomy

1. The cervical spine is unique in its variable anatomical configuration from vertebra to vertebra, particularly C1 and C2.

E. Positioning

1. Position patients undergoing a ventral approach as described for ventral slot procedure.
2. Place the neck in a slightly extended position and fix in mild linear traction. This position reduces the subluxation and decompresses the spinal cord and nerve roots
3. Aseptically prepare an area from the intermandibular space to the caudal cervical region, including the heads of the humeri.
4. Position patients undergoing a dorsal approach in sternal recumbency with the head and neck slightly flexed. Aseptically prepare an area from the occiput to the caudal cervical region.

F. Surgical Techniques

1. Dorsal stabilization.
   a. General considerations.
      i. The dorsal approach allows reduction of the subluxation

and fixation of the dorsal lamina of C1 to the dorsal spine of C2.

ii. Bony decompression is provided by hemilaminectomy or reduction of the subluxation.

iii. Hemilaminectomy provides dorsal spinal cord decompression, but it does not correct the instability or relieve ventral spinal cord compression; in fact, it reduces stability of the fixation. Thus it is not recommended.

iv. Rigid immobilization using dorsal lamina of C1 and C2 is often unrewarding.

v. Reduction of the luxation and immobilization of the vertebra, without hemilaminectomy, provide adequate decompression.

vi. Provide dorsal fixation by a loop of orthopedic wire, synthetic suture material, or autogenous graft (i.e., nuchal ligament). Regardless of the material chosen, pass it under the lamina of C1, over the spinal cord, and tie it to two holes drilled in the dorsal spine of C2. The fixation relies on fibrous tissue to form a solid union.

vii. Frequent postoperative complications with this technique, include: breakdown of the suture or bone, tearing out of the suture with minimal strain because the dorsal arch of the atlas and dorsal spinous process of the axis in young toy-breed dogs have the consistency and strength of wet cardboard, and continued micromotion at the atlantoaxial joint causing the wire to fatigue and break. Additionally, improper placement of fixation material may result in spinal cord trauma.

viii. Inadequate reduction of the subluxation and inappropriate stabilization, especially if used in conjunction with hemilaminectomy, are possible.

b. Technique.

Perform a dorsal approach to the cranial cervical spine as described under General Principles and Techniques. Periosteally elevate epaxial muscle from the dorsal lamina of the atlas and dorsal spine, lamina, and pedicles of the axis. Carefully incise the atlantoaxial fascia caudal to the arch of the atlas and enter the epidural space. Incise the atlantooccipital fascia cranial to the arch of the atlas and enter the epidural space. Gently thread a loop of 25-gauge orthopedic wire under the arch of the atlas in a cranial-to-caudal direction. Thread the suture material through this loop of orthopedic wire and gently pull it under the arch of the atlas. Drill two holes in the dorsal spinous process of the axis and pass the ends of the suture material through the holes; one from right to left and the other from left to right. Reduce the atlantoaxial joint and tie the suture ends to maintain reduction. Close muscle, subcutaneous tissue, and skin routinely.

2. Ventral stabilization.

a. General considerations.

i. The ventral approach allows accurate anatomical reduction for decompression, use of transarticular pins for stability (placed in the most solid portion of the atlas and axis), placement of an autogenous cancellous bone graft to encourage atlantoaxial arthrodesis, and odontoidectomy if indicated (i.e., malformed dens).

ii. The technique is easy, fast, safe, and effective and involves the placement of Kirschner wires or screws across the C1-C2 articulation.

iii. Placement of Kirschner wires is described in the following text. Screws may be used instead of pins, especially in large-breed dogs with traumatic subluxation.

iv. The most common complication has been pin migration. This is effectively prevented by applying methylmethacrylate bone cement to the exposed portion of the Kirschner pins.

b. Technique.

Approach to the ventral aspect of C1 and C2 is as described for ventral slot. Periosteally elevate longus coli muscles from the ventral aspect of the atlas and axis. Be careful not to cause excessive motion of the atlantoaxial joint during exposure. Identify and open the paired atlantoaxial joints. Dissect the joint capsule from the ventral aspect of the vertebral bodies with a No. 15 scalpel blade to visualize articular cartilage. Use an ASIF small fragment forceps or towel clamp to grasp the midbody of C2. Place caudal traction on C2 to open the atlantoaxial joint, enabling safe removal of articular cartilage. Use a bone curette or high-speed pneumatic drill to remove approximately 50% of the articular surface, bilaterally. Expose the head of the humerus, drill a 1/8-in Steinmann pin through the outer cortex, and introduce a size 0 curette to harvest cancellous bone. Transfer the bone graft to the scarified atlantoaxial joints and reduce the subluxation, using the reduction forceps or towel clamps. Select two appropriately sized nonthreaded Kirschner wires (0.625 in or 0.45 in). Start the first pin close to the midline on the caudoventral body of the axis. Direct the pin medial toward the alar notch on the cranial edge of the atlas, with the point of the pin angled ventrally. An air-driven or electric drill facilitates accurate and easy pin placement. Place the second pin through the opposite joint, using similar landmarks. Cut the pins, leaving approximately 5 to 7 mm protruding from the body of C2 and notch or slightly bend the exposed pin. Carefully mold methylmethacrylate bone cement to incorporate both pins. Lavage the bone cement with cool saline to dissipate the heat of polymerization. Close muscle, subcutaneous tissue, and skin routinely.

VI. Suture Materials/Special Instruments

A. When using the dorsal approach, use braided polyester suture, nonabsorbable monofilament suture, or orthopedic wire as fixation materials.

B. For the ventral approach, use methylmethacrylate bone cement to prevent pin migration. Small fragment forceps or towel clamps aid in reduction and stabilization during pin placement.

VII. Postoperative Care and Assessment

A. Evaluate patients with atlantoaxial instability postoperatively in a similar fashion as patients with other cervical spinal disorders.

B. Because of the anatomical configuration of C1 and C2 in young toy breeds, consider any form of fixation marginal.

C. Regardless of whether a dorsal or ventral approach is used, support all forms of internal fixation with a neck brace and strict cage confinement until there is radiographic evidence of union.

VIII. Prognosis

A. Generally, prognosis for patients treated medically is unfavorable because of recurrence of clinical signs.

B. Prognosis for patients treated surgically using a dorsal approach is related to implant success or failure. If implants fail, prognosis is unfavorable. If implants succeed, prognosis is favorable.

C. Prognosis for patients treated using a ventral approach is favorable to excellent; even patients that present with weakly ambulatory or nonambulatory tetraparesis have favorable return to an ambulatory status.

Fractures and Luxations of the Cervical Spine (*SAS*, pp. 1088-1096)

I. Definitions

A. Traumatic or pathologic disruption of osseous and supporting soft tissue structures of the cervical spine may result in vertebral fracture or luxation and subsequent spinal cord and nerve root compression.

II. General Considerations and Clinically Relevant Pathophysiology

A. Cervical vertebral fractures and luxations occur less frequently than fractures and luxations of the thoracolumbar spine.

B. The most common cause of cervical fracture/luxation is automobile trauma. Less common causes include dog fights, gunshot injuries, running head first into a solid object, hanging by a leash or collar, and underlying metabolic or neoplastic disorders resulting in bone demineralization (e.g., nutritional secondary hyperparathyroidism, osteosarcoma).

C. Traumatic spinal fractures/luxations are induced by forces resulting in severe hyperextension, hyperflexion, compression, or rotation. They generally occur at or near the junction of a movable (kinetic) and immovable (static) vertebral segment.

D. In the cervical spine, the skull, atlas, and dens and body of the axis form a unit called the cervicocranium. The dorsal spinous process of the axis is secured to the lower cervical spine by caudal articular facets, spinalis and semispinalis muscles, and nuchal ligament. This produces a static-kinetic relationship between the cervicocranium and lower cervical spine; the axis (C2) is the point of stress concentration.

E. Traumatic forces applied to the cervical spine therefore culminate at the axis.

F. Failure of supporting structures of the spine to resist such stress results in mechanical discontinuity (i.e., fracture or luxation) with resultant spinal cord and nerve root compression.

G. Proposed areas of the spine with a static-kinetic relationship include craniocervical, cervicothoracic, thoracolumbar, and lumbosacral junctions.

H. The most frequent anatomical location of cervical fracture/luxation is the cranial cervical region with approximately 80% occurring at C1-C2.

I. Pathologic fractures generally occur when the integrity of bone is compromised because of an underlying disease process. Chronic calcium/phosphorus imbalances, primary and secondary neoplasia (e.g., multiple myeloma, osteosarcoma, metastatic neoplasia), and osteoporosis are examples of systemic disorders that can result in pathologic fracture. The cause of the underlying disorder must be determined and therapy instituted before spinal fracture/luxation repair.

III. Diagnosis

A. Clinical Presentation

1. Signalment.
   a. There is no breed or sex predilection.
   b. Cervical spinal fractures may occur in any age dog or cat; however, it is most common in patients younger than 5 years of age.
2. History.
   a. Patients with fracture or luxation of the cervical spine typically have a history of trauma. The majority have been hit by an automobile.
   b. They may appear to be in pain; hold their neck in a stiff, protected position; or present with varying degrees of tetraparesis, depending on the amount of spinal cord contusion/compression.
   c. Occasionally, patients may have no significant neurologic deficits on initial presentation; however, deficits may occur several days after injury.
   d. Perform careful physical and neurologic examinations to detect subtle deficits.

B. Physical Examination Findings

1. Handle animals suspected of suffering from cervical fracture/luxation with extreme caution.
2. Because trauma is the most common etiology, carefully examine all systems and treat for shock.
3. In patients with no obvious neurologic deficits, perform a careful cervical spinal examination. Perform gentle palpation for an area of hyperpathia (i.e., increased sensitivity to pain) by grasping the ventral aspect of the neck with thumb and fingers and gently squeezing each vertebral body. Discomfort on palpation suggests a lesion and warrants further diagnostics.
4. Carefully palpate the spine, also, to reveal information as to the type of injury sustained. Crepitus, excessive movement, or anatomical discontinuity of the spine suggests an unstable fracture/luxation.
5. In patients with neurologic deficits, perform a careful neurologic examination to localize the fracture or luxation and to determine severity of spinal cord and nerve root compression.
6. Characteristic findings of the neurologic examination (UMN or

LMN signs to the front limbs, UMN signs to the hind limbs) allow accurate localization of the fracture/luxation.

7. Because the most common location of cervical spinal fracture/luxation is C1-C2, the most likely sign is varying degrees of acute neck pain, with or without upper motor neuron tetraparesis.

C. Radiography/Myelography

1. Use survey and contrast radiography to accurately diagnose spinal fractures and luxations.
2. Take survey radiographs of conscious or anesthetized animals. Conscious patients may protect the fracture/luxation during positioning; however, an uncooperative patient may cause unpredictable radiographic detail.
3. If surgery is necessary or closer radiographic evaluation is needed, anesthetize the patient. Advantages of anesthetizing the patient for radiographs include excellent positioning and quality radiographs. The disadvantage is loss of inherent support and increased instability of the spine during transport and positioning.
4. Always handle anesthetized patients with possible neurologic abnormalities very carefully.
5. Typical radiographic findings in patients with cervical spinal fracture/luxation include any combination of these: discontinuity of bony structures (i.e., spinous process, lamina, pedicle, vertebral body), malalignment of intervertebral space or articular facets, fracture lines in the body or spinous processes of involved vertebrae, and loss of continuity or malalignment of the spinal canal.
6. Radiographs of the cervical spine may be difficult to interpret; oblique views are often necessary in addition to standard lateral and ventrodorsal views.
7. Radiograph the entire spine; 20% of patients with traumatic spinal injury have a spinal fracture/luxation at a second location.
8. Fractures may be classified as stable or unstable according to radiographic appearance and the force that caused the injury.
9. Forces resulting in laminar or pedicle fracture, dorsal spinous process fracture, articular facet fracture, and supraspinous/interspinous ligament rupture (dorsal compartment) are generally considered unstable.
10. Forces resulting in disk rupture, ventral longitudinal ligament rupture, and avulsion fracture of the ventral vertebral body (ventral compartment) are generally considered stable.
11. Forces resulting in a combination of dorsal and ventral compartment injury are generally considered unstable.
12. Radiographs reveal the status of spinal displacement only at the time they are taken. It is possible that spinal displacement during the traumatic episode was greater than that seen on radiographs. Evaluate the severity of spinal fracture or luxation radiographically and with neurologic examination findings.
13. Use myelography if there is suspicion of herniated intervertebral disk material (i.e., annulus fibrosus or nucleus pulposus), bone fragments in the spinal canal, no evidence of spinal discontinuity, or when radiographic findings do not correlate with neurologic examination.

D. Laboratory Findings

1. Patients with cervical fracture/luxation rarely have abnormalities on CBC and biochemical profile unless the fracture is secondary to a metabolic disorder (e.g., nutritional secondary hyperparathyroidism).
2. Because most patients present with severe neck pain, a stress leukogram may be seen.

3. Patients with a history of trauma or those that have undergone recent treatment with corticosteroids may have elevated concentrations of hepatic enzymes.

IV. Differential Diagnosis

A. Base presumptive diagnosis of cervical fracture/luxation on a young dog presenting with a history of trauma and physical and neurologic examination findings consistent with neck pain and tetraparesis.

B. Eliminate other differentials by physical, hematologic, serum biochemical, cerebrospinal fluid, or radiographic evaluations.

C. Confirm diagnosis of cervical fracture/luxation by radiography.

V. Medical Management

A. Patient stabilization is the initial objective. Treat patients with severe trauma for shock.

B. Stabilize the neck with a padded neck brace.

C. Give analgesics to control neck pain.

D. After patient stabilization, use physical and neurologic examination to localize the fracture/luxation.

E. Take radiographs of the cervical spine while the patient is conscious, for initial assessment.

F. Base the decision for conservative or surgical management on initial neurologic status, radiographic assessment of spinal stability, and serial neurologic examinations.

G. Manage stable fractures in patients with strong voluntary motor movements by conservative means, including strict age confinement, neck brace, and antiinflammatory agents.

H. Recommended drug treatment regimens are listed in Table 34-2.

I. Perform serial neurologic examinations twice daily to determine response to therapy.

J. If the patient does not remain quiet and causes further displacement of the fracture/luxation, is ambulatory but shows severe instability (palpation of a crepitant "click" over the fracture/luxation site while ambulating), remains unacceptably static, or deteriorates neurologically, consider surgical therapy.

K. Perform surgery if the fracture/luxation appears unstable, if the patient presents weakly ambulatory or nonambulatory tetraparetic, or if conservative therapy is unsuccessful.

VI. Surgical Treatment

A. General Considerations

1. Objectives of surgery in a patient with traumatic or pathologic cervical spinal fracture/luxation are spinal cord and nerve root decompression and vertebral stabilization.
2. In patients with pathologic fracture, determine the cause of the underlying disorder and institute medical therapy before surgical fracture/luxation repair. Once the underlying disorder has been controlled, perform treatment as described for traumatic fracture/luxation.
3. When selecting a stabilization technique, consider the following.
   a. Location of the fracture/luxation.
   b. Special anatomical considerations, because implant selection will be based on specific holding power in various regions of the cervical spine.
   c. Presence of a compressive lesion within the spinal canal; if a compressive lesion is identified within the spinal canal the removal technique is dictated by lesion location.
   d. Patient size, which affects the size and type of implant used to stabilize the fracture/luxation (the larger the patient, the larger the implant).
   e. Patient age, which may influence the surgical technique chosen. Younger animals usually have softer, more cancellous bone, whereas older animals have harder, more compact bone.
   f. Equipment available.
   g. Surgeon's experience.
4. Facilitate and maintain reduction of the fracture/luxation by two techniques: (1) by drilling holes in the ventral bodies of the vertebrae cranial and caudal to the fracture/luxation and placing ASIF small fragment reduction forceps in the holes, and (2) by fenestrating adjacent intervertebral disks or drilling holes into adjacent vertebral bodies to accommodate a vertebral distractor to gently distract affected vertebral bodies.
5. Approach C1-C7 body fractures/luxations, traumatic cervical disk extrusions, and atlantoaxial subluxation ventrally, as described for ventral slot.
6. Use Steinmann pins and methylmethacrylate (bone cement) for selected cervical spinal fractures or luxations. Generally, vertebral body subluxation or body fractures occurring from C1 to C7 can be adequately stabilized with this technique.
7. Appropriate exposure for pin and bone cement placement generally requires one or two vertebral bodies cranial and caudal to the fracture/luxation to be visible.
8. In patients with vertebral luxations it is advisable to prepare a ventral slot and pack it with autogenous cancellous bone to encourage interbody fusion.
9. Do not use ventral interbody screw fixation to stabilize vertebral body fracture or luxation because of an unacceptably high incidence of implant failure and vertebral body fracture.
10. Approach fractures of the lamina of C1 and dorsal spine and lamina and pedicles of C2 dorsally and stabilize with orthopedic wire, monofilament or nonabsorbable suture material, or methylmethacrylate to reestablish continuity of displaced fragments.
11. Perform decompressive hemilaminectomy only if bone fragments in the spinal canal cause spinal cord compression.

12. Because laminectomy and hemilaminectomy decrease the stability of an already unstable spine, do not routinely perform these procedures.

B. Preoperative Management

1. Give patients intravenous fluids and steroids (methylprednisolone sodium succinate, 30 mg/kg IV) before surgery; the latter are given to protect the spinal cord from effects of surgical manipulation.
2. Patients with open fractures (e.g., gunshot wounds, bite wounds) require antibiotics (see General Principles and Techniques).
3. Fracture/luxation of the cervical spine frequently causes laceration of vertebral venous sinuses. Surgical manipulation encourages further hemorrhage. Because venous sinus hemorrhage can be severe and life threatening, have blood readily available for transfusion.
4. Evaluate thoracic films in trauma patients for evidence of pneumothorax/pneumomediastinum and diaphragmatic herniation.

C. Anesthesia

1. The patient's neurologic status and positioning for surgery are important preanesthetic considerations.
2. Those with motor weakness (i.e., weakly ambulatory or nonambulatory tetraparesis) or those that require special positioning may be predisposed to respiratory compromise.
3. Reduction of cranial cervical fracture/luxations (C1–C3) may also traumatize the cranial cervical spinal cord, causing transient respiratory arrest; therefore support ventilation during surgery.

D. Surgical Anatomy

1. The cervical spine has a unique configuration from vertebra to vertebra, particularly C1 and C2.
2. Refer to *Small Animal Surgery* or an anatomy text.

E. Positioning

1. Place patients undergoing a ventral approach in dorsal recumbency with their chest in a V-trough and secure carefully with sandbags or a rigid vacuum type of apparatus to prevent lateral motion.
2. Tape front legs caudally and tie a loop of rope around the muzzle caudal to the maxillary canine teeth. Use the rope and tape to apply traction or countertraction (based on radiographic evaluation) resulting in complete or partial fracture/luxation reduction and stabilization.
3. Prepare an area from the laryngeal cartilages to caudal to the manubrium sterni for midline cervical incision.
4. Position patients undergoing a dorsal approach in sternal recumbency with the head and cervical spine positioned to encourage fracture/luxation reduction and stabilization.
5. Cranial cervical, midcervical, and caudal cervical exposures require slight variation in patient position.

F. Surgical Technique

1. Stabilization with pins and methylmethacrylate.
   a. The limiting factor of this procedure is the amount of pin purchase in the relatively narrow vertebral bodies of the cranial cervical vertebrae.
   b. In patients with a C2 body fracture, pin purchase cranially is established by placing cross pins bilaterally through the atlantoaxial joints, and caudally by placing pins in the caudal aspect of the C2 vertebral body.

c. This fixation is generally adequate for mid-C2 body fractures. However, if the caudal aspect of the C2 body is fractured, caudal pins are placed in the body of C3.

After fracture/luxation reduction, place two appropriately sized Steinmann pins at a 20- to 25-degree angle to the midline on the ventral surface of the vertebral bodies cranial and caudal to the fracture/luxation. Drive each pin into the vertebral body to engage two cortices. Cut the pins to protrude 3 to 4 cm from the vertebral body. Notch each pin with a pin cutter and place methylmethacrylate bone cement on the protruding pins, taking care to ensure that each pin is completely surrounded and covered with bone cement. Use cool saline lavage to dissipate the heat of polymerization. Close longus colli muscles cranial and caudal to the bone cement mass. Close sternohyoideus-thyroideus muscle, subcutaneous tissues, and skin routinely.

2. Stabilization with ventral cross pins.
   a. Perform ventral cross-pin or screw stabilization in patients with C1–C2 luxations or subluxations (refer to the section on atlantoaxial instability).
3. Stabilization with ventral spinal plates.

Fracture/luxations of C2–C7 may be stabilized by the use of ventral spinal plates. The fracture/luxation is exposed as described for ventral slot; however, the vertebral body cranial and caudal to the fracture/luxation is also exposed. Reduce the fracture/luxation. Fashion an appropriate size plastic or metal plate to the ventral aspect of the vertebral bodies, allowing for two screws cranial and caudal to the fracture/luxation. Determine screw length by evaluating vertebral body size from preoperative radiographs. Drill screw holes 20 to 25 degrees from midline to engage two cortices. Tap the holes and apply the plate across the fracture/luxation. It is impossible to safely engage two cortices unless screws are placed at an angle. Harvest autogenous cancellous bone from the heads of the humeri and place it in the fracture defect. Close longus colli muscles over the plate and graft. Close subcutaneous tissues and skin routinely.

4. Stabilization using articular facet screws.
   a. Fractures and luxations rarely occur from C3 to C7. As small dorsal spinous processes in this region preclude the use of dorsal spinous process plates, the only dorsal technique for C3–C7 stabilization is articular facet screwing.

Identify the articular facets of the articular processes of the fractured or luxated vertebrae. Remove the articular surface of each facet with a curette or high-speed pneumatic drill. Reduce the fracture/luxation by grasping the dorsal spinous process cranial and caudal to the fracture/luxation with towel forceps. Bring the articular facets into apposition. Drill and tap appropriate size holes in each facet. Place one screw in each facet joint in lag screw fashion. Harvest autogenous corticocancellous bone from the dorsal spinous processes of exposed vertebrae. Place the bone graft in and around the stabilized articular facets. Close epaxial muscles, subcutaneous tissues, and skin routinely.

VII. Suture Materials/Special Instruments

A. Facilitate careful reduction and stabilization of cervical fractures by the use of ASIF small reduction forceps and modified Gelpi retractors.

VIII. Postoperative Care and Assessment

A. Evaluate patients with cervical spinal fracture/luxation postoperatively in a similar fashion as patients with other cervical spinal disorders.

B. Because of the anatomic configuration of cervical vertebrae, particularly C1 and C2, any form of fixation is marginal at best. Support all forms of internal fixation with a neck brace and strict cage confinement until radiographic evidence of union.

IX. Prognosis

A. Prognosis depends on appropriate case management, including assessment of presenting neurologic examination, radiographic classification of the fracture/luxation, repair method, and postoperative care.

B. If adequate and early stabilization is performed (conservative or surgical), a favorable prognosis is possible.

Neoplasia of the Cervical Vertebrae, Spinal Cord, and Nerve Roots (*SAS*, pp. 1096-1099)

I. Definitions

A. **Neurofibromas** and **neurofibrosarcoma** arise from nerve connective tissue (medullary layer of a nerve fiber).

B. **Schwannomas** are benign tumors of the neurilemma (Schwann cells).

C. **Meningiomas** are slow-growing tumors that arise from arachnoidal tissue.

D. **Astrocytomas** and **ependymomas** arise from spinal cord parenchymal cells.

II. General Considerations and Clinically Relevant Pathophysiology

A. Tumors may arise from numerous sites in and around the spinal cord and may be classified as primary bone, primary spinal cord, primary peripheral nerve root, primary paraspinal soft tissue, or metastatic tumors.

B. Spinal tumors are also classified, according to their location relative to the dura, as extradural, intradural-extramedullary, or intramedullary.
   1. Determine the location myelographically.

2. The majority of canine cervical vertebral and spinal cord tumors occur extradurally and generally arise from bone (e.g., multiple cartilaginous exostoses, osteosarcoma, fibrosarcoma, multiple myeloma, chondrosarcoma).

C. Tumors may metastasize to the vertebra, causing spinal cord compression (e.g., hemangiosarcoma, undifferentiated sarcoma, lymphosarcoma).

D. Lymphosarcoma is the most common canine soft tissue extradural spinal tumor.

E. The majority of canine intradural-extramedullary tumors are nerve sheath tumors (e.g., neurofibroma, neurofibrosarcoma, schwannoma) and meningiomas.

F. Nerve sheath tumors arise from nerve roots, but often cause spinal cord compression because of their close proximity.

G. Meningiomas can arise from any location along the spinal cord, but they are generally near the nerve roots.

H. Intramedullary tumors are rare and include astrocytomas and ependymomas.

I. Lymphosarcoma is the most common spinal tumor in cats and generally occurs extradurally.

J. Intradural-extramedullary and intramedullary tumors are rare in cats.

III. Diagnosis

A. Clinical Presentation

1. Signalment.
   a. There does not appear to be a sex or breed predilection for cervical vertebral, spinal cord, or nerve root tumors.
   b. The majority of patients with cervical spinal tumors are older than 5 years of age.
   c. Benign solitary or multiple cartilaginous exostoses most often occur in patients younger than 1 year of age.
   d. When considering differentials in patients with neurologic disorders remember that "tumors know no age."
2. History.
   a. The classic history of patients with cervical spinal neoplasia is slowly progressing tetraparesis.
   b. However, some patients have an acute onset of neurologic abnormalities preceded by insidious, slowly progressing signs.
   c. Careful historical evaluation often reveals that subtle neurologic abnormalities occurred before the acute episode.
   d. Historical features may also vary, depending on location of the neoplasm with respect to the dura (i.e., extradural, intradural-extramedullary, or intramedullary).

B. Physical Examination Findings

1. Physical and neurologic examination findings associated with vertebral, spinal cord, and nerve root tumors depend on tumor location, degree of spinal cord compression, rate of tumor growth, and associated secondary effects of the tumor.

2. Pain is often associated with cervical spinal tumors, especially if they involve a nerve root (i.e., intradural-extramedullary), cause bone destruction or destruction of adjoining soft tissues, or are extradural.
3. Tumors involving nerve roots of the brachial plexus (spinal cord segments C6-T1) often produce forelimb lameness (i.e., monoparesis), progressing to hemiparesis or tetraparesis.
4. Neurologic examination may reveal UMN signs to the hindlimbs and LMN signs to the forelimbs.
5. Patients with an intramedullary tumor have acute paresis but no pain because there are no sensitive pain fibers within spinal cord parenchyma.
6. The presence of Horner's syndrome (i.e., miosis, ptosis, enophthalmos, and third-eyelid protrusion) localizes the tumor to spinal cord segments C7 through T2.
7. Diagnosis and lesion localization depend on performance and interpretation of the neurologic examination.

C. Radiography/Myelography

1. Use survey radiography in evaluating spinal neoplasia.
2. Osteoproduction and osteolysis from vertebral tumors may be seen on survey radiographs.
3. Some peripheral nerve tumors cause lysis of the intervertebral foramen.
4. Diagnosis of vertebral, spinal cord, and nerve root neoplasms requires myelography.
5. Myelography identifies the lesion as extradural, intradural-extramedullary, or intramedullary.
6. Occasionally, CT scans or MRI may be necessary to accurately determine extent of a vertebral or spinal cord lesion.

D. Laboratory Findings

1. Laboratory findings in patients with vertebral and spinal cord neoplasia are generally normal.
2. May reflect abnormalities caused by a paraneoplastic syndrome.
3. Changes in cerebrospinal fluid are usually noncontributory; however, cell type or evidence of an inflammatory process may suggest neoplasia.

IV. Differential Diagnosis

A. A list of differential diagnoses that mimic cervical vertebral and spinal cord neoplasia is provided in Table 34-3.

V. Medical Management

A. Direct medical management of cervical spinal tumors at both the primary lesion and secondary effects of the tumor.

B. Use corticosteroids to decrease peritumoral edema. The steroid of choice is methylprednisolone sodium succinate.

C. Definitive medical treatment, without surgery, is rarely recommended

Table 34-3
Differential diagnoses that mimic cervical vertebral and spinal cord neoplasia using the DAMNIT-V scheme

Classification	Examples	Diagnostic differentials
Degenerative	Cervical disk disease	Plain and contrast radiography
	Wobbler syndrome	History; plain and stress myelography
Anomalous	Atlantoaxial instability	Plain and stress radiography
	Congenital malformation	Plain and stress radiography
Metabolic	Any disorder causing generalized weakness (e.g., Addison's disease)	History; neurologic exam; laboratory findings
Nutritional	Nutritional secondary hyperparathyroidism (may cause pathologic fractures)	Dietary history; plain radiography
Neoplastic	—	—
Immunologic	Polyarthritis	Neurologic exam; laboratory data
	Polymyositis	Neurologic exam; laboratory data
Infectious	Cervical diskospondylitis	History; plain and contrast radiographs
	Vertebral osteomyelitis	History; plain and contrast radiographs
	Paraspinal abscess	History; plain and contrast radiographs
	Meningitis	History; CSF analysis
Traumatic	Cervical spinal fracture/luxation	History; plain radiographs
Vascular	Fibrocartilaginous embolism	History; CSF analysis; myelography

unless the tumor is inaccessible or the tumor type can be more effectively treated with chemotherapy or irradiation alone.

D. Surgical exposure and incisional or excisional biopsy are usually necessary to determine tumor type and plan adjunct therapy.

VI. Surgical Treatment

A. Preoperative Management

1. Before surgery, give the animal intravenous fluids and give steroids (methylprednisolone sodium succinate, 30 mg/kg IV) to protect the spinal cord from the effects of surgical manipulation.

B. Anesthesia

1. Consider the patient's neurologic status and positioning required for surgery.
2. If motor weakness (i.e., ambulatory tetraparesis, weakly ambulatory tet-

raparesis, or nonambulatory tetraparesis) is present or if positioning may cause respiratory compromise (i.e., sternal recumbency, flexed neck, or lateral chest wall compression), consider mechanical ventilatory support.

C. Surgical Anatomy

1. The cervical spine has a unique and variable anatomical configuration from vertebra to vertebra, particularly C1 and C2 (see General Principles and Techniques).

D. Positioning

1. Generally, patients with cervical vertebral, spinal cord, or nerve root tumors require a dorsal approach because ventral approaches do not provide sufficient exposure for tumor resection.
2. Position patients in sternal recumbency with the head and cervical spine gently flexed.
3. Choice of cranial cervical, midcervical, or caudal cervical laminectomy is based on tumor location and may require slight variation in patient positioning.

E. Surgical Technique

1. General considerations.
   a. Surgical objectives include exposure of the vertebral, spinal cord, or nerve root tumor; wide resection of neoplastic tissue; spinal cord and nerve root decompression; and vertebral stabilization.
   b. If wide resection is not possible, attempt biopsy and decompression.
   c. Definitive diagnosis of tumor type may suggest appropriate adjunct therapy.
   d. Patients with tumors of the cranial cervical, midcervical, or caudal cervical vertebrae, spinal cord, or nerve roots are approached via cranial cervical, midcervical, or caudal cervical laminectomy, respectively.
   e. Wide laminectomy, laminotomy, facetectomy, and foramenotomy are required for adequate exposure of most extradural and intradural-extramedullary tumors.
   f. Dorsal laminectomy and durotomy are necessary for exposure and removal of intramedullary tumors.

VII. Suture Materials/Special Instruments

A. Ultrasonic aspirators use high-frequency ultrasonic vibration to fragment (phacoemulsify) tissue; they reduce dense masses to a nearly liquid state that can be atraumatically aspirated. Ultrasonic aspirators are an invaluable addition to neurosurgical instrumentation, especially in removing neoplastic tissue; however, cost may be prohibitive ($25,000 to $70,000).

VIII. Postoperative Care and Assessment

A. Evaluate patients with cervical spinal neoplasia postoperatively in a similar fashion as patients with other cervical spinal disorders.

B. Base adjunct chemotherapy, irradiation, immunotherapy, or combination therapy on results of histopathology and surgical margins.

IX. Prognosis

A. Prognosis for patients with cervical vertebral, spinal cord, and nerve root tumors depends on tumor type, degree of surgical resection, and sensitivity to adjunct chemotherapy, radiation, immunotherapy, or a combination of any of these factors.

B. Malignant extradural neoplasms usually have an unfavorable prognosis.

C. Benign extradural neoplasms have a favorable prognosis.

D. Malignant and benign intramedullary neoplasms have an unfavorable to grave prognosis.

E. Extradural-intramedullary neoplasms have a guarded prognosis.

35

Surgery of the Thoracolumbar Spine (*SAS*, pp. 1101-1130)

General Principles and Techniques (*SAS*, pp. 1101-1109)

I. Definitions

A. **Dorsal laminectomy** is the removal of the dorsal spinous processes and portions of the lamina, articular facets, and pedicles of affected vertebrae.
   1. **Funkquist A dorsal laminectomy** refers to the removal of the vertebral lamina, articular facets, and pedicle to a level corresponding to the middle of the dorsoventral diameter of the spinal cord.
   2. **Funkquist B dorsal laminectomy** is the removal of the lamina above the dorsal aspect of the spinal cord (articular facets and pedicles are not removed).
   3. **Modified dorsal laminectomy** is similar to a Funkquist B procedure; however, the entire caudal articular processes are removed and the laminectomy edges undercut, causing additional exposure of the spinal canal.
   4. **Deep dorsal laminectomy** involves the removal of dorsal lamina, articular facets, and pedicles to the ventral aspect of the vertebral canal.

B. **Hemilaminectomy** is the unilateral removal of lamina, articular facets, and portions of the pedicle of affected vertebrae.
   1. **Minihemilaminectomy** or **pediculectomy** is the removal of portions of the pedicle at the level of the intervertebral foramen.

II. Preoperative Concerns

A. Perform serial neurologic examinations to determine surgical urgency.
   1. Patients with severe neurologic deficits, deterioration, or unacceptably static neurologic examinations may require immediate surgery.

B. Immobilize patients with possible unstable spinal fractures or luxations on a rigid platform or place in a back brace until definitively diagnosed.

C. Spinal surgery generally requires spinal cord and/or nerve root manipulation.

D. Preoperative corticosteroid administration may partially protect the spinal cord and nerve roots during surgical manipulation; however, steroids may predispose to gastrointestinal ulceration/perforation.

III. Anesthetic Considerations

A. Anesthetic management for thoracolumbar spinal cord surgery is similar to that described for animals with cervical lesions.

IV. Surgical Anatomy

A. The dorsal longitudinal ligament lies directly on the ventral floor of the spinal canal with venous sinuses running on each side.

B. This is also the location of the intervertebral foramen, its exiting nerve root, and radicular artery.

V. Surgical Techniques

A. General Considerations

1. Treat patients with surgical disorders of the thoracolumbar spine by dorsal laminectomy, hemilaminectomy, fenestration, or thoracolumbar spinal stabilization via a dorsal approach.
2. Properly position the patient.
   a. Position patients with spinal fracture/luxation to encourage reduction of the fracture/luxation and spinal cord decompression.
   b. Avoid placing towels or sandbags under the abdomen, which may divert venous return through vertebral venous sinuses.
   c. Avoid hyperextending the spine during positioning.
   d. Gently flex the backs of patients undergoing dorsal laminectomy to open articular facets and interarcuate spaces.
   e. For hemilaminectomy, gently rotate the affected side dorsally (about 15 degrees) to facilitate lateral exposure of vertebral lamina and articular facets.
3. Dorsal laminectomy allows entrance to all areas of the thoracolumbar spinal canal and spinal cord (i.e., dorsal, lateral, and ventral) for removal of herniated disk fragments, resection of vertebral, spinal cord, and nerve root tumors, and exposure of fracture/luxations.

B. Modified Dorsal Laminectomy

1. General considerations.
   a. Perform a modified dorsal laminectomy for exposure of compressive masses in the ventrolateral and dorsal aspect of the spinal canal (i.e., disk fragments, fracture fragments, vertebral and spinal cord neoplasms).
   b. Do not perform laminectomy of more than two consecutive vertebrae using this technique.

Make an incision over the dorsal midline to include two spinous processes cranial and caudal to the lesion. Use a periosteal elevator or small osteotome to subperiosteally elevate epaxial muscles from dorsal spinous processes, lamina,

articular facets, and pedicles of affected vertebrae. Use Gelpi retractors to facilitate gentle retraction of epaxial musculature during dissection. Control soft-tissue hemorrhage with bipolar cautery. Remove the exposed dorsal spinous processes to the level of the dorsal lamina with large, single-action duckbill rongeurs. Use a pneumatic air drill to begin burring the outer cortical (white) layer of bone from the lamina of both vertebrae. Remove articular processes of the cranial vertebrae with the drill, working carefully so as much of the cranial articular processes are left intact as possible. Continue drilling the dorsal lamina until the medullary layer of bone is encountered (it is red in appearance, soft, and easily drilled). Carefully burr this layer until the white inner cortical layer is visualized. The inner cortical layer is easily recognized in the midlaminar portion of each vertebral body; however, it becomes more difficult to recognize at the intervertebral space, where bone appears white throughout drilling. Before drilling over the intervertebral space, remove the interarcuate ligament (also known as ligamentum flavum and yellow ligament) using sharp dissection with a No. 11 Bard-Parker scalpel blade. Do not use a pneumatic bone drill because it tends to grab soft tissue and force the drill downward toward the spinal canal. Estimate drilling depth at the intervertebral space first by reaching the inner cortical layer at the midlaminar portion of the vertebral body cranial and caudal to the interspace. Drill remaining bone at the intervertebral space to the same level. Once the inner cortical layers of both laminae have been reached, use careful paintbrushlike burring until soft periosteum can be palpated with a dental spatula. Continue to burr until periosteum is palpable over both vertebrae and the intervertebral space. Use a dental tool and Lempert rongeurs to gently penetrate periosteum, and carefully pry the remaining inner cortical layer away. If necessary, undercut the dorsal laminae to gain additional exposure. Use a 2- to 3-mm diameter carbide or diamond burr to carefully drill away the inner layer of laminar bone. This is the recommended modification, because it provides greater exposure, ensuring atraumatic removal of compressive lesions. If hemorrhage from soft tissue occurs, use suction and bipolar cautery for control. If hemorrhage from bone occurs, apply bone wax to the tip of a periosteal elevator and gently press it on the bleeding surface. Lesions near the vertebral venous sinus should be manipulated with great care. Occasionally, venous sinus hemorrhage is incurred. Proper use of hemostatic agents (e.g., Gelfoam, Surgicel, Avistat) with cottonoid and suction helps control hemorrhage. Before closure, irrigate the wound with room temperature physiologic saline solution to dislodge any remaining bone fragments from soft tissues. Span the dorsal spinous processes cranial and caudal to the laminectomy site with 20-gauge, stainless steel orthopedic wire (wire is used for cosmetic purposes only). Harvest a piece of subcutaneous fat and place it over the laminectomy site to help prevent dural adhesions. Debride any devitalized muscle and close fascia and epaxial muscles with a simple interrupted pattern over the spanning wire. Close subcutaneous tissues and skin routinely.

C. Funkquist A Dorsal Laminectomy

1. General considerations
   a. Funkquist A dorsal laminectomy provides improved exposure of the lateral aspect of the spinal canal and spinal cord compared to a modified dorsal or Funkquist B laminectomy.
   b. Perform this procedure when compressive masses are located in the dorsal, lateral, or ventrolateral aspect of the spinal canal (i.e., lateral disk extrusions, lateral vertebral, spinal cord, nerve root neoplasms, lateral fracture fragments).
   c. Exposure of the spinal canal is limited to two consecutive vertebrae (one intervertebral space).

The approach is as previously described for modified dorsal laminectomy to the level of laminar and facet exposure. Remove exposed dorsal lamina and

cranial and caudal articular facets with rongeurs or pneumatic drill. Identify outer cortical, medullary, and inner cortical layers of exposed lamina. Enter the spinal canal by carefully penetrating periosteum with a dental spatula or Lempert rongeur. Use double action duckbill and Lempert rongeurs to remove remnants of the lamina, articular facets, and pedicles to a level corresponding to that of a dorsal plane through the middle of the dorsoventral diameter of the spinal cord. Carefully explore the dorsal, lateral, and ventrolateral aspect of the spinal canal, spinal cord, and nerve roots. Close as previously described for modified dorsal laminectomy.

D. Funkquist B Dorsal Laminectomy

1. General considerations.
   a. Funkquist B dorsal laminectomy exposes the dorsal aspect of the spinal canal and spinal cord.
   b. Perform this technique when compressive masses are located in the dorsal aspect of the spinal canal (i.e., dorsal disk extrusion, dorsal extradural neoplasia, dorsal laminar neoplasia).
   c. Laminectomy of up to three consecutive vertebrae can be performed using this technique.

The approach is as previously described for modified dorsal laminectomy to the level of laminar exposure. Remove laminar bone with a pneumatic bone drill, taking care to preserve the cranial and caudal articular facets. Identify the outer cortical, medullary, and inner cortical layers as you drill. Remove periosteum from the dorsal lamina with a dental spatula or Lempert rongeurs. Carefully explore the dorsal aspect of the spinal canal and spinal cord. Close as previously described for modified dorsal laminectomy.

E. Deep Dorsal Laminectomy

1. General considerations.
   a. Deep dorsal laminectomy provides excellent exposure of the dorsal, lateral, and ventral aspects of the spinal canal, spinal cord, and nerve roots.
   b. Perform this technique when maximal decompression within the limits of one vertebral length is required (e.g., vertebral, spinal cord, or nerve root tumors, and severe disk herniation).

This procedure is performed as described for Funkquist A laminectomy to the level of articular facet and pedicle removal. Carefully rongeur the remaining pedicles to the level of the ventral aspect of the spinal canal. Identify vertebral venous sinuses bilaterally and avoid them if possible. Control venous sinus hemorrhage. Gently manipulate beneath the spinal cord to remove ventrally located masses. Close as previously described for modified dorsal laminectomy.

F. Hemilaminectomy

1. General considerations.
   a. Perform a hemilaminectomy when the spinal cord is compressed by mass lesions in the lateral, dorsolateral, or ventrolateral spinal canal (e.g., disk extrusion, extradural mass, intradural-extramedullary mass, nerve root tumor, fracture fragment).
   b. Hemilaminectomy is preferable to dorsal laminectomy because it best preserves the structural and mechanical integrity of the spine, is less traumatic, is more cosmetic, and reduces the chance of scars causing spinal cord compression.
   c. Lesions that are lateralized on the myelogram are most apt to be completely removed via this approach.

d. Bilateral hemilaminectomy may be performed when the compressive lesion is on both sides of the spinal cord.
e. Unilateral hemilaminectomy can be performed along three consecutive vertebrae without producing clinically significant spinal instability, whereas bilateral hemilaminectomy can be performed along two consecutive vertebrae.

Make a dorsal midline incision to include two dorsal spinous processes cranial and caudal to the affected intervertebral space or vertebral body. Use a periosteal elevator or small osteotome to elevate epaxial muscles from their attachments on the lateral aspect of the dorsal spinous processes, lamina, articular facet, and pedicle to the level of the accessory process. Use a Gelpi retractor to maintain muscle retraction. Use a drill or rongeur to enter the spinal canal. Regardless of technique used to enter the spinal canal, be careful when manipulating lesions involving the ventral and ventrolateral aspect of the spinal canal, because the vertebral venous sinuses are in close proximity. Control soft-tissue hemorrhage with bipolar cautery and hemorrhage from bone with bone wax. Lavage the surgical site with room temperature physiologic saline solution to dislodge any loose bone fragments. Harvest a fat graft from the subcutaneous area and place it over the laminectomy site. Close epaxial muscles to the dorsal midline. Close subcutaneous tissues and skin routinely. If a drill is used, remove articular processes of the involved intervertebral space with a high-speed drill. Visualize a rectangular area from the base of the dorsal spinous processes dorsally, accessory process ventrally, articular facet of the cranial vertebra, and articular facet of the caudal vertebra. Drill the outer cortical bone of this rectangle, beginning cranially and working caudally. Continue to drill through the soft, red, medullary layer to the inner cortical layer. Once the inner cortical layer is reached, use a paintbrush action to expose the soft inner periosteum. Use a dental spatula or Lempert rongeu r to carefully enter the spinal canal. If rongeurs are used, remove articular processes of the involved intervertebral space with rongeurs. Have an assistant grasp and elevate the dorsal spinous process of the vertebra cranial to the involved intervertebral space with towel forceps. This maneuver will open the intervertebral space and facilitate exposure of the foramen. Place one blade of a Lempert rongeur into the opening and remove a small amount of bone. Continue to enlarge the opening cranially and caudally with rongeurs until the laminectomy defect is an appropriate size to allow adequate decompression.

G. Pediculectomy

1. General considerations.
   a. Perform a pediculectomy (modified lateral hemilaminectomy) for lesions confined to the lateral and ventral aspects of the spinal canal (e.g., ventrolateral intervertebral disk extrusion).

The initial surgical approach is as described for hemilaminectomy. Continue epaxial muscle dissection to the level of the caudomedial one fourth of the transverse process at the affected intervertebral space. This allows complete exposure of the intervertebral foramen and associated structures. Using the accessory process as a landmark, drill the slot defect just dorsal and ventral to the accessory process and extend it half the vertebral lengths cranial and caudal. If the radicular artery is encountered, control hemorrhage with bipolar cautery. Determine depth of drilling by identifying outer cortical, medullary, and inner cortical layers. Use caution when drilling the inner cortical layer and removing inner periosteum. Identify the spinal nerve from its origin within the spinal canal and its exit from the intervertebral foramen. Retract the nerve with a small blunt hook and remove the remaining portion of the pedicle to extend the defect to the floor of the spinal canal. After removal of disk fragments, harvest a fat graft from the subcutaneous area and place it over the

pediculectomy site. Close epaxial muscle, subcutaneous tissues, and skin as described for hemilaminectomy.

VI. Healing of the Spinal Cord

A. Healing of the thoracolumbar spinal cord is similar to that described for the cervical spinal cord.

VII. Suture Materials/Special Instruments

A. Special instrumentation necessary to perform dorsal laminectomy, fenestration, and spinal stabilization is shown by technique in Table 35-1.

VIII. Postoperative Care and Assessment

A. Determine the patient's neurologic status when the animal has fully recovered from anesthesia, and perform complete neurologic examinations daily until discharge.

B. Discharge ambulatory patients 24 to 48 hours postoperatively.

Table 35-1
Special instruments necessary to perform thoracolumbar and lumbosacral spinal surgery

Special instruments needed for most procedures	High-speed pneumatic or electric drill Drill burrs: carbide and diamond tip Cautery unit (monopolar and bipolar) Periosteal elevator/osteotome Suction Hemostatic sponge (Gelfoam) Cottonoid felt sponge Bone wax Dental spatula Dural hook
Dorsal laminectomy, hemilaminectomy, facetectomy, foramenotomy	Duck-bill, double action ronguers Lempert ronguers Microsuction tip Dental spatula Iris spatula Tartar scraper Ophthalmic forceps
Fenestration	Tartar scraper Ear curette No. 7 Bard-Parker scalpel handle 14- to 20-gauge hypodermic needle
Spinal stabilization	Steinmann pins Methylmethacrylate bone cement Plating equipment Dorsal spinous process plates External skeletal fixator

C. For nonambulatory patients, perform frequent hydrotherapy, physiotherapy, and bladder expression three to four times a day, and provide elevated padded cage racks.

D. Avoid indwelling urinary catheters to help reduce urinary tract infections.

E. Keep patients clean and dry to prevent decubital ulcers.

F. Use a supporting cart or sling to help patients return to an ambulatory status.

G. Nonambulatory patients should remain in the hospital until recovery of bladder function, or until clients can provide appropriate aftercare.

IX. Special Age Considerations

A. Take care when performing laminectomy procedures on young dogs because their cortical and cancellous bone is much softer.

Thoracolumbar Disk Disease (*SAS*, pp. 1109-1118)

I. Definitions

A. **Thoracolumbar (T-L) disk disease** is associated with chondroid degeneration of the nucleus pulposus of intervertebral disks producing extrusion, spinal cord compression, and nerve root entrapment.

B. **Fenestration** is creation of a window in the lateral or ventral annulus fibrosus to gain access to the nucleus pulposus.

C. **Durotomy** is an incision through dura mater to expose spinal cord parenchyma.

II. General Considerations

A. Management methodology is controversial and generally determined by clinical experience, rather than critically analyzed data.

B. Pathophysiology and pathogenesis of thoracolumbar disk disease are identical to cervical disk disease, as discussed in Chapter 34.

C. The most commonly involved sites of T-L disk extrusion are intervertebral disk spaces between T11 and L2.

III. Diagnosis

A. Clinical Presentation

1. Signalment
   a. T-L disk disease primarily occurs in chondrodystrophoid breeds of dogs such as dachshunds, Pekingese, beagles, miniature and toy poodles, cocker spaniels, shih tzus, Lhasa apsos, and Welsh corgis.
   b. Most disk problems occur between 3 and 7 years of age.
   c. Disk protrusion is rare in cats.
2. History
   a. The classic presentation is acute to subacute back pain only, or back pain in addition to varying degrees of paraparesis.
   b. Acute, rapid extrusions tend to be more deleterious than slow extrusions (i.e., days to weeks).
   c. Signs may be rapidly progressive, slowly progressive, remain static, or disappear and then later recur.

B. Physical Examination

1. Physical examination findings are usually normal.
2. The most common presenting neurologic abnormalities are varying degrees of back pain and upper motor neuron (UMN) ambulatory or nonambulatory paraparesis.
3. Perform a careful neurologic examination (see Chapter 33) for accurate localization of the affected intervertebral space.
4. The presence or absence of deep pain perception is an important prognostic tool.
   a. Patients with deep pain perception generally have a favorable prognosis.
   b. Patients without deep pain perception have an unfavorable to grave prognosis.

C. Radiography/Myelography

1. Obtain highly collimated lateral, ventrodorsal, and oblique radiographic projections of the entire T-L spine under general anesthesia to confirm the location of an extruded T-L disk.
2. Survey radiographs.
   a. Findings indicative of disk extrusion include narrow or wedged intervertebral space, narrow or "fogged" (i.e., radiodense disk material) intervertebral foramen, collapse of articular facets, and calcified material in the spinal canal.
   b. Survey films are rarely diagnostic.
3. Myelography.
   a. Myelography is indicated if there are no visible narrowed interspaces, disk material is not visible in the spinal canal or intervertebral foramen, a lesion is found that is incompatible with the neurologic examination, or when precise localization of the disk is necessary.
   b. Myelographic signs are consistent with an extradural mass.

IV. Differential Diagnosis

A. Differential diagnoses for extradural masses are intervertebral disk extrusion, fracture/luxation, diskospondylitis, congenital malformation, neoplasia, vertebral body and osteomyelitis.

B. Evaluate history and serial neurologic examinations to formulate appropriate management plans.
1. A staging system may help determine the most appropriate therapy (nonsurgical or surgical) (Table 35-2).

V. Medical Management

A. Ambulatory Patients

1. Manage ambulatory patients with strict cage confinement for 3 to 4 weeks. Gradually return the animal to normal activity over the next 3 to 4 weeks.
2. Medical management is successful approximately 80% to 90% of the time in patients with just back pain.

B. Nonambulatory Patients

1. Perform bladder expression three to four times daily, bowel management, and physiotherapy to maintain muscle mass and joint range of motion.
2. Provide easy access to water and food, and a soft, dry area to lie down.
3. A cart may speed recovery by allowing freedom of movement and by improving the patient's attitude.

C. Analgesics

1. Do not administer analgesics or antiinflammatories without concurrent strict cage confinement.
2. Monitor patients for gastrointestinal side effects, because ulceration associated with antiinflammatory medication, spinal cord injury, and stress can be catastrophic.

VI. Surgical Treatment

A. General Considerations

1. Consider surgery if presenting signs warrant surgical intervention, or if the patient fails to respond to appropriate medical management (Table 35-3).
2. The objectives include gaining access to the spinal canal and removal of disk fragments causing spinal cord and nerve root compression.
   a. It is generally accepted that patients with even mild paraparesis (i.e., motor weakness) should be treated by early decompression and mass removal via dorsal laminectomy, hemilaminectomy, or pediculectomy.
   b. Decompression in addition to prophylactic fenestration to prevent recurrent disk extrusion at a second site is also controversial. Recurrence of disk extrusion at an adjacent intervertebral space after decompression of the active disk is rare; thus prophylactic fenestration is probably not warranted.
3. The earlier spinal cord decompression is undertaken, the better the chance for complete neural recovery.
   a. Operate on patients requiring surgery within 24 to 48 hours of disk extrusion.
   b. Surgery is still a viable option in patients with severe neurologic deficits that have been treated medically for 72 to 96 hours; however, they may not recover to a normal neural status.
   c. Patients with several weeks to months of weakly ambulatory or nonambulatory paraparesis may benefit from surgical intervention

Table 35-2
Staging system to help determine medical vs. surgical treatment and prognosis in animals with thoracolumbar disk disease

Stage	Clinical signs	Radiography/lesion location	Treatment	Prognosis
I	Single or occasional episodes of mild, moderate, or severe back pain, +/– slight CP* deficits, no motor weakness	Radiographs not taken	Conservative	Favorable
		Incidental finding of degenerate disks	Conservative +/– fenestration	Favorable
II	Second episode or persistent and severe back pain, +/– CP deficits, +/– ambulatory paraparesis†	Radiographs not taken	Conservative +/– fenestration	Favorable/guarded
		Extruded disk in canal	Decompression	Excellent
III	Uncontrolled, severe back pain, +/– CP deficits, +/– ambulatory paraparesis	Extruded disk in canal	Decompression	Excellent
	Weakly ambulatory‡ or nonambulatory§ paraparesis, +/– back pain	Extruded disk in canal	Decompression	Excellent/favorable
IV	Paraplegia,‖ +/– back pain			
	Duration <48 hrs	Extruded disk in canal	Decompression	Unfavorable
	Duration >48 hrs	Extruded disk in canal	Conservative or decompression	Unfavorable/grave

*CP, conscious proprioception; †ambulatory paraparesis, patients with hindlimb motor weakness that can rise and ambulate without assistance, ‡weakly ambulatory paraparesis, patients that can rise without assistance, take several steps, tire easily, and assume a sitting or recumbent position; §nonambulatory paraparesis, patients that have lost the ability for unassisted hindlimb ambulation (voluntary motor movements may or may not be present); ‖ paraplegia, patients that have complete loss of both motor and sensory function.

Table 35-3
Recommended therapy* for patients with thoracolumbar disk disease based on neurologic signs

Clinical presentation	Initial treatment†	Result	Second treatment†	Result	Third treatment†
Mild to moderate back pain only; first episode or multiple episodes	No drug therapy; cage rest only	No improvement in 5 to 7 days	Muscle relaxant; follow daily	No improvement in 2 to 3 days	Steroids‡ and muscle relaxant; follow daily
Severe back pain only; first episode or multiple episodes	Muscle relaxant; follow daily	No improvement in 2 to 3 days	Steroids‡ and muscle relaxant; follow daily	No improvement in 2 to 3 days	Repeat second treatment or consider surgery
+/− Back pain and ambulatory paraparesis	Steroids for 1 day	Improvement	Continue steroids for 6 days	Improvement	Observe
		Static	Steroids 1 day	Improvement	Observe, consider surgery
		Deterioration	Consider surgery	Deterioration	Consider surgery
+/− Back pain and weakly ambulatory or nonambulatory paraparesis	Recommend early surgery; administer steroids preoperatively				
Recurrent mild, moderate, or severe back pain; unresponsive to medical management	Recommend surgery; administer steroids preoperatively				

*See *SAS*, Table 34-9 (p. 1068) for drug dosages and variations on duration of therapy. †All patients are placed in strict confinement for 3 to 4 weeks as part of their medical management regardless of the drug used or duration of drug therapy. ‡NSAIDs can be substituted for corticosteroids; however, the use of corticosteroids and NSAIDs in combination should not be considered.

if there is myelographic evidence of a compressive mass that can be surgically removed.

4. Do not perform laminectomy, hemilaminectomy, or pediculectomy alone without removing the compressive mass lesion.

B. Preoperative Management

1. Administer intravenous fluids and steroids before surgery. The steroid of choice is methylprednisolone sodium succinate (30 mg/kg IV).

C. Surgical Anatomy

1. The tough intercapital ligament from T1-2 to T9-10 attaches to each rib head and extends over the dorsal annulus fibrosus, acting as a natural dorsal buttress that helps prevent disk extrusion.
2. Disk extrusions generally occur at the junction of the vertebral venous sinus and dorsal longitudinal ligament (i.e., area of least resistance) resulting in a ventrolateral location of extruded disk fragments.

D. Positioning

1. Position patients for dorsal laminectomy, hemilaminectomy, pediculectomy, or dorsolateral fenestration in sternal recumbency.
2. Position patients for lateral or ventral fenestration in lateral recumbency.

E. Surgical Technique

1. Spinal cord decompression.
   a. The most common procedures used to decompress spinal cord and nerve roots are hemilaminectomy, pediculectomy, modified dorsal laminectomy, Funkquist B laminectomy, Funkquist A laminectomy, and deep dorsal laminectomy.

Regardless of decompression procedure chosen, enter the spinal canal by carefully lifting off periosteum with a dental spatula, iris spatula, or Lempert rongeur. At this point, disk material, black venous blood ("crankcase oil"), swollen spinal cord, or epidural fat will be visible.

   b. Acute disk protrusions.
      i. Acutely extruded disk material may be white flecks of disk incorporated in an organized clot, that when incised looks like crankcase oil. This type of disk is often easily suctioned and removal results in full decompression.
      ii. Extruded material may include portions of the dorsal annulus fibrosus. These fragments are white, firm, and cartilaginous in nature, easy to grasp with ophthalmic forceps, and often can be completely removed as a long continuous strand resulting in full decompression.
      iii. Occasionally, hard, white chalky disk material is found. Removal is accomplished by continual chipping away at the mass with a dental or iris spatula. Take care to protect the spinal cord, nerve root, and venous sinus during dissection because the majority of disks extrude ventral and lateral.
      iv. Mild to moderate shifts of the dural tube back to its normal position following laminectomy and disk removal indicate appropriate decompression.
   c. Chronic disk protrusions.
      i. Patients with a chronic history (i.e., months) of medically treated pain and ambulatory paraparesis that finally develop severe motor weakness and require surgery, often have a firm, encapsulated, protruded mass that may be adherent to venous sinus and dura mater (i.e., Hansen type II).

ii. Disk removal is difficult because of its hard, encapsulated nature, ventrolateral location (i.e., venous sinus), and adhesions to dura and venous sinus.

If the disk can be lateralized, perform a hemilaminectomy, including complete removal of the pedicle. If the disk cannot be lateralized, perform a deep dorsal laminectomy and visualize the protruded disk. Remove the entire pedicle to the level of the floor of the spinal canal. Expose the vertebral venous sinus at the level of the affected intervertebral space and transect the sinus, if necessary, to expose the encapsulated disk. Once the disk is adequately exposed, use a No. 11 scalpel blade to incise the disk capsule. Use a dental spatula, iris spatula, and tartar scraper to evacuate the firm disk material. It is rarely necessary to place dural sutures to manipulate the spinal cord and allow adequate visualization and removal of the disk. If the protruded disk is located on the ventral midline and cannot be adequately removed as described above, transect the nerve root at the site of extrusion (permissible only at T3-L3 spinal cord segments). Gently expose the nerve root and radicular vessels and cauterize them with bipolar cautery. As the spinal cord releases, gently roll it off the offending disk for better visualization and less traumatic disk removal. Remove disk material as previously described. Do not attempt to reattach the severed nerve root.

2. Durotomy.
   a. Durotomy is rarely indicated.
   b. Patients with complete loss of motor function and sensory perception generally have a poor prognosis. Consider a durotomy to evaluate presence or absence of myelomalacia to help in deciding patient outcome.

Carefully tent the dura with fine ophthalmic forceps. Use a gentle longitudinal stroke along the dura with a No. 11 or No. 12 scalpel blade. Penetration of the dura is obviated by the flow of CSF. A 1.5- to 2-cm long incision allows adequate visualization of spinal cord parenchyma. Observe the spinal cord for evidence of central hemorrhagic necrosis, loss of anatomic integrity, and a toothpastelike consistency. These findings are compatible with complete functional loss. Leave the dural incision open. Harvest a subcutaneous fat graft and place it over the laminectomy site.

3. Disk fenestration.
   a. Ventral approach.

Place the patient in right lateral recumbency and make a paracostal incision. Enter the abdominal cavity, identify the left kidney, and retract it ventrally. Pack off abdominal viscera caudally with moistened laparotomy pads. Elevate the iliopsoas muscle and locate the short transverse process of L1 for orientation. Digitally depress the aorta and sympathetic trunk to expose the ventral annulus fibrosus of intervertebral disks L1-2 through L5-6. Using a No. 11 scalpel blade or high-speed pneumatic or electric drill, create a window in the ventral annulus. Use a hypodermic needle (14 to 20 gauge), tartar scraper, or curved spatula to remove as much nucleus pulposus as possible. Place the patient through positional changes (i.e., lateral flexion and extension) to encourage evacuation of nuclear material. After all disks have been fenestrated, close abdominal musculature with absorbable suture material. Move the skin incision to the tenth intercostal space and make a thoracotomy incision. Place self-retaining retractors to hold the ribs apart, pack the lungs cranially with moistened laparotomy pads, and dissect parietal pleura from intervertebral disks T9-10 through T13-L1. Avoid aorta, sympathetic trunk, and intercostal vessels. Perform disk fenestration as previously described. Close the thoracotomy incision routinely.

b. Lateral approach.
   i. This approach is satisfactory for exposing disks T13-L1 through L5-L6.
   ii. Fenestration of disks T10-11 through T12-13 is more difficult.

Clip and aseptically prepare an area from T6 cranially to the greater trochanter caudally, dorsal spinous processes dorsally to midabdomen ventrally. Place the patient in right lateral recumbency if you are right handed, and left lateral recumbency if you are left handed. Place a 4-inch diameter sandbag or rolled towel under the L2-L6 vertebrae to create an arch effect that helps open the intervertebral spaces. Make a skin incision from the dorsal spine of T9 to the ventral aspect of the ilial wing. Continue the incision through subcutaneous fat, lumbar fascia, a second layer of fat, and to the longissimus dorsi, and iliocostalis lumborum muscles. Palpate the short transverse process of L1 for orientation, and with a pair of Kelly forceps, dissect overlying muscle fibers to expose its dorsocranial surface. Identify the lateral annulus fibrosus, located just cranial and slightly ventral to the junction of the transverse process and vertebral body. Use a blunt retractor to expose the lateral surface of the annulus fibrosus; retract muscle fibers dorsally and muscle fibers, spinal nerve, and spinal vessels ventrally. Use a No. 11 scalpel blade to make a window in the lateral aspect of the annulus fibrosus. Be careful not to incise dorsal to the junction of the transverse process and vertebral body because this may result in spinal cord damage. Perform disk fenestration as described for ventral fenestration. To fenestrate disks T10-11 through T12-13, elevate the iliocostalis lumborum muscle off the craniodorsal aspect of the rib to the level of the vertebral body and retract it craniodorsally. Retract the remaining musculature on the cranial aspect of the rib ventrally, exposing the lateral annulus. The thoracic pleura is just ventral to this dissection. Visualization is limited; be careful to stay below the arch of the rib when incising the annulus fibrosus. After all disks have been fenestrated, use positional changes to encourage further evacuation of nuclear material. Close muscle, subcutaneous tissues, and skin routinely.

c. Dorsolateral approach.

Place the patient in ventral recumbency with the spine gently arched dorsally. Make a dorsal midline skin incision from the dorsal spinous process of T9 to the dorsal spinous process of L6. Continue dissection to the level of the thoracolumbar fascia. Incise the thoracolumbar fascia along the dorsal spinous processes on the side toward the surgeon. Using a periosteal elevator or small osteotome, elevate epaxial muscles from the lateral aspect of the dorsal spinous processes, working in a caudal to cranial direction. Elevate a second level of epaxial muscle from articular facets. Begin by elevating musculature from the caudal aspect of the articular process and progress to the cranial aspect. Use curved scissors to sever muscular attachments close to their tendon of origin to minimize hemorrhage. Place Gelpi retractors to hold muscles apart and improve exposure. Elevate remaining musculature from the dorsal aspect of the transverse processes of lumbar vertebrae and cranial surface of the ribs of thoracic vertebrae. Identify muscular attachments to the accessory process, spinal nerve, and vessels. Retract these structures cranially to expose the lateral surface of the annulus fibrosus. Perform fenestration as described for ventral fenestration. Close muscle, subcutaneous tissues, and skin routinely.

VII. Postoperative Care and Assessment

A. Encourage physiotherapy as soon as the patient has recovered from postoperative discomfort, generally in 24 to 48 hours.

B. Instruct clients in home management and send these patients home within 72 hours of surgery, even if they are weakly ambulatory or nonambulatory paraparetic.
  1. Express the bladder three to four times daily until voluntary urination occurs.

VIII. Prognosis

A. Inform owners that prognosis for patients treated medically or surgically for T-L disk disease is generally favorable and depends on neurologic signs and the medical or surgical management selected.

Fractures and Luxations of the Thoracolumbar Spine (*SAS*, pp. 1118-1128)

I. General Considerations

A. The thoracolumbar spine is the most common site for spinal fractures and luxations, with the majority occurring between T11 and L6.

B. Fractures involving T1 through T9 are relatively uncommon; when they do occur, they are generally stable and nondisplaced because of the inherent stability gained by massive epaxial muscle mass, rib attachments, ligamentous support, and intercostal muscle attachments.

C. Perform a complete physical examination because patients with vertebral fractures often have concurrent injuries.

D. Approximately 20% of patients have a second spinal fracture/luxation.

E. Pathologic fractures/luxations generally occur when hereditary or congenital ligamentous instability decreases spinal support (e.g., atlantoaxial instability) or when bone integrity is compromised because of an underlying disease process (e.g., metabolic bone disease, neoplasia).

II. Diagnosis

A. Clinical Presentation

1. Signalment.
   a. There is no breed or sex predisposition; however, dogs more commonly sustain vertebral fracture/luxation than cats.
   b. Vertebral fractures may occur at any age, but are more common in younger animals (i.e., 1 to 2 years of age).
2. History.
   a. Patients with thoracolumbar vertebral fractures typically present because of trauma associated with automobiles.
   b. They usually have varying degrees of back pain and paraparesis, but occasionally have subtle neurologic deficits.

B. Physical Examination

1. Examine for concurrent injuries.
2. Take extreme care during physical examination to avoid exacerbating the spinal injury by excessive movement.
   a. Secure patients with profound neurologic deficits to a rigid platform during examination and preoperative management.
3. Carefully palpate the spine for a depression over its dorsal aspect, or for a displaced or fractured dorsal spinous process.
4. If the patient is ambulatory, palpate the back for crepitus or excessive movement as the patient moves.
5. Perform a thorough neurologic examination.

C. Radiography

1. Take survey radiographs (lateral and cross-table ventrodorsal projections) on the awake or anesthetized patient.
   a. Because up to 20% have a second spinal fracture/luxation obtain a complete spinal series for all patients with traumatic spinal injury.
2. Radiographs may not show the maximum displacement at the time of injury.
   a. Spontaneous reduction of subluxations, luxations, and fractures often occurs before radiography.
3. Neurologic examination findings are more useful than radiographic findings in discerning extent of injury and prognosis.
   a. Markedly displaced fractures may be found in ambulatory animals and no discernible radiographic lesion may be evident in animals without deep pain.
   b. Radiographs may help determine prognosis when vertebral displacement is severe enough to reduce spinal canal diameter more than 80% in the lateral and ventrodorsal projections; these patients generally have irreversible spinal cord and nerve root compression.
4. Perform myelography if there is a suspicion of herniated intervertebral disk material, bone fragments in the spinal canal, no evidence of vertebral discontinuity, or when radiographic findings do not correlate with neurologic examination.

III. Medical Management

A. Provide medical management, including strict confinement, a back brace, antiinflammatory medication, and serial neurologic examinations.
1. Restrict ambulatory patients to a cage, or a small room or kennel for 2 to 3 weeks.
2. Use a comfortable, well-padded back brace or body splint constructed from basswood or light-weight, moldable fiberglass to support the spine.
   a. Although the efficacy of a back brace may be questioned, it appears useful to counteract excessive ventral and lateral flexion of the torso while the patient is confined.
3. Provide nonambulatory patients with easy access to water and food and a soft, dry area to lie down.
4. Perform bladder expression three to four times a day, bowel management, and physiotherapy to maintain muscle mass and joint range of motion.
   a. Do not use a cart because the supporting bars place pressure on the thoracolumbar spine.

IV. Surgical Treatment

A. General Considerations

1. Perform surgery on patients that fail to respond to an appropriate course of medical management or present with profound neurologic deficits.
2. Objectives of surgical treatment include the following.
   a. Spinal cord and nerve root decompression by fracture/luxation reduction.
      i. Laminectomy and mass removal are rarely needed.
   b. Vertebral fracture/luxation stabilization.
      i. Select technique by location of the fracture, size, age, and disposition of the patient, equipment available, and experience of the surgeon.

B. Preoperative Management

1. Administer intravenous fluids and steroids before surgery. The steroid of choice is methylprednisolone sodium succinate (30 mg/kg IV).

C. Positioning

1. In general, position the patient in sternal recumbency.

D. Surgical Technique

1. Steinmann pins and bone cement.
   a. General considerations.
      i. This technique can be performed on any area of the spine (i.e., thoracic, thoracolumbar, lumbar, lumbosacral) and in any age or size animal of any disposition; it is performed easily and requires a minimum of special equipment.

Approach the spine as described for modified dorsal laminectomy. Place towel forceps in the dorsal spinous processes of the vertebrae cranial and caudal to the fracture/luxation; apply traction and countertraction during epaxial muscle elevation from lamina and pedicles. This helps avoid fracture/luxation displacement during dissection. Continue dissection ventrally to the level of the costal fovea of the transverse processes if a thoracic vertebra is involved, or the base of the transverse processes if a lumbar vertebra is involved. If a dorsal laminectomy or hemilaminectomy is indicated, perform one as described previously. Reduce the vertebral fracture/luxation using bone-holding forceps or towel clamps applied to the dorsal spinous processes. Facilitate reduction by having two nonsterile assistants apply gentle traction on the head and tail. Maintain reduction of the fracture/luxation with traction on towel clamps, or if a dorsal laminectomy is not performed, place a 0.45-inch Kirschner wire across each articular facet. Use an electric or air driven drill to place Steinmann pins into the vertebral bodies on each side of the fracture/luxation. In the thoracic vertebrae, place pins into the pedicle and drive them into the vertebral body, using the tubercle of the ribs and base of the accessory processes as anatomic landmarks. In the lumbar vertebrae, place pins into the vertebral bodies, using the accessory processes and transverse processes as landmarks. Direct the Steinmann pins cranioventrally and from lateral to medial in the vertebral body cranial to the fracture/luxation, and caudoventrally and from lateral to medial in the vertebral body caudal to the fracture/luxation. Drive each Steinmann pin to exit 2 to 3 mm from the ventral aspect of the vertebral body. Cut the pins 3 to 4 mm below the level of the dorsal spinous processes. Notch each pin at its dorsal aspect with a pin cutter. If a laminectomy was performed, cover the defect with an autogenous fat graft. Thoroughly mix the liquid monomer with polymer powder. Once the

methylmethacrylate can be handled without sticking to the surgeon's gloves, pack it around the Steinmann pins, making sure it contacts all surfaces of each pin and covers the dorsal aspects. If a dorsal laminectomy or hemilaminectomy has been performed, mold the methylmethacrylate into the shape of a doughnut as it is packed around the Steinmann pins. Take care not to allow methylmethacrylate to contact spinal cord or nerve roots. If a laminectomy was not performed, apply a circular mass of methylmethacrylate, incorporating Steinmann pins, articular facets, lamina, pedicles, and adjacent dorsal spinous process. If a fractured vertebral body must be spanned, place pins in the body cranial and caudal to the fractured body. Use the same technique as previously described. Lavage the methylmethacrylate with cool saline for 5 minutes to dissipate the heat of polymerization. If necessary, excise portions of epaxial muscles adjacent to methylmethacrylate, to facilitate closure. Close lumbodorsal fascia to the dorsal midline with nonabsorbable monofilament suture material in a simple interrupted pattern. Rarely, relief incisions in the lumbodorsal fascia lateral to the methylmethacrylate are necessary to facilitate closure. Close subcutaneous tissues and skin routinely.

2. Dorsolateral vertebral body plating.
   a. General considerations.
      i. Dorsolateral vertebral body plating requires dorsolateral exposure of lamina, pedicles, facet, and transverse process of lumbar vertebrae or lamina, pedicle, facet and rib head of thoracic vertebrae; the approach is as described for hemilaminectomy.
      ii. Obtain exposure of articular processes of the vertebra to be plated and articular processes of vertebrae cranial and caudal to these.
      iii. If the luxation, subluxation, or fracture is close to the intervertebral space, stabilization of the two adjacent vertebrae is adequate. If a midbody fracture exists, span three vertebral bodies by the plate.

Identify and protect spinal nerve roots encountered cranial and caudal to the fracture/luxation. Using bipolar cautery, carefully cauterize the vessels and nerve root emerging from the intervertebral foramen between the vertebrae to be plated. Carefully sever the vessels and nerve root. If a hemilaminectomy is indicated, perform it now. Select a bone plate that will allow placement of two screws in each vertebral body cranial and caudal to the affected intervertebral space (luxation, subluxation) or affected vertebral body (fracture). Reduce and stabilize the fracture/luxation by placing towel clamps in the dorsal spinous processes of the vertebrae cranial and caudal to the fracture/luxation to provide a means of traction and countertraction. If a laminectomy is not performed, place a 0.45-inch Kirschner wire through the reduced articular facet to maintain reduction. Lay the plate on the dorsolateral surface of the reduced vertebral body, ventral to the articular facet or laminectomy defect. Drill and tap screw holes to ensure four cortices are engaged cranial and caudal to the involved fracture/luxation. Judge the proper angle for each hole by referring to an anatomic specimen. If a laminectomy is performed, use the anatomic location of the spinal cord and spinal canal as reference points to determine proper drill angle. After the hole is drilled, measure the depth with a depth gauge, tap the hole, select an appropriate length screw, and secure the plate to the vertebral body. For thoracic vertebrae, expose the rib heads of the vertebral bodies to be plated. Use a bone-cutting forceps to cut the rib head from its attachment to the vertebral body. Contour the transverse process with rongeurs until the plate lies flat against the vertebral body. Secure the plate as previously described. Reattach the severed ribs to the dorsal spinous processes with orthopedic wire. Lavage the surgical site with sterile saline solution, harvest an autogenous fat graft and place it over the laminectomy site, appose epaxial muscles with

nonabsorbable monofilament suture, and close subcutaneous tissues and skin routinely.

3. Dorsal spinous process plating.
   a. General considerations.
      i. Dorsal spinous process plating uses plastic plates, which come in various sizes designed to conform to the normal curvature of the spine.
      ii. Plate application requires exposure of the dorsal spinous processes and articular facets as described for modified dorsal laminectomy.
      iii. The technique for reducing and maintaining reduction of the fracture/luxation is as previously described.

Make an incision on each side of the dorsal spinous processes, being careful to preserve supraspinous and interspinous ligaments. Elevate epaxial muscles from the dorsal spines and articular facets of at least three vertebrae cranial and caudal to the fracture/luxation. Do not sever muscle attachments from the lateral aspect of the articular processes. Select two appropriately sized plates and lay them along the space between the dorsal spine and articular facet on each side of the vertebrae. Be sure the plates are long enough to grip spinous processes of three vertebrae on each side of the fracture/luxation. Place them such that the roughened surface lies against the dorsal spinous processes. Identify areas of contact that will keep the plates from lying uniformly on the lamina. Remove the plates and use a high-speed air drill to deepen these areas. Replace the plates, pass stainless steel bolts through predrilled holes in each plate and between spinous processes, and place washers and nuts on each bolt. Hold the fracture/luxation reduced, and tighten the nuts until plates are in contact between the spinous processes. Lavage the surgical site with sterile saline, debride any devitalized muscle, close epaxial muscles with a non-absorbable monofilament suture, and close subcutaneous tissues and skin routinely.

4. Modified segmental spinal fixation.
   a. Pin and wire application requires exposure of dorsal spinous processes and articular facets as described for dorsal laminectomy procedures.
   b. The number and size of longitudinal and central pins (explained later in this chapter) used depends on the size and activity of the patient and relative stability of the fracture/luxation.
      i. Generally, large patients with an unstable fracture/luxation are stabilized with relatively large central pins and a greater number of longitudinal pins (i.e., three to six pins).
      ii. If further stiffness is desired, muscular and tendinous attachments lateral to the articular facets are dissected free and a second set of pins is placed in a similar fashion lateral to the facets.

Expose two to three spinous processes and articular facets cranial and caudal to the fracture/luxation, depending on patient size and activity, and inherent stability of the fracture/luxation. Perform a dorsal laminectomy if indicated. Reduce the fracture/luxation and maintain reduction as previously described above. Drill holes through the bases of articular facets (do not cross the articulation), bases of dorsal spinous processes, and tangentially through the dorsal lamina. Make the holes large enough to accommodate 18- or 20-gauge orthopedic wire. Preplace orthopedic wire through each hole, leaving the ends long enough to wrap around several Steinmann pins. Select two Steinmann pins long enough to include at least two vertebrae cranial and

caudal to the affected vertebra (fracture) or intervertebral space (luxation, subluxation), called longitudinal pins. Bend the ends of the longitudinal pins at right angles to extend either into the interspinous space or through holes drilled transversely through the base of the dorsal spinous process. Place longitudinal pins in the space between dorsal spinous processes and articular facets. Place one central pin on each side of the dorsal spinous processes nearest the fracture/luxation. Bend the ends of the central pins to hook around the base of the dorsal spinous processes. Wire the central and longitudinal pins to the base of the articular facets, dorsal lamina, and dorsal spinous processes with the preplaced stands of orthopedic wire. Lavage the surgical site with sterile saline, debride any devitalized muscle, close epaxial muscles with a nonabsorbable monofilament suture, and close subcutaneous tissue and skin routinely.

V. Prognosis

A. Inform owners that the prognosis for patients treated medically or surgically for thoracic and lumbar fracture/luxation is generally favorable and depends on assessment of apparent neurologic signs and subsequent medical or surgical management chosen.

Neoplasia of Thoracolumbar Vertebrae, Spinal Cord, and Nerve Roots (*SAS*, pp. 1128-1130)

I. General Considerations

A. Most canine thoracolumbar vertebral, spinal cord, and nerve root tumors are extradural, generally arising from bone.

B. Lymphosarcoma is the most common spinal tumor in cats and generally occurs extradurally.

C. Intradural-extramedullary and intramedullary tumors in cats are rare.

II. Diagnosis

A. Clinical Presentation

1. Signalment.
   a. Any age, breed, or sex can be affected by thoracolumbar vertebral, spinal cord, or nerve root neoplasia.
   b. Most patients are older than 5 years of age.
   c. An exception is benign, solitary or multiple cartilaginous exostoses that usually occur in patients younger than 1 year of age.
2. History.
   a. Historical findings depend on location of the neoplasm relative to the dura.

i. Animals with extradural neoplasia generally present because of acute pain and varying degrees of upper or lower motor neuron paraparesis.
ii. Those with intradural-extramedullary neoplasia present with a chronic history (months to years) of dull back pain or hindlimb lameness plus varying degrees of monoparesis or paraparesis.
iii. Patients with intramedullary neoplasia present with acute paraparesis (often after a long insidious onset), with or without back pain.

B. Physical Examination

1. Patients with tumors involving spinal cord segments T3 to L3 present with varying degrees of back pain and UMN paraparesis, whereas those with tumors involving spinal cord segments L4 to S3 have varying degrees of low back pain and LMN paraparesis (see Chapter 33).

C. Radiography/Myelography

1. Assess survey radiographs for signs of vertebral, spinal cord, or nerve root neoplasia, including osteoproduction, osteolysis, or lysis of the intervertebral foramen.
2. Diagnosis of most spinal cord and paraspinal vertebral neoplasms requires myelography (see Chapter 33).
3. Determination of the extent of the tumor may require CT scan or MRI.

III. Medical Management

A. In general, definitive medical treatment requires surgical exposure and incisional or excisional biopsy to determine tumor type and plan adjunct chemotherapy, irradiation, or combination therapy.

IV. Surgical Treatment

A. Preoperative Management

1. Administer intravenous fluids and steroids before surgery. The steroid of choice is methylprednisolone sodium succinate (30 mg/kg IV).

B. Positioning

1. Position patients requiring dorsal laminectomy with the back gently flexed to open articular facets and interarcuate spaces, facilitating exposure.
2. Position patients requiring hemilaminectomy with the affected side gently rotated (about 15 degrees) to facilitate dorsolateral exposure of affected vertebrae.

C. Surgical Technique

1. Surgical objectives include exposure of the tumor, wide resection or biopsy of the tumor, spinal cord and nerve root decompression, and occasionally vertebral stabilization.
2. Thoracolumbar vertebral, spinal cord, or nerve root tumors are generally approached via dorsal laminectomy or hemilaminectomy.
   a. Wide laminectomy, facetectomy, and foramenotomy are required for adequate exposure of extradural and intradural-extramedullary tumors.

b. Dorsal or hemilaminectomy and durotomy are necessary for exposure and removal of intramedullary tumors.

V. Suture Materials/Special Instruments

A. Ultrasonic aspirators are invaluable, especially when removing neoplastic tissue closely associated with, or invading, neural tissues.

VI. Postoperative Care and Assessment

A. Evaluate patients with thoracic and lumbar vertebral, spinal cord, and nerve root neoplasia postoperatively just like patients with other thoracolumbar spinal disorders.

B. Base adjunct chemotherapy, irradiation, immunotherapy, or combination therapy on tumor type and surgical margins.

VII. Prognosis

A. Prognosis depends on tumor location (i.e., spine, spinal cord, or nerve root), myelographic classification (i.e., extradural, intradural-extramedullary, or intramedullary), tumor type (i.e., biologic activity), degree of surgical resection, and tumor sensitivity to adjunct therapy. In general:

1. Malignant extradural neoplasms have an unfavorable prognosis.
2. Benign extradural neoplasms have a favorable prognosis.
3. Malignant and benign intramedullary neoplasms have an unfavorable to grave prognosis.
4. Extradural-intramedullary neoplasms have a guarded to unfavorable prognosis.

36

Surgery of the Lumbosacral Spine (*SAS*, pp. 1131-1149)

General Principles and Techniques (*SAS*, pp. 1131-1134)

I. Definitions

A. **Dorsal laminectomy** of the lumbosacral spine is the removal of dorsal spinous processes, lamina, pedicles, and articular facets of L7 and S1, S2, and/or S3.

B. **Hemilaminectomy** is the removal of lamina and pedicles on the right or left side.

C. **Facetectomy** is the removal of articular facets, either unilaterally (hemilaminectomy) or bilaterally (dorsal laminectomy), to increase exposure to the spinal canal and intervertebral foramen.

D. **Cauda equina** refers to the nerve roots that course through the lumbosacral spinal canal (i.e., L7, S1-3, and Cd 1-5).

E. **Dysesthesia** is the sensation of burning or tingling in areas supplied by entrapped nerve roots.

II. Preoperative Concerns

A. Stabilize traumatized patients, and examine them for concurrent trauma.

B. Determine surgical urgency by initial and serial neurologic examinations.
   1. Perform surgery as quickly as possible on patients with acute signs and severe neurologic deficits.
   2. Carefully evaluate and stage patients with chronic signs before medical or surgical treatment.

C. Steroids are generally not administered because their efficacy in nerve root injury is uncertain.

III. Anesthesia

A. Appendix G-29 lists anesthetic protocols for patients with spinal disorders.

IV. Surgical Techniques

A. General Considerations

1. Treat patients with surgical lumbosacral disorders by dorsal laminectomy, hemilaminectomy, facetectomy, or dorsal lumbosacral spinal stabilization.
   a. Dorsal laminectomy is most commonly used for decompressing lumbosacral stenosis (i.e., cauda equina syndrome) and exposing and removing herniated disk material, fracture fragments, neoplasms, or paraspinal abscesses at L6-L7 or L7-S1.
   b. Perform a unilateral or bilateral facetectomy with laminectomy, if the compressive lesion is located laterally.
   c. Hemilaminectomy is most commonly used to expose extradural or intradural-extramedullary lesions involving L6-L7.

B. Positioning

1. Position animals with lumbosacral stenosis (i.e., cauda equina syndrome) with the hind legs tucked under the abdomen, thus stretching the interarcuate ligament and accentuating the dorsal lumbosacral space.
2. Position patients with lumbosacral fracture/luxation to encourage fracture/luxation reduction.

C. Dorsal Laminectomy

Position the patient in sternal recumbency. Make a dorsal midline incision from the dorsal spinous process of L6 to the first caudal vertebra. Incise the superficial and deep sacral fascia parallel to the skin incision. Using a periosteal elevator or small osteotome, elevate epaxial muscles from their attachments on dorsal spinous processes, lamina, articular facets, pedicles, and accessory processes of L7-S3. Remove the dorsal spinous process of L7 and S1 with rongeurs. Identify the wide interarcuate space of L7-S1; carefully incise and remove associated soft-tissue structures (i.e., remaining muscle attachments, interarcuate ligament) with a No. 11 scalpel blade. Use a high-speed pneumatic or electric drill to remove the outer cortical and softer medullary layer and identify the inner cortical layer from midbody of L7 to midbody of S2-S3. The dorsal laminar thickness of L7 and S1 varies greatly; L7 is two to three times thicker than S1. Carefully drill through the inner cortical layer until it becomes soft. Penetrate and remove the inner periosteum with a dental or iris spatula until the entire laminectomy site is exposed. Structures present include nerve roots of L7, S1, S2, S3, and caudal nerve roots, vertebral venous sinus, dorsal longitudinal ligament, and dorsal annulus fibrosus. If the L7 or S1 nerve roots appear to be compressed within the foramen or by enlarged facets, perform a facetectomy and/or foramenotomy, respectively, to establish complete nerve root decompression. Using a high-speed drill, remove the cranial articular process of S1 and caudal articular process of L7. Use the drill to approach the intervertebral foramen and Lempert rongeurs to enter the foramen by removing any remaining articular facet. This exposure allows visualization of the intervertebral foramen and exiting L7 nerve root. Lavage the surgical site with warm saline. Harvest a free subcutaneous fat graft and position it over the laminectomy site. Close epaxial muscles with interrupted, monofilament, nonabsorbable suture. Close subcutaneous tissues and skin routinely.

D. Hemilaminectomy

1. General considerations.
    a. Hemilaminectomy and facetectomy are indicated for exposure of the lateral aspects of the lumbosacral spinal canal.
    b. Position the patient as for dorsal laminectomy.

Make a dorsal midline skin incision from the dorsal spinous process of L6 to the first caudal vertebra, and continue it through the dorsal sacral fascia. Elevate epaxial muscles from the right or left lateral aspect of the dorsal spinous process, lamina, articular facet, pedicle, and accessory process of the L7-S1 intervertebral space. Visualize the dorsal aspect of the transverse process of L7. Use a high-speed drill to remove lamina, articular facet, and pedicle to the level of the accessory process. Identify outer cortical, medullary, and inner cortical layers while drilling. Carefully break through the inner periosteal layer with rongeurs and a dental or iris spatula to enter the spinal canal. Identify the vertebral venous sinus located on the floor of the spinal canal. Be careful not to lacerate the sinus while manipulating lesions within the spinal canal. After complete decompression and mass removal, lavage the surgical site with warm saline. Harvest a free subcutaneous fat graft and position it over the laminectomy site. Close epaxial muscles to the dorsal sacral fascia with interrupted, monofilament, nonabsorbable suture. Close subcutaneous tissues and skin routinely.

E. Spinal Stabilization

1. General considerations.
    a. Accomplish spinal stabilization by one of various techniques, including: transilial pins, transilial pins and plastic dorsal spinous process plates, Steinmann pins and methylmethacrylate bone cement, a combination of external skeletal fixation and dorsal spinous process plates, or modified segmental spinal fixation.

V. Healing of the Cauda Equina

A. Nerve roots of the cauda equina respond to injury in a fashion similar to peripheral nerves.

B. Healing of peripheral nerves depends on the extent of injury.

1. Mild injury.
    a. Mild injury results in neuropraxia, a transient physiologic dysfunction without anatomic disruption of axons.
    b. The nerve regains normal function within 3 months or less (peripheral nerve regeneration occurs at approximately 1 mm per day).
2. Severe injury.
    a. Severe injury results in axonotmesis or neurotmesis, partial or complete nerve severing, causing immediate degeneration at the site of injury.
    b. Nerve processes distal to the injury degenerate completely.
    c. Neuron regeneration and return of function depend on several factors.
        i. If continuity of the nerve is maintained, the distance from injury site to end-organ is the most important variable.
            (a) The best chance for functional regeneration is a distance of less than 10 to 15 cm.
        ii. Clean lacerations heal better than avulsion or crush injuries.
        iii. Nerves repaired earlier with anatomic alignment have a better chance for functional regeneration.

iv. Young, healthy patients usually have faster nerve regeneration.

VI. Postoperative Care and Assessment

A. Specific care requirements are similar to patients with thoracolumbar spinal disorders.

VII. Special Age Considerations

A. Take care when performing laminectomy procedures on young patients because their cortical and cancellous bone is much softer than in older patients.

Cauda Equina Syndrome (*SAS*, pp. 1134-1141)

I. Definitions

A. **Cauda equina** is the termination or most caudal portion of the spinal cord and adjacent spinal roots.

B. **Cauda equina syndrome** is a complex of neurologic signs caused by compression of the nerve roots (i.e., cauda equina) coursing through the lumbosacral spinal canal.

C. **Transitional vertebrae** are vertebrae that possess properties of lumbar and sacral vertebrae.

II. General Considerations

A. Congenital or acquired defects (Table 36-1) causing abnormalities in the skeletal or soft-tissue boundaries of the cauda equina may produce cauda equina compression and cauda equina syndrome.
   1. The nerve roots involved are L7, S1-3, and Cd 1-5.
   2. Vertebral bodies that contain the cauda equina are L5-L7, S1-S3, and Cd 1-5.

III. Diagnosis

A. Clinical Presentation

1. Signalment.
   a. Most dogs are middle-aged when clinical signs become apparent.
   b. There is no breed or sex predilection for congenital cauda equina stenosis.
   c. Acquired cauda equina syndrome most commonly affects large-breed dogs (particularly German shepherds).
2. History.

Table 36-1
Causes of cauda equina syndrome

Acquired
Vertebral fracture or luxation
Diskospondylitis
Vertebral osteomyelitis
Chronic IVD disease
Acute IVD extrusion
Fibrocartilaginous emboli
Neoplasia of the L7-S1 vertebra, surrounding soft tissues, or nerve roots
Congenital
Transitional vertebra
Congenital spinal canal stenosis
Breed-influenced spinal canal stenosis
Developmental sacral osteochondrosis

a. Dogs with cauda equina syndrome typically present with a chronic history of back pain and hindlimb lameness, with or without hindlimb weakness.
b. Other historical findings may include scuffing hindlimb toenails, difficulty climbing stairs, a reluctance to jump or sit up on hind legs, urinary or fecal incontinence, abnormal tail carriage, hindlimb muscle atrophy, and excessive chewing on the tail and/or lateral aspect of the hind feet.

B. Physical Examination

1. General physical examination findings vary depending on the cause of cauda equina compression.
2. Neurologic signs vary depending on cause and severity of compression and may be acute or chronic, intermittent or persistent, static or progressive (Table 36-2).
3. The most common neurologic abnormality is lumbosacral hyperpathia (i.e., pain on deep palpation of the lumbosacral junction).
4. Unilateral or bilateral pelvic limb lameness caused by referred pain from attenuation of the L7 and/or S1 nerve root is common.
   a. This finding often progresses to loss of conscious proprioception, development of motor weakness, and hind limb atrophy as nerve root ischemia and compression increase.
   b. Patellar reflexes may be normal or exaggerated because of loss of antagonism from sciatic innervation (i.e., attenuation of L7, S1-2 nerve roots). Do not misinterpret this as an UMN sign.
5. Urinary and anal sphincter disturbances may accompany back pain and paraparesis when S2 and S3 nerve roots become compressed.
6. Tail carriage or function may be affected as the caudal nerve roots are affected.
7. Paresthesia and dysesthesia (i.e., burning or tingling sensations in areas supplied by entrapped nerve roots) may occur in the tail, lateral digits, perineum, or genitals.
   a. Patients may constantly lick and chew the affected area.

C. Radiography

1. Survey radiographs.

Table 36-2
Neurologic deficits possible with cauda equina compression

Nerve involved	Nerve roots involved	Neurologic examination findings possible
Cauda equina*	L6, L7, S1-3, Cd1-5	Back pain with or without any of the findings below
Sciatic nerve	L6, L7, S1, +/– S2	Sensory: loss of sensation on lateral digit; licking and chewing of lateral digit; knuckling Motor: decreased withdrawal reflex, especially hock flexion; hindlimb atrophy; motor weakness
Perineal nerve	S1, S2, S3	Sensory: decreased sensation to perineum and caudal thigh; licking perineum
Caudal rectal nerve	S2, S3	Motor: decreased to absent anal sphincter tone on rectal exam
Pelvic nerve	S1, S2, S3	Parasympathetic: loss of bladder control
Pudendal nerve	S1, S2, S3	Motor: varying degrees of urinary incontinence
Caudal nerves	Cd 1-5	Sensory: decreased sensation to the tail; pain upon tail manipulation; excessive tail linking Motor: change in tail carriage and tail wag
Femoral nerve†	L4, L5, L6	Sensory: no change expected Motor: patellar reflex appears brisk because of absence of sciatic innervated antagonist muscles

*All neurologic abnormalities involving cauda equina ischemia and/or compression are LMN.
†Although the femoral nerve is not supplied by nerve roots of the cauda equina, when the patellar reflex is performed, it appears brisk (UMN); this is due to loss of antagonist muscles innervated by sciatic nerve and is not a UMN sign.

a. Assess patients with fracture/luxation with survey radiographs.
b. Assess patients with neoplasia with survey radiographic and myelographic studies based on tumor location.
c. Patients with infectious cauda equina compression (diskospondylitis, vertebral osteomyelitis) may have osteolysis and/or osteoproduction of the vertebral body, intervertebral space, or both.

2. Additional imaging
   a. Imaging the lumbosacral spine to diagnose cauda equina compression secondary to chronic degenerative disk disease, intervertebral disk extrusion, or congenital lumbosacral stenosis is often a challenge.
   b. Consider performing survey radiography, stress radiography, myelography, diskography, epidurography, CT and/or MRI.

D. Differential Diagnosis

1. Disorders not associated with the lumbosacral junction that mimic cauda equina syndrome include hip dysplasia, metabolic disorders causing weakness, and degenerative myelopathy.

IV. Medical Management

A. Manage patients with cauda equina compression based on etiology.

B. Select medical management of patients with cauda equina compression secondary to chronic degenerative disk disease, intervertebral disk extrusion, and congenital lumbosacral stenosis based on severity and duration of neurologic signs, as well as serial neurologic examinations (Table 36-3).

1. Prescribe strict confinement for 4 to 6 weeks and nonsteroidal antiinflammatory drug (NSAID) therapy.
   a. Inform owners of potential side effects of NSAIDs.
   b. Steroids are of little benefit to patients with nerve root injury.

V. Surgical Treatment

A. General Considerations

1. Surgical objectives include nerve root decompression and vertebral stabilization.
2. Specific surgical procedures for patients with cauda equina compression depend on the etiology.
3. The surgical treatment of patients with cauda equina compression secondary to chronic degenerative disk disease, intervertebral disk extrusion, and congenital lumbosacral stenosis is based on severity and duration of neurologic signs, outcome of medical management, results of imaging, EMG findings, and serial neurologic examinations (see Table 36-3).

B. Preoperative Management

1. Preoperative management of patients with cauda equina compression is similar to that described for patients with other lumbosacral compressive lesions.
2. Preoperative steroids are not recommended.

C. Positioning

1. Positions patients for laminectomy in sternal recumbency with the hind legs tucked under the abdomen to encourage flexion and facilitate exposure of the dorsal lumbosacral intervertebral space.

D. Surgical Techniques

1. Surgical techniques for dorsal laminectomy, hemilaminectomy, facetectomy, and foramenotomy are previously described.
2. Patients with chronic degenerative disk disease.
   a. Adequate decompression involves dorsal laminectomy, with or without foramenotomy and facetectomy.

Perform a dorsal laminectomy on patients with dorsal compression from lamina and interarcuate ligament. Use a No. 11 scalpel blade and ophthalmic forceps to carefully resect the ligament. In patients with lateral compression, perform a facetectomy to decompress the L7 and S1 nerve roots from the bulbous articular facets. In patients requiring further lateral decompression of the L7 nerve root, perform a foramenotomy to establish complete decompression. Perform unilateral or bilateral facetectomy/foramenotomy based on neurologic examination findings, results of imaging, and surgical findings. Approach nerve root compression from the ventral floor of the spinal canal (i.e., protrusion of dorsal annulus fibrosus) through careful retraction of nerve roots, sharp annular incision, and mass removal. Patients may require all or a variety of the above decompressive techniques. Spinal stabilization is not indicated unless spinal instability is documented.

3. Patients with acute intervertebral disk herniation.

In patients with herniated intervertebral disk material, perform a dorsal laminectomy if disk fragments are located on the midline or bilaterally, or a

Table 36-3

Recommended therapy* for patients with cauda equina compression (i.e., chronic degenerative disk disease, intervertebral disk herniation, congenital lumbosacral stenosis, lumbosacral fracture/luxation, of diskospondylitis/vertebral osteomyelitis†) based on clinical presentation

Initial treatment§	Result	Second treatment§	Result	Third treatment§
Back pain only, with or without paresthesia or dysesthesia				
Cage rest only	Improvement Static Deteriorating	Continue cage rest NSAIDs‡ Consider surgery¶	Improvement Static/deteriorating	Follow Consider surgery
Back pain; mild paraparesis; no urinary incontinence				
NSAIDs	Improvement Static Deteriorating	Cage rest/NSAIDs Continue NSAIDs Consider surgery	Improvement Static/deteriorating	Cage rest/follow Consider surgery
Back pain; mild paraparesis; early urinary incontinence				
NSAIDs	Improvement Static Deteriorating	Cage rest/NSAIDs Consider surgery Consider surgery	Improvement	Cage rest/follow

Back pain; moderate paraparesis; no urinary incontinence				
NSAIDs	Improvement	Cage rest/NSAIDs	Improvement	Cage rest/follow
	Static	Consider surgery		
	Deteriorating	Consider surgery		
Back pain; severe parapares s; no urinary incontinence				
Consider surgery				
Back pain; moderate or severe paraparesis; urinary incontinence				
Consider surgery				

*All patients are strictly confined (4 to 6 weeks) as part of their medical management regardless of the drug used or duration of drug therapy.
†Patients suspected of having L7-S1 diskospondylitis or vertebral osteomyelitis should also be treated with antimicrobials (see *SAS,* Tables 34-5 and 34-6)
‡*NSAIDs,* nonsteroidal antiinflammatory drugs; specific drugs, dosages, and duration of therapy are listed in Table 36-8.
§Initial treatment may be the first 24 to 48 hours or 3 to 5 days depending on results of serial neurologic examinations. Second and third treatments also depend on neurologic status.
¶Regardless of clinical presentation, if a client cannot afford surgery, a course of cage rest and NSAID therapy should be attempted.

hemilaminectomy if neurologic signs and imaging results lateralize disk fragments to one side. Adequately expose the spinal canal to achieve complete mass removal. Spinal stabilization is generally not indicated unless spinal instability is documented.

4. Patients with congenital lumbosacral stenosis.

In patients with congenital lumbosacral stenosis, perform a dorsal laminectomy with unilateral or bilateral facetectomy based on neurologic signs, imaging results, and surgical findings. If stenosis is radiographically or surgically demonstrated extending from L6 to S1, perform a multilevel dorsal laminectomy and bilateral facetectomy from L6 to S1. Remove interarcuate ligaments dorsally and facets laterally to provide complete decompression. Place a free fat graft over the entire laminectomy defect. Spinal stabilization is generally indicated because spinal instability is likely.

VI. Prognosis

A. Medical management.
   1. For medically managed patients with mild to moderate back pain, mild lameness, absent or mild paraparesis, and/or no urinary incontinence the prognosis is favorable to excellent.
   2. For medically managed patients with severe back pain, moderate to severe lameness, moderate to severe paraparesis, and/or urinary incontinence the prognosis is guarded to unfavorable.
   3. If patients with mild neurologic deficits show static or deteriorating signs or loss of urinary continence during medical management, early surgical decompression has a better prognosis.

B. Surgical management.
   1. Generally, prognosis for surgically treated patients with acute back pain, mild to moderate lameness, mild to moderate paraparesis, and no urinary incontinence is favorable to excellent.

C. Prognosis for patients with chronic back pain, severe lameness, severe paraparesis, and urinary incontinence is guarded to unfavorable.

Fractures and Luxations of the Lumbosacral Spine (*SAS*, pp. 1141-1147)

I. General Considerations

A. Fractures are usually oblique or short oblique, involving the vertebral body of L6 or L7, and may be accompanied by luxation of articular facets.
   1. Cranioventral displacement of the caudal segment typically occurs.

B. The spinal cord terminates in the body of L6; therefore neurologic signs are usually associated with trauma to nerve roots of the cauda equina (i.e., L6-7, S1-3, and Cd 1-5) instead of the spinal cord.

1. Because of the ability of nerve roots to resist traumatic injury, substantial displacement of the fracture or luxation may still leave the patient neurologically intact.
2. Conversely, tethering or avulsion of nerve roots will occasionally produce trauma to the caudal spinal cord; neurologic deficits in these patients are often profound.

II. Diagnosis

A. Clinical Presentation

1. Signalment.
   a. Any age, sex, or breed cat or dog can be affected.
   b. Dogs are more likely to sustain this injury than cats.
2. History.
   a. Typically there is a history of recent vehicular trauma.
   b. Patients generally present with varying degrees of lumbar pain, ambulatory or nonambulatory paraparesis, and decreased anal and tail tone.

B. Physical Examination

1. Assess the patient for concurrent injuries.
2. Secure patients that have profound neurologic deficits to a rigid platform to prevent further nerve root trauma until definitive treatment is taken.
3. Lumbosacral fracture/luxation may cause trauma to the cauda equina.
   a. The most commonly involved nerve roots are L6-7, S1-3, and Cd1-5.
   b. Major nerves associated with these nerve roots include the sciatic nerve (L6, L7, S1, and/or S2), perineal nerve (S1, S2, S3), caudal rectal nerve (S2, S3), pelvic nerve (S1, S2, S3), pudendal nerve (S1, S2, S3), and caudal nerves of the tail (Cd1-5).
4. The most common presentation is lumbosacral hyperpathia (i.e., pain on deep palpation of the lumbosacral junction), LMN ambulatory or nonambulatory paraparesis, varying degrees of anal sphincter atonia, and abnormalities in tail carriage and sensation.

C. Radiography

1. Survey radiographs generally reveal an oblique or short oblique fracture through the vertebral body of L6 or L7, or a luxation or subluxation between L6 and L7 or L7 and S1.
   a. The caudal vertebral body is characteristically displaced cranioventral to the cranial vertebral body.
2. Base prognosis on neurologic examination findings, not radiologic findings.
3. Up to 20% of patients with spinal fracture/luxation have a second fracture/luxation; therefore obtain a complete series of spinal radiographs.

III. Medical Management

A. Objectives of medical management include immobilization of the spine and patient confinement until fracture/luxation stabilization and union occur.

B. Observe strict confinement for 4 to 6 weeks in a dry, elevated padded cage.

C. Administer analgesics/NSAIDs as needed.

D. Perform urinary bladder expression four times daily, and passive physical therapy of the hind legs two to three times daily

E. Evaluate the patient with serial neurologic examinations twice daily to assess response to therapy.

IV. Surgical Treatment

A. General Considerations

1. Objectives of surgical management are decompression of the cauda equina, followed by adequate spinal stabilization.
2. Infrequently, patients may require dorsal laminectomy for complete decompression (i.e., when bone fragments are present in the spinal canal) or for its prognostic value in evaluating the severity of cauda equina damage.
3. Select surgical versus medical treatment based on the patient's neurologic status at presentation, response to medical management, and serial neurologic examinations (see Table 36-3).
4. Select a technique for stabilization of the lumbosacral junction based on the surgeon's experience and equipment available.

B. Positioning

1. Position the patient in sternal recumbency with the hind legs tucked under the abdomen to encourage flexion of the dorsal lumbosacral region and facilitate fracture reduction and cauda equina decompression.

C. Surgical Technique

1. L7 Fracture and L7-S1 luxation.
   a. Transilial pins.

Expose dorsal spinous processes and lamina of L6, L7, and the entire median sacral crest as described for dorsal laminectomy. Because of the cranioventral displacement of the sacrum, visualization of the cranial aspect of the sacral crest is obscured by the lamina of L7. L7 laminectomy is not compatible with this technique. Use a periosteal elevator or small osteotome to elevate epaxial muscles and expose the articular processes of L7. Use the tip of a Kelly or Carmalt forceps and carefully place it in the lumbosacral junction. Visually monitor the depth of placement of the forceps to avoid injuring nerve roots. Hook the tip of the forceps under the cranial lamina of the sacrum to act as a lever against the caudal lamina of L7. Adequate exposure of the lumbosacral junction is facilitated by reducing the fracture/luxation. Before attempting reduction, place a bone forceps or towel clamp in the wing of each ilium. Have an unsterile assistant available to provide cranial traction on the patient's head or front legs. Reduce the fracture/luxation. These manipulations force the sacrum caudodorsally, to reduce the fracture/luxation. Visualize the lumbosacral articular facets; when the articular processes of L7 and S1 are reapposed, reduction is anatomic. Place an 0.062-inch Kirschner wire through each L7-S1 articular facet to maintain fracture/luxation reduction. Next, incise gluteal fascia on the dorsolateral crest of the wings of each ilium, elevate the middle gluteal musculature, and expose the dorsolateral aspect of each ilial crest. Place an appropriate size Steinmann pin through the lateral aspect of the ilial wing,

across the dorsal lamina of L7, and through the opposite ilial wing. Place a second pin in a similar fashion starting from the opposite side. Be sure both pins cross over the dorsal lamina of L7. Prevent pin migration by employing one of the following techniques: (1) bend the ends of each pin at a 90-degree angle; (2) connect the pins on each side with double Kirschner clamps of the appropriate size; or (3) notch the pins' ends with a pin cutter and incorporate them with methylmethacrylate bone cement. If indicated, remove the interarcuate ligament and perform sacral laminectomy to visualize nerve roots. Lavage the surgical wound with sterile physiologic saline solution, cover the ends of the pins by closing gluteal fascia, and close epaxial muscles by apposing dorsal midline fascia. Close subcutaneous tissue and skin routinely.

2. Fractures of the body of L6 and L7, and luxation of L7-S1.
   a. Transilial pins with dorsal spinous process plates.
      i. General considerations.
         (a) This technique incorporates the caudal lumbar spine to help counteract flexion (i.e., plastic plate) and uses multiple points of fixation to prevent rotational instability (i.e., transilial pins).
         (b) It is compatible with dorsal laminectomy.

Prepare the dorsum of the back, from the midthoracic region to the base of the tail, for aseptic surgery. Make a dorsal midline skin incision such that three dorsal spinous processes cranial to the fracture/luxation can be exposed, and caudally to a point midway between the tuber ischii. Preserve the interspinous and supraspinous ligaments cranial to the lumbosacral junction by making two parallel lumbosacral fascial incisions on either side of the dorsal spinous processes. Elevate epaxial muscles to the level of the articular facets bilaterally. Carefully expose dorsal spinous processes, lamina, and articular facets of L6, L7, and/or sacrum, depending on location of the fracture. Reduce the fracture/luxation and maintain reduction with transarticular pins. Perform a dorsal laminectomy at this time, if indicated. Select the appropriate size of plastic plates and secure them along each side of the dorsal spinous processes. Include a minimum of three dorsal spinous processes in length cranial to the fracture/luxation. Place two transilial Steinmann pins as described. Be sure to place each pin through predrilled holes in each plastic plate. Prevent pin migration by placing Kirschner clamps on the pin ends, bending the pin ends to 90-degree angles, or notching and covering the pin ends with bone cement as described. Place a final bolt, washer, and nut through the plates caudal to the transilial pins. Lavage the surgical wound and close dorsal lumbar fascia, gluteal fascia, subcutaneous tissue, and skin routinely.

   b. Modified segmental spinal fixation.
      i. General considerations.
         (a) Use modified segmental spinal fixation in patients of all sizes.
         (b) It does not require deep exposure, is compatible with dorsal laminectomy, simple to perform, and versatile (i.e., can be used in combination with other techniques).

Approach the dorsal aspect of the lumbar and lumbosacral spine as described for transilial pins and dorsal spinous process plates. Expose three dorsal spinous processes cranial to the fracture/luxation. Expose, carefully reduce, and maintain fracture/luxation reduction as described for transilial pinning. Perform a dorsal laminectomy at this time, if indicated. Drill holes in the caudal articular processes and bases of dorsal spinous processes of at least two to three vertebrae cranial to the fracture/luxation. Drill holes in the cranial sacral articular facets to ensure a minimum of two points of fixation per pin in

the sacroiliac segment. Preplace 3- to 4-inch lengths of 18- to 20-gauge stainless steel wire through each hole. Drill two holes transversely through each ilial wing at the level of the dorsal lamina of the sacrum. Bend four appropriate size and length Steinmann pins at a 90-degree angle, remove the points, and pass the pins through the holes drilled in the wings of the ilia. Place the pins alongside the lamina and attach them to the articular facets and dorsal spinous processes using the preplaced stainless steel wire.

3. Fracture of L6 or L7 vertebral bodies and luxation of L6-L7 or L7-S.
   a. Steinmann pins and methylmethacrylate bone cement.
      i. General considerations.
         (a) Use Steinmann pins and methylmethacrylate bone cement in patients of all sizes.
         (b) This technique requires exposure of the dorsal surface of the transverse processes of L6 and L7, is compatible with dorsal laminectomy, and is versatile (i.e., can be used in combination with other techniques).

Adequately expose the vertebrae cranial and caudal to the fracture or luxation. Incise muscle attachments to articular facets and periosteally elevate epaxial muscles until the dorsal aspect of the transverse processes of L6 and L7 and dorsal lamina of the sacrum are identified. Reduce the fracture/luxation and maintain reduction as described for transilial pinning. If the fracture involves the body of L6, place two pins in the body of L5 and two pins in the body of L7. If an L6-L7 luxation is being repaired, place two pins in the body of L6 and two pins in the body of L7. Place pins and apply bone cement using the technique described in Chapter 35. If the fracture involves the vertebral body of L7 or is an L7-S1 luxation, place two pins in the body of L6, two pins in the body of L7, and two pins in the cranial articular process of S1 with penetration through the ilium. If the fracture involves the vertebral body of L7, pin placement in L7 is dictated by the type of fracture present (i.e., avulsion fracture of the endplate, place two pins in L7; transverse fracture, place one or two smaller pins depending on the size of the fracture fragments; comminuted fracture, no pins should be placed in L7). Insert pins directly into the vertebral bodies of L6 or L7 using the accessory process and transverse process as landmarks. Insert pins into the center of the cranial articular processes of S1. Drive the pin until it penetrates the gluteal surface of the wing of the ilium. Direct the L6 and L7 pins cranioventral and from lateral to medial, and the S1 pins caudoventral and from lateral to medial. Drive pins to exit 2 to 3 mm from the ventral aspect of the vertebral bodies and wings of the ilia. Cut pins to leave 2 cm protruding and notch the exposed pin heads with a pin cutter. Thoroughly lavage and dry the surgical field. Apply methylmethacrylate bone cement as described. If necessary, excise portions of epaxial muscles adjacent to the methyl methacrylate to facilitate closure. Rarely, relief incisions in the lumbodorsal fascia lateral to the methylmethacrylate are necessary to allow closure of the primary incision. Close subcutaneous tissues and skin routinely.

   b. Transilial pins with dorsal spinous process plates and external skeletal fixation.
      i. General considerations.
         (a) Use transilial pins in patients of all sizes.
         (b) This technique is compatible with dorsal laminectomy, offers dorsal and ventral compartment fixation, and requires minimal special equipment.

Performing a dorsal approach, expose three dorsal spinous processes cranial to the fracture/luxation. Expose dorsal lamina and articular facets of affected vertebrae, reduce the fracture/luxation, maintain reduction, and place a dorsal

spinous process plate as described. Pull skin and muscle to the center of the incision and percutaneously place a Steinmann pin through skin, muscle, wing of the ilium, holes in the dorsal spinous process plates, opposite ilial wing, and muscle and skin of the opposite side. Place a second Steinmann pin through the vertebral body cranial to the fracture/luxation. Start the pin just caudal to the junction of the transverse process and vertebral body. Pull skin and muscle to the center of the incision and percutaneously insert the pin through skin, epaxial and body wall muscle mass, vertebral body (i.e., just caudal to the junction of the transverse process and vertebral body), and through muscles and skin on the opposite side. Place single clamps on both ends of each Steinmann pin, and attach connecting bars to each side. Close dorsal lumbar and sacral fascia, subcutaneous tissues, and skin routinely.

V. Postoperative Care and Assessment

A. Monitor postoperatively as with other lumbosacral disorders.
   1. Provide strict confinement, analgesics as needed, short walks using an abdominal sling, frequent urinary bladder evacuation, and daily neurologic examinations.

VI. Prognosis

A. Cauda equina nerve roots withstand considerably more trauma than the spinal cord.

B. Patients with 100% lumbosacral spinal canal compromise may retain neurologic function of the hind limbs, anus, urinary bladder, perineum, and tail; their prognosis is favorable.

C. However, give patients with profound neurologic deficits (i.e., complete loss of motor function and deep pain perception) a guarded prognosis, regardless of the percentage of spinal canal compromise.

D. Do not use the amount of spinal canal compromise observed on lateral radiographs as a prognostic indicator.

Neoplasia of the Lumbosacral Spine and Nerve Roots (*SAS*, pp. 1147-1149)

I. General Considerations

A. Tumors of the lumbosacral vertebrae and nerve roots are rare.

B. Tumor type, location (i.e., spine, surrounding soft tissue, or nerve root), and classification (i.e., extradural, intradural-extramedullary, or intramedullary) are similar to neoplasms of the cervical, thoracic, and lumbar spine.

II. Diagnosis

A. Clinical Presentation

1. Signalment.
   a. Any sex or breed animal may be affected.
   b. Patients are typically older than 5 years of age.
   c. An exception is solitary or multiple cartilaginous exostoses, which usually occur in patients less than 1 year of age.
2. History.
   a. Patients may present with variable degrees of back pain, with or without LMN ambulatory paraparesis.
   b. Anal sphincter atonia and urinary incontinence are inconsistent, but occur.
   c. Patients with nerve root tumors usually have a chronic history of dull hind leg lameness (i.e., monoparesis from root signature).
   d. Patients with vertebral body or surrounding soft-tissue (i.e., extradural) tumors have an acute history of back pain and ambulatory or nonambulatory paraparesis.

B. Physical Examination

1. Generally, patients present with any combination of LMN signs associated with cauda equina compression.

C. Radiography

1. Survey radiographs.
   a. Radiographic findings suggestive of vertebral neoplasia include vertebral body osteolysis and/or osteoproduction.
   b. Lysis of an intervertebral foramen suggests a nerve root tumor (i.e., neurofibroma, meningioma).
2. Diagnosis of lumbosacral neoplasms may require stress radiography, myelography, or epidurography.
3. Occasionally, CT scan, MRI or exploratory laminectomy is needed for a definitive diagnosis.

III. Medical Management

A. With most lumbosacral neoplasms, definitive medical treatment requires surgical exposure and incisional or excisional biopsy to determine tumor type and to plan appropriate adjunct chemotherapy, immunotherapy, irradiation, or combination therapy.

B. Corticosteroid therapy is generally not recommended for primary treatment of nerve root injury. However, steroids may be used for their antitumor effects.

IV. Surgical Treatment

A. General Considerations

1. Surgical treatment objectives include the definitive diagnosis of cauda equina compression (i.e., neoplasia, herniated disk, abscess), decompression and mass removal, incisional or excisional biopsy (wide surgical excision is preferred if possible), tumor staging, and, if necessary, spinal stabilization.

B. Preoperative Management

1. Preoperative management of patients with lumbosacral neoplasia is similar to that described for patients with any lumbosacral compressive lesion.
2. Preoperative steroids are not indicated because they do not protect nerve roots.

C. Positioning

1. Position the patient in sternal recumbency with the hind legs tucked under the abdomen to gently flex the lumbosacral junction.

D. Surgical Technique

1. Nerve root tumors.
   a. General considerations.
      i. Approach tumors as they course through the lumbosacral spinal canal using dorsal laminectomy, facetectomy, and foramenotomy.
      ii. Identify the specific nerve root or roots to be resected, and know their effect on the patient's neurologic function.
         (a) Single or multiple nerve root resection may incapacitate the patient to an unacceptable degree.
         (b) In such cases, biopsy for histopathologic diagnosis.
      iii. If possible, excise the tumor with 2-cm margins.

Enter the spinal canal by carefully elevating the inner periosteal layer with a dental or iris spatula and ophthalmic forceps. Remove any remaining epidural fat. Identify cauda equina nerve roots on the floor of the spinal canal. Use a dural hook, dental spatula, or iris spatula to carefully follow the S1 and L7 nerve roots as they course along the floor of the spinal canal. Identify the L7 nerve root as it lies against the caudal aspect of the L7 pedicle, and follow it as it disappears through the L7-S1 intervertebral foramen. Carefully examine each nerve root for evidence of diffuse enlargement or localized bulging. If the lesion is resectable, identify the nerve root involved, carefully cauterize the root cranial to the lesion using bipolar cautery, transect the root with a No. 11 scalpel blade, and carefully elevate the transected portion of the root. Follow the affected nerve root caudal to the lesion and complete the resection as previously described. Reexamine the cauda equina to rule out multiple nerve root tumors. Lavage the surgical wound and close tissues routinely.

2. Tumors involving the vertebral body or surrounding soft tissues.
   a. General considerations.
      i. Approach tumors involving the vertebral body or surrounding soft tissues via dorsal laminectomy.
      ii. Remove affected bone and provide cauda equina decompression.
         (a) If bony involvement is nonresectable, biopsy and perform a dorsal laminectomy to provide cauda equina decompression.
         (b) If neoplastic tissue is abscessed, obtain samples for anaerobic and aerobic culture and susceptibility testing.
      iii. If spinal instability is diagnosed or occurs as a result of decompression, perform spinal stabilization.

V. Postoperative Care and Assessment

A. Monitor postoperatively as with other lumbosacral disorders.
   1. Provide strict confinement, analgesics as needed, short walks using

an abdominal sling, frequent urinary bladder evacuation, and daily neurologic examinations.

B. Long-term monitoring and medical therapy depend on tumor type and surgical margins.

VI. Prognosis

A. Prognosis depends on tumor type (i.e., biologic activity), surgical margins (i.e., percent of tumor resection), and sensitivity to adjunct therapy (i.e., chemotherapy, immunotherapy, radiation therapy, or combination therapy).

B. Malignant extradural neoplasms tend to have an unfavorable prognosis, benign extradural neoplasms have a favorable prognosis, and extradural-intramedullary neoplasms (i.e., nerve root tumors) have a guarded to unfavorable prognosis.

37

Nonsurgical Diseases of the Spine (*SAS*, pp. 1151-1159)

Diskospondylitis (*SAS*, pp. 1151-1154)

I. Definitions

A. **Diskospondylitis** is infection of the intervertebral disk with concurrent osteomyelitis of adjacent vertebral endplates and vertebral bodies.

B. Infection confined to the vertebral body is referred to as **vertebral osteomyelitis.**

II. General Considerations

A. Infection generally originates in a nonvertebral location (e.g., UTI, pyogenic dermatitis, valvular endocarditis, dental disease) and spreads hematogenously.
   1. *Staphylococcus aureus* and *Staphylococcus intermedius* are the most common organisms associated with diskospondylitis.
   2. Because of the public health hazard, test animals with diskospondylitis for *Brucella canis* infection.

B. Infrequently, diskospondylitis is caused by foreign body migration or postoperative sequelae to disk fenestration.

C. Areas of the spine most commonly affected include lumbosacral junction, cervicothoracic junction, thoracolumbar junction, and midthoracic disks.
   1. Vertebral infection usually begins in the endplate, where sludging blood in sinusoidal veins is predisposed to bacterial colonization.
   2. Rarely, bacteria migrate dorsally and cause epidural abscess formation.

III. Diagnosis

A. Clinical Presentation

1. Signalment.
   a. Largebreed dogs (i.e., 30 to 35 kg or greater) are typically affected, with males outnumbering females approximately 2 to 1.

b. Age at presentation is generally less than 4 years; however, a significant number of patients may be middle aged or older.

2. History.
   a. The hallmark of patients with diskospondylitis is spinal hyperpathia (i.e., neck or back pain on deep palpation) associated with systemic disease.
   b. Typically the onset of symptoms is insidious, with subtle lameness, difficulty jumping, anorexia, depression, and/or weight loss for weeks to months previously.
   c. Varying degrees of chronic paraparesis or tetraparesis may occur later.

B. Physical Examination

1. Early findings.
   a. Systemic signs (i.e., depression, weight loss, fever) are common.
   b. Signs of spinal involvement include hyperpathia without paresis.
   c. Less frequently, patients may have an acute onset of back pain and ambulatory or nonambulatory paraparesis or tetraparesis, with or without systemic signs.
2. Later findings.
   a. Usually, subtle signs of systemic involvement are coupled with profound neurologic signs (i.e., severe, single or multilevel hyperpathia, with varying degrees of paresis caudal to the lesion).
3. Specific neurologic signs depend on location of the lesion (see Chapter 33).

C. Radiography

1. Confirm the diagnosis by survey radiographs.
   a. The hallmark of diskospondylitis is intradiskal lysis.
   b. The earliest signs, evident at 10 to 14 days after infection, include lysis of one or both vertebral endplates, followed by collapse of the intervertebral disk space.
   c. As the infection progresses, proliferative bony changes adjacent to the disk space, sclerotic margins, and ventral osseous proliferation with varying degrees of bridging spondylosis result.
2. Consider bone scintigraphy to diagnose early cases of diskospondylitis (i.e., as early as 3 days).
3. Perform myelography in patients requiring surgical intervention.

D. Laboratory Findings

1. Complete blood count.
   a. A leukocytosis does not occur unless other systemic abnormalities are present (i.e., UTI, endocarditis, pyoderma, prostatic abscess).
2. Cultures.
   a. Blood cultures are positive in 50% to 70% of patients.
   b. UTI has been reported in up to 40% of cases; occasionally the same organism is identified in blood and bone cultures.
   c. A bone culture is usually not performed. Results are generally unrewarding, but may identify the same organism in urine and blood cultures.
   d. Positive *Brucella* titers are occasionally found.
3. CSF.
   a. Analysis is usually normal but may show mild protein elevation.

IV. Differential Diagnosis

A. Differentiate diskospondylitis from spondylosis deformans and spinal neoplasia.

1. Spondylosis and sclerosis are common findings in both spondylosis deformans and diskospondylitis; however, vertebral endplate lysis is only seen with infection.
2. Similarly, endplate lysis of adjacent or multiple vertebrae is uncommon in spinal neoplasia.

V. Medical Management

A. In general, treat patients that present with pain alone or pain and mild paresis, regardless of the number of vertebra affected, with analgesics, antibiotics, and 4 to 6 weeks of strict confinement.

1. Select antibiotic therapy based on results of a urine, blood, and/or bone culture and susceptibility testing and *Brucella* titer.
2. If cultures and titers are negative, select an antibiotic based on the most likely causative agent (i.e., *S. intermedius* or *S. aureus*) (Table 37-1).
3. Treat for 6 to 8 weeks, at least 2 weeks after resolution of clinical signs.
4. For *Brucella canis,* treat patients until the titer is negative.
5. Most patients (i.e., 80% to 90%) respond to an appropriate course of medical management.

B. If patients are unresponsive (i.e., continued hyperpathia without paresis) to medical therapy within 7 to 10 days, treat with a different antibiotic.

Table 37-1
Antibiotics for use in diskospondylitis*

Amikacin (Amiglyde-V)
10 mg/kg IV, IM, SC, TID
Cephradine (Veslosef)
20 mg/kg PO, TID
Clindamycin (Antirobe)
11 mg/kg PO, BID
Cloxacillin (Cloxapen, Orbenin, Tegopen)
10 mg/kg PO, QID
Doxycycline (Vibramycin)
5 mg/kg PO, BID
Enrofloxacin (Baytril)
5-10 mg/kg PO or IV, BID
Gentamicin (Gentocin)
2 mg/kg IM, BID for 1 week; monitor renal function
Minocycline (Minocin)
10 mg/kg PO, BID
Streptomycin
20 mg/kg BID, IM, for 1 week

*Duration of therapy may be based on one or a combination of the following guidelines:

- Treat for 6 to 8 weeks
- Treat for 2 weeks after resolution of clinical signs
- Treat until radiographic evidence of ankylosing spondylosis
- Treat until Brucella titer is negative

C. If pain persists, attempt a third antibiotic, or perform surgical curettage to obtain bone samples for culture and susceptibility testing, and debride intradiskal lesions.

D. Provide analgesics as necessary.

VI. Surgical Treatment

A. Consider surgical treatment if a medically treated patient shows neurologic deterioration (i.e., paraparesis or tetraparesis) or if a patient presents with an acute onset of spinal hyperpathia and weakly ambulatory or nonambulatory paraparesis or tetraparesis.
   1. Use myelography to determine the specific location of the compressive lesion.
   2. Perform spinal cord decompression via a dorsal laminectomy or hemilaminectomy; hemilaminectomy is preferred because it creates the least spinal instability.
   3. Additionally, you may collect bone samples for culture and susceptibility testing, and debride intradiskal lesions.
   4. Perform spinal stabilization if decompression and debridement result in spinal instability, or if instability is documented radiographically before surgery.

B. Preoperative management.
   1. See preoperative management for each specific location of the spine affected.

C. Positioning.
   1. Refer to the surgical procedure chosen for appropriate surgical positioning.

D. Surgical technique.
   1. See surgical technique descriptions for each specific location of the spine affected (i.e., cervical, thoracolumbar, and lumbosacral).

VII. Suture Materials/Special Instruments

A. Avoid using nonabsorbable multifilament sutures (e.g., silk) in infected surgical sites.

VIII. Postoperative Care and Assessment

A. Continue antibiotics for a minimum of 4 to 6 weeks.

IX. Prognosis

A. Patients with spinal hyperpathia only or spinal hyperpathia plus ambulatory paresis have a favorable to excellent prognosis.

B. Those with spinal hyperpathia and weakly ambulatory paresis, particularly if weakness is a result of spinal pain, have a favorable prognosis.

C. Patients with either of the above neurologic findings that do not respond to an initial course of medication have a guarded to favorable prognosis for responding to either a different antibiotic or surgical bone culture and intradiskal debridement.

D. Patients with an acute onset of spinal hyperpathia, weakly ambulatory or nonambulatory paraparesis or tetraparesis, evidence of an extradural lesion, and no evidence of spinal instability have a guarded prognosis when treated surgically. If these patients have evidence of spinal instability, the prognosis is guarded to unfavorable.

Granulomatous Meningoencephalitis (*SAS*, pp. 1154-1156)

I. Definition

A. **Granulomatous meningoencephalitis (GME)** is an acute, progressive disorder of the central nervous system (CNS), characterized histologically by focal or disseminated perivascular granulomas in the meninges, brain, and spinal cord.

II. General Considerations

A. GME is a neurologic disorder that may affect any portion of the CNS (i.e., meninges, brain, and spinal cord).

B. Disseminated, focal, and ocular forms have been described.
   1. Clinical signs may differ depending on the form (Table 37-2).

C. The cause of GME is currently unknown.

III. Diagnosis

A. Clinical Presentation

1. Signalment.
   a. Typically young to middle-aged dogs (i.e., 2 to 6 years) are affected.
   b. Female and toy breeds are more often affected than males, mixed breeds, and larger breeds.
   c. GME is rarely diagnosed in cats.
2. History.
   a. Patients generally present with an acute history of continuous or episodic progression of multifocal neurologic disease that may involve the brain, meninges, and/or cervical spinal cord.

B. Physical Examination

1. Physical and neurologic examination findings depend on lesion localization and the form of disease present (i.e., disseminated, focal, or ocular) (see Table 37-2).

Table 37-2
Clinical signs associated with various forms of GME

Form*	Lesion location†	Clinical signs‡	Duration of signs	Prognosis
Disseminated	Lower brainstem Cervical spinal cord Meninges	Acute onset; rapidly progressive; fever may occur early	1 to 8 weeks (25% are dead in 1 week)	Grave; may live 12 to 16 weeks
Focal	Brainstem Cerebral cortex Cerebellum Cervical spine cord	Insidious onset; signs consistent with a space-occupying mass	3 to 6 months	Unfavorable; may live up to 12 months
Ocular	Ocular nerve	Sudden blindness; anisocoria	3 to 6 months§	Unfavorable may live 12 to 18 months

*The disseminated and focal forms frequently occur together; the ocular form may occur alone or accompanied by the disseminated or focal forms. †Although lesions can occur anywhere in the CNS, each form of the disease seems to have a predilection for specific locations. ‡Specific clinical signs are associated with lesion location; see Chapter 33 for a description of signs expected in each location. §If the ocular form is present with the disseminated form, duration of signs and prognosis usually follow the disseminated form.

2. Findings include cervical pain evidenced by nuchal rigidity (i.e., suggesting meningeal involvement) or nystagmus, head tilt, blindness, and facial and trigeminal palsy (i.e., suggesting brainstem involvement).
3. Ataxia, paraparesis or tetraparesis, seizures, circling, altered states of consciousness, and behavioral changes are also common.
4. Patients with the disseminated form may present with fever.
5. Animals with the ocular form may be blind or have pupillary abnormalities.

C. Radiography/Myelography/Computed Tomography

1. Survey radiographs are normal.
2. Myelography is generally normal, but occasionally reveals diffuse spinal cord swelling. Analyze the CSF before injecting contrast media.
3. A CT scan (particularly when contrast-enhanced) may be helpful in the diagnosis of focal GME.

D. Laboratory Findings

1. CSF.
   a. CSF analysis often reveals a mild to marked pleocytosis consisting of lymphocytes, monocytes, and occasional plasma cells.
   b. Neutrophils may be seen in up to two thirds of affected animals. They generally make up less than 20% of the total cell count, but occasionally predominate.
   c. Protein concentrations are usually mildly to moderately elevated.

IV. Differential Diagnosis

A. Suspect GME in any mature small-breed dog with acute, progressive, multifocal disease involving the brain, meninges, or cervical spinal cord.

B. Diagnose GME based on history, signalment, onset and progression of clinical signs, CSF analysis, results of imaging techniques, and postmortem examination of CNS tissue.

V. Medical Management

A. Treat GME with corticosteroids (Table 37-3).

1. Treat patients with moderate to severe clinical signs initially with dexamethasone at 2 mg/kg IV. Decrease this dosage to 0.2 mg/kg daily over 3 to 4 days or until neurologic improvement is noted. Discharge the patient on prednisone.
2. Treat patients with mild clinical signs initially with oral prednisone.

B. Continue patients on a maintenance dose indefinitely.

C. If therapy is discontinued, rapid exacerbation of clinical signs often occurs and it may be difficult to achieve a second remission.

D. Treat patients with seizures with anticonvulsant medications.

VI. Surgical Treatment

A. GME is not a surgical disorder.

Table 37-3
Corticosteroid therapy of dogs with GME

Moderate to Severe Clinical Signs
Dexamethasone
0.2-2 mg/kg IV
Prednisone
1-2 mg/kg PO BID, for 2 to 3 weeks; taper over a 3- to 4-week period to 2.5 to 5 mg total dose EOD
Mild Clinical Signs
Prednisone
1-2 mg/kg PO, BID for 2 to 3 weeks; taper as described above

VII. Prognosis

A. Prognosis for GME is generally unfavorable to grave (see Table 37-2).

B. Duration of remission with corticosteroid therapy varies with the form of disease (see Table 37-3).

Degenerative Myelopathy (*SAS*, pp. 1156-1157)

I. Definition

A. **Degenerative myelopathy** is a neurologic disorder of unknown etiology causing progressive demyelination of long-tract fibers, which begins in the thoracolumbar spinal cord.

II. General Considerations

A. Degenerative myelopathy is a progressive disorder causing varying degrees of paraparesis.

B. Pathologic findings include loss of myelin in the spinal cord white matter, a process that generally begins in the thoracic region.

C. The cause is currently unknown.

III. Diagnosis

A. Clinical Presentation

1. Signalment.
   a. Degenerative myelopathy generally occurs in middle-aged to older (i.e., 5 to 7 years) large-breed dogs, particularly German shepherds.

2. History.
   a. There is usually a history of slowly progressive hindlimb weakness without back pain; signs may have been present for months.
   b. Owners may complain that the dog has difficulty rising, or that they hear scuffing or clicking of the hind toenails during ambulation.

B. Physical Examination

1. A neurologic examination generally reveals UMN, ambulatory or weakly ambulatory paraparesis without spinal hyperpathia (i.e., back pain).
2. Patients generally have symmetric or asymmetric loss of conscious proprioception, exaggerated patellar reflexes, and crossed extensor reflexes.
3. Occasionally, patients show LMN (i.e., decreased patellar reflex) and UMN signs.
4. Pain perception and urinary and fecal continence are not lost, even late in the disorder.
5. Thoracic limbs are spared, unless the patient is maintained long after complete paraplegia.

C. Radiography

1. Survey radiographs and myelography are normal in patients with degenerative myelopathy.

D. Laboratory Findings

1. CSF analysis may show mild increases in protein; however, this finding can be consistent with chronic disk protrusion or spinal neoplasia.

IV. Differential Diagnosis

A. Make a strong presumptive diagnosis based on compatible history and neurologic examination combined with normal survey radiographs and a myelogram.

V. Medical Management

A. Although corticosteroids, NSAIDs, vitamins, immune modifiers, interferon and enzyme inhibitors have been tried, no therapy has consistently been effective.

VI. Surgical Treatment

A. Degenerative myelopathy is not a surgical disorder.

VII. Prognosis

A. Inform owners that patients with degenerative myelopathy have an unfavorable prognosis.

B. Progression of this condition to a nonambulatory paraparesis may take months to years.

Spinal Cord Ischemia (*SAS*, pp. 1157-1159)

I. Definition

A. **Fibrocartilaginous embolization (FCE)** is the ischemic necrosis of a segment of spinal cord caused by herniation of intervertebral disk material into the spinal cord microvasculature.

II. General Considerations

A. The pathogenesis of canine FCE is poorly understood.

B. Although other material such as parasites or neoplasia could embolize the spinal cord, fibrocartilaginous material is most commonly associated with canine embolic myelopathy.

III. Diagnosis

A. Clinical Presentation

1. Signalment.
   a. FCE most commonly affects large nonchondrodystrophoid breeds (e.g., Great Danes, St. Bernards, Labrador retrievers, and German shepherds).
   b. The disease is most common in young adults (3 to 7 years).
   c. FCE has also been reported in cats.
2. History.
   a. Patients typically present with an acute, nonprogressive, ambulatory or nonambulatory, tetraparesis, paraparesis, hemiparesis, or monoparesis without spinal hyperpathia (i.e., back or neck pain).
   b. Frequently, history reveals the dog was running or jumping when clinical dysfunction was detected.

B. Physical Examination

1. Neurologic examination findings include an acute onset of nonprogressive UMN or LMN, lateralizing, ambulatory or nonambulatory, tetraparesis, paraparesis, hemiparesis, or monoparesis, without spinal hyperpathia.
2. A loss of deep pain perception occurs in severe cases of spinal cord ischemia.

C. Radiography

1. Survey radiographs are generally normal, although mild collapse of an intervertebral space may be seen.
2. If myelography is performed within 12 to 24 hours of the injury, mild spinal cord swelling, suggestive of an intramedullary mass, is seen.

D. Laboratory Findings

1. CSF.
   a. CSF analysis is often normal, but may reveal mild protein elevation with normal numbers of leukocytes.

b. Mild xanthochromia (i.e., a yellowish appearance caused by hemolyzed blood) sometimes occurs.

IV. Differential Diagnosis

A. Base a presumptive diagnosis on a compatible history and neurologic examination, combined with normal survey spinal radiographs, and characteristic myelographic findings (i.e., normal or mild spinal cord swelling), and by eliminating other causes of spinal cord disease.

V. Medical Management

A. Treat patients presented within 72 hours of the onset of clinical signs with corticosteroids (Dexamethasone 0.2-0.4 mg/kg PO, TID, then BID for 2 days and SID for 2 days), physiotherapy, and confinement for 2 to 3 weeks in an elevated cage with dry soft bedding and easy access to food and water. Perform frequent bladder expressions (i.e., QID).

B. Treat patients presented after 72 hours with supportive care only.

VI. Surgical Treatment

A. Fibrocartilaginous embolism is not a surgical disorder.

VII. Prognosis

A. Prognosis for recovery depends on the site of embolism (i.e., UMN versus LMN), degree of improvement within 14 days, and the extent of spinal cord damage.

B. Generally, patients with UMN deficits are more likely to recover than patients with LMN deficits. Patients showing improvement within 14 days and those with less extensive spinal cord damage (i.e., based on neurologic examination) are more likely to recover.

Appendixes

Appendix A
Calculation of volumes needed for blood transfusions

$$\text{Blood needed (ml)} = \text{recipient's weight (kg)} \times \frac{\text{Desired PCV} - \text{recipient's PCV}}{\text{Donor's PCV}} \times 70[\text{cat}] \text{ or } 90\ [\text{dog}]^*$$

Note: A rough estimate is that 2.2 ml of blood/kg of body weight increases the recipient's PCV by 1%.
*Total blood volume is estimated at 90 ml/kg for dogs and 70 ml/kg for cats.

Appendix B
Shock treatment

Lactated Ringer's Solution or Physiologic Saline Solution

Dogs

Up to 90 ml/kg/hr (to effect)

Cats

Up to 60 ml/kg/hr (to effect)

OR

Hetastarch

5-10 ml/kg (up to 20 ml/kg/day)

OR

7% Hypertonic Saline

4-5 ml/kg (up to 10 ml/kg/day), then isotonic crystalloids at 10-20 ml/kg/hr (to effect)

OR

7% Saline and Dextran 70

3-5 ml/kg (up to 10 ml/kg/day), then isotonic crystalloids at 10-20 ml/kg/hr (to effect)

Flunixin Meglumine (Banamine)

1 mg/kg IV, once or twice if in septic shock

50% Dextrose

1-2 ml/kg IV

Appendix C
Calculation of volumes needed for bicarbonate therapy

Bicarbonate needed (mEq) = 0.3 × base deficit† (mEq) × body weight (kg)
(Give one half IV over 10-15 minutes and reevaluate. Give the remainder over 4-6 hours if necessary, or give 1-2 mEq/kg IV; repeat only if indicated based on assessment of acid-base balance and potassium concentration.)

Note: Because CO_2 is an end product of bicarbonate administration, adequate ventilation should be ensured.
†Some calculate the base deficit as the difference between the desired bicarbonate and the actual bicarbonate (versus normal bicarbonate and actual bicarbonate). Animals that are acidotic enough to require bicarbonate therapy need repeated monitoring.

Appendix D
Commonly used systemic opioid analgesics

Drugs	Sample surgeries	Dosage (mg/kg)*†	Route	Duration*
Butorphanol	Elective reproductive surgery, caudal abdominal procedures, gall bladder surgery, bile peritonitis, distal limb fractures	0.2-0.4	IV, SC, IM	2-3 hr
Buprenorphine	Elective reproductive surgery, caudal abdominal procedures, distal limb fractures	0.005-0.015	IV, IM	4-6 hr
Fentanyl	Used as premedicant, too short acting for analgesia	0.005	IV, SC, IM	<1 hr
Morphine	Thoracotomies, amputations, pelvic fractures, ear ablations	0.1-0.4	IV‡, SC, IM	3-4 hr
Oxymorphone	Thoracotomies, amputations, pelvic fractures, ear ablations	0.05-0.1	IV, SC§, IM	3-4 hr

Modified from Carroll GL: How to manage perioperative pain, *Vet Med* 91:353, 1996.
*Dosages and duration are based on clinical experience and may need to be individualized for a given situation and patient. Higher dosages may be needed for recalcitrant pain.
†The lower dosages are used for intravenous routes and cats.
‡Morphine may be associated with hypotension when administered intravenously; morphine may be associated with excitement in cats.
§Subcutaneous administration may be less efficacious.

Appendix E
Epidural drugs in dogs*

Drug	Uses	Dosage	Onset	Duration
Lidocaine 2%†	Motor and sensory block; abdominal and hindlimb procedures	1 ml/3.4 kg (T_5)‡ 1 ml/4.5 kg (T_{13}-L_1)‡	10 min	1-1.5 hr
Bupivacaine 0.25% or 0.5%†	Motor and sensory block; abdominal and hindlimb procedures	1 ml/4.5 kg‡	20-30 min	4-6 hr
Fentanyl	Sensory block: abdominal and hindlimb procedures	0.001 mg/kg	4-10 min	6 hr
Morphine	Sensory block: thoracotomies, forelimb and hindlimb amputations, cranial and caudal abdominal procedures, hindlimb and pelvic fractures	0.1 mg/kg§ (preservative free)	25 min	~20 hr
Buprenorphine	Sensory block: abdominal and hindlimb procedures	0.003-0.005 mg/kg diluted with saline	—	12-18 hr
Oxymorphone	Sensory block: abdominal, pelvic, and hindlimb procedures	0.1 mg/kg	—	~10 hr

Modified from Carroll GL: How to manage perioperative pain, *Vet Med* 91:353, 1996.
*Dosages, onset, and duration are based on clinical experience; each patient should be evaluated individually.
†Avoid head down position after epidural with local anesthetic.
‡A block to T_1 leads to intercostal nerve paralysis; a block to C_7-C_5 leads to phrenic nerve paralysis.
§The dose for epidural morphine in cats is 0.03 mg/kg.

Appendix F
Postoperative analgesics

Oxymorphone (Numorphan)

0.05-0.1 mg/kg IV, IM every 4 hr (as needed)

Butorphanol (Torbutrol, Torbugesic)

0.2-0.4 mg/kg IV, IM, or SC every 2-4 hr (as needed)

Buprenorphine (Buprenex)

5-15 μg/kg IV, IM every 6 hr (as needed)

Appendix G
Anesthetic Protocols

G-1 Ear Surgery
G-2 Abdominal Surgery
G-3 Peritonitis with Debilitation or Shock
G-4 Oral Disease
G-5 Cervical Esophageal Disorders
G-6 Stable Animals with Gastric Disorders
G-7 Animals That Are Hypovolemic, Dehydrated, or Shocky
G-8 Dogs with Gastric Dilatation-Volvulus
G-9 Stable Animals with Intestinal Disorders
G-10 Dogs with Intestinal Volvulus/Torsion
G-11 Perineal, Rectal, or Anal Surgery
G-12 Hepatic Disease
G-13 Portosystem Shunt
G-14 Dogs with Biliary Disease
G-15 Stable Dogs and Cats with Pancreatic Disease
G-16 Hypovolemic, Dehydrated, or Shocky Animals with Pancreatic Disease
G-17 Stable Dogs and Cats with Renal Disease
G-18 Decompensated Patients in Renal Failure or in Hypovolemic, Dehydrated, or Shocky Animals
G-19 Stable Dogs and Cats with Urinary Abnormalities
G-20 Decompensated Patients in Renal Failure or Hypovolemic, Dehydrated, or Shocky Animals with Urinary Abnormalities
G-21 Elective Reproductive Surgery in Healthy Animals Older Than 6 Months of Age
G-22 Cesarean Section
G-23 Debilitated or Shocky Animals with Pyometra
G-24 Stable Animals with Cardiovascular Disease
G-25 Animals with Heart Failure, Hypovolemia, Dehydration, or Those in Shock
G-26 Respiratory Dysfunction
G-27 Repair of Pectus Excavation in Young Animals That Are Not Dyspneic
G-28 Orthopedic Disease

Appendix G-1
Selected anesthetic protocols for ear surgery

DOGS

Premedication

Give atropine (0.02-0.04 mg/kg SC or IM) or glycopyrrolate (0.005-0.011 mg/kg SC or IM) plus oxymorphone (0.05-0.1 mg/kg SC or IM; see text)

Induction

Thiopental sodium (10-12 mg/kg IV) or propofol (4-6 mg/kg IV)

Maintenance

Isoflurane or halothane

CATS

Premedication

Give atropine (0.02-0.04 mg/kg SC or IM) or glycopyrrolate (0.005-0.011 mg/kg SC or IM) plus butorphanol (0.2-0.4 mg/kg SC or IM) or buprenorphine (5-15 μg/kg IM)

Induction

Use chamber induction with isoflurane; or thiopental sodium or propofol at dose given above for dogs; or diazepam plus ketamine (see text) (0.27 mg/kg and 5.5 mg/kg, respectively) combined and administered IV to effect

Maintenance

Isoflurane or halothane

Appendix G-2
Selected anesthetic protocols for abdominal surgery

Premedication

Atropine (0.02-0.04 mg/kg SC or IM) or glycopyrrolate (0.005-0.011 mg/kg SC or IM) plus oxymorphone (0.05-0.1 mg/kg SC or IM) or butorphanol (0.2-0.4 mg/kg SC or IM) or buprenorphine (5-15 μg/kg IM)

Induction

Thiopental sodium (10-12 mg/kg IV) or propofol (4-6 mg/kg IV) or diazepam plus ketamine (0.27 mg/kg and 5.5 mg/kg, respectively) combined and administered IV to effect

Maintenance

Isoflurane or halothane

Appendix G-3
Selected anesthetic protocols for use in animals with peritonitis that are debilitated or in shock

DOGS

Induction

Oxymorphone (0.1 mg/kg IV) plus diazepam (0.2 mg/kg IV). Give in incremental dosages. Intubate if possible. If necessary, give etomidate (0.5-1.5 mg/kg IV). Alternately, if there is no vomiting, use mask induction or give thiopental or propofol at reduced doses.

Maintenance

Isoflurane

CATS

Premedication

Butorphanol (0.2-0.4 mg/kg SC or IM) or buprenorphine (5-15 μg/kg IM) or oxymorphone (0.05 mg/kg SC or IM)

Induction

Diazepam (0.2 mg/kg IV) followed by etomidate (0.5-1.5 mg/kg IV). Alternately, if there is no vomiting, use mask or chamber induction or give thiopental or propofol at reduced dosages. If there are no contraindications to ketamine, reduced dosages of diazepam and ketamine may also be used.

Maintenance

Isoflurane

Appendix G-4
Selected anesthetic protocols for use in animals with oral disease

Premedication

Give atropine (0.02-0.04 mg/kg SC or IM) or glycopyrrolate (0.005-0.011 mg/kg SC or IM) plus oxymorphone* (0.05-0.1 mg/kg SC or IM) or butorphanol (0.2-0.4 mg/kg SC or IM), or buprenorphine (5-15 μg/kg IM)

Induction

Thiopental (10-12 mg/kg IV) or propofol (4-6 mg/kg IV) to effect or a combination of diazepam and ketamine (diazepam 0.27 mg/kg plus 5.5 mg/kg ketamine IV) titrated to effect

Maintenance

Isoflurane or halothane

*Use 0.05 mg/kg in cats.

Appendix G-5
Selected anesthetic protocols for use in animals with cervical esophageal disorders

Premedication

Give atropine (0.02-0.04 mg/kg SC or IM) or glycopyrrolate (0.005-0.011 mg/kg SC or IM) plus oxymorphone* (0.05-0.1 mg/kg SC or IM) or butorphanol (0.2-0.4 mg/kg SC or IM), or buprenorphine (5-15 μg/kg IM).

Induction

Thiopental (10-12 mg/kg IV) or propofol (4-6 mg/kg IV). Alternately, use a combination of diazepam and ketamine (diazepam 0.27 mg/kg plus 5.5 mg/kg ketamine IV) titrated to effect.

Maintenance

Give isoflurane or halothane.

*Use 0.05 mg/kg in cats.

Appendix G-6
Selected anesthetic protocols for use in stable animals with gastric disorders

Premedication

Give atropine (0.02-0.04 mg/kg SC, IM) or glycopyrrolate (0.005-0.011 mg/kg SC, IM) plus oxymorphone (0.05-0.1 mg/kg SC, IM) or butorphanol (0.2-0.4 mg/kg SC, IM), or buprenorphine (5-15 μg/kg IM).

Induction

Thiopental (10-12 mg/kg IV) or propofol (4-6 mg/kg IV) or a combination of diazepam and ketamine (diazepam 0.27 mg/kg plus 5.5 mg/kg ketamine IV, titrated to effect)

Maintenance

Isoflurane or halothane

Appendix G-7
Selected anesthetic protocols for use in patients that are hypovolemic, dehydrated, or shocky*

DOGS

Induction

Oxymorphone (0.1 mg/kg IV) plus diazepam (0.2 mg/kg IV). Give in incremental dosages. Intubate if possible. If necessary give etomidate (0.5-1.5 mg/kg IV). Alternatively, give thiopental or propofol at extremely reduced dosages.

Maintenance

Isoflurane

CATS

Premedication

Butorphanol (0.2-0.4 mg/kg SC, IM) or buprenorphine (5-15 μg/kg IM) or oxymorphone (0.05 mg/kg SC, IM)

Induction

Diazepam (0.2 mg/kg IV) followed by etomidate (0.5-1.5 mg/kg IV) Alternatively, give thiopental or propofol at reduced dosages. If there are no contraindications to ketamine, reduced dosages of diazepam and ketamine may also be used.

Maintenance

Isoflurane

*Anticholinergics may be administered if indicated.

Appendix G-8
Selected anesthetic protocols for dogs with gastric dilatation volvulus

Induction

Give oxymorphone (0.1 mg/kg IV) plus diazepam (0.2 mg/kg IV). Give in incremental dosages as necessary to intubate. If intubation is not possible, give etomidate (0.5-1.5 mg/kg IV) or thiopental or propofol (at reduced dosages) or (after diazepam and oxymorphone) use a combination of lidocaine and thiobarbiturates (see text).

Maintenance

Isoflurane

Appendix G-9
Selected anesthetic protocols for use in stable animals with intestinal disorders

Premedication

Give atropine (0.02-0.04 mg/kg SC or IM) or glycopyrrolate (0.005-0.011 mg/kg SC or IM) plus oxymorphone* (0.05-0.1 mg/kg SC or IM) or butorphanol (0.2-0.4 mg/kg SC or IM) or buprenorphine (5-15 μg/kg IM).

Induction

Thiopental (10-12 mg/kg IV) or propofol (4-6 mg/kg IV) or a combination of diazepam and ketamine (diazepam 0.27 mg/kg plus 5.5 mg/kg ketamine IV; titrated to effect)

Maintenance

Isoflurane or halothane

*Use 0.05 mg/kg in cats.

Appendix G-10
Selected anesthetic protocols for use in dogs with intestinal volvulus/torsion

Induction

Oxymorphone (0.1 mg/kg IV) plus diazepam (0.2 mg/kg IV). Give in incremental dosages. Intubate if possible. If necessary, give etomidate (0.5-1-5 mg/kg IV). Alternately give thiopental or propofol at reduced doses.

Maintenance

Isoflurane

Appendix G-11
Selected anesthetic protocols for use in animals undergoing perineal, rectal, or anal surgery

DOGS

Premedication

Atropine (0.02-0.04 mg/kg IV, IM, SC) or glycopyrrolate (0.005-0.011 mg/kg IV, IM SC) plus butorphanol (0.2-0.4 mg/kg SC or IM) or buprenorphine (5-15 μg/kg IM) or oxymorphone (0.05-0.1 mg/kg SC or IM)

Induction

Thiopental (10-12 mg/kg) or propofol (4-6 mg/kg) administered IV to effect

Maintenance

Isoflurane or halothane

CATS

Premedication

Atropine (0.02-0.04 mg/kg IV, IM, SC) or glycopyrrolate (0.005-0.011 mg/kg IV, IM, SC) plus ketamine (5 mg/kg IM) plus butorphanol (0.2-0.4 mg/kg SC, IM)

Induction

Diazepam (0.27 mg/kg) plus ketamine (5.5 mg/kg) combined and administered IV to effect or thiopental (10-12 mg/kg) or propofol (4-6 mg/kg) administered IV to effect or mask or chamber induction

Maintenance

Isoflurane or halothane

Appendix G-12
Selected anesthetic agents for animals with hepatic disease*

Premedication

Give atropine (0.02-0.04 mg/kg SC or IM) or glycopyrrolate (0.005-0.011 mg/kg SC or IM) plus oxymorphone† (0.05-0.1 mg/kg SC or IM) or butorphanol (0.2-0.4 mg/kg SC or IM) or buprenorphine (5-15 μg/kg IM).

Induction

Diazepam (0.2 mg/kg IV) plus etomidate (0.5-1.5 mg/kg IV). Alternatively, if not vomiting, mask induction can be used or give thiopental or propofol at reduced doses.

Maintenance

Isoflurane

*See Appendix G-13 for recommendations for patients with portosystemic shunts.
†Use 0.05 mg/kg in cats.

Appendix G-13
Selected anesthetic protocols for animals with portosystemic shunt

DOGS

Premedication

Give atropine (0.02-0.04 mg/kg SC or IM) or glycopyrrolate (0.005-0.011 mg/kg SC or IM) plus oxymorphone (0.05-0.1 mg/kg SC or IM).

Induction

Mask induce with isoflurane.

Maintenance

Isoflurane

CATS

Premedication

Give atropine (0.02-0.04 mg/kg SC or IM) or glycopyrrolate (0.005-0.011 mg/kg SC or IM) plus butorphanol (0.2-0.4 mg/kg SC or IM) or buprenorphine (5-15 μg/kg IM) or oxymorphone (0.05 mg/kg SC or IM).

Induction

Chamber induce with isoflurane.

Maintenance

Isoflurane

Appendix G-14
Selected anesthetic protocol for dogs with biliary disease

Induction

Oxymorphone (0.1 mg/kg IV) plus diazepam (0.2 mg/kg IV). Give in incremental dosages. Intubate if possible. If necessary, give etomidate (0.5-1.5 mg/kg IV) to effect.

Maintenance

Isoflurane

Appendix G-15
Selected anesthetic protocols for use in stable dogs and cats with pancreatic disease

Premedication

Give atropine (0.02-0.04 mg/kg SC or IM) or glycopyrrolate (0.005-0.011 mg/kg SC or IM) plus oxymorphone* (0.05-0.1 mg/kg SC or IM) or butorphanol (0.2-0.4 mg/kg SC or IM) or buprenorphine (5-15 μg/kg IM).

Induction

Thiopental (10-12 mg/kg IV) or propofol (4-6 mg/kg IV)

Maintenance

Isoflurane or halothane

*Use 0.05 mg/kg in cats.

Appendix G-16
Selected anesthetic protocols for use in hypovolemic, dehydrated, or shocky animals with pancreatic disease

DOGS

Induction

Oxymorphone (0.1 mg/kg IV) plus diazepam (0.2 mg/kg IV). Give in incremental dosages. Intubate if possible. If necessary, give etomidate (0.5-1.5 mg/kg IV). (See text also.)

Maintenance

Isoflurane

CATS

Premedication

Butorphanol (0.2-0.4 mg/kg SC or IM) or buprenorphine (5-15 μg/kg IM) or oxymorphone (0.05 mg/kg SC or IM)

Induction

Diazepam (0.2 mg/kg IV) followed by etomidate (0.5-1.5 mg/kg IV). (See text also.)

Maintenance

Isoflurane

Appendix G-17
Selected anesthetic protocols for use in stable dogs and cats with renal disease

Premedication

Give atropine (0.02-0.04 mg/kg SC or IM) or glycopyrrolate (0.005-0.011 mg/kg SC or IM) plus oxymorphone* (0.05-0.1 mg/kg SC or IM); or butorphanol (0.2-0.4 mg/kg SC or IM); or buprenorphine (5-15 μg/kg IM).

Induction

Thiopental (10-12 mg/kg IV) or propofol (4-6 mg/kg IV) (See text also.)

Maintenance

Isoflurane or halothane

*Use 0.05 mg/kg in cats.

Appendix G-18
Selected anesthetic protocols for use in decompensated patients in renal failure or in hypovolemic, dehydrated, or shocky animals

DOGS

Induction

Oxymorphone (0.1 mg/kg IV) plus diazepam (0.2 mg/kg IV). Give in incremental dosages. Intubate if possible. If necessary, give etomidate (0.5-1.5 mg/kg IV).

Maintenance

Isoflurane

CATS

Premedication

Butorphanol (0.2-0.4 mg/kg SC or IM) or buprenorphine (5-15 μg/kg IM) or oxymorphone (0.05 mg/kg SC or IM)

Induction

Diazepam (0.2 mg/kg IV) followed by etomidate (0.5-1.5 mg/kg IV) (See text also.)

Maintenance

Isoflurane

Appendix G-19
Selected anesthetic protocols for use in stable dogs and cats with urinary abnormalities

Premedication

Oxymorphone* (0.05-0.1 mg/kg SC or IM) or butorphanol (0.2-0.4 mg/kg SC or IM) or buprenorphine (5-15 μg/kg IM)

Induction

Thiopental (10-12 mg/kg IV) or propofol (4-6 mg/kg IV) (see text also)

Maintenance

Isoflurane or halothane

*Use 0.05 mg/kg in cats

Appendix G-20
Selected anesthetic protocols for use in decompensated patients in renal failure or hypovolemic, dehydrated, or shocky animals with urinary abnormalities

DOGS

Induction

Oxymorphone (0.1 mg/kg IV) plus diazepam (0.2 mg/kg IV). Give in incremental dosages. Intubate if possible. If necessary, give etomidate (0.5-1.5 mg/kg IV). (See text also.)

Maintenance

Isoflurane

CATS

Premedication

Butorphanol (0-2-0.4 mg/kg SC or IM) or buprenorphine (5-15 μg/kg IM) or oxymorphone (0.05 mg/kg SC or IM)

Induction

Diazepam (0.2 mg/kg IV) followed by etomidate (0.5-1.5 mg/kg IV). (See text also.)

Maintenance

Isoflurane

Appendix G-21
Selected anesthetic protocols for elective reproductive surgery in healthy animals older than 6 months of age

DOGS

Premedication

Atropine (0.02-0.04 mg/kg SC or IM) or glycopyrrolate (0.005-0.011 mg/kg SC, IM) plus acepromazine (0.05 mg/kg SC or IM; not to exceed 1 mg) and butorphanol* (0.2-0.4 mg/kg SC, IM)

Induction

Thiopental (10-12 mg/kg) administered IV to effect

Maintenance

Isoflurane or halothane

CATS

Premedication

Atropine (0.02-0.04 mg/kg SC or IM) or glycopyrrolate (0.005-0.011 mg/kg SC, IM) plus ketamine (5 mg/kg IM) and butorphanol (0.2-0.4 mg/kg SC, IM)

Induction

Diazepam (0.27 mg/kg) plus ketamine (5.5 mg/kg) combined and administered IV to effect or thiopental (10-12 mg/kg) administered IV to effect or mask or chamber induction

Maintenance

Isoflurane or halothane

*Other opioids may be substituted for butorphanol (see text).

Appendix G-22
Selected anesthetic protocols for cesarean section

GENERAL PRINCIPLES

1. Place an IV catheter
2. Immediately begin volume replacement with IV crystalloids (10-20 ml/kg)
3. Preoxygenate before induction

DOGS

Premedication

Glycopyrrolate (0.005-0.011 mg/kg SC, IM)

Induction

Oxymorphone (0.1 mg/kg IV) plus diazepam (0.2 mg/kg IV); intubate if possible. If necessary, give etomidate (0.5-1.5 mg/kg IV). Alternatively, small doses of thiopental or propofol may be used.

Maintenance

Isoflurane

CATS

Premedication

Glycopyrrolate (0.005-0.011 mg/kg SC, IM) and butorphanol (0.2-0.4 mg/kg SC, IM)

Induction

Diazepam (0.2 mg/kg IV) followed by etomidate (0.5-1.5 mg/kg IV). Alternately, a combination of diazepam (0.27 mg/kg) plus ketamine (5.5 mg/kg) may be administered IV to effect or reduced dosages of thiopental or propofol may be used.

Maintenance

Isoflurane

Appendix G-23
Selected anesthetic protocols for debilitated or shocky animals with pyometra

DOGS

Induction

Oxymorphone (0.1 mg/kg IV) plus diazepam (0.2 mg/kg IV). Give in incremental dosages. Intubate if possible. If necessary, give etomidate (0.5-1.5 mg/kg IV). Alternatively, if not vomiting, mask induction can be used or give thiopental or propofol at reduced doses.

Maintenance

Isoflurane

CATS

Premedication

Butorphanol (0.2-0.4 mg/kg SC or IM) or buprenorphine (5-15 μg/kg IM) or oxymorphone (0.05 mg/kg SC or IM)

Induction

Diazepam (0.2 mg/kg IV) followed by etomidate (0.5-1.5 mg/kg IV). Alternatively, if not vomiting, mask or chamber induction can be used or give thiopental or propofol at reduced dosages. If there are no contraindications to ketamine (i.e., renal dysfunction), reduced dosages of diazepam and ketamine may also be used.

Maintenance

Isoflurane

Appendix G-24
Selected anesthetic protocols for use in stable animals with cardiovascular disease

Premedication

Give atropine (0.02-0.04 mg/kg SC or IM) or glycopyrrolate (0.005-0.011 mg/kg SC or IM) if indicated plus oxymorphone* (0.05-0.1 mg/kg SC or IM) or butorphanol (0.2-0.4 mg/kg SC or IM) or buprenorphine (5-15 μg/kg IM).

Induction

Thiopental (10-12 mg/kg IV) or propofol (4-6 mg/kg IV)

Maintenance

Isoflurane or halothane

*Use 0.05 mg/kg in cats.

Appendix G-25
Selected anesthetic protocols for use in animals with heart failure, hypovolemia, dehydration, or those in shock

DOGS

Induction

Oxymorphone (0.1 mg/kg IV) plus diazepam (0.2 mg/kg IV). Give in incremental dosages. Intubate if possible. If necessary, give etomidate (0.5-1.5 mg/kg IV). Alternately, give thiopental or propofol at reduced dosages. If there are no contraindications to ketamine, reduced dosages of diazepam and ketamine may also be used.

Maintenance

Isoflurane

CATS

Premedication

Butorphanol (0.2-0.4 mg/kg SC or IM) or buprenorphine (5-15 μg/kg IM) or oxymorphone (0.05 mg/kg SC or IM)

Induction

Diazepam (0.2 mg/kg IV) followed by etomidate (0-5-1.5 mg/kg IV). Alternately, if not vomiting, mask or chamber induction can be used or give thiopental or propofol at reduced dosages. If there are no contraindications to ketamine, reduced dosages of diazepam and ketamine may also be used.

Maintenance

Isoflurane

Appendix G-26
Selected anesthetic protocols for use in animals with respiratory dysfunction

For Stable (Nonarrhythmic, Nondyspneic) Animals

Premedication

Oxymorphone* (0.05-0.1 mg/kg SC or IM)

Induction

Thiopental (10-12 mg/kg IV) or propofol (4-6 mg/kg IV) or give diazepam (0.27 mg/kg IV) and ketamine (5.5 mg/kg IV) combined and titrated to effect

Maintenance

Isoflurane or halothane

For Dyspneic, Nonarrhythmic Animals

Induction

Diazepam (0.2 mg/kg IV) followed immediately with thiopental (10-12 mg/kg IV)† or propofol (4-6 mg/kg IV) or give diazepam (0.27 mg/kg IV) and ketamine (5.5 mg/kg IV) combined and titrated to effect

Maintenance

Isoflurane or halothane

For Very Sick or Arrhythmic Animals

Induction

Diazepam (0.2 mg/kg IV) followed by etomidate (1-3 mg/kg IV)†

Maintenance

Isoflurane

*Use 0.05 mg/kg in cats.
†Can add oxymorphone (0.05-0.1 mg/kg IV) in dogs as part of the induction and decrease the etomidate or barbiturate dose.

Appendix G-27
Selected anesthetic protocols for repair of pectus excavation in young animals that are not dyspneic

DOGS

Premedication

Atropine (0.02-0.04 mg/kg, SC or IM) or glycopyrrolate (0.005-0.01 mg/kg SC or IM) plus oxymorphone (0.05-0.1 mg/kg IM or SC) or butorphanol (0.2-0.4 mg/kg IM or SC)

Induction

Use mask induction with isoflurane after 5 min of preoxygenation

CATS

Premedication

Atropine (0.02-0.04 mg/kg, SC or IM) or glycopyrrolate (0.005-0.01 mg/kg SC or IM) plus butorphanol at dose above or buprenorphine (5-15 μg/kg IM or SC)

Induction

Use chamber induction with isoflurane after preoxygenating for 5 min

Appendix G-28
Suggested protocols for the anesthetic management of patients with orthopedic disease

For Stable Patients and Those Presented for Elective Procedures

Premedication

Glycopyrrolate (0.005-0.011 mg/kg SC or IM) or atropine (0.02-0.04 mg/kg SC or IM) plus oxymorphone (0.05-0.1 mg/kg SC or IM) or butorphanol (0.2-0.4 mg/kg SC or IM) or buprenorphine (5-15 μg/kg IM) and acepromazine 0.05 mg/kg, not to exceed 1 mg SC or IM

Induction

Thiopental (10-12 mg/kg IV) or propofol (4-6 mg/kg IV)

Maintenance

Isoflurane or halothane

For Unstable Animals that Have Recently Had Trauma

Induction

Oxymorphone (0.1 mg/kg IV) plus diazepam (0.2 mg/kg IV). Give in incremental dosages. Intubate if possible. If necessary, give etomidate (0.5-1.5 mg/kg IV). Alternatively, mask induction or thiopental or propofol at extremely reduced dosages may be used.

Maintenance

Isoflurane

Appendix G-29
Selected anesthetic protocols for dogs undergoing spinal surgery

Premedication

Methylprednisolone sodium succinate (30 mg/kg IV) or dexamethasone (1.5 mg/kg IV) plus oxymorphone (0.05-0.1 mg/kg SC or IM), or butorphanol (0.2-0.4 mg/kg SC or IM), or buprenorphine (5-15 μg/kg IM)

Induction

Thiopental (10-12 mg/kg IV) or propofol (4-6 mg/kg IV)

Maintenance

Isoflurane or halothane

Appendix H
Intravenous potassium supplementation guidelines

Serum potassium* (mEq/L)	mEq KCl/L of fluid	Maximal infusion rate† (ml/kg/hr)
<2.0	80	6
2.1-2.5	60	8
2.6-3.0	40	12
3.1-3.5	28	16

*If serum potassium not available, add potassium to a total concentration of 20 mEq/L.
†Do not exceed 0.5 mEq/kg/hr

Appendix I
Drug index

Drug name	Brand name	Dosage and route	Species	Use; indication	*SAS* reference
50% Dextrose		1-2 ml/kg IV	Dogs and cats	Medical treatment; shock	Table 23-34, p. 556
Acepromazine		0.02-0.05 mg/kg IV, IM, or SC; max 1 mg	Dogs	Sedation; severely dyspneic dogs	Table 25-2, p. 609
		0.05 mg/kg IM with butorphanol	Cats	Sedation; orthopedic disease	Table 28-8, p. 723
		0.05 mg/kg IV, IM, or SC, max 1 mg	Dogs and cats	Premedication; healthy animals undergoing elective surgery	Table 23-5, p. 519
				Sedation; severely dyspneic cats	Table 25-3, p. 609
				Sedation; nasal surgery	Table 25-18, p. 643
				Premedication; stable with orthopedic disease	Table 28-2, p. 708
		0.05 mg/kg IV, IM, or SC; max 1 mg with oxymorphone	Dogs	Sedation; orthopedic disease	Table 28-7, p. 723
Allopurinol	Zyloprim	7-10 mg/kg PO, SID to TID	Dogs and cats	Medical management; urinary calculi	Table 22-9, p. 502
Amikacin	Amiglyde-V	10 mg/kg IV, IM, or SC, TID or 30 mg/kg SID	Dogs and cats	Treatment of aspiration pneumonia	Table 16-18, p. 233
				Antibiotic; upper respiratory infection	Table 25-9, p. 611
				Antibiotic; orthopedic infection	Table 28-5, p. 710
				Antibiotic; diskospondylitis	Table 37-2, p. 1153
		30 mg/kg IV, SID	Dogs and cats	Antibiotic; peritonitis	Table 15-6, p. 195
				Antibiotic; septic shock	Table 23-35, p. 556
				Antibiotic; pyothorax	Table 27-17, p. 700
Aminophylline		11 mg/kg PO, IM, or IV, TID	Dogs	Treatment of aspiration pneumonia	Table 16-18, p. 233
				Medical therapy; tracheal collapse	Table 25-16, p. 634
		5 mg/kg PO, BID	Cats	Treatment of aspiration pneumonia	Table 16-18, p. 233
				Medical therapy; tracheal collapse	Table 25-16, p. 634
Amoxicillin	Amoxi-tabs, Amoxi-drops, Amoxi-inject	22 mg/kg PO, IM, or SC, BID to TID	Dogs and cats	Antibiotic; oral surgery	Table 16-2, p. 201
				Antibiotic; esophagitis	Table 16-22, p. 262
				Antibiotic; biliary disease	Table 18-3, p. 390
		22-30 mg/kg IV, IM, SC, or PO, TID to QID	Dog and cats	Antibiotic; orthopedic infection	Table 28-5, p. 710

Amoxicillin plus clavulanate	Clavamox	12.5-25 mg/kg PO, BID	Dogs	Antibiotic; hepatic abscess	Table 17-9, p. 385
				Antibiotic; renal disease	Table 21-4, p. 463
				Antibiotic; reproductive disorder	Table 23-8, p. 521
				Antibiotic; pyometra	Table 23-23, p. 548
				Antibiotic; cervical spinal surgery	Table 34-6, p. 1051
		22 mg/kg PO, TID to QID	Dogs and cats	Antibiotic; orthopedic infection	Table 28-5, p. 710
		62.5 mg PO, BID	Cats	Antibiotic; hepatic abscess	Table 17-9, p. 385
				Antibiotic; renal disease	Table 21-4, p. 463
				Antibiotic; reproductive disorder	Table 23-8, p. 521
				Antibiotic; pyometra	Table 23-23, p. 548
				Antibiotic; cervical spinal surgery	Table 34-6, p. 1051
Ampicillin		20-40 mg/kg IM, SC, PO or IV, QID	Dogs and cats	Antibiotic; pyothorax	Table 27-17, p. 700
		22 mg/kg IV, IM, SC, or PO, TID to QID	Dogs and cats	Antibiotic; aspiration pneumonia	Table 16-6, p. 212
				Treatment of aspiration pneumonia	Table 16-18, p. 233
				Antibiotic; esophagitis	Table 16-22, p. 262
				Antibiotic; postoperative peritonitis	Table 16-50, p. 304
				Antibiotic; hepatocellular compromise	Table 17-3, p. 368
				Medical management; portosystemic shunt	Table 17-6, p. 377
				Antibiotic; renal disease	Table 21-4, p. 463
				Antibiotic; reproductive disorder	Table 23-8, p. 521
				Antibiotic; pyometra	Table 23-23, p. 548
				Antibiotic; upper respiratory infection	Table 25-9, p. 611
				Medical therapy; tracheal collapse	Table 25-16, p. 634
				Antibiotic; orthopedic infection	Table 28-5, p. 710
		22 mg/kg IV, TID or QID	Dogs and cats	Antibiotic; peritonitis	Table 15-6, p. 195
				Antibiotic; septic shock	Table 23-35, p. 556
				Medical treatment; Lyme disease	Table 30-9, p. 894

Continued

Appendix I
Drug index—cont'd

Drug name	Brand name	Dosage and route	Species	Use; indication	*SAS* reference
Apomorphine		0.02 mg/kg IV or 0.04 mg/kg SC	Dogs	Induction of vomiting	Table 16-30, p. 276
Aspirin		1 regular strength tablet per 25 lb b.w., not to exceed 3 tablets/dose, PO with food, BID to TID	Dogs	Medical management; degenerative joint disease	Table 30-5, p. 890
				Medical treatment; panosteitis	Table 32-1, p. 1011
		10 mg/kg BID for 2-3 days	Dogs and cats	Medical management; cauda equina syndrome	Table 36-8, p. 1140
		10 mg/kg PO, BID for 7 days	Dogs	Medical management; cervical or thoracolumbar disk disease	Table 34-9, p. 1068
				Medical management; wobbler syndrome	Table 34-20, p. 1078
Aspirin		25 mg/kg PO with food, BID to TID	Dogs	Medical management; degenerative joint disease	Table 30-5, p. 890
				Medical treatment; panosteitis	Table 32-1, p. 1011
Aspirin, buffered	Ascriptin	1 regular strength tablet per 25 lb b.w., not to exceed 3 tablets/dose, PO with food, BID to TID	Dogs	Analgesic; osteochondritis dissecans of scapulohumeral joint	Table 30-14, p. 905
		25 mg/kg PO with food, BID to TID	Dogs	Medical management; degenerative joint disease	Table 30-5, p. 890
				Analgesic; osteochondritis dissecans of scapulohumeral joint	Table 30-14, p. 905
				Medical managment; hip dysplasia	Table 30-20, p. 944
				Medical treatment; panosteitis	Table 32-1, p. 1011
				Analgesic; craniomandibular osteopathy	Table 32-2, p. 1012

Atenolol	Tenormin	6.25-12.5 mg/cat PO, SID to BID	Cats	Medical management; cardiac disease	Table 24-1, p. 575
				β-Adrenergic therapy; aortic stenosis	Table 24-8, p. 589
				β-Adrenergic therapy; tetralogy of fallot	Table 24-10, p. 595
		6.25-50 mg/dog PO, SID to BID	Dogs	Medical management; cardiac disease	Table 24-1, p. 575
				β-Adrenergic therapy; aortic stenosis	Table 24-8, p. 589
				β-Adrenergic therapy; tetralogy of fallot	Table 24-10, p. 595
Atropine		0.02 mg/kg IV or 0.04 mg/kg IM or SC with butorphanol or diazepam	Dogs	Sedation; orthopedic disease	Table 28-7, p. 723
		0.02-0.04 mg/kg SC or IM	Dogs and cats	Premedication; ear surgery	Table 14-2, p. 154
				Premedication; abdominal surgery	Table 15-1, p. 180
				Anticholinergic	Table 15-10, p. 197
				Premedication; oral disease	Table 16-1, p. 201
				Premedication; cervical esophageal disorder	Table 16-19, p. 234
				Premedication; stable with gastric disorder	Table 16-23, p. 262
					Table 16-47, p. 294
				Premedication; perineal, rectal, or anal surgery	Table 16-68, p. 337
				Premedication; hepatic disease	Table 17-2, p. 368
				Premedication; portosystemic shunt	Table 17-7, p. 378
				Premedication; cats with pancreatic disease	Table 19-12, p. 415
				Premedication; cats with renal disease	Table 21-2, p. 462
				Premedication; healthy animals	Table 23-5, p. 519
				Premedication; stable with cardiovascular disease	Table 24-2, p. 576

Continued

Appendix I
Drug index—cont'd

Drug name	Brand name	Dosage and route	Species	Use; indication	*SAS* reference
Atropine—cont'd				Atropine response test; sinus bradycardia	Table 24-13, p. 604
				Premedication; canine laryngeal examination	Table 25-6, p. 610
				Premedication; not dyspneic, pectus excavatum	Table 26-9, p. 670
				Premedication; stable with orthopedic disease	Table 28-2, p. 708
		0.04 mg/kg IM with butorphanol	Cats	Sedation; orthopedic disease	Table 28-8, p. 723
Aurothioglucose (gold salts)		1 mg/kg IM once weekly for 10 wk or until remission	Dogs and cats	Medical treatment; rheumatoid arthritis	Table 30-12, p. 897
Azathioprine	Imuran	0.3 mg/kg EOD, give with extreme care	Cats	Medical management; colitis	Table 16-62, p. 331
				Medical treatment; feline chronic progressive polyarthritis	Table 30-13, p. 898
		2.2 mg/kg PO SID, for 2-3 wk, reduce to EOD	Dogs	Medical management; colitis	Table 16-62, p. 331
				Medical treatment, idiopathic immune-mediated polyarthritis	Table 30-10, p. 894
				Medical treatment; rheumatoid arthritis	Table 30-12, p. 897
Bethanechol	Urecholine	1.25-5 mg/cat PO, BID to TID	Cats	Improve urination; urethral surgery	Table 22-6, p. 499
		5-15 mg/dog PO, BID to TID	Dogs	Improve urination; urethral surgery	Table 22-6, p. 499
Bisacodyl	Dulcolax	2.5-5 mg/kg PO, SID to BID	Cats	Bowel preparation; large intestinal or rectal surgery	Table 16-56, p. 320
				Stool softener, laxative	Table 16-61, p. 327
		5-20 mg PO, SID to BID	Dogs	Bowel preparation; large intestine, or rectal surgery	Table 16-56, p. 320
				Stool softener, laxative	Table 16-61, p. 327

Bupivacaine		2 mg/kg intrapleural, intercostal, or split	Dogs	Local anesthesia; thoracotomy	Table 26-2, p. 650
		1 ml/4.5 kg epidural (0.25%-0.5%)	Dogs	Epidural anesthesia/analgesia	Table 12-2, p. 88 Table 23-6, p. 520 Table 28-4, p. 709
Buprenorphine	Buprenex	0.003-0.005 mg/kg epidural, diluted with saline	Dogs	Epidural anesthesia/analgesia	Table 12-2, p. 88
				Epidural anesthesia	Table 23-6, p. 520
		0.005 mg/kg epidural	Dogs	Epidural anesthesia	Table 28-4, p. 709
		0.005-0.015 mg/kg IM	Dogs and cats	Premedication; debilitated/shocky with peritonitis	Table 15-9, p. 197
				Premedication; hypovolemic, dehydrated, or shocky	Table 16-24, p. 263
				Premedication; hypovolemic, dehydrated, or shocky with pancreatic disease	Table 19-13, p. 415
				Premedication; hypovolemic, dehydrated, or shocky with decompensated renal failure	Table 21-3, p. 462
				Premedication; stable dogs, cats with urinary abnormalities	Table 22-3; p. 482
				Premedication; hypovolemic, dehydrated, or shocky with decompensated renal failure or urinary abnormalities	Table 22-4, p. 483
				Premedication; shocky, dehydrated, or hypovolemic cats with sterile cystitis	Table 22-12, p. 513
				Premedication; debilitated or shocky with pyometra	Table 23-24, p. 548

Continued

Appendix I
Drug index—cont'd

Drug name	Brand name	Dosage and route	Species	Use; indication	*SAS* reference
Buprenorphine	Buprenex	0.005-0.015 mg/kg IM	Dogs and cats	Premedication; hypovolemia, dehydration, shock, or heart failure	Table 24-3, p. 576
				Premedication; canine laryngeal examination	Table 25-6, p. 610
				Premedication; stable with orthopedic disease	Table 28-2, p. 708
				Premedication; spinal surgery	Table 34-3, p. 1050
		0.005-0.015 mg/kg IM with glycopyrrolate	Stable dogs or cats with disease condition	Premedication; ear surgery	Table 14-2, p. 154
				Premedication; abdominal surgery	Table 15-1, p. 180
				Premedication; oral disease	Table 16-1, p. 201
				Premedication; cervical esophageal disorder	Table 16-19, p. 234
				Premedication; stable with gastric disorder	Tables 16-23, p. 262 and 16-47, p. 294
				Premedication; perineal, rectal, or anal surgery	Table 16-68, p. 337
				Premedication; hepatic disease	Table 17-2, p. 368
				Premedication; portosystemic shunt	Table 17-7, p. 378
				Premedication; cats with pancreatic disease	Table 19-12, p. 415
				Premedication; cats with renal disease	Table 21-2, p. 462
				Premedication; stable with cardiovascular disease	Table 24-2, p. 576
				Premedication; not dyspneic, pectus excavatum	Table 26-9, p. 670
		0.005-0.015 mg/kg IV or IM	Dogs and cats	Systemic opioid analgesic	Table 12-1, p. 87

Buprenorphine—cont'd	Buprenex—cont'd	0.005-0.015 mg/kg IV or IM every 6 hr as needed	Dogs and cats	Analgesic; digestive surgery	Table 16-4, p. 209
				Analgesic; hepatic surgery	Table 17-4, p. 373
				Analgesic; renal surgery	Table 21-5, p. 469
				Analgesic; urinary tract surgery	Table 22-5, p. 495
				Analgesic; ovariohysterectomy	Table 23-25, p. 548
				Analgesic; cardiac surgery	Table 24-6, p. 581
				Analgesic; upper respiratory surgery	Table 25-10, p. 618
				Analgesic; thoracotomy	Tables 26-3, p. 650 and 27-22, p. 704
				Analgesic; orthopedic surgery	Table 28-3, p. 708
				Analgesic; cervical spinal surgery	Table 34-13, p. 1070
Butorphanol	Torbutrol, Torbugesic	0.2 mg/kg IM with acepromazine or xylazine and atropine or glycopyrrolate	Cats	Sedation; orthopedic disease	Table 28-8, p. 723
		0.2 mg/kg IV or IM with atropine or glycopyrrolate	Dogs	Sedation; orthopedic disease	Table 28-7, p. 723
		0.2-0.4 mg/kg IV, SC, or IM	Dogs; use low end doses for cats and IV	Systemic opioid analgesic	Table 12-1, p. 87
				Preanesthetic; biliary disease	Table 18-2, p. 390
				Premedication; stable dogs, cats with urinary abnormalities	Table 22-3, p. 482
				Sedation; severely dyspneic dogs	Table 25-2, p. 609

Continued

Appendix I
Drug index—cont'd

Drug name	Brand name	Dosage and route	Species	Use; indication	*SAS* reference
Butorphanol—cont'd	Torbutrol, Torbugesic—cont'd	0.2-0.4 mg/kg IV, SC, or IM every 2 to 4 hr as needed	Dogs and cats	Analgesic; digestive surgery	Table 16-4, p. 209
				Analgesic; hepatic surgery	Table 17-4, p. 373
				Analgesic; biliary disease	Table 18-2, p. 390
				Analgesic; bile peritonitis	Table 18-5, p. 399
				Analgesic; renal surgery	Table 21-5, p. 469
				Analgesic; urinary tract surgery	Table 22-5, p. 495
				Analgesic; ovariohysterectomy	Table 23-25, p. 548
				Analgesic; cardiac surgery	Table 24-6, p. 581
				Analgesic; upper respiratory surgery	Table 25-10, p. 618
				Analgesic; thoracotomy	Tables 26-3, p. 650 and 27-22, p. 704
				Analgesic; orthopedic surgery	Table 28-3, p. 708
				Analgesic; cervical spine surgery	Table 34-13, p. 1070
		0.2-0.4 mg/kg SC or IM	Dogs and cats	Premedication; debilitated/shocky with peritonitis	Table 15-9, p. 197
				Premedication; hypovolemic, dehydrated, or shocky	Table 16-24, p. 263
				Premedication; hypovolemic, dehydrated, or shocky with pancreatic disease	Table 19-13, p. 415
				Premedication; hypovolemic, dehydrated, or shocky with decompensated renal failure	Table 21-3, p. 462
				Premedication; hypovolemic, dehydrated, or shocky with decompensated renal failure or urinary abnormalities	Table 22-4, p. 483
				Premedication; shocky, dehydrated, or hypovolemic cats with sterile cystitis	Table 22-12, p. 513
				Premedication; healthy animals	Table 23-5, p. 519

Butorphanol—cont'd	Torbutrol, Torbugesic—cont'd			
				Premedication; cesarean section	Table 23-7, p. 521
				Premedication; debilitated/shocky, pyometra	Table 23-24, p. 548
				Premedication; canine laryngeal examination	Table 25-6, p. 610
				Premedication; stable with orthopedic disease	Table 28-2, p. 708
				Premedication; spinal surgery	Table 34-3, p. 1050
		0.2-0.4 mg/kg SC or IM with glycopyrrolate	Stable dogs, cats with disease condition	Premedication; ear surgery	Table 14-2, p. 154
				Premedication; abdominal surgery	Table 15-1, p. 180
				Premedication; oral disease	Table 16-1, p. 201
				Premedication; cervical esophageal disorder	Table 16-19, p. 234
				Premedication; stable with gastric disorder	Table 16-23, p. 262 Table 16-47, p. 294
				Premedicatipn; perineal, rectal, or anal surgery	Table 16-68, p. 337
				Premedication; hepatic disease	Table 17-2, p. 368
				Premedication; portosystemic shunt	Table 17-7, p. 378
				Premedication; cats with pancreatic disease	Table 19-12, p. 415
				Premedication; cats with renal disease	Table 21-2, p. 462
				Premedication; stable with cardiovascular disease	Table 24-2, p. 576
				Premedication; hypovolemia, dehydration, shock, or heart failure	Table 24-3, p. 576
				Premedication; not dyspneic, pectus excavatum	Table 26-9, p. 670
		0.5-1.0 mg/kg PO, BID to TID	Dogs and cats	Medical therapy; tracheal collapse	Table 25-16, p. 634

Continued

Appendix I
Drug index—cont'd

Drug name	Brand name	Dosage and route	Species	Use; indication	*SAS* reference
Calcium gluconate		0.5-1.0 ml/kg IV over 5 min; use with extreme caution	Dogs and cats	Medical therapy; hyperkalemia	Table 24-15, p. 605
		10 ml, 10% CaGl in 250 ml LRS IV drip	Dogs and cats	Correction of hypocalcemia; thyroidectomy	Table 19-32, p. 436
		5-15 mg Ca/kg IV slowly (10-20 min) bolus	Dogs and cats	Correction of hypocalcemia; thyroidectomy	Table 19-32, p. 436
		5-15 mg/kg Ca in equal amounts saline SC, in multiple sites	Dogs and cats	Correction of hypocalcemia; thyroidectomy	Table 19-32, p. 436
Calcium lactate		0.2-0.5 mg/cat/day divided, PO with vitamin D	Cats	Correction of hypocalcemia; thyroidectomy	Table 19-32, p. 436
Canned pumpkin		1-4 tablespoons PO, SID	Dogs and cats	Stool softener, laxative	Table 16-61, p. 327
Carbenicillin	Geocillin	10 mg/kg PO, TID	Dogs and cats	Antibiotic; reproductive disorder	Table 23-8, p. 521
Carprofen	Rimadyl	2.2 mg/kg PO, BID	Dogs	Medical management; degenerative joint disease	Table 30-5, p. 890
				Medical management; hip dysplasia	Table 30-20, p. 944
Cefadroxil	Cefa-tab	22 mg/kg PO, BID to TID	Dogs and cats	Antibiotic; orthopedic infection	Table 28-5, p. 710
				Medical treatment; Lyme disease	Table 30-9, p. 894
Cefazolin	Ancef, Kefzol	20 mg/kg IV	Dogs and cats	Antibiotic; oral surgery	Table 16-2, p. 201
				Antibiotic; intestinal surgery	Table 16-48, p. 294
				Antibiotic; postoperative peritonitis	Table 16-50, p. 304
				Antibiotic; prophylactic, cardiac surgery	Table 24-5, p. 577
		20 mg/kg IV or IM, TID to QID	Dogs and cats	Treatment of aspiration pneumonia	Table 16-18, p. 233
				Antibiotic; esophagitis	Table 16-22, p. 262
				Antibiotic; hepatocellular compromise	Table 17-3, p. 368
				Antibiotic; hepatic abscess	Table 17-9, p. 385
				Antibiotic; biliary disease	Table 18-3, p. 390

Cefazolin—cont'd	Ancef, Kefzol—cont'd			Antibiotic; renal disease	Table 21-4, p. 463
				Antibiotic; reproductive disorder	Table 23-8, p. 521
				Antibiotic; pyometra	Table 23-23, p. 548
				Antibiotic; upper respiratory infection	Table 25-9, p. 611
				Medical therapy; tracheal collapse	Table 25-16, p. 634
				Antibiotic; cervical spine surgery	Table 34-6, p. 1051
		20 mg/kg IV, repeat once or twice at 4-6 hr intervals	Dogs and cats	Antibiotic; perioperative, gastric surgery	Table 16-25, p. 263 Table 16-40, p. 285
				Antibiotic; prophylactic, pancreatic surgery	Table 19-14, p. 415
				Antibiotic; perioperative, upper respiratory surgery	Table 25-8, p. 611
				Antibiotic; perioperative, thoracotomy	Table 26-4, p. 651
		20 mg/kg IV; QID for 24 hr	Dogs and cats	Antibiotic; prophylactic, perineal, rectal, or colonic surgery	Table 16-57, p. 321
				Antibiotic; perioperative, cervical spine surgery	Table 34-5, p. 1051
				Antibiotic; perioperative, thoracolumbar spine surgery	Table 35-1, p. 1101
		22 mg/kg IV, IM, or SC, TID to QID	Dogs and cats	Antibiotic; orthopedic infection	Table 28-5, p. 710
Cefmetazole	Zefazone	15 mg/kg IV	Dogs and cats	Antibiotic; prophylactic, intestinal surgery	Table 16-48, p. 294
				Antibiotic; postoperative peritonitis	Table 16-50, p. 304
		15 mg/kg IV, repeat 2-3 times at 1.5-2 hr intervals	Dogs and cats	Antibiotic; prophylactic, perineal, rectal, or colonic surgery	Table 16-57, p. 321
Cefotamine		20-40 mg/kg IV, IM, or SC, TID to QID	Dogs and cats	Antibiotic; orthopedic infection	Table 28-5, p. 710
Cefotetan	Cefotan	30 mg/kg IV; repeat every 8 hr for 24 hr	Dogs and cats	Antibiotic; prophylactic, perineal, rectal, or colonic surgery	Table 16-57, p. 321

Continued

Appendix I
Drug index—cont'd

Drug name	Brand name	Dosage and route	Species	Use; indication	*SAS* reference
Cefoxitin	Mefoxin	15-30 mg/kg IV	Dogs and cats	Antibiotic; intestinal surgery	Table 16-48, p. 294
				Antibiotic; postoperative peritonitis	Table 16-50, p. 304
		15-30 mg/kg IV, TID to QID	Dogs and cats	Antibiotic; reproductive disorder	Table 23-8, p. 521
				Antibiotic; pyometra	Table 23-23, p. 548
				Antibiotic; septic shock	Table 23-35, p. 556
		15-30 mg/kg IV; repeat 2-3 times at 1.5-2 hr intervals	Dogs and cats	Antibiotic; prophylactic, perineal, rectal, or colonic surgery	Table 16-57, p. 321
		22 mg/kg IV or IM, TID to QID	Dogs and cats	Antibiotic; orthopedic infection	Table 28-5, p. 710
		30 mg/kg IV at induction	Dogs and cats	Antibiotic; prophylactic, cardiac surgery	Table 24-5, p. 577
		30 mg/kg IV, QID	Dogs and cats	Antibiotic; peritonitis	Table 15-6, p. 195
				Antibiotic; hepatic abscess	Table 17-9, p. 385
Ceftazidime		25 mg/kg IV or IM, BID to TID	Dogs and cats	Antibiotic; orthopedic infection	Table 28-5, p. 710
Cephadrine	Veslosef	22 mg/kg IV, IM, SC, or PO, TID to QID	Dogs and cats	Antibiotic; orthopedic infection	Table 28-5, p. 710
Cephalexin		22-30 mg/kg PO, TID to QID	Dogs and cats	Antibiotic; orthopedic infection	Table 28-5, p. 710
Cephalothin	Keflin	20 mg/kg IV or IM, TID to QID	Dogs and cats	Antibiotic; cervical spine surgery	Table 34-6, p. 1051
		22-30 mg/kg IV, IM, or SC, TID to QID	Dogs and cats	Antibiotic; orthopedic infection	Table 28-5, p. 710
Cephapirin	Cefadyl	22 mg/kg IV at induction	Dogs and cats	Antibiotic; prophylactic, cardiac surgery	Table 24-5, p. 577
		22 mg/kg IV, IM, or SC, TID to QID	Dogs and cats	Antibiotic; orthopedic infection	Table 28-5, p. 710
Cephradine	Veslosef	20 mg/kg PO, TID	Dogs and cats	Antibiotic; diskospondylitis	Table 37-2, p. 1153

Chlorambucil	Leukeran	1 mg twice/wk, reduce after 6 wk if effective	Cats <3 kg	Medical management; colitis	Table 16-62, p. 331
		2 mg twice/wk, reduce after 6 wk if effective	Cats >3 kg	Medical management; colitis	Table 16-62, p. 331
Chloram-phenicol	Chloromycetin	50 mg/kg PO, BID, warn owners about handling tabs	Cats	Antibiotic; aspiration pneumonia	Table 16-6, p. 212
		50 mg/kg PO, TID to QID, warn owners about handling tabs	Dogs	Antibiotic; aspiration pneumonia	Table 16-6, p. 212
				Medical management; rickettsial polyarthritis	Table 30-8, p. 893
				Medical treatment; Lyme disease	Table 30-9, p. 894
Chlorpromazine	Thorazine	0.2-0.4 mg/kg IM, SC, or PO, TID to QID	Dogs and cats	Treatment of vomiting	Table 16-31, p. 277
Cimetidine	Tagamet	5-10 mg/kg PO, IV, or SC, TID to QID	Dogs and cats	Treatment of esophagitis	Tables 16-17, p. 233 and 16-21, p. 262
				H_2 receptor blocker	Table 16-36, p. 282
				H_2 receptor blocker, protein pump inhibitor	Table 16-39, p. 285
				Medical therapy; gastric ulcers	Table 16-43, p. 288
				Medical treatment; short-bowel syndrome	Table 16-52, p. 305
				Medical therapy; gastroduodenal ulcers	Table 23-42, p. 564
				Medical treatment or prevention; gastrointestinal complications of corticosteroids or NSAIDs	Table 34-12, p. 1070
Ciprofloxacin		11 mg/kg PO, BID	Dogs and cats	Antibiotic; orthopedic infection	Table 28-5, p. 710

Continued

Appendix I
Drug index—cont'd

Drug name	Brand name	Dosage and route	Species	Use; indication	*SAS* reference
Cisapride	Propulsid	0.25-0.5 mg/kg PO, BID to TID	Dogs	Treatment of esophagitis	Tables 16-17, p. 233 and 16-21, p. 262
				Prokinetic	Table 16-26, p. 269
				Medical treatment; constipation	Table 16-63, p. 333
		2.5-5 mg/cat PO, BID to TID	Cats	Treatment of esophagitis	Tables 16-17, p. 233 and 16-21, p. 262
				Prokinetic	Table 16-26, p. 269
				Medical treatment; constipation	Table 16-63, p. 333
Clindamycin	Antirobe, Cleocin	11 mg/kg IV, IM, or PO, BID to TID	Dogs and cats	Antibiotic; orthopedic infection	Table 28-5, p. 710
		11 mg/kg IV, TID	Dogs and cats	Antibiotic; peritonitis	Table 15-6, p. 195
				Antibiotic; septic shock	Table 23-35, p. 556
		11 mg/kg PO or IV, BID	Dogs and cats	Antibiotic; aspiration pneumonia	Table 16-6, p. 212
				Treatment of aspiration pneumonia	Table 16-18, p. 233
				Antibiotic; esophagitis	Table 16-22, p. 262
		11 mg/kg PO, BID	Dogs and cats	Antibiotic; oral surgery	Table 16-2, p. 201
				Antibiotic; hepatocellular compromise	Table 17-3, p. 368
				Antibiotic; reproductive disorder	Table 23-8, p. 521
				Antibiotic; diskospondylitis	Table 37-2, p. 1153
		11 mg/kg PO, IV, IM, BID	Dogs and cats	Medical therapy; tracheal collapse	Table 25-16, p. 634
Cloxacillin	Cloxapen, Orbenin, Tegopen	10 mg/kg PO, QID	Dogs and cats	Antibiotic; diskospondylitis	Table 37-2, p. 1153
		10-15 mg/kg IV, IM, PO, TID to QID	Dogs and cats	Antibiotic; orthopedic infection	Table 28-5, p. 710
Coarse Wheat Bran		1-2 tablespoons PO, SID	Dogs	Stool softener, laxative	Table 16-61, p. 327
Colloid fluids (hetastarch, dextrans)		20 ml/kg/day total; 7-10 mg/kg as a surgical dose	Dogs and cats	Preoperative fluids; intestinal volvulus/torsion	Table 16-54, p. 318

Cortisone		2.5 mg/kg BID for 7-14 days; then 0.5 mg/kg BID	Dogs	Postoperative management; canine adrenalectomy	Table 19-3, p. 404
Cortisone acetate		2.5 mg/kg BID	Dogs and cats	Preoperative management; adrenocortical insufficiency	Table 19-2, p. 402
Cyclophosphamide	Cytoxan	50 mg/m^2, up to 4 days/wk for up to 4 mo	Dogs	Medical treatment; idiopathic immune-mediated polyarthritis	Table 30-10, p. 894
			Dogs and cats	Medical treatment; rheumatoid arthritis	Table 30-12, p. 897
		6.25-12.5 mg/cat PO, up to 4 days/wk up to 4 mo	Cats	Medical treatment; feline chronic progressive polyarthritis	Table 30-13, p. 898
Cyproheptadine	Periactin	2 mg/cat PO	Cats	Appetite stimulant	Table 11-4, p. 69
		2.0 mg/cat PO, BID	Cats	Appetite stimulant	Table 16-64, p. 334
Desmopressin acetate		0.002 mg/dog (2-4 drops 100 mg/ml) intranasally or in conjunctiva SID to BID	Dogs and cats	Postoperative management; hypophysectomy	Table 19-11, p. 414
Dexamethasone	Azium	0.1 mg/kg SID	Dogs and cats	Preoperative management; adrenocortical insufficiency	Table 19-2, p. 402
		0.1-0.2 mg/kg IV, 1 hr preoperatively; repeat postoperatively	Dogs and cats	Preoperative management; adrenocortical insufficiency	Table 19-1, p. 401
		0.2 mg/kg IV, IM or SC, BID, up to 6 mg/kg for emergency treatment	Dogs and cats	Medical therapy; tracheal collapse	Table 25-16, p. 634
		0.2 mg/kg PO or IM, BID for 3 days; SID for 3 days; repeat 1-2 times if necessary	Dogs	Medical management; cervical or thoracolumbar disk disease	Table 34-9, p. 1068
				Medical management; wobbler syndrome	Table 34-20, p. 1078

Continued

Appendix I
Drug index—cont'd

Drug name	Brand name	Dosage and route	Species	Use; indication	*SAS* reference
Dexamethasone—cont'd	Azium—cont'd	0.2 mg/kg PO, IM, or IV, BID for 1 day; SID for 1 day	Dogs and cats	Antiinflammatory; cervical or thoracic fracture or luxation	Table 34-25, p. 1091
		0.2-0.4 mg/kg PO, TID; BID for 2 days; SID for 2 days	Dogs and cats	Medical management; spinal cord ischemia	Table 37-5, p. 1159
		0.2-0.5 mg/kg IV once; 0.2 mg/kg PO BID for 2 days; SID for 2 days	Dogs and cats	Antiinflammatory; cervical or thoracic fracture or luxation	Table 34-25, p. 1091
		0.2-1.1 mg/kg IM, BID	Dogs and cats	Medical management; atlantoaxial instability	Table 34-23, p. 1085
		0.2-2.0 mg/kg IV	Dogs	Medical management; granulomatous meningoencephalitis	Table 37-4, p. 1156
		0.5-2 mg/kg IV, IM or SC	Dogs and cats	Preoperative management; upper respiratory surgery	Table 25-5, p. 610
		1.5 mg/kg IV with oxymorphone, butorphanol or buprenorphine	Dogs	Premedication; spinal surgery	Table 34-3, p. 1050
Diazepam	Valium	0.1-0.2 mg/kg IV, with oxymorphone and atropine or glycopyrrolate	Dogs	Sedation; orthopedic disease	Table 28-7, p. 723
		0.2 mg/kg IV	Dogs and cats	Appetite stimulant for dogs Sedation; severely dyspneic cats Induction; debilitated/shocky with peritonitis	Table 11-4, p. 69 Table 25-3, p. 609 Table 15-9, p. 197

Diazepam—cont'd	Valium—cont'd	0.2 mg/kg IV with etomidate	Dogs and cats	Induction; hypovolemic, dehydrated, or shocky	Table 16-24, p. 263
				Induction; hepatic disease	Table 17-2, p. 368
				Induction; hypovolemic, dehydrated, or shocky with pancreatic disease	Table 19-13, p. 415
				Induction; hypovolemic, dehydrated, or shocky with decompensated renal failure	Table 21-3, p. 462
				Induction; hypovolemic, dehydrated, or shocky with decompensated renal failure or urinary abnormalities	Table 22-4, p. 483
				Induction; shocky, dehydrated or hypovolemic cats with sterile cystitis	Table 22-12, p. 513
				Induction; cesarean section	Table 23-7, p. 521
				Induction; debilitated or shocky with pyometra	Table 23-24, p. 548
				Induction; hypovolemia, dehydration, shock, or heart failure	Table 24-3, p. 576
				Induction; very sick or arrhythmic with upper respiratory disorder	Table 25-7, p. 610
				Induction; very sick or arrhythmic with respiratory dysfunction	Table 26-1, p. 650
		0.2 mg/kg IV with oxymorphone	Dogs	Induction; gastric dilation-volvulus	Table 16-34, p. 281
				Induction; intestinal volvulus/torsion	Table 16-53, p. 318
				Induction; biliary disease	Table 18-4, p. 399
				Induction; orthopedic disease and unstable or with trauma	Table 28-2, p. 708

Continued

Appendix I
Drug index—cont'd

Drug name	Brand name	Dosage and route	Species	Use; indication	*SAS* reference
Diazepam—cont'd	Valium—cont'd	0.2 mg/kg IV with thiopental or propofol	Dogs and cats	Induction; dyspneic, nonarrhythmic with respiratory dysfunction	Table 25-7, p. 610 Table 26-1, p. 650
		0.2 mg/kg PO, TID	Dogs	Improve urination; urethral surgery	Table 22-6, p. 499
		0.27 mg/kg IV with ketamine	Dogs and cats	Induction; ear surgery	Table 14-2, p. 154
				Induction; abdominal surgery	Table 15-1, p. 180
				Induction; oral disease	Table 16-1, p. 201
				Induction; cervical esophageal disorder	Table 16-19, p. 234
				Induction; stable with gastric disorder	Tables 16-23, p. 262 and 16-47, p. 294
				Induction; perineal, rectal, or anal surgery	Table 16-68, p. 337
				Induction; healthy animals	Table 23-5, p. 519
				Induction; cesarean section	Table 23-7, p. 521
				Induction; dyspneic, nonarrhythmic with upper respiratory disorder	Table 25-7, p. 610
				Induction; dyspneic, nonarrhythmic with respiratory dysfunction	Table 26-1, p. 650
				Induction; stable with respiratory dysfunction	Table 26-1, p. 650
		0.5 mg/cat IV	Cats	Appetite stimulant	Table 16-64, p. 334
		1.1 mg/kg PO, BID; max 20 mg/day; for 10 days; repeat 1-2 times if needed	Dogs	Medical management; cervical or thoracolumbar disk disease	Table 34-9, p. 1068
		2-5 mg/cat PO or 0.2 mg/kg IV	Cats	Appetite stimulant	Table 11-4, p. 69
		2-5 mg/cat PO, BID to TID	Cats	Improve urination; urethral surgery	Table 22-6, p. 499

Diazoxide	Proglycem	5 mg/kg BID with food; gradually increase to 30 mg/kg BID	Dogs and cats	Medical management, prevent hypoglycemia; islet cell tumors	Table 19-19, p. 423
Diethylstilbestrol	DES	0.1-1.0 mg PO, SID for 3-5 days, then 0.1-1 mg PO once/week	Dogs	Medical management; urinary incontinence	Table 22-11, p. 509 Table 23-14, p. 537
		0.5-1.0 mg SID for 2-3 wk	Dogs and cats	Medical treatment; perianal gland adenoma	Table 16-72, p. 346
Digoxin	Lanoxin	$0.22\ mg/m^2$ PO, BID	Dogs and cats	Medical management; congestive heart failure	Table 24-9, p. 592
Diltiazem	Cardiazem	1.0-1.5 mg/kg PO, TID	Dogs and cats	Medical management; cardiac disease	Table 24-1, p. 575
Dioctyl sodium sulfosuccinate	Colace	50 mg PO, SID to BID	Cats	Stool softener, laxative Stool softeners; prostatic or perineal surgery	Table 16-61, p. 327 Table 23-11, p. 536
		50-200 mg PO, BID to TID	Dogs	Stool softener, laxative Stool softeners; prostatic or perineal surgery	Table 16-61, p. 327 Table 23-11, p. 536
Diphenoxylate hydrochloride	Lomotil	0.05-0.1 mg/kg PO, BID 0.1-0.2 mg/kg PO, BID to TID	Cats Dogs	Reduce bowel transit time; fecal incontinence	Table 16-81, p. 365
Dobutamine		0.002-0.010 mg/kg/min IV	Dogs and cats	Inotropic support; hypotension Operative management; inflow occlusion Medical therapy; perioperative, hypotension	Table 15-8, p. 197 Table 24-4, p. 577 Table 34-2, p. 1050
Dopamine		0.002-0.010 mg/kg/min IV	Dogs and cats	Inotropic support; hypotension Diuretic; ovariohysterectomy Medical therapy; perioperative, hypotension	Table 15-8, p. 197 Table 23-26, p. 548 Table 34-2, p. 1050

Continued

Appendix I
Drug index—cont'd

Drug name	Brand name	Dosage and route	Species	Use; indication	*SAS* reference
Doxycycline	Vibramycin	10 mg/kg PO, SID	Dogs and cats	Medical management; rickettsial polyarthritis	Table 30-8, p. 893
				Medical treatment; Lyme disease	Table 30-9, p. 894
		5 mg/kg PO, BID	Dogs and cats	Antibiotic; reproductive disorder	Table 23-8, p. 521
				Antibiotic; diskospondylitis	Table 37-2, p. 1153
D-penicillamine	Cuprimine	10-15 mg/kg PO, BID	Dogs and cats	Medical management; urinary calculi	Table 22-9, p. 502
Ducosate sodium	Colace	50 mg PO, SID to BID	Cats	Stool softener, laxative	Table 16-61, p. 327
		50-200 mg PO, BID to TID	Dogs		
Edrophonium chloride	Tensilon	0.1-2.0 mg, with caution	Dogs	Tensilon test; laryngeal paralysis	Table 25-14, p. 629
				Tensilon test; myasthenia gravis	Table 27-20, p. 703
		0.5-1.0 mg, with caution	Cats	Tensilon test; laryngeal paralysis	Table 25-14, p. 629
				Tensilon test; myasthenia gravis	Table 27-20, p. 703
Enalapril	Vasotec, Enacard	0.25-0.5 mg/kg PO, SID to BID	Dogs and cats	Medical management; cardiac disease	Table 24-1, p. 575
				Medical management; congestive heart failure	Table 24-9, p. 592
Enrofloxacin	Baytril	2.5-10 mg/kg PO, BID	Dogs and cats	Antibiotic; cervical spine surgery	Table 34-6, p. 1051
		5-10 mg/kg PO or IV, BID	Dogs and cats	Antibiotic; peritonitis	Table 15-6, p. 195
				Treatment of aspiration pneumonia	Table 16-18, p. 233
				Antibiotic; esophagitis	Table 16-22, p. 262
				Antibiotic; postoperative peritonitis	Table 16-50, p, 304
				Antibiotic; biliary disease	Table 18-3, p. 390
				Antibiotic; renal disease	Table 21-4, p. 463
				Antibiotic; reproductive disorder	Table 23-8, p. 521
				Antibiotic; pyometra	Table 23-23, p. 548
				Antibiotic; septic shock	Table 23-35, p. 556
				Antibiotic; upper respiratory infection	Table 25-9, p. 611
				Medical therapy; tracheal collapse	Table 25-16, p. 634
				Antibiotic; diskospondylitis	Table 37-2, p. 1153
		5-11 mg/kg PO, BID	Dogs and cats	Antibiotic; orthopedic infection	Table 28-5, p. 710

Ephedrine		2-4 mg/kg PO, BID to TID	Cats	Medical management; urinary incontinence	Table 22-11, p. 509 Table 23-14, p. 537
		4 mg/kg or 12.5-50 mg/dog PO, BID to TID	Dogs	Medical management; urinary incontinence	Table 22-11, p. 509 Table 23-14, p. 537
Epinephrine		0.1-0.4 µg/kg/min IV	Dogs and cats	Operative management; inflow occlusion	Table 24-4, p. 577
Ergonovine maleate		0.02-0.1 mg/kg IM	Dogs and cats	Initiate uterine contraction	Table 23-9, p. 531
Erythromycim		10-20 mg/kg PO, BID to TID	Dogs and cats	Antibiotic; prophylactic, perineal, rectal, or colonic surgery	Table 16-57, p. 321
				Antibiotic; reproductive disorder	Table 23-8, p. 521
				Medical treatment; Lyme disease	Table 30-9, p. 894
Esmolol	Brevibloc	0.05-0.1 mg/kg slow IV boluses every 5 min up to 0.5 mg/kg	Dogs and cats	Medical management; pheochromocytoma	Table 19-9, p. 409
				Medical management; cardiac disease	Table 24-1, p. 575
		0.05-0.2 mg/kg/min IV continuous drip	Dogs and cats	Medical management; pheochromocytoma	Table 19-9, p. 409
		0.075-0.7 mg/kg slow IV bolus, then 0.025-0.15 mg/kg/min IV drip	Dogs and cats	Antiarrhythmic; surgery of thyroid or parathyroid	Table 19-31, p. 434
		0.1 mg/kg/min continuous IV drip	Dogs and cats	Medical management; cardiac disease	Table 24-1, p. 575
Etidronate disodium	Didronel	10 mg/kg/day 5 mg/kg/day PO	Cats Dogs	Medical treatment; hypercalcemia	Table 16-73, p. 346

Continued

Appendix I
Drug index—cont'd

Drug name	Brand name	Dosage and route	Species	Use; indication	*SAS* reference
Etomidate		0.5-1.5 mg/kg IV	Dogs and cats	Induction; hypovolemic, dehydrated, or shocky	Table 16-24, p. 263
				Induction; gastric dilation-volvulus	Table 16-34, p. 281
				Induction; intestinal volvulus/torsion	Table 16-53, p. 318
				Induction; hepatic disease	Table 17-2, p. 368
				Induction; biliary disease	Table 18-4, p. 399
				Induction; hypovolemic, dehydrated, or shocky with pancreatic disease	Table 19-13, p. 415
				Induction; hypovolemic, dehydrated, or shocky, decompensated renal failure	Table 21-3, p. 462
				Induction; hypovolemic, dehydrated, or shocky with decompensated renal failure or urinary abnormalities	Table 22-4, p. 483
				Induction; shocky, dehydrated or hypovolemic cats with sterile cystitis	Table 22-12, p. 513
				Induction; cesarean section	Table 23-7, p. 521
				Induction; debilitated/shocky, pyometra	Table 23-24, p. 548
				Induction; hypovolemia, dehydration, shock, or heart failure	Table 24-3, p. 576
				Induction; orthopedic disease and unstable or with trauma	Table 28-2, p. 708
		0.5-1.5 mg/kg IV with diazepam	Dogs and cats	Induction; debilitated/shocky with peritonitis	Table 15-9, p. 197
		1-3 mg/kg IV	Dogs and cats	Induction; very sick or arrhythmic with upper respiratory disorder	Table 25-7, p. 610
				Induction; very sick or arrhythmic with respiratory dysfunction	Table 26-1, p. 650

Famotidine	Pepcid	0.5 mg/kg PO, SID to BID	Dogs and cats	Treatment of esophagitis	Table 16-17, p. 233 Table 16-21, p. 262
				H_2 receptor blocker, protein pump inhibitor	Table 16-36, p. 282 Table 16-39, p. 285
				Medical therapy; gastric ulcers	Table 16-43, p. 288
				Medical treatment; short-bowel syndrome	Table 16-52, p. 305
				Medical therapy; gastrinoma	Table 19-23, p. 426
				Medical therapy; gastroduodenal ulcers	Table 23-42, p. 564
				Medical treatment or prevention; gastrointestinal complications of corticosteroids or NSAIDs	Table 34-12, p. 1070
Fentanyl	Sublimaze	0.001 mg/kg epidural	Dogs	Epidural anesthesia/analgesia	Table 12-2, p. 88 Table 23-6, p. 520 Table 28-4, p. 709
		0.005 mg/kg IV or 0.01 mg/kg SC or IM	Dogs	Sedation; canine pericardiocentesis	Table 24-11, p. 598
		0.005 mg/kg IV, SC, or IM	Dogs; use low end doses for cats and IV	Systemic opioid analgesic	Table 12-1, p. 87
Fentanyl plus droperidol	Innovar-Vet	1 ml/20-40 kg IV or 1 ml/10-15 kg IM	Dogs	Sedation; severely dyspneic dogs	Table 25-2, p. 609
Fludrocortisone acetate	Florinef	0.02 mg/kg PO, SID to BID	Dogs	Postoperative management; canine adrenalectomy	Table 19-3, p. 404

Continued

Appendix I
Drug index—cont'd

Drug name	Brand name	Dosage and route	Species	Use; indication	*SAS* reference
Flunixin meglumine	Banamine	0.5 mg/kg IV, IM, or SC, BID for 2 days	Dogs	Medical management; cervical or thoracolumbar disk disease	Table 34-9, p. 1068
				Medical management; wobbler syndrome	Table 34-20, p. 1078
		0.5-1.0 mg/kg IV, IM, or SC; max 2 days	Dogs and cats	Medical management; cauda equina syndrome	Table 36-8, p. 1140
		1 mg/kg IV, once or twice if in septic shock	Dogs	Adjunctive therapy; peritonitis	Table 15-7, p. 195
				Medical treatment; shock	Table 23-34, p. 556
Furosemide	Lasix	2-4 mg/kg IM or IV, QID	Dogs and cats	Diuretic; pulmonary edema	Table 24-7, p. 583
		2-4 mg/kg IV, BID to TID	Dogs	Diuresis; canine hypercalcemia	Table 19-34, p. 438
		2-4 mg/kg IV, PO, or SC, BID to TID	Dogs and cats	Medical treatment; hypercalcemia	Table 16-73, p. 346
		2-4 mg/kg PO, IV, IM, or SC, SID to QID as needed	Dogs and cats	Diuretic; ovariohysterectomy	Table 23-26, p. 548
				Medical management; cardiac disease	Table 24-1, p. 575
				Medical management; congestive heart failure	Table 24-9, p. 592
Gentamicin	Gentocin	2 mg/kg IM, BID for 1 wk; monitor renal function	Dogs and cats	Antibiotic; diskospondylitis	Table 37-2, p. 1153
		2.2 mg/kg IV, IM, or SC, BID to TID	Dogs and cats	Antibiotic; orthopedic infection	Table 28-5, p. 710
		6 mg/kg IV, SID	Dogs and cats	Antibiotic; prophylactic, perineal, rectal, or colonic surgery	Table 16-57, p. 321

Glycopyrrolate	0.005-0.011 mg/kg IM with butorphanol	Cats	Sedation; orthopedic disease	Table 28-8, p. 723
	0.005-0.011 mg/kg IV, SC, or IM with butorphanol or diazepam	Dogs	Sedation; orthopedic disease	Table 28-7, p. 723
	0.005-0.011 mg/kg SC or IM	Dogs and cats	Premedication; ear surgery	Table 14-2, p. 154
			Premedication; abdominal surgery	Table 15-1, p. 180
			Anticholinergic	Table 15-10, p. 197
			Premedication; oral disease	Table 16-1, p. 201
			Premedication; cervical esophageal disorder	Table 16-19, p. 234
			Premedication; stable with gastric disorder	Table 16-23, p. 262 Table 16-47, p. 294
			Premedication; perineal, rectal, or anal surgery	Table 16-68, p. 337
			Premedication; hepatic disease	Table 17-2, p. 368
			Premedication; portosystemic shunt	Table 17-7, p. 378
			Premedication; cats with renal disease	Table 21-2, p. 462
			Premedication; healthy animals	Table 23-5, p. 519
			Premedication; cesarean section	Table 23-7, p. 521
			Premedication; stable with cardiovascular disease	Table 24-2, p. 576
			Premedication; canine laryngeal examination	Table 25-6, p. 610
			Premedication; pectus excavatum	Table 26-9, p. 670
			Premedication; stable with orthopedic disease	Table 28-2, p. 708

Continued

Appendix I
Drug index—cont'd

Drug name	Brand name	Dosage and route	Species	Use; indication	*SAS* reference
Heparin		50-100 units/kg SC, BID	Dogs	Adjunctive therapy; peritonitis	Table 15-7, p. 195
				Preoperative management; hyperadrenocorticism, hypercoagulopathy	Table 19-8, p. 409
				Preoperative management; dessiminated intravascular hemolysis, splenic surgery	Table 20-3, p. 450
		75 IU/kg SC, TID	Dogs	Postoperative management, canine adrenalectomy	Table 19-3, p. 404
Heparin activated plasma		10 ml/kg IV of 5-10 units/kg heparin in 125 ml blood, incubated 30 min.	Dogs	Adjunctive therapy; peritonitis	Table 15-7, p. 195
				Preoperative management; hyperadrenocorticism, hypercoagulopathy	Table 19-8, p. 409
				Preoperative management; dessiminated intravascular hemolysis, splenic surgery	Table 20-3, p. 450
Hetastarch		5-10 ml/kg (up to 10 ml/kg/day)	Dogs and cats	Medical treatment; shock	Table 23-34, p. 556
Hydrocodone bitartrate	Hycodan	0.2 mg/kg TID to QID	Dogs and cats	Medical therapy; tracheal collapse	Table 25-16, p. 634
Hydrocortisone (soluble)		4-5 mg/kg IV, 1 hr preoperatively; repeat postoperatively	Dogs and cats	Preoperative management; adrenocortical insufficiency	Table 19-1, p. 401
Hypertonic saline	7% NaCl solution	4-5 ml/kg (up to 10 ml/kg/day), then isotonic crystalloids	Dogs and cats	Medical treatment; shock	Table 23-34, p. 556
Hypertonic saline and Dextran 70		3-5 ml/kg (up to 10 ml/kg/day), then isotonic crystalloids	Dogs and cats	Medical treatment; shock	Table 23-34, p. 556

Imipenem	Primaxin	3-10 mg/kg, slow IV, TID or QID	Dogs and cats	Antibiotic; peritonitis	Table 15-6, p. 195
				Antibiotic; septic shock	Table 23-35, p. 556
Iohexol	Omnipaque	0.25-0.45 ml/kg, 180-300 mgI/ml	Dogs and cats	Myelograph contrast agent	Table 33-8, p. 1044
Iopamidol	Isovue	0.25-0.45 ml/kg, 180-300 mgI/ml	Dogs and cats	Myelograph contrast agent	Table 33-8, p. 1044
Isoproterenol	Isuprel	0.01 μg/kg/min IV	Dogs and cats	Increase heart rate; unresponsive bradycardia	Table 24-16, p. 605
Isotonic crystalloids		10-20 ml/kg/hr to effect	Dogs and cats	Medical treatment; shock	Table 23-34, p. 556
Isotonic saline	0.9% NaCl Solution	90 ml/kg/day	Dogs	Diuresis; canine hypercalcemia	Table 19-34, p. 438
		To effect to dilute potassium	Dogs and cats	Medical therapy; hyperkalemia	Table 24-15, p. 605
		Up to 60 ml/kg/hr, to effect	Cats	Medical treatment; shock	Table 23-34, p. 556
		Up to 90 ml/kg/hr, to effect	Dogs	Medical treatment; shock	Table 23-34, p. 556
Kanamycin	Kantrim	11 mg/kg PO, TID	Dogs and cats	Antibiotic; prophylactic, perineal, rectal, or colonic surgery	Table 16-57, p. 321
Ketamine		5 mg/kg IM	Cats	Premedication; healthy animals undergoing elective surgery	Table 23-5, p. 519
			Cats	Sedation; orthopedic disease	Table 28-8, p. 723

Continued

Appendix I
Drug index—cont'd

Drug name	Brand name	Dosage and route	Species	Use; indication	*SAS* reference
Ketamine—cont'd		5.5 mg/kg IV with diazepam	Dogs and cats	Induction; ear surgery in cats	Table 14-2, p. 154
				Induction; abdominal surgery	Table 15-1, p. 180
				Induction; oral disease	Table 16-1, p. 201
				Induction; cervical esophageal disorder	Table 16-19, p. 234
				Induction; stable with gastric disorder	Tables 16-23, p. 262 and 16-47, p. 294
				Induction; perineal, rectal or anal surgery	Table 16-68, p. 337
				Induction; healthy cats	Table 23-5, p. 519
				Induction; cesarean section	Table 23-7, p. 521
				Induction; dyspneic, nonarrhythmic with upper respiratory disorder	Table 25-7, p. 610
				Induction; dyspneic, nonarrhythmic with respiratory dysfunction	Table 26-1, p. 650
				Induction; stable with respiratory dysfunction	Table 26-1, p. 650
Ketoconazole		5 mg/kg BID with food for first 7 days 10 mg/kg BID with food for second 7 days Continue at 10-15 mg/kg BID with food after 2 wk	Dogs and cats	Medical management; adrenal tumor	Table 19-7, p. 408
Lactated Ringer's solution	LRS	Up to 60 ml/kg/hr, to effect	Cats	Medical treatment; shock	Table 23-34, p. 556
		Up to 90 ml/kg/hr, to effect	Dogs	Medical treatment; shock	Table 23-34, p. 556

Lactulose	Chronulac, Cephulac	0.5 ml/kg PO, TID	Dogs	Medical management; portosystemic shunt	Table 17-6, p. 377
		1 ml/4.5 kg PO, TID to effect	Dogs	Stool softener, laxative	Table 16-61, p. 327
				Medical treatment; constipation	Table 16-63, p. 333
				Stool softeners; prostatic or perineal surgery	Table 23-11, p. 536
		2.5 to 25 ml PO, TID; goal of 2-3 soft stools/day	Dogs and cats	Medical management; portosystemic shunt	Table 17-6, p. 377
		2.5-5 ml/cat PO, TID	Cats	Medical management; portosystemic shunt	Table 17-6, p. 377
		5 ml/cat, PO, TID	Cats	Stool softener, laxative	Table 16-61, p. 327
				Medical treatment; constipation	Table 16-63, p. 333
				Stool softeners; prostatic or perineal surgery	Table 23-11, p. 536
Levothyroxine	Soloxine	0.022 mg/kg PO, BID	Dogs	Medical treament; canine hypothyroidism	Table 19-24, p. 429
Lidocaine	Xylocaine	0.05-0.075 mg/kg/min IV infusion	Dogs and cats	Operative management; inflow occlusion	Table 24-4, p. 577
		2-8 mg/kg IV bolus, then 0.05 mg/kg/min (500 mg in 500 ml fluid) IV	Dogs	Antiarrhythmic	Table 16-37, p. 282
				Antiarrhythmic; hyperadrenocorticism	Table 19-10, p. 409
				Medical management; cardiac disease	Table 24-1, p. 575
		9 mg/kg IV, incrementally to effect, with thiobarbituate	Dogs	Induction; arrhythmic with gastric dilation-volvulus	Text p. 280
Lidocaine 2%	Xylocaine	1 ml/3.4 kg (T5) or 1 ml/4.5 kg (T13-L1) epidural	Dogs	Epidural anesthesia/analgesia	Table 12-2, p. 88
					Table 23-6, p. 520
					Table 28-4, p. 709

Continued

Appendix I
Drug index—cont'd

Drug name	Brand name	Dosage and route	Species	Use; indication	*SAS* reference
Liothyronine	T3, Cytobin or Cytomel	0.004-0.006 mg/kg PO, TID to QID	Dogs	Medical treament; canine hypothyroidism	Table 19-24, p. 429
Lisinopril	Prinvil, Zestril	0.25-0.5 mg/kg PO, SID	Dogs	Medical management; cardiac disease	Table 24-1, p. 575
Loperamide	Imodium	0.08-0.16 mg/kg PO, BID	Cats	Medical treatment; short-bowel syndrome	Table 16-52, p. 305
				Reduce bowel transit time: fecal incontinence	Table 16-81, p. 365
		0.1-0.2 mg/kg PO, BID to TID	Dogs	Medical treatment; short-bowel syndrome	Table 16-52, p. 305
				Reduce bowel transit time; fecal incontinence	Table 16-81, p. 365
L-thyroxine		0.02-0.04 mg/kg IV bolus	Dogs	Medical treament; canine hypothyroidism	Table 19-24, p. 429
Magnesium hydroxide	Milk of Magnesia	15-50 ml/dog PO, SID (cathartic dose)	Dogs	Stool softener, laxative	Table 16-61, p. 327
		2-6 ml/cat PO, SID (cathartic dose)	Cats		
Meclofenamic acid	Arquel	1.1 mg/kg PO SID after eating for 5 days, then decrease dose	Dogs	Medical management; degenerative joint disease	Table 30-5, p. 890
Medroxy-progesterone acetate	Depo-Provera	3 mg/kg (minimum dose 50 mg) SC, repeat in 4-6 wk if needed	Dogs	Medical management; benign prostatic enlargement	Table 23-27, p. 553
Mesalamine	Asacol, Mesasal	10-20 mg/kg PO, BID to TID	Dogs and cats	Medical management; colitis	Table 16-62, p. 331

Methimazole	Tapazole	5 mg PO, BID to TID; then 2.5-5 mg PO, BID to TID	Cats	Preoperative therapy; feline hyperthyroidism	Table 19-30, p. 433
Methylene blue 1%		3 mg/kg in 250 ml of isotonic saline; IV over 30 min	Dogs and cats	Neoplastc cell differentiation; insulinoma	Table 19-20, p. 424
Methylprednisolone sodium succinate	Solu-Medrol	30 mg/kg IV	Dogs	Premedication-spinal surgery	Table 34-3, p. 1050
				Medical management; cervical or thoracolumbar disk disease	Table 34-9, p. 1068
				Medical management; wobbler syndrome	Table 34-20, p. 1078
				Antiinflammatory; cervical or thoracic fracture or luxation	Table 34-25, p. 1091
		30 mg/kg IV, repeat after 12 hr needed, max 2 doses	Dogs and cats	Medical management; cervical spinal peritumoral edema	Table 34-30, p. 1099
Methyocarbamol	Robaxin-V	22 mg/kg PO once, then 11 mg/kg PO, TID for 10 days, repeat 1-2 times if needed	Dogs	Medical management; cervical or thoracolumbar disk disease	Table 34-9, p. 1068
Metoclopramide	Reglan	0.25-0.5 mg/kg PO, IV, or SC, SID to QID	Dogs and cats	Prokinetic	Table 16-26, p. 269
		1-2 mg/kg/day via continuous IV infusion		Treatment of vomiting	Table 16-31, p. 277

Continued

Appendix I
Drug index—cont'd

Drug name	Brand name	Dosage and route	Species	Use; indication	*SAS* reference
Metronidazole	Flagyl	10 mg/kg IV or PO, TID	Dogs and cats	Antibiotic; prophylactic, perineal, rectal, or colonic surgery	Table 16-57, p. 321
				Medical management; portosystemic shunt	Table 17-6, p. 377
				Antibiotic; hepatic abscess	Table 17-9, p. 385
		10 mg/kg IV, QID	Dogs and cats	Antibiotic; peritonitis	Table 15-6, p. 195
		10 mg/kg IV, TID	Dogs and cats	Antibiotic; septic shock	Table 23-35, p. 556
		10 mg/kg PO, TID	Dogs and cats	Antibiotic; oral surgery	Table 16-2, p. 201
				Antibiotic; hepatocellular compromise	Table 17-3, p. 368
		10-15 mg/kg PO, BID	Dogs and cats	Medical management; colitis	Table 16-62, p. 331
Minocycline	Minocin	10 mg/kg PO, BID	Dogs and cats	Antibiotic; diskospondylitis	Table 37-2, p. 1153
Misoprostol	Cytotec	0.001-0.005 mg/kg PO, TID to QID	Dogs and cats	Medical therapy; gastric ulcers	Table 16-43, p. 288
				Medical treatment; canine cystic transitional cell carcinoma	Table 22-10, p. 507
				Medical treatment or prevention; gastrointestinal complications of corticosteroids or NSAIDs	Table 34-12, p. 1070
		0.002-0.005 mg/kg PO, BID to TID	Dogs	Prevention of NSAID-induced gastrointestinal erosions	Table 30-6, p. 891
Mitotane	Lysodren	50-75 mg/kg/day for first 14 days Increase by 50 mg/kg/day for 14 days; repeat increase as needed	Dogs and cats	Medical management; adrenal tumor	Table 19-6, p. 408

Morphine		0.03 mg/kg (preservative free) epidural	Cats	Epidural anesthesia/analgesia	Table 12-2, p. 88 Table 23-6, p. 520 Table 28-4, p. 709
		0.1 mg/kg (preservative free) epidural	Dogs	Epidural anesthesia/analgesia	Table 12-2, p. 88 Table 23-6, p. 520 Table 28-4, p. 709
		0.1-0.4 mg/kg IV, SC, or IM	Dogs; use low end doses for cats and IV	Systemic opioid analgesic	Table 12-1, p. 87
		0.4-mg/kg SC or IM, every 4-6 hr as needed	Dogs and cats	Analgesic; orthopedic surgery	Table 28-3, p. 708
N-(2-mercaptopropionyl)-glycine	MPG	15 mg/kg PO, BID	Dogs and cats	Medical management; urinary calculi	Table 22-9, p. 502
Naloxone	Narcan	0.02 mg/kg IV	Dogs	Reversal of oxymorphone	Table 28-7, p. 723
Naproxen	Naprosyn, Anaprox	2.2 mg/kg PO with food, SID or EOD; not approved for use in dogs	Dogs	Medical management; degenerative joint disease	Table 30-5, p. 890
				Medical management; hip dysplasia	Table 30-20, p. 944
Neomycin	Biosol	10-20 mg/kg PO, BID to TID	Dogs and cats	Medical management; portosystemic shunt	Table 17-6, p. 377
		20 mg/kg PO, TID	Dogs and cats	Antibiotic; prophylactic, perineal, rectal, or colonic surgery	Table 16-57, p. 321
Nitroprusside sodium	Nipride	0.0005-0.005 mg/kg/min IV	Dogs and cats	Medical management; pheochromocytoma	Table 19-9, p. 409

Continued

Appendix I
Drug index—cont'd

Drug name	Brand name	Dosage and route	Species	Use; indication	*SAS* reference
Ocreotide		0.001-0.002 mg/kg SC preoperatively	Dogs and cats	Prevention of pancreatitis	Table 19-15, p. 418
Omeprazole	Prilosec	0.7-1.5 mg/kg PO, SID to BID	Dogs and cats	Treatment of esophagitis	Table 16-17, p. 233
					Table 16-21, p. 262
				H_2 receptor blocker, protein pump inhibitor	Table 16-39, p. 285
				Medical therapy; gastric ulcers	Table 16-43, p. 288
				Medical therapy; gastrinoma	Table 19-23, p. 426
				Medical therapy; gastroduodenal ulcers	Table 23-42, p. 564
				Medical treatment or prevention; gastrointestinal complications of corticosteroids or NSAIDs	Table 34-12, p. 1070
Ondansetron	Zofran	0.1-0.3 mg/kg IV or SC, SID to BID	Dogs and cats	Treatment of vomiting	Table 16-31, p. 277
Osalazine	Dipentum	10-20 mg/kg PO, BID to TID	Dogs and cats	Medical management; colitis	Table 16-62, p. 331
Oxacillin		22 mg/kg IV, IM, SC, or PO, TID to QID	Dogs and cats	Antibiotic; orthopedic infection	Table 28-5, p. 710
Oxazepam	Serax	2.5 mg/cat PO	Cats	Appetite stimulant	Table 11-4, p. 69
Oxtriphylline elixir	Choledyl SA	14-15 mg/kg PO, TID	Dogs	Treatment of aspiration pneumonia	Table 16-18, p. 233
			Dogs and cats	Medical therapy; tracheal collapse	Table 25-16, p. 634
		6-8 mg/kg PO, BID to TID	Cats	Treatment of aspiration pneumonia	Table 16-18, p. 233

Oxymorphone	Numorphan	0.05 mg/kg IV, IM, or SC; max 4 mg	Dogs	Sedation; severely dyspneic dogs	Table 25-2, p. 609
		0.05 mg/kg SC or IM	Cats	Premedication; debilitated/shocky with peritonitis	Table 15-9, p. 197
				Premedication; hypovolemic, dehydrated, or shocky	Table 16-24, p. 263
			Dogs and cats	Premedication; portosystemic shunt	Table 17-7, p. 378
			Cats	Premedication; hypovolemic, dehydrated, or shocky, with pancreatic disease	Table 19-13, p. 415
				Premedication; hypovolemic, dehydrated, or shocky with decompensated renal failure	Table 21-3, p. 462
				Premedication; hypovolemic, dehydrated, or shocky, decompensated renal failure or urinary abnormalities	Table 22-4, p. 483
				Premedication; shocky, dehydrated or hypovolemic cats with sterile cystitis	Table 22-12, p. 513
				Premedication; debilitated/shocky, pyometra	Table 23-24, p. 548
				Premedication; hypovolemia, dehydration, shock, or heart failure	Table 24-3, p. 576
		0.05-0.1 mg/kg IV or IM, every 4 hr as needed	Dogs and cats	Analgesic; digestive surgery	Table 16-4, p. 209
				Analgesic; hepatic surgery	Table 17-4, p. 373
				Analgesic; bile peritonitis	Table 18-5, p. 399
				Analgesic; renal surgery	Table 21-5, p. 469
				Analgesic; urinary tract surgery	Table 22-5, p. 495
				Analgesic; ovariohysterectomy	Table 23-25, p. 548
				Analgesic; cardiac surgery	Table 24-6, p. 581
				Analgesic; upper respiratory surgery	Table 25-10, p. 618
				Analgesic; thoracotomy	Table 26-3, p. 650
					Table 27-22, p. 704
				Analgesic; orthopedic surgery	Table 28-3, p. 708
				Analgesic; cervical spinal surgery	Table 34-13, p. 1070

Continued

Appendix I
Drug index—cont'd

Drug name	Brand name	Dosage and route	Species	Use; indication	*SAS* reference
Oxymorphone—cont'd	Numorphan—cont'd	0.05-0.1 mg/kg IV, SC, or IM with acepromazine or diazepam	Dogs	Sedation: orthopedic disease	Table 28-7, p. 723
		0.05-0.1 mg/kg IV, SC, or IM	Dogs; use low end doses for cats and IV	Systemic opioid analgesic	Table 12-1, p. 87
				Premedication; cats with urinary abnormalities	Table 22-3, p. 482
				Sedation; canine pericardiocentesis	Table 24-11, p. 598
				Premedication; canine laryngeal examination	Table 25-6, p. 610
				Premedication; stable with respiratory dysfunction	Table 26-1, p. 650
				Premedication; stable with orthopedic disease	Table 28-2, p. 708
				Premedication; spinal surgery	Table 34-3, p. 1050
		0.05-0.1 mg/kg SC or IM with glycopyrrolate	Dogs	Premedication; ear surgery	Table 14-2, p. 154
			Dogs and cats	Premedication; abdominal surgery	Table 15-1, p. 180
			Dogs and cats	Premedication; oral disease	Table 16-1, p. 201
			Dogs	Premedication; cervical esophageal disorder	Table 16-19, p. 234
				Premedication; stable with gastric disorder	Table 16-23, p. 262 Table 16-47, p. 294
				Premedication; perineal, rectal, or anal surgery	Table 16-68, p. 337
				Premedication; hepatic disease	Table 17-2, p. 368
				Premedication; portosystemic shunt	Table 17-7, p. 378
				Premedication; cats with pancreatic disease	Table 19-12, p. 415
				Premedication; cats with renal disease	Table 21-2, p. 462
				Premedication; stable with cardiovascular disease	Table 24-2, p. 576
				Premedication; pectus excavatum	Table 26-9, p. 670

Oxymorphone—cont'd	Numorphan—cont'd	0.1 mg/kg epidural	Dogs and cats	Epidural anesthesia/analgesia	Table 12-2, p. 88 Table 23-6, p. 520 Table 28-4, p. 709
		0.1 mg/kg IV with diazepam	Dogs	Induction; debilitated/shocky with peritonitis	Table 15-9, p. 197
				Induction; hypovolemic, dehydrated, or shocky	Table 16-24, p. 263
				Induction; gastric dilation-volvulus	Table 16-34, p. 281
				Induction; intestinal volvulus/torsion	Table 16-53, p. 318
				Induction; biliary disease	Table 18-4, p. 399
				Induction; hypovolemic, dehydrated, or shocky with pancreatic disease	Table 19-13, p. 415
				Induction; hypovolemic, dehydrated, or shocky, decompensated renal failure	Table 21-3, p. 462
				Induction; hypovolemic, dehydrated, or shocky with decompensated renal failure or urinary abnormalities	Table 22-4, p. 483
				Induction; cesarean section	Table 23-7, p. 521
				Induction; debilitated/shocky, pyometra	Table 23-24, p. 548
				Induction; hypovolemia, dehydration, shock, or heart failure	Table 24-3, p. 576
				Induction; orthopedic disease and unstable or with trauma	Table 28-2, p. 708
Oxytocin		0.5 units IM or IV; can repeat but do not exceed 3 units	Cats	Initiate uterine contraction	Table 23-9, p. 531
		1-5 units IM or IV	Dogs		
Pancrelipase	Festal II	1 tablet PO, SID, with food; do not break tablet	Dogs and cats	Medical treatment; exocrine pancreatic insufficiency	Table 19-16, p. 418
Penicillin G (aqueous)		20,000-40,000 IU/kg IV, QID	Dogs and cats	Antibiotic; orthopedic infection	Table 28-5, p. 710

Continued

Appendix I
Drug index—cont'd

Drug name	Brand name	Dosage and route	Species	Use; indication	*SAS* reference
Phenoxy-benzamine	Dibenzyline	0.2-0.4 mg/kg PO, BID	Dogs and cats	Medical management; pheochromocytoma	Table 19-9, p. 409
		0.25 mg/kg PO, BID to TID	Dogs	Improve urination; urethral surgery	Table 22-6, p. 499
		0.5 mg/kg PO, BID (may cause hypotension)	Cats		
Phentolamine	Regitine	0.02-0.1 mg/kg IV	Dogs and cats	Medical management; pheochromocytoma	Table 19-9, p. 409
Phenylbutazone	Butazolidin	15 mg/kg PO, BID to TID, max 800 mg/day	Dogs	Medical management; degenerative joint disease	Table 30-5, p. 890
				Medical management; hip dysplasia	Table 30-20, p. 944
				Medical treatment; panosteitis	Table 32-1, p. 1011
				Medical management; cauda equina syndrome	Table 36-8, p. 1140
		22 mg/kg PO, TID; max 800 mg/day; for 7 days	Dogs	Medical management; cervical or thoracolumbar disk disease	Table 34-9, p. 1068
				Medical management; wobbler syndrome	Table 34-20, p. 1078
Phenylpro-panolamine	Propagest, Dexatrim	1.5 mg/kg PO, TID	Cats	Medical management; urinary incontinence	Table 21-6, p. 472 Table 22-11, p. 509 Table 23-14, p. 537
		1.5-2.0 mg/kg PO, BID to TID	Dogs	Medical management; urinary incontinence	Table 21-6, p. 472 Table 22-11, p. 509 Table 23-14, p. 537
Piroxicam	Feldene	0.3 mg/kg PO, EOD to SID	Dogs	Medical treatment; canine cystic transitional cell carcinoma	Table 22-10, p. 507
		10 mg/day PO	Dogs	Medical management; hip dysplasia	Table 30-20, p. 944

Polyethylene glycol electrolyte solution	Colyte or GoLytely	25-40 ml/kg PO via stomach tube 24 and 18-20 hr preoperatively	Dogs and cats	Bowel preparation; large intestinal/rectal surgery	Table 16-56, p. 320
Prednisolone		0.2 mg/kg SID	Dogs and cats	Postoperative management; hypophysectomy	Table 19-11, p. 414
		0.25-2 mg/kg BID	Dogs and cats	Medical management, prevent hypoglycemia; islet cell tumors	Table 19-19, p. 423
		0.5 mg/kg BID	Dogs and cats	Preoperative management; adrenocortical insufficiency	Table 19-2, p. 402
		0.5 mg/kg BID for 7-14 days; then 0.5 mg/kg BID	Dogs	Postoperative management; canine adrenalectomy	Table 19-3, p. 404
		0.5-1.0 mg/kg PO, BID for 3 days; SID for 3 days; repeat 1-2 times if necessary	Dogs	Medical management; cervical or thoracolumbar disk disease	Table 34-9, p. 1068
				Medical management; wobbler syndrome	Table 34-20, p. 1078
		1-2 mg/kg SID	Dogs and cats	Medical management; colitis	Table 16-62, p. 331
Prednisolone sodium		1.0-2.0 mg/kg IV, 1 hr preoperatively; repeat postoperatively	Dogs and cats	Preoperative management; adrenocortical insufficiency	Table 19-1, p. 401
Prednisone		0.2 mg/kg SID	Dogs and cats	Postoperative management; hypophysectomy	Table 19-11, p. 414
		0.25-2 mg/kg BID	Dogs and cats	Medical management, prevent hypoglycemia; islet cell tumors	Table 19-19, p. 423
		0.5 mg/kg BID	Dogs and cats	Preoperative management; adrenocortical insufficiency	Table 19-2, p. 402
		0.5 mg/kg BID for 7-14 days; then 0.5 mg/kg BID	Dogs	Postoperative management; canine adrenalectomy	Table 19-3, p. 404

Continued

Appendix I
Drug index—cont'd

Drug name	Brand name	Dosage and route	Species	Use; indication	*SAS* reference
Prednisone—cont'd		1 mg/kg PO, BID; gradually discontinue over 2-3 wk	Dogs	Medical management; idiopathic pericardial effusion	Table 24-12, p. 599
		1-2 mg/kg IV, PO, or SC, BID	Dogs and cats	Medical treatment; hypercalcemia	Table 16-73, p. 346
		1-2 mg/kg PO, BID for 2-3 wk; reduce gradually to 2.5-5 mg total dose EOD	Dogs	Medical management; granulomatous meningoencephalitis	Table 37-4, p. 1156
		1-2 mg/kg PO, SID to BID	Dogs and cats	Medical therapy; tracheal collapse	Table 25-16, p. 634
		1-2 mg/kg/day	Dogs	Medical management; myasthenia gravis	Table 27-21, p. 703
		2-4 mg/kg/day for first 2 wk, 1-2 mg/kg for next 2 wk, reduce to EOD for another 4 wk	Dogs	Medical treatment; idiopathic immune-mediated polyarthritis	Table 30-10, p. 894
			Dogs and cats	Medical treatment; rheumatoid arthritis	Table 30-12, p. 897
		4-6 mg/kg/day IV for 2 wk, 2 mg/kg/day for 2 wk, reduce to 1-2 mg/kg EOD	Cats	Medical treatment; feline chronic progressive polyarthritis	Table 30-13, p. 898
Procainamide	Pronestyl	0.025-0.06 mg/kg continuous IV drip, or 10-15 mg/kg slow IV bolus, or	Dogs	Antiarrhythmic	Table 16-37, p. 282
		15 mg/kg IM or PO, BID to QID		Medical management; cardiac disease	Table 24-1, p. 575
Propantheline bromide	Pro-Banthine	0.25-0.5 mg/kg PO, TID to QID	Dogs and cats	Increase heart rate; unresponsive bradycardia	Table 24-16, p. 605

Propofol		4-6 mg/kg IV	Dogs and cats	Induction; ear surgery	Table 14-2, p. 154
				Induction; abdominal surgery	Table 15-1, p. 180
				Induction; oral disease	Table 16-1, p. 201
				Induction; cervical esophageal disorder	Table 16-19, p. 234
				Induction; stable with gastric disorder	Table 16-23, p. 262
					Table 16-47, p. 294
				Induction; perineal, rectal, or anal surgery	Table 16-68, p. 337
				Induction; cats with pancreatic disease	Table 19-12, p. 415
				Induction; cats with renal disease	Table 21-2, p. 462
				Induction; feline urinary abnormalities	Table 22-3, p. 482
				Induction; stable with cardiovascular disease	Table 24-2, p. 576
				Induction; stable with respiratory dysfunction	Table 26-1, p. 650
				Induction; stable with orthopedic disease	Table 28-2, p. 708
				Induction; spinal surgery	Table 34-3, p. 1050
		4-6 mg/kg IV with diazepam	Dogs and cats	Induction; dyspneic, nonarrhythmic with upper respiratory disorder	Table 25-7, p. 610
			Dogs	Induction; dyspneic, nonarrhythmic with respiratory dysfunction	Table 26-1, p. 650
Propranolol	Inderal	0.2-2.0 mg/kg PO, BID to TID	Dogs and cats	Medical management; cardiac disease	Table 24-1, p. 575
				β-Adrenergic therapy; aortic stenosis	Table 24-8, p. 589
				β-Adrenergic therapy; tetralogy of fallot	Table 24-10, p. 595
		2.5-5 mg/cat (0.4-1.5 mg/kg) PO, BID to TID	Cats	Preoperative therapy; feline hyperthyroidism	Table 19-30, p. 433

Continued

Appendix I
Drug index—cont'd

Drug name	Brand name	Dosage and route	Species	Use; indication	*SAS* reference
Prostaglandin	$PGF_{2\alpha}$	0.1-0.25 mg/kg SC, SID to BID for 3-5 days	Dogs and cats	Medical therapy; pyometra	Table 23-22, p. 547
Psyllium	Metamucil	1-4 g PO, SID to BID, or 1 tsp/10 kg PO, BID in food	Cats	Stool softener, laxative	Table 16-61, p. 327
				Stool softeners; prostatic or perineal surgery	Table 23-11, p. 536
		2-10 g PO, SID to BID, or 1 tsp/10 kg PO, BID in food	Dogs	Stool softener, laxative	Table 16-61, p. 327
				Stool softeners; prostatic or perineal surgery	Table 23-11, p. 536
Pyridostigmine bromide	Mestinon, Regonol	0.02-0.04 mg/kg IV every 2 hr or 0.5-3.0 mg/kg PO, BID to TID	Dogs	Medical management; myasthenia gravis	Table 27-21, p. 703
Ranitidine	Zantac	2 mg/kg PO, SC, IV, or IM, BID	Dogs and cats	Treatment of esophagitis	Table 16-17, p. 233 Table 16-21, p. 262
				H_2 receptor blocker, protein pump inhibitor	Table 16-36, p. 282 Table 16-39, p. 285
				Medical therapy; gastric ulcers	Table 16-43, p. 288
				Medical treatment; short-bowel syndrome	Table 16-52, p. 305
				Medical therapy; gastroduodenal ulcers	Table 23-42, p. 564
				Medical treatment or prevention; gastrointestinal complications of corticosteroids or NSAIDs	Table 34-12, p. 1070
Rutin		50 mg/kg	Dogs and cats	Medical treatment; lymphedema	Table 20-1, p. 447
		50 mg/kg PO, TID	Dogs and cats	Medical management; chylothorax	Table 27-12, p. 695
Salmon calcitonin		4 U/kg IV; then 4-8 U/kg SC, SID to BID	Dogs and cats	Medical treatment; hypercalcemia	Table 16-73, p. 346

Sodium bicarbonate		0.3 × base deficit (mEq) × b.w. (kg); IV, give half and reevaluate	Dogs and cats	Correction of base deficit	Table 15-5, p. 195
		0.5-2 mEq/kg in IV fluids; check blood gas	Dogs and cats	Medical treatment; hypercalcemia	Table 16-73, p. 346
		1-2 mEq/kg, IV	Dogs and cats	Correction of base deficit	Table 15-5, p. 195
				Medical therapy; hyperkalemia	Table 24-15, p. 605
Solotol	Betapace	1.0-2.0 mg/kg PO, BID	Dogs	Antiarrhythmic	Table 16-37, p. 282
Streptokinase		5000 IU/kg IV over 30 min; then 2000 IU/kg/hr for 24 hr	Dogs	Postoperative management; canine adrenalectomy	Table 19-3, p. 404
Streptomycin		20 mg/kg IM, BID for 1 wk	Dogs and cats	Antibiotic; diskospondylitis	Table 37-2, p. 1153
Sucralfate	Carafate	0.5-1.0 g PO, TID to QID; give 1 hr after other meds	Dogs and cats	Treatment of esophagitis	Table 16-17, p. 233 Table 16-21, p. 262
				Medical therapy; gastric ulcers	Table 16-43, p. 288
				Medical therapy; gastrinoma	Table 19-23, p. 426
				Medical therapy; gastroduodenal ulcers	Table 23-42, p. 564
				Medical treatment or prevention; gastrointestinal complications of corticosteroids or NSAIDs	Table 34-12, p. 1070
Sulfasalazine	Azulfidine	25 mg/kg PO, BID	Dogs and cats	Medical management; colitis	Table 16-62, p. 331
Terbutaline	Brethine, Bricanyl	1.25 mg/cat SC or PO, BID	Cats	Treatment of aspiration pneumonia	Table 16-18, p. 233
		1.25-2.5 mg/dog SC or PO, BID to TID	Dogs		
Testosterone cypionate	Depo-testosterone	2.2 mg/kg IM every 30 days	Dogs	Medical management; urinary incontinence	Table 22-11, p. 509
Tetracycline	Panmycin, Achromycin	22 mg/kg PO, BID	Dogs and cats	Medical management; rickettsial polyarthritis	Table 30-8, p. 893
				Medical treatment; Lyme disease	Table 30-9, p. 894

Continued

Appendix I
Drug index—cont'd

Drug name	Brand name	Dosage and route	Species	Use; indication	*SAS* reference
Thiobarbituate		9 mg/kg IV, incrementally to effect, with lidocaine	Dogs	Induction; arrhythmic with gastric dilation-volvulus	Text, p. 280
Thiopental sodium		10-12 mg/kg IV	Dogs and cats	Induction; ear surgery	Table 14-2, p. 154
				Induction; abdominal surgery	Table 15-1, p. 180
				Induction; oral disease	Table 16-1, p. 201
				Induction; cervical esophageal disorder	Table 16-19, p. 234
				Induction; stable with gastric disorder	Tables 16-23, p. 262 and 16-47, p. 294
				Induction; perineal, rectal or anal surgery	Table 16-68, p. 337
				Induction; stable dogs, cats with pancreatic disease	Table 19-12, p. 415
				Induction; cats with renal disease	Table 21-2, p. 462
				Induction; feline urinary abnormalities	Table 22-3, p. 482
				Induction; healthy animals	Table 23-5, p. 519
				Induction; stable, cardiovascular disease	Table 24-2, p. 576
				Induction; stable with respiratory dysfunction	Table 26-1, p. 650
				Induction; stable with orthopedic disease	Table 28-2, p. 708
				Induction; spinal surgery	Table 34-3, p. 1050
		10-12 mg/kg IV with diazepam	Dogs and cats	Induction; dyspneic, nonarrhythmic with upper respiratory disorder	Table 25-7, p. 610
				Induction; dyspneic, nonarrhythmic with respiratory dysfunction	Table 26-1, p. 650
Thyroid hormone	Soloxine, Thyrotabs, Synthyroid	0.022 mg/kg PO, BID	Dogs and cats	Postoperative management; hypophysectomy	Table 19-11, p. 414

Tolazoline		1.0-2.0 mg/kg IM or IV	Dogs and cats	Reversal of xylazine	Table 28-7, p. 723 Table 28-8, p. 723
Trimethoprim-sulfadiazine	Tribrissen	15 mg/kg PO or IM, BID	Dogs	Antibiotic; aspiration pneumonia	Table 16-6, p. 212
				Treatment of aspiration pneumonia	Table 16-18, p. 233
				Antibiotic; prophylactic, perineal, rectal, or colonic surgery	Table 16-57, p. 321
				Antibiotic; renal disease	Table 21-4, p. 463
				Antibiotic; reproductive disorder	Table 23-8, p. 521
				Antibiotic; pyometra	Table 23-23, p. 548
			Dogs and cats	Antibiotic; upper respiratory infection	Table 25-9, p. 611
		15 mg/kg PO, BID	Cats	Antibiotic; aspiration pneumonia	Table 16-6, p. 212
				Treatment of aspiration pneumonia	Table 16-18, p. 233
				Antibiotic; prophylactic, perineal, rectal, or colonic surgery	Table 16-57, p. 321
				Antibiotic; renal disease	Table 21-4, p. 463
				Antibiotic; reproductive disorder	Table 23-8, p. 521
				Antibiotic; pyometra	Table 23-23, p. 548
		45 mg/kg PO, BID, watch for side effects	Dogs and cats	Antibiotic; pyothorax	Table 27-17, p. 700
Viokase		1-2 teaspoons with food	Dogs and cats	Medical treatment; exocrine pancreatic insufficiency	Table 19-16, p. 418
Vitamin D	Dihydrochysterol	0.02-0.03 mg/kg/day for 1 wk, half for 1 wk, half again for 4 mo	Cats	Correction of hypocalcemia; thyroidectomy	Table 19-32, p. 436
Vitamin K_1	AquaMephyton, Mephyton	0.1-0.2 mg/kg SC, SID; do not give IV or IM	Dogs and cats	Preoperative management; prolonged biliary obstruction	Table 18-1, p. 389
Xylazine	Rompun	0.2 mg/kg IM with butorphanol	Cats	Sedation; orthopedic disease	Table 28-8, p. 723
		0.2 mg/kg IV or IM	Dogs	Sedation; orthopedic disease	Table 28-7, p. 723
		0.4 mg/kg IV or 0.5 mg/kg SC	Cats	Induction of vomiting	Table 16-30, p. 276

Appendix J
Treatment of hyperkalemia in cats

1. Dilute by giving 0.9% saline IV
2. If necessary give sodium bicarbonate (see *SAS,* Table 22-2) or insulin (0.5 units/kg regular insulin IV) plus dextrose (2 g per unit of insulin)
3. If hyperkalemia is life threatening may give 10% calcium gluconate (0.5-1.0 ml/kg) for transient cardiac protection. Give slowly (over 5-10 min) while monitoring the patient's ECG

Appendix K
Premedicants for laryngeal examination in dogs

Atropine

0.02-0.04 mg/kg IM, or SC

Glycopyrrolate

0.005-0.011 mg/kg IM, or SC

Oxymorphone (Numorphan)

0.05-0.1 mg/kg IM

Butorphanol (Torbutrol, Torbugesic)

0.2-0.4 mg/kg IM, or SC

Buprenorphine (Buprenex)

5-15 μg/kg IM

Appendix L
Normal pH and blood gas values on room air

Value	Range
pH = 7.4	(7.35-7.45)
Pao_2 = 95 mm Hg	(80-110)
Pvo_2 = 40 mm Hg	(35-45)
$Paco_2$ = 40 mm Hg	(35-45)
$Pvco_2$ = 45 mm Hg	(40-48)
HCO_3 = 24 mEq/L	(22-27)

Appendix M
Sedation for palpation and radiographs

Dogs*

Drug/combination	Dose	Route	Comments
Acepromazine	0.05 mg/kg, max of 1 mg	IV, SC, IM	Acepromazine is not reversible
plus			
Oxymorphone	0.05-0.1 mg/kg	IV, SC, IM	Animal will require restraint if acepromazine is used alone
or			
Butorphanol	0.2-0.4 mg/kg	IV, SC, IM	Acepromazine is contraindicated with seizure history
plus			
Atropine	0.02 mg/kg	IV	Oxymorphone can be reversed with 0.02 mg/kg naloxone (Narcan) IV
or	0.04 mg/kg	SC, IM	
Glycopyrrolate	0.005-0.011 mg/kg	IV, SC, IM	Auditory hypersensitivity/panting with oxymorphone
Xylazine	0.2 mg/kg	IV, IM	Xylazine can be reversed with 1.0-2.0 mg/kg tolazoline, IM or IV
plus			
Butorphanol	0.2 mg/kg	IV, IM	Total dose of xylazine may vary with route of administration and weight of the patient
plus			
Atropine	0.02 mg/kg	IV	
or	0.04 mg/kg	SC, IM	
Glycopyrrolate	0.005-0.011 mg/kg	IV, SC, IM	
Oxymorphone	0.05-0.1 mg/kg	IV, SC, IM	Oxymorphone can be reversed with 0.02 mg/kg naloxone (Narcan) IV
plus			
Diazepam	0.1-0.2 mg/kg	IV	
plus			
Atropine	0.02 mg/kg	IV	Auditory hypersensitivity/panting
or	0.04 mg/kg	SC, IM	
Glycopyrrolate	0.005-0.011 mg/kg	IV, SC, IM	

*Acepromazine (0.05 mg/kg IM or SC; max of 2 mg) may be used alone for radiographs and palpation; however, it provides minimal restraint.

Continued

Appendix M
Sedation for palpation and radiographs—cont'd
Cats

Drug/combination	Dose	Route†	Comments
Acepromazine	0.05 mg/kg	IM	Acepromazine is not reversible
plus			
Butorphanol	0.2 mg/kg	IM	Animal will require restraint if acepromazine is used alone
plus			
Atropine	0.04 mg/kg	IM	
or			
Glycopyrrolate	0.005-0.011 mg/kg	IM	Acepromazine is contraindicated with seizure history
Xylazine	0.2 mg/kg	IM	Xylazine can be reversed with 1.0-2.0 mg/kg tolazoline, IM or IV
plus			
Butorphanol	0.2 mg/kg	IM	
plus			
Atropine	0.04 mg/kg	IM	
or			
Glycopyrrolate	0.005-0.011 mg/kg	IM	
Ketamine	5 mg/kg	IM	Provides little to no muscle relaxation

†Other routes of administration may be appropriate for some drugs (e.g., IV if a catheter is in place).

INDEX

P

Q

R

T

U